Health, United States, 2010

With Special Feature on Death and Dying

U.S. DEPARTMENT OF HEALTH AND HUMAN SERVICES
Centers for Disease Control and Prevention
National Center for Health Statistics

March 2011
DHHS Publication No. 2011–1232

U.S. Department of Health and Human Services

Kathleen Sebelius
Secretary

Centers for Disease Control and Prevention

Thomas R. Frieden, M.D., M.P.H.
Director

National Center for Health Statistics

Edward J. Sondik, Ph.D.
Director

For sale by the Superintendent of Documents, U.S. Government Printing Office
Internet: bookstore.gpo.gov Phone: toll free (866) 512-1800; DC area (202) 512-1800
Fax: (202) 512-2104 Mail: Stop IDCC, Washington, DC 20402-0001

ISBN 978-0-16-087942-5

Preface

Health, United States, 2010 is the 34th report on the health status of the Nation and is submitted by the Secretary of the Department of Health and Human Services to the President and the Congress of the United States in compliance with Section 308 of the Public Health Service Act. This report was compiled by the Centers for Disease Control and Prevention's (CDC) National Center for Health Statistics (NCHS). The National Committee on Vital and Health Statistics served in a review capacity.

The *Health, United States* series presents national trends in health statistics. The report contains a Chartbook that assesses the Nation's health by presenting trends and current information on selected measures of morbidity, mortality, health care utilization, health risk factors, prevention, health insurance, and personal health care expenditures. This year's Chartbook includes a special feature on death and dying. The report also contains 148 trend tables organized around four major subject areas: health status and determinants, health care utilization, health care resources, and health care expenditures. A companion product to *Health, United States—Health, United States: In Brief*—features information extracted from the full report. The complete report, *In Brief*, and related data products are available on the *Health, United States* website at: http://www.cdc.gov/nchs/hus.htm.

The 2010 Edition

Health, United States, 2010 includes a summary "At a Glance" table that displays selected indicators of health and their determinants, cross-referenced to charts and tables in the report. It also contains a Highlights section, a Chartbook, detailed trend tables, extensive appendixes, and an index. Major sections of the 2010 report are described below.

Chartbook

The 2010 Chartbook has been reformatted to present data in a more concise, user-friendly format. The Chartbook section contains 41 charts, including 18 charts on this year's special feature on death and dying. The special feature includes charts (Figures 24–41) on the leading causes of death by age group; changes in place of death by race and ethnicity; preventable death (motor-vehicle traffic death rates); characteristics of hospice care patients and the types of services and medications they use; use of advance directives by nursing home, hospice care, and home health care patients; and geographic patterns in the utilization of the ICU/CCU in the last 6 months of life.

Trend Tables

The Chartbook section is followed by 148 trend tables organized around four major subject areas: health status and determinants, health care utilization, health care resources, and health care expenditures. The tables present data for selected years to highlight major trends in health statistics. Additional years of data may be available in Excel spreadsheet files on the *Health, United States* website. Tables for which additional data years are available are listed in Appendix III. Comparability across years in *Health, United States* is fostered by including similar trend tables in each volume, and timeliness is maintained by improving the content of ongoing tables and adding new tables each year to reflect emerging topics in public health. A key criterion used in selecting these tables is the availability of comparable national data over a period of several years.

Health, United States, 2010 includes six new trend tables on the following subjects: selected health conditions among children (Table 46), based on the National Health Interview Survey; respondent-reported heart disease, cancer, and stroke prevalence (Table 49), based on the National Health Interview Survey; adolescent risk behaviors (Table 63), based on the Youth Risk Behavior Survey; adolescent vaccination (Table 83), based on the National Immunization Survey; prescription drug use (Table 95), based on the National Health and Nutrition Examination Survey; and certified intermediate care facilities and specialty hospitals (Table 118), based on the Online Survey Certification and Reporting Database (OSCAR).

Appendixes

Appendix I. Data Sources describes each data source used in the report and provides references for further information about the sources. Data sources are listed alphabetically within two broad categories: Government Sources, and Private and Global Sources.

Appendix II. Definitions and Methods is an alphabetical listing of terms used in the report. It also contains information on the methods used in the report.

Appendix III. Additional Data Years Available lists tables for which additional years of trend data are available in Excel spreadsheet files on the *Health, United States* website.

Index

The Index to the trend tables and charts is a useful tool for locating data by topic. Tables and figures are cross-referenced by such topics as child and adolescent health; older population aged 65 years and over; women's health; men's health; state data; American Indian and Alaska Native, Asian, black or African American, and Hispanic-origin populations; education; injury; disability; and metropolitan and nonmetropolitan data. Many of the index topics are available as conveniently grouped data packages on the *Health, United States* website.

Data Considerations

Racial and Ethnic Data

Many tables in *Health, United States* present data according to race and Hispanic origin, consistent with a Department-wide emphasis on expanding racial and ethnic detail when presenting health data. Trend data on race and ethnicity are presented in the greatest detail possible after taking into account the quality of the data, the amount of missing data, and the number of observations. These issues significantly affect the availability of reportable data for certain populations, such as the Native Hawaiian and Other Pacific Islander population and the American Indian and Alaska Native population. Standards for the classification of federal data on race and ethnicity are described in Appendix II, Race.

Education and Income Data

Many tables in *Health, United States* present data according to socioeconomic status, using education and family income as proxy measures. Education and income data are generally obtained directly from survey respondents and are not generally available from records-based data collection systems. Categories shown for income data were expanded in *Health, United States, 2010*. State vital statistics systems currently report mother's education on the birth certificate and (based on an informant) decedent's education on the death certificate. See Appendix II, Education; Family income; and Poverty.

Disability Data

Disability can include the presence of physical or mental impairments that limit a person's ability to perform an important activity and affect the use of or need for supports, accommodations, or interventions required to improve functioning. Information on disability in the U.S. population is critical to health planning and policy. Several current initiatives are under way to coordinate and standardize measurement of disability across federal data systems. *Health, United States, 2009* introduced the first detailed trend table using data from the National Health Interview Survey to create disability measures consistent with two of the conceptual components that have been indentified in disability models and in disability legislation: basic actions difficulty and complex activity limitation. Basic actions difficulty captures limitations or difficulties in movement and sensory, emotional, or mental functioning that are associated with some health problem. Complex activity limitation describes limitations or restrictions in a person's ability to participate fully in social role activities such as working or maintaining a household. This year's report expands the use of the basic actions difficulty and complex activity limitation measures to include additional tables from the National Health Interview Survey (Tables 52, 53, 56, 60, 64, 65, 70, 75, 76, 79, 84–87, 89, 93, 98, and 135–138). *Health, United States* also includes the following disability-related information for the civilian noninstitutionalized population: vision and hearing limitations for adults (Table 55) and disability-related information for Medicare enrollees (Table 142), Medicaid recipients (Table 143), and veterans with service-connected disabilities (Table 145). For more information on disability statistics, see: Altman B, Bernstein A. Disability and health in the United States, 2001–2005. Hyattsville, MD: NCHS. 2008. Available from: http://www.cdc.gov/nchs/data/misc/disability2001-2005.pdf.

Statistical Significance

All differences between estimates noted in the Highlights section of *Health, United States* were determined to be statistically significant at the 0.05 level using two-sided significance tests (z tests). In the Chartbook, weighted least squares regression was performed to test for the presence of a statistically significant increase or decrease in the estimates during the time period (see Technical Notes accompanying the Chartbook). Terms such as "similar," "stable," and "no difference" indicate that the statistics being compared were not significantly different. Lack of comment regarding the difference between statistics does not necessarily suggest that the difference was tested and found to be not significant. Because statistically significant differences or trends are partly a function of sample size (the larger the sample size, the smaller the change that can be detected), statistically significant differences or trends do not necessarily have public health significance (1).

Overall estimates generally have relatively small standard errors, but estimates for certain population subgroups may be based on small numbers and have relatively large standard errors. Although numbers of births and deaths from the U.S. Vital Statistics System represent complete counts (except for births in those states where data are based on a 50% sample for selected years) and are not subject to sampling error, the counts are subject to random variation, which means that the number of events that actually occur in a given year may be considered as one of a large series of possible results that could have arisen under the same circumstances. When the number of events is small and the probability of such an event is small, considerable caution must be observed in interpreting the conditions described by the figures. Estimates that are unreliable because of large standard errors or small numbers of events have been noted with an asterisk. The criteria used to designate or suppress unreliable estimates are indicated in the notes to the applicable tables.

For NCHS surveys, point estimates and their corresponding variances were calculated using the SUDAAN software package (2), which takes into consideration the complex survey design. Standard errors for other surveys or datasets were computed using the methodology recommended by the programs providing the data or were provided directly by those programs. Standard errors are available for selected tables in the Excel spreadsheet version on the *Health, United States* website at: http://www.cdc.gov/nchs/hus.htm.

Access to *Health, United States*

Health, United States may be accessed in its entirety at: http://www.cdc.gov/nchs/hus.htm. The website is a user-friendly resource for *Health, United States* and related products. In addition to the report, it contains the *In Brief* companion report, data conveniently grouped by topic, as well as the Chartbook figures as PowerPoint slides, and trend tables and Chartbook data tables as Excel spreadsheet files. Many Excel spreadsheet files include additional years of data not shown in the printed report, as well as standard errors where available. Visitors to the website can also join the *Health, United States* listserv to receive announcements about release dates and notices of updates to tables. Spreadsheet files for selected tables will be updated on the website if more current data become available near the time when the printed report is released. Previous editions of *Health, United States*, and their chartbooks, can also be accessed from the website.

Printed copies of *Health, United States* can be purchased from the Government Printing Office (GPO) at: http://bookstore.gpo.gov.

Questions?

If you have questions about *Health, United States* or related data products, please contact:

Office of Information Services
Information Dissemination Staff
National Center for Health Statistics
Centers for Disease Control and Prevention
3311 Toledo Road, Fifth Floor
Hyattsville, MD 20782
Phone: 1–800–232–4636
E-mail: nchsquery@cdc.gov
Internet: http://www.cdc.gov/nchs/

References

1. Interpretation of YRBS trend data [online]. CDC, Youth Risk Behavior Survey (YRBS). 2010. Available from: http://www.cdc.gov/HealthyYouth/yrbs/pdf/YRBS_trend_interpretation.pdf.
2. Shah B. SUDAAN [computer software]. Research Triangle Park, NC: RTI, International. Available from: http://www.rti.org/sudaan/index.cfm.

Acknowledgments

Overall responsibility for planning and coordinating the content of this volume rested with the National Center for Health Statistics' (NCHS) Office of Analysis and Epidemiology, under the direction of Amy B. Bernstein, Diane M. Makuc, and Linda T. Bilheimer.

Production of **Health, United States, 2010**, including highlights, trend tables, and appendixes, was managed by Amy B. Bernstein, Sheila Franco, and Virginia M. Freid. Trend tables were prepared by Mary Ann Bush, La-Tonya D. Curl, Anne K. Driscoll, Catherine R. Duran, Sheila Franco, Virginia M. Freid, Tamyra C. Garcia, Ji-Eun Kim, Patricia N. Pastor, Rebecca A. Placek, Cynthia A. Reuben, and Henry Xia, with assistance from Anita L. Powell and Ilene B. Rosen. Appendix II tables and the index were assembled by Anita L. Powell. Production planning and coordination of trend tables were managed by Rebecca A. Placek. Review and clearance books were assembled by Ilene B. Rosen. Administrative and word processing assistance was provided by Lillie C. Featherstone and Danielle Wood.

Production of the **Chartbook** was managed by Virginia M. Freid. Data and analysis for specific charts were provided by Amy B. Bernstein, Anne K. Driscoll, Sheila Franco, Virginia M. Freid, Tamyra C. Garcia, Deborah D. Ingram, and Ji-Eun Kim. Graphs were drafted by La-Tonya D. Curl, and data tables were prepared by Rebecca A. Placek. Technical assistance and programming were provided by Mary Ann Bush, La-Tonya D. Curl, Catherine R. Duran, Xiang Liu, and Henry Xia.

Publication production was performed by the NCHS Office of Information Services, Information Design and Publishing Staff. Project management and editorial review were provided by Barbara J. Wassell. Oversight review for publications and electronic products was provided by Demarius V. Miller, Tommy C. Seibert, Jr., and Linda B. Torian. The designer was Sarah M. Hinkle. Layout and production were done by Zung T. Le and Jacqueline M. Davis. Artwork and production for Health, United States, 2010: In Brief were provided by Sarah M. Hinkle and Kyung M. Park. Printing was managed by Patricia L. Wilson, CDC/OCOO/MASO.

Electronic access through the NCHS Internet site was provided by Christine J. Brown, Jacqueline M. Davis, Zung T. Le, Anthony Lipphardt, Anita L. Powell, Sharon L. Ramirez, Ilene B. Rosen, and Barbara J. Wassell.

Data and technical assistance were provided by staff of the following NCHS organizations: *Division of Health Care Statistics*: Vladislav Beresovsky, Frederic H. Decker, Carol J. DeFrances, Lisa L. Dwyer, Marni J. Hall, Lauren Harris-Kojetin, Maria F. Owings, Susan M. Schappert, and Ingrid Vassanelli; *Division of Health Examination Statistics*: Vicki L. Burt, Margaret D. Carroll, Bruce A. Dye, Mark Eberhardt, Jaime J. Gahche, Quiping Gu, Clifford L. Johnson, David A. Lacher, Cynthia L. Ogden, Susan E. Schober, Jacqueline D. Wright, and Sarah Yoon; *Division of Health Interview Statistics*: Patricia F. Adams, Patricia Barnes, Veronica E. Benson, Barbara Bloom, Robin A. Cohen, Susan S. Jack, John Pleis, Charlotte A. Schoenborn, and Brian W. Ward; *Division of Vital Statistics*: Joyce C. Abma, Robert N. Anderson, Elizabeth Arias, Anjani Chandra, Brady Hamilton, Donna L. Hoyert, Kenneth D. Kochanek, Joyce A. Martin, T. J. Mathews, Sherry L. Murphy, Michelle Osterman, and Stephanie J. Ventura; *Office of Analysis and Epidemiology*: Lara Akinbami, Barbara Altman, Li-Hui Chen, Deborah D. Ingram, Ellen A. Kramarow, Mitch Loeb, Susan Lukacs, Andrea P. MacKay, Laura A. Pratt, Cheryl V. Rose, Rashmi Tandon, Margaret Warner, and Julie Dawson Weeks; *Office of the Center Director*: Patricia Markovich and Francis C. Notzon; and *Office of Research and Methodology*: Meena Khare.

Additional data and technical assistance were provided by the following organizations of the Centers for Disease Control and Prevention (CDC): *Epidemiology Program Office*: Samuel L. Groseclose, Patsy A. Hall, and Michael Wodajo; *National Center for Chronic Disease Prevention and Health Promotion*: Sonya Gamble and Steve Kinchen; *National Center for HIV, Viral Hepatitis, STD, and TB Prevention*: Michael Campsmith, Delicia Carey, Rachel S. Wynn, Annemarie Wasley, and Jill Wasserman; *National Center for Immunization and Respiratory Diseases*: Christina Dorell, Gary Euler, and James A. Singleton; *National Institute for Occupational Safety and Health*: Roger Rosa; by the following organizations within the Department of Health and Human Services: *Agency for Healthcare Research and Quality*: David Kashihara and Steven R. Machlin; *Centers for Medicare & Medicaid Services*: Dovid Chaifetz, Cathy A. Cowan, Karen Edrington, Denise Franz, Christopher Kessler, Deborah W. Kidd, Maggie S. Murgolo, Olivia Nuccio, Joseph S. Regan, Loan Swisher, and Lekha Whittle; *National Institutes of Health*: Kathy Cronin, Brenda Edwards, Paul W. Eggars, and Marsha Lopez;

Substance Abuse and Mental Health Services Administration: Jeffrey Buck, James Colliver, Laura Milazzo-Sayre, and Rita Vandivort-Warren; and by the following governmental and nongovernmental organizations: *U.S. Census Bureau*: Bernadette D. Proctor; *Bureau of Labor Statistics*: Daniel Ginsburg, George Long, Stephen Pegula, Elizabeth Rogers, Swati Patel, and Peter Horner; *Department of Veterans Affairs*: Pheakdey Lim and Dat Tran; *American Association of Colleges of Pharmacy*: Jennifer M. Patton and Danielle Taylor; *American Association of Colleges of Osteopathic Medicine*: Wendy Fernando and Tom Levitan; *American Association of Colleges of Podiatric Medicine*: Moraith G. North; *American Osteopathic Association*: Mark Dvorak and Margaret Harrison; *American Dental Education Association*: Jon D. Ruesch; *Association of American Medical Colleges*: Franc Slapar and Amber Sterling; *Association of Schools and Colleges of Optometry*: Ginny Pickles and Joanne Zuckerman; *Association of Schools of Public Health*: Kristin Dolinski; *Cowles Research Group*: C. McKeen Cowles; *The Guttmacher Institute*: Rachel Jones; *The Dartmouth Institute for Health Policy and Clinical Practice*: Kristen K. Bronner; *NOVA Research Company*: Shilpa Bengeri; and *Thomson Reuters:* Rosanna Coffey and Katharine Levit.

Contents

Contents

At a Glance Table and Highlights

Chartbook With Special Feature on Death and Dying

Trend Tables

Appendixes

Index

List of Chartbook Figures

Introduction

Morbidity

Health Care Utilization

Health Risk Factors

Prevention

Access to Care

Health Insurance Coverage

Personal Health Care Expenditures

Special Feature on Death and Dying

List of Trend Tables

Health Status and Determinants

Population

Fertility and Natality

Mortality

Utilization of Health Resources

Ambulatory Care

Health Care Expenditures and Payors

National Health Expenditures

Health Care Coverage and Major Federal Programs

State Health Expenditures and Health Insurance

Health, United States, 2010: At a Glance Table

	Value (year)			Health, United States Figure/Table no.
Life Expectancy and Mortality				
Life expectancy in years				Figure 1/Table 22
At birth	76.8 (2000)	77.7 (2006)	77.9 (2007)	
At age 65 years	17.6 (2000)	18.5 (2006)	18.6 (2007)	
Infant deaths per 1,000 live births				Figure 25
All infants	6.91 (2000)	6.69 (2006)	6.75 (2007)	
Deaths per 100,000, age-adjusted				Table 24
All causes	869.0 (2000)	776.5 (2006)	760.2 (2007)	
Heart disease	257.6 (2000)	200.2 (2006)	190.9 (2007)	
Cancer	199.6 (2000)	180.7 (2006)	178.4 (2007)	
Stroke	60.9 (2000)	43.6 (2006)	42.2 (2007)	
Chronic lower respiratory diseases	44.2 (2000)	40.5 (2006)	40.8 (2007)	
Unintentional injuries	34.9 (2000)	39.8 (2006)	40.0 (2007)	
Motor-vehicle	15.4 (2000)	15.0 (2006)	14.4 (2007)	
Diabetes	25.0 (2000)	23.3 (2006)	22.5 (2007)	
Morbidity and Risk Factors				
Fair or poor health, percent				Table 56
All ages	8.9 (2000)	9.9 (2008)	9.9 (2009)	
65 years and over	26.9 (2000)	24.9 (2008)	24.0 (2009)	
Heart disease, percent				Table 49
18 years and over	10.9 (1999–2000)	11.4 (2005–2006)	11.8 (2008–2009)	
65 years and over	29.6 (1999–2000)	31.2 (2005–2006)	31.7 (2008–2009)	
Cancer (ever had), percent				Table 49
18 years and over	4.9 (1999–2000)	5.7 (2005–2006)	6.1 (2008–2009)	
65 years and over	15.2 (1999–2000)	17.1 (2005–2006)	17.7 (2008–2009)	
Diabetes,[1] percent				Figure 5/Table 66
20 years and over	8.5 (1999–2000)	10.7 (2005–2006)	11.9 (2007–2008)	
Hypertension,[2] percent				Figure 15/Table 66
20 years and over	28.9 (1999–2000)	31.7 (2005–2006)	32.6 (2007–2008)	
High serum total cholesterol,[3] percent				Figure 16/Table 66
20 years and over	17.7 (1999–2000)	15.9 (2005–2006)	14.6 (2007–2008)	
Obese, percent				Figures 13 and 14/Table 66
Obese,[4] 20 years and over	29.9 (1999–2000)	34.2 (2005–2006)	33.7 (2007–2008)	
Obese (BMI at or above sex- and age-specific 95th percentile)				
2–5 years	10.3 (1999–2000)	11.0 (2005–2006)	10.4 (2007–2008)	
6–11 years	15.1 (1999–2000)	15.1 (2005–2006)	19.6 (2007–2008)	
12–19 years	14.8 (1999–2000)	17.8 (2005–2006)	18.1 (2007–2008)	
Cigarette smoking, percent				Figure 11/Table 58
18 years and over	23.2 (2000)	20.6 (2008)	20.6 (2009)	
Aerobic activity and muscle strengthening,[5] percent				Figure 12/Table 70
18 years and over	15.1 (2000)	18.1 (2008)	18.8 (2009)	
Health Care Utilization				
No health care visit in past 12 months, percent				Table 79
Under 18 years	12.3 (2000)	10.1 (2008)	9.1 (2009)	
18–44 years	23.5 (2000)	22.7 (2008)	22.7 (2009)	
45–64 years	15.0 (2000)	14.4 (2008)	15.4 (2009)	
65 years and over	7.5 (2000)	5.6 (2008)	4.7 (2009)	

	Value (year)			Health, United States Figure/Table no.
Emergency room visit in past 12 months, percent				Tables 88 and 89
Under 18 years	20.3 (2000)	20.9 (2008)	20.8 (2009)	
18–44 years	20.5 (2000)	21.5 (2008)	22.0 (2009)	
45–64 years	17.6 (2000)	17.6 (2008)	18.4 (2009)	
65 years and over	23.7 (2000)	23.4 (2008)	24.9 (2009)	
Dental visit in past year, percent				Table 93
2–17 years	74.1 (2000)	77.3 (2008)	78.4 (2009)	
18–64 years	65.1 (2000)	60.4 (2008)	62.0 (2009)	
65 years and over	56.6 (2000)	57.6 (2008)	59.6 (2009)	
Prescription drug in past month, percent				Table 94
Under 18 years	24.1 (1999–2000)	23.9 (2001–2004)	25.3 (2005–2008)	
18–44 years	34.7 (1999–2000)	37.6 (2001–2004)	37.8 (2005–2008)	
45–64 years	62.1 (1999–2000)	66.2 (2001–2004)	64.8 (2005–2008)	
65 years and over	83.9 (1999–2000)	87.3 (2001–2004)	90.1 (2005–2008)	
Hospitalization in past year, percent				Table 98
18–44 years	7.0 (2000)	6.4 (2008)	6.7 (2009)	
45–64 years	8.4 (2000)	7.9 (2008)	8.5 (2009)	
65 years and over	18.2 (2000)	17.5 (2008)	17.1 (2009)	
Insurance and Access to Care				
Uninsured, percent				Figures 21 and 22/Table 138
Under 65 years	17.0 (2000)	16.8 (2008)	17.5 (2009)	
Under 18 years	12.6 (2000)	9.0 (2008)	8.2 (2009)	
18–44 years	22.4 (2000)	24.4 (2008)	25.9 (2009)	
45–64 years	12.6 (2000)	13.6 (2008)	14.6 (2009)	
Delayed or did not receive needed medical care due to cost, percent				Figure 19/Table 76
Under 18 years	4.6 (2000)	5.4 (2008)	5.2 (2009)	
18–44 years	9.5 (2000)	13.6 (2008)	15.1 (2009)	
45–64 years	8.8 (2000)	13.5 (2008)	15.1 (2009)	
65 years and over	4.5 (2000)	4.5 (2008)	5.1 (2009)	
Health Care Resources				
Physicians in patient care per 10,000 population				Table 106
United States	22.7 (2000)	25.3 (2007)	25.7 (2008)	
Highest state (postal code)	34.4 (MA) (2000)	39.1 (MA) (2007)	39.7 (MA) (2008)	
Lowest state (postal code)	14.4 (ID) (2000)	17.0 (ID) (2007)	17.0 (ID) (2008)	
Community hospital beds per 1,000 population				Table 115
United States	2.9 (2000)	---	2.7 (2008)	
Highest state (postal code)	6.0 (ND) (2000)	---	5.4 (ND) (2008)	
Lowest state (postal code)	1.9 (NM,NV, OR,UT,WA) (2000)	---	1.7 (WA) (2008)	
Expenditures				
Personal health care expenditures, dollars				Figure 23/Table 126
Total in trillions	$1.1 (2000)	$1.9 (2007)	$2.0 (2008)	
Per capita	$4,032 (2000)	$6,186 (2007)	$6,411 (2008)	

---Data not available. [1]Diabetes prevalence is based on report of a physician diagnosis, or a fasting blood glucose of 126 mg/dL or higher, or a hemoglobin A1c of 6.5% or higher. [2]Having elevated blood pressure (measured) and/or taking antihypertensive medications. [3]Having cholesterol of 240 mg/dL or greater. [4]Obesity is a body mass index greater than or equal to 30 kg/m². Height and weight are measured. [5]Meeting 2008 federal guidelines for aerobic activity and muscle strengthening.

NOTES: Some estimates are from the Excel spreadsheet version of the cited table and are not shown in the PDF version or in the printed version. For more information, data sources, notes, and the Excel version of the spreadsheet, see the complete report, *Health, United States, 2010*, available from: http://www.cdc.gov/nchs/hus.htm.

Special Feature on Death and Dying

In 2007, heart disease was the first **leading cause of death** and cancer was the second. One-quarter of all deaths were from heart disease, and 23% were from cancer, in 2007 (Figure 24).

In 2007, the **infant mortality** rate was 6.75 infant deaths per 1,000 live births—2% lower than in 2000 (Figure 25).

The unintentional injury death rate among **children 1–14 years** of age—the leading cause of death in this age group—dropped 30% from 1997 to 2007 (7 deaths per 100,000 population) (Figure 27).

Unintentional injuries accounted for nearly one-half of deaths among **persons 15–24 years** of age. Between 1997 and 2007, the unintentional injury death rate among this age group increased 5%, to 37 deaths per 100,000 population (Figure 28).

Between 1997 and 2007, the death rate among **adults 25–44 years** of age declined 7% due to a decrease in cancer and HIV-related deaths. Unintentional injuries were the leading cause of death for this age group, accounting for one-quarter of deaths in 2007 (Figure 29).

Cancer, the leading cause of death for adults **45–64 years** of age, accounted for one-third of deaths among this age group in 2007. Between 1997 and 2007, the cancer death rate in this age group decreased 14%, to 200 deaths per 100,000 population (Figure 30).

Between 1997 and 2007, the heart disease death rate for **adults 65 years** of age and over—the leading cause of death in this age group—decreased 26%, to 1,309 deaths per 100,000 population. In 2007, heart disease accounted for 28% of deaths for adults in this age group (Figure 31).

In 2000–2007, **motor-vehicle traffic death rates** varied more than fourfold by state, ranging from 31 per 100,000 population in Mississippi to 7 per 100,000 population in Massachusetts (Figure 32).

On average in 2005, Medicare decedents spent 3.5 **days in the ICU/CCU** in the last 6 months of life. The average ranged from 5.7 days in New Jersey to 1.3 days in North Dakota (Figure 35).

One-quarter of deaths occurred at home in 2007—more than in previous years. This shift in place of death was found both for decedents under age 65 and those 65 and over. In 2007, most deaths still occurred in facilities such as hospitals (36%) and nursing homes (22%) (Figure 33).

Place of death varied by race and Hispanic origin. In 2007, among decedents 65 years of age and over, non-Hispanic white decedents were less likely to die while hospital inpatients and more likely to die in nursing homes than Hispanic, non-Hispanic black, American Indian or Alaska Native, or Asian or Pacific Islander decedents (Figure 34).

Nearly all discharged hospice care patients, 70% of current nursing home residents, and one-third of current home health care patients 65 years of age and over had **advance directives** in place in recent years (Figure 36).

Between 1998 and 2007, the percentage of discharged **hospice care patients with a primary admission diagnosis other than cancer** increased from 35% to 57% (Figure 38).

In 2007, **bereavement services** were offered or provided to 85% of hospice care patients' family members or friends, and **spiritual services and medication management** were offered or provided to two-thirds of family members or friends. **Caregiver health or wellness services** were offered or provided to one-quarter of family members or friends (Figure 39).

One-half of **hospice care patients** had difficulty breathing, and one-third had pain at the last hospice care visit before death (Figure 40).

Ninety-one percent of **hospice care patients** had a narcotic analgesic (for severe pain), and 79% had an antiemetic drug (for vomiting or dizziness), prescribed for them in the last week of life (Figure 41).

Life Expectancy

Between 2000 and 2007, **life expectancy at birth** increased 1.3 years for **males** and 1.1 years for **females**. The gap in life expectancy between males and females narrowed from 5.2 years in 2000 to 5.0 years in 2007 (Table 22).

Between 2000 and 2007, **life expectancy at birth** increased more for the **black** than for the **white** population, thereby narrowing the gap in life expectancy between these two racial groups. In 2000, life expectancy at birth for the white population was 5.5 years longer than for the black population. By 2007, the difference had narrowed to 4.8 years (Table 22).

Fertility and Natality

The **birth rate among teenagers** 15–19 years of age fell 2% in 2008 (preliminary data), to 41.5 live births per 1,000 females, reversing a brief 2-year increase that had halted the long-term decline in births to teenagers from 1991 to 2005, when rates fell 34% (Table 3).

Low birthweight is associated with elevated risk of death and disability in infants. In 2008 (preliminary data), the percentage of low birthweight births (infants weighing less than 2,500 grams (5.5 pounds) at birth) was 8.2%, unchanged from 2007. The 2008 percentage is 18% higher than for 1990 (Table 9).

Health Risk Factors

Between 1988–1994 and 2007–2008, the prevalence of **obesity among preschool-age children** 2–5 years of age increased from 7% to 10% (Table 66 and Figure 13).

The prevalence of **obesity among school-age children and adolescents** increased between 1988–1994 and 2007–2008. The prevalence of obesity almost doubled, from 11% to 20%, among children 6–11 years of age, and increased from 11% to 18% among adolescents 12–19 years of age (Table 66 and Figure 13).

From 1988–1994 to 2007–2008, the percentage of adults 20 years of age and over who were **obese** increased from 22% to 34% (Table 66).

In 2009, 21% of U.S. adults were current **cigarette smokers**, unchanged in recent years. Men were more likely to be current cigarette smokers than women (Figure 11 and Table 58).

Between 1999 and 2009, the percentage of men and women who met the 2008 federal guidelines for **aerobic activity and muscle strengthening** increased for most age groups. In 2009, 19% of adults 18 years of age and over met the guidelines (Figure 12 and Table 70).

Between 1991 and 2009, the percentage of high school students who reported **rarely or never using a seat belt** declined from 26% to 10%. In 2009, 12% of high school boys and 8% of high school girls rarely or never used a seat belt (Table 63).

In 2009, the percentage of **sexually active high school students who reported using a condom** the most recent time they had sexual intercourse was 61%, up from 46% in 1991. In 2009, 69% of high school boys and 54% of high school girls used a condom at last sexual intercourse (Table 63).

Measures of Health and Disease Prevalence

In 2007–2009, 5% of children under 18 years of age had an **asthma attack** in the past year, 11% had a **skin allergy**, and 6% had three or more **ear infections** in the past year. Among school-age children 5–17 years of age, 9% had **attention deficit hyperactivity disorder** and 6% had **serious emotional or behavioral difficulties** (Table 46 and Figure 2).

In 2009, the percentage of noninstitutionalized adults who reported their **health as fair or poor** ranged from 6% of those 18–44 years of age to 29% of those 75 years and over. The proportion of all persons with fair or poor health was five times as high among persons living in poverty as among those with family income at least four times the poverty level (Table 56).

The prevalence of **hypertension** (defined as high blood pressure or taking antihypertensive medication) increases with age. In 2005–2008, 33%–34% of men and women 45–54 years of age had hypertension, compared with 67% of men and 80% of women 75 years of age and over (Table 67).

In 2005–2008, 11% of adults 20 years of age and over had **diabetes** (diagnosed and undiagnosed). In 2005–2008, the percentage of adults with diabetes increased with age from 4% of persons 20–44 years of age to 27% of adults 65 years of age and over (Table 50 and Figure 5).

In 2009, 46% of men and 31% of women 75 years of age and over had ever been told by a physician or other health professional that they had **heart disease**. Among those 75 years of age and over, prevalence rose between 1999 and 2009 among men but not among women (Figure 3).

In 2009, 23% of men and 17% of women 75 years of age and over had ever been told by a physician or other health professional that they had **cancer** (excluding the common types of skin cancers) (Figure 4).

Between 1988–1994 and 2005–2008, the percentage of adults 20 years of age and over with **high serum total cholesterol level** (defined as greater than or equal to 240 mg/dL) declined from 20% to 15% (Figure 16).

In 2008–2009, 3% of the noninstitutionalized population 18 years of age and over was classified as having had **serious psychological distress** in a 30-day period. Adults with a family income below the poverty threshold were more than eight times as likely to report serious psychological distress as adults in families with an income at least four times the poverty level (Table 57).

Health Care Utilization

Use of Health Care Services

In 2008, there were about 1.2 billion **visits to physician offices, hospital outpatient departments, and hospital emergency departments**. There were 956 million visits to physician offices, 110 million visits to hospital outpatient departments, and 124 million visits to hospital emergency departments (Table 91).

In 2009, 21% of adults 18 years of age and over had at least one **emergency department visit** in the past year, and 8% had two or more visits. Emergency department utilization was 93% higher among persons with a family income below the poverty level compared with those with a family income at least four times the poverty level (Table 89).

Between 1997 and 2009, two-thirds of persons 2 years of age and over **had seen a dentist in the past year**. Dental visit rates were higher among children 2–17 years of age than among adults, with about three-quarters of children having had a recent dental visit during this period (Table 93).

Between 2000 and 2007, nonfederal short-stay **hospital discharge rates** were stable after declining sharply during the 1980s. During this period, the average length of a hospital stay was 5 days (Table 99).

The percentage of the population with at least one **prescription drug** during the previous month increased from 38% in 1988–1994 to 48% in 2005–2008. During the same period, the percentage taking three or more prescription drugs increased from 11% to 21% (Table 94).

Use of Preventive Medical Care Services

In 2009, 27% of females 13–17 years of age had received three or more doses of **human papillomavirus (HPV)** vaccine (Table 83).

In 2009, one-half of noninstitutionalized **adults 50 years of age and over** had received **influenza vaccination** in the past year, ranging from 41% of those 50–64 years of age to 73% of those 75 years of age and over (Figure 18 and Table 84).

Between 1989 and 2009, the percentage of noninstitutionalized **adults 65 years of age and over** who ever received a **pneumococcal vaccination** quadrupled (from 14% to 61%). In 2009, 55% of those 65–74 years of age and 68% of those 75 years of age and over ever had a pneumococcal vaccination (Table 85).

The percentage of women 40 years of age and over who had a **mammogram** in the past 2 years more than doubled from 1987 to 1999, increasing from 29% to 70%. Between 1999 and 2008, 67%–70% of women 40 years of age and over had a mammogram within the past 2 years (Table 86).

Unmet Need for Medical Care, Prescription Drugs, and Dental Care Due to Cost

Between 1997 and 2009, among adults 18–64 years of age, the percentage who reported **not receiving, or delaying, needed medical care** in the past 12 months **due to cost** increased from 11% to 15%; the percentage not receiving needed **prescription drugs** due to cost rose from 6% to 11%; and the percentage not receiving needed **dental care** due to cost grew from 11% to 17% (Table 76 and Figure 19).

In 2009, 37% of adults 18–64 years of age who were uninsured **did not receive, or delayed, needed medical care** in the past 12 months **due to cost**, compared with 9% of adults with private coverage and 14% of adults with Medicaid (Figure 19).

In 2009, 19%–21% of adults 18–64 years of age in families with income below 200% of poverty **did not receive needed prescription drugs due to cost** in the past 12 months, compared with 12% of those with a family income 200%–399% of poverty and 4% of those with a family income 400% of poverty or higher (Table 76).

In 2009, 28% of adults 18–64 years of age with any basic actions difficulty or complex activity limitation reported they did not receive needed **dental care due to cost** in the past 12 months, compared with 13% of adults with no disability (Table 76).

Health Care Resources

Between 2000 and 2008, the number of **physicians in patient care** increased 13%, to 26 per 10,000 population. In 2008, the number of patient care physicians per 10,000 population ranged from 17 in Idaho and Mississippi to 40 in Massachusetts (Table 106).

Between 2000 and 2008, there were about 5,000 **community hospitals** and 800,000 **community hospital beds**. During that period, the community hospital occupancy rate ranged from 64% to 67% (Table 113).

In 2009, there were about 1.7 million **nursing home beds** in 16,000 certified nursing homes. Between 1995 and 2009, nursing home bed occupancy for the United States was relatively stable at 82%–85%. **Occupancy rates** were 90% or higher in 14 states and the District of Columbia in 2009 (Table 117).

The number of beds in **intermediate care facilities** for persons with mental retardation declined nationwide by 31% from 1995 to 2009 (Table 118).

Since their creation as part of the Balanced Budget Act of 1997, the number of **critical access hospitals** (small rural hospitals that are certified to receive cost-based reimbursement from Medicare) has grown to more than 1,300 in 2009. Four states (Iowa, Kansas, Minnesota, and Texas) each had more than 75 critical access hospitals in 2009 (Table 118).

Health Care Expenditures and Payors

Health Care Expenditures

The United States spends a larger share of its **gross domestic product (GDP) on health** than does any other major industrialized country. In 2007, the United States devoted 16% of its GDP to health, compared with 11% in France and 10.8% in Switzerland—the countries with the next highest shares (Table 121).

In 2008, **national health care expenditures** in the United States totaled $2.3 trillion, a 4.4% increase from 2007. The average per capita expenditure on health in the United States was $7,700 in 2008 (Table 122).

Expenditures for hospital care accounted for 31% of all national health expenditures in 2008. Physician and clinical services accounted for 21% of the total in 2008, prescription drugs for 10%, and nursing home care for 6% (Table 125).

Prescription drug expenditures increased 3.2% between 2007 and 2008, compared with a 4.5% increase between 2006 and 2007 (Table 125).

Health Care Payors

In 2008, 35% of **personal health care expenditures** were paid by private health insurance, consumers paid 14% out of pocket, and 47% were paid by public funds. The majority of public funds went toward Medicare and Medicaid expenditures (Figure 23 and Table 126).

In 2008, the **Medicare** program had 45 million **enrollees and expenditures** of $468 billion, up from $432 billion the previous year. Expenditures for the Medicare drug program (Part D) were $49 billion in 2008, accounting for 11% of Medicare expenditures in that year (Table 140).

Of the 35 million **Medicare enrollees in the fee-for-service program** in 2008, 18% were under 65 years of age, compared with 12% in 1994 (Table 141).

In 2008, children under 21 years of age accounted for 48% of **Medicaid recipients** but only 19% of expenditures. Aged, blind, and persons with disabilities accounted for 22% of recipients and 64% of expenditures (Table 143).

In 2008, the **Children's Health Insurance Program (CHIP)** accounted for less than 1% of personal health care expenditures (Table 126).

Health Insurance Coverage

Between 2000 and 2009, the percentage of the population under 65 years of age with **private health insurance obtained through the workplace** declined from 67% to 58% (Table 136).

In 2009, 18% of the **population under 65 years of age had no health insurance coverage** (public or private) **at the time of interview**. Between 2000 and 2009, this percentage was 16% to 18% (Table 138).

Among the under-65 population, persons with a family income less than 400% of the poverty level were 3.1 to 5.3 times as likely to be **uninsured at the time of interview** as persons in higher income families in 2009 (Table 138).

In 2009, 8% of **children** under 18 years of age were **uninsured at the time of interview**. Between 2000 and 2009, among children in families with income just above the poverty level (100%–199% of poverty), the percentage uninsured dropped from 22% to 12%, whereas the percentage with coverage through Medicaid or CHIP increased from 28% to 54% (Tables 137 and 138).

Chartbook With Special Feature on Death and Dying

Introduction
Life Expectancy at Birth

The gap in life expectancy at birth between white persons and black persons persists but has narrowed since 1990.

Life expectancy is a measure often used to gauge the overall health of a population. As a summary measure of mortality, life expectancy represents the average number of years of life that could be expected if current death rates were to remain constant. Shifts in life expectancy are often used to describe trends in mortality. Life expectancy at birth is strongly influenced by infant and child mortality.

From 1980 through 2007, life expectancy at birth in the United States increased from 70 years to 75 years for men and from 77 years to 80 years for women (Table 22). Women have had longer life expectancy at birth in all decennial periods since 1900–1902, with white females having the longest life expectancy (1).

Racial disparities in life expectancy at birth persisted in 2007 but had narrowed since 1990. During this period, the gap in life expectancy between white males and black males narrowed from 8 years to

6 years and the gap in life expectancy between white females and black females decreased from 6 years to 4 years.

Reference

1. Arias E, Curtin LR, Wei R, Anderson RN. U.S. Decennial life tables for 1999–2001, United States life tables. National vital statistics reports; vol 57 no 1. Hyattsville, MD: NCHS; 2008. Available from: http://www.cdc.gov/nchs/data/nvsr/nvsr57/nvsr57_01.pdf.

Figure 1. Life expectancy at birth, by race and sex: United States, 1980–2007

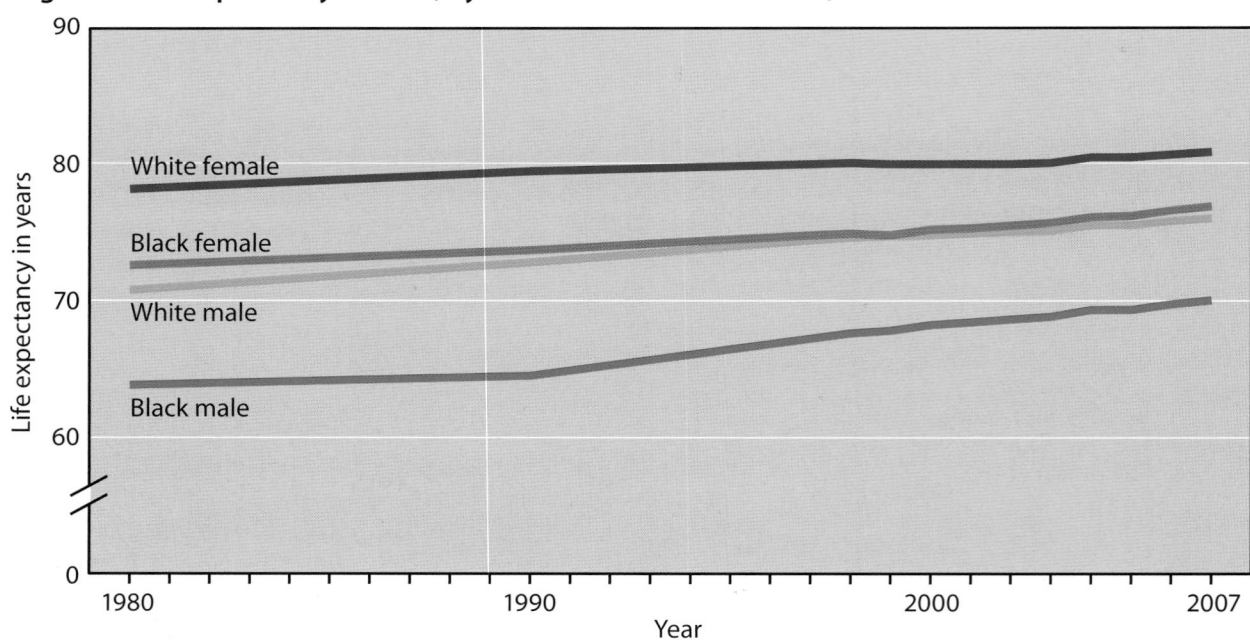

NOTE: See data table for Figure 1.

SOURCE: CDC/NCHS, National Vital Statistics System.

Morbidity
Health Conditions Among Children

Between 1997–1999 and 2007–2009, the percentage of children with reported food or skin allergies and with attention deficit hyperactivity disorder (ADHD or ADD) increased, while the percentage with a recent asthma attack was unchanged.

Most children enjoy good health, with only 2% of children having their health status reported as fair or poor (Table 56). Yet, this is a period when concerns about growth and development emerge and access to diagnostic and treatment services from professionals in health care, mental health, and the school system is critical. Both chronic health and developmental conditions have important consequences for children's ability to participate in school (1).

Between 1997–1999 and 2007–2009, the percentage of children with respondent-reported food allergies increased from 3% to 5%, and the percentage with skin allergies increased from 7% to 11%. The prevalence of reported skin allergies among children was twice as high as that of food allergies. Children with food allergies were more likely to have asthma and other allergies (2).

During this period, 5% of children were reported to have had an asthma attack in the past year. Asthma attacks were more common among boys than girls

and among non-Hispanic black children than among non-Hispanic white children (3) (Table 46).

The percentage of school-age children with ADHD or ADD increased from 7% to 9% during this period. School-age boys (12%) were twice as likely as girls (6%) to have ever been diagnosed with ADHD or ADD (4) (Table 46). In 2005–2008, 5% of boys 5–17 years of age and 3% of girls in that age group had recently used prescription central nervous system stimulants; these drugs are commonly prescribed for ADHD or ADD (5).

References

1. Van Cleave J, Gortmaker SL, Perrin JM. Dynamics of obesity and chronic health conditions among children and youth. JAMA 2010;303(7):623–30.
2. Branum AM, Lukacs SL. Food allergy among U.S. children: Trends in prevalence and hospitalizations. NCHS data brief no 10. Hyattsville, MD: NCHS; 2008. Available from: http://www.cdc.gov/nchs/data/databriefs/db10.pdf.
3. Akinbami LJ. The state of childhood asthma, United States, 1980–2005. Advance data from vital and health statistics; no 381. Hyattsville, MD: NCHS; 2006 Available from: http://www.cdc.gov/nchs/data/ad/ad381.pdf.
4. Pastor PN, Reuben CA. Diagnosed attention deficit hyperactivity disorder and learning disability: United States, 2004–2006. NCHS. Vital health stat 2008;10(237). Available from: http://www.cdc.gov/nchs/data/series/sr_10/Sr10_237.pdf.
5. CDC/NCHS. National Health and Nutrition Examination Survey [unpublished analysis].

Figure 2. Respondent-reported selected conditions among children under 18 years of age: United States, 1997–1999 and 2007–2009

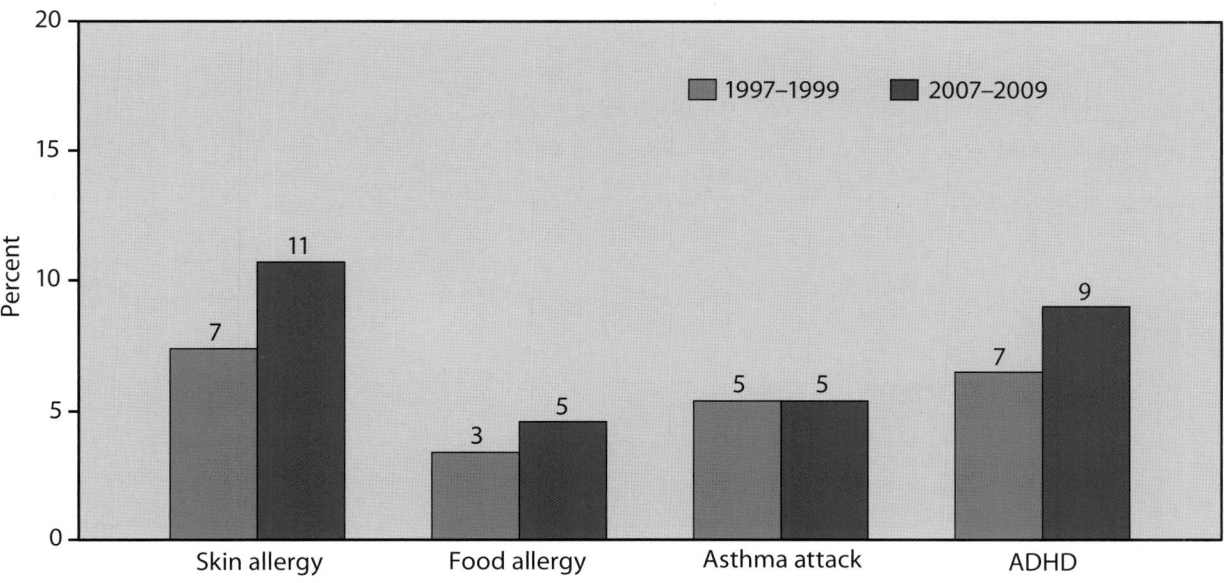

NOTES: ADHD is attention deficit hyperactivity disorder. See data table for Figure 2.

SOURCE: CDC/NCHS, National Health Interview Survey.

Heart Disease Prevalence

From 1999 to 2009, heart disease prevalence rates have remained stable among adult women in all age groups and among adult men younger than 75 years of age.

Heart disease is the leading cause of death in the United States. In 2007, one-quarter of all deaths (616,000) were from diseases of the heart (Figure 24). The majority (81%) of heart disease deaths were among people 65 years of age and over (1).

Risk factors for heart disease include obesity, lack of regular physical activity, and smoking (2–4). Over the past 40 years, smoking rates have declined and obesity rates have increased (Tables 60 and 71). Physical activity rates increased only modestly over the last decade (Figure 12). High serum total cholesterol and uncontrolled high blood pressure rates—also risk factors for cardiovascular disease—have declined among older men and women (Tables 67 and 68). The prevalence of diabetes has increased since 1988–1994 (Table 50). Among heart disease patients, medical care and preventive drug treatments have contributed to continued decreases in death rates.

Between 1999 and 2009, the prevalence of lifetime respondent-reported heart disease differed by sex and age. The proportion of adults 18–64 years of age who reported ever being diagnosed with heart disease was similar for men and women. Among older adults 65 years of age and over, respondent-reported prevalence rates were higher for men than women. Among adult women in all age groups, and among men under age 75, prevalence rates remained steady from 1999 to 2009. Among men 75 years of age and over, prevalence rates rose from 38% in 1999 to 46% in 2009. Although prevalence rates overall showed little change, age-adjusted death rates from heart disease declined by 28% from 1999 to 2007 (Table 30).

References

1. Xu JQ, Kochanek KD, Murphy SL, Tejada-Vera B. Deaths: Final data for 2007. National vital statistics reports; vol 58 no 19. Hyattsville, MD: NCHS; 2010. Available from: http://www.cdc.gov/nchs/data/nvsr/nvsr58/nvsr58_19.pdf.
2. Flegal KM, Graubard BI, Williamson DF, Gail MH. Cause-specific excess deaths associated with underweight, overweight, and obesity. JAMA 2007;298(17):2028–37.
3. CDC. The health consequences of smoking: A report of the Surgeon General. Washington, DC: U.S. Government Printing Office. 2004. Available from: http://www.cdc.gov/tobacco/data_statistics/sgr/sgr_2004/index.htm.
4. 2008 Physical activity guidelines for Americans [online]. 2008. U.S. Department of Health and Human Services, Office of Disease Prevention and Health Promotion (ODPHP) pub no U0036. Available from: http://www.health.gov/paguidelines/guidelines/default.aspx.

Figure 3. Respondent-reported lifetime heart disease prevalence among adults 18 years of age and over, by sex and age: United States, 1999–2009

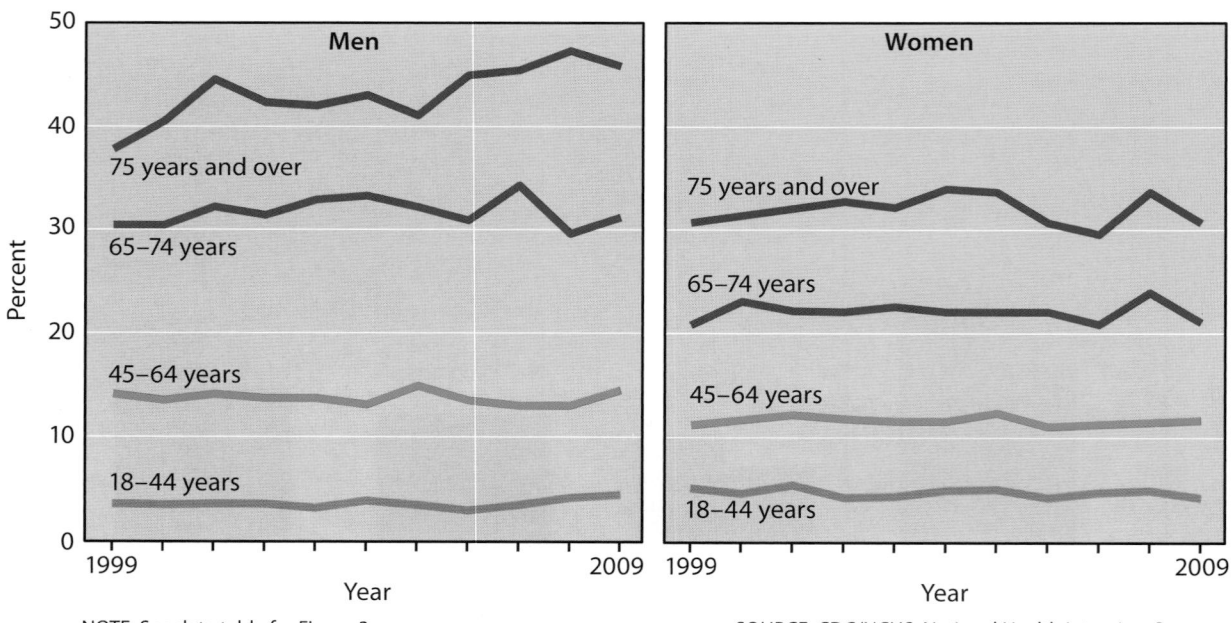

NOTE: See data table for Figure 3.

SOURCE: CDC/NCHS, National Health Interview Survey.

Cancer Prevalence

Cancer prevalence rates increased among women 45 years of age and over and among men 75 years of age and over from 1999 to 2009.

Cancer (also called malignant neoplasm) is the second leading cause of death in the United States after heart disease. In 2007, there were 560,000 deaths from all sites of cancer combined, accounting for 23% of all deaths (Figure 24). Seven in ten (69%) cancer deaths were to persons 65 years of age and over. Cancer is the leading cause of death for persons ages 45–64 and the second leading cause of death for 25–44 year olds (1) (Table 27 and Figures 29 and 30).

Between 1999 and 2009, the percentage of adults 18 years of age and over who reported ever having been told they had cancer (excluding nonmelanoma skin cancers) increased from 5% to 6% (data table for Figure 4). This increase in lifetime prevalence was largely driven by increases in cancer prevalence among men 75 years of age and over and among women 45 years of age and over.

In 2009, lifetime cancer prevalence increased with age, from 1% to 2% among men and women 18–44 years of age to 17% to 23% among men and women 75 years of age and over. Among adults under 65 years of age, lifetime cancer prevalence rates were higher for women than men; rates were lower for older women than men. Cancer prevalence was three times as high among women 18–44 years of age as men in that age group and nearly twice as high among women 45–64 years of age as men in that age group.

Reference

1. Xu JQ, Kochanek KD, Murphy SL, Tejada-Vera B. Deaths: Final data for 2007. National vital statistics reports; vol 58 no 19. Hyattsville, MD: NCHS; 2010. Available from: http://www.cdc.gov/nchs/data/nvsr/nvsr58/nvsr58_19.pdf.

Figure 4. Respondent-reported lifetime cancer prevalence among adults 18 years of age and over, by sex and age: United States, 1999–2009

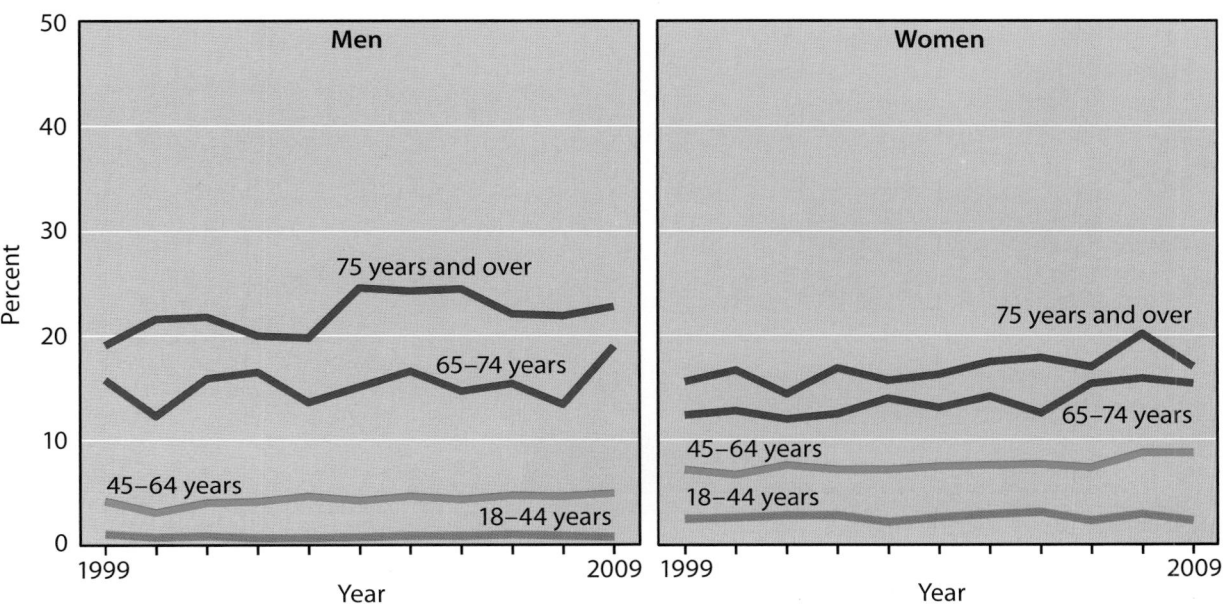

NOTE: See data table for Figure 4.

SOURCE: CDC/NCHS, National Health Interview Survey.

Diabetes Prevalence

Diabetes prevalence among adults 20 years of age and over was 11% in 2005–2008, up from 8% in 1988–1994.

Long-term complications of diabetes include cardiovascular disease, renal failure, nerve damage, and retinal damage (1,2). Treatment guidelines for diabetes recommend dietary modifications, physical activity, weight loss (if overweight), and the possible use of medication (2,3).

Among adults 20 years of age and over, the prevalence of diabetes (including physician-diagnosed and undiagnosed diabetes) has increased from 8% in 1988–1994 to 11% in 2005–2008 (see data table for Figure 5 for definition of diabetes). The increase in diabetes prevalence was due primarily to an increase in physician-diagnosed diabetes (Table 50). The prevalence of undiagnosed diabetes has held steady from 1988–1994 to 2005–2008 at 3%.

Diabetes prevalence increases with age. In 2005–2008, 4% of adults 20–44 years, 14% of those 45–64 years, and 27% of those 65 years of age and over had diabetes. Diabetes is more common among non-Hispanic black adults (20%) and Mexican-origin adults (17%) than among non-Hispanic white adults (9%), after age-adjusting the data (Table 50). This disparity has persisted over time.

From 1988–1994 to 2005–2008, diabetes prevalence increased among adults 20–44 years and 65 years of age and over and held steady among adults 45–64 years of age. In the past two decades, diabetes has also been reported among U.S. children and adolescents with increasing frequency. It is estimated that in 2007, almost 200,000 persons under 20 years of age had diabetes (4).

References

1. Beers MH, Fletcher AJ, Porter R, eds. Merck manual of medical information. 2nd home edition. Whitehouse Station, NJ: Merck Research Laboratories; 2003.
2. Masharani U. Diabetes mellitus and hypoglycemia. In: McPhee SJ, Papadakis MA, eds. Current medical diagnosis and treatment, 49th ed. New York, NY: McGraw-Hill; 2010:1079–117.
3. American Diabetes Association. Standards of medical care in diabetes—2010. Diabetes Care 2010;33(suppl 1):S11–S61.
4. CDC. National diabetes fact sheet: General information and national estimates on diabetes in the United States, 2007. Atlanta, GA: CDC; 2008. Available from: http://www.cdc.gov/diabetes/pubs/pdf/ndfs_2007.pdf.

Figure 5. Diabetes prevalence among adults 20 years of age and over, by age: United States, 1988–1994 and 2005–2008

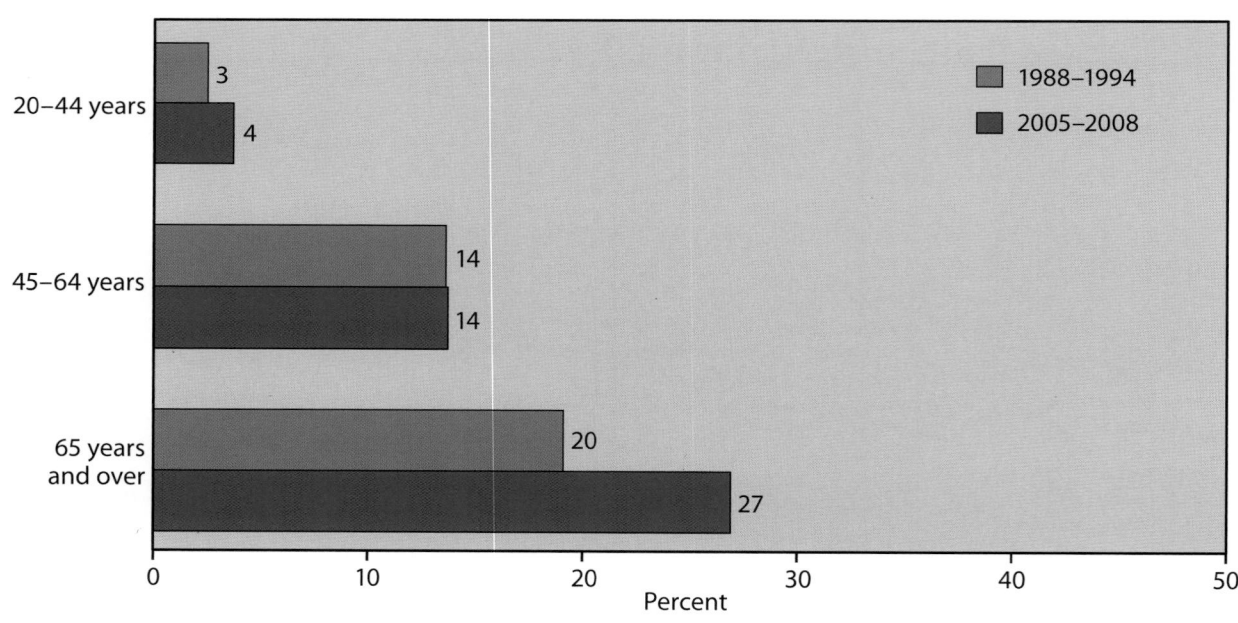

NOTE: See data table for Figure 5.

SOURCE: CDC/NCHS, National Health and Nutrition Examination Survey.

Poor Diabetes Control (Hemoglobin A1c Levels Above 9%)

The prevalence of poor diabetes control among persons diagnosed with diabetes has declined by 45% since 1988–1994 for adults 45–64 years of age and by 72% for adults 65 years of age and over.

Treatment and control of diabetes are necessary to reduce the likelihood of its complications, which include cardiovascular disease, renal failure, nerve damage, and retinal damage (1,2). Control of diabetes is generally measured by the degree of glycemic control. Good glycemic control significantly decreases retinopathy, nephropathy, and neuropathic complications. Hemoglobin A1c levels (one measure of glycemic control for persons with diabetes) help assess a patient's average blood glucose control over several months, help indicate whether glucose control goals are being met, and evaluate whether changes in the patient's treatment plan are needed (2). Elevated A1c values are strongly predictive of complications from diabetes. Lowering A1c values to around 7% has been shown to reduce complications; however, the target A1c value for individual patients depends on the patient's characteristics, comorbidities, and history. In general,

A1c values exceeding 9% indicate poor glycemic control (3).

From 1988–1994 to 2005–2008, the percentage of persons with diabetes who have poor glycemic control declined by 45% for adults 45–64 years of age and by 72% for older adults. There was no decline in the percentage with poor glycemic control for those 20–44 years of age. In 2005–2008, the percentage of persons with diabetes who have poor glycemic control was 26% for those 20–44 years, 14% for those 45–64 years, and 5% for those 65 years of age and over.

References

1. Masharani U. Diabetes mellitus and hypoglycemia. In: McPhee SJ, Papadakis MA, eds. Current medical diagnosis and treatment, 49th ed. New York, NY: McGraw-Hill; 2010:1079–117.
2. American Diabetes Association. Standards of medical care in diabetes—2010. Diabetes Care 2010;33(suppl 1):S11–S61.
3. Diabetes mellitus: Percent of patients with a diagnosis of diabetes mellitus having hemoglobin A1c (HbA1c) greater than 9 or not done during the past year [online]. National Quality Measures Clearinghouse, Agency for Healthcare Research and Quality. Available from: http://www.qualitymeasures.ahrq.gov/content.aspx?id=14624&search=a1c.

Figure 6. Poor diabetes control (hemoglobin A1c levels greater than 9%) among adults 20 years of age and over with diagnosed diabetes, by age: United States, 1988–1994 and 2005–2008

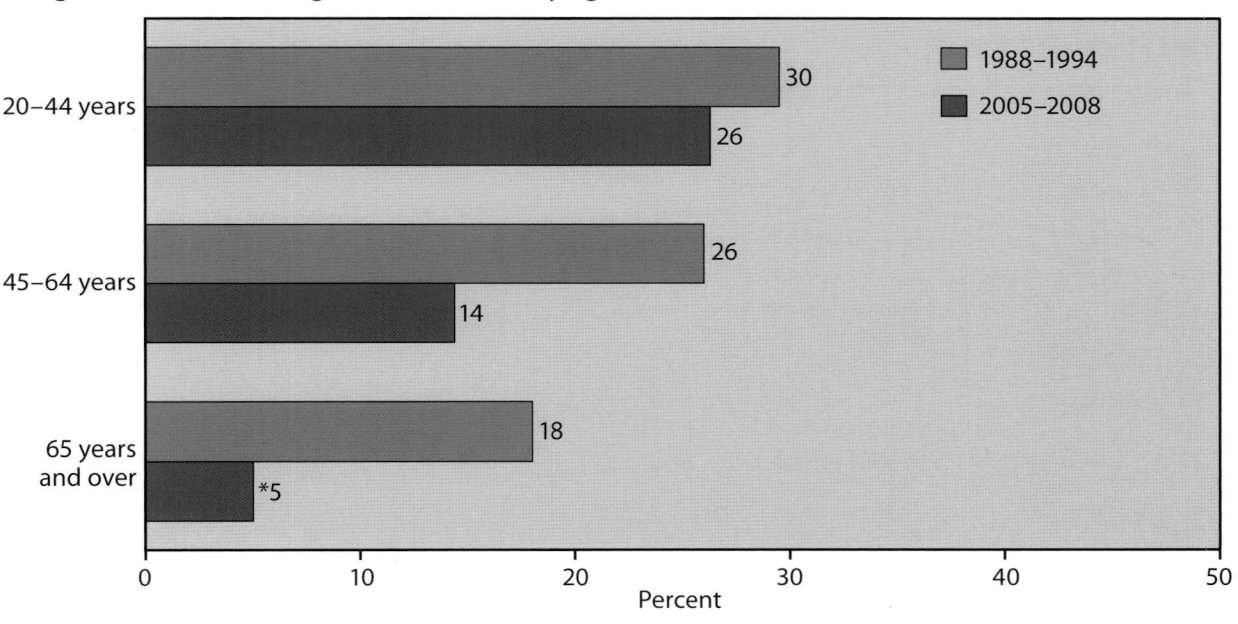

* Estimates are considered unreliable. Data preceded by an asterisk have a relative standard error of 20%–30%.

NOTE: See data table for Figure 6.

SOURCE: CDC/NCHS, National Health and Nutrition Examination Survey.

Joint Pain

Between 2002 and 2009, the prevalence of joint pain among adults was unchanged.

Pain affects physical and mental functioning and impacts quality of life. Pain perception and reporting are subjective and are influenced by a host of psychological and cultural factors (1). Joint pain can be caused by many types of conditions and by injury. Osteoarthritis is a common cause of joint pain (2). Factors associated with osteoarthritis include overweight, older age, and injury to a joint. Therapies that manage osteoarthritis pain and improve function include exercise, weight control, rest, over-the-counter and prescription medications, alternative therapies, and surgery (Figure 8).

Between 2002 and 2009, about 30% of adults 18 years of age and over reported recent (in the past 30 days) symptoms of pain, aching, or swelling around a joint. The knee was the most common painful joint reported (Table 53). During this period, the percentage of adults of all ages who reported recent joint pain was unchanged. Reported joint pain was strongly associated with age. In 2009, one in five adults 18–44 years, 42% of adults 45–64 years, and

about one-half of adults 65–74 years and 75 years of age and over had recent joint pain. Joint pain was more common among middle-aged and older women than among men in those age categories (Table 53).

References

1. NCHS. Health, United States, 2006: With chartbook on trends in the health of Americans. Special feature: Pain. Hyattsville, MD; 2006:68–87. Available from: http://www.cdc.gov/nchs/data/hus/hus06.pdf.
2. Osteoarthritis [online]. Medline Plus. National Institutes of Health, National Library of Medicine. Available from: http://www.nlm.nih.gov/medlineplus/osteoarthritis.html.

Figure 7. Joint pain in the past 30 days among adults 18 years of age and over, by age: United States, 2002–2009

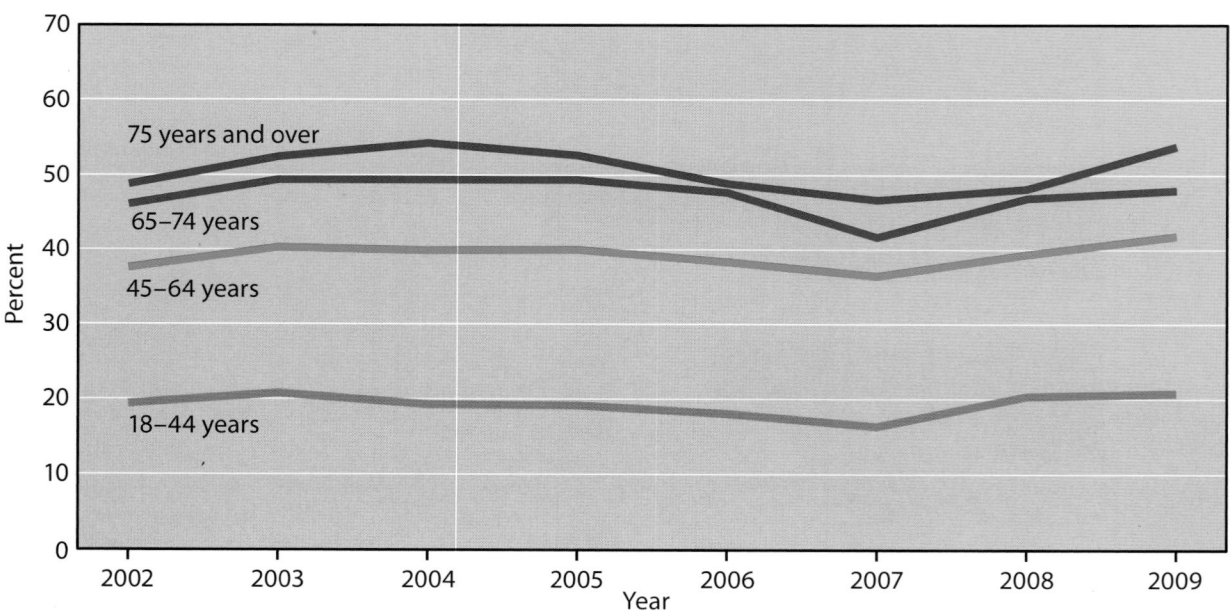

NOTE: See data table for Figure 7.

SOURCE: CDC/NCHS, National Health Interview Survey.

Health Care Utilization
Selected Back and Joint Procedures

Between 1996–1997 and 2006–2007, total knee replacement rates increased among adults 45 years of age and over.

Knee, back, and hip pain are common conditions among middle-aged and older persons (Table 53 and Figure 7). Methods to alleviate joint and low back pain include the use of over-the-counter and prescription medications, weight loss if needed, exercise, physical therapy, and surgical procedures (1,2). Total knee replacement is one of the most commonly performed orthopedic procedures and has been shown to improve functional status and relieve the pain often associated with osteoarthritis (3). Total hip replacement procedures are commonly performed to relieve pain from osteoarthritis, whereas partial hip replacements are generally performed to repair hip fractures (4). The evidence is mixed on the efficacy of disc removal and spinal fusion to relieve back pain (5).

Between 1996–1997 and 2006–2007, inpatient procedure rates among persons 45–64 years of age doubled for total knee replacements (from 12 to 26 per 10,000 population) and increased 80%, from 7 to 12 per 10,000 population, for total hip replacements. During this period, inpatient procedure rates for

excision of intervertebral disc and spinal fusion, which are typically not performed on an outpatient basis, were unchanged among this age group.

Among persons 65 years of age and over, excision of intervertebral disc and spinal fusion procedure rates increased 67%, from 17 to 28 per 10,000 population, and total knee replacement procedures increased 60%, from 51 to 82 per 10,000 population, during this period.

References

1. Osteoarthritis [online]. Medline Plus. National Institutes of Health, National Library of Medicine. Available from: http://www.nlm.nih.gov/medlineplus/osteoarthritis.html.
2. Joint disorders [online]. Medline Plus. National Institutes of Health, National Library of Medicine. Available from: http://www.nlm.nih.gov/medlineplus/jointdisorders.html.
3. Kane RL, Saleh KJ, Wilt TJ, Bershadsky B, Cross WW III, MacDonald RM, Rutks I. Total knee replacement. Evidence report/technology assessment no 86. AHRQ pub no 04–E006–1. Rockville, MD: Agency for Healthcare Research and Quality; 2003. Available from: http://www.ahrq.gov/clinic/epcsums/kneesum.pdf.
4. Zhan C, Kaczmarek R, Loyo-Berrios N, Sangl J, Bright RA. Incidence and short-term outcomes of primary and revision hip replacement in the United States. J Bone Joint Surg Am 2007; 89(3):526–33.
5. Deyo RA, Nachemson A, Mirza SK. Spinal-fusion surgery—The case for restraint. N Engl J Med 2004;350(7):722–6.

Figure 8. Selected back and joint procedures among adults 45 years of age and over, by age: United States, 1996–1997 through 2006–2007

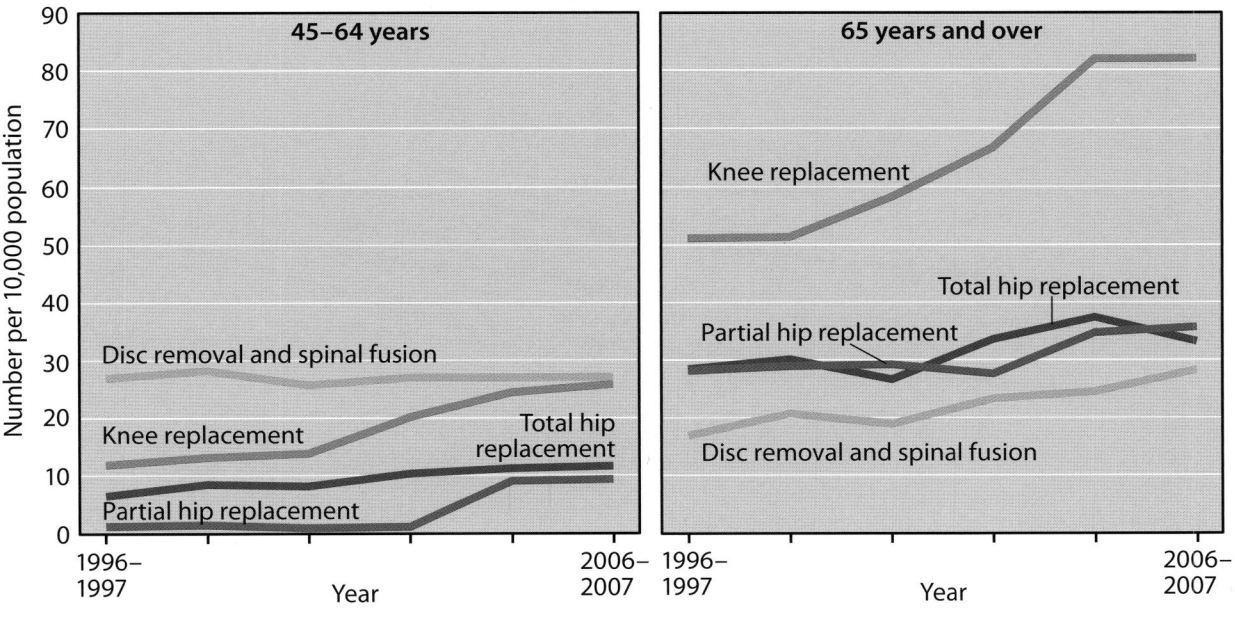

NOTE: See data table for Figure 8.

SOURCE: CDC/NCHS, National Hospital Discharge Survey.

Colorectal Tests and Procedures

Between 2000 and 2008, reported colorectal tests and procedures increased for adults 50–75 years of age among all racial and ethnic groups.

Colorectal cancer is the third most common cancer (excluding skin cancers) diagnosed in both men and women in the United States, accounting for an estimated 143,000 new cases in 2010 (1). Modifiable risk factors include a diet high in red meat, obesity, smoking, physical inactivity, and heavy alcohol consumption (1). Since 1990, age-adjusted colon cancer death rates have declined 31% overall but at a slower rate among black persons (Table 24). Declining colon cancer death rates were primarily associated with increased screening (2). Black persons have higher incidence and poorer survival for colon cancer than other racial groups (Tables 47 and 48).

In 1995, the U.S. Preventive Services Task Force first recommended screening for colorectal cancer for all persons age 50 and over (3). These recommendations were further refined in 2002 and again in 2008 (4). The task force now strongly urges adults 50–75 years of age to undergo high-sensitivity fecal occult blood testing (FOBT) annually, sigmoidoscopy every 5 years accompanied by FOBT every 3 years, or colonoscopy every 10 years.

Between 2000 and 2008, the percentage of adults 50–75 years of age who reported having colorectal procedures increased 55%, from 33% to 51% (see data table for Figure 9 for definition of colorectal procedures). Increases were noted among all racial and ethnic groups. However, Hispanic adults were less likely than adults in other racial and ethnic groups to have had colorectal procedures in 2008. Between 2000 and 2008, growth in reported colorectal procedures was fueled mainly by increased colonoscopy procedures (5).

References

1. Cancer facts and figures, 2010 [online]. American Cancer Society. Available from: http://www.cancer.org/Research/CancerFactsFigures/CancerFactsFigures/cancer-facts-and-figures-2010.
2. Edwards BK, Ward E, Kohler BA, Eheman C, Zauber AG, Anderson RN, et al. Commentary. Annual report to the Nation on the status of cancer, 1975–2006, featuring colorectal cancer trends and impact of interventions (risk factors, screening, and treatment) to reduce future rates. Cancer 2010;116:544–73. Available from: http://www3.interscience.wiley.com/cgi-bin/fulltext/123206036/PDFSTART.
3. Guide to clinical preventive services. 2nd ed. Report of the U.S. Preventive Services Task Force. Ch 8, Screening for colorectal cancer. Washington, DC: Department of Health and Human Services. 1995;89–103. Available from: http://odphp.osophs.dhhs.gov/pubs/guidecps/PDF/CH08.pdf.

(References continue on data table for Figure 9)

Figure 9. Respondent-reported colorectal tests and procedures among adults 50–75 years of age, by race and Hispanic origin: United States, 2000–2008

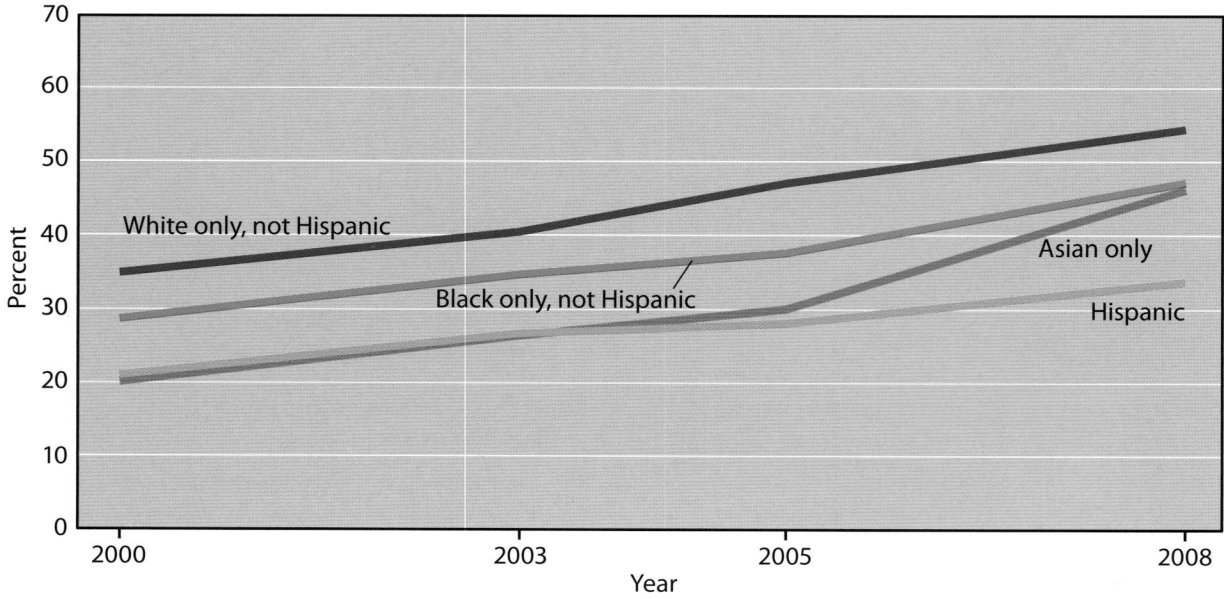

NOTE: See data table for Figure 9.

SOURCE: CDC/NCHS, National Health Interview Survey.

Antidepressant and Antianxiety Prescription Drug Use

Between 1988–1994 and 2005–2008, the percentage of adults taking prescription antidepressants increased almost fivefold to 11%, while the percentage taking antianxiety medications increased from 4% to 6%.

In their lifetimes, about one-half of Americans will have a serious mental health condition (1). Almost 30% of Americans will experience an anxiety disorder, and 17% will have a major depressive disorder (1). Research suggests that fewer than one-half of people with serious mental illness receive treatment (2–5). For many with mental illness, drugs are a helpful treatment option.

In addition to their use to treat depression, antidepressants are used to treat eating, anxiety, and posttraumatic stress disorders. Antianxiety medications are used for anxiety disorders and sedation. Drugs in these classes are also sometimes prescribed for subsyndromal mental health conditions and a variety of physical disorders (6,7).

From 1988–1994 to 2005–2008, the use of antidepressants increased almost fivefold among adults 18 years of age and over. In 2005–2008, 11% of adults reported taking a prescription antidepressant in the past month. Women were more than twice as

likely as men to take antidepressants (16% compared with 6%). Use was higher for women 45–64 years of age, compared with younger and older women.

Use of antianxiety drugs grew by about 50% from 1988–1994 to 2005–2008. In 2005–2008, 6% of adults 18 years of age and over reported taking a prescription antianxiety drug in the past month. Women 65 years of age and over were 66% more likely to report taking antianxiety drugs than men in the same age group (12% compared with 7%). The use of antianxiety drugs is higher for those 45 years of age and over, compared with younger adults.

References

1. Kessler RC, Berglund P, Demler O, Jin R, Merikangas KR, Walters EE. Lifetime prevalence and age-of-onset distributions of DSM–IV disorders in the National Comorbidity Survey Replication. Arch Gen Psychiatry 2005;62(6):593–602.
2. Kessler RC, Berglund PA, Bruce ML, Koch JR, Laska EM, Leaf PJ, et al. The prevalence and correlates of untreated serious mental illness. Health Serv Res 2001;36(6):987–1007.
3. Colman I, Wadsworth ME, Croudace TJ, Jones PB. Three decades of antidepressant, anxiolytic and hypnotic use in a national population birth cohort. Br J Psychiatry. 2006;189(2):156–60.

(References continue on data table for Figure 10)

Figure 10. Adults 18 years of age and over reporting prescription antidepressant and antianxiety drug use in the past month, by age and sex: United States, 1988–1994 and 2005–2008

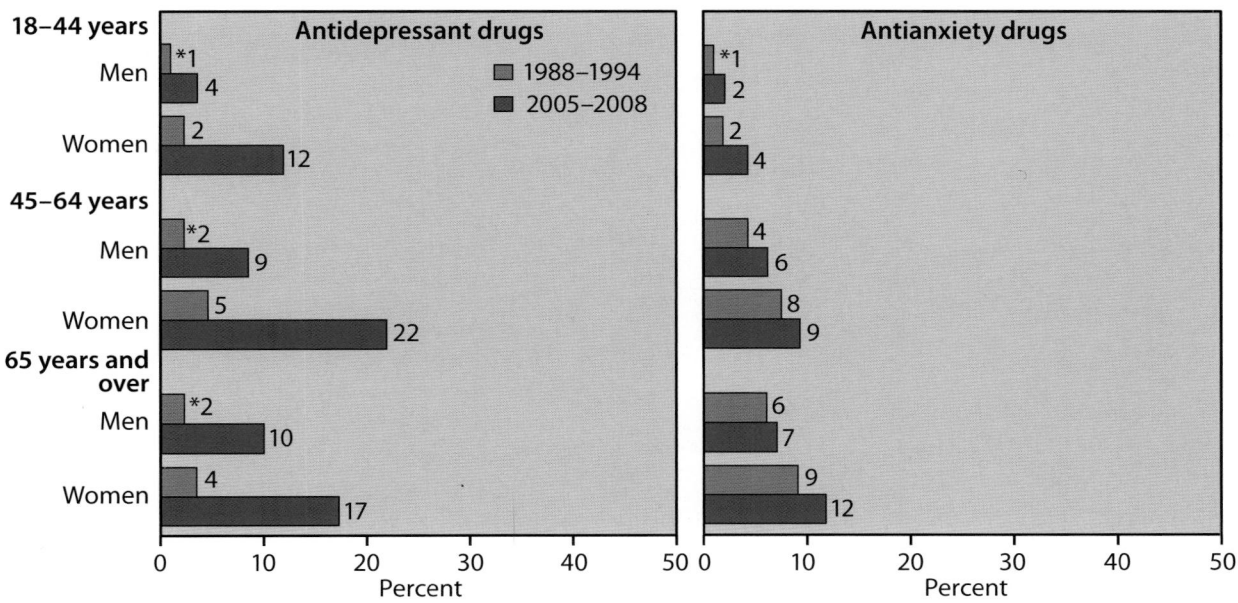

* Estimates are considered unreliable. Data preceded by an asterisk have a relative standard error of 20%–30%.
NOTE: See data table for Figure 10.

SOURCE: CDC/NCHS, National Health and Nutrition Examination Survey.

Health Risk Factors
Cigarette Smoking

Since 2004, little progress has been made in lowering the percentage of high school students and adults who smoke cigarettes.

Smoking is associated with an increased risk of heart disease, stroke, lung and other types of cancer, and chronic lung diseases (1). Smoking during pregnancy is an important preventable cause of poor pregnancy outcomes (1). Tobacco use, primarily cigarette smoking, remains the single largest preventable cause of death in the United States (2). Each year, an estimated 443,000 people die prematurely from smoking or exposure to secondhand smoke, and another 8.6 million have a serious illness caused by smoking (2). Decreasing cigarette smoking is a major public health objective. Preventing smoking among teenagers and young adults is critical because smoking usually begins in adolescence (3).

Between 1999 and 2009, cigarette smoking among males and females in grades 9–12 decreased from 35% to 19%–20%. Males and females in these grades were equally likely to smoke cigarettes in 2009.

The percentage of adults 18 years of age and over who smoked cigarettes declined between 1999 and 2004 and then stabilized at about 21%. Cigarette smoking decreased the most for younger men and women 18–44 years of age. Men under 65 years of age were more likely to smoke cigarettes than women of a similar age.

References

1. CDC. The health consequences of smoking: A report of the Surgeon General. National Center for Chronic Disease Prevention and Health Promotion, Office on Smoking and Health. Washington, DC: U.S. Government Printing Office; 2004. Available from: http://www.cdc.gov/tobacco/data_statistics/sgr/sgr_2004/index.htm.
2. Tobacco use: Targeting the Nation's leading killer—At a glance 2010 [online]. CDC, National Center for Chronic Disease Prevention and Health Promotion. Available from: http://www.cdc.gov/chronicdisease/resources/publications/aag/pdf/2010/tobacco_2010.pdf.
3. CDC. Preventing tobacco use among young people: A report of the Surgeon General. Office on Smoking and Health. Washington, DC: U.S. Government Printing Office; 1994. Available from: http://www.cdc.gov/tobacco/data_statistics/sgr/1994/index.htm.

Figure 11. Cigarette smoking among students in grades 9–12 and adults 18 years of age and over, by sex, grade, and age: United States, 1999–2009

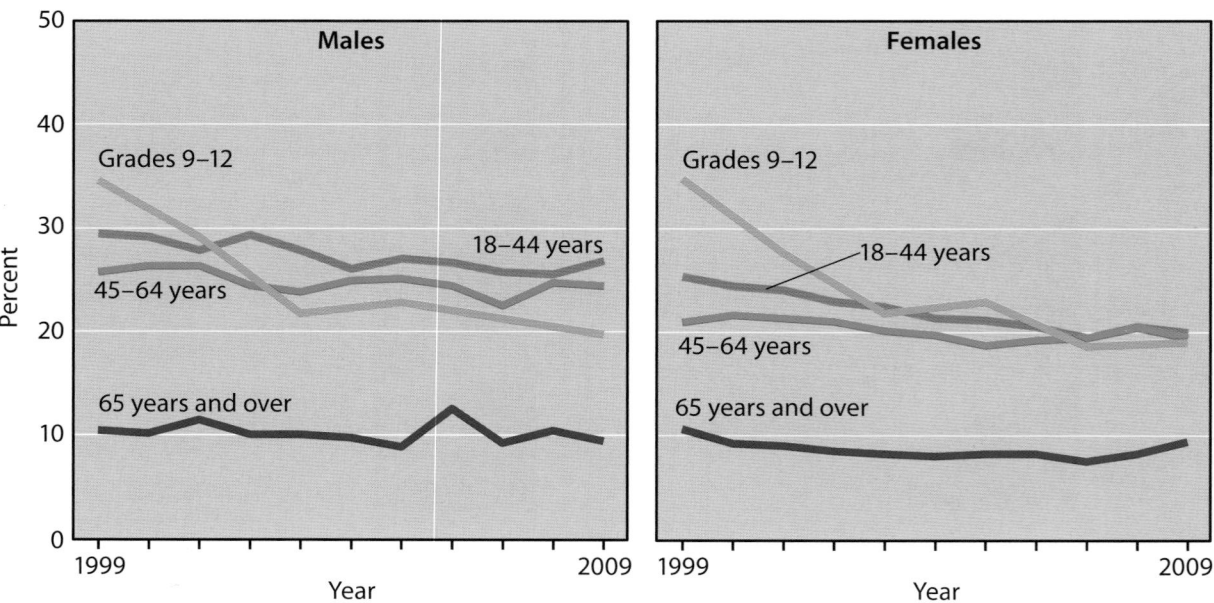

NOTE: See data table for Figure 11.

SOURCE: CDC/NCHS, National Health Interview Survey and CDC, Youth Risk Behavior Survey.

Participation in Leisure-time Aerobic and Muscle-strengthening Activities

Between 1999 and 2009, the percentage of men and women who met the 2008 federal guidelines for aerobic activity and muscle-strengthening increased among middle-age and older age groups, but the overall level remained below 20%.

Physical activity has been shown to have significant positive health effects, including lowering the risk of chronic illness (heart disease, stroke, type 2 diabetes, high blood pressure, and certain cancers), preventing falls, avoiding weight gain, and reducing depression (1). Since 1995, the Dietary Guidelines for Americans (2) have included advice on physical activity. In 2008, the Department of Health and Human Services released updated guidelines for aerobic activity and muscle-strengthening activities for Americans (1).

Between 1999 and 2009, the percentage of men 18 years of age and over who met the 2008 federal aerobic activity and muscle-strengthening guidelines increased from 19% to 22%. Among men, the percentage who met the guidelines for those 45–64 years and 65 years of age and over increased during this period, although their levels were lower than

among younger men. In 2009, 12% of men 65 years of age and over met the guidelines, compared with 28% of men 18–44 years of age.

Throughout this period, women were generally less likely to meet the guidelines than men in the same age group. The percentage of women 18 years of age and over who met the guidelines increased during this period, from 12% to 16%. As with men, the percentage who met the guidelines increased during this period for women 45–64 years and 65 years of age and over. The percentage of women who met the guidelines decreased with age (9% of women 65 years of age and over compared with 19% of women 18–44 years in 2009).

References

1. 2008 Physical activity guidelines for Americans [online]. U.S. Department of Health and Human Services. Available from: http://www.health.gov/paguidelines/default.aspx.
2. Nutrition and your health: Dietary guidelines for Americans, 4th ed [online]. U.S. Department of Agriculture and U.S. Department of Health and Human Services. 1995. Available from: http://www.cnpp.usda.gov/Publications/DietaryGuidelines/1995/1995DGConsumerBrochure.pdf.

Figure 12. Participation in leisure-time aerobic and muscle-strengthening activities that meet the 2008 federal physical activity guidelines for adults 18 years of age and over, by sex and age: United States, 1999–2009

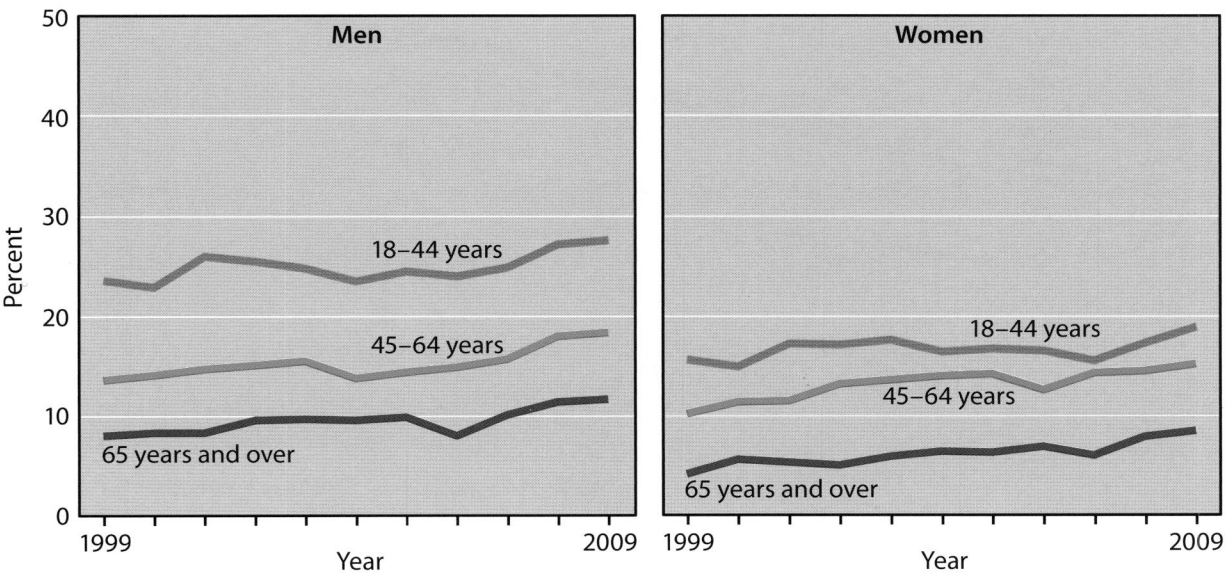

NOTE: See data table for Figure 12.

SOURCE: CDC/NCHS, National Health Interview Survey.

Obesity Among Children

The percentage of children who were obese rose in the 1980s and 1990s and has plateaued since then; in 2007–2008, almost one in five children older than 5 years of age was obese.

Excess body weight in children is associated with excess morbidity in childhood and adulthood (1). Obesity among children and teens 2–19 years of age is defined as a body mass index (BMI) for age and sex at or above the 95th percentile of the CDC growth charts (2). Obese children are more likely than their normal weight counterparts to become obese adults (3,4). Evidence suggests that the morbidity associated with obesity may increase with longer duration of obesity (5,6). Therefore, obesity trends among children may portend higher morbidity and mortality rates among future adults. Diet, physical inactivity, genetic factors, environment, and health conditions contribute to overweight and obesity. Changes in children's physical activity and eating habits over time appear to contribute to increases in prevalence of obesity (7–9).

Between 1988–1994 and 1999–2000, the percentage of obese children increased in all age groups. Young children (2–5 years of age) are less likely to be obese than older children. The percentage of young children who were obese rose from 7% in 1988–1994 to 10% in 1999–2000 and has held steady since that time (10). The prevalence of obesity among 6–11 year olds increased from 11% in 1988–1994 to 15% in 1999–2000 and has not increased significantly since then. The increase was similar among adolescents (12–19 years of age) for whom the prevalence of obesity rose from 11% to 15% between 1988–1994 and 1999–2000 before leveling off during the 2000s.

References

1. Dietz WH. Health consequences of obesity in youth: Childhood predictors of adult disease. Pediatrics 1998;101(3 pt 2):518–25.
2. Ogden CL, Flegal KM. Changes in terminology for childhood overweight and obesity. National health statistics reports; no 25. Hyattsville, MD: NCHS; 2010. Available from: http://www.cdc.gov/nchs/data/nhsr/nhsr025.pdf.
3. Singh AS, Mulder C, Twisk JW, van Mechelen W, Chinapaw MJ. Tracking of childhood overweight into adulthood: A systematic review of the literature. Obes Rev 2008;9(5): 474–88.
4. Freedman DS, Mei Z, Srinivasan SR, Berenson GS, Dieta WH. Cardiovascular risk factors and excess adiposity among overweight children and adolescents: The Bogalusa Heart Study. J Pediatr 2007 150(1):12–17.
5. Gregg EW, Cheng YJ, Cadwell BL, Imperatore G, Williams DE, Flegal KM, et al. Secular trends in cardiovascular disease risk factors according to body mass index in U.S. adults. JAMA 2005;293(15):1868–74.

(References continue on data table for Figure 13)

Figure 13. Obesity among children, by age: United States, 1988–1994 through 2007–2008

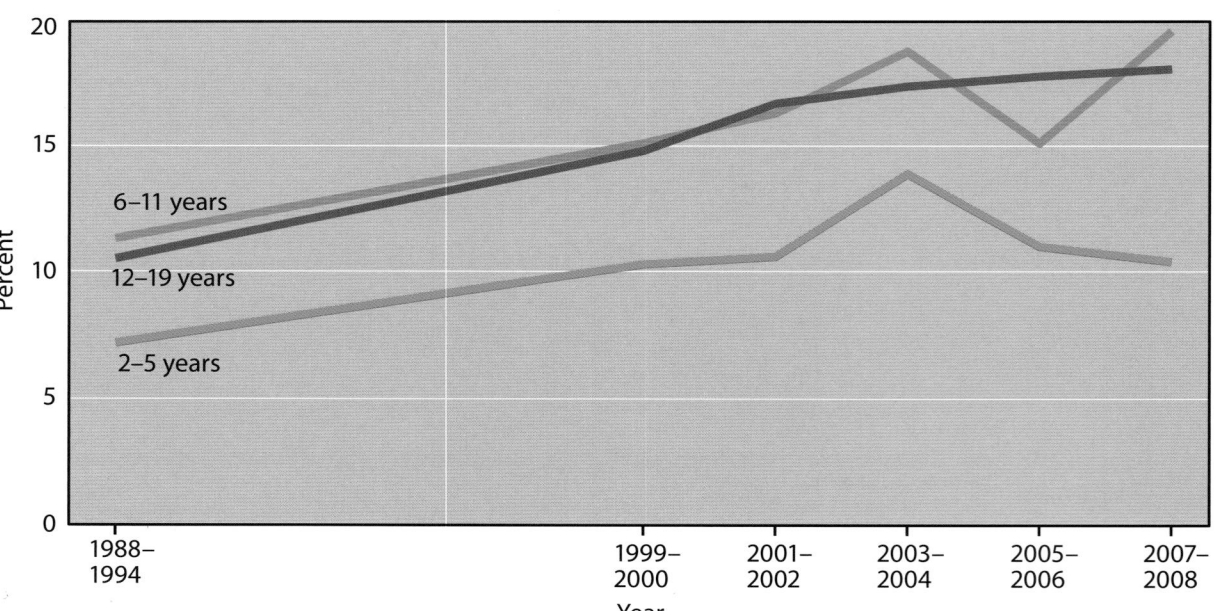

NOTE: See data table for Figure 13.

SOURCE: CDC/NCHS, National Health and Nutrition Examination Survey.

Overweight and Obesity Among Adults

The proportion of American adults 20 years of age and over who were obese rose in the 1980s and 1990s. In 2007–2008, about one-third of adults were obese and about two-thirds were overweight or obese.

Excess body weight is associated with excess morbidity and mortality (1,2). Obesity (body mass index (BMI) of 30.0 or higher) is correlated with excess mortality; Grade 2+ obesity (BMI of 35.0 or higher), in particular, significantly increases the risk of death (3). Obesity is also associated with increased risk of heart disease, stroke, some cancers, diabetes, osteoarthritis, and disability (1,2,4–7). Diet, physical inactivity, genetic factors, environment, and health conditions contribute to overweight and obesity.

The proportion of men who are obese grew from 19% in 1988–1994 to 32% in 2007–2008 although there was no increase after 2005–2006. For women, this proportion increased from 25% to 35% during this period; obesity rates did not rise between 1999–2000 and 2007–2008. The proportion of men with Grade 2+ obesity doubled from 5% to 11%; the proportion of women in this category grew from 11% to 18%. In 2007–2008, 4% of men and 7% of women had a BMI of 40 or higher (Grade 3 obesity) (8). The proportion of adults who were overweight but not

obese (BMI between 25 and 29.9) remained stable between 1988–1994 and 2007–2008.

Obesity patterns vary by race and ethnicity. Among women, non-Hispanic black women had the highest obesity rates, followed by Mexican-origin women (Table 71). There was less racial and ethnic variation in obesity among men.

References

1. National Heart, Lung, and Blood Institute and National Institute of Diabetes and Digestive and Kidney Diseases. Clinical guidelines on the identification, evaluation, and treatment of overweight and obesity in adults: The evidence report. NIH pub no 98–4083. Bethesda, MD: National Institutes of Health; 1998. Available from: http://www.nhlbi.nih.gov/guidelines/obesity/ob_gdlns.pdf.
2. National Task Force on the Prevention and Treatment of Obesity. Overweight, obesity, and health risk. Arch Intern Med 2000; 160(7):898–904.
3. Flegal KM, Graubard BI, Williamson DF, Gail MH. Excess deaths associated with underweight, overweight, and obesity. JAMA 2005; 293(15):1861–7.
4. Ogden CL, Yanovski SZ, Carroll MD, Flegal KM. The epidemiology of obesity. Gastroenterology 2007; 132(6):2087–102.
5. Gregg EW, Guralnik JM. Is disability obesity's price of longevity? JAMA 2007; 298(17):2066–7.
6. Alley DE, Chang VW. The changing relationship of obesity and disability, 1988–2004. JAMA 2007; 298(17):2020–7.

(References continue on data table for Figure 14)

Figure 14. Overweight and obesity among adults 20 years of age and over, by sex: United States, 1988–1994 through 2007–2008

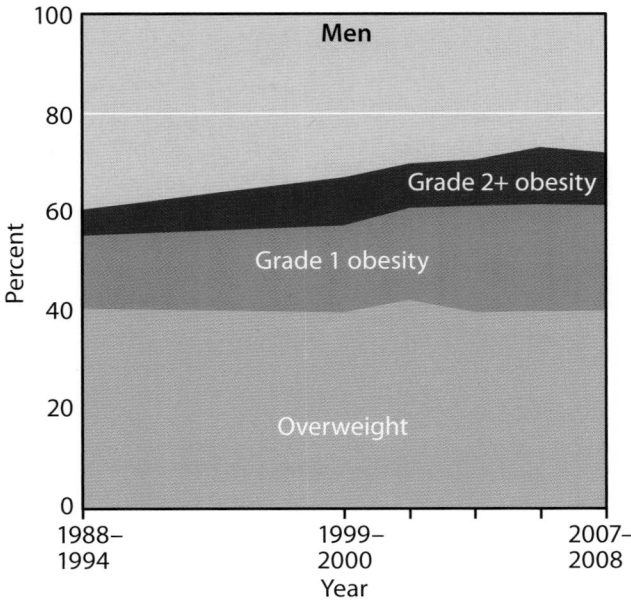

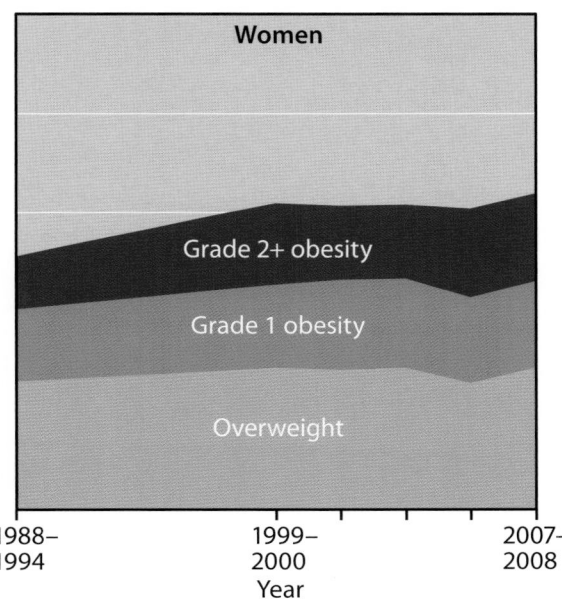

NOTE: See data table for Figure 14.

SOURCE: CDC/NCHS, National Health and Nutrition Examination Survey.

Hypertension Prevalence

Hypertension prevalence increased among all age groups for men and women 45 years of age and over.

Hypertension increases the risk for cardiovascular disease, heart attack, and stroke (1). Treatment of hypertension may include lifestyle modifications such as weight loss and a modified diet, as well as medication. Between 1988–1994 and 2005–2008, the prevalence of hypertension (defined in this figure as having an average systolic blood pressure reading of at least 140 mmHg or an average diastolic reading of at least 90 mmHg or taking antihypertensive medication) among adults 20 years of age and over increased from 24% to 32%.

During this period, the prevalence of hypertension was stable among men and women 20–44 years of age. Hypertension prevalence increased among men and women 45–64 years, 65–74 years, and 75 years of age and over. The largest increases were among women 45–64 and 65–74 years of age. Hypertension was more common among men than women 20–44 years of age, was similar among those 45–74 years, and was more common among women than men 75 years and over.

The prevalence of hypertension was higher among non-Hispanic black adults 20 years of age and over than among non-Hispanic white and Mexican-origin adults, even after age-adjusting the data (2) (Table 67). This racial disparity has persisted over time.

Between 1988–1994 and 2005–2008, the overall prevalence of uncontrolled high blood pressure (average systolic pressure of at least 140 mmHg or diastolic pressure of at least 90 mmHg among those previously told they had hypertension) among adults 20 years of age and over decreased from 74% to 54% (Table 67). The use of antihypertensive medications increased during this period (Table 95).

References

1. National High Blood Pressure Education Program. Seventh report of the Joint National Committee on Prevention, Detection, Evaluation, and Treatment of High Blood Pressure: Complete report. NIH pub no 04–5230. Bethesda, MD: National Heart, Lung, and Blood Institute, National Institutes of Health; 2004. Available from: http://www.nhlbi.nih.gov/guidelines/hypertension/jnc7full.htm.
2. CDC/NCHS. National Health and Nutrition Examination Survey [unpublished analysis].

Figure 15. Hypertension among adults 20 years of age and over, by sex and age: United States, 1988–1994, 1999–2002, and 2005–2008

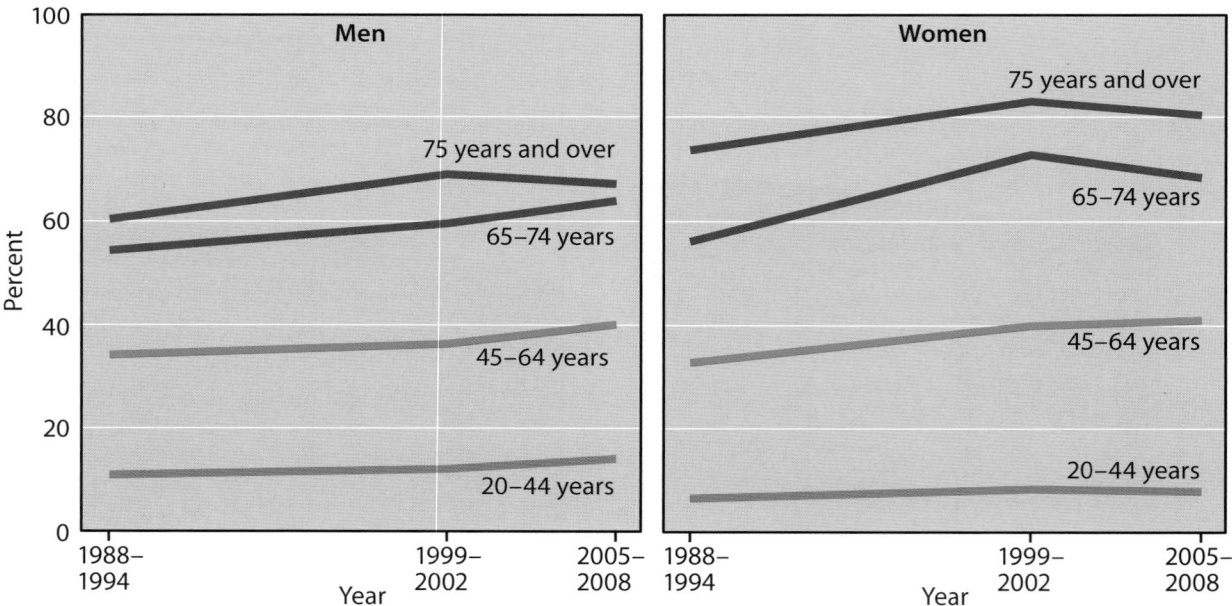

NOTE: See data table for Figure 15.

SOURCE: CDC/NCHS, National Health and Nutrition Examination Survey.

High Serum Total Cholesterol (240 mg/dL or Higher)

Between 1988–1994 and 2005–2008, the percentage of the population 45 years of age and over with high serum total cholesterol levels (240 mg/dL or higher) declined among all age groups of men and women.

High serum (blood) total cholesterol is a major risk factor for heart disease—the leading cause of death in the United States (1,2). Cholesterol levels may be reduced by dietary modifications and increased physical activity. Additionally, cholesterol-lowering medication may be recommended (2).

The percentage of adults 20 years of age and over with a high serum total cholesterol level (defined as measured serum total cholesterol of 240 mg/dL or higher) decreased from 20% in 1988–1994 to 15% in 2005–2008. During this period, about 10% of men and women 20–44 years of age had high serum total cholesterol. The percentage of men and women with high serum total cholesterol levels declined among those 45–64 years, 65–74 years, and 75 years of age and over. These declines may be a result of improved awareness and increased use of cholesterol-lowering medications (3) (Figure 17).

In 2005–2008, women 65–74 years and 75 years of age and over were more than twice as likely as men in those age groups to have high serum total cholesterol and were less likely to use cholesterol-lowering medications (Figure 17). The higher serum total cholesterol levels among older women may also be due to hormonal changes after menopause and because women often have higher levels of high-density lipoprotein (HDL), a component of total cholesterol (3,4).

References

1. American Heart Association. Heart disease and stroke statistics—2010 update. Circulation 2010;121:e46–e215. Available from: http://circ.ahajournals.org/cgi/content/full/121/7/e46.
2. National Cholesterol Education Program. Third Report of the Expert Panel on Detection, Evaluation, and Treatment of the High Blood Cholesterol in Adults (Adult Treatment Panel III): Executive Summary. NIH pub no 01–3670. Bethesda, MD: National Heart, Lung, and Blood Institute, National Institutes of Health. 2001. Available from: http://www.nhlbi.nih.gov/guidelines/cholesterol/atp3xsum.pdf.
3. Schober SE, Carroll MD, Lacher DA, Hirsch R. High serum total cholesterol—An indicator for monitoring cholesterol lowering efforts: U.S. adults, 2005–2006. NCHS data brief no 2. Hyattsville, MD: NCHS; 2007. Available from: http://www.cdc.gov/nchs/data/databriefs/db02.pdf.
4. Carroll MD, Lacher DA, Sorlie PD, Cleeman JI, Gordon DJ, Wolz M, et al. Trends in serum lipids and lipoproteins of adults, 1960–2002. JAMA 2005;294(14):1773–81.

Figure 16. High serum total cholesterol (240 mg/dL or higher) among adults 20 years of age and over, by sex and age: United States, 1988–1994, 1999–2002, and 2005–2008

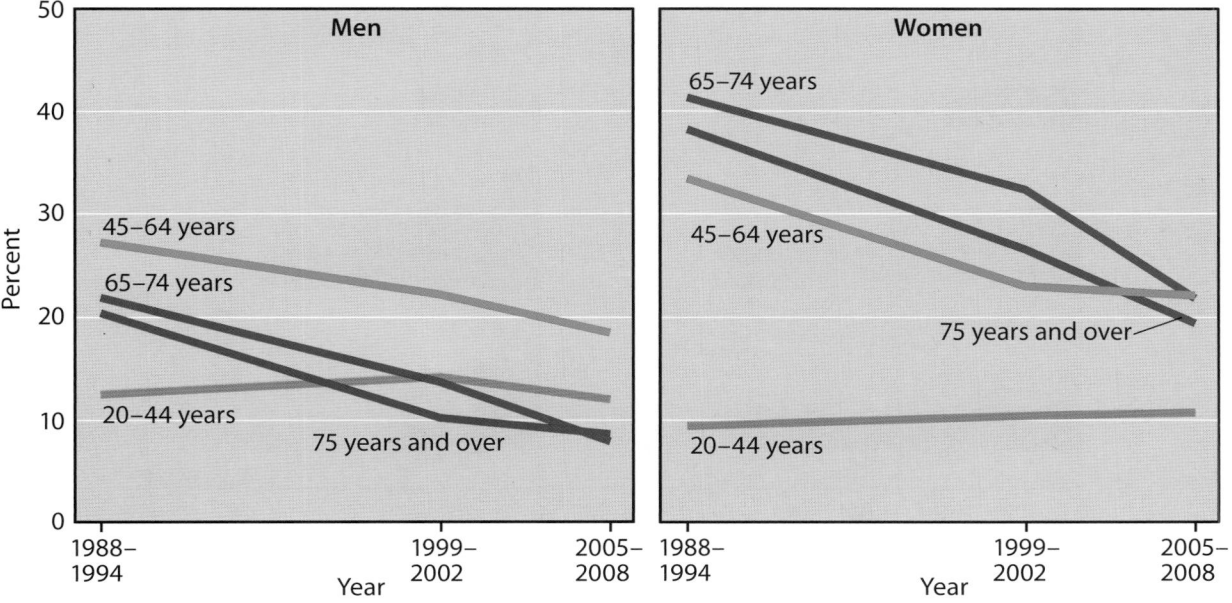

NOTE: See data table for Figure 16.

SOURCE: CDC/NCHS, National Health and Nutrition Examination Survey.

Prevention
Statin Drug Use

The percentage of adults 45 years of age and over using statin drugs has increased from 2% in 1988–1994 to 25% in 2005–2008.

High cholesterol is a risk factor for heart disease (Figure 3). Although cholesterol levels may be reduced by dietary modifications and increased physical activity, these lifestyle changes are often difficult to maintain or not sufficiently effective (1). In those cases, or for persons with other risk factors for heart disease, the use of cholesterol-lowering medications is often suggested.

Widespread belief in the value of drug therapy to lower cholesterol—and consequently to reduce mortality from heart disease—began with the introduction of statin drugs in 1987 and published studies that proved their effectiveness (2,3). There are several classes of cholesterol-lowering drugs (3,4), but statins have become the drug class of choice because of their demonstrated efficacy and safety (3,5).

From 1988–1994 to 2005–2008, the use of statin drugs by adults 45 years of age and over increased 10-fold, from 2% to 25%. There was a concurrent decline in the percentage of Americans with high serum total cholesterol (greater than or equal to 240 mg/dL) over this time period, which may be attributable to increased use of cholesterol-lowering medications, especially statins (6) (Figure 16 and Table 68).

Both men and women are increasingly taking statin drugs. However, in 2005–2008 one-half of men 65–74 years of age took a statin drug in the past 30 days, compared with just over one-third of women in that age group.

References

1. National Cholesterol Education Program. Third Report of the Expert Panel on Detection, Evaluation, and Treatment of the High Blood Cholesterol in Adults (Adult Treatment Panel III): Executive Summary. NIH pub no 01–3670. Bethesda, MD: National Heart, Lung, and Blood Institute, National Institutes of Health. 2001. Available from: http://www.nhlbi.nih.gov/guidelines/cholesterol/atp3xsum.pdf.
2. Knopp RH. Drug treatment of lipid disorders. N Eng J Med 1999;341(7):498–511.
3. Steinberg D, Gotto AM Jr. Preventing coronary artery disease by lowering cholesterol levels: Fifty years from bench to bedside. JAMA 1999;282(21):2043–50.

(References continue on data table for Figure 17)

Figure 17. Statin drug use in the past 30 days among adults 45 years of age and over, by sex and age: United States, 1988–1994, 1999–2002, and 2005–2008

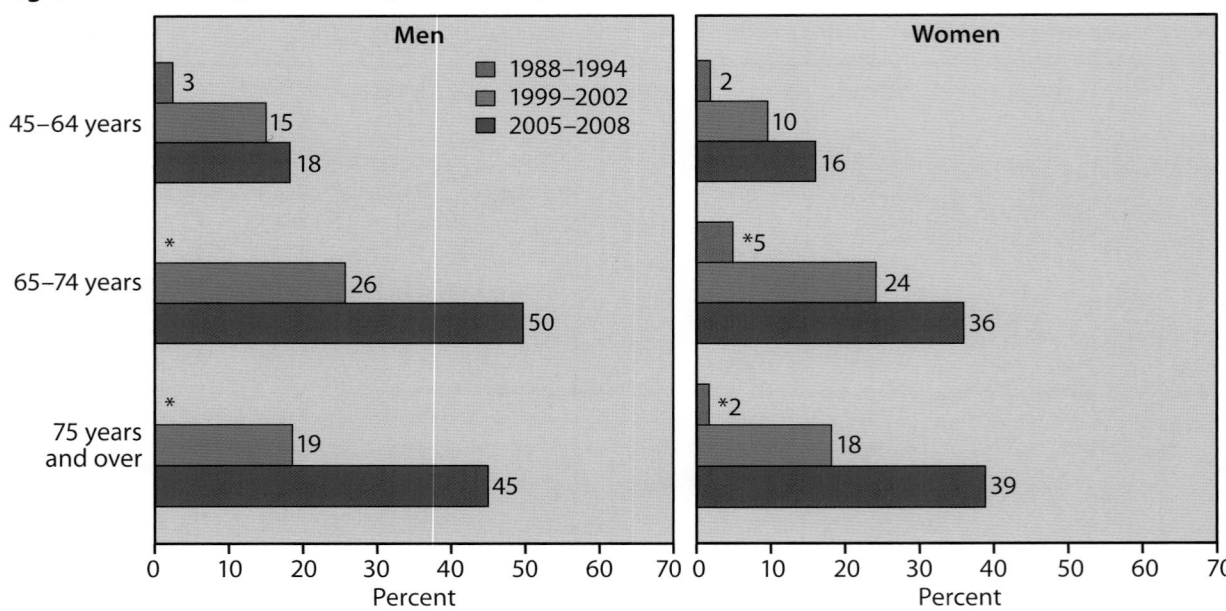

* Estimates are considered unreliable. Data preceded by an asterisk have a relative standard error (RSE) of 20%–30%. Data not shown have an RSE greater than 30%.
NOTE: See data table for Figure 17.

SOURCE: CDC/NCHS, National Health and Nutrition Examination Survey.

Influenza Vaccination

Between 1999 and 2009, influenza vaccination increased among adults 50–64 years of age and those 85 years and over.

Vaccination of persons at risk for complications from influenza is an important public health strategy for preventing morbidity and mortality in the United States. Thousands of deaths each year are associated with influenza (1).

In April 2000, the Advisory Committee on Immunization Practices (ACIP) recommended that all adults 50 years of age and over receive an annual influenza vaccination (2). In response to the unexpected shortfall in the 2000–2001 and 2004–2005 influenza vaccine supply, ACIP and CDC modified the universal recommendation and established vaccine priority groups. These groups included persons 65 years of age and over and children and adults with chronic underlying health conditions (3,4). In February 2010, ACIP voted to expand the influenza recommendation for the 2010–2011 season to include all persons 6 months of age and over (5).

Between 1999 and 2009, influenza vaccination in the past 12 months among noninstitutionalized adults

increased among adults 50–64 years of age and among those 85 years and over and was stable among other age groups. Among those under age 85, a decrease in coverage in 2005 was related to the influenza vaccine shortage (6).

Receipt of influenza vaccination increased with age. In 2009, 77% of adults 85 years of age and over reported an influenza vaccination in the past 12 months—nearly twice the level of those 50–64 years (41%) and four times the level of those 18–49 years (23%).

References

1. CDC. Estimates of deaths associated with seasonal influenza—United States, 1976–2007. MMWR 2010;59(33):1057–62. Available from: http://www.cdc.gov/mmwr/preview/mmwrhtml/mm5933a1.htm.
2. CDC. Prevention and control of influenza: Recommendations of the Advisory Committee on Immunization Practices (ACIP), 2007. MMWR 2007;56(RR-06):1–60. Available from: http://www.cdc.gov/mmwr/PDF/rr/rr5606.pdf.
3. CDC. Notice to readers: Delayed supply of influenza vaccine and adjunct ACIP influenza vaccine recommendations for the 2000–01 influenza season. MMWR 2000;49(27);619–22. Available from: http://www.cdc.gov/mmwr/preview/mmwrhtml/mm4927a4.htm.

(References continue on data table for Figure 18)

Figure 18. Influenza vaccination in the past 12 months among adults 18 years of age and over, by age: United States, 1999–2009

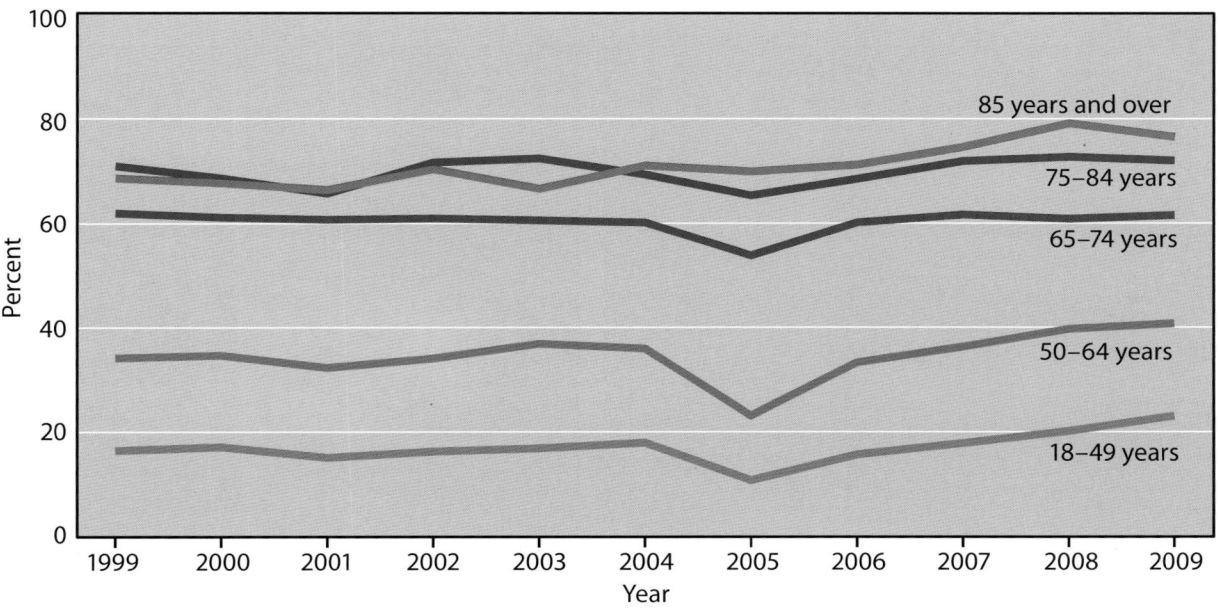

NOTE: See data table for Figure 18.

SOURCE: CDC/NCHS, National Health Interview Survey.

Access to Care
Delay or Nonreceipt of Needed Medical Care Due to Cost

Between 1999 and 2009, the percentage of working-age adults who delayed or did not receive needed medical care due to cost increased among persons with private coverage and among the uninsured.

Delaying or not receiving needed medical care may result in more serious illness, increased complications, and longer hospital stays (1,2). Persons with limited access to medical care, such as the uninsured, are more likely to delay or fail to obtain medical care when needed (3).

Among adults 18–64 years of age, the percentage who reported delaying or not receiving needed medical care in a 12-month period due to cost increased from 9% in 1999 to 15% in 2009. This increase was driven by a 72% increase in reported delay or nonreceipt of needed care among those with private insurance and a 41% increase among the uninsured.

Throughout this time period, delay or nonreceipt of needed medical care due to cost was highest among the uninsured and lowest among those with private coverage. In 2009, 37% of uninsured adults 18–64 years of age reported delay or nonreceipt of needed medical care due to cost, compared with 14% of

those with Medicaid and 9% of privately insured adults.

Delay or nonreceipt of needed medical care due to cost also varied by age for adults with different types of coverage. Older working-age adults 45–64 years of age with Medicaid coverage or without insurance were more likely to report delaying or not receiving needed medical care due to cost than adults 18–44 years of age in the same insurance categories. Among those with private insurance coverage, older working-age adults did not report more problems in accessing care due to cost than younger adults.

References

1. Diamant AL, Hays RD, Morales LS, Ford W, Clames D, Asch S, et al. Delays and unmet need for health care among adult primary care patients in a restructured urban public health system. Am J Public Health 2004;94(5):783–9.
2. Baker DW, Shapiro MF, Schur CL. Health insurance and access to care for symptomatic conditions. Arch Intern Med 2000;160(9):1269–74.
3. Institute of Medicine (U.S.). Coverage matters: Insurance and health care. Washington, DC: National Academy Press; 2001. Available from: http://www.nap.edu/catalog.php?record_id=10188.

Figure 19. Adults 18–64 years of age who delayed or did not receive needed medical care in the past 12 months due to cost, by age and type of health insurance coverage: United States, 1999–2009

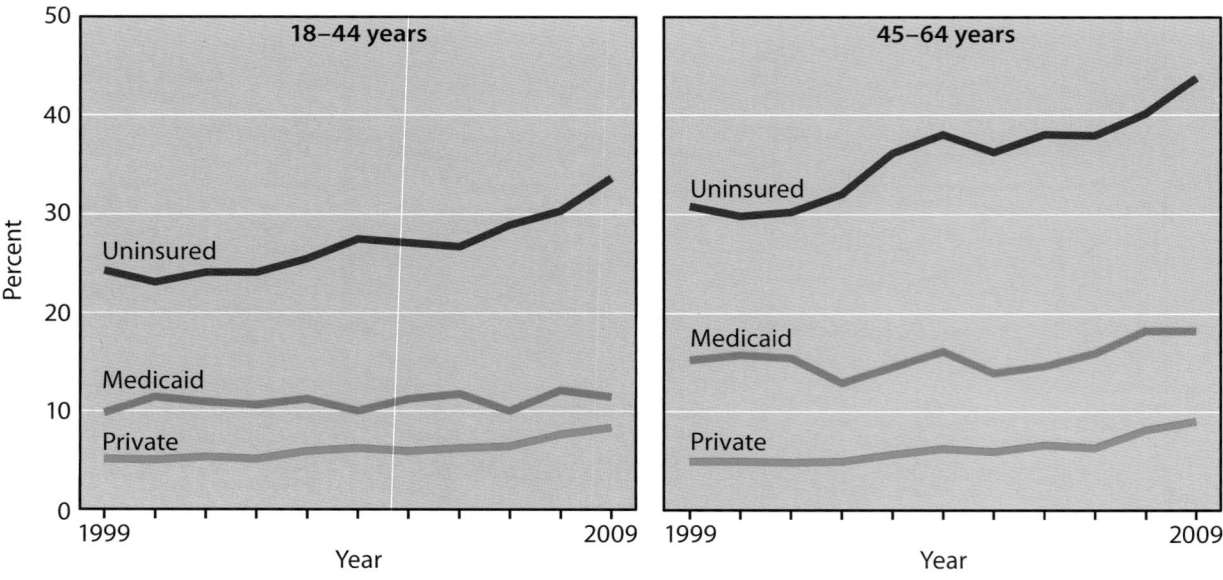

NOTE: See data table for Figure 19.

SOURCE: CDC/NCHS, National Health Interview Survey.

Dental Health Services Needs Unmet Due to Cost

From 1999 to 2009, the percentage of adults 18 years of age and over reporting unmet dental health care needs due to cost increased from 8% to 15%.

Oral health is integral to overall health. Poor oral health is associated with heart disease, stroke, and preterm, low-birthweight births (1). Poor oral health and its consequences may affect people's daily lives by interfering with eating, sleeping, working, and learning. Many diseases and conditions manifest themselves with oral symptoms, and these early signs may be initially noted by dental care providers.

In 2009, working-age adults 18–44 and 45–64 years of age were more likely than children or older adults to report having unmet dental health care needs in the past 12 months because they could not afford care. Among working-age adults, women were more likely to report unmet dental health care needs than men. For children and older adults, the reported rates of unmet dental health care were similar for males and females.

Since 1999, there has been a significant increase in the percentage of adults reporting unmet dental health care needs due to cost. In 1999, 8% of adults reported that they did not receive needed dental health services within the past 12 months because they could not afford them. By 2009, this percentage had increased to 15% (data table for Figure 20).

Reference

1. U.S. Department of Health and Human Services. Oral health in America: A report of the Surgeon General—Executive summary. Rockville, MD: U.S. Department of Health and Human Services, National Institute of Dental and Craniofacial Research, National Institutes of Health; 2000. Available from: http://www.surgeongeneral.gov/library/oralhealth/.

Figure 20. Persons who did not receive needed dental services in the past 12 months due to cost, by sex and age: United States, 1999–2009

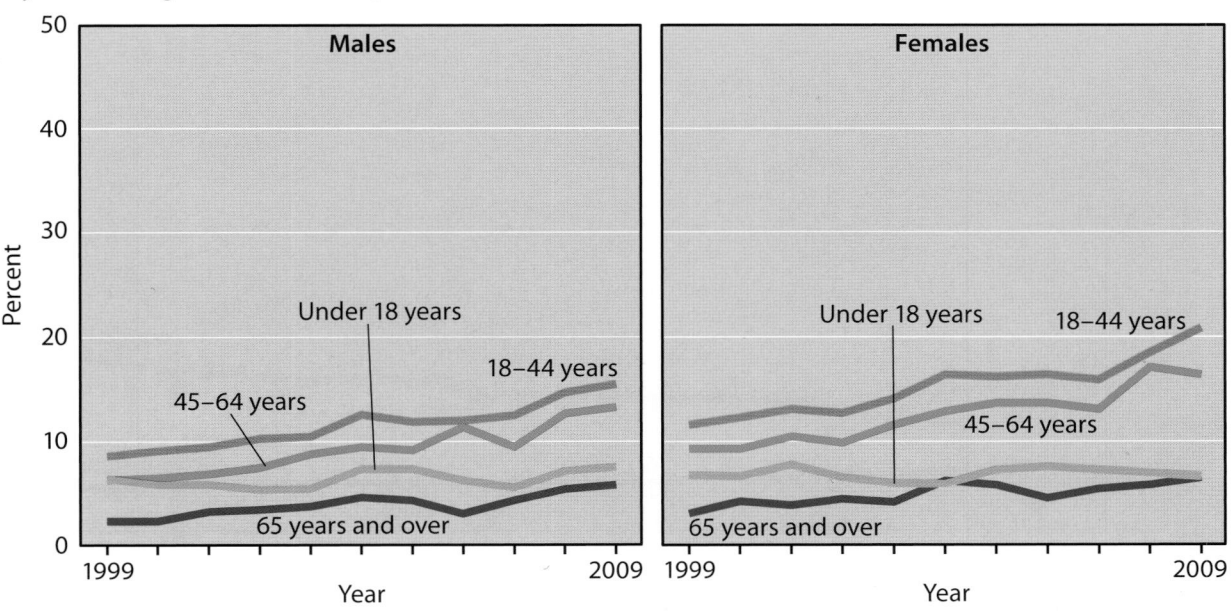

NOTE: See data table for Figure 20.

SOURCE: CDC/NCHS, National Health Interview Survey.

Health Insurance Coverage
Health Insurance Coverage Among Children

Between 1999 and 2009, the percentage of children with private coverage declined but Medicaid coverage grew at a faster rate, resulting in a decline in the percentage who were uninsured.

Children need access to the health care system for diagnosis and treatment of acute and chronic illnesses, treatment of injuries, and for preventive care such as vaccinations and health promotion teaching and counseling. Health insurance is a major determinant of access to care. Uninsured children are three times as likely as insured children to have not had a doctor's visit in the past year (Table 79).

The Children's Health Insurance Program (CHIP) provides coverage to eligible low-income, uninsured children who do not qualify for Medicaid. CHIP was originally enacted by the Balanced Budget Act of 1997 (BBA) (1). The Children's Health Insurance Program Reauthorization Act of 2009 (CHIPRA, P.L. 111–3) reauthorized CHIP through fiscal year 2013. CHIP is jointly financed by federal and state governments and is administered by the states.

Between 1999 and 2009, the percentage of children under 18 years of age with private health insurance declined from 69% to 56%. During this period, Medicaid coverage (which includes the CHIP category) increased from 18% to 35%. This led to a decline in the percentage of children who were uninsured, from 12% in 1999 to 8% in 2009.

In 2009, children 6–17 years of age were more likely to be uninsured than younger children, and children with a family income below 200% of the poverty level were more likely to be uninsured than children in higher-income families (Table 138).

Reference

1. National CHIP policy: Overview [online]. Centers for Medicare & Medicaid Services. Available from: http://www.cms.hhs.gov/NationalCHIPPolicy.

Figure 21. Health insurance coverage among children under 18 years of age, by type of coverage: United States, 1999–2009

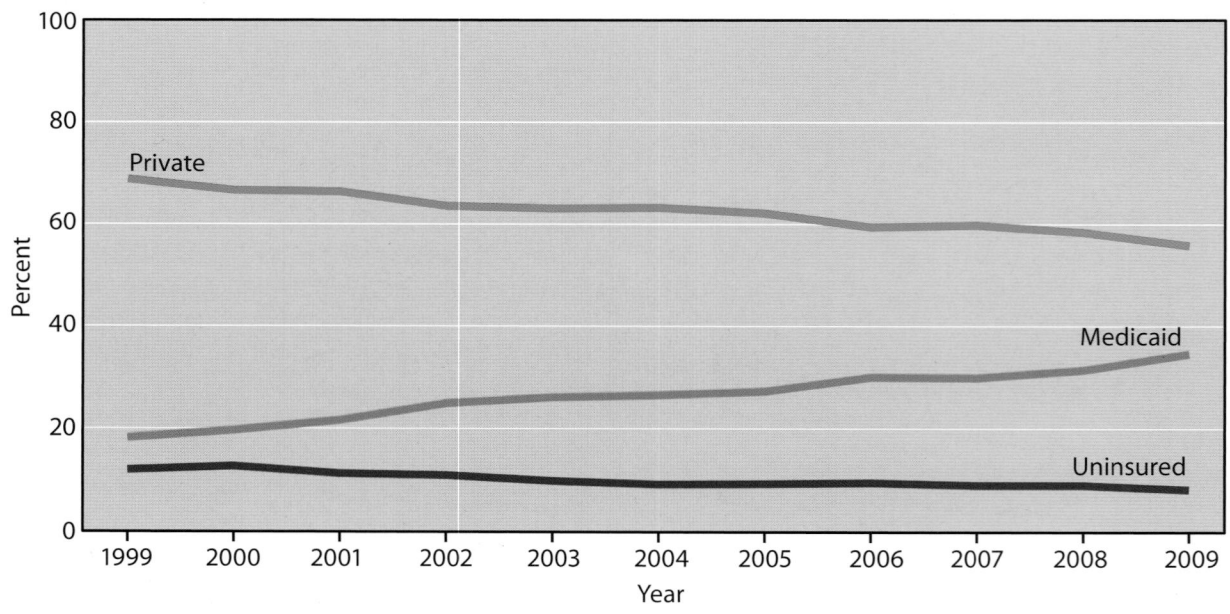

NOTE: See data table for Figure 21.

SOURCE: CDC/NCHS, National Health Interview Survey.

Health Insurance Coverage Among Adults 18–64 Years of Age

Between 1999 and 2009, the percentage of working-age adults with private health insurance coverage decreased while the percentage who were uninsured increased.

The major source of health insurance coverage for working-age adults is private employer-sponsored group health insurance (Table 136). Private health insurance may also be purchased on an individual basis but is generally more costly and tends to provide less adequate coverage than group health insurance. Health insurance is a major determinant of access to health care (1). Uninsured working-age adults were less likely to have a usual source of care or a recent health care visit (Tables 75 and 79) and were more likely to forego or delay needed medical care, prescription drugs, or preventive care because of cost (Tables 76, 86, and 87; and Figure 19).

Among adults 18–44 years of age, the percentage with private coverage declined from 72% in 1999 to 62% in 2009, while Medicaid coverage increased from 6% to 10%, resulting in an increase in the percentage of persons 18–44 years of age who

were uninsured. In 2009, more than one-quarter of adults 18–44 years of age were uninsured. In this age group, the percentage of adults without coverage is higher among those 18–34 years than those 35–44 years (Table 138).

Similar to the trend for younger working-age adults, the percentage of adults 45–64 years of age with private coverage declined, Medicaid coverage increased, and the percentage without coverage increased from 1999 to 2009. Although lack of health insurance coverage is less common among this age group than among those 18–44 years of age (15% compared with 26% in 2009), chronic illness is more prevalent in this older working-age group (Tables 49, 50, 67, and 68).

Reference

1. The uninsured and the difference health insurance makes [online]. Kaiser Commission on Medicaid and the Uninsured. 2010. Available from: http://www.kff.org/uninsured/upload/1420-12.pdf.

Figure 22. Health insurance coverage among adults 18–64 years of age, by age and type of coverage: United States, 1999–2009

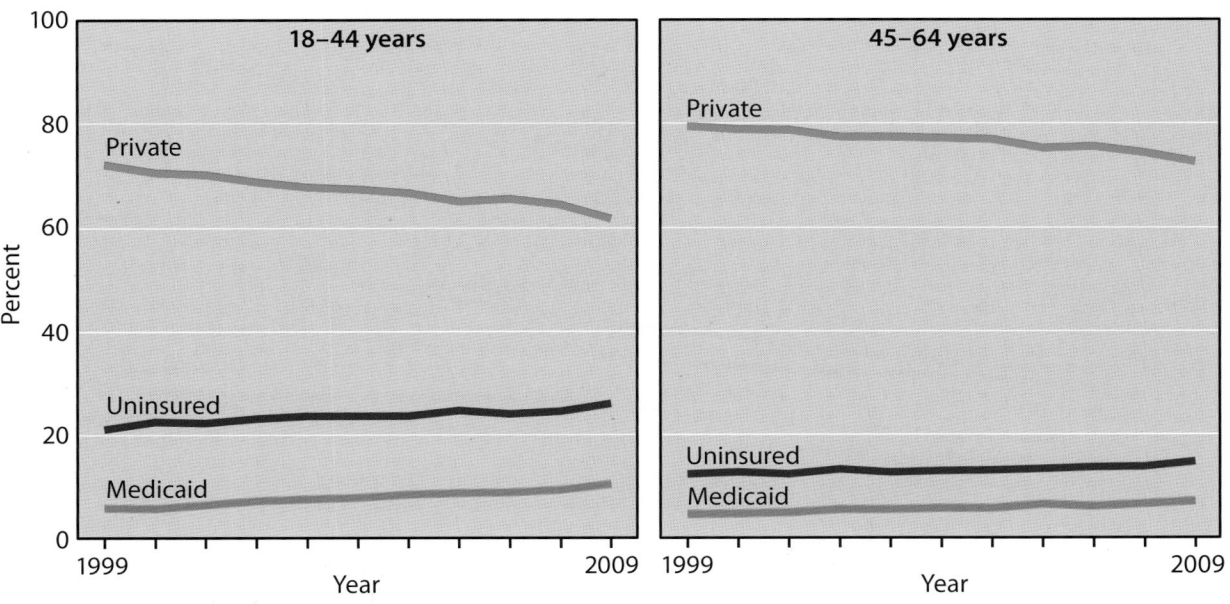

NOTE: See data table for Figure 22.

SOURCE: CDC/NCHS, National Health Interview Survey.

Personal Health Care Expenditures

Out-of-pocket spending for personal health care expenditures grew less rapidly than Medicare, Medicaid, and private insurance spending from 1998–2008.

Between 1998 and 2008, total personal health expenditures (PHCE) nearly doubled, growing from $1.0 trillion to nearly $2.0 trillion. During this period, the average annual growth for Medicare was 9%, for Medicaid and private health insurance 8%, and for out-of-pocket expenditures 5%.

In 2008, more than one-half of PHCE were paid by private funds (data table for Figure 23). The bulk of private expenditures were paid by private health insurance, for which the portion of private spending increased from 60% in 1998 to 66% in 2008. The share of private spending paid out of pocket declined from 30% in 1998 to 27% in 2008.

Government funds paid for 47% of PHCE in 2008. About one-half of government funds spent on PHCE was from Medicare, which is largely financed by the federal government. Medicaid expenditures are shared by the federal and state governments; the federal contribution varies by state (1). Medicaid accounted for about one-third of government funds spent on PHCE in 2008. The Children's Health Insurance Program, included with

Medicaid funds, was less than 1% of total PHCE (Table 127).

Much of the increase in government expenditures was due to increased enrollment and use of services (2). Medicare Part D prescription drug coverage, begun in 2006, and increased enrollment since 2004 in Medicare Advantage plans (private health plan options that are part of the Medicare program) accounted for much of the increase in Medicare expenditures (3). In contrast, enrollment in private health insurance plans has declined in recent years but expenditures continue to rise.

References

1. Office of the Actuary, Centers for Medicare & Medicaid Services (CMS). 2008 Actuarial report on the financial outlook for Medicaid. Baltimore, MD: CMS; 2008. Available from: http://www.cms.hhs.gov/ActuarialStudies/downloads/MedicaidReport2008.pdf.
2. Zuckerman S, McFeeters J. Recent growth in health expenditures. Report prepared for the Commonwealth Fund/Alliance for Health Reform 2006 Bipartisan Congressional Health Policy Conference. Commonwealth Fund pub no 914. New York, NY: The Commonwealth Fund; 2006. Available from: http://www.commonwealthfund.org/~/media/Files/Publications/Fund%20Report/2006/Mar/Recent%20Growth%20in%20Health%20Expenditures/Zuckerman_recentgrowth_914%20pdf.pdf.

(References continue on data table for Figure 23)

Figure 23. Personal health care expenditures, by source of funds: United States, 1998–2008

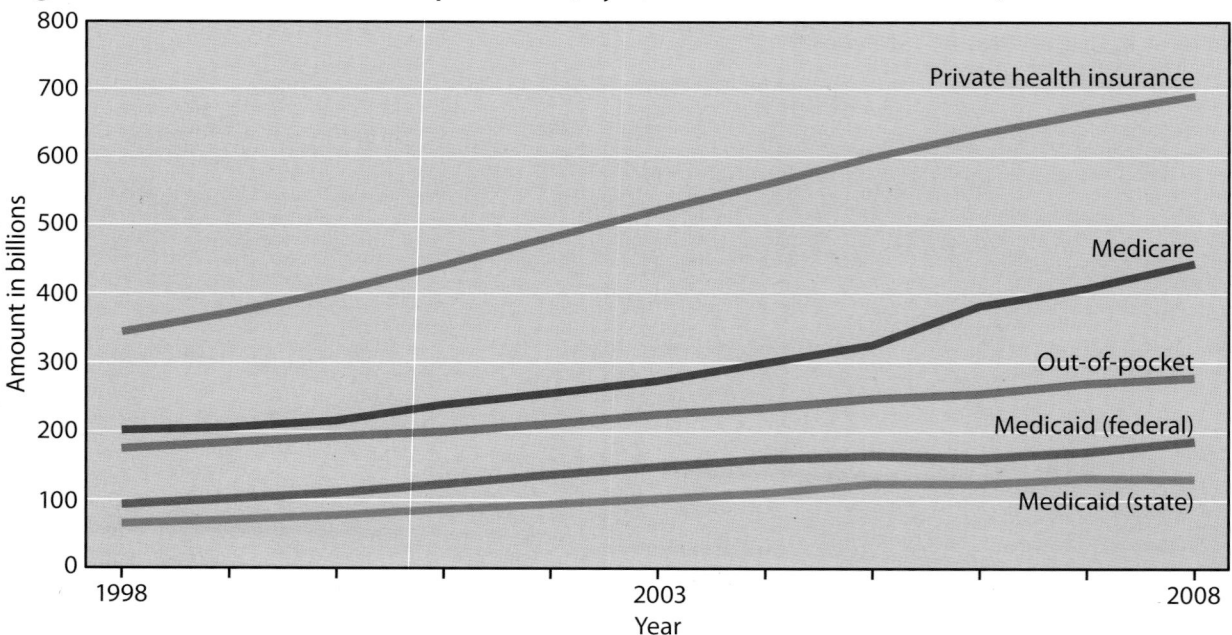

NOTE: See data table for Figure 23.

SOURCE: Centers for Medicare & Medicaid Services, Office of the Actuary, National Health Statistics Group, National Health Expenditure Accounts.

Special Feature on Death and Dying
Introduction

This year's Chartbook includes 18 charts on our Special Feature: Death and Dying.

Death and dying are complex processes with implications for individuals, their families and friends, their care providers, and the health care system. In 2007 in the United States, nearly 2.5 million people died. Those 85 years of age and over accounted for 29% of deaths, but people of all ages died and from various causes. Adequate preparation for death, and appropriate end-of-life care, may be hampered by the difficulty in predicting when death will occur, even for those with serious or terminal illnesses.

For persons who are dying, and their families and friends, the circumstances surrounding the event can result in a more (or less) comfortable and dignified experience. Death can be instantaneous, or dying can be a drawn-out process that is either relatively comfortable ("a good death") or painful and undignified. Dying can also be a great emotional and financial burden on families and caregivers. Because it can be associated with both physical and emotional pain and discomfort—which may be mitigated with proper support for the individual and those close to them—dying can be considered a major public health issue (1).

Dealing with death and dying is a personal process, influenced by culture, one's beliefs, how different health care providers communicate information and advice about prognosis, and many other individual and societal factors (2,3). Some people and cultures discourage talk about the possibility of dying, even when faced with a terminal illness, perhaps because they, their families, or their care providers do not want to give up hope of recovery (2). Others diagnosed with a terminal illness assertively seek out information to help them plan their end-of-life medical care and other needed services. Research suggests that end-of-life discussions may be associated with less aggressive medical care near death and with earlier referral to hospice services. Aggressive care for some terminal conditions, on the other hand, has been associated with worse patient quality of life and worse bereavement adjustment (2).

When asked, most terminally ill patients, their families, and their medical care providers agree that the most important aspects of dying include having a designated decision maker, knowing what to expect about prognosis and physical condition, maintaining dignity, having one's financial affairs in order, and being free of pain (4). Yet even for patients

Figure 24. Deaths for all ages, by age and cause of death: United States, 2007

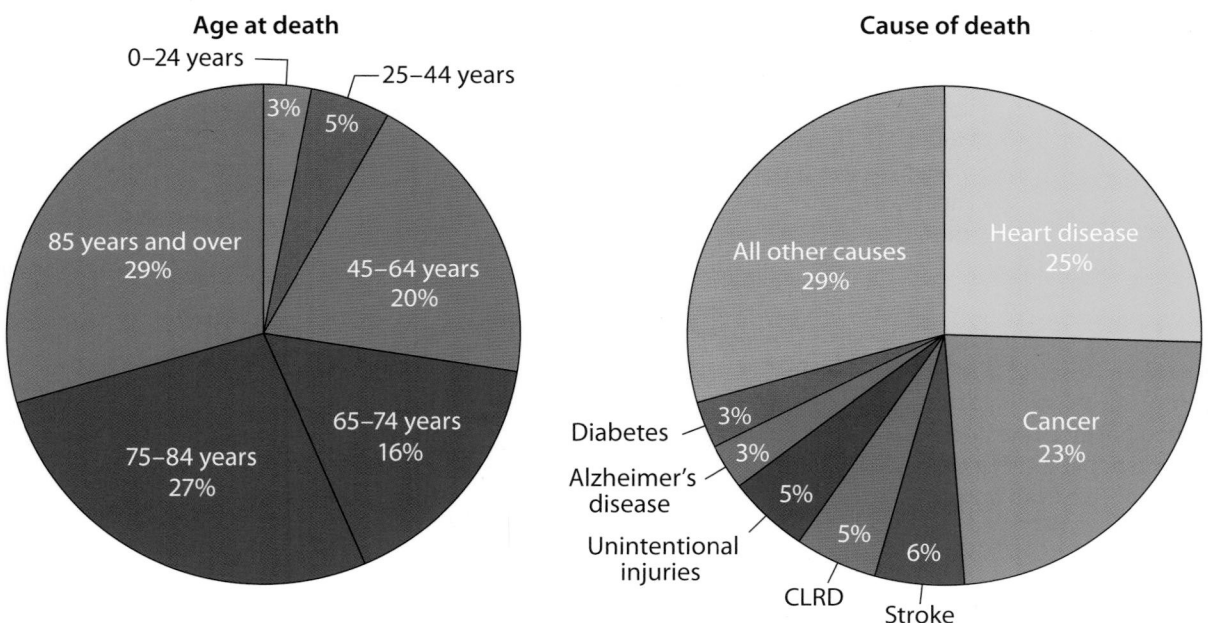

NOTE: CLRD is chronic lower respiratory diseases. See data table for Figure 24.

SOURCE: CDC/NCHS, National Vital Statistics System.

enrolled in a hospice care program that has the stated purpose of making the dying process more comfortable, one-third of decedents had pain near the time of death (Figure 40). Nine-tenths of hospice care patients had on file some form of advance directive that stated their preferences in case of incapacitation, particularly immediately before death. The use of advance directives was less common among nursing home residents, with just over two-thirds of residents 65 years of age and over having some form of advance directive (Figure 36).

The emphasis in the United States on conquering disease—combined with the uncertainty of predicting when death will occur—can lead to intense and costly efforts to prolong life, sometimes resulting in great discomfort, loss of function, and diminished quality of life for the dying person (1). Medical technology has helped save lives, but it also can prolong life for the critically ill, unresponsive patient who has little or no chance of recovery. Services such as mechanical ventilation, dialysis, parenteral (tube) feeding, and other means can keep even comatose and "brain dead" patients alive, making the very definition of death controversial (5,6).

For the health care system, dying can be extremely expensive, particularly when hospital intensive care unit (ICU) or critical care services are used. About one in five Americans died during a hospitalization that involved the use of ICU services (7). The average length of stay for terminal ICU hospitalizations was 12.0 days, with costs of $24,541—compared with 8.9 days and $8,548 for non-ICU terminal hospitalizations (7). Many studies have found that health care expenditures are concentrated at the end of life and are often interpreted as "the high cost of dying" (8,9).

This Special Feature focuses on death and dying in the United States. Data are presented on trends in the leading causes of death by age group and place of death, as well as characteristics of patients receiving hospice care and the services received by hospice care patients' families. Types of medications patients receive from hospice care are also highlighted. State data include preventable deaths (e.g., motor-vehicle traffic fatalities) and average number of intensive care days in the last 6 months of life for Medicare beneficiaries. Knowing more about the circumstances surrounding death, including who dies, and when, where, and how, can help policymakers, practitioners, and others target resources to reduce preventable deaths and to improve the quality of the dying process for patients and their families and friends.

References

1. Rao JK, Anderson LA, Smith SM. End of life is a public health issue. Am J Prev Med 2002;23(3):215–20.
2. Wright AA, Zhang B, Ray A, Mack JW, Trice E, Balboni T, et al. Associations between end-of-life discussions, patient mental health, medical care near death, and caregiver bereavement adjustment. JAMA 2008;300(14):1665–73.
3. Gruenewald DA, White EJ. The illness experience of older adults near the end of life: A systematic review. Anesthesiol Clin 2006;24:163–80.
4. Steinhauser KE, Christakis NA, Clipp EC, McNeilly M, McIntyre L, Tulsky JA. Factors considered important at the end of life by patients, family, physicians, and other care providers. JAMA 2000;284(19):2476–82.
5. Thomas AG. Continuing the definition of death debate: The report of the President's Council on Bioethics on controversies in the determination of death. Bioethics 2010; ISSN 0269–9702 (print); ISSN 1467–8519 (online).
6. Controversies in the Determination of Death: A White Paper by the President's Council on Bioethics [online]. The President's Council on Bioethics, Washington, DC. 2008. Available from: http://www.thenewatlantis.com/docLib/20091130_ determination_of_death.pdf.
7. Angus DC, Barnato AE, Linde-Zwirble WT, Weissfeld LA, Watson RS, Rickert T, Rubenfeld GD. Use of intensive care at the end of life in the United States: An epidemiologic study. Crit Care Med 2004;32(3):638–43.
8. Scitovsky AA. The high cost of dying: What do the data show? 1984. Milbank Q 2005;83(4):825–41.
9. Levinsky NG, Yu W, Ash A, Moskowitz M, Gazelle G, Saynina O, Emanuel EJ. Influence of age on Medicare expenditures and medical care in last year of life. JAMA 2001;286:1349–55.

Infant Mortality

Infant mortality rates declined by 5%–8% between 1997 and 2007.

The infant mortality rate—the risk of death during the first year of life—is related to the underlying health of the mother, public health practices, socioeconomic conditions, and availability and use of appropriate health care for infants and pregnant women. The 2007 infant mortality rate of 6.75 per 1,000 live births was 7% lower than in 1997. During the same period, the neonatal mortality rate (deaths under 28 days of age) decreased 8%, to 4.41 per 1,000 live births, and the postneonatal mortality rate (deaths from 28 days to 11 months of age) decreased 5%, to 2.33 per 1,000 live births. In 2007, congenital malformations, low birthweight, and sudden infant death syndrome (SIDS) were the three leading causes of infant deaths, accounting for 45% of the 29,000 infant deaths that occurred (1).

Large disparities in infant mortality rates by race and Hispanic origin of the mother persist. In the past 10 years, the infant mortality rate was consistently highest for infants of non-Hispanic black mothers (Table 15). Infant mortality rates were also higher among infants of American Indian or Alaska Native mothers and mothers of Puerto Rican descent than for other racial and ethnic groups. Infants of Central and South American mothers, Asian or Pacific Islander mothers, and Cuban mothers had lower infant mortality rates than other racial and ethnic groups (2). However, substantial variation in birth outcomes exists within subgroups of the Asian or Pacific Islander population (3). During this period, infant mortality rates for non-Hispanic black mothers were three times the rates for Cuban mothers (Table 15).

References

1. Xu JQ, Kochanek KD, Murphy SL, Tejada-Vera B. Deaths: Final data for 2007. National vital statistics reports; vol 58 no 19. Hyattsville, MD: NCHS; 2010. Available from: http://www.cdc.gov/nchs/data/nvsr/nvsr58/nvsr58_19.pdf.
2. Mathews TJ, MacDorman MF. Infant mortality statistics from the 2006 period linked birth/infant death data set. National vital statistics reports; vol 58 no 17. Hyattsville, MD: NCHS; 2010. Available from: http://www.cdc.gov/nchs/data/nvsr/nvsr58/nvsr58_17.pdf.
3. Schempf AH, Mendola P, Hamilton BE, Hayes DK, Makuc DM. Perinatal outcomes for Asian, Native Hawaiian, and Other Pacific Islander mothers of single and multiple race/ethnicity: California and Hawaii, 2003–2005. Am J Public Health 2010;100(5):877–87.

Figure 25. Infant, neonatal, and postneonatal mortality rates: United States, 1997–2007

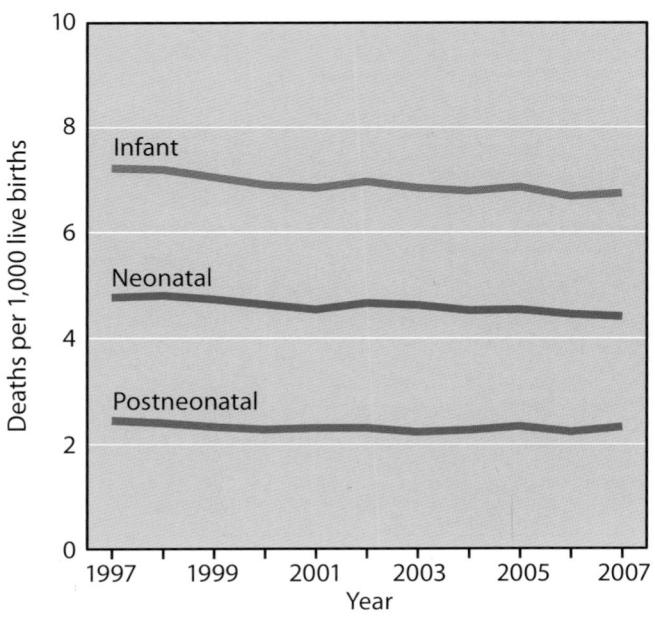

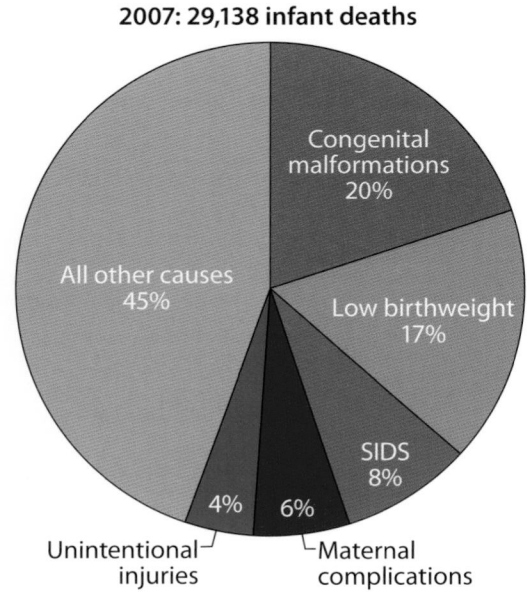

2007: 29,138 infant deaths

NOTES: SIDS is sudden infant death syndrome. See data table for Figure 25.

SOURCE: CDC/NCHS, National Vital Statistics System.

Child Mortality Rates by Organisation for Economic Co-operation and Development (OECD) Country

The United States has a higher child mortality rate than most other OECD member countries.

Child mortality (deaths at 1–19 years of age) rates are lower than for any other age group. However, they vary considerably across countries. The U.S. child mortality rate (32.7 per 100,000 children) was the second highest among the member countries of OECD (1). Rates for other OECD countries ranged from 14.8 per 100,000 children in Luxembourg (average annual 2003–2005) to 34.6 per 100,000 children in Portugal (average annual 2001–2003).

Child mortality rates exclude infants because most neonatal and postneonatal deaths are due to different causes than those of children and adolescents. Unintentional injuries (accidents) were the leading cause of death among children in the United States and Europe (2,3). Among 1–4 year olds, motor-vehicle accidents were the leading cause of unintentional injury death in the United States, whereas drownings were the most common cause of unintentional injury death in Europe (4). Motor-vehicle injuries are the leading cause of unintentional injury deaths among older children in both the United States and Europe. Among the other top

causes of death to children in the United States and Europe were birth defects (congenital malformations, deformations, and chromosomal abnormalities), homicide, cancer, and heart disease. Among adolescents (15–24 years of age), suicide was a leading cause of death (Figure 28).

The vast majority of child deaths occur in the developing world, where the leading causes differ from those in OECD countries. They include diarrhea, pneumonia, measles, malaria, human immunodeficiency virus (HIV)/AIDS, and malnutrition (5,6).

References

1. Child well-being [online]. OECD StatExtracts. Organisation for Economic Co-operation and Development. Available from: http://stats.oecd.org/Index.aspx.
2. Xu JQ, Kochanek KD, Murphy SL, Tejada-Vera B. Deaths: Final data for 2007. National vital statistics reports; vol 58 no 19. Hyattsville, MD: NCHS; 2010. Available from: http://www.cdc.gov/nchs/data/nvsr/nvsr58/nvsr58_19.pdf.
3. Sethi D, Towner E, Vicenten J, Segui-Gomez M, Racioppi F. European report on child injury prevention. Copenhagen: World Health Organization; 2008. Available from: http://www.euro.who.int/__data/assets/pdf_file/0003/83757/E92049.pdf.

(References continue on data table for Figure 26)

Figure 26. Death rates among children 1–19 years of age, by OECD country: 3-year average of most recent data, 2001–2006

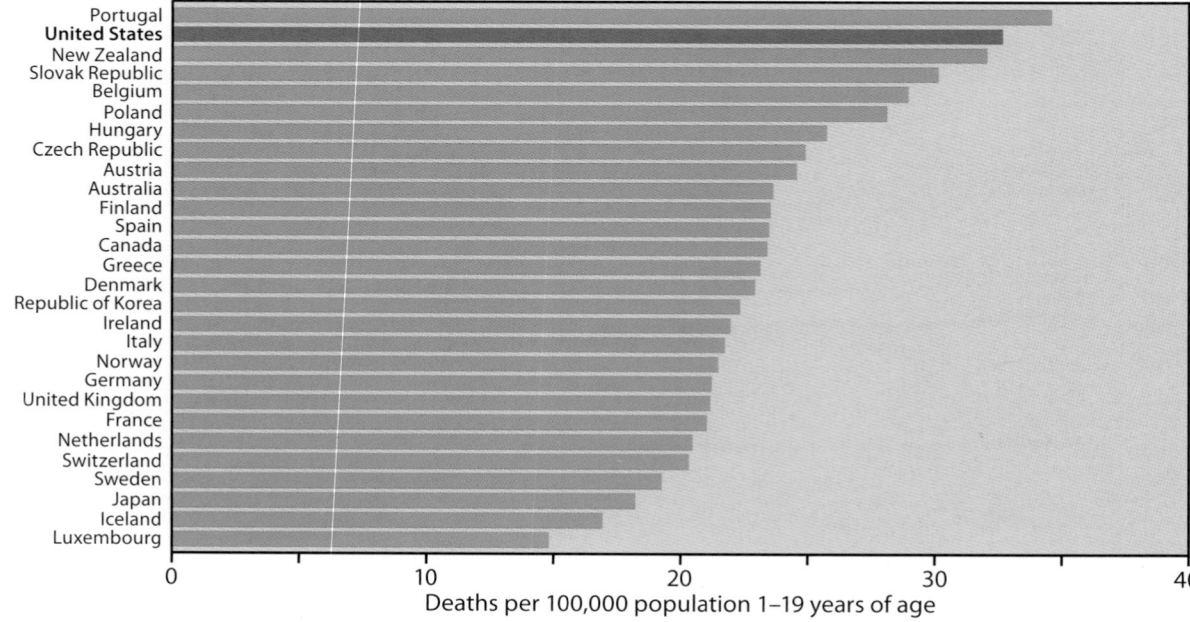

NOTES: OECD is Organisation for Economic Co-operation and Development. Data for Belgium are for 1995–1997; data for Denmark are for 1999–2001. See data table for Figure 26.

SOURCE: World Health Organization.

Deaths Among Children 1–14 Years of Age

The death rate among children 1–14 years of age decreased 22% from 1997 to 2007.

Almost 11,000 U.S. children 1–14 years of age died in 2007. Unintentional injuries were the leading cause of death, accounting for 35% of deaths in this age group in 2007. The unintentional injury death rate dropped 30%, from 9.6 per 100,000 children in 1997 to 6.7 per 100,000 children in 2007.

Cancer was the second leading cause of death for 1–14 year olds. In 2007, about 1,300 children 1–14 years of age died from cancer, representing 12% of deaths in this age group. In 2007, the cancer death rate was 2.3 per 100,000 children, 15% lower than in 1997. Congenital malformations, deformations, and chromosomal abnormalities were the third leading cause of death in this age group, representing 9% of deaths. About three-fifths (59%) of deaths in this age group from congenital malformations were among children 1–4 years of age (1). Death rates from congenital malformations decreased 16% between 1997 and 2007.

Homicide was the fourth leading cause of death, accounting for 7% of deaths in this age group. Children 1–4 years of age accounted for 53% of homicide deaths in this age group (1). Homicide rates among children 1–14 years decreased 13% between 1997 and 2007.

Heart disease was the fifth leading cause of death for children in this age group in 2007, accounting for 414 deaths—4% of all deaths to children 1–14 years of age.

Reference

1. Xu JQ, Kochanek KD, Murphy SL, Tejada-Vera B. Deaths: Final data for 2007. National vital statistics reports; vol 58 no 19. Hyattsville, MD: NCHS; 2010. Available from: http://www.cdc.gov/nchs/data/nvsr/nvsr58/nvsr58_19.pdf.

Figure 27. Death rates for leading causes of death among children 1–14 years of age: United States, 1997–2007

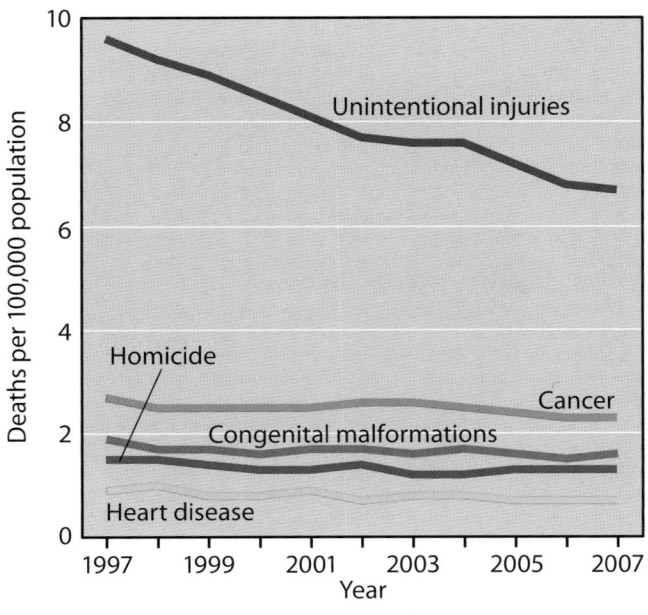

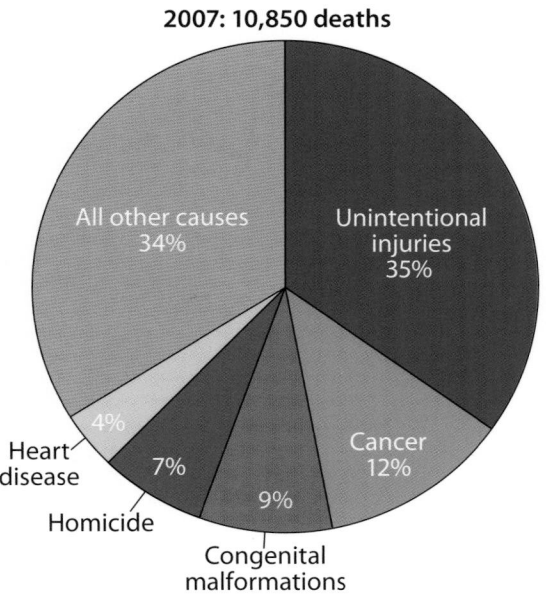

2007: 10,850 deaths

NOTE: See data table for Figure 27.

SOURCE: CDC/NCHS, National Vital Statistics System.

Deaths Among Persons 15–24 Years of Age

Death rates from unintentional injuries—the leading cause of death for persons 15–24 years of age—increased 5% between 1997 and 2007.

In 2007, there were about 34,000 deaths among persons 15–24 years of age (1). The overall death rate for this age group was stable from 1997 to 2007. Unintentional injuries were the leading cause of death for teens and young adults throughout this period, accounting for almost one-half of deaths in 2007. Between 1997 and 2007, the death rate for unintentional injuries increased 5% for this age group. The majority of unintentional injury deaths resulted from motor-vehicle traffic injuries (Table 37). Motor-vehicle traffic-related death rates were more than twice as high among males as females.

Homicide was the second leading cause of death in this age group during this period, accounting for 16% of deaths in 2007. Between 1997 and 2000, the homicide rate declined and then stabilized. In 2007, the homicide death rate was six times as high for males as for females ages 15–24 years and was higher among African American males and Hispanic males than among non-Hispanic white males in this age group (Table 38).

Since 1997, the suicide death rate—the third leading cause among this age group—declined from 11 to 10 per 100,000 population. Suicide death rates were five times as high among males as females in this age group in 2007 (Table 39).

Death rates for the next leading causes of death, cancer and heart disease, decreased about 10% for this age group between 1997 and 2007.

Reference

1. Xu JQ, Kochanek KD, Murphy SL, Tejada-Vera B. Deaths: Final data for 2007. National vital statistics reports; vol 58 no 19. Hyattsville, MD: NCHS; 2010. Available from: http://www.cdc.gov/nchs/data/nvsr/nvsr58/nvsr58_19.pdf.

Figure 28. Death rates for leading causes of death among persons 15–24 years of age: United States, 1997–2007

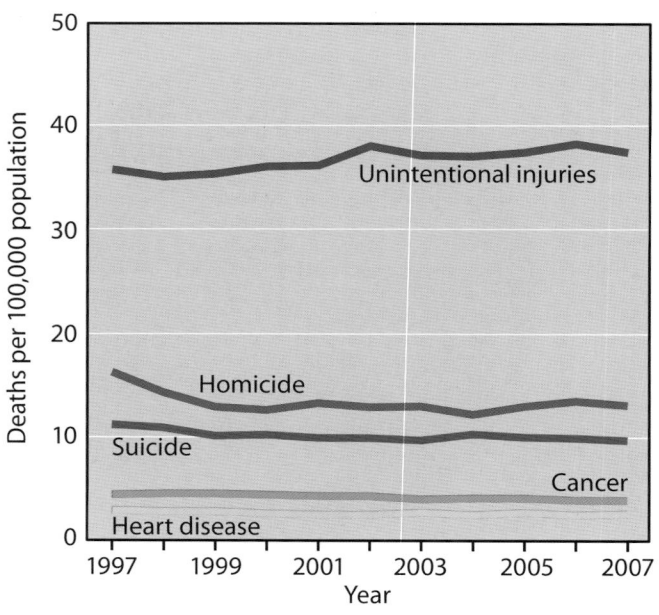

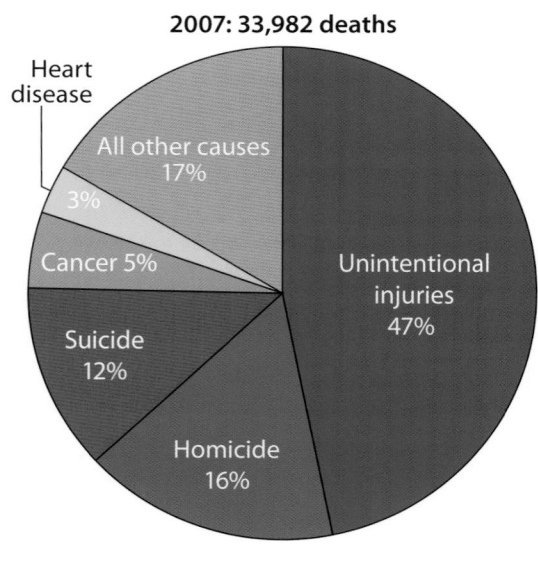

NOTE: See data table for Figure 28.

SOURCE: CDC/NCHS, National Vital Statistics System.

Deaths Among Persons 25–44 Years of Age

Between 1997 and 2007, the death rate among persons 25–44 years of age declined 7%, primarily due to a reduction in cancer and HIV-related deaths.

In 2007, there were 122,000 deaths among persons 25–44 years of age. Between 1997 and 2007, the overall death rate among persons in this age group declined 7%. During this period, the death rate for unintentional injuries—the leading cause of death for this age group—increased 21%, from 31 to 38 deaths per 100,000 population. In 2007, 42% of unintentional injury deaths were from poisoning (1).

Death rates for cancer—the second leading cause of death during this period—decreased 21%, from 25 to 20 deaths per 100,000 population. Lung, brain, and colon cancers were the leading causes of cancer death among men in this age group, and breast, lung, and cervical cancers were the leading causes of cancer death among women in this age group (2) (Tables 33 and 34). Death rates for the third leading cause of death, heart disease, were stable during this period (Table 30).

Death rates for suicide (the fourth leading cause) and homicide (the fifth leading cause) were stable for persons 25–44 years of age between 1997 and 2007. Suicide and homicide death rates were generally three times higher among men than women in this age group (Tables 38 and 39).

Death rates for human immunodeficiency virus (HIV) disease, the sixth leading cause of death in 2007, decreased by more than one-half, from 13 to 6 per 100,000 population in 2007. After rising rapidly in the late 1980s and early 1990s, the HIV disease death rate fell sharply in the mid- to late 1990s with the introduction of antiretroviral therapies (3,4). In 2007, HIV accounted for 4% of deaths among this age group.

References

1. Xu JQ, Kochanek KD, Murphy SL, Tejada-Vera B. Deaths: Final data for 2007. National vital statistics reports; vol 58 no 19. Hyattsville, MD: NCHS; 2010. Available from: http://www.cdc.gov/nchs/data/nvsr/nvsr58/nvsr58_19.pdf.
2. CDC/NCHS. Compressed Mortality File: Underlying cause of death—Mortality for 1999–2006 with ICD–10 codes [online]. WONDER online database. Compiled from Compressed Mortality File 1999–2006, Series 20 no 2L; 2009. Available from: http://wonder.cdc.gov/cmf-icd10.html.
3. CDC. HIV and AIDS—United States, 1981–2000. MMWR 2001;50(21): 430–4. Available from: http://www.cdc.gov/mmwr/preview/mmwrhtml/mm5021a2.htm.
4. CDC. HIV/AIDS surveillance report. Atlanta, GA: CDC 2000;12(2):3–41. 2001. Available from: http://www.cdc.gov/hiv/surveillance/resources/reports/2000report_no2/.

Figure 29. Death rates for leading causes of death among persons 25–44 years of age: United States, 1997–2007

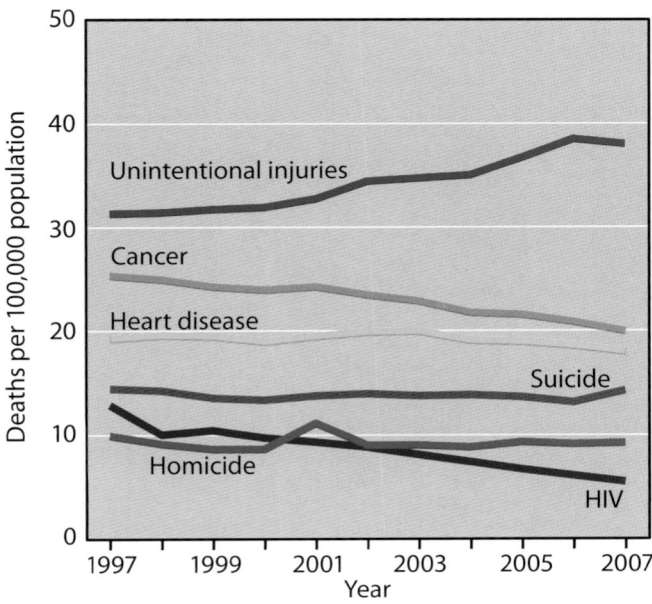

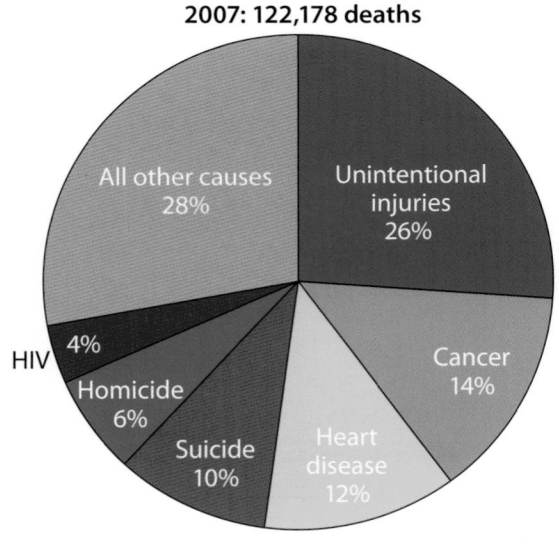

NOTE: See data table for Figure 29.

SOURCE: CDC/NCHS, National Vital Statistics System.

Deaths Among Persons 45–64 Years of Age

The death rate among adults 45–64 years of age decreased 8% from 1997 to 2007. Cancer and heart disease accounted for 54% of deaths in this age group in 2007.

In 2007, there were 472,000 deaths among 45–64 year olds in the United States (1). Chronic diseases accounted for five of the six leading causes of death in this age group. The first and second leading causes of death were cancer and heart disease, which accounted for 54% of deaths in this age group. Between 1997 and 2007, cancer death rates decreased 15%, to 200 per 100,000 population. Heart disease death rates declined even more, by 25%, to 134 per 100,000 population.

Unintentional injury was the third leading cause of death in this age group, accounting for 7% of deaths in 2007. Between 1997 and 2007, death rates for unintentional injuries rose 42%. Unintentional poisoning accounted for 37% of unintentional injury deaths for this age group in 2007 (1).

Diabetes, stroke, and chronic lower respiratory diseases (CLRD), the fourth, fifth, and sixth leading causes of death, respectively, each accounted for 4% of deaths to persons in this age group in 2007. Diabetes and CLRD death rates remained stable between 1997 and 2007, while the stroke death rate for 45–64 year olds decreased 19% during this period, from 27 to 22 per 100,000 population.

Reference

1. Xu JQ, Kochanek KD, Murphy SL, Tejada-Vera B. Deaths: Final data for 2007. National vital statistics reports; vol 58 no 19. Hyattsville, MD: NCHS; 2010. Available from: http://www.cdc.gov/nchs/data/nvsr/nvsr58_19.pdf.

Figure 30. Death rates for leading causes of death among persons 45–64 years of age: United States, 1997–2007

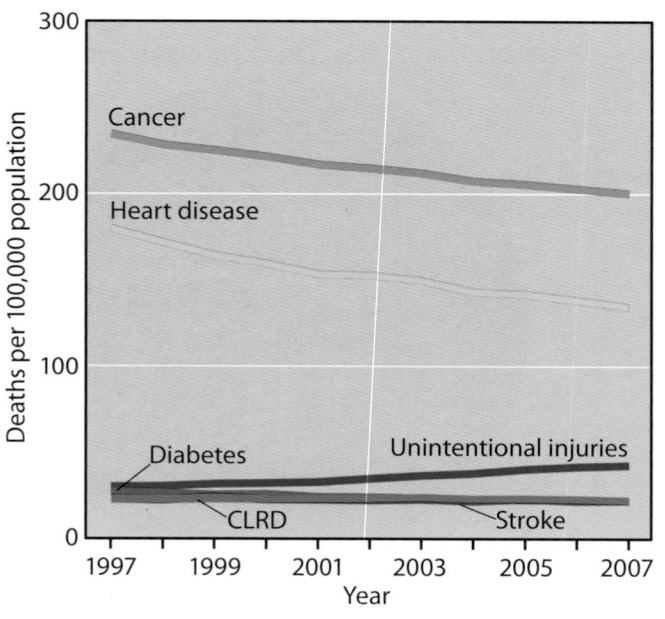

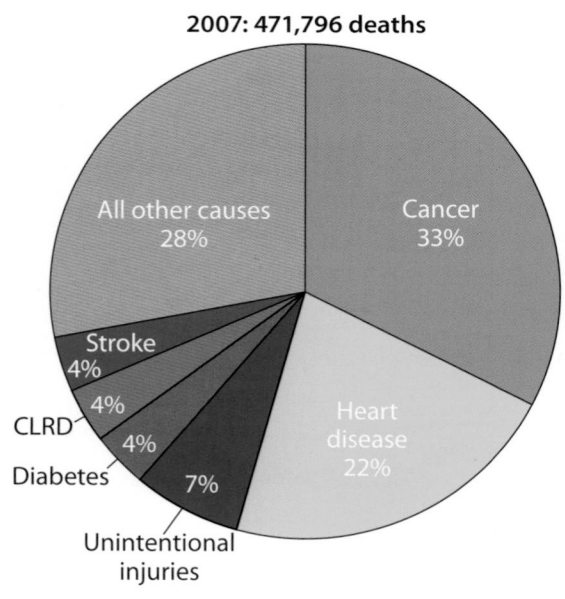

NOTES: CLRD is chronic lower respiratory diseases. See data table for Figure 30.

SOURCE: CDC/NCHS, National Vital Statistics System.

Deaths Among Persons 65 Years of Age and Over

Heart disease, cancer, stroke, and influenza and pneumonia death rates decreased over the past decade among older adults, while death rates due to Alzheimer's disease increased.

Almost three-quarters of all deaths in the United States occur among persons 65 years of age and over, accounting for about 1.8 million deaths in 2007 (1). During the past decade, overall death rates have declined by 8% for this age group.

The death rate for heart disease—the leading cause of death for persons 65 years of age and over—and stroke, the third leading cause, declined by one-quarter between 1997 and 2007. The death rate for cancer, the second leading cause of death for this age group, decreased by 8%. The death rate for the fourth leading cause of death, chronic lower respiratory diseases (CLRD), was stable in the past decade.

In 2007, the fifth leading cause of death among persons 65 years of age and over was Alzheimer's disease, which accounted for 4% of deaths in this age group. Between 1999 and 2007, the death rate for Alzheimer's disease increased more than 50%, from 127 to 195 per 100,000 population.

In 2007, diabetes, the sixth leading cause of death, and influenza and pneumonia, the seventh leading cause of death, each accounted for about 3% of deaths in persons 65 years and over. Since 1999, influenza and pneumonia deaths decreased 26%.

Reference

1. Xu JQ, Kochanek KD, Murphy SL, Tejada-Vera B. Deaths: Final data for 2007. National vital statistics reports; vol 58 no 19. Hyattsville, MD: NCHS; 2010. Available from: http://www.cdc.gov/nchs/data/nvsr/nvsr58/nvsr58_19.pdf.

Figure 31. Death rates for leading causes of death among persons 65 years of age and over: United States, 1997–2007

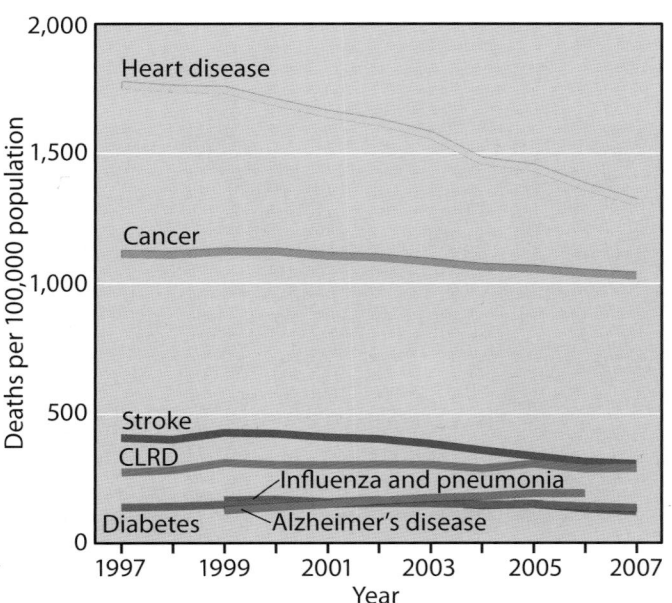

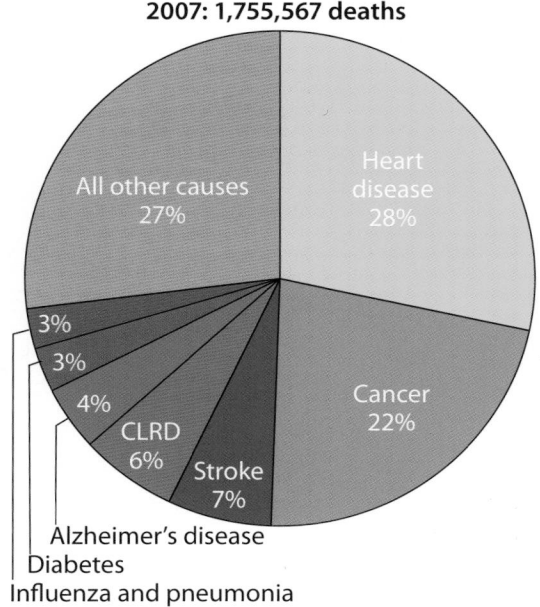

NOTE: CLRD is chronic lower respiratory diseases. See data table for Figure 31.

SOURCE: CDC/NCHS, National Vital Statistics System.

Motor-vehicle Traffic Fatalities

During 2000–2007, average annual age-adjusted motor-vehicle traffic death rates ranged from 31 per 100,000 population in Mississippi to 7 per 100,000 population in Massachusetts.

Motor-vehicle traffic deaths—a significant cause of preventable death—accounted for about 42,000 deaths in the United States in 2007 (1). Between 2000 and 2007, the age-adjusted motor-vehicle traffic death rate was stable at about 15 per 100,000 population (1,2).

Nationwide, alcohol-impaired driving is a major risk behavior associated with motor-vehicle traffic fatalities and accounted for 32% of motor-vehicle traffic fatalities in the United States in 2008 (3). Alcohol-impaired driving fatality rates declined 7%, from 0.43 to 0.40 per 100 million vehicle miles traveled, between 2007 and 2008 (3).

Lap and shoulder seat belts, when used, reduce the risk of fatal injuries to front-seat passenger car occupants and the risk of moderate-to-critical injury (4). Over one-half (55%) of passenger vehicle occupant fatalities were among unrestrained occupants in 2008 (4). Seat belt use was lower in rural than urban areas (5).

In 2000–2007, the average annual age-adjusted motor-vehicle traffic death rate varied fourfold by state (6). The five states with the highest age-adjusted rates (25–31 per 100,000 population) were Mississippi, Wyoming, Montana, Arkansas, and Alabama. Age-adjusted motor-vehicle traffic death rates were higher in the most rural areas (non-metropolitan, noncore areas) compared with the most urban areas (large central metropolitan areas) (2). Even after controlling for vehicle miles traveled, motor-vehicle fatality rates in rural areas were greater than in urban areas (5).

References

1. Xu JQ, Kochanek KD, Murphy SL, Tejada-Vera B. Deaths: Final data for 2007. National vital statistics reports; vol 58 no 19. Hyattsville, MD: NCHS; 2010. Available from: http://www.cdc.gov/nchs/data/nvsr/nvsr58/nvsr58_19.pdf.
2. CDC/NCHS. Compressed Mortality File: Underlying cause of death—Mortality for 1999–2006 with ICD–10 codes [online]. WONDER online database. Compiled from Compressed Mortality File 1999–2006, Series 20 no 2L; 2009. Available from: http://wonder.cdc.gov/cmf-icd10.html.
3. National Highway Traffic Safety Administration (NHTSA). Alcohol-impaired driving. Traffic safety facts, 2008 data. DOT HS 811 155. Washington, DC: NHTSA. Available from: http://www-nrd.nhtsa.dot.gov/Pubs/811155.pdf.

(References continue on data table for Figure 32)

Figure 32. Unintentional motor-vehicle traffic death rates, by state: United States, 2000–2007

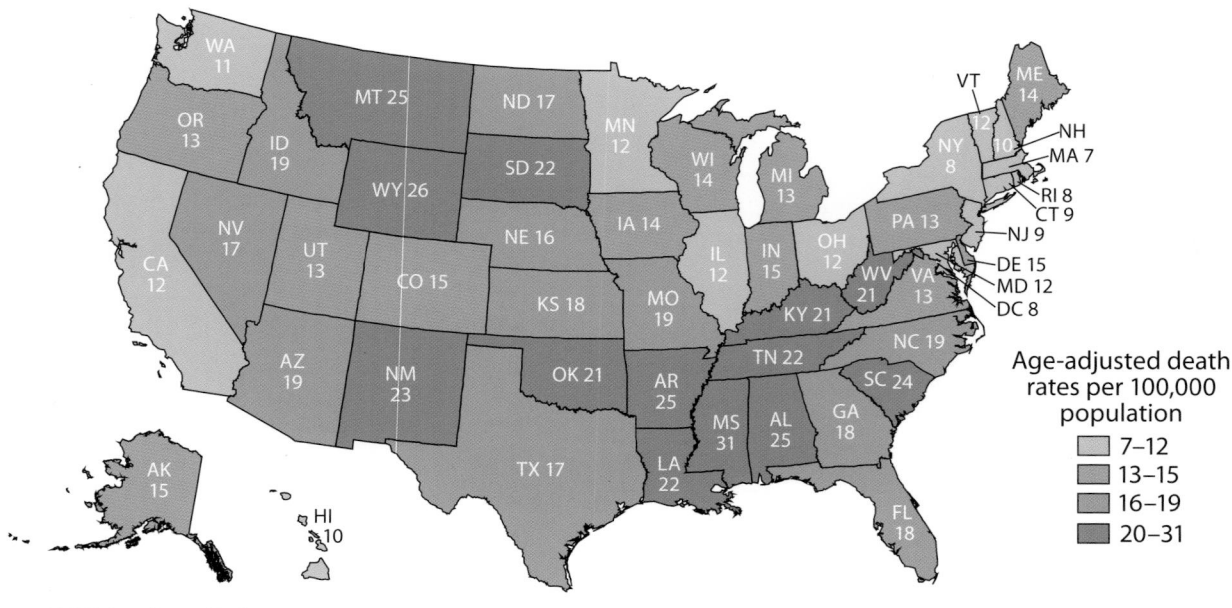

NOTE: See data table for Figure 32.

SOURCE: CDC/NCHS, National Vital Statistics System.

Place of Death, Over Time

Between 1989 and 2007, there was a shift in the places where Americans die, with more people dying at home and fewer dying in institutional settings.

When surveyed, most Americans express a preference to die in their homes (1), yet most die in institutional settings. Factors that affect the place of death include individual preference, cultural beliefs, access to care, age, cause of death, social support, and race and ethnicity (1–4). Health insurance coverage, and policies and services used around the time of death—such as hospice care services or nursing home care—are also related to the place of death.

Since 1989, there has been a shift in where Americans die. Although most still are pronounced dead while in nursing homes or hospitals, in 2007 one-quarter died at home—up from one-sixth in 1989. Between 1989 and 2007, more people died in nursing homes or long-term care settings. These increases have been met by a decline in the percentage of Americans dying while hospital inpatients, down to 36% in 2007 from 49% in 1989. This shift in place of death was found both for decedents under age 65 and those 65 and over. From 1989 to 2007, there was an increase of more than 50% in the percentage of deaths at home and a

decline of more than 20% in the percentage while hospital inpatients for both age groups.

Age is a significant factor related to where Americans die (3). Older persons may have had greater opportunity to plan for their deaths, and place of death is related to the location of recent care. In 2007, decedents under age 65 were more likely to die at home (30%) than those 65 and over (24%). Older decedents were five times more likely to die in nursing homes than those under age 65.

References

1. Grunier A, Mor V, Weitzen S, Truchil R, Teno J, Roy J. Where people die: A multilevel approach to understanding influences on site of death in America. Med Care Res Rev 2007;64(4):351–78.
2. Johnson KS, Kuchibhatala M, Sloane RJ, Tanis D, Galanos AN, Tulsky JA. Ethnic differences in the place of death of elderly hospice enrollees. J Am Geriatr Soc 2005;53(12):2209–15.
3. Flory J, Yinong YX, Gurol I, Levinsky N, Ash A, Emanuel E. Place of death: U.S. trends since 1980. Health Aff (Millwood) 2004;23(3):194–200.
4. Institute of Medicine. Field MJ, Cassel CK, eds. Approaching death: Improving care at the end of life. Washington, DC: National Academy Press; 1997. Available from: http://www.nap.edu/catalog.php?record_id=5801.

Figure 33. Place of death, over time: United States, 1989, 1997, and 2007

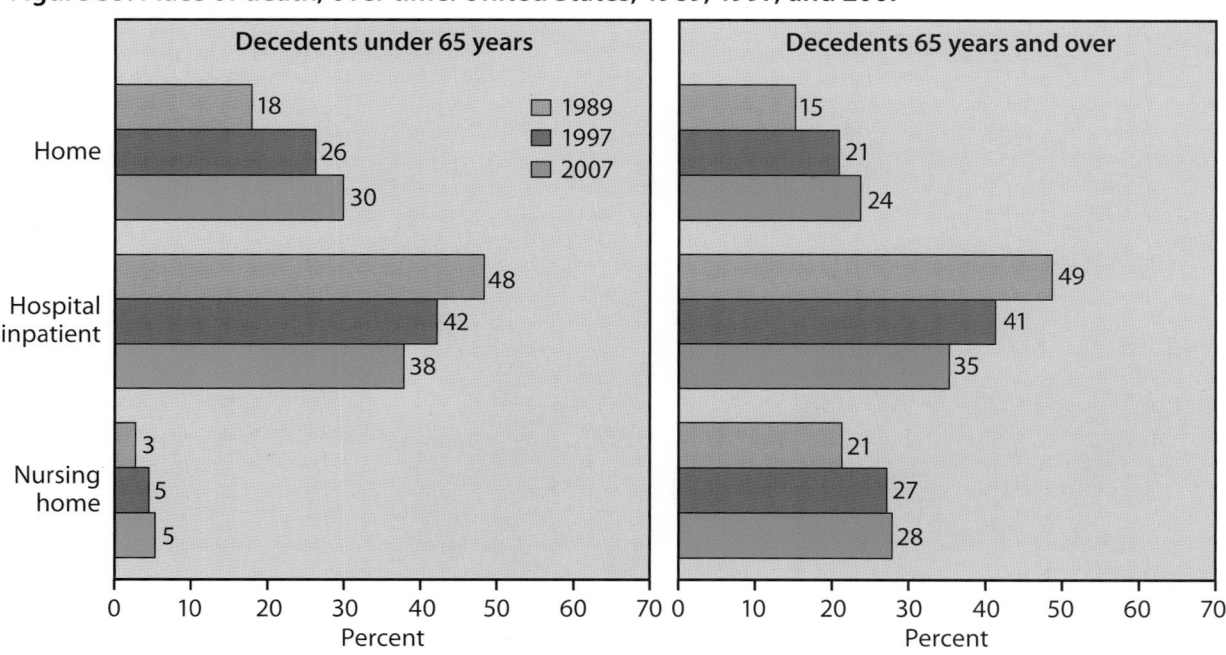

NOTE: See data table for Figure 33.

SOURCE: CDC/NCHS, National Vital Statistics System.

Place of Death, by Age and Race and Hispanic Origin

Among decedents 65 years of age and over, non-Hispanic white decedents were less likely to die while hospitalized and more likely to die in nursing homes than decedents in other racial and ethnic groups.

Race and ethnicity have been identified as factors affecting end-of-life care and place of death (1–7). When surveyed, white persons are more likely to have expressed a preference to die at home compared with black and Hispanic persons (4,6). Hispanic and black persons are less likely to use hospice care than white persons, and Hispanic survey respondents express a preference not to place relatives in nursing homes. Previous studies have shown that non-Hispanic white decedents are less likely to die while hospitalized than decedents of other racial and ethnic groups (1,3–5). Although cultural beliefs of racial and ethnic groups affect where people die, place of death is decided by a complex interplay of many factors, including individual preferences, social support, access to care, age at death, cause of death, and the services being used around the time of death.

Place of death varied by race and Hispanic origin in 2007. Among decedents 65 years of age and over, non-Hispanic white decedents were less likely to die while hospitalized and more likely to die in nursing homes than Hispanic or non-Hispanic black,

American Indian or Alaska Native, or Asian or Pacific Islander decedents. Among decedents under age 65, non-Hispanic white decedents were more likely to die at home and less likely to die while hospitalized than the other racial and ethnic groups examined.

References

1. Weitzen S, Teno JM, Fennell M, Mor V. Factors associated with site of death: A national study of where people die. Med Care 2003;41(2):323–35.
2. Hopp FP, Duffy SA. Racial variations in end-of-life care. J Am Geriatr Soc 2000;48(6):658–63.
3. Grunier A, Mor V, Weitzen S, Truchil R, Teno J, Roy J. Where people die: A multilevel approach to understanding influences on site of death in America. Med Care Res Rev 2007;64(4):351–78.
4. Johnson KS, Kuchibhatala M, Sloane RJ, Tanis D, Galanos AN, Tulsky JA. Ethnic differences in the place of death of elderly hospice enrollees. J Am Geriatr Soc 2005;53(12):2209–15.
5. Flory J, Yinong YX, Gurol I, Levinsky N, Ash A, Emanuel E. Place of death: U.S. trends since 1980. Health Aff (Millwood) 2004;23(3):194–200.
6. Duffy SA, Jackson FC, Schim SM, Ronis DL, Fowler KE. Racial/ethnic preferences, sex preferences, and perceived discrimination related to end-of-life care. J Am Geriatr Soc 2006;54(1):150–7.
7. Steinhauser KE, Christakis NA, Clipp EC, McNeilly M, McIntyre L, Tulsky JA. Factors considered important at the end of life by patients, family, physicians, and other care providers. JAMA 2000;284(19):2476–82.

Figure 34. Place of death, by age and race and Hispanic origin: United States, 2007

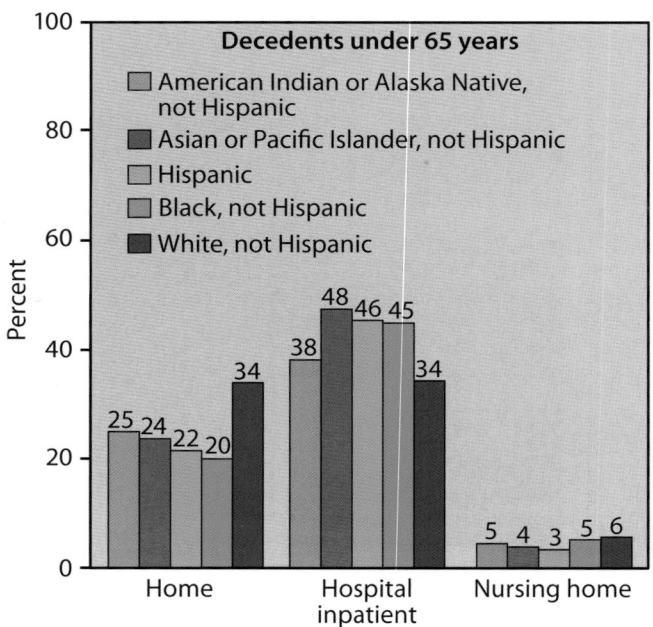

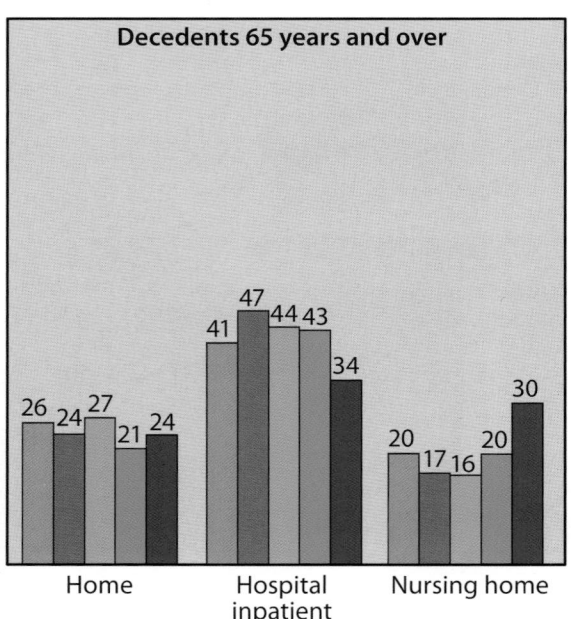

NOTE: See data table for Figure 34.

SOURCE: CDC/NCHS, National Vital Statistics System.

Intensive Care Unit (ICU) Days in the Last 6 Months of Life

The mean number of days Medicare decedents spent in an ICU during the last 6 months of life in 2005 varied from 1.3 days in North Dakota to 5.7 days in New Jersey.

A disproportionate percentage of health care dollars are spent in the last 6 months of life, and ICU stays are a significant portion of these health care costs. In the United States, 17% of deaths in 2001 followed a stay in the ICU, and 47% of hospital deaths were preceded by an ICU stay (1). In 2005, intensive and critical care medicine accounted for 13% of hospital costs and 4% of national health expenditures. Daily costs averaged $3,518, compared with daily average non-critical care costs of $1,153; total annual critical care medical costs were $81.7 billion in 2005 (2). Use of ICU/CCU care is determined by supply, provider practice patterns and preferences, patient preferences, and case mix or "need" (3,4).

The mean number of days that people spend in an ICU or a cardiac care unit in their last 6 months of life varied widely by state of residence in 2005. Medicare decedents who were residents of states in upper New England and the upper Midwest averaged fewer days in the ICU/CCU than the U.S. mean of 3.5 days. Decedents who were residents of 12 states averaged

less than 2 days in an ICU/CCU: North Dakota, Vermont, Oregon, Idaho, Wisconsin, New Hampshire, Maine, Wyoming, Iowa, South Dakota, Minnesota, and Montana. Medicare decedents who were residents of four states (Texas, Illinois, Nevada, and California) averaged between 4 and 5 days in the ICU/CCU in their last 6 months of life. Decedents who were residents of New Jersey and Florida averaged more than 5 days in an ICU/CCU in their last 6 months of life.

References

1. Wunsch H, Linde-Zwirble WT, Harrison DA, Barnato AE, Rowan KM, Angus DC. Use of intensive care services during terminal hospitalizations in England and the United States. Am J Respir Crit Care Med 2009;180(9):875–80.
2. Halpern NA, Pastores SM. Critical care medicine in the United States 2000–2005: An analysis of bed numbers, occupancy rates, payer mix, and costs. Crit Care Med 2010;38(1):65–71.
3. Fisher E, Goodman D, Skinner J, Bronner K. Health care spending, quality, and outcomes: More isn't always better [online]. Dartmouth Atlas Project Topic Brief. 2009. Available from: http://www.dartmouthatlas.org/downloads/reports/Spending_Brief_022709.pdf.
4. Barnato AE, Herndon MB, Anthony DL, Gallagher PM, Skinner JS, Bynum JP, Fisher ES. Are regional variations in end-of-life care intensity explained by patient preferences? A study of the U.S. Medicare population. Med Care 2007;45(5):386–93.

Figure 35. Average number of days in ICU/CCU for Medicare decedents in the last 6 months of life, by state of residence: United States, 2005

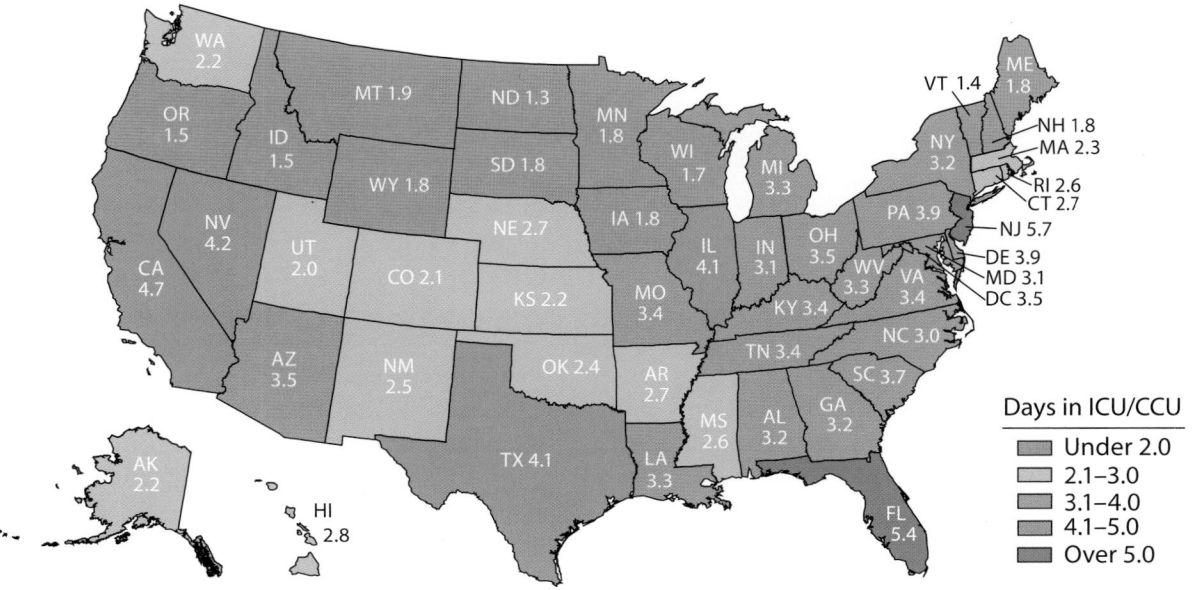

NOTE: See data table for Figure 35.

SOURCE: Dartmouth Atlas of Health Care.

Advance Directives

Discharged hospice care patients were more likely to have advance directives than current nursing home and home health care patients 65 years of age and over.

Advance directives are legal documents that establish guidelines for what treatments patients wish to receive and not receive (including life-sustaining treatments or procedures such as cardiac resuscitation) and who will make treatment decisions for them if they are unable to communicate informed decisions (1–4). Many people—even those who are seriously or terminally ill—do not enact directives. The decision to have advance directives depends on individual preference, cultural and religious beliefs, and medical condition and prognosis (3).

Among persons 65 years of age and over, 92% of discharged hospice care patients had some form of advance directive on file, compared with 70% of nursing home and 35% of home health care patients. Non-Hispanic white nursing home and home health care patients were more likely to have directives than Hispanic and non-Hispanic black patients. Non-Hispanic white and Hispanic discharged hospice care patients were more likely to have some directive prepared than

non-Hispanic black patients. Although the life expectancy of nursing home and home health care patients varies considerably, hospice care is generally available only to persons whom a physician has determined have less than 6 months to live.

Among the 92% of hospice care patients 65 years and over with some directive in place, the most common forms were do not resuscitate (84%), power of attorney (38%), living will (27%), health care proxy (17%), and comfort measures only (13%) directives (5).

References

1. Advance directives [online]. National Cancer Institute Fact Sheet. 2000. Available from: http://www.cancer.gov/cancertopics/factsheet/support/advance-directives.
2. Gaeta S, Price KJ. End-of-life issues in critically ill cancer patients. Crit Care Clin 2010;26(1):219–27.
3. Prendergast TJ. Advance care planning: Pitfalls, progress, promise. Crit Care Med 2001;29(2 suppl):N34–N39.
4. Silveira MJ, Kim SYH, Langa KM. Advance directives and outcomes of surrogate decision making before death. N Engl J Med 2010;362(13):1211–8.
5. CDC/NCHS. National Home and Hospice Care Survey [unpublished analysis].

Figure 36. Advance directives among adults 65 years of age and over, by type of care and race and Hispanic origin: United States, selected years

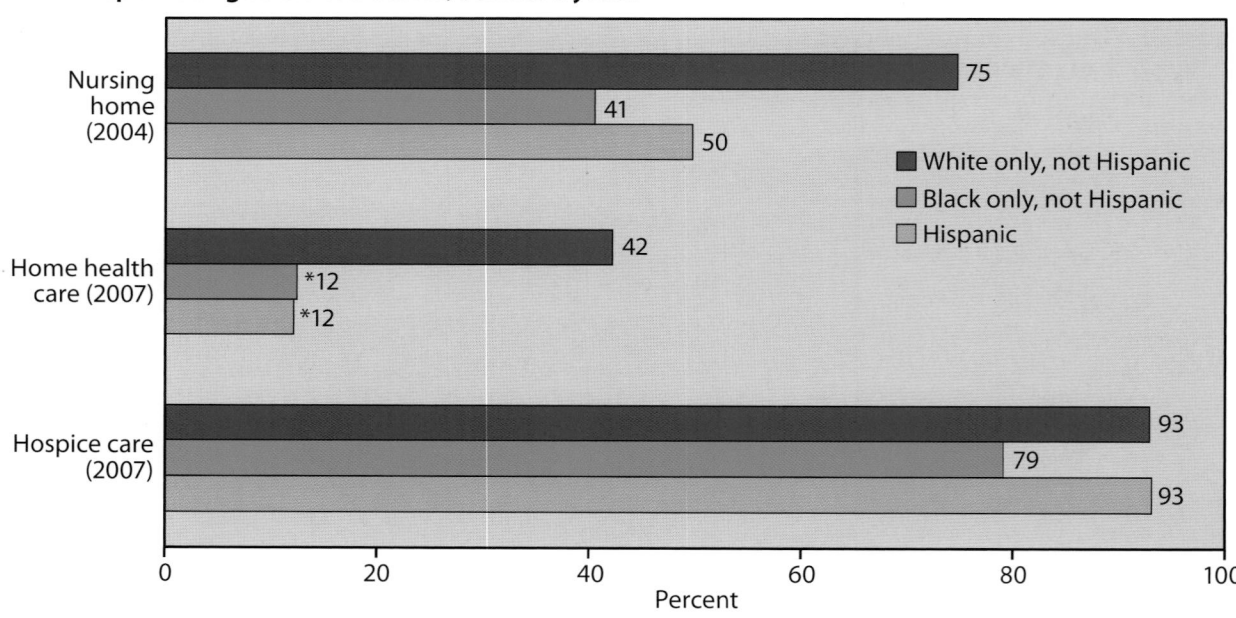

* Estimates are considered unreliable. Data preceded by an asterisk have a relative standard error of 20%–30%.

NOTE: See data table for Figure 36.

SOURCE: CDC/NCHS, National Nursing Home Survey and National Home and Hospice Care Survey.

Selected Characteristics of Discharged Hospice Care Patients

In 2007, discharged hospice care patients were predominantly 65 years of age and over and non-Hispanic white, and most received hospice care in their homes.

Hospice care involves the provision of palliative care and support services for persons with terminal illnesses (1,2). In 1983, Medicare introduced a hospice care program. Since 1985, the number of certified hospice care agencies has grown 20-fold (Table 119). Medicare's hospice program covers an assortment of medical and support services, some of which are not covered by traditional Medicare. Covered services include spiritual, psychosocial, and family bereavement counseling; pain medications; homemaker services; and respite care (2–4). To be eligible for hospice care, Medicare and most other insurers require that a physician certify that the patient is expected to die within 6 months if their illness follows its anticipated course, and the patient must forego curative treatment. Recently passed health care reform legislation requires that Medicare study the impact of relaxing the requirement that hospice care patients forego curative treatment.

The vast majority of discharged hospice care patients in 2007 were 65 years of age and over, Medicare beneficiaries, and non-Hispanic white. Just over one-half were female. Two-fifths were widowed, 45% were married or living with a partner, and the remainder were single, divorced, or separated. Over one-half received hospice care while in their own homes, and another one-fifth received care in nursing homes. Most died while receiving hospice care, but 16% were discharged alive.

References

1. U.S. General Accounting Office (GAO). Hospice care—A growing concept in the United States. Report to the Congress by the Comptroller General of the United States. HRD–79–50. Washington, DC: GAO; 1979. Available from: http://archive.gao.gov/f0302/108711.pdf.
2. Medicare Payment Advisory Commission (MedPAC). Hospice care in Medicare: Recent trends and a review of the issues. In: Report to the Congress: New approaches in Medicare. Washington, DC: MedPAC; 2004:139–54. Available from: http://www.medpac.gov/documents/June04_Entire_Report.pdf.
3. Iglehart JK. A new era of for-profit hospice care—The Medicare benefit. N Engl J Med 2009;360(26):2701–3.
4. Huskamp HA, Stevenson DG, Chernew ME, Newhouse JP. A new Medicare end-of-life benefit for nursing home residents. Health Aff (Millwood) 2010;29(1):130–5.

Figure 37. Selected characteristics of discharged hospice care patients: United States, 2007

Hospice care discharges: 1.0 million

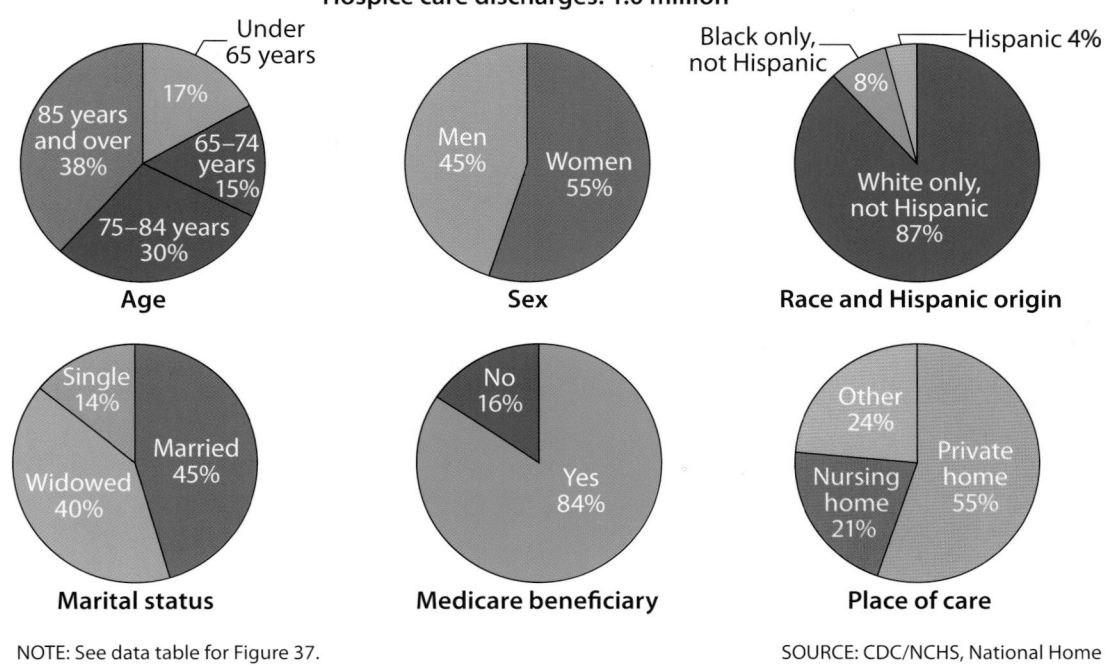

NOTE: See data table for Figure 37.

SOURCE: CDC/NCHS, National Home and Hospice Care Survey.

Primary Admission Diagnosis of Discharged Hospice Care Patients

The percentage of discharged hospice patients with a primary diagnosis of cancer declined by one-third from 1998 to 2007.

The first formal hospice care agency in the United States opened in 1971 (1). At that time, hospice care was almost exclusively for terminally ill cancer patients for whom curative treatment was no longer reasonable (1). The goal of hospice care was to provide end-of-life care, as well as support services for patients and their families (1,2). Medicare introduced a hospice care program in 1983 that covered some services not included in traditional Medicare (2,3). In the last decade, the use of Medicare's hospice benefit has increased rapidly, due to increased knowledge and appreciation among providers and patients and Medicare's promotion of this benefit (2).

In 1998, 65% of discharged hospice care patients had a primary admission diagnosis of cancer. In 2007, cancer remained the most common diagnosis but had declined to 43% of patients. Increasingly, persons with other diagnoses are using hospice care. The top five diagnoses in 2007 were cancer, Alzheimer's disease and other dementia, heart disease, chronic lower respiratory diseases, and stroke.

The use of hospice care has almost doubled in the past decade, from 182 discharges per 100,000 population in 1998 to 348 in 2007 (4). Despite greater use of hospice, the majority of hospice care patients have short stays. Although the median length of stay among discharged hospice care patients was 17 days in 2007, length of stay varied greatly. About one-third had hospice care for a week or less, while almost one-fifth had hospice care for longer than 90 days (4).

References

1. U.S. General Accounting Office (GAO). Hospice care—A growing concept in the United States. Report to the Congress by the Comptroller General of the United States. HRD–79–50. Washington, DC: GAO; 1979. Available from: http://archive.gao.gov/f0302/108711.pdf.
2. Medicare Payment Advisory Commission (MedPAC). Hospice care in Medicare: Recent trends and a review of the issues. In: Report to the Congress: New approaches in Medicare. Washington, DC: MedPAC; 2004:139–54. Available from: http://www.medpac.gov/documents/June04_Entire_Report.pdf.
3. Iglehart JK. A new era of for-profit hospice care—The Medicare benefit. N Engl J Med 2009;360(26):2701–3.
4. CDC/NCHS. National Home and Hospice Care Survey [unpublished analysis].

Figure 38. Primary admission diagnosis of discharged hospice care patients: United States, 1998 and 2007

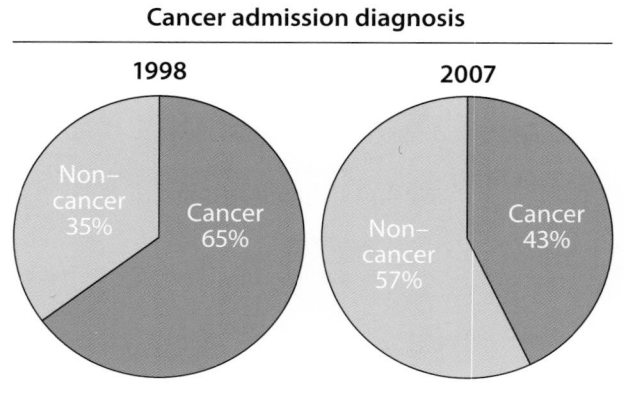

Cancer admission diagnosis

1998
- Non-cancer 35%
- Cancer 65%

2007
- Non-cancer 57%
- Cancer 43%

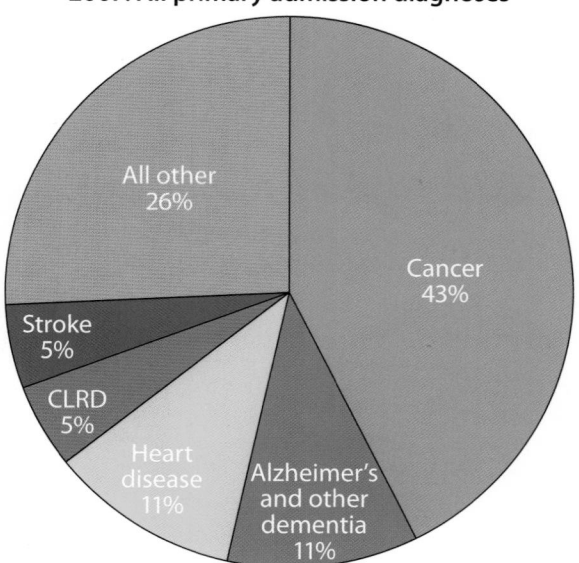

2007: All primary admission diagnoses
- All other 26%
- Cancer 43%
- Stroke 5%
- CLRD 5%
- Heart disease 11%
- Alzheimer's and other dementia 11%

NOTES: CLRD is chronic lower respiratory diseases. See data table for Figure 38.

SOURCE: CDC/NCHS, National Home and Hospice Care Survey.

Services to Hospice Care Patients' Family Members or Friends

Bereavement, spiritual services, and medication management were the most common types of services offered or provided to hospice care patients' family members or friends.

A critical function of hospice care is the provision of palliative care to those with a terminal prognosis of 6 months or less. According to the National Consensus Project for Quality Palliative Care (1), the goal of palliative care is to "prevent and relieve suffering and to support the best possible quality of life for patients and their families. . ." Palliative care services should be comprehensive in nature and may require the expertise of various types of providers, such as physicians, nurses, social workers, nutritionists, and clergy, in order to adequately assess and treat the complex needs of seriously ill patients and their families (1). In 2007, 84% of hospice care patients were Medicare beneficiaries (Figure 37), and from its inception the Medicare hospice benefit was designed to be broad in scope and include grief counseling, respite care, and other services for caregivers and family members (2). Caregiver stress and burnout are increasingly recognized areas of concern (3–5).

In 2007, bereavement services were offered or provided to 85% of hospice care patients' family members or friends; spiritual services and medication management information were offered or provided to two-thirds of family members or friends. Information about activities of daily living, safety training, and equipment use were offered to one-half of family members or friends. Caregiver health and wellness services were offered or provided to one-quarter of family members or friends.

References

1. National Consensus Project for Quality Palliative Care. Clinical practice guidelines for quality palliative care, 2nd ed. Pittsburgh, PA: National Consensus Project; 2009. Available from: http://www.nationalconsensusproject.org/guideline.pdf.
2. Centers for Medicare & Medicaid Services (CMS). Hospice payment system. Medicare Learning Network Payment System Fact Sheet. Baltimore, MD: CMS; 2009. Available from: http://www.cms.gov/MLNProducts/downloads/hospice_pay_sys_fs.pdf.
3. Ybema JF, Kuijer RG, Hagedoorn M, Buunk BP. Caregiver burnout among intimate partners of patients with a severe illness: An equity perspective. Pers Relat 2002;9:73–88.
4. DuBenske LL, Wen KY, Gustafson DH, Guarnaccia CA, Cleary JF, Dinauer SK, McTavish FM. Caregivers' differing needs across key experiences of the advanced cancer disease trajectory. Palliat Support Care 2008;6(3):265–72.
5. Harding R, Higginson IJ. What is the best way to help caregivers in cancer and palliative care? A systematic literature review of interventions and their effectiveness. Palliat Med 2003;17(1):63–74.

Figure 39. Services offered or provided to hospice care patients' family members or friends: United States, 2007

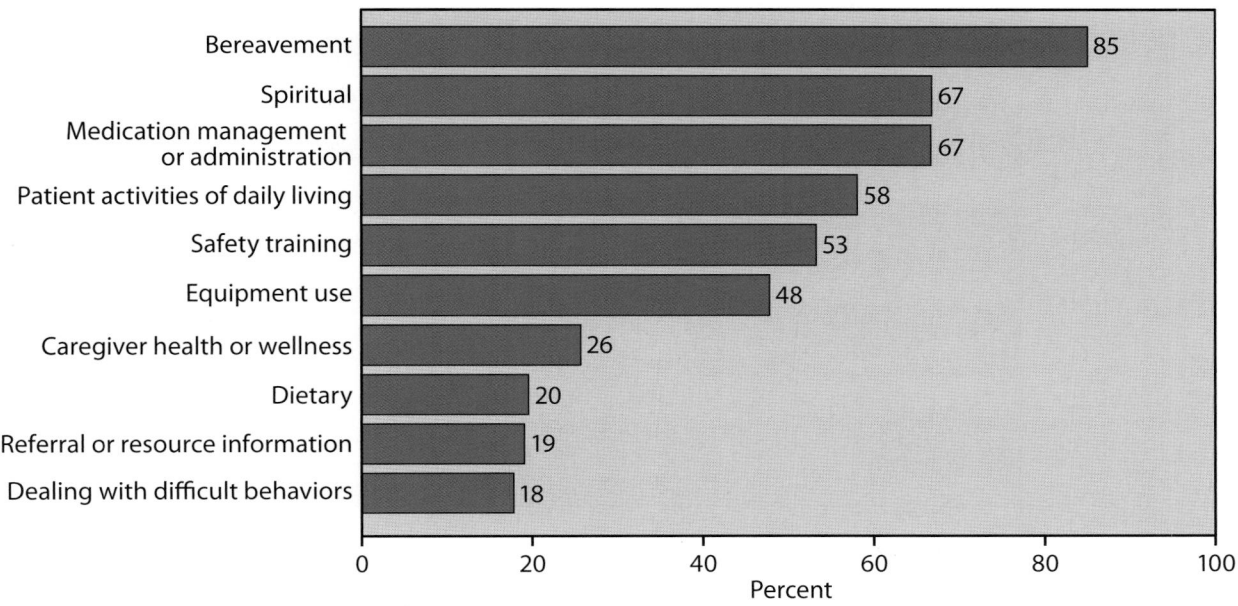

NOTE: See data table for Figure 39.

SOURCE: CDC/NCHS, National Home and Hospice Care Survey.

Hospice Care Patients' Symptoms at the Last Hospice Visit Before Death

One-third of hospice care patients had pain near the time of their death.

Controlling pain and other distressing symptoms near the end of life is a major concern identified by hospice care patients and their family members and by hospice care personnel (1–4). Nearly 90% of hospice care patients in 2007 had their level of pain assessed at the time of their admission to hospice care services (5).

Recognition of the onset of the acute phase of dying is important in order to initiate appropriate symptom control measures such as medication use, and comfort measures such as positioning, distraction, and guided imagery (4,6). Many family members and some health care professionals express concern that prescription narcotic pain medications, such as morphine, may hasten death or lead to addiction (4,7). Several studies refute the fear of hastened death associated with prescription narcotics use (4). Prescription narcotics are safe and effective for the treatment of patients with moderate to severe pain, and their side effects can be managed effectively (6). Constipation is the most frequent side effect of narcotic drugs (7). While many dying patients can have their pain controlled with

manageable side effects, others experience breakthrough pain (4,8).

Based on information from agency personnel who were familiar with the care received, as well as information in the medical record for patients who died while under hospice care, one-half of hospice care patients had difficulty breathing at the time of their last hospice visit, one-third had pain, one-quarter had restlessness, nearly one-quarter had anorexia, and one-tenth had constipation.

References

1. National Consensus Project for Quality Palliative Care. Clinical practice guidelines for quality palliative care, 2nd ed. Pittsburgh, PA: National Consensus Project; 2009. Available from: http://www.nationalconsensusproject.org/guideline.pdf.
2. Shugarman LR, Lorenz K, Lynn J. End-of-life care: An agenda for policy improvement. Clin Geriatr Med 2005;21(1): 255–72.
3. Steinhauser KE, Clipp EC, McNeilly M, Christakis NA, McIntyre LM, Tulsky JA. In search of a good death: Observations of patients, families, and providers. Ann Intern Med 2000;132(10): 825–32.
4. National Cancer Institute (NCI). Last days of life (PDQ): Symptom management. Bethesda, MD: NCI; 2010. Available from: http://www.cancer.gov/cancertopics/pdq/supportivecare/lasthours/HealthProfessional/page2.

(References continue on data table for Figure 40)

Figure 40. Hospice care patients' symptoms at the last hospice care visit before death: United States, 2007

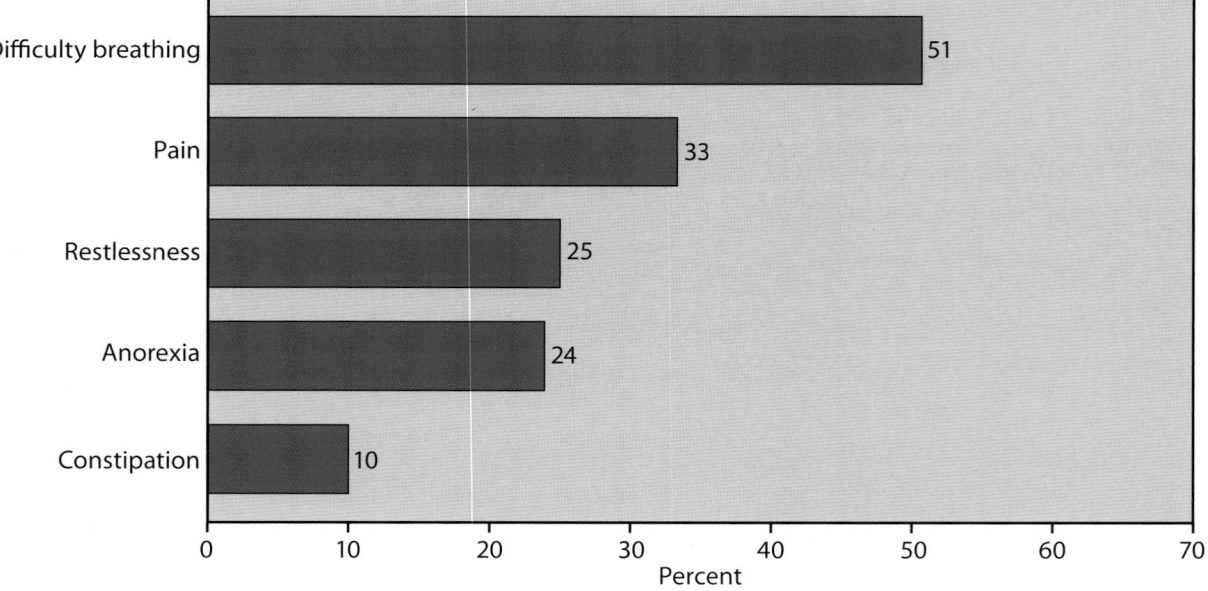

NOTE: See data table for Figure 40.

SOURCE: CDC/NCHS, National Home and Hospice Care Survey.

Hospice Care Patients' Drugs in the Last Week of Life

Ninety percent of hospice care patients had a narcotic analgesic (for severe pain) prescribed to them in the last week of life.

A fundamental goal of hospice care is the relief of pain and management of symptoms in those with a life expectancy of 6 months or less (1). Methods for pain and symptom relief can include relaxation techniques, imagery, distraction, skin stimulation, acupuncture, and over-the-counter and prescription medications (2). As the course of a terminal illness progresses, questions arise as to whether to continue to treat comorbid medical conditions with drugs or to only use drugs to manage symptoms related to dying (3,4).

In a national sample of hospice care providers, medication information was obtained from patients' records and included drugs prescribed in the last 7 days of life. The most commonly prescribed medications were related to symptoms often present near the time of death (Figure 40). Ninety percent of hospice care patients had a narcotic analgesic for pain control prescribed to them in the last week of life. Three-quarters of hospice care patients had an antiemetic for vomiting, and one-half of patients had a laxative for constipation. One-third of hospice care

patients had an antipsychotic drug to treat restlessness or agitation that may be present in the final phase of life. One-quarter of hospice care patients had an antidepressant drug prescribed for treatment of depression or pain. Seven percent of hospice care patients had a cholesterol-lowering (antihyperlipidemia) drug, and 3% of hospice care patients had baby aspirin or clopidogrel (Plavix) for clot prevention.

References

1. Medicare Payment Advisory Commission (MedPAC). Hospice care in Medicare: Recent trends and a review of the issues. In: Report to the Congress: New approaches in Medicare. Washington, DC: MedPAC; 2004:139–54. Available from: http://www.medpac.gov/documents/June04_Entire_Report.pdf.
2. Symptoms during a fatal illness [online]. Merck Manuals Online Medical Library. 2007. Available from: http://www.merck.com/mmhe/sec01/ch008/ch008f.html.
3. Tanvetyanon T, Choudhury AM. Physician practice in the discontinuation of statins among patients with advanced lung cancer. J Palliat Care 2006;22(4):281–5.
4. Currow DC, Stevenson JP, Abernethy AP, Plummer J, Shelby-James TM. Prescribing in palliative care as death approaches. J Am Geriatr Soc 2007;55(4):590–5.

Figure 41. Selected drugs prescribed to hospice care patients in the last week of life: United States, 2007

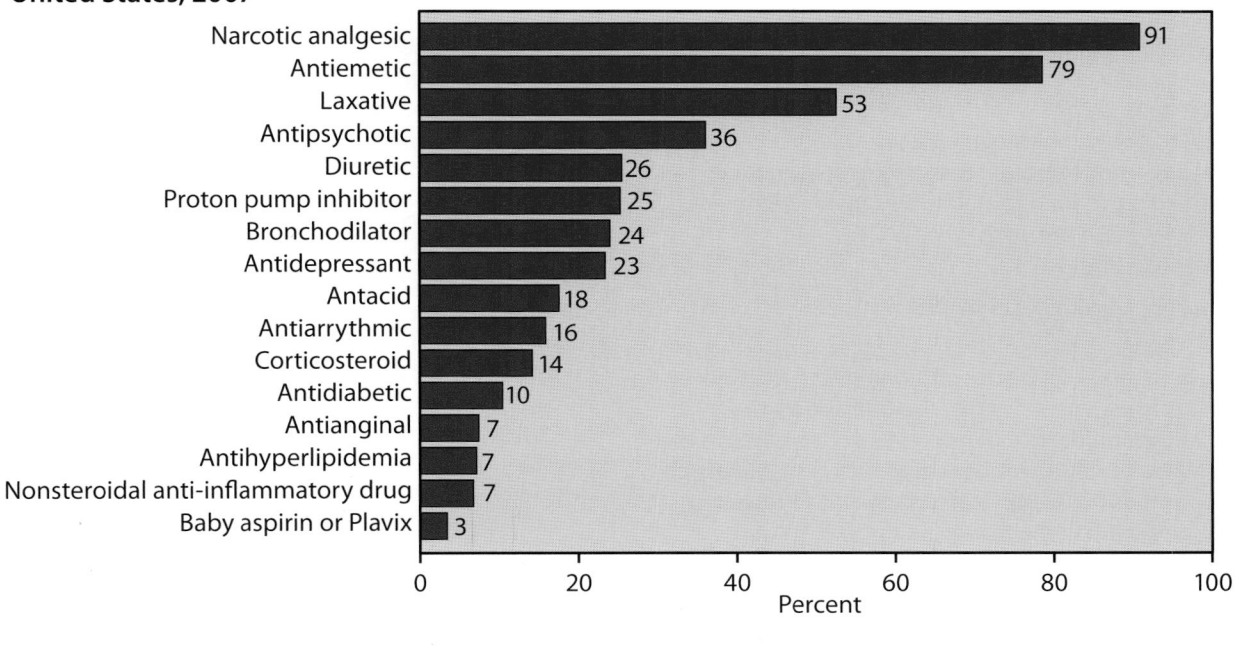

NOTE: See data table for Figure 41.

SOURCE: CDC/NCHS, National Home and Hospice Care Survey.

Data Sources and Comparability

Data for the *Health, United States, 2010 Chartbook* come from many surveys and data systems and cover a broad range of years. Detailed descriptions of the data sources included in the Chartbook are provided in Appendix I—Data Sources. Additional information clarifying and qualifying the data are included in the table notes and in Appendix II—Definitions and Methods.

Data Presentation

Many measures in the Chartbook section are shown for people in specific age groups because of the strong effect of age on most health outcomes. Some estimates are age-adjusted using the age distribution of the 2000 standard population, and this is noted in the data tables that accompany each chart (see Appendix II, Age adjustment). Age-adjusted rates are computed to eliminate differences in observed rates that result from age differences in population composition. For some charts, data years are combined to increase sample size and the reliability of the estimates. Some charts present time trends, and others focus on differences in estimates among population subgroups for the most recent time point available. Trends are shown on a linear scale to emphasize absolute differences over time. The linear scale is the scale most frequently used and recognized, and it emphasizes the absolute changes between data points over time (1). Data tables accompany each chart and present the data points graphed. Some data tables contain additional data that were not graphed because of space considerations. Standard errors for data points are provided for many measures presented in the data tables.

Statistical Testing

Trends in rates can be described in many ways. For trend analyses presented in the Chartbook, the statistical significance of increases or decreases in the estimates during the time period was assessed at the 0.05 level using weighted least squares regression, performed using the National Cancer Institute's Joinpoint software. The regression models were fit to the log of the estimates, with the number of joinpoints limited to zero. For more information on Joinpoint, see: http://srab.cancer.gov/joinpoint.

For analyses that show two time periods, differences between the two periods were assessed for statistical significance at the 0.05 level using two-sided significance tests (z test).

Terms such as "similar," "stable," and "no difference" indicate that the statistics being compared were not significantly different. Lack of comment regarding the difference between statistics does not necessarily suggest that the difference was tested and found to be not significant. Because statistically significant differences or trends are partly a function of sample size (the larger the sample, the smaller the change that can be detected), even statistically significant differences or trends do not necessarily have public health significance (1).

Overall estimates generally have relatively small sampling errors, but estimates for certain population subgroups may be based on small numbers and have relatively large sampling errors. Numbers of deaths from the National Vital Statistics System represent complete counts and therefore are not subject to sampling error. However, they are subject to random variation, which means that the number of events that actually occur in a given year may be considered as one of a large series of possible results that could have arisen under the same circumstances. When the number of events is small and the probability of such an event is small, considerable caution must be observed in interpreting the conditions described by the figures. Estimates that are unreliable because of large sampling errors or small numbers of events have been noted with an asterisk. The criteria used to designate or suppress unreliable estimates are indicated in the notes to the applicable tables or charts.

For NCHS surveys, point estimates and their corresponding variances were calculated using the SUDAAN software package, which takes into consideration the complex survey design (2). Standard errors for other surveys or datasets were computed using the methodology recommended by the programs providing the data or were provided directly by those programs.

References

1. Interpretation of YRBS trend data [online]. CDC, Youth Risk Behavior Survey (YRBS). 2010. Available from: http://www.cdc.gov/HealthyYouth/yrbs/pdf/YRBS_trend_interpretation.pdf.
2. Shah BV. SUDAAN [computer software]. Research Triangle Park, NC: RTI International.

Data Tables for Figures 1–41

Data table for Figure 1. Life expectancy at birth, by race and sex: United States, 1980–2007

Year	All races			Male		Female	
	Both sexes	Male	Female	White	Black	White	Black
	Life expectancy in years						
1980	73.7	70.0	77.4	70.7	63.8	78.1	72.5
1990	75.4	71.8	78.8	72.7	64.5	79.4	73.6
1997	76.5	73.6	79.4	74.3	67.2	79.9	74.7
1998	76.7	73.8	79.5	74.5	67.6	80.0	74.8
1999	76.7	73.9	79.4	74.6	67.8	79.9	74.7
2000	76.8	74.1	79.3	74.7	68.2	79.9	75.1
2001	76.9	74.2	79.4	74.8	68.4	79.9	75.2
2002	76.9	74.3	79.5	74.9	68.6	79.9	75.4
2003	77.1	74.5	79.6	75.0	68.8	80.0	75.6
2004	77.5	74.9	79.9	75.4	69.3	80.4	76.0
2005	77.4	74.9	79.9	75.4	69.3	80.4	76.1
2006	77.7	75.1	80.2	75.7	69.7	80.6	76.5
2007	77.9	75.4	80.4	75.9	70.0	80.8	76.8

NOTES: Populations for computing life expectancy are 1990-based postcensal estimates of U.S. resident population for 1991–1999 and 2000-based postcensal estimates for 2001–2007. See Appendix I, Population Census and Population Estimates. Life table values for 2000 and later years were computed using a slight modification of the new life table method due to a change in the age detail of populations received from the U.S. Census Bureau. Values for data years 2000–2007 are based on a newly revised methodology that uses vital statistics death rates for ages under 66 years and modeled probabilities of death for ages 66–100 years based on blended vital statistics and Medicare probabilities of dying and may differ from figures previously published. The revised methodology is similar to that developed for the 1999–2001 decennial life tables. Starting with 2003 data, some states allowed the reporting of more than one race on the death certificate. The multiple-race data for these states were bridged to the single-race categories of the 1977 Office of Management and Budget Standards, for comparability with other states. See Appendix II, Race; Table 22.

SOURCE: CDC/NCHS, National Vital Statistics System. Arias E, Rostron BL, Tejada-Vera B. United States life tables, 2005. National vital statistics reports; vol 58 no 10. Hyattsville, MD: NCHS. 2010. Available from: http://www.cdc.gov/nchs/data/nvsr/nvsr58/nvsr58_10.pdf. Xu JQ, Kochanek KD, Murphy SL, Tejada-Vera B. Deaths: Final data for 2007. National vital statistics reports; vol 58 no 19. Hyattsville, MD: NCHS; 2010. Available from: http://www.cdc.gov/nchs/data/nvsr/nvsr58/nvsr58_19.pdf.

Data table for Figure 2. Respondent-reported selected conditions among children under 18 years of age: United States, 1997–1999 and 2007–2009

Condition	1997–1999		2007–2009	
	Percent	SE	Percent	SE
Skin allergy	7.4	0.2	10.7	0.3
Food allergy	3.4	0.1	4.6	0.2
Asthma attack	5.4	0.1	5.4	0.2
ADHD or ADD (ever diagnosed, 5–17 years of age)	6.5	0.2	9.0	0.3

SE is standard error.

NOTES: ADHD is attention deficit hyperactivity disorder, and ADD is attention deficit disorder; based on the parent's or knowledgable household adult's report of having ever been told by a doctor or other health professional that the child has ADHD or ADD. Food allergy includes digestive allergy; skin allergy includes eczema. Food allergy is based on asking "During the past 12 months has your child had any kind of food or digestive allergy?" Skin allergy is based on asking "During the past 12 months has your child had eczema or any kind of skin allergy?" Asthma attack is based on the parent's or knowledgable household adult's report of having ever been told by a doctor or other health professional that [child] had asthma and that [child] had an episode of asthma or an asthma attack in the past 12 months. Also see Table 46.

SOURCE: CDC/NCHS, National Health Interview Survey, sample child questionnaire.

Data table for Figure 3. Respondent-reported lifetime heart disease prevalence among adults 18 years of age and over, by sex and age: United States, 1999–2009

Sex and age	1999	2000	2001	2002	2003	2004	2005	2006	2007	2008	2009
						Percent					
Total											
18 years and over, age-adjusted	11.0	11.1	11.7	11.2	11.1	11.5	11.6	10.8	11.1	11.5	11.4
18 years and over, crude.	10.8	11.0	11.6	11.1	11.1	11.5	11.8	11.0	11.2	11.8	11.8
Men											
18 years and over, age-adjusted	11.9	11.9	12.6	12.2	12.1	12.4	12.5	12.0	12.4	12.5	13.1
18 years and over, crude.	11.0	11.0	11.7	11.4	11.4	11.7	12.0	11.4	11.9	12.1	12.9
18–44 years	3.6	3.5	3.6	3.6	3.2	3.9	3.5	3.0	3.5	4.2	4.5
45–64 years	14.1	13.5	14.1	13.7	13.7	13.1	14.9	13.5	13.0	13.0	14.5
65–74 years	30.4	30.4	32.2	31.4	32.9	33.3	32.2	30.9	34.3	29.6	31.2
75 years and over	37.8	40.5	44.5	42.3	42.0	43.0	41.1	44.9	45.4	47.3	45.8
Women											
18 years and over, age-adjusted	10.4	10.6	11.2	10.4	10.4	10.8	11.1	10.0	10.1	10.9	10.1
18 years and over, crude.	10.6	10.9	11.5	10.8	10.8	11.3	11.6	10.5	10.7	11.6	10.8
18–44 years	5.2	4.7	5.5	4.3	4.4	5.0	5.1	4.3	4.8	5.0	4.3
45–64 years	11.2	11.7	12.2	11.8	11.6	11.6	12.4	11.1	11.3	11.5	11.7
65–74 years	20.8	23.1	22.2	22.1	22.6	22.1	22.1	22.1	20.9	24.0	21.1
75 years and over	30.7	31.4	32.1	32.8	32.2	34.0	33.7	30.7	29.6	33.7	30.7
						Standard error					
Total											
18 years and over, age-adjusted	0.2	0.2	0.2	0.2	0.2	0.2	0.2	0.2	0.2	0.2	0.2
18 years and over, crude.	0.2	0.2	0.2	0.2	0.2	0.2	0.2	0.2	0.3	0.3	0.3
Men											
18 years and over, age-adjusted	0.3	0.3	0.3	0.3	0.3	0.3	0.3	0.3	0.4	0.4	0.4
18 years and over, crude.	0.3	0.3	0.3	0.3	0.3	0.3	0.3	0.4	0.4	0.4	0.4
18–44 years	0.2	0.3	0.3	0.2	0.3	0.3	0.3	0.3	0.3	0.4	0.4
45–64 years	0.6	0.6	0.6	0.6	0.6	0.6	0.6	0.7	0.7	0.7	0.7
65–74 years	1.5	1.4	1.4	1.5	1.6	1.5	1.5	1.7	1.8	1.6	1.6
75 years and over	1.7	1.7	1.7	1.8	1.8	1.8	1.7	2.1	2.2	2.2	2.1
Women											
18 years and over, age-adjusted	0.3	0.2	0.3	0.3	0.3	0.3	0.3	0.3	0.3	0.3	0.3
18 years and over, crude.	0.3	0.3	0.3	0.3	0.3	0.3	0.3	0.3	0.3	0.3	0.3
18–44 years	0.3	0.3	0.3	0.3	0.3	0.3	0.3	0.3	0.3	0.3	0.3
45–64 years	0.5	0.5	0.5	0.5	0.5	0.5	0.5	0.6	0.7	0.6	0.6
65–74 years	1.0	1.2	1.1	1.1	1.1	1.2	1.1	1.6	1.4	1.4	1.2
75 years and over	1.3	1.2	1.2	1.3	1.2	1.2	1.2	1.4	1.3	1.3	1.4

NOTES: Data are for the civilian noninstitutionalized population. Heart disease prevalence is ascertained by a "yes" answer to at least one of the following four questions: "Have you EVER been told by a doctor or other health professional that you had coronary heart disease?" "Have you EVER been told by a doctor or other health professional that you had angina, also called angina pectoris?" "Have you EVER been told by a doctor or other health professional that you had a heart attack (also called myocardial infarction)?" "Have you EVER been told by a doctor or other health professional that you had any kind of heart condition or heart disease (other than the ones I asked about)?" Estimates are age-adjusted to the year 2000 standard population using five age groups: 18–44 years, 45–54 years, 55–64 years, 65–74 years, and 75 years and over. See Appendix II, Age adjustment; Table 49.

SOURCE: CDC/NCHS, National Health Interview Survey, sample adult questionnaire.

Data table for Figure 4. Respondent-reported lifetime cancer prevalence among adults 18 years of age and over, by sex and age: United States, 1999–2009

Sex and age	1999	2000	2001	2002	2003	2004	2005	2006	2007	2008	2009
						Percent					
Total											
18 years and over, age-adjusted	5.2	4.9	5.3	5.3	5.1	5.4	5.7	5.6	5.4	5.9	5.8
18 years and over, crude.	5.1	4.8	5.2	5.2	5.1	5.4	5.7	5.7	5.5	6.1	6.1
Men											
18 years and over, age-adjusted	4.0	4.1	4.8	4.6	4.5	4.9	5.2	4.9	4.9	4.7	5.3
18 years and over, crude.	4.2	3.6	4.3	4.1	4.1	4.4	4.7	4.5	4.6	4.5	5.1
18–44 years	1.0	0.7	0.8	0.6	0.6	0.7	0.8	0.8	0.9	*0.8	*0.7
45–64 years	4.1	3.0	3.9	4.0	4.5	4.1	4.5	4.2	4.6	4.5	4.8
65–74 years	15.7	12.2	15.8	16.4	13.5	15.0	16.5	14.6	15.3	13.3	18.9
75 years and over	19.0	21.5	21.7	19.9	19.7	24.5	24.2	24.4	22.0	21.8	22.7
Women											
18 years and over, age-adjusted	5.8	5.8	5.9	6.0	5.7	6.0	6.4	6.4	5.9	7.1	6.5
18 years and over, crude.	5.8	5.9	6.0	6.2	6.0	6.3	6.6	6.7	6.3	7.6	7.0
18–44 years	2.4	2.5	2.7	2.7	2.1	2.5	2.8	3.0	2.2	2.8	2.2
45–64 years	7.1	6.6	7.5	7.1	7.1	7.4	7.5	7.6	7.3	8.7	8.7
65–74 years	12.3	12.7	11.9	12.4	13.9	13.0	14.1	12.5	15.3	15.8	15.3
75 years and over	15.5	16.6	14.3	16.8	15.6	16.2	17.4	17.8	16.9	20.1	16.9
						Standard error					
Total											
18 years and over, age-adjusted	0.1	0.1	0.1	0.1	0.1	0.1	0.1	0.2	0.2	0.2	0.2
18 years and over, crude.	0.1	0.1	0.1	0.1	0.1	0.1	0.1	0.2	0.2	0.2	0.2
Men											
18 years and over, age-adjusted	0.2	0.2	0.2	0.2	0.2	0.2	0.2	0.2	0.2	0.2	0.2
18 years and over, crude.	0.2	0.2	0.2	0.2	0.2	0.2	0.2	0.3	0.2	0.2	0.2
18–44 years	0.1	0.1	0.1	0.1	0.1	0.1	0.1	0.1	0.2	*0.2	*0.1
45–64 years	0.4	0.3	0.3	0.3	0.4	0.3	0.3	0.4	0.4	0.4	0.4
65–74 years	1.1	1.0	1.1	1.3	1.1	1.1	1.1	1.4	1.2	1.2	1.3
75 years and over	1.5	1.5	1.5	1.4	1.5	1.5	1.4	1.8	1.8	1.9	1.6
Women											
18 years and over, age-adjusted	0.2	0.2	0.2	0.2	0.2	0.2	0.2	0.2	0.2	0.2	0.2
18 years and over, crude.	0.2	0.2	0.2	0.2	0.2	0.2	0.2	0.3	0.2	0.3	0.3
18–44 years	0.2	0.2	0.2	0.2	0.2	0.2	0.2	0.3	0.2	0.3	0.2
45–64 years	0.4	0.4	0.4	0.4	0.4	0.4	0.4	0.5	0.5	0.5	0.5
65–74 years	0.9	0.8	0.8	0.9	0.9	0.9	1.0	1.4	1.0	1.3	1.1
75 years and over	1.0	1.0	0.9	1.0	0.9	1.0	1.0	1.2	1.2	1.3	1.3

* Estimates are considered unreliable. Data preceded by an asterisk have a relative standard error of 20%–30%.

NOTES: Data are for the civilian noninstitutionalized population. Cancer prevalence is ascertained by a "yes" answer to the question: "Have you EVER been told by a doctor or other health professional that you had a cancer or malignancy of any kind?" Excludes nonmelanoma skin carcinomas. Estimates are age-adjusted to the year 2000 standard population using five age groups: 18–44 years, 45–54 years, 55–64 years, 65–74 years, and 75 years and over. See Appendix II, Age adjustment; Table 49.

SOURCE: CDC/NCHS, National Health Interview Survey, sample adult questionnaire.

Data table for Figure 5. Diabetes prevalence among adults 20 years of age and over, by age: United States, 1988–1994 and 2005–2008

Age	1988–1994 Percent	1988–1994 SE	2005–2008 Percent	2005–2008 SE
20 years and over, age-adjusted	9.1	0.4	10.9	0.5
20 years and over, crude	8.4	0.3	11.3	0.6
20–44 years.	2.6	0.3	3.7	0.4
45–64 years.	13.9	0.8	13.7	1.2
65 years and over	19.6	1.0	26.9	1.5

SE is standard error.

NOTES: Diabetes prevalence estimates include physician-diagnosed and undiagnosed diabetes. Physician-diagnosed diabetes was defined by respondents answering "yes" to the question, "Have you ever been told by a doctor or health professional that you have diabetes or sugar diabetes?" and excludes women who reported having diabetes only during pregnancy. Undiagnosed diabetes is defined as a fasting blood glucose (FBG) of at least 126 mg/dL and/or a hemoglobin A1c of at least 6.5% and no reported physician diagnosis. Respondents had fasted for at least 8 hours and less than 24 hours. The definition of undiagnosed diabetes in previous editions of *Health, United States* did not consider hemoglobin A1c. See Appendix II, Diabetes. In 2005–2006 and 2007–2008, FBG and hemoglobin A1c testing were performed at different laboratories and using different instruments than testing in earlier years. As a result, the National Health and Nutrition Examination Survey recommended that 2005–2008 data be adjusted to be compatible with earlier years. Diabetes estimates in *Health, United States* were produced after adjusting the 2005–2008 laboratory data as recommended. For more information, see: http://www.cdc.gov/nchs/nhanes/nhanes2007-2008/GLU_E.htm. Estimates are age-adjusted to the year 2000 standard population using three age groups: 20–44 years, 45–64 years, and 65 years and over. See Appendix II, Age adjustment; Table 50.

SOURCE: CDC/NCHS, National Health and Nutrition Examination Survey.

Data table for Figure 6. Poor diabetes control (hemoglobin A1c levels greater than 9%) among adults 20 years of age and over with diagnosed diabetes, by age: United States, 1988–1994 and 2005–2008

Age	1988–1994		2005–2008	
	Percent	SE	Percent	SE
20 years and over, crude	23.3	1.9	12.7	1.3
20–44 years.	29.5	5.7	26.3	4.4
45–64 years.	26.0	3.4	14.4	1.9
65 years and over	18.0	2.5	*5.0	1.0

SE is standard error.

* Estimates are considered unreliable. Data preceded by an asterisk have a relative standard error of 20%–30%.

NOTES: Poorly controlled diabetes is defined as hemoglobin A1c (glycohemoglobin) laboratory values greater than 9%, among adults with diagnosed diabetes (based on self-report). In 2005–2006 and 2007–2008, hemoglobin A1c testing was performed at different laboratories and using different instruments than testing in earlier years. As a result, the National Health and Nutrition Examination Survey recommended that 2005–2008 data be adjusted to be compatible with earlier years. Poorly controlled diabetes estimates in *Health, United States* were produced after adjusting the 2005–2008 laboratory data as recommended. For more information, see: http://www.cdc.gov/nchs/nhanes/nhanes2007-2008/GHB_E.htm.

SOURCE: CDC/NCHS, National Health and Nutrition Examination Survey.

Data table for Figure 7. Joint pain in the past 30 days among adults 18 years of age and over, by age: United States, 2002–2009

Age	2002	2003	2004	2005	2006	2007	2008	2009
				Percent				
18 years and over, age-adjusted	29.5	31.6	30.8	30.7	29.2	27.0	30.5	32.0
18 years and over, crude	29.5	31.8	31.1	31.1	29.7	27.6	31.3	33.0
18–44 years.	19.3	20.7	19.2	19.1	18.0	16.3	20.3	20.7
45–64 years.	37.5	40.2	39.8	39.9	38.3	36.4	39.3	41.8
65–74 years.	46.0	49.3	49.3	49.3	47.6	41.6	46.8	47.9
75 years and over	48.7	52.4	54.2	52.6	48.8	46.6	48.1	53.8
				Standard error				
18 years and over, age-adjusted	0.3	0.3	0.3	0.3	0.4	0.4	0.4	0.4
18 years and over, crude	0.3	0.4	0.3	0.3	0.4	0.4	0.4	0.4
18–44 years.	0.4	0.4	0.4	0.4	0.4	0.4	0.5	0.5
45–64 years.	0.6	0.6	0.6	0.6	0.7	0.7	0.7	0.7
65–74 years.	1.0	1.1	1.1	1.0	1.3	1.2	1.3	1.1
75 years and over	1.1	1.1	1.1	1.1	1.2	1.3	1.4	1.3

NOTES: Respondents were asked, "During the past 30 days, have you had any symptoms of pain, aching, or stiffness in or around a joint?" Respondents were instructed to not include the back or neck because other questions focused on those areas. To facilitate their response, respondents were shown a card illustrating the body joints. Estimates are age-adjusted to the year 2000 standard population using five age groups: 18–44 years, 45–54 years, 55–64 years, 65–74 years, and 75 years and over. See Appendix II, Age adjustment; Table 53.

SOURCE: CDC/NCHS, National Health Interview Survey, sample adult questionnaire.

Data table for Figure 8. Selected back and joint procedures among adults 45 years of age and over, by age: United States, 1996–1997 through 2006–2007

Age and type of procedure	1996–1997	1998–1999	2000–2001	2002–2003	2004–2005	2006–2007
	Number per 10,000 population					
45–64 years						
Excision of intervertebral disc and spinal fusion.	27.0	28.3	25.8	27.1	27.1	27.2
Total knee replacement.	11.9	13.2	13.9	20.2	24.5	25.9
Total hip replacement	6.5	8.5	8.2	10.4	11.3	11.7
Partial hip replacement	1.3	1.5	1.0	1.2	9.1	9.4
65 years and over						
Excision of intervertebral disc and spinal fusion.	17.0	20.8	19.0	23.4	24.6	28.4
Total knee replacement.	51.2	51.4	58.3	66.8	82.0	82.1
Total hip replacement	28.5	30.2	26.7	33.7	37.5	33.3
Partial hip replacement	28.2	29.0	29.3	27.7	34.8	35.8
	Standard error					
45–64 years						
Excision of intervertebral disc and spinal fusion.	2.0	2.1	1.9	1.9	1.9	1.8
Total knee replacement.	0.9	0.9	1.0	1.6	2.0	1.8
Total hip replacement	0.5	0.6	0.8	0.9	1.0	0.9
Partial hip replacement	0.2	0.2	0.2	0.2	1.3	1.3
65 years and over						
Excision of intervertebral disc and spinal fusion.	1.4	2.0	1.8	2.0	2.1	2.3
Total knee replacement.	4.2	3.3	5.0	4.5	6.6	5.7
Total hip replacement	1.9	2.1	2.1	2.7	3.1	2.5
Partial hip replacement	2.0	2.2	2.3	2.2	2.8	2.8

NOTES: Procedures are any-listed. Up to four procedures were coded for each hospital discharge. Procedure categories are based on the *International Classification of Diseases, 9th Revision, Clinical Modification* (ICD–9–CM). See Appendix II, Table XI for ICD–9–CM codes. Rates are based on the civilian population as of July 1. Rates for 2000 and beyond are based on the 2000 census. Rates for 1996–1999 use population estimates based on the 1990 census adjusted for net underenumeration using the 1990 National Population Adjustment Matrix from the U.S. Census Bureau. Also see Table 103.

SOURCE: CDC/NCHS, National Hospital Discharge Survey.

Data table for Figure 9. Respondent-reported colorectal tests and procedures among adults 50–75 years of age, by race and Hispanic origin: United States, selected years 2000–2008

Race and Hispanic origin	2000 Percent	2000 SE	2003 Percent	2003 SE	2005 Percent	2005 SE	2008 Percent	2008 SE
Total, 50–75 years	33.2	0.6	38.6	0.6	44.0	0.6	51.4	0.7
White only, not Hispanic	35.0	0.7	40.5	0.7	47.1	0.7	54.5	0.8
Black only, not Hispanic.	28.8	1.7	34.8	1.6	37.7	1.6	47.2	2.0
Asian only	20.2	3.4	26.5	3.6	30.1	3.4	46.2	3.3
Hispanic.	21.1	1.6	26.8	1.7	28.2	1.8	33.8	2.0

SE is standard error.

NOTES: Asian only race includes persons of Hispanic and non-Hispanic origin. Persons of Hispanic origin may be of any race. In this analysis, colorectal tests and procedures include reports of home fecal occult blood test (FOBT) in the past year, sigmoidoscopy procedure in the past 5 years with FOBT in the past 3 years, or colonoscopy in the past 10 years. Colorectal procedures are performed for diagnostic and screening purposes.

SOURCE: CDC/NCHS, National Health Interview Survey.

References (continued from page 18)

4. Screening for colorectal cancer: Topic page [online]. U.S. Preventive Services Task Force, Agency for Healthcare Research and Quality. 2008. Available from: http://www.uspreventiveservicestaskforce.org/uspstf/uspscolo.htm.
5. CDC/NCHS. National Health Interview Survey [unpublished analysis].

Data table for Figure 10. Adults 18 years of age and over reporting prescription antidepressant and antianxiety drug use in the past month, by sex and age: United States, 1988–1994 and 2005–2008

	Multum Lexicon Plus therapeutic drug class							
	Antidepressant drugs				Antianxiety drugs (anxiolytics, sedatives, and hypnotics)			
	1988–1994		2005–2008		1988–1994		2005–2008	
Sex and age	Percent	SE	Percent	SE	Percent	SE	Percent	SE
Total								
18 years and over, age-adjusted	2.4	0.2	11.1	0.4	3.9	0.2	5.7	0.3
18 years and over, crude.	2.3	0.2	11.4	0.5	3.6	0.2	5.8	0.3
Men								
18 years and over.	1.5	0.2	6.2	0.4	2.6	0.3	4.3	0.4
18–44 years	*1.0	0.2	3.6	0.6	*1.0	0.2	2.1	0.4
45–64 years	*2.3	0.5	8.5	0.8	4.3	0.8	6.2	0.9
65 years and over	*2.3	0.5	10.0	0.9	6.1	0.9	7.1	0.9
Women								
18 years and over.	3.1	0.3	16.2	0.7	4.6	0.3	7.3	0.5
18–44 years	2.3	0.4	11.9	0.8	1.9	0.3	4.3	0.4
45–64 years	4.6	0.7	21.9	1.2	7.5	0.8	9.3	0.9
65 years and over	3.5	0.4	17.3	1.1	9.1	0.7	11.8	1.1

SE is standard error.

* Estimates are considered unreliable. Data preceded by an asterisk have a relative standard error of 20%–30%.

NOTES: The drug therapeutic class is based on Lexicon Plus, a proprietary database of Cerner Multum, Inc. Lexicon Plus is a comprehensive database of all prescription and some nonprescription drug products available in the U.S. drug market. In the National Health and Nutrition Examination Survey, data on prescription drug use only are collected. Up to four classes are assigned to drugs. All four classes were included in this analysis. Drugs classified into more than one class were counted in each class. For more information, see: http://www.cdc.gov/nchs/nhanes/nhanes2007-2008/RXQ_DRUG.htm. Estimates are age-adjusted to the year 2000 standard population using three age groups: 18–44 years, 45–64 years, and 65 years and over. See Appendix II, Age adjustment; Table 94.

SOURCE: CDC/NCHS, National Health and Nutrition Examination Survey.

References *(continued from page 19)*

4. Kessler RC, Chiu WT, Demler O, Merikangas KR, Walters EE. Prevalence, severity, and comorbidity of 12-month DSM–IV disorders in the National Comorbidity Survey Replication. Arch Gen Psychiatry 2005;62(6):617–27.
5. Timonen M, Liukkonen T. Management of depression in adults. BMJ 2008;336(7641):435–9.
6. Stone KJ, Viera AJ, Parman CL. Off-label applications for SSRIs. Am Fam Physician 2003;68(3):498–504.
7. Chouinard G. The search for new off-label indications for antidepressant, antianxiety, antipsychotic and anticonvulsant drugs. J Psychiatry Neurosci 2006;31(3):168–76.

Data table for Figure 11. Cigarette smoking among students in grades 9–12 and adults 18 years of age and over, by sex, grade, and age: United States, 1999–2009

Sex, grade, and age	1999	2000	2001	2002	2003	2004	2005	2006	2007	2008	2009
						Percent					
Sex and grade											
Total, grades 9–12.	34.8	- - -	28.5	- - -	21.9	- - -	23.0	- - -	20.0	- - -	19.5
Males, grades 9–12.	34.7	- - -	29.2	- - -	21.8	- - -	22.9	- - -	21.3	- - -	19.8
Females, grades 9–12.	34.9	- - -	27.7	- - -	21.9	- - -	23.0	- - -	18.7	- - -	19.1
Sex and age											
Total:											
18 years and over, age-adjusted	23.3	23.1	22.6	22.3	21.5	20.8	20.8	20.8	19.7	20.6	20.6
18 years and over, crude	23.5	23.2	22.7	22.4	21.6	20.9	20.9	20.8	19.8	20.6	20.6
Men:											
18 years and over, age-adjusted	25.2	25.2	24.6	24.6	23.7	23.0	23.4	23.6	22.0	22.8	23.2
18 years and over, crude	25.7	25.6	25.1	25.1	24.1	23.4	23.9	23.9	22.3	23.1	23.5
18–44 years.	29.5	29.2	27.9	29.4	27.9	26.1	27.1	26.7	25.8	25.6	26.9
45–64 years.	25.8	26.4	26.4	24.5	23.9	25.0	25.2	24.5	22.6	24.8	24.5
65 years and over.	10.5	10.2	11.5	10.1	10.1	9.8	8.9	12.6	9.3	10.5	9.5
Women:											
18 years and over, age-adjusted	21.6	21.1	20.7	20.0	19.4	18.7	18.3	18.1	17.5	18.5	18.1
18 years and over, crude	21.5	20.9	20.6	19.8	19.2	18.5	18.1	18.0	17.4	18.3	17.9
18–44 years.	25.4	24.5	24.1	23.0	22.5	21.4	21.2	20.6	19.5	20.6	20.0
45–64 years.	21.0	21.7	21.4	21.1	20.2	19.8	18.8	19.3	19.5	20.5	19.5
65 years and over.	10.7	9.3	9.1	8.6	8.3	8.1	8.3	8.3	7.6	8.3	9.5
						Standard error					
Sex and grade											
Total, grades 9–12.	1.3	- - -	1.0	- - -	1.1	- - -	1.2	- - -	1.2	- - -	0.8
Males, grades 9–12.	1.5	- - -	1.3	- - -	1.1	- - -	1.1	- - -	1.5	- - -	1.0
Females, grades 9–12.	1.3	- - -	1.1	- - -	1.4	- - -	1.3	- - -	1.1	- - -	0.9
Sex and age											
Total:											
18 years and over, age-adjusted	0.3	0.3	0.3	0.3	0.3	0.3	0.3	0.3	0.4	0.4	0.4
18 years and over, crude	0.3	0.3	0.3	0.3	0.3	0.3	0.3	0.3	0.4	0.4	0.4
Men:											
18 years and over, age-adjusted	0.5	0.4	0.4	0.4	0.4	0.4	0.5	0.5	0.5	0.6	0.5
18 years and over, crude	0.5	0.5	0.4	0.5	0.4	0.4	0.5	0.5	0.6	0.6	0.5
18–44 years.	0.7	0.6	0.6	0.7	0.6	0.6	0.7	0.8	0.8	0.8	0.8
45–64 years.	0.8	0.8	0.8	0.7	0.8	0.8	0.8	0.9	0.9	1.0	0.9
65 years and over.	0.7	0.7	0.7	0.7	0.7	0.7	0.6	0.9	0.8	0.9	0.7
Women:											
18 years and over, age-adjusted	0.4	0.4	0.4	0.4	0.4	0.4	0.4	0.4	0.5	0.5	0.4
18 years and over, crude	0.4	0.4	0.4	0.4	0.4	0.4	0.4	0.4	0.5	0.5	0.4
18–44 years.	0.6	0.5	0.6	0.6	0.6	0.6	0.6	0.6	0.7	0.7	0.7
45–64 years.	0.7	0.7	0.6	0.6	0.6	0.6	0.6	0.7	0.7	0.8	0.8
65 years and over.	0.6	0.5	0.5	0.5	0.5	0.5	0.5	0.6	0.6	0.6	0.7

- - - Data not available.

NOTES: Data are for men and women 18 years of age and over in the civilian noninstitutionalized population. Estimates are age-adjusted to the 2000 standard population using five age groups: 18–24 years, 25–34 years, 35–44 years, 45–64 years, and 65 years and over. Age-adjusted estimates in this table may differ from other age-adjusted estimates presented elsewhere if different age groups are used in the adjustment procedure. Cigarette smoking is defined as: among men and women 18 years of age and over, those who ever smoked 100 cigarettes in their lifetime and now smoke every day or some days; among high school students in grades 9–12, those who smoked cigarettes on one or more of the 30 days preceding the survey. See Appendix II, Age adjustment; Cigarette smoking; Tables 58–60.

SOURCE: CDC/NCHS, National Health Interview Survey (data for men and women); National Center for Chronic Disease Prevention and Health Promotion, Youth Risk Behavior Survey (data for students).

Data table for Figure 12. Participation in leisure-time aerobic and muscle-strengthening activities that meet the 2008 federal physical activity guidelines for adults 18 years of age and over, by sex and age: United States, 1999–2009

Sex and age	1999	2000	2001	2002	2003	2004	2005	2006	2007	2008	2009
						Percent					
Total											
18 years and over, age-adjusted.	15.0	15.0	16.6	16.8	17.0	16.2	16.6	16.2	16.6	18.4	19.1
18 years and over, crude	15.2	15.1	16.6	16.8	16.9	16.1	16.5	16.0	16.5	18.1	18.8
Men											
18 years and over, age-adjusted.	18.0	17.9	19.7	19.7	19.5	18.3	19.1	18.7	19.7	21.9	22.2
18 years and over, crude	18.5	18.2	20.1	20.0	19.7	18.5	19.2	18.7	19.7	21.8	22.1
18–44 years	23.7	23.0	26.1	25.6	24.9	23.6	24.6	24.1	25.0	27.3	27.7
45–64 years	13.7	14.2	14.8	15.2	15.6	13.9	14.5	15.0	15.8	18.1	18.5
65 years and over	8.1	8.4	8.4	9.7	9.8	9.7	10.0	8.1	10.2	11.5	11.8
Women											
18 years and over, age-adjusted.	12.1	12.3	13.6	14.0	14.6	14.1	14.3	13.8	13.7	15.0	16.2
18 years and over, crude	12.1	12.2	13.4	13.8	14.4	14.0	14.1	13.6	13.5	14.7	15.8
18–44 years	15.7	15.0	17.3	17.2	17.7	16.5	16.8	16.6	15.6	17.4	19.0
45–64 years	10.3	11.5	11.6	13.3	13.7	14.1	14.3	12.7	14.4	14.6	15.3
65 years and over	4.2	5.7	5.4	5.1	6.0	6.5	6.4	7.0	6.1	8.0	8.6
						Standard error					
Total											
18 years and over, age-adjusted.	0.3	0.3	0.3	0.3	0.3	0.3	0.3	0.4	0.4	0.4	0.4
18 years and over, crude	0.3	0.3	0.3	0.3	0.3	0.3	0.3	0.4	0.4	0.4	0.4
Men											
18 years and over, age-adjusted.	0.4	0.4	0.4	0.4	0.4	0.4	0.4	0.5	0.5	0.6	0.5
18 years and over, crude	0.4	0.4	0.4	0.4	0.5	0.4	0.4	0.5	0.5	0.6	0.5
18–44 years	0.6	0.6	0.6	0.7	0.7	0.7	0.7	0.9	0.8	0.9	0.8
45–64 years	0.7	0.6	0.6	0.6	0.7	0.6	0.6	0.8	0.8	0.9	0.8
65 years and over	0.7	0.7	0.7	0.7	0.7	0.7	0.7	0.8	0.9	1.0	0.9
Women											
18 years and over, age-adjusted.	0.3	0.3	0.3	0.3	0.4	0.3	0.4	0.4	0.4	0.5	0.4
18 years and over, crude	0.3	0.3	0.3	0.3	0.4	0.3	0.3	0.4	0.4	0.4	0.4
18–44 years	0.5	0.5	0.5	0.5	0.5	0.5	0.5	0.7	0.6	0.7	0.7
45–64 years	0.5	0.6	0.5	0.6	0.6	0.6	0.6	0.7	0.7	0.7	0.7
65 years and over	0.4	0.5	0.4	0.4	0.5	0.5	0.5	0.7	0.6	0.6	0.7

NOTES: Starting with *Health, United States, 2010*, measures of physical activity changed to reflect the 2008 federal physical activity guidelines for Americans (available from: http://www.health.gov/PAGuidelines/). This new table presents the percentage of adults who fully met the 2008 federal guidelines for both aerobic activity and muscle strengthening. The 2008 federal guidelines recommend that for substantial health benefits, adults perform at least 150 minutes (2 hours and 30 minutes) a week of moderate-intensity, or 75 minutes (1 hour and 15 minutes) a week of vigorous-intensity aerobic physical activity, or an equivalent combination of moderate- and vigorous-intensity aerobic activity. Aerobic activity should be performed in episodes of at least 10 minutes, and preferably it should be spread throughout the week. The 2008 guidelines also recommend that adults perform muscle-strengthening activities that are moderate or high intensity and involve all major muscle groups on two or more days a week because these activities provide additional health benefits. See Table 70; Appendix II, Physical activity, leisure-time. Estimates are age-adjusted to the year 2000 standard population using five age groups: 18–44 years, 45–54 years, 55–64 years, 65–74 years, and 75 years and over. Age-adjusted estimates in this table may differ from other age-adjusted estimates based on the same data and presented elsewhere if different age groups are used in the adjustment procedure. See Appendix II, Age adjustment.

SOURCE: CDC/NCHS, National Health Interview Survey.

Data table for Figure 13. Obesity among children, by age: United States, 1988–1994 through 2007–2008

Age	1988–1994	1999–2000	2001–2002	2003–2004	2005–2006	2007–2008
	Percent					
2–5 years	7.2	10.3	10.6	13.9	11.0	10.4
6–11 years	11.3	15.1	16.3	18.8	15.1	19.6
12–19 years	10.5	14.8	16.7	17.4	17.8	18.1
	Standard error					
2–5 years	0.7	1.7	1.8	1.6	1.2	1.3
6–11 years	1.0	1.4	1.6	1.3	2.1	1.2
12–19 years	0.9	0.9	1.1	1.7	1.8	1.7

NOTES: Obesity among children and youth is defined as a body mass index (BMI) at or above the sex- and age-specific 95th percentile BMI cut points from the 2000 CDC Growth Charts. Also see Table 72.

SOURCE: CDC/NCHS, National Health and Nutrition Examination Survey.

References *(continued from page 22)*

6. Flegal KM, Graubard BI, Williamson DF, Gail MH. Cause-specific excess deaths associated with underweight, overweight, and obesity. JAMA 2007;298(17):2028–37.
7. Danner FW. A national longitudinal study of the association between hours of TV viewing and the trajectory of BMI growth among U.S. children. J Pediatr Psychol 2008; 33(10):1100–7.
8. Gortmaker SL, Must A, Sobol AM, Peterson K, Colditz GA, Dietz WH. Television viewing as a cause of increasing obesity among children in the United States, 1986–1990. Arch Pediatr Adolesc Med 1996;150(4):356–62.
9. McMurray RG, Harrell JS, Deng S, Bradley CB, Cox LM, Bangdiwala SI. The influence of physical activity, socioeconomic status, and ethnicity on the weight status of adolescents. Obes Res 2000;8(3):130–9.
10. Ogden CL, Carroll MD, Curtin LR, Lamb MM, Flegal KM. Prevalence of high body mass index in U.S. children and adolescents, 2007–2008. JAMA 2010;303(3):242–9.

Data table for Figure 14. Overweight and obesity among adults 20 years of age and over, by sex: United States, 1988–1994 to 2007–2008

Sex and obesity/overweight	1988–1994	1999–2000	2001–2002	2003–2004	2005–2006	2007–2008
20 years and over, age-adjusted	Percent					
Total:						
Grade 2+ obesity	8.1	13.2	12.1	12.2	14.8	14.3
Grade 1 obesity	14.8	17.3	18.5	19.9	19.6	19.5
Overweight (not including obese)	33.0	34.0	35.1	34.1	32.6	34.2
Men:						
Grade 2+ obesity	5.3	9.8	9.0	9.4	11.6	10.7
Grade 1 obesity	14.9	17.7	18.8	21.7	21.8	21.5
Overweight (not including obese)	40.5	39.7	42.2	39.7	39.9	40.0
Women:						
Grade 2+ obesity	10.7	16.5	15.0	15.0	18.0	17.8
Grade 1 obesity	14.7	16.9	18.3	18.1	17.4	17.6
Overweight (not including obese)	25.8	28.6	28.2	28.6	25.5	28.6
20 years and over, crude						
Total:						
Grade 2+ obesity	8.0	13.1	12.1	12.3	15.0	14.3
Grade 1 obesity	14.4	17.2	18.5	20.0	19.7	19.6
Overweight (not including obese)	32.6	33.9	35.0	34.2	32.6	34.4
Men:						
Grade 2+ obesity	5.3	9.7	9.1	9.4	11.7	10.7
Grade 1 obesity	14.3	17.5	18.7	21.8	21.8	21.5
Overweight (not including obese)	39.9	39.4	42.2	39.7	39.8	40.1
Women:						
Grade 2+ obesity	10.5	16.4	15.0	15.1	18.1	17.7
Grade 1 obesity	14.5	16.9	18.3	18.3	17.6	17.8
Overweight (not including obese)	25.7	28.6	28.1	29.0	25.7	28.9
20 years and over, age-adjusted	Standard error					
Total:						
Grade 2+ obesity	0.5	0.9	0.9	0.7	1.0	0.8
Grade 1 obesity	0.4	0.8	0.8	0.8	0.7	0.6
Overweight (not including obese)	0.6	1.0	1.2	1.1	0.8	0.8
Men:						
Grade 2+ obesity	0.5	1.1	1.2	0.5	1.0	0.8
Grade 1 obesity	0.7	1.0	0.8	1.1	1.4	0.9
Overweight (not including obese)	0.8	1.4	1.4	1.5	1.3	1.4
Women:						
Grade 2+ obesity	0.7	1.2	1.0	1.1	1.3	1.0
Grade 1 obesity	0.6	1.0	1.3	1.3	0.6	0.8
Overweight (not including obese)	0.7	1.6	1.7	1.2	1.2	1.2
20 years and over, crude						
Total:						
Grade 2+ obesity	0.5	0.9	0.9	0.7	1.0	0.8
Grade 1 obesity	0.4	0.8	0.8	0.8	0.7	0.6
Overweight (not including obese)	0.6	1.0	1.2	1.1	0.8	0.7
Men:						
Grade 2+ obesity	0.5	1.1	1.3	0.5	1.1	0.8
Grade 1 obesity	0.6	1.0	0.8	1.1	1.5	0.9
Overweight (not including obese)	0.8	1.4	1.4	1.4	1.3	1.3
Women:						
Grade 2+ obesity	0.7	1.2	1.0	1.0	1.3	0.9
Grade 1 obesity	0.6	1.0	1.3	1.3	0.6	0.8
Overweight (not including obese)	0.7	1.6	1.7	1.2	1.3	1.2

NOTES: Data are for the civilian noninstitutionalized population. Overweight (not including obese) is defined as a body mass index (BMI) equal to or greater than 25 but less than 30. Grade 1 obesity is defined as a BMI equal to or greater than 30 but less then 35, and Grade 2+ obesity is defined as a BMI of 35 or greater. Pregnant women 18 years of age and over were excluded in all years. See Appendix II, Body mass index (BMI). Estimates are age-adjusted to the year 2000 standard population using three age groups: 20–39 years, 40–59 years, and 60 years and over. See Appendix II, Age adjustment; Table 71.
SOURCE: CDC/NCHS, National Health and Nutrition Examination Survey.

References (continued from page 23)

7.   World Cancer Research Fund/American Institute for Cancer Research (AICR). Food, nutrition, physical activity, and the prevention of cancer: A global perspective. Washington, DC: AICR; 2007.

8.   Flegal KM, Carroll MD, Ogden CL, Curtin LR. Prevalence and trends in obesity among US adults, 1999–2008. JAMA 2010; 303(3):235–41.

Data table for Figure 15. Hypertension among adults 20 years of age and over, by sex and age: United States, 1988–1994, 1999–2002, and 2005–2008

Sex and age	1988–1994		1999–2002		2005–2008	
	Percent	SE	Percent	SE	Percent	SE
Total						
20 years and over, age-adjusted	25.5	0.6	30.0	0.8	30.9	0.7
20 years and over, crude	24.1	0.8	30.2	1.0	32.1	0.7
20–44 years.	8.7	0.6	10.3	0.8	11.1	0.7
45–64 years.	33.5	1.1	38.3	1.7	40.6	1.2
65–74 years.	55.4	1.5	66.8	1.9	66.5	1.8
75 years and over	68.8	1.5	77.6	1.2	75.0	1.0
Men						
20 years and over, age-adjusted	26.4	0.9	28.8	1.2	31.6	0.9
20 years and over, crude	23.8	1.0	27.6	1.2	31.4	0.9
20–44 years.	10.9	1.0	12.1	1.3	14.1	1.0
45–64 years.	34.2	1.6	36.4	2.0	40.2	1.6
65–74 years.	54.4	2.8	59.6	3.1	64.0	2.6
75 years and over	60.4	2.2	69.0	1.9	67.2	2.1
Women						
20 years and over, age-adjusted	24.4	0.6	30.6	0.7	29.8	0.7
20 years and over, crude	24.4	0.9	32.7	1.1	32.8	0.9
20–44 years.	6.5	0.5	8.3	0.8	7.9	0.7
45–64 years.	32.8	1.5	40.0	1.8	41.1	1.9
65–74 years.	56.2	1.7	72.7	2.2	68.4	2.4
75 years and over	73.6	1.8	83.1	1.4	80.4	1.9

SE is standard error.

NOTES: Estimates are age-adjusted to the year 2000 standard population using five age groups: 20–34 years, 35–44 years, 45–64 years, 55–64 years, and 65 years and over. Hypertension is defined as having an average measured systolic blood pressure of at least 140 mmHg or an average measured diastolic of at least 90 mmHg or taking antihypertensive drugs. See Appendix II, Age adjustment; Blood pressure, high; Table 67.

SOURCE: CDC/NCHS, National Health and Nutrition Examination Survey.

Data table for Figure 16. High serum total cholesterol (240 mg/dL or higher) among adults 20 years of age and over, by sex and age: United States, 1988–1994, 1999–2002, and 2005–2008

Sex and age	1988–1994 Percent	1988–1994 SE	1999–2002 Percent	1999–2002 SE	2005–2008 Percent	2005–2008 SE
Total						
20 years and over, age-adjusted	20.8	0.6	17.3	0.6	14.9	0.6
20 years and over, crude	19.6	0.6	17.3	0.7	15.2	0.6
20–44 years.	10.9	0.6	12.3	0.8	11.3	0.7
45–64 years.	30.4	1.2	22.6	1.1	20.3	1.1
65–74 years.	32.3	1.8	24.0	1.6	15.6	1.1
75 years and over	31.6	1.7	20.2	1.2	14.9	1.6
Men						
20 years and over, age-adjusted	19.0	0.7	16.4	0.9	13.4	0.7
20 years and over, crude	17.7	0.7	16.5	0.9	13.8	0.7
20–44 years.	12.5	0.7	14.2	1.0	12.0	1.0
45–64 years.	27.2	1.6	22.2	1.7	18.5	1.4
65–74 years.	21.9	2.2	13.7	1.8	7.9	1.3
75 years and over	20.4	1.8	10.2	1.3	8.6	1.2
Women						
20 years and over, age-adjusted	22.0	0.8	17.8	0.7	16.0	0.7
20 years and over, crude	21.3	0.9	18.0	0.8	16.6	0.7
20–44 years.	9.4	0.8	10.4	0.9	10.7	0.9
45–64 years.	33.4	1.6	23.0	1.5	22.1	1.5
65–74 years.	41.3	2.4	32.3	2.3	21.8	1.6
75 years and over	38.2	2.2	26.5	1.8	19.4	2.3

SE is standard error.

NOTES: Estimates are age-adjusted to the year 2000 standard population using five age groups: 20–34 years, 35–44 years, 45–64 years, 55–64 years, and 65 years and over. See Appendix II, Cholesterol. Two measures of high cholesterol are presented in *Health, United States*: high serum total cholesterol (presented here) and high cholesterol, which includes both those with high serum total cholesterol and those taking medication to control their cholesterol levels. Also see Table 68 for data on the prevalence of high cholesterol.

SOURCE: CDC/NCHS, National Health and Nutrition Examination Survey.

Data table for Figure 17. Statin drug use in the past 30 days among adults 45 years of age and over, by sex and age: United States, 1988–1994, 1999–2002, and 2005–2008

Sex and age	1988–1994		1999–2002		2005–2008	
	Percent	SE	Percent	SE	Percent	SE
Total						
45 years and over	2.4	0.3	15.6	0.7	25.1	0.7
45–64 years.	2.2	0.3	12.2	1.0	17.2	0.9
65–74 years.	3.7	0.7	24.9	1.6	42.0	1.5
75 years and over	*1.4	0.4	18.4	1.2	41.4	1.3
Men						
45 years and over	2.3	0.3	17.5	1.1	26.9	0.9
45–64 years.	2.5	0.5	15.1	1.4	18.3	1.2
65–74 years.	*	*	25.7	1.5	49.7	2.1
75 years and over	*	*	18.6	1.7	45.0	1.4
Women						
45 years and over	2.6	0.5	13.9	0.8	23.6	1.1
45–64 years.	1.9	0.5	9.6	1.0	16.1	1.2
65–74 years.	*4.9	1.0	24.2	2.6	36.0	2.2
75 years and over	*1.7	0.5	18.2	1.9	38.9	2.1

SE is standard error.

* Estimates are considered unreliable. Data preceded by an asterisk have a relative standard error (RSE) of 20%–30%. Data not shown have an RSE greater than 30%.

NOTES: Respondents reporting use of a prescription drug containing any of the following ingredients—atorvastatin, cerivastatin, fluvastatin, lovastatin, pravastatin, rosuvastatin, or simvastatin—were classified as taking a statin drug. Also see Figure 16, Table 68.

SOURCE: CDC/NCHS, National Health and Nutrition Examination Survey.

References (continued from page 26)

4. LaRosa JC. Unresolved issues in early trials of cholesterol lowering. Am J Cardiol 1995;76(9):5C–9C.
5. Evans M, Roberts A, Davies S, Rees A. Medical lipid-regulating therapy: Current evidence, ongoing trials, and future developments. Drugs 2004;64(11):1181–96.
6. Carroll MD, Lacher DA, Sorlie PD, Cleeman JI, Gordon DJ, Wolz M, et al. Trends in serum lipids and lipoproteins of adults, 1960–2002. JAMA 2005;294(14):1773–81.

Data table for Figure 18. Influenza vaccination in the past 12 months among adults 18 years of age and over, by age: United States, 1999–2009

| | 18 years and over | | | | 18–49 years | | 50–64 years | | 65–74 years | | 75–84 years | | 85 years and over | |
| | Age-adjusted | | Crude | | | | | | | | | | | |
Year	Percent	SE	Percent	SE	Percent	SE	Percent	SE	Percent	SE	Percent	SE	Percent	SE
1999	28.4	0.3	27.9	0.3	16.4	0.3	34.1	0.7	61.9	1.0	70.9	1.2	68.6	2.1
2000	28.7	0.3	28.4	0.3	17.1	0.3	34.6	0.7	61.1	1.0	68.6	1.1	67.7	2.2
2001	26.7	0.3	26.4	0.3	15.0	0.3	32.2	0.7	60.7	1.0	65.7	1.1	66.4	2.1
2002	28.3	0.3	28.0	0.3	16.2	0.3	34.0	0.7	60.9	1.0	71.6	1.1	70.3	2.0
2003	29.2	0.3	29.0	0.3	16.8	0.3	36.8	0.7	60.5	1.0	72.4	1.1	66.6	2.1
2004	29.5	0.3	29.4	0.3	17.9	0.4	35.9	0.7	60.1	1.0	69.3	1.1	71.0	2.0
2005	21.6	0.3	21.4	0.3	10.7	0.3	23.0	0.6	53.7	1.0	65.3	1.2	69.9	1.9
2006	27.4	0.3	27.6	0.4	15.6	0.4	33.2	0.8	60.1	1.3	68.5	1.3	71.2	2.3
2007	29.9	0.4	30.1	0.4	17.8	0.4	36.2	0.9	61.6	1.2	71.9	1.3	74.6	2.4
2008	32.1	0.4	32.6	0.4	20.1	0.5	39.6	0.8	60.9	1.2	72.7	1.4	79.1	2.2
2009	34.1	0.4	34.7	0.4	23.0	0.5	40.7	0.7	61.5	1.1	72.0	1.3	76.5	1.8

SE is standard error.

NOTES: Data are for the civilian noninstitutionalized population. Estimates are based on the question: "During the past 12 months, have you had a flu shot? A flu shot is usually given in the fall and protects against influenza for the flu season." Beginning in September 2003, respondents were asked about influenza vaccination by nasal spray (sometimes called by the brand name FluMist) during the past 12 months, in addition to the question regarding the flu shot. Starting with 2005 data, receipt of nasal spray or flu shot were included in the calculation of influenza vaccination estimates. Annual influenza vaccination has been recommended for all adults 50 years and over since 2000. Due to the shortfall in the 2000–2001 and 2004–2005 influenza vaccine supply, CDC recommended vaccine be reserved for priority groups, including those 65 years of age and over and those 2–64 years with chronic underlying health conditions. For more information, see: CDC. Prevention and control of influenza: Recommendations of the Advisory Committee on Immunization Practices (ACIP). MMWR 2000;49(RR–03):1–38. Available from: http://www.cdc.gov/mmwr/PDF/rr/rr4903.pdf. Interim influenza vaccination recommendations, 2004–05 influenza season. MMWR 2004; 53(39):923–4. Available from: http://www.cdc.gov/mmwr/preview/mmwrhtml/mm5339a6.htm.
CDC. Notice to readers: Updated recommendations from the Advisory Committee on Immunization Practices in response to delays in supply of influenza vaccine for the 2000–01 season. MMWR 2000;49(39);888–92. Available from: http://www.cdc.gov/mmwr/preview/mmwrhtml/mm4927a4.htm. Estimates are age-adjusted to the year 2000 standard population using four age groups: 18–49 years, 50–64 years, 65–74 years, and 75 years and over. See Appendix II, Age adjustment; Table 84.

SOURCE: CDC/NCHS, National Health Interview Survey.

References (continued from page 27)

4. CDC. Interim influenza vaccination recommendations, 2004–05 influenza season. MMWR 2004;53(39);923–4. Available from: http://www.cdc.gov/mmwr/preview/mmwrhtml/mm5339a6.htm.
5. CDC. CDC's Advisory Committee on Immunization Practices (ACIP) recommends universal annual influenza vaccination [press release]. Atlanta, GA; 2010 February 24. Available from: http://www.cdc.gov/media/pressrel/2010/r100224.htm.
6. CDC. Experiences with obtaining influenza vaccination among persons in priority groups during a vaccine shortage—United States, October–November, 2004. MMWR 2004;53(49):1153–5. Available from: http://www.cdc.gov/mmwr/preview/mmwrhtml/mm5349a2.htm.

Data table for Figure 19. Adults 18–64 years of age who delayed or did not receive needed medical care in the past 12 months due to cost, by age and type of health insurance coverage: United States, 1999–2009

Age and type of insurance	1999	2000	2001	2002	2003	2004	2005	2006	2007	2008	2009
						Percent					
18–64 years											
Total.	9.2	9.2	9.5	9.7	10.6	11.4	11.0	11.7	11.8	13.6	15.1
Private	5.0	5.0	5.1	5.1	5.8	6.2	5.9	6.4	6.3	7.8	8.6
Medicaid.	11.4	12.7	12.3	11.3	12.2	11.9	12.0	12.6	11.9	14.1	13.6
Uninsured.	25.8	24.7	25.5	26.1	28.1	30.2	29.5	29.7	31.4	33.1	36.5
18–44 years											
Total.	9.4	9.5	9.8	9.9	10.8	11.4	11.3	11.7	12.0	13.6	15.1
Private	5.1	5.0	5.3	5.1	5.9	6.2	5.9	6.2	6.4	7.6	8.3
Medicaid.	9.8	11.4	10.9	10.6	11.2	10.0	11.2	11.7	10.0	12.1	11.4
Uninsured.	24.3	23.1	24.1	24.1	25.5	27.5	27.1	26.7	28.9	30.3	33.6
45–64 years											
Total.	8.9	8.8	8.9	9.4	10.3	11.2	10.6	11.7	11.6	13.5	15.1
Private	4.9	4.9	4.8	4.9	5.6	6.2	5.9	6.6	6.3	8.1	9.0
Medicaid.	15.2	15.7	15.4	12.9	14.5	16.1	13.9	14.6	15.9	18.2	18.2
Uninsured.	30.8	29.8	30.2	32.0	36.1	38.0	36.2	38.0	37.9	40.1	43.7
						Standard error					
18–64 years											
Total	0.2	0.2	0.2	0.2	0.2	0.2	0.2	0.2	0.2	0.3	0.3
Private	0.1	0.1	0.1	0.1	0.2	0.2	0.2	0.2	0.2	0.2	0.2
Medicaid.	0.7	0.7	0.7	0.6	0.6	0.6	0.6	0.7	0.7	0.7	0.7
Uninsured.	0.6	0.6	0.5	0.5	0.6	0.5	0.5	0.7	0.7	0.7	0.7
18–44 years											
Total	0.2	0.2	0.2	0.2	0.2	0.2	0.2	0.3	0.3	0.3	0.3
Private	0.2	0.2	0.2	0.2	0.2	0.2	0.2	0.3	0.2	0.3	0.3
Medicaid.	0.8	0.8	0.8	0.7	0.7	0.7	0.7	0.9	0.8	0.8	0.7
Uninsured.	0.6	0.6	0.6	0.6	0.6	0.6	0.6	0.8	0.8	0.8	0.7
45–64 years											
Total.	0.3	0.2	0.2	0.3	0.3	0.3	0.2	0.3	0.3	0.4	0.4
Private	0.2	0.2	0.2	0.2	0.2	0.2	0.2	0.3	0.3	0.3	0.3
Medicaid.	1.4	1.2	1.2	1.2	1.1	1.1	1.0	1.2	1.3	1.4	1.2
Uninsured.	1.1	1.0	1.0	1.1	1.1	1.0	0.9	1.4	1.2	1.1	1.1

NOTES: Totals include other types of insurance coverage not shown and unknown health insurance status. Based on persons responding "yes" to at least one of the following questions: "During the past 12 months was there any time when person needed medical care but did not get it because person couldn't afford it?" or "During the past 12 months has medical care been delayed because of worry about the cost?" Health insurance categories are mutually exclusive. Persons who reported both Medicaid and private coverage are classified as having private coverage. State-sponsored health plan coverage is included as Medicaid coverage. Starting with 1999, coverage by the Children's Health Insurance Program (CHIP) is included with Medicaid coverage. Persons not covered by private insurance, Medicaid, CHIP, state-sponsored health plans, Medicare, or military plans are considered to to have no health insurance coverage. Adults with Indian Health Service coverage only are considered to have no coverage. See Appendix II, Health insurance coverage; Tables 76 and 77.

SOURCE: CDC/NCHS, National Health Interview Survey, family core questionnaire.

Data table for Figure 20. Persons who did not receive needed dental services in the past 12 months due to cost, by sex and age: United States, 1999–2009

Sex and age	1999	2000	2001	2002	2003	2004	2005	2006	2007	2008	2009
						Percent					
Total...................	7.9	8.1	8.7	8.6	9.2	10.7	10.7	10.8	10.5	12.6	13.3
Under 18 years............	6.5	6.2	6.7	5.9	5.6	6.6	7.3	6.9	6.3	7.0	7.1
18 years and over..........	8.3	8.7	9.3	9.4	10.3	12.0	11.8	12.0	11.7	14.2	15.1
18–44 years.............	10.2	10.7	11.3	11.5	12.3	14.5	14.1	14.2	14.2	16.6	18.2
45–64 years.............	7.9	7.9	8.7	8.7	10.2	11.3	11.5	12.6	11.3	14.9	14.9
65 years and over	2.7	3.4	3.5	4.0	4.0	5.5	5.2	3.9	5.0	5.6	6.2
Male....................	6.9	6.9	7.3	7.6	8.1	9.7	9.3	9.5	9.2	11.3	12.0
Under 18 years............	6.4	5.8	5.8	5.3	5.4	7.3	7.3	6.2	5.5	7.1	7.5
18 years and over..........	7.0	7.3	7.8	8.4	9.0	10.5	9.9	10.5	10.3	12.6	13.3
18–44 years.............	8.6	9.1	9.5	10.3	10.5	12.6	11.9	12.0	12.5	14.7	15.5
45–64 years.............	6.3	6.5	6.9	7.5	8.8	9.5	9.2	11.4	9.5	12.7	13.3
65 years and over	2.3	2.3	3.2	3.4	3.7	4.6	4.3	3.0	4.3	5.4	5.8
Female..................	8.8	9.2	10.0	9.4	10.3	11.8	12.1	12.1	11.8	13.8	14.5
Under 18 years............	6.7	6.6	7.7	6.5	5.9	5.9	7.2	7.5	7.2	6.9	6.6
18 years and over..........	9.4	9.9	10.6	10.3	11.5	13.4	13.5	13.4	13.1	15.7	16.7
18–44 years.............	11.6	12.3	13.1	12.7	14.1	16.4	16.2	16.4	15.9	18.5	20.8
45–64 years.............	9.3	9.3	10.5	9.9	11.6	12.9	13.7	13.7	13.1	17.1	16.4
65 years and over	3.0	4.2	3.8	4.4	4.1	6.2	5.8	4.5	5.4	5.8	6.5
						Standard error					
Total...................	0.2	0.2	0.2	0.2	0.2	0.2	0.2	0.3	0.3	0.3	0.3
Under 18 years............	0.3	0.3	0.3	0.3	0.3	0.3	0.3	0.4	0.4	0.3	0.3
18 years and over..........	0.2	0.2	0.2	0.2	0.2	0.2	0.2	0.3	0.3	0.3	0.3
18–44 years.............	0.3	0.3	0.3	0.3	0.3	0.4	0.4	0.4	0.5	0.5	0.5
45–64 years.............	0.4	0.3	0.3	0.3	0.4	0.4	0.4	0.4	0.4	0.5	0.5
65 years and over	0.2	0.3	0.3	0.3	0.3	0.4	0.3	0.3	0.4	0.4	0.4
Male....................	0.3	0.2	0.2	0.2	0.2	0.3	0.3	0.3	0.3	0.4	0.4
Under 18 years............	0.4	0.4	0.4	0.3	0.3	0.4	0.4	0.4	0.4	0.5	0.5
18 years and over..........	0.3	0.3	0.3	0.3	0.3	0.3	0.3	0.4	0.4	0.4	0.4
18–44 years.............	0.4	0.4	0.4	0.4	0.4	0.5	0.5	0.6	0.6	0.6	0.6
45–64 years.............	0.5	0.5	0.4	0.4	0.5	0.5	0.5	0.6	0.5	0.7	0.7
65 years and over	0.3	0.3	0.4	0.5	0.4	0.5	0.5	0.4	0.6	0.6	0.6
Female..................	0.2	0.3	0.3	0.3	0.3	0.3	0.3	0.3	0.3	0.4	0.4
Under 18 years............	0.4	0.4	0.5	0.4	0.4	0.4	0.4	0.6	0.5	0.5	0.5
18 years and over..........	0.3	0.3	0.3	0.3	0.3	0.3	0.3	0.4	0.4	0.4	0.4
18–44 years.............	0.4	0.4	0.4	0.4	0.5	0.5	0.5	0.6	0.6	0.7	0.7
45–64 years.............	0.5	0.5	0.5	0.5	0.5	0.5	0.5	0.6	0.6	0.7	0.7
65 years and over	0.3	0.4	0.3	0.4	0.4	0.5	0.5	0.4	0.5	0.5	0.5

NOTES: Data are for the civilian noninstitutionalized population. Based on persons responding "yes" to the question, "During the past 12 months was there any time when [person] needed dental care (including check-ups) but did not get it because [person] couldn't afford it?" Also see Tables 76 and 77.

SOURCE: CDC/NCHS, National Health Interview Survey.

Data table for Figure 21. Health insurance coverage among children, by type of coverage and age: United States 1999–2009

Type of coverage and age	1999	2000	2001	2002	2003	2004	2005	2006	2007	2008	2009
						Percent					
Private											
Under 19 years	68.9	66.7	66.4	63.7	63.2	63.3	62.3	59.5	59.9	58.6	56.1
Under 18 years	68.8	66.6	66.3	63.5	63.0	63.2	62.1	59.4	59.8	58.4	55.8
Medicaid											
Under 19 years	17.7	19.2	21.0	24.3	25.4	25.8	26.6	29.4	29.3	30.6	33.9
Under 18 years	18.1	19.6	21.5	24.8	26.0	26.4	27.2	29.9	29.8	31.3	34.5
Uninsured											
Under 19 years	12.2	12.9	11.6	11.2	10.2	9.6	9.7	9.8	9.4	9.5	8.5
Under 18 years	11.9	12.6	11.2	10.9	9.8	9.2	9.3	9.5	9.0	9.0	8.2
						Standard error					
Private											
Under 19 years	0.5	0.5	0.5	0.5	0.6	0.6	0.6	0.7	0.7	0.7	0.8
Under 18 years	0.5	0.5	0.6	0.6	0.6	0.6	0.6	0.7	0.7	0.7	0.8
Medicaid											
Under 19 years	0.4	0.5	0.4	0.5	0.5	0.5	0.5	0.7	0.6	0.7	0.7
Under 18 years	0.4	0.5	0.5	0.5	0.5	0.5	0.5	0.7	0.6	0.7	0.7
Uninsured											
Under 19 years	0.3	0.3	0.3	0.3	0.3	0.3	0.3	0.3	0.4	0.4	0.4
Under 18 years	0.3	0.3	0.4	0.3	0.3	0.3	0.3	0.3	0.4	0.4	0.4

NOTES: Data are for the civilian noninstitutionalized population. State-sponsored health plan coverage is included with Medicaid. Starting with 1999, coverage by the Children's Health Insurance Program (CHIP) is included with Medicaid. Uninsured children are not covered by private insurance, Medicaid, CHIP, state-sponsored or other government-sponsored health plans, Medicare, or military plans. Children with only Indian Health Service coverage are considered to have no coverage. Percents do not add to 100 because the percentage of children with Medicare, military plans, and other government-sponsored plans is not shown and because children with both private insurance and Medicaid appear in both categories. Starting with data from the third quarter of 2004, persons under 65 years of age with no reported coverage were asked explicitly about Medicaid coverage. Estimates for Medicaid coverage shown in this table include the additional information. Estimates for 2000–2002 were calculated using 2000-based sample weights and may differ from estimates in other reports that used 1990-based sample weights for 2000–2002 estimates. See Appendix II, Health insurance coverage; Tables 135, 137, and 138.

SOURCE: CDC/NCHS, National Health Interview Survey.

Data table for Figure 22. Health insurance coverage among adults 18–64 years of age, by type of coverage and age: United States, 1999–2009

Type of coverage and age	1999	2000	2001	2002	2003	2004	2005	2006	2007	2008	2009
	Percent										
Private											
18–44 years..................	72.0	70.5	70.1	68.7	67.7	67.3	66.6	65.0	65.5	64.4	61.7
45–64 years..................	79.3	78.7	78.6	77.3	77.3	77.1	76.9	75.2	75.5	74.3	72.6
Medicaid											
18–44 years..................	5.7	5.6	6.3	7.1	7.4	7.7	8.3	8.6	8.7	9.2	10.3
45–64 years..................	4.4	4.5	4.7	5.3	5.3	5.5	5.5	6.3	5.9	6.4	6.9
Uninsured											
18–44 years..................	21.0	22.4	22.2	23.0	23.5	23.5	23.5	24.6	23.9	24.4	25.9
45–64 years..................	12.2	12.6	12.2	13.1	12.5	12.8	12.9	13.2	13.5	13.6	14.6
	Standard error										
Private											
18–44 years..................	0.4	0.4	0.4	0.4	0.4	0.4	0.4	0.5	0.5	0.5	0.5
45–64 years..................	0.4	0.4	0.4	0.4	0.4	0.4	0.4	0.5	0.5	0.5	0.5
Medicaid											
18–44 years..................	0.2	0.2	0.2	0.2	0.2	0.2	0.2	0.3	0.3	0.3	0.3
45–64 years..................	0.2	0.2	0.2	0.2	0.2	0.2	0.2	0.2	0.2	0.3	0.2
Uninsured											
18–44 years..................	0.3	0.3	0.3	0.3	0.4	0.3	0.4	0.4	0.4	0.4	0.4
45–64 years..................	0.3	0.3	0.3	0.3	0.3	0.3	0.3	0.3	0.4	0.3	0.4

NOTES: Data are for the civilian noninstitutionalized population. The category Medicaid includes state-sponsored plans and Children's Health Insurance Program (CHIP) (starting in 1999). Uninsured adults are not covered by private insurance, Medicaid, CHIP, state-sponsored or other government-sponsored health plans, Medicare, or military plans. Adults with only Indian Health Service coverage are considered to have no coverage. Percents do not add to 100 because the percentage of adults with Medicare, military plans, and other government-sponsored plans is not shown and because adults with both private insurance and Medicaid appear in both categories. Starting with data from the third quarter of 2004, persons under 65 years of age with no reported coverage were asked explicitly about Medicaid coverage. Estimates for Medicaid coverage shown in this table include the additional information. Estimates for 2000–2002 were calculated using 2000-based sample weights and may differ from estimates in other reports that used 1990-based sample weights for 2000–2002 estimates. See Appendix II, Health insurance coverage; Tables 135, 137, and 138.

SOURCE: CDC/NCHS, National Health Interview Survey.

Data table for Figure 23. Personal health care expenditures, by source of funds: United States, 1998–2008

Source of funds	1998	1999	2000	2001	2002	2003	2004	2005	2006	2007	2008	1998–2008 AAPC
	Amount in billions											AAPC
Total (PHCE)	$1,010	$1,068	$1,139	$1,238	$1,340	$1,448	$1,550	$1,655	$1,763	$1,866	$1,952	7.1
Private funds	575	612	652	697	752	810	860	916	964	1,016	1,044	6.9
Out-of-pocket	175	184	193	200	211	225	235	248	255	270	278	5.3
Private insurance	344	371	403	441	482	522	560	600	635	665	691	8.0
Public funds	435	456	487	541	588	637	689	739	799	850	908	8.5
Federal funds	332	346	370	412	448	486	527	562	620	661	718	8.9
Medicare	202	206	216	239	256	274	300	326	382	408	444	9.1
Medicaid (including CHIP)	93	101	110	123	137	149	160	165	162	171	186	7.9
State and local funds	103	109	117	130	140	151	162	177	179	189	190	7.1
Medicaid (including CHIP)	65	70	77	86	94	102	110	124	124	132	131	8.2

NOTES: AAPC is average annual percent change. This rate assumes that the change is at the same rate from 1998 to 2008. PHCE is personal health care expenditures, which are outlays for goods and services relating directly to patient care. CHIP is Children's Health Insurance Program. CHIP expenditures started in 1998. See Appendix II, Average annual rate of change (percent change); Health expenditures, national; Table 126.

SOURCE: Centers for Medicare & Medicaid Services, Office of the Actuary, National Health Statistics Group, National Health Expenditure Accounts. National health expenditures, 2008. Available from: http://www.cms.hhs.gov/NationalHealthExpendData/ and unpublished data.

References *(continued from page 32)*

3. Hartman M, Martin A, Nuccio O, Catlin A; National Health Expenditure Accounts Team. Health spending growth at a historic low in 2008. Health Aff (Millwood) 2010;29(1):147–55.

Data table for Figure 24. Deaths for all ages, by age and cause of death: United States, 2007

Age and cause of death	Number of deaths	Percent distribution
All ages	2,423,712	100.0
Under 25 years	73,970	3.1
25–44 years	122,178	5.0
45–64 years	471,796	19.5
65–74 years	389,238	16.1
75–84 years	652,682	26.9
85 years and over	713,647	29.4
All causes.	2,423,712	100.0
Heart disease	616,067	25.4
Cancer.	562,875	23.2
Stroke	135,952	5.6
Chronic lower respiratory diseases (CLRD)	127,924	5.3
Unintentional injuries	123,706	5.1
Alzheimer's disease.	74,632	3.1
Diabetes.	71,382	2.9
All other causes.	711,174	29.3

NOTES: Cancer refers to malignant neoplasms; stroke refers to cerebrovascular diseases; and unintentional injuries is preferred to "accidents" in the public health community. See Appendix II, Cause of death.

SOURCE: CDC/NCHS, National Vital Statistics System. Xu JQ, Kochanek KD, Murphy SL, Tejada-Vera B.
Deaths: Final data for 2007. National vital statistics reports; vol 58 no 19. Hyattsville, MD: NCHS; 2010. Available from:
http://www.cdc.gov/nchs/data/nvsr/nvsr58/nvsr58_19.pdf.

Data table for Figure 25. Infant, neonatal, and postneonatal mortality rates: United States, 1997–2007

Year	Infant	Neonatal	Postneonatal
	Deaths per 1,000 live births		
1997	7.23	4.77	2.45
1998	7.20	4.80	2.40
1999	7.06	4.73	2.33
2000	6.91	4.63	2.28
2001	6.85	4.54	2.31
2002	6.97	4.66	2.31
2003	6.85	4.62	2.23
2004	6.79	4.52	2.27
2005	6.87	4.54	2.34
2006	6.69	4.45	2.24
2007	6.75	4.41	2.33

Cause of infant death, 2007	Number	Percent distribution
All causes	29,138	100.0
Congenital malformations	5,785	19.9
Low birthweight	4,857	16.7
Sudden infant death syndrome	2,453	8.4
Maternal complications	1,769	6.1
Unintentional injuries	1,285	4.4
All other causes	12,989	44.6

NOTES: Infant is defined as under 1 year of age, neonatal as under 28 days of age, and postneonatal as 28 days through 11 months of life. See related Table 21.

SOURCE: CDC/NCHS, National Vital Statistics System: Xu JQ, Kochanek KD, Murphy SL, Tejada-Vera B.
Deaths: Final data for 2007. National vital statistics reports; vol 58 no 19. Hyattsville, MD: NCHS; 2010. Available from:
http://www.cdc.gov/nchs/data/nvsr/nvsr58/nvsr58_19.pdf.

Data table for Figure 26. Death rates among children 1–19 years of age, by OECD country: 3-year average of most recent data, 2001–2006

OECD Country	Child mortality rate	Years (average annual)
Portugal	34.60	2001–2003
United States	32.67	2003–2005
New Zealand	32.05	2002–2004
Slovak Republic	30.15	2003–2005
Belgium	28.97	1995–1997
Poland	28.13	2003–2005
Hungary	25.75	2003–2005
Czech Republic	24.92	2003–2005
Austria	24.57	2004–2006
Australia	23.66	2001–2003
Finland	23.54	2004–2006
Spain	23.49	2003–2005
Canada	23.43	2002–2004
Greece	23.15	2004–2006
Denmark	22.93	1999–2001
Republic of Korea	22.36	2004–2006
Ireland	21.97	2003–2005
Italy	21.76	2001–2003
Norway	21.49	2003–2005
Germany	21.23	2002–2004
United Kingdom	21.17	2003–2005
France	21.04	2003–2005
Netherlands	20.49	2002–2004
Switzerland	20.33	2003–2005
Sweden	19.27	2002–2004
Japan	18.23	2004–2006
Iceland	16.95	2003–2005
Luxembourg	14.84	2003–2005

NOTES: OECD is Organisation for Economic Co-operation and Development. Child mortality rates are the number of deaths among children 1–19 years of age per 100,000 children. Data for Belgium and Denmark were the most current available.

SOURCE: World Health Organization mortality database 2008. Available from: http://stats.oecd.org/Index.aspx.

References (continued from page 36)

4. World Health Organization, Europe. Tackling injuries, the leading killers of children. Fact sheet. Copenhagen and Rome: WHO; 2008. Available from: http://www.euro.who.int/__data/assets/pdf_file/0006/98601/FS_TacklingInjuries_Children.pdf.

5. Patten GC, Coffey C, Sawyer SM, Viner RM, Haller DM, Bose K, et al. Global patterns of mortality in young people: A systematic analysis of population health data. Lancet 2009:374(9693);881–92.

6. Bryce J, Boschi-Pinto C, Shibuya K, Black RE, WHO Child Health Epidemiology Reference Group. WHO estimates of the causes of death in children. Lancet 2005:365(9465);1147–52.

Data table for Figure 27. Death rates for leading causes of death among children 1–14 years of age: United States, 1997–2007

Year	All causes	Unintentional injuries	Cancer	Congenital malformations	Homicide	Heart disease
			Deaths per 100,000 population			
1997	24.5	9.6	2.7	1.9	1.5	0.9
1998	23.4	9.2	2.5	1.7	1.5	1.0
1999	22.9	8.9	2.5	1.7	1.4	0.8
2000	22.0	8.5	2.5	1.6	1.3	0.8
2001	21.6	8.1	2.5	1.7	1.3	0.9
2002	21.2	7.7	2.6	1.7	1.4	0.7
2003	21.0	7.6	2.6	1.6	1.2	0.8
2004	20.5	7.6	2.5	1.7	1.2	0.8
2005	20.1	7.2	2.4	1.6	1.3	0.7
2006	19.0	6.8	2.3	1.5	1.3	0.7
2007	19.2	6.7	2.3	1.6	1.3	0.7
			Standard error			
1997	0.21	0.13	0.07	0.06	0.05	0.04
1998	0.20	0.13	0.07	0.05	0.05	0.04
1999	0.20	0.13	0.07	0.06	0.05	0.04
2000	0.20	0.12	0.07	0.05	0.05	0.04
2001	0.20	0.12	0.07	0.05	0.05	0.04
2002	0.19	0.12	0.07	0.05	0.05	0.04
2003	0.19	0.12	0.07	0.05	0.05	0.04
2004	0.19	0.12	0.07	0.05	0.05	0.04
2005	0.19	0.11	0.07	0.05	0.05	0.04
2006	0.18	0.11	0.06	0.05	0.05	0.04
2007	0.18	0.11	0.06	0.05	0.05	0.04

Cause of death, 2007	Number	Percent distribution
All causes	10,850	100.0
Unintentional injuries	3,782	34.8
Cancer	1,323	12.2
Congenital malformations	920	8.5
Homicide	744	6.8
Heart disease	414	3.8
All other causes	3,667	33.8

NOTES: Causes of death shown are the five leading causes of death among persons 1–14 years of age in 2007. Death rates for 1997–1998 are based on *International Classification of Diseases, 9th Revision*. Starting in 1999, death rates are based on *International Classification of Diseases, 10th Revision*. Comparability ratios for selected revisions are available from: http://www.cdc.gov/nchs/nvss/mortality/comparability_icd.htm. Homicide refers to deaths due to assault. Cancer refers to malignant neoplasms. See Appendix II, Cause of death; Comparability ratio; Tables 35, 36, 38, 45, and 46.

SOURCE: CDC/NCHS, National Vital Statistics System. Xu JQ, Kochanek KD, Murphy SL, Tejada-Vera B. Deaths: Final data for 2007. National vital statistics reports; vol 58 no 19. Hyattsville, MD: NCHS; 2010. Available from: http://www.cdc.gov/nchs/data/nvsr/nvsr58/nvsr58_19.pdf.

Data table for Figure 28. Death rates for leading causes of death among persons 15–24 years of age: United States, 1997–2007

Year	All causes	Unintentional injuries	Homicide	Suicide	Cancer	Heart disease
			Deaths per 100,000 population			
1997	84.6	35.7	16.3	11.2	4.4	2.9
1998	80.6	35.0	14.3	10.9	4.5	2.8
1999	79.3	35.3	12.9	10.1	4.5	2.8
2000	79.9	36.0	12.6	10.2	4.4	2.6
2001	80.7	36.1	13.3	9.9	4.3	2.5
2002	81.4	38.0	12.9	9.9	4.3	2.5
2003	81.5	37.1	13.0	9.7	4.0	2.7
2004	80.1	37.0	12.2	10.3	4.1	2.5
2005	81.4	37.4	13.0	10.0	4.1	2.7
2006	82.2	38.2	13.5	9.9	3.9	2.5
2007	79.9	37.4	13.1	9.7	3.9	2.6
			Standard error			
1997	0.48	0.31	0.21	0.17	0.11	0.09
1998	0.46	0.30	0.19	0.17	0.11	0.09
1999	0.45	0.30	0.18	0.16	0.11	0.08
2000	0.45	0.30	0.18	0.16	0.11	0.08
2001	0.45	0.30	0.18	0.16	0.10	0.08
2002	0.45	0.31	0.18	0.16	0.10	0.08
2003	0.44	0.30	0.18	0.15	0.10	0.08
2004	0.44	0.30	0.17	0.16	0.10	0.08
2005	0.44	0.30	0.18	0.15	0.10	0.08
2006	0.44	0.30	0.18	0.15	0.10	0.08
2007	0.43	0.30	0.18	0.15	0.10	0.08

Cause of death, 2007	Number	Percent distribution
All causes	33,982	100.0
Unintentional injuries	15,897	46.8
Homicide	5,551	16.3
Suicide	4,140	12.2
Cancer	1,653	4.9
Heart disease	1,084	3.2
All other causes	5,657	16.6

NOTES: Causes of death shown are the five leading causes of death among persons 15–24 years of age in 2007. Death rates for 1997–1998 are based on the *International Classification of Diseases, 9th Revision.* Starting in 1999, death rates are based on the *International Classification of Diseases, 10th Revision.* Comparability ratios for selected revisions are available from: http://www.cdc.gov/nchs/nvss/mortality/comparability_icd.htm. Homicide refers to deaths due to assault. Suicide refers to deaths from intentional self-harm. Cancer refers to malignant neoplasms. See Appendix II, Cause of death; Comparability ratio; Tables 35, 36, 38, 45, and 46.

SOURCE: CDC/NCHS, National Vital Statistics System. Xu JQ, Kochanek KD, Murphy SL, Tejada-Vera B. Deaths: Final data for 2007. National vital statistics reports; vol 58 no 19. Hyattsville, MD: NCHS; 2010. http://www.cdc.gov/nchs/data/nvsr/nvsr58/nvsr58_19.pdf.

Data table for Figure 29. Death rates for leading causes of death among persons 25–44 years of age: United States, 1997–2007

Year	All causes	Unintentional injuries	Cancer	Heart disease	Suicide	Homicide	HIV
	Deaths per 100,000 population						
1997.	157.7	31.4	25.4	19.3	14.5	10.0	12.9
1998.	153.7	31.5	25.0	19.6	14.3	9.2	10.1
1999.	152.9	31.8	24.3	19.5	13.6	8.7	10.5
2000.	153.2	32.0	24.0	19.0	13.4	8.7	9.8
2001.	157.6	32.8	24.3	19.5	13.8	11.2	9.4
2002.	156.2	34.5	23.5	19.9	14.0	9.1	8.9
2003.	155.2	34.8	22.9	20.0	13.8	9.1	8.2
2004.	150.0	35.1	21.8	19.1	13.9	8.9	7.5
2005.	150.8	36.8	21.6	19.0	13.7	9.4	6.8
2006.	149.8	38.6	20.9	18.6	13.8	9.2	6.2
2007.	145.9	38.1	20.0	18.0	14.3	9.3	5.6
	Standard error						
1997.	0.43	0.19	0.17	0.15	0.13	0.11	0.12
1998.	0.42	0.19	0.17	0.15	0.13	0.10	0.11
1999.	0.42	0.19	0.17	0.15	0.13	0.10	0.11
2000.	0.42	0.19	0.17	0.15	0.13	0.10	0.11
2001.	0.43	0.20	0.17	0.15	0.13	0.12	0.11
2002.	0.43	0.20	0.17	0.15	0.13	0.10	0.10
2003.	0.43	0.20	0.16	0.15	0.13	0.10	0.10
2004.	0.42	0.20	0.16	0.15	0.13	0.10	0.09
2005.	0.42	0.21	0.16	0.15	0.13	0.11	0.09
2006.	0.42	0.21	0.16	0.15	0.13	0.10	0.09
2007.	0.42	0.21	0.15	0.15	0.13	0.11	0.08

Cause of death, 2007	Number	Percent distribution
All cause.	122,178	100.0
Unintentional injuries.	31,908	26.1
Cancer.	16,751	13.7
Heart disease	15,062	12.3
Suicide.	12,000	9.8
Homicide	7,810	6.4
HIV	4,663	3.8
All other causes.	33,984	27.8

NOTES: Causes of death shown are the six leading causes of death among persons 25–44 years of age in 2007. Death rates for 1997–1998 are based on the *International Classification of Diseases, 9th Revision*. Starting in 1999, death rates are based on the *International Classification of Diseases, 10th Revision*. Comparability ratios for selected revisions are available from: http://www.cdc.gov/nchs/nvss/mortality/comparability_icd.htm. Cancer refers to malignant neoplasms. Suicide refers to deaths from intentional self-harm. Homicide refers to deaths due to assault. HIV is human immunodeficiency virus (HIV) disease. See Appendix II, Cause of death; Comparability ratio; Tables 35, 36, 38, 45, and 46.

SOURCE: CDC/NCHS, National Vital Statistics System. Xu JQ, Kochanek KD, Murphy SL, Tejada-Vera B. Deaths: Final data for 2007. National vital statistics reports; vol 58 no 19. Hyattsville, MD: NCHS; 2010. Available from: http://www.cdc.gov/nchs/data/nvsr/nvsr58/nvsr58_19.pdf.

Data table for Figure 30. Death rates for leading causes of death among persons 45–64 years of age: United States, 1997–2007

Year	All causes	Cancer	Heart disease	Unintentional injuries	Diabetes	Stroke	Chronic lower respiratory diseases (CLRD)
				Deaths per 100,000 population			
1997	669.7	234.1	179.9	29.9	22.6	27.3	23.0
1998	652.8	228.0	171.9	30.2	22.5	26.3	22.3
1999	649.4	224.9	164.3	31.4	22.9	25.2	23.9
2000	647.6	221.2	159.6	31.9	22.8	25.8	22.6
2001	639.1	216.7	153.3	32.6	23.1	24.1	22.5
2002	638.4	214.5	152.7	34.5	23.3	23.9	22.1
2003	639.4	211.8	149.6	36.4	23.9	23.4	22.7
2004	625.8	207.2	143.1	37.6	23.1	22.8	21.6
2005	629.9	205.4	141.8	40.1	23.3	22.5	23.0
2006	623.0	202.7	138.3	41.6	22.9	22.5	21.8
2007	616.0	200.2	134.4	42.4	22.3	22.0	22.1
				Standard error			
1997	1.09	0.64	0.57	0.23	0.20	0.22	0.20
1998	1.06	0.63	0.54	0.23	0.20	0.21	0.20
1999	1.04	0.61	0.52	0.23	0.19	0.20	0.20
2000	1.02	0.60	0.51	0.23	0.19	0.20	0.19
2001	1.00	0.58	0.49	0.22	0.19	0.19	0.19
2002	0.98	0.57	0.48	0.23	0.19	0.19	0.18
2003	0.96	0.56	0.47	0.23	0.19	0.18	0.18
2004	0.94	0.54	0.45	0.23	0.18	0.18	0.17
2005	0.93	0.53	0.44	0.23	0.18	0.18	0.18
2006	0.91	0.52	0.43	0.24	0.17	0.17	0.17
2007	0.90	0.51	0.42	0.24	0.17	0.17	0.17

Cause of death, 2007	Number	Percent distribution
All causes	471,796	100.0
Cancer.	153,338	32.5
Heart disease	102,961	21.8
Unintentional injuries	32,508	6.9
Diabetes	17,057	3.6
CLRD	16,930	3.6
Stroke	16,885	3.6
All other causes.	132,117	28.0

NOTES: CLRD is chronic lower respiratory diseases. Causes of death shown are the six leading causes of death among persons 45–64 years of age in 2007. Death rates for 1997–1998 are based on the *International Classification of Diseases, 9th Revision*. Starting in 1999, death rates are based on the *International Classification of Diseases, 10th Revision*. Comparability ratios for selected revisions are available from: http://www.cdc.gov/nchs/nvss/mortality/comparability_icd.htm. Cancer refers to malignant neoplasms. Stroke refers to cerebrovascular diseases. See Appendix II, Cause of death; Comparability ratio; Tables 35, 36, 38, 45, and 46.

SOURCE: CDC/NCHS, National Vital Statistics System. Xu JQ, Kochanek KD, Murphy SL, Tejada-Vera B. Deaths: Final data for 2007. National vital statistics reports; vol 58 no 19. Hyattsville, MD: NCHS; 2010. Available from: http://www.cdc.gov/nchs/data/nvsr/nvsr58/nvsr58_19.pdf.

Data table for Figure 31. Death rates for leading causes of death among persons 65 years of age and over: United States, 1997–2007

Year	All causes	Heart disease	Cancer	Stroke	Chronic lower respiratory diseases (CLRD)	Alzheimer's disease	Diabetes	Influenza and pneumonia
					Deaths per 100,000 population			
1997	5,025.6	1,764.2	1,113.1	406.9	274.4	†	137.5	†
1998	5,064.3	1,749.5	1,109.7	400.8	282.7	†	141.5	†
1999	5,165.1	1,745.1	1,121.1	427.0	310.7	126.5	149.0	164.6
2000	5,143.6	1,696.7	1,121.3	423.1	304.0	140.0	149.8	167.3
2001	5,096.0	1,651.2	1,105.7	409.4	302.9	150.9	152.2	157.3
2002	5,088.8	1,618.7	1,098.3	402.5	304.2	163.7	153.7	165.2
2003	5,023.4	1,568.5	1,082.7	384.6	303.8	174.9	152.9	160.6
2004	4,837.4	1,469.4	1,063.1	359.7	289.8	180.0	148.7	145.4
2005	4,860.5	1,443.1	1,055.5	336.7	306.4	192.6	150.1	150.7
2006	4,722.0	1,370.2	1,040.0	314.0	286.8	192.3	140.5	132.4
2007	4,633.6	1,309.4	1,028.6	306.1	289.2	194.8	136.0	121.3
					Standard error			
1997	3.82	2.26	1.80	1.09	0.89	†	0.63	†
1998	3.82	2.25	1.79	1.08	0.90	†	0.64	†
1999	3.85	2.24	1.79	1.11	0.94	0.60	0.65	0.69
2000	3.83	2.20	1.79	1.10	0.93	0.63	0.65	0.69
2001	3.80	2.16	1.77	1.08	0.93	0.65	0.66	0.67
2002	3.78	2.13	1.76	1.06	0.92	0.68	0.66	0.68
2003	3.74	2.09	1.74	1.03	0.92	0.70	0.65	0.67
2004	3.65	2.01	1.71	1.00	0.89	0.70	0.64	0.63
2005	3.63	1.98	1.69	0.96	0.91	0.72	0.64	0.64
2006	3.56	1.92	1.67	0.92	0.88	0.72	0.61	0.60
2007	3.50	1.86	1.65	0.90	0.87	0.72	0.60	0.57

Cause of death, 2007	Number	Percent distribution
All causes	1,755,567	100.0
Heart disease	496,095	28.3
Cancer.	389,730	22.2
Stroke	115,961	6.6
CLRD	109,562	6.2
Alzheimer's disease	73,797	4.2
Diabetes	51,528	2.9
Influenza and pneumonia	45,941	2.6
All other causes.	472,953	26.9

† Data not comparable.

NOTES: Causes of death shown are the seven leading causes of death among persons 65 years of age and over in 2007. Death rates for 1997–1998 are based on the *International Classification of Diseases, 9th Revision (ICD–9)*. Starting in 1999, death rates are based on the *International Classification of Diseases, 10th Revision* (ICD–10). Comparability ratios for selected revisions are available from: http://www.cdc.gov/nchs/nvss/mortality/comparability_icd.htm. Data for 1997–1998 for Alzheimer's disease and Influenza and pneumonia are not presented due to large differences in death rates caused by changes in the coding of these causes between ICD–9 and ICD–10. Stroke refers to cerebrovascular diseases. See Appendix II, Cause of death; Comparability ratio; Tables 35, 36, 38, 45, and 46.

SOURCE: CDC/NCHS, National Vital Statistics System. Xu JQ, Kochanek KD, Murphy SL, Tejada-Vera B. Deaths: Final data for 2007. National vital statistics reports; vol 58 no 19. Hyattsville, MD: NCHS; 2010. Available from: http://www.cdc.gov/nchs/data/nvsr/nvsr58/nvsr58_19.pdf.

Data table for Figure 32. Unintentional motor-vehicle traffic death rates by state: United States, average annual 2000–2007

State	2000–2007	State	2000–2007
	Deaths per 100,000 population		Deaths per 100,000 population
United States...............	14.7	Alaska.....................	14.9
		Indiana	14.9
Mississippi.................	30.6	Colorado	14.7
Wyoming...................	25.7	Wisconsin	14.2
Montana	24.9	Iowa	14.1
Arkansas..................	24.7	Maine	13.8
Alabama	24.6	Utah	13.2
South Carolina.............	23.8	Oregon	13.2
New Mexico................	22.5	Virginia	12.9
South Dakota..............	21.9	Michigan	12.6
Louisiana.................	21.9	Pennsylvania..............	12.5
Tennessee.................	21.8	Vermont	12.3
Kentucky..................	20.9	Maryland..................	12.1
West Virginia	20.9	Ohio	12.0
Oklahoma	20.6	Minnesota	12.0
North Carolina	19.3	California.................	11.7
Missouri..................	19.2	Illinois...................	11.5
Idaho	19.0	Washington	11.2
Arizona	19.0	New Hampshire	10.4
Florida...................	18.4	Hawaii....................	10.3
Georgia...................	17.8	Connecticut	9.1
Kansas	17.7	New Jersey	8.7
Texas	17.2	District of Columbia	8.3
Nevada...................	16.7	Rhode Island	8.1
North Dakota	16.5	New York..................	7.8
Nebraska..................	15.6	Massachusetts..............	7.4
Delaware..................	15.2		

NOTES: Rates are per 100,000 population and are age-adjusted to the year 2000 standard population. States listed are where the deaths occurred, not state of residence. Rates are rounded to whole numbers and plotted as quartiles.

SOURCE: CDC/NCHS. National Vital Statistics System.

References (continued from page 42)

4. National Highway Traffic Safety Administration (NHTSA). Occupant protection. Traffic safety facts, 2008 data. DOT HS 811 160. Washington, DC: NHTSA. Available from: http://www-nrd.nhtsa.dot.gov/Pubs/811160.pdf.
5. National Highway Traffic Safety Administration (NHTSA). Rural/Urban comparison. Traffic Safety Facts, 2007 data. DOT HS 810 996. Washington, DC: NHTSA. Available from: http://www-nrd.nhtsa.dot.gov/Pubs/810996.pdf.
6. Web-based Injury Statistics Query and Reporting System (WISQARS) [online]. CDC, National Center for Injury Control and Prevention. Available from: http://www.cdc.gov/injury/wisqars/index.html.

Data table for Figure 33. Place of death, over time: United States, 1989, 1997, and 2007

Age and year	Place of death				
	Nursing home	Hospital inpatient	Hospital outpatient or emergency department	Home	All other places
	Percent				
All ages					
1989	16.0	48.6	7.9	15.9	11.6
1997	21.4	41.5	8.1	22.3	6.8
2007	21.7	36.0	7.0	25.4	9.9
Under 65 years					
1989	2.7	48.3	12.4	17.9	18.8
1997	4.5	42.1	13.5	26.2	13.7
2007	5.3	37.8	12.1	29.9	14.9
65 years and over					
1989	21.3	48.7	6.2	15.2	8.7
1997	27.2	41.3	6.2	20.9	4.4
2007	27.9	35.3	5.0	23.7	8.0
	Standard error				
All ages					
1989	0.02	0.03	0.02	0.02	0.02
1997	0.03	0.03	0.02	0.03	0.02
2007	0.03	0.03	0.02	0.03	0.02
Under 65 years					
1989	0.02	0.09	0.04	0.05	0.06
1997	0.03	0.06	0.04	0.06	0.04
2007	0.03	0.06	0.04	0.06	0.04
65 years and over					
1989	0.04	0.06	0.02	0.03	0.02
1997	0.03	0.04	0.02	0.03	0.02
2007	0.03	0.04	0.02	0.03	0.02

NOTES: Persons were classified based on where death was pronounced and on the physical location of death, not the services they were receiving at the time of death. "All other places" includes dead on arrival, hospice facility, other, and unknown. Place of death was unknown for fewer than 2% of all deaths. Place of death data were collected using two different versions of the death certificate. The U.S. Standard Certificate of Death (which is used as a model by the states) was revised in 2003. This table includes 2007 data for the 23 states and the District of Columbia (representing about 50% of all deaths) that used the 2003 revision of the U.S. Standard Certificate of Death, and 2007 data for the remaining 27 states that collected and reported death data based on the 1989 revision of the U.S. Standard Certificate of Death. Data for 1989 and 1997 were collected using the 1989 revision of the Certificate of Death. The 2003 Certificate added "Hospice facility" as a check box item for place of death and "Long-term care facility" was added to the "Nursing home" check box. "Long-term care facility" and "Hospice facility" reflect changes in terminology and place of care. See Appendix I, Population Census and Population Estimates.

SOURCE: CDC/NCHS, National Vital Statistics System.

Data table for Figure 34. Place of death, by age and race and Hispanic origin: United States, 2007

Age and race and Hispanic origin	Place of death				
	Nursing home	Hospital inpatient	Hospital outpatient or emergency department	Home	All other places
Age	Percent				
All ages:					
Hispanic or Latino	10.6	44.4	8.9	24.4	11.7
Not Hispanic or Latino:					
White	24.0	33.9	6.1	26.2	9.8
Black or African American	13.6	43.9	11.7	20.7	10.1
Asian or Pacific Islander	12.7	46.9	8.3	23.9	8.2
American Indian or Alaska Native.	12.2	39.4	9.2	25.5	13.7
Under 65 years:					
Hispanic or Latino	3.4	45.5	12.8	21.5	16.8
Not Hispanic or Latino:					
White	5.7	34.4	11.0	34.0	14.8
Black or African American	5.2	45.0	15.7	20.0	14.0
Asian or Pacific Islander	3.9	47.5	12.2	23.7	12.6
American Indian or Alaska Native.	4.5	38.2	11.8	25.0	20.5
65 years and over:					
Hispanic or Latino	16.4	43.6	5.6	26.9	7.5
Not Hispanic or Latino:					
White	29.6	33.8	4.6	23.8	8.3
Black or African American	20.3	43.0	8.5	21.3	6.8
Asian or Pacific Islander	16.8	46.6	6.6	23.9	6.1
American Indian or Alaska Native.	20.4	40.7	6.5	26.0	6.4
Race and Hispanic origin	Standard error				
All ages:					
Hispanic or Latino	0.08	0.13	0.08	0.12	0.09
Not Hispanic or Latino:					
White	0.03	0.03	0.02	0.03	0.02
Black or African American	0.06	0.09	0.06	0.08	0.06
Asian or Pacific Islander	0.16	0.24	0.13	0.20	0.13
American Indian or Alaska Native.	0.28	0.42	0.25	0.37	0.29
Under 65 years:					
Hispanic or Latino	0.07	0.20	0.14	0.17	0.15
Not Hispanic or Latino:					
White	0.03	0.07	0.05	0.07	0.05
Black or African American	0.06	0.14	0.10	0.11	0.10
Asian or Pacific Islander	0.16	0.42	0.28	0.36	0.28
American Indian or Alaska Native.	0.25	0.58	0.36	0.51	0.48
65 years and over:					
Hispanic or Latino	0.14	0.18	0.08	0.16	0.10
Not Hispanic or Latino:					
White	0.04	0.04	0.02	0.03	0.02
Black or African American	0.10	0.12	0.07	0.10	0.06
Asian or Pacific Islander	0.21	0.28	0.14	0.24	0.14
American Indian or Alaska Native.	0.50	0.60	0.30	0.54	0.30

NOTES: Persons were classified based on where death was pronounced and on the physical location of death, not the services they were receiving at the time of death. "All other places" includes dead on arrival, hospice facility, other, and unknown. Place of death was unknown for fewer than 2% of all deaths. Place of death data were collected using two different versions of the death certificate. The U.S. Standard Certificate of Death (which is used as a model by the states) was revised in 2003. This table includes 2007 data for the 23 states and the District of Columbia (representing about 50% of all deaths) that used the 2003 revision of the U.S. Standard Certificate of Death, and 2007 data for the remaining 27 states that collected and reported death data based on the 1989 revision of the U.S. Standard Certificate of Death. The 2003 Certificate added "Hospice facility" as a check box item for place of death and "Long-term care facility" was added to the "Nursing home" check box. "Long-term care facility" and "Hospice facility" reflect changes in terminology and place of care. See Appendix I, Population Census and Population Estimates.

SOURCE: CDC/NCHS, National Vital Statistics System.

Data table for Figure 35. Average number of days in ICU/CCU for Medicare decedents in the last 6 months of life, by state of residence: United States, 2005

State of residence	Mean	State of residence	Mean
United States	3.47	Hawaii	2.83
New Jersey	5.71	Arkansas	2.73
Florida	5.42	Connecticut	2.72
California	4.69	Nebraska	2.72
Nevada	4.19	Mississippi	2.61
Illinois	4.09	Rhode Island	2.60
Texas	4.08	New Mexico	2.47
Delaware	3.92	Oklahoma	2.42
Pennsylvania	3.86	Massachusetts	2.30
South Carolina	3.74	Kansas	2.20
Arizona	3.51	Alaska	2.18
District of Columbia	3.51	Washington	2.18
Ohio	3.51	Colorado	2.06
Virginia	3.37	Utah	2.02
Kentucky	3.36	Montana	1.88
Missouri	3.36	Minnesota	1.84
Tennessee	3.36	South Dakota	1.81
Louisiana	3.32	Iowa	1.78
Michigan	3.28	Maine	1.77
West Virginia	3.25	Wyoming	1.77
Alabama	3.22	New Hampshire	1.76
Georgia	3.20	Wisconsin	1.69
New York	3.17	Idaho	1.53
Maryland	3.13	Oregon	1.51
Indiana	3.11	Vermont	1.41
North Carolina	3.02	North Dakota	1.34

NOTES: Includes Medicare enrollees who had full Part A and Part B entitlement throughout the last 6 months of life. Persons enrolled in managed care organizations (HMOs) were excluded. Restricted to those whose age on the date of death was 65–99 years. Geographic location is based on decedent's residence, not place of care. Estimates were adjusted for differences in age, sex, and race.

SOURCE: The Dartmouth Atlas of Health Care. Available from: http://www.dartmouthatlas.org/.

Data table for Figure 36. Advance directives among adults 65 years of age and over, by type of care and race and Hispanic origin: United States, selected years

Race and Hispanic origin	Type of care					
	Nursing home residents		Home health care patients		Discharged hospice care patients	
	2004		2007		2007	
	Percent	SE	Percent	SE	Percent	SE
Total.................................	69.9	0.8	35.0	2.2	91.7	1.0
Hispanic or Latino........................	49.7	3.5	*12.1	*3.4	93.1	3.3
Not Hispanic or Latino:						
White only............................	74.8	0.7	42.2	2.6	92.9	1.0
Black or African American only.............	40.5	2.1	*12.4	*2.7	79.1	5.3

SE is standard error.

* Estimates are considered unreliable. Data preceded by an asterisk have a relative standard error of 20%–30%.

NOTES: For nursing home residents, advance directives include any of these orders: living will, do not resuscitate (dnr), do not hospitalize, feeding restrictions, medication restrictions, organ donation, or other. For home health care and discharged hospice care patients, advance directives include any of these orders: living will, do not resuscitate (dnr), do not hospitalize/do not send to emergency department, feeding restrictions, medication restrictions, comfort measures only, durable power of attorney, health care proxy/surrogate, organ donation, or other. The 2007 National Home and Hospice Care Survey data were collected through interviews with agency directors and their designated staffs; no interviews were conducted directly with patients or their families or friends. Data collected on home health care and hospice care patients are taken from medical records. For more information see: http://www.cdc.gov/nchs/data/nhhcsd/NHHCS_NHHAS_web_documentation.pdf. The 2004 National Nursing Home Survey data were collected through interviews with designated staff familiar with the residents and their care. The interviewed staff were asked to use the residents' medical records to answer the data items. No interviews were conducted with residents. For more information see: http://www.cdc.gov/nchs/data/nnhsd/2004NNHS_DesignCollectionEstimates_072706tags.pdf. See Appendix I, National Home and Hospice Care Survey; National Nursing Home Survey; Appendix II, Resident, health facility.

SOURCE: CDC/NCHS, National Nursing Home Survey and National Home and Hospice Care Survey.

Data table for Figure 37. Selected characteristics of discharged hospice care patients: United States, 2007

Characteristic	2007	
	Percent	SE
Age		
Under 65 years	16.9	0.8
65 years and over	83.1	0.8
65–74 years.	15.4	1.1
75–84 years.	29.5	1.2
85 years and over	38.2	1.3
Sex		
Male.	44.9	1.4
Female.	55.1	1.4
Race and Hispanic origin		
Hispanic or Latino	4.1	0.7
Not Hispanic or Latino:		
White	86.6	1.2
Black or African American	7.6	1.0
Marital status		
Married or living with partner.	45.4	1.6
Single, divorced, or separated.	14.2	0.9
Widowed	40.4	1.5
Vital status at discharge		
Deceased.	84.4	1.1
Alive.	15.6	1.1
Medicare beneficiary		
Yes	84.3	0.9
No	15.7	0.9
Place of care on first day		
Private home.	55.3	1.7
Nursing home/skilled nursing facility	21.1	1.4
Other place.	23.6	1.6

SE is standard error.

NOTES: There were 1.0 million hospice care discharges (weighted) in 2007. The 2007 National Home and Hospice Care Survey data were collected through interviews with agency directors and their designated staffs; no interviews were conducted directly with patients or their families or friends. Data collected on home health care patients and hospice care discharges are taken from medical records. For more information, see: http://www.cdc.gov/nchs/nhhcs/nhhcs_questionnaires.htm. Race and ethnicity of fewer than 2% of hospice care patient discharges were non-Hispanic Asian or American Indian or Alaska Native. These discharges are included in tabulations for characteristics other than race and Hispanic origin. The place of hospice care may change over the course of treatment. Data presented here are based on the place on the first day of hospice care. Other place includes residential care facility, inpatient hospice care agency, hospital, and other locations.

SOURCE: CDC/NCHS, National Home and Hospice Care Survey.

Data table for Figure 38. Primary admission diagnosis of discharged hospice care patients: United States, 1998 and 2007

Admission diagnosis	1998		2007		ICD–9–CM code
	Percent	SE	Percent	SE	
Cancer (malignant neoplasms)	64.8	2.5	42.9	1.5	140–208
Noncancer.	35.2	2.5	57.1	1.5	All noncancer
Alzheimer's, mental disorders, and other dementia.	*3.1	0.6	11.2	0.9	290–319 or 331
Heart disease.	8.6	1.6	11.1	0.9	390–398, 402, 404, 410–429
CLRD (chronic lower respiratory diseases)	*3.5	0.9	4.8	0.5	490–494, 496
Stroke (cerebrovascular diseases)	*2.6	0.6	4.5	0.6	430–434, 436–438
All other.	17.4	2.0	25.6	1.1	All other

SE is standard error.

* Estimates are considered unreliable. Data preceded by an asterisk have a relative standard error of 20%–30%.

NOTES: ICD–9–CM is *International Classification of Diseases, 9th Revision, Clinical Modification.* The 2007 National Home and Hospice Care Survey data were collected through interviews with agency directors and their designated staffs; no interviews were conducted directly with patients or their families or friends. Data collected on home health care patients and hospice care discharges are taken from medical records. For more information see: http://www.cdc.gov/nchs/nhhcs/nhhcs_questionnaires.htm.

SOURCE: CDC/NCHS, National Home and Hospice Care Survey.

Data table for Figure 39. Services offered or provided to hospice care patients' family members or friends: United States, 2007

Type of service	Percent	SE
Bereavement	85.1	1.3
Spiritual	66.8	2.2
Medication management or administration	66.7	2.3
Patient activities of daily living	58.1	2.2
Safety training	53.3	2.5
Equipment use	47.8	2.4
Caregiver health or wellness	25.7	2.4
Dietary	19.6	2.0
Referral or resource information	19.1	2.2
Dealing with difficult behaviors	17.8	1.9

SE is standard error.

NOTES: Data were collected through in-person interviews with agency directors and their designated staffs who were familiar with the patients and the care they received. Information was also abstracted from patients' medical records. No information was obtained from family members or friends. Hospice staff were asked: "Did this agency offer or provide the patient's family members or friends any of the services listed on this card? Which ones?"

SOURCE: CDC/NCHS, National Home and Hospice Care Survey.

Data table for Figure 40. Hospice care patients' symptoms at the last hospice care visit before death: United States, 2007

Type of symptom	Percent	SE
Difficulty breathing	50.7	2.0
Pain	33.3	1.8
Restlessness	25.0	1.7
Anorexia	23.9	2.3
Constipation	10.0	1.2

SE is standard error.

NOTES: Data were collected through in-person interviews with agency directors and their designated staffs who were familiar with the patients and the care they received. Information was also abstracted from patients' medical records. No information was obtained from family members or friends. Data are based on the question: "When this agency last provided care to the patient did (he/she) have any of these symptoms before (his/her) death? Select all symptoms that apply." This analysis is limited to those who died while under hospice care.

SOURCE:CDC/NCHS, National Home and Hospice Care Survey.

References (continued from page 50)

5. CDC/NCHS. National Home and Hospice Care Survey [unpublished analysis].

6. Sykes N. End of life issues. Eur J Cancer 2008;44(8):1157–62.

7. Leleszi JP, Lewandowski JG. Pain management in end-of-life care. J Am Osteopath Assoc 2005;105(3 suppl):S6–S11. Available from: http://www.jaoa.org/cgi/content/full/105/3_suppl/6S.

8. Hanks GW, de Conno F, Cherny N, Hanna M, Kalso E, McQuay HJ, et al. Morphine and alternative opioids in cancer pain: The EAPC recommendations. Expert Working Group of the Research Network of the European Association for Palliative Care (EAPC). Br J Cancer 2001;84(5): 587–93. Available from: http://www.ncbi.nlm.nih.gov/pmc/articles/PMC2363790/pdf/84–6691680a.pdf.

Data table for Figure 41. Selected drugs prescribed to hospice care patients in the last week of life: United States, 2007

Multum Lexicon Plus therapeutic class (common reasons for hospice use)	Percent	SE
Narcotic analgesic (severe pain)	90.9	0.8
Antiemetic (vomiting or dizziness)	78.6	1.5
Laxative (constipation)	52.6	1.9
Antipsychotic (restlessness, agitation)	36.1	1.8
Diuretic (fluid retention, high blood pressure, cardiac, kidney conditions)	25.5	1.3
Proton pump inhibitor (antiulcer, antiitch)	25.3	1.4
Bronchodilator (breathing difficulties)	24.0	1.3
Antidepressant (depression, pain)	23.4	1.3
Antacid (stomach acid, antiulcer)	17.6	1.2
Antiarrythmic (heart rhythm disturbances)	15.9	1.1
Corticosteroid (antiinflammatory, pain)	14.2	1.0
Antidiabetic (elevated blood sugar)	10.4	0.8
Antianginal (chest pain)	7.4	0.7
Antihyperlipidemia (elevated cholesterol)	7.1	0.7
Nonsteroidal antiinflammatory drug (inflammation, mild pain)	6.7	0.7
Baby aspirin or Plavix (clopidogrel) (clot prevention)	3.4	0.5

SE is standard error.

NOTES: Information is collected from the patient's medical record based on the question: "What are the names of all the medications and drugs he/she was taking the 7 days prior to and on the the day of his/her death? Please include any standing routine, or PRN (as needed) medications." Up to 25 medication names could be recorded. Information on dosage, strength, route, and frequency of administration was not recorded. Drug therapeutic class is based on Lexicon Plus, a proprietary database of Cerner Multum, Inc. Lexicon Plus is a comprehensive database of all prescription and some nonprescription drug products available in the U.S. drug market. Up to four classes are assigned to each drug. Data presented here are based on the second-level classification of prescription drugs except as noted: the category for narcotic analgesics is based on the first level, and the category for baby aspirin or Plavix is based on the third level. This analysis is limited to those patients who died while under hospice care.

SOURCE: CDC/NCHS, National Home and Hospice Care Survey.

Table 1 (page 1 of 3). Resident population, by age, sex, race, and Hispanic origin: United States, selected years 1950–2008

[Data are based on the decennial census updated with data from multiple sources]

Sex, race, Hispanic origin, and year	Total resident population	Under 1 year	1–4 years	5–14 years	15–24 years	25–34 years	35–44 years	45–54 years	55–64 years	65–74 years	75–84 years	85 years and over
All persons						Number in thousands						
1950	150,697	3,147	13,017	24,319	22,098	23,759	21,450	17,343	13,370	8,340	3,278	577
1960	179,323	4,112	16,209	35,465	24,020	22,818	24,081	20,485	15,572	10,997	4,633	929
1970	203,212	3,485	13,669	40,746	35,441	24,907	23,088	23,220	18,590	12,435	6,119	1,511
1980	226,546	3,534	12,815	34,942	42,487	37,082	25,635	22,800	21,703	15,581	7,729	2,240
1990	248,710	3,946	14,812	35,095	37,013	43,161	37,435	25,057	21,113	18,045	10,012	3,021
2000	281,422	3,806	15,370	41,078	39,184	39,892	45,149	37,678	24,275	18,391	12,361	4,240
2006	299,398	4,130	16,287	40,337	42,435	40,416	43,667	43,278	31,587	18,917	13,047	5,297
2007	301,621	4,257	16,467	40,164	42,506	40,591	43,161	43,875	32,712	19,352	13,024	5,512
2008	304,060	4,313	16,693	40,120	42,573	40,932	42,501	44,372	33,686	20,123	13,025	5,722
Male												
1950	74,833	1,602	6,634	12,375	10,918	11,597	10,588	8,655	6,697	4,024	1,507	237
1960	88,331	2,090	8,240	18,029	11,906	11,179	11,755	10,093	7,537	5,116	2,025	362
1970	98,912	1,778	6,968	20,759	17,551	12,217	11,231	11,199	8,793	5,437	2,436	542
1980	110,053	1,806	6,556	17,855	21,419	18,382	12,570	11,009	10,152	6,757	2,867	682
1990	121,239	2,018	7,581	17,971	18,915	21,564	18,510	12,232	9,955	7,907	3,745	841
2000	138,054	1,949	7,862	21,043	20,079	20,121	22,448	18,497	11,645	8,303	4,879	1,227
2006	147,512	2,113	8,329	20,640	21,845	20,565	21,850	21,290	15,224	8,670	5,298	1,688
2007	148,659	2,179	8,424	20,549	21,860	20,683	21,619	21,595	15,775	8,887	5,313	1,777
2008	149,925	2,208	8,540	20,522	21,873	20,900	21,314	21,853	16,251	9,265	5,336	1,864
Female												
1950	75,864	1,545	6,383	11,944	11,181	12,162	10,863	8,688	6,672	4,316	1,771	340
1960	90,992	2,022	7,969	17,437	12,114	11,639	12,326	10,393	8,036	5,881	2,609	567
1970	104,300	1,707	6,701	19,986	17,890	12,690	11,857	12,021	9,797	6,998	3,683	969
1980	116,493	1,727	6,259	17,087	21,068	18,700	13,065	11,791	11,551	8,824	4,862	1,559
1990	127,471	1,928	7,231	17,124	18,098	21,596	18,925	12,824	11,158	10,139	6,267	2,180
2000	143,368	1,857	7,508	20,034	19,105	19,771	22,701	19,181	12,629	10,088	7,482	3,013
2006	151,886	2,017	7,959	19,697	20,590	19,851	21,817	21,989	16,363	10,247	7,748	3,609
2007	152,962	2,078	8,043	19,615	20,646	19,908	21,543	22,280	16,937	10,465	7,711	3,735
2008	154,135	2,105	8,153	19,598	20,701	20,032	21,187	22,519	17,436	10,858	7,689	3,858
White male												
1950	67,129	1,400	5,845	10,860	9,689	10,430	9,529	7,836	6,180	3,736	1,406	218
1960	78,367	1,784	7,065	15,659	10,483	9,940	10,564	9,114	6,850	4,702	1,875	331
1970	86,721	1,501	5,873	17,667	15,232	10,775	9,979	10,090	7,958	4,916	2,243	487
1980	94,976	1,487	5,402	14,773	18,123	15,940	11,010	9,774	9,151	6,096	2,600	621
1990	102,143	1,604	6,071	14,467	15,389	18,071	15,819	10,624	8,813	7,127	3,397	760
2000	113,445	1,524	6,143	16,428	15,942	16,232	18,568	15,670	10,067	7,343	4,419	1,109
2006	119,950	1,635	6,479	16,064	17,146	16,307	17,723	17,751	13,055	7,530	4,740	1,520
2007	120,734	1,679	6,533	16,002	17,130	16,396	17,472	17,969	13,502	7,712	4,742	1,598
2008	121,605	1,691	6,591	15,995	17,104	16,569	17,171	18,144	13,872	8,047	4,749	1,672
White female												
1950	67,813	1,341	5,599	10,431	9,821	10,851	9,719	7,868	6,168	4,031	1,669	314
1960	80,465	1,714	6,795	15,068	10,596	10,204	11,000	9,364	7,327	5,428	2,441	527
1970	91,028	1,434	5,615	16,912	15,420	11,004	10,349	10,756	8,853	6,366	3,429	890
1980	99,835	1,412	5,127	14,057	17,653	15,896	11,232	10,285	10,325	7,951	4,457	1,440
1990	106,561	1,524	5,762	13,706	14,599	17,757	15,834	10,946	9,698	9,048	5,687	2,001
2000	116,641	1,447	5,839	15,576	14,966	15,574	18,386	15,921	10,731	8,757	6,715	2,729
2006	122,147	1,560	6,178	15,261	16,042	15,358	17,285	17,929	13,741	8,727	6,826	3,239
2007	122,849	1,600	6,223	15,209	16,069	15,415	16,997	18,131	14,185	8,904	6,770	3,347
2008	123,635	1,613	6,279	15,211	16,084	15,536	16,652	18,284	14,555	9,247	6,725	3,450
Black or African American male												
1950	7,300	- - -	[1]944	1,442	1,162	1,105	1,003	772	459	299	[2]113	- - -
1960	9,114	281	1,082	2,185	1,305	1,120	1,086	891	617	382	137	29
1970	10,748	245	975	2,784	2,041	1,226	1,084	979	739	461	169	46
1980	12,585	269	967	2,614	2,807	1,967	1,235	1,024	854	567	228	53
1990	14,420	322	1,164	2,700	2,669	2,592	1,962	1,175	878	614	277	66
2000	17,407	313	1,271	3,454	2,932	2,586	2,705	1,957	1,090	683	330	87
2006	18,890	347	1,343	3,345	3,381	2,722	2,682	2,399	1,438	752	370	112
2007	19,121	365	1,370	3,316	3,422	2,767	2,667	2,452	1,504	768	374	118
2008	19,293	366	1,368	3,256	3,464	2,829	2,644	2,500	1,570	791	381	124

See footnotes at end of table.

[Data are based on the decennial census updated with data from multiple sources]

Sex, race, Hispanic origin, and year	Total resident population	Under 1 year	1–4 years	5–14 years	15–24 years	25–34 years	35–44 years	45–54 years	55–64 years	65–74 years	75–84 years	85 years and over
Black or African American female						Number in thousands						
1950	7,745	- - -	[1]941	1,446	1,300	1,260	1,112	796	443	322	[2]125	- - -
1960	9,758	283	1,085	2,191	1,404	1,300	1,229	974	663	430	160	38
1970	11,832	243	970	2,773	2,196	1,456	1,309	1,134	868	582	230	71
1980	14,046	266	951	2,578	2,937	2,267	1,488	1,258	1,059	776	360	106
1990	16,063	316	1,137	2,641	2,700	2,905	2,279	1,416	1,135	884	495	156
2000	19,187	302	1,228	3,348	2,971	2,866	3,055	2,274	1,353	971	587	233
2006	20,669	333	1,298	3,240	3,293	2,932	3,024	2,793	1,784	1,051	650	274
2007	20,907	351	1,325	3,212	3,331	2,953	3,005	2,852	1,867	1,073	656	283
2008	21,074	349	1,320	3,154	3,373	2,981	2,975	2,910	1,949	1,104	666	293
American Indian or Alaska Native male												
1980	702	17	59	153	161	114	75	53	37	22	9	2
1990	1,024	24	88	206	192	183	140	86	55	32	13	3
2000	1,488	28	109	301	271	229	229	165	88	45	18	5
2006	1,599	23	88	273	306	254	232	203	126	60	28	8
2007	1,615	24	90	263	307	259	231	208	132	64	29	9
2008	1,709	35	130	281	306	266	230	213	139	67	31	10
American Indian or Alaska Native female												
1980	718	16	57	149	158	118	79	57	41	27	12	4
1990	1,041	24	85	200	178	186	148	92	61	41	21	6
2000	1,496	26	106	293	254	219	236	174	95	54	28	10
2006	1,602	22	85	265	293	234	229	216	136	70	37	16
2007	1,620	23	87	255	295	240	227	221	143	73	39	18
2008	1,713	34	127	273	296	246	225	225	150	77	40	19
Asian or Pacific Islander male												
1980	1,814	35	130	321	334	366	252	159	110	72	30	6
1990	3,652	68	258	598	665	718	588	347	208	133	57	12
2000	5,713	84	339	861	934	1,073	947	705	399	231	112	27
2006	7,073	108	419	958	1,012	1,281	1,214	938	605	328	162	48
2007	7,188	111	431	967	1,002	1,261	1,248	966	637	344	168	53
2008	7,318	115	451	989	999	1,235	1,270	996	671	360	175	58
Asian or Pacific Islander female												
1980	1,915	34	127	307	325	423	269	192	126	71	33	9
1990	3,805	65	247	578	621	749	664	371	264	166	65	17
2000	6,044	81	336	817	914	1,112	1,024	812	451	305	152	41
2006	7,468	103	398	931	963	1,327	1,279	1,051	702	399	235	80
2007	7,586	105	409	940	952	1,301	1,314	1,075	741	415	246	88
2008	7,714	109	427	960	947	1,268	1,335	1,101	782	430	258	96

See footnotes at end of table.

Table 1 (page 3 of 3). Resident population, by age, sex, race, and Hispanic origin: United States, selected years 1950–2008

[Data are based on the decennial census updated with data from multiple sources]

Sex, race, Hispanic origin, and year	Total resident population	Under 1 year	1–4 years	5–14 years	15–24 years	25–34 years	35–44 years	45–54 years	55–64 years	65–74 years	75–84 years	85 years and over
Hispanic or Latino male						Number in thousands						
1980	7,280	187	661	1,530	1,646	1,256	761	570	364	200	86	19
1990	11,388	279	980	2,128	2,376	2,310	1,471	818	551	312	131	32
2000	18,162	395	1,506	3,469	3,564	3,494	2,653	1,551	804	474	203	50
2006	22,925	496	1,906	4,109	3,905	4,456	3,526	2,287	1,218	617	316	89
2007	23,524	528	1,983	4,188	3,910	4,503	3,630	2,414	1,295	643	331	98
2008	24,254	567	2,135	4,322	3,927	4,514	3,729	2,542	1,379	680	348	112
Hispanic or Latina female												
1980	7,329	181	634	1,482	1,546	1,249	805	615	411	257	117	30
1990	10,966	268	939	2,039	2,028	2,073	1,448	868	632	403	209	59
2000	17,144	376	1,441	3,318	3,017	3,016	2,476	1,585	907	603	303	101
2006	21,396	475	1,828	3,923	3,470	3,636	3,134	2,230	1,323	759	452	167
2007	21,981	505	1,900	4,000	3,527	3,665	3,212	2,336	1,397	787	471	181
2008	22,689	542	2,045	4,132	3,587	3,668	3,280	2,441	1,475	826	494	201
White, not Hispanic or Latino male												
1980	88,035	1,308	4,772	13,317	16,554	14,739	10,284	9,229	8,803	5,906	2,519	603
1990	91,743	1,351	5,181	12,525	13,219	15,967	14,481	9,875	8,303	6,837	3,275	729
2000	96,551	1,163	4,761	13,238	12,628	12,958	16,088	14,223	9,312	6,894	4,225	1,062
2006	98,540	1,171	4,679	12,263	13,526	12,128	14,418	15,615	11,915	6,949	4,439	1,436
2007	98,774	1,190	4,676	12,113	13,509	12,174	14,069	15,714	12,291	7,106	4,427	1,504
2008	99,085	1,181	4,663	12,011	13,472	12,342	13,673	15,769	12,583	7,407	4,419	1,566
White, not Hispanic or Latina female												
1980	92,872	1,240	4,522	12,647	16,185	14,711	10,468	9,700	9,935	7,707	4,345	1,411
1990	96,557	1,280	4,909	11,846	12,749	15,872	14,520	10,153	9,116	8,674	5,491	1,945
2000	100,774	1,102	4,517	12,529	12,183	12,778	16,089	14,446	9,879	8,188	6,429	2,633
2006	102,252	1,116	4,451	11,635	12,839	11,981	14,375	15,857	12,506	8,013	6,399	3,080
2007	102,418	1,132	4,443	11,496	12,815	12,011	14,013	15,961	12,882	8,164	6,325	3,175
2008	102,659	1,125	4,432	11,405	12,778	12,130	13,605	16,017	13,179	8,471	6,258	3,259

- - - Data not available.

[1]Population for age group under 5 years.

[2]Population for age group 75 years and over.

NOTES: The race groups, white, black, American Indian or Alaska Native, and Asian or Pacific Islander, include persons of Hispanic and non-Hispanic origin. Persons of Hispanic origin may be of any race. Starting with *Health, United States, 2003*, intercensal population estimates for the 1990s and 2000 are based on the 2000 census. Population estimates for 2001 and later years are 2000-based postcensal estimates. Population figures are census counts as of April 1 for 1950, 1960, 1970, 1980, 1990, and 2000; estimates as of July 1 are for other years. See Appendix I, Population Census and Population Estimates. Populations for age groups may not sum to the total due to rounding. Unrounded population figures are available in the spreadsheet version of this table. Available from: http://www.cdc.gov/nchs/hus.htm. Data for additional years are available. See Appendix III.

SOURCE: U.S. Census Bureau: 1950 Nonwhite Population by Race. Special Report P-E, No. 3B. Washington, DC: U.S. Government Printing Office, 1951; U.S. Census of Population: 1960, Number of Inhabitants, PC(1)-A1, United States Summary, 1964; 1970, Number of Inhabitants, Final Report PC(1)-A1, United States Summary, 1971; U.S. population estimates, by age, sex, race, and Hispanic origin: 1980 to 1991. Current population reports, series P–25, no 1095. Washington, DC: U.S. Government Printing Office, Feb. 1993; NCHS. Estimates of the July 1, 1991–July 1, 1999, April 1, 2000, and July 1, 2001–July 1, 2008 United States resident population by age, sex, race, and Hispanic origin, prepared under a collaborative arrangement with the U.S. Census Bureau, Population Estimates Program. Available from: http://www.cdc.gov/nchs/nvss/bridged_race.htm.

Table 2 (page 1 of 2). **Persons and families below poverty level, by selected characteristics, race, and Hispanic origin: United States, selected years 1973–2008**

[Data are based on household interviews of the civilian noninstitutionalized population]

Selected characteristics, race, and Hispanic origin[1]	1973	1980	1985	1990	1995	2000[2]	2004[3]	2007	2008
All persons				Percent below poverty					
All races	11.1	13.0	14.0	13.5	13.8	11.3	12.7	12.5	13.2
White only	8.4	10.2	11.4	10.7	11.2	9.5	10.8	10.5	11.2
Black or African American only	31.4	32.5	31.3	31.9	29.3	22.5	24.7	24.5	24.7
Asian only	- - -	- - -	- - -	12.2	14.6	9.9	9.8	10.2	11.8
Hispanic or Latino	21.9	25.7	29.0	28.1	30.3	21.5	21.9	21.5	23.2
Mexican	- - -	- - -	28.8	28.1	31.2	22.9	- - -	- - -	- - -
Puerto Rican	- - -	- - -	43.3	40.6	38.1	25.6	- - -	- - -	- - -
White only, not Hispanic or Latino	7.5	9.1	9.7	8.8	8.5	7.4	8.7	8.2	8.6
Related children under 18 years of age in families									
All races	14.2	17.9	20.1	19.9	20.2	15.6	17.3	17.6	18.5
White only	9.7	13.4	15.6	15.1	15.5	12.4	14.3	14.4	15.3
Black or African American only	40.6	42.1	43.1	44.2	41.5	30.9	33.4	34.3	34.4
Asian only	- - -	- - -	- - -	17.0	18.6	12.5	9.4	11.8	14.2
Hispanic or Latino	27.8	33.0	39.6	37.7	39.3	27.6	28.6	28.3	30.3
Mexican	- - -	- - -	37.4	35.5	39.3	29.5	- - -	- - -	- - -
Puerto Rican	- - -	- - -	58.6	56.7	53.2	32.1	- - -	- - -	- - -
White only, not Hispanic or Latino	- - -	11.3	12.3	11.6	10.6	8.5	9.9	9.7	10.0
Related children under 18 years of age in families with female householder and no spouse present									
All races	- - -	50.8	53.6	53.4	50.3	40.1	41.9	43.0	43.5
White only	- - -	41.6	45.2	45.9	42.5	33.9	38.2	39.0	39.3
Black or African American only	- - -	64.8	66.9	64.7	61.6	49.3	49.2	50.4	51.9
Asian only	- - -	- - -	- - -	32.2	42.4	38.0	18.7	32.3	25.0
Hispanic or Latino	- - -	65.0	72.4	68.4	65.7	49.8	51.9	51.6	51.9
Mexican	- - -	- - -	64.4	62.4	65.9	51.4	- - -	- - -	- - -
Puerto Rican	- - -	- - -	85.4	82.7	79.6	55.3	- - -	- - -	- - -
White only, not Hispanic or Latino	- - -	- - -	- - -	39.6	33.5	28.0	31.5	32.4	31.7
All persons				Number below poverty in thousands					
All races	22,973	29,272	33,064	33,585	36,425	31,581	37,040	37,276	39,829
White only	15,142	19,699	22,860	22,326	24,423	21,645	25,327	25,120	26,990
Black or African American only	7,388	8,579	8,926	9,837	9,872	7,982	9,014	9,237	9,379
Asian only	- - -	- - -	- - -	858	1,411	1,258	1,201	1,349	1,576
Hispanic or Latino	2,366	3,491	5,236	6,006	8,574	7,747	9,122	9,890	10,987
Mexican	- - -	- - -	3,220	3,764	5,608	5,460	- - -	- - -	- - -
Puerto Rican	- - -	- - -	1,011	966	1,183	814	- - -	- - -	- - -
White only, not Hispanic or Latino	12,864	16,365	17,839	16,622	16,267	14,366	16,908	16,032	17,024
Related children under 18 years of age in families									
All races	9,453	11,114	12,483	12,715	13,999	11,005	12,473	12,802	13,507
White only	5,462	6,817	7,838	7,696	8,474	6,834	7,876	8,002	8,441
Black or African American only	3,822	3,906	4,057	4,412	4,644	3,495	3,702	3,838	3,781
Asian only	- - -	- - -	- - -	356	532	407	265	345	430
Hispanic or Latino	1,364	1,718	2,512	2,750	3,938	3,342	3,985	4,348	4,888
Mexican	- - -	- - -	1,589	1,733	2,655	2,537	- - -	- - -	- - -
Puerto Rican	- - -	- - -	535	490	610	329	- - -	- - -	- - -
White only, not Hispanic or Latino	- - -	5,174	5,421	5,106	4,745	3,715	4,190	3,996	4,059

See footnotes at end of table.

Table 2 (page 2 of 2). Persons and families below poverty level, by selected characteristics, race, and Hispanic origin: United States, selected years 1973–2008

[Data are based on household interviews of the civilian noninstitutionalized population]

Selected characteristics, race, and Hispanic origin[1]	1973	1980	1985	1990	1995	2000[2]	2004[3]	2007	2008
Related children under 18 years of age in families with female householder and no spouse present				Number below poverty in thousands					
All races.	- - -	5,866	6,716	7,363	8,364	6,300	7,152	7,546	7,587
White only	- - -	2,813	3,372	3,597	4,051	3,090	3,782	3,931	3,926
Black or African American only	- - -	2,944	3,181	3,543	3,954	2,908	2,963	3,114	3,123
Asian only	- - -	- - -	- - -	80	145	162	55	100	88
Hispanic or Latino	- - -	809	1,247	1,314	1,872	1,407	1,840	2,092	2,218
Mexican	- - -	- - -	553	615	1,056	938	- - -	- - -	- - -
Puerto Rican	- - -	- - -	449	382	459	242	- - -	- - -	- - -
White only, not Hispanic or Latino	- - -	- - -	- - -	2,411	2,299	1,832	2,114	2,101	1,985

- - - Data not available.

[1]The race groups, white, black, and Asian, include persons of Hispanic and non-Hispanic origin. Persons of Hispanic origin may be of any race. Starting with 2002 data, race-specific estimates are tabulated according to the 1997 Revisions to the Standards for the Classification of Federal Data on Race and Ethnicity and are not strictly comparable with estimates for earlier years. The three single-race categories shown in the table conform to the 1997 Standards. For 2002 and subsequent years, race-specific estimates are for persons who reported only one racial group. Estimates for single-race categories prior to 2002 are based on answers to the Current Population Survey question which asked respondents to choose only a single race. Prior to data year 2002, data were tabulated according to the 1977 Standards in which the Asian only category included Native Hawaiian and Other Pacific Islander. See Appendix II, Hispanic origin; Race.
[2]Estimates are consistent with 2001 data through implementation of the 2000 census-based population controls and a 28,000 household sample expansion.
[3]The 2004 data have been revised to reflect a correction to the weights in the 2005 Annual Social and Economic Supplements (ASEC) of the Current Population Survey. See Appendix I, Current Population Survey (CPS).

NOTES: Estimates of poverty for 1991–1998 are based on 1990 postcensal population estimates. Estimates for 1999 and subsequent years are based on 2000 census population controls. Poverty level is based on family income and family size using U.S. Census Bureau poverty thresholds. See Appendix II, Poverty. The Current Population Survey is not large enough to produce reliable annual estimates for American Indian or Alaska Native persons, or for Native Hawaiians. The 2006–2008 average poverty rate for American Indian or Alaska Natives only was 26.7%, representing 721,000 persons. Data for additional years are available. See Appendix III.

SOURCE: U.S. Census Bureau, Current Population Survey, Annual Social and Economic Supplements; DeNavas-Walt C, Proctor BD, Smith JC. Income, poverty, and health insurance coverage in the United States: 2008. Current Population Reports, P–60–236. Washington, DC: U.S. Government Printing Office. 2009. Available from: http://www.census.gov/prod/2009pubs/p60-236.pdf.

Table 3 (page 1 of 3). Crude birth rates, fertility rates, and birth rates, by age, race, and Hispanic origin of mother: United States, selected years 1950–2007

[Data are based on birth certificates]

Race, Hispanic origin, and year	Crude birth rate[1]	Fertility rate[2]	10–14 years	15–19 years Total	15–17 years	18–19 years	20–24 years	25–29 years	30–34 years	35–39 years	40–44 years	45–54 years[3]
All races				Live births per 1,000 women								
1950	24.1	106.2	1.0	81.6	40.7	132.7	196.6	166.1	103.7	52.9	15.1	1.2
1960	23.7	118.0	0.8	89.1	43.9	166.7	258.1	197.4	112.7	56.2	15.5	0.9
1970	18.4	87.9	1.2	68.3	38.8	114.7	167.8	145.1	73.3	31.7	8.1	0.5
1980	15.9	68.4	1.1	53.0	32.5	82.1	115.1	112.9	61.9	19.8	3.9	0.2
1985	15.8	66.3	1.2	51.0	31.0	79.6	108.3	111.0	69.1	24.0	4.0	0.2
1990	16.7	70.9	1.4	59.9	37.5	88.6	116.5	120.2	80.8	31.7	5.5	0.2
1995	14.6	64.6	1.3	56.0	35.5	87.7	107.5	108.8	81.1	34.0	6.6	0.3
2000	14.4	65.9	0.9	47.7	26.9	78.1	109.7	113.5	91.2	39.7	8.0	0.5
2005	14.0	66.7	0.7	40.5	21.4	69.9	102.2	115.5	95.8	46.3	9.1	0.6
2006	14.2	68.5	0.6	41.9	22.0	73.0	105.9	116.7	97.7	47.3	9.4	0.6
2007	14.3	69.5	0.6	42.5	22.1	73.9	106.3	117.5	99.9	47.5	9.5	0.6
Race of child:[4] White												
1950	23.0	102.3	0.4	70.0	31.3	120.5	190.4	165.1	102.6	51.4	14.5	1.0
1960	22.7	113.2	0.4	79.4	35.5	154.6	252.8	194.9	109.6	54.0	14.7	0.8
1970	17.4	84.1	0.5	57.4	29.2	101.5	163.4	145.9	71.9	30.0	7.5	0.4
1980	14.9	64.7	0.6	44.7	25.2	72.1	109.5	112.4	60.4	18.5	3.4	0.2
Race of mother:[5] White												
1980	15.1	65.6	0.6	45.4	25.5	73.2	111.1	113.8	61.2	18.8	3.5	0.2
1985	15.0	64.1	0.6	43.3	24.4	70.4	104.1	112.3	69.9	23.3	3.7	0.2
1990	15.8	68.3	0.7	50.8	29.5	78.0	109.8	120.7	81.7	31.5	5.2	0.2
1995	14.1	63.6	0.8	49.5	29.6	80.2	104.7	111.7	83.3	34.2	6.4	0.3
2000	13.9	65.3	0.6	43.2	23.3	72.3	106.6	116.7	94.6	40.2	7.9	0.4
2005	13.4	66.3	0.5	37.0	18.9	64.7	99.2	118.3	99.3	47.3	9.0	0.6
2006	13.7	68.0	0.5	38.2	19.4	67.5	102.5	119.1	100.9	48.2	9.2	0.6
2007	13.7	68.8	0.5	38.8	19.7	68.1	102.8	119.4	102.7	48.1	9.4	0.6
Race of child:[4] Black or African American												
1960	31.9	153.5	4.3	156.1	- - -	- - -	295.4	218.6	137.1	73.9	21.9	1.1
1970	25.3	115.4	5.2	140.7	101.4	204.9	202.7	136.3	79.6	41.9	12.5	1.0
1980	22.1	88.1	4.3	100.0	73.6	138.8	146.3	109.1	62.9	24.5	5.8	0.3
Race of mother:[5] Black or African American												
1980	21.3	84.7	4.3	97.8	72.5	135.1	140.0	103.9	59.9	23.5	5.6	0.3
1985	20.4	78.8	4.5	95.4	69.3	132.4	135.0	100.2	57.9	23.9	4.6	0.3
1990	22.4	86.8	4.9	112.8	82.3	152.9	160.2	115.5	68.7	28.1	5.5	0.3
1995	17.8	71.0	4.1	94.4	68.5	135.0	133.7	95.6	63.0	28.4	6.0	0.3
2000	17.0	70.0	2.3	77.4	49.0	118.8	141.3	100.3	65.4	31.5	7.2	0.4
2005	16.2	69.0	1.7	62.0	35.5	104.9	129.9	105.9	70.3	35.3	8.5	0.5
2006	16.8	72.1	1.5	64.6	36.6	110.2	135.8	109.4	74.0	36.6	8.5	0.5
2007	16.9	72.7	1.5	64.9	36.1	110.7	135.9	109.6	75.4	36.9	8.8	0.6
American Indian or Alaska Native mothers[5]												
1980	20.7	82.7	1.9	82.2	51.5	129.5	143.7	106.6	61.8	28.1	8.2	*
1985	19.8	78.6	1.7	79.2	47.7	124.1	139.1	109.6	62.6	27.4	6.0	*
1990	18.9	76.2	1.6	81.1	48.5	129.3	148.7	110.3	61.5	27.5	5.9	*
1995	15.3	63.0	1.6	72.9	44.6	122.2	123.1	91.6	56.5	24.3	5.5	*
2000	14.0	58.7	1.1	58.3	34.1	97.1	117.2	91.8	55.5	24.6	5.7	0.3
2005	14.2	59.9	0.9	52.7	30.5	87.6	109.2	93.8	60.1	27.0	6.0	0.3
2006	14.9	63.1	0.9	55.0	30.7	93.0	115.4	97.8	61.8	28.4	6.1	0.4
2007	15.3	64.9	0.9	59.3	31.8	101.6	116.8	96.4	64.0	29.5	6.1	0.3

See footnotes at end of table.

Table 3 (page 2 of 3). Crude birth rates, fertility rates, and birth rates, by age, race, and Hispanic origin of mother: United States, selected years 1950–2007

[Data are based on birth certificates]

Race, Hispanic origin, and year	Crude birth rate[1]	Fertility rate[2]	10–14 years	15–19 years Total	15–17 years	18–19 years	20–24 years	25–29 years	30–34 years	35–39 years	40–44 years	45–54 years[3]
Asian or Pacific Islander mothers[5]					Live births per 1,000 women							
1980	19.9	73.2	0.3	26.2	12.0	46.2	93.3	127.4	96.0	38.3	8.5	0.7
1985	18.7	68.4	0.4	23.8	12.5	40.8	83.6	123.0	93.6	42.7	8.7	1.2
1990	19.0	69.6	0.7	26.4	16.0	40.2	79.2	126.3	106.5	49.6	10.7	1.1
1995	16.7	62.6	0.7	25.5	15.6	40.1	64.2	103.7	102.3	50.1	11.8	0.8
2000	17.1	65.8	0.3	20.5	11.6	32.6	60.3	108.4	116.5	59.0	12.6	0.8
2005	16.5	66.6	0.2	17.0	8.2	30.1	61.1	107.9	115.0	61.8	13.8	1.0
2006	16.6	67.5	0.2	17.0	8.8	29.5	63.2	108.4	116.9	63.0	14.1	1.0
2007	17.2	71.3	0.2	16.9	8.2	29.9	65.5	118.0	125.4	66.3	14.4	1.1
Hispanic or Latina mothers[5,6]												
1980	23.5	95.4	1.7	82.2	52.1	126.9	156.4	132.1	83.2	39.9	10.6	0.7
1990	26.7	107.7	2.4	100.3	65.9	147.7	181.0	153.0	98.3	45.3	10.9	0.7
1995	24.1	98.8	2.6	99.3	68.3	145.4	171.9	140.4	90.5	43.7	10.7	0.6
2000	23.1	95.9	1.7	87.3	55.5	132.6	161.3	139.9	97.1	46.6	11.5	0.6
2005	23.1	99.4	1.3	81.7	48.5	134.6	170.0	149.2	106.8	54.2	13.0	0.8
2006	23.4	101.5	1.3	83.0	47.9	139.7	177.0	152.4	108.5	55.6	13.3	0.8
2007	23.4	102.2	1.2	81.8	47.9	137.2	178.6	155.7	111.0	56.5	13.4	0.8
White, not Hispanic or Latina mothers[5,6]												
1980	14.2	62.4	0.4	41.2	22.4	67.7	105.5	110.6	59.9	17.7	3.0	0.1
1990	14.4	62.8	0.5	42.5	23.2	66.6	97.5	115.3	79.4	30.0	4.7	0.2
1995	12.5	57.5	0.4	39.3	22.0	66.2	90.2	105.1	81.5	32.8	5.9	0.3
2000	12.2	58.5	0.3	32.6	15.8	57.5	91.2	109.4	93.2	38.8	7.3	0.4
2005	11.5	58.3	0.2	25.9	11.5	48.0	81.4	109.1	96.9	45.6	8.3	0.5
2006	11.6	59.5	0.2	26.6	11.8	49.3	83.4	109.1	98.1	46.3	8.4	0.6
2007	11.6	60.1	0.2	27.2	11.8	50.4	83.2	108.6	99.5	45.8	8.6	0.6
Black or African American, not Hispanic or Latina mothers[5,6]												
1980	22.9	90.7	4.6	105.1	77.2	146.5	152.2	111.7	65.2	25.8	5.8	0.3
1990	23.0	89.0	5.0	116.2	84.9	157.5	165.1	118.4	70.2	28.7	5.6	0.3
1995	18.2	72.8	4.2	97.2	70.4	139.2	137.8	98.5	64.4	28.8	6.1	0.3
2000	17.3	71.4	2.4	79.2	50.1	121.9	145.4	102.8	66.5	31.8	7.2	0.4
2005	15.7	67.2	1.7	60.9	34.9	103.0	126.8	103.0	68.4	34.3	8.2	0.5
2006	16.5	70.6	1.6	63.7	36.2	108.4	133.2	107.1	72.6	36.0	8.3	0.5
2007	16.6	71.6	1.5	64.2	35.8	109.3	133.6	107.5	74.3	36.4	8.6	0.6

See footnotes at end of table.

Table 3 (page 3 of 3). Crude birth rates, fertility rates, and birth rates, by age, race, and Hispanic origin of mother: United States, selected years 1950–2007

[Data are based on birth certificates]

- - - Data not available.

* Rates based on fewer than 20 births are considered unreliable and are not shown.

[1]Live births per 1,000 population.

[2]Total number of live births regardless of age of mother per 1,000 women 15–44 years of age.

[3]Prior to 1997, data are for live births to mothers 45–49 years of age per 1,000 women 45–49 years of age. Starting with 1997 data, rates are for live births to mothers 45–54 years of age per 1,000 women 45–49 years of age. See Appendix II, Age.

[4]Live births are tabulated by race of child. See Appendix II, Race, Birth file.

[5]Live births are tabulated by race and/or Hispanic origin of mother. See Appendix II, Race, Birth file.

[6]Prior to 1993, data from states lacking an Hispanic-origin item on the birth certificate were excluded. See Appendix II, Hispanic origin. Rates in 1985 were not calculated because estimates for the Hispanic and non-Hispanic populations were not available.

NOTES: Data are based on births adjusted for underregistration for 1950 and on registered births for all other years. Starting with 1970 data, births to persons who were not residents of the 50 states and the District of Columbia are excluded. Starting with *Health, United States, 2003,* rates for 1991–1999 were revised using intercensal population estimates based on the 2000 census. Rates for 2000 were computed using the 2000 census counts and starting in 2001 rates were computed using 2000-based postcensal estimates. See Appendix I, Population Census and Population Estimates. The race groups white, black, American Indian or Alaska Native, and Asian or Pacific Islander include persons of Hispanic and non-Hispanic origin. Persons of Hispanic origin may be of any race. Starting with 2003 data, some states reported multiple-race data. The multiple-race data for these states were bridged to the single-race categories of the 1977 Office of Management and Budget standards for comparability with other states. See Appendix II, Race. Interpretation of trend data should take into consideration expansion of reporting areas and immigration. Some data have been revised and differ from previous editions of *Health, United States.* Data for additional years are available. See Appendix III.

SOURCE: CDC/NCHS, National Vital Statistics System, Birth File. Martin JA, Hamilton BE, Sutton PD, Ventura SJ, Mathews TJ, Kirmeyer S, Osterman MJK. Births: Final data for 2007. National vital statistics reports; vol 58 no 24. Hyattsville, MD: NCHS. 2010; Hamilton BE, Sutton PD, Ventura SJ. Revised birth and fertility rates for the 1990s and new rates for Hispanic populations, 2000 and 2001: United States. National vital statistics reports; vol 51 no 12. Hyattsville, MD: NCHS. 2003; Ventura SJ. Births of Hispanic parentage, 1980 and 1985. Monthly vital statistics report; vol 32 no 6 and vol 36 no 11, suppl. Public Health Service. Hyattsville, MD. 1983 and 1988; Internet release of: Vital statistics of the United States, 2000, vol 1, Natality, Tables 1–1 and 1–7; available from: http://www.cdc.gov/nchs/products/vsus.htm#electronic.

Table 4. Live births, by plurality and detailed race and Hispanic origin of mother: United States, selected years 1970–2007

[Data are based on birth certificates]

Plurality of birth and race and Hispanic origin of mother	1970	1971	1975	1980	1985	1990	1995	2000	2006	2007
All births					Number of live births					
All races	3,731,386	3,555,970	3,144,198	3,612,258	3,760,561	4,158,212	3,899,589	4,058,814	4,265,555	4,316,233
White	3,109,956	2,939,568	2,576,818	2,936,351	3,037,913	3,290,273	3,098,885	3,194,005	3,310,308	3,336,626
Black or African American	561,992	553,750	496,829	568,080	581,824	684,336	603,139	622,598	666,481	675,676
American Indian or Alaska Native	22,264	23,254	22,690	29,389	34,037	39,051	37,278	41,668	47,721	49,443
Asian or Pacific Islander[1]	- - -	27,004	28,884	74,355	104,606	141,635	160,287	200,543	241,045	254,488
Hispanic or Latina[2]	- - -	- - -	- - -	- - -	- - -	- - -	679,768	815,868	1,039,077	1,062,779
Mexican	- - -	- - -	- - -	- - -	- - -	- - -	469,615	581,915	718,146	722,055
Puerto Rican	- - -	- - -	- - -	- - -	- - -	- - -	54,824	58,124	66,932	68,488
Cuban	- - -	- - -	- - -	- - -	- - -	- - -	12,473	13,429	16,936	16,981
Central and South American	- - -	- - -	- - -	- - -	- - -	- - -	94,996	113,344	165,321	169,851
Other and unknown Hispanic or Latina	- - -	- - -	- - -	- - -	- - -	- - -	47,860	49,056	71,742	85,404
Not Hispanic or Latina:[2]										
White	- - -	- - -	- - -	- - -	- - -	- - -	2,382,638	2,362,968	2,308,640	2,310,333
Black or African American	- - -	- - -	- - -	- - -	- - -	- - -	587,781	604,346	617,247	627,191
Twin births										
All races	- - -	63,298	59,192	68,339	77,102	93,865	96,736	118,916	137,085	138,961
White	- - -	49,972	46,715	53,104	60,351	72,617	76,196	93,235	105,224	106,409
Black or African American	- - -	12,452	11,375	13,638	14,646	18,164	17,000	20,626	24,004	24,432
American Indian or Alaska Native	- - -	362	348	491	537	699	769	900	1,148	1,186
Asian or Pacific Islander[1]	- - -	320	505	1,045	1,536	2,320	2,771	4,155	6,709	6,934
Hispanic or Latina[2]	- - -	- - -	- - -	- - -	- - -	- - -	12,685	16,470	22,698	23,405
Mexican	- - -	- - -	- - -	- - -	- - -	- - -	8,341	11,130	14,532	14,754
Puerto Rican	- - -	- - -	- - -	- - -	- - -	- - -	1,248	1,461	1,999	2,097
Cuban	- - -	- - -	- - -	- - -	- - -	- - -	312	371	496	525
Central and South American	- - -	- - -	- - -	- - -	- - -	- - -	1,769	2,361	3,828	3,792
Other and unknown Hispanic or Latina	- - -	- - -	- - -	- - -	- - -	- - -	1,015	1,147	1,843	2,237
Not Hispanic or Latina:[2]										
White	- - -	- - -	- - -	- - -	- - -	- - -	62,370	76,018	83,108	83,632
Black or African American	- - -	- - -	- - -	- - -	- - -	- - -	16,622	20,173	22,702	23,101
Triplet and higher-order multiple births										
All races	- - -	1,034	1,066	1,337	1,925	3,028	4,973	7,325	6,540	6,427
White	- - -	834	909	1,104	1,648	2,639	4,505	6,551	5,613	5,404
Black or African American	- - -	196	151	211	240	321	352	521	620	660
American Indian or Alaska Native	- - -	0	2	9	13	4	20	18	27	39
Asian or Pacific Islander[1]	- - -	0	4	9	23	61	96	235	280	324
Hispanic or Latina[2]	- - -	- - -	- - -	- - -	- - -	- - -	355	659	787	857
Mexican	- - -	- - -	- - -	- - -	- - -	- - -	202	391	491	523
Puerto Rican	- - -	- - -	- - -	- - -	- - -	- - -	35	73	67	69
Cuban	- - -	- - -	- - -	- - -	- - -	- - -	24	15	15	30
Central and South American	- - -	- - -	- - -	- - -	- - -	- - -	59	122	143	176
Other and unknown Hispanic or Latina	- - -	- - -	- - -	- - -	- - -	- - -	35	58	71	59
Not Hispanic or Latina:[2]										
White	- - -	- - -	- - -	- - -	- - -	- - -	4,050	5,821	4,805	4,559
Black or African American	- - -	- - -	- - -	- - -	- - -	- - -	340	506	580	612

- - - Data not available.

[1]Starting with 2003 data, estimates are not available for Asian or Pacific Islander subgroups during the transition from single-race to multiple-race reporting. See Appendix II, Race, Birth file.

[2]Prior to 1993, data from states lacking an Hispanic-origin item on the birth certificate were excluded. See Appendix II, Hispanic origin.

NOTES: The race groups white, black, American Indian or Alaska Native, and Asian or Pacific Islander include persons of Hispanic and non-Hispanic origin. Persons of Hispanic origin may be of any race. Starting with 2003 data, some states reported multiple-race data. The multiple-race data for these states were bridged to the single-race categories of the 1977 Office of Management and Budget standards for comparability with other states. See Appendix II, Race. Interpretation of trend data should take into consideration expansion of reporting areas and immigration. Prior to 1993, only a portion of the states reported Hispanic origin on birth certificates. Starting in 1993, Hispanic origin of mother was reported by all 50 states and D.C. Therefore, before 1993, the total number of live births reported for Hispanics and Hispanic subgroups, as well as non-Hispanic whites and blacks, does not include live births in many states. Data for additional years are available. See Appendix III.

SOURCE: CDC/NCHS, National Vital Statistics System, Birth File. Martin JA, Hamilton BE, Sutton PD, Ventura SJ, Mathews TJ, Kirmeyer S, Osterman MJK. Births: Final data for 2007. National vital statistics reports; vol 58 no 24. Hyattsville, MD: NCHS. 2010; Births: Final data for each data year 1997–2005. National vital statistics reports. Hyattsville, MD; Final natality statistics for each data year 1970–1996. Monthly vital statistics report. Hyattsville, MD.

Table 5. Prenatal care for live births, by detailed race and Hispanic origin of mother: United States, selected years 1970–2000 and selected states 2006–2007

[Data are based on birth certificates]

Prenatal care, race, and Hispanic origin of mother	1970	1980	1990	2000	28 reporting areas (1989 revision) 2006[1]	28 reporting areas (1989 revision) 2007[1]	18 reporting areas (2003 revision) 2006[2]	18 reporting areas (2003 revision) 2007[2]
Prenatal care began during 1st trimester				Percent of live births[3]				
All races	68.0	76.3	75.8	83.2	82.4	82.0	69.0	67.5
White	72.3	79.2	79.2	85.0	84.4	84.0	70.9	69.5
Black or African American	44.2	62.4	60.6	74.3	75.6	75.0	58.3	57.0
American Indian or Alaska Native	38.2	55.8	57.9	69.3	68.9	68.3	54.3	53.2
Asian or Pacific Islander[4]	- - -	73.7	75.1	84.0	82.0	82.6	71.4	69.8
Hispanic or Latina[5]	- - -	60.2	60.2	74.4	72.3	72.4	57.7	56.1
Mexican	- - -	59.6	57.8	72.9	70.5	70.7	53.4	51.5
Puerto Rican	- - -	55.1	63.5	78.5	78.7	78.3	68.1	66.1
Cuban	- - -	82.7	84.8	91.7	83.3	83.6	80.4	78.9
Central and South American	- - -	58.8	61.5	77.6	71.8	71.7	61.0	59.0
Other and unknown Hispanic or Latina	- - -	66.4	66.4	75.8	78.3	79.0	63.5	63.7
Not Hispanic or Latina:[5]								
White	- - -	81.2	83.3	88.5	88.0	87.7	76.2	74.9
Black or African American	- - -	60.8	60.7	74.3	75.7	75.0	58.4	57.1
Prenatal care began during 3rd trimester or no prenatal care								
All races	7.9	5.1	6.1	3.9	3.9	3.9	7.9	8.4
White	6.3	4.3	4.9	3.3	3.3	3.2	7.2	7.6
Black or African American	16.6	8.9	11.3	6.7	5.8	6.0	11.8	12.6
American Indian or Alaska Native	28.9	15.2	12.9	8.6	8.2	8.5	13.2	14.0
Asian or Pacific Islander[4]	- - -	6.5	5.8	3.3	3.9	3.6	7.1	7.7
Hispanic or Latina[5]	- - -	12.0	12.0	6.3	6.4	6.2	12.2	12.9
Mexican	- - -	11.8	13.2	6.9	6.8	6.5	14.2	15.1
Puerto Rican	- - -	16.2	10.6	4.5	4.1	3.9	6.7	7.8
Cuban	- - -	3.9	2.8	1.4	3.7	3.2	3.1	3.4
Central and South American	- - -	13.1	10.9	5.4	6.9	6.7	10.1	11.0
Other and unknown Hispanic or Latina	- - -	9.2	8.5	5.9	4.9	5.0	9.5	9.4
Not Hispanic or Latina:[5]								
White	- - -	3.5	3.4	2.3	2.3	2.3	5.2	5.5
Black or African American	- - -	9.7	11.2	6.7	5.8	6.0	11.8	12.6

- - - Data not available.

[1]Data are for the 28 reporting areas that used the 1989 Revision of the U.S. Standard Certificate of Live Birth for data on prenatal care in 2006 and 2007. Reporting areas that have implemented the 2003 Revision of the U.S. Standard Certificate of Live Birth are excluded because prenatal care data based on the 2003 revision are not comparable with data based on the 1989 and earlier revisions of the U.S. Standard Certificate of Live Birth. See Appendix II, Prenatal care.

[2]Data are for the 18 reporting areas that used the 2003 Revision of the U.S. Standard Certificate of Live Birth for data on prenatal care in 2006 and 2007. Reporting areas that used the 1989 Revision of the U.S. Standard Certificate of Live Birth are excluded because prenatal care data based on the 2003 revision are not comparable with data based on the 1989 or earlier revisions.

[3]Excludes live births where trimester when prenatal care began is unknown.

[4]Starting with 2003 data, estimates are not available for Asian or Pacific Islander subgroups during the transition from single-race to multiple-race reporting. See Appendix II, Race, Birth file.

[5]Prior to 1993, data from states lacking an Hispanic-origin item on the birth certificate were excluded. See Appendix II, Hispanic origin. Data for non-Hispanic white and non-Hispanic black women for years prior to 1989 are not nationally representative and are provided for comparison with Hispanic data.

NOTES: Prior to 2003, all data are based on the 1989 and earlier revisions of the U.S. Standard Certificate of Live Birth. See Appendix II, Prenatal care. Data for 1970 and 1975 exclude births that occurred in states not reporting prenatal care. Starting in 2003 some states have implemented the 2003 Revision of the U.S. Standard Certificate of Live Birth on a voluntary basis. Data are not shown for 2006 and 2007 for the six states that implemented the 2003 revision mid-year 2006 or during 2007. California implemented a partial revision of the 2003 Revision of the U.S. Standard Certificate of Live Birth in 2006 but continued to use the 1989 revision format for data on prenatal care. See Appendix II, Prenatal care for a listing of states that used the 1989 and 2003 revisions in both 2006 and 2007. The race groups white, black, American Indian or Alaska Native, and Asian or Pacific Islander include persons of Hispanic and non-Hispanic origin. Persons of Hispanic origin may be of any race. Starting with 2003 data, some states reported multiple-race data. The multiple-race data for these states were bridged to the single-race categories of the 1977 Office of Management and Budget standards for comparability with other states. See Appendix II, Race. Interpretation of trend data should take into consideration changes in reporting areas and immigration. Data for additional years are available. See Appendix III.

SOURCE: CDC/NCHS, National Vital Statistics System, Birth File. Martin JA, Hamilton BE, Sutton PD, Ventura SJ, Mathews TJ, Kirmeyer S, Osterman MJK. Births: Final data for 2007. National vital statistics reports; vol 58 no 24. Hyattsville, MD: NCHS. 2010; Births: Final data for each data year 1997–2005. National vital statistics reports. Hyattsville, MD; Final natality statistics for each data year 1970–1996. Monthly vital statistics report. Hyattsville, MD.

Table 6. Teenage childbearing, by detailed race and Hispanic origin of mother: United States, selected years 1970–2007

[Data are based on birth certificates]

Maternal age, race, and Hispanic origin of mother	1970	1975	1980	1985	1990	1995	2000	2004	2005	2006	2007
Age of mother under 18 years					Percent of live births						
All races	6.3	7.6	5.8	4.7	4.7	5.3	4.1	3.4	3.4	3.4	3.4
White	4.8	6.0	4.5	3.7	3.6	4.3	3.5	3.0	2.9	3.0	3.0
Black or African American	14.8	16.3	12.5	10.6	10.1	10.8	7.8	6.4	6.2	6.2	6.1
American Indian or Alaska Native	7.5	11.2	9.4	7.6	7.2	8.7	7.3	6.4	6.5	6.2	6.1
Asian or Pacific Islander[1]	- - -	- - -	1.5	1.6	2.1	2.2	1.5	1.1	1.0	1.0	0.9
Hispanic or Latina[2]	- - -	- - -	7.4	6.4	6.6	7.6	6.3	5.4	5.3	5.2	5.3
Mexican	- - -	- - -	7.7	6.9	6.9	8.0	6.6	5.8	5.7	5.6	5.7
Puerto Rican	- - -	- - -	10.0	8.5	9.1	10.8	7.8	6.8	6.5	6.3	6.2
Cuban	- - -	- - -	3.8	2.2	2.7	2.8	3.1	2.4	2.4	2.5	2.3
Central and South American	- - -	- - -	2.4	2.4	3.2	4.1	3.3	2.8	2.9	2.9	3.0
Other and unknown Hispanic or Latina	- - -	- - -	6.5	7.0	8.0	9.0	7.6	6.3	6.6	6.5	6.7
Not Hispanic or Latina:[2]											
White	- - -	- - -	4.0	3.2	3.0	3.4	2.6	2.0	2.0	2.0	2.0
Black or African American	- - -	- - -	12.7	10.7	10.2	10.8	7.8	6.5	6.3	6.3	6.1
Age of mother 18–19 years											
All races	11.3	11.3	9.8	8.0	8.1	7.9	7.7	6.8	6.8	7.0	7.1
White	10.4	10.3	9.0	7.1	7.3	7.2	7.1	6.4	6.5	6.5	6.5
Black or African American	16.6	16.9	14.5	12.9	13.0	12.4	11.9	10.7	10.6	10.8	11.1
American Indian or Alaska Native	12.8	15.2	14.6	12.4	12.3	12.7	12.4	11.5	11.3	11.4	12.2
Asian or Pacific Islander[1]	- - -	- - -	3.9	3.4	3.7	3.5	3.0	2.3	2.3	2.2	2.2
Hispanic or Latina[2]	- - -	- - -	11.6	10.1	10.2	10.3	9.9	8.9	8.8	9.0	8.9
Mexican	- - -	- - -	12.0	10.6	10.7	10.8	10.4	9.4	9.2	9.4	9.2
Puerto Rican	- - -	- - -	13.3	12.4	12.6	12.7	12.2	10.8	10.9	11.4	11.0
Cuban	- - -	- - -	9.2	4.9	5.0	4.9	4.4	5.4	5.3	5.5	5.9
Central and South American	- - -	- - -	6.0	5.8	5.9	6.5	6.5	5.6	5.7	6.0	6.1
Other and unknown Hispanic or Latina	- - -	- - -	10.8	10.5	11.1	11.1	11.3	9.9	10.5	10.4	10.5
Not Hispanic or Latina:[2]											
White	- - -	- - -	8.5	6.5	6.6	6.4	6.1	5.4	5.3	5.4	5.5
Black or African American	- - -	- - -	14.7	12.9	13.0	12.4	12.0	10.8	10.7	10.9	11.1

- - - Data not available.

[1]Starting with 2003 data, estimates are not available for Asian or Pacific Islander subgroups during the transition from single-race to multiple-race reporting. See Appendix II, Race, Birth file.

[2]Prior to 1993, data from states lacking an Hispanic-origin item on the birth certificate were excluded. See Appendix II, Hispanic origin. Data for non-Hispanic white and non-Hispanic black women for years prior to 1989 are not nationally representative and are provided for comparison with Hispanic data.

NOTES: The race groups, white, black, American Indian or Alaska Native, and Asian or Pacific Islander, include persons of Hispanic and non-Hispanic origin. Persons of Hispanic origin may be of any race. Starting with 2003 data, some states reported multiple-race data. The multiple-race data for these states were bridged to the single-race categories of the 1977 Office of Management and Budget standards for comparability with other states. See Appendix II, Race. Interpretation of trend data should take into consideration expansion of reporting areas and immigration. Data for additional years are available. See Appendix III.

SOURCE: CDC/NCHS, National Vital Statistics System, Birth File.

Table 7. Nonmarital childbearing, by detailed race and Hispanic origin of mother, and maternal age: United States, selected years 1970–2007

[Data are based on birth certificates]

Race, Hispanic origin of mother, and maternal age	1970	1975	1980	1985	1990	1995	2000	2004	2005	2006	2007
	Live births per 1,000 unmarried women 15–44 years of age[1]										
All races and origins	26.4	24.5	29.4	32.8	43.8	44.3	44.1	46.1	47.5	50.6	52.3
White[2]	13.9	12.4	18.1	22.5	32.9	37.0	38.2	41.6	43.0	46.1	48.1
Black or African American[2]	95.5	84.2	81.1	77.0	90.5	74.5	70.5	67.2	67.8	71.5	72.6
Asian or Pacific Islander	- - -	- - -	- - -	- - -	- - -	- - -	20.9	23.6	24.9	25.9	27.3
Hispanic or Latina[3]	- - -	- - -	- - -	- - -	89.6	88.8	87.2	95.7	100.3	106.1	108.4
White, not Hispanic or Latina	- - -	- - -	- - -	- - -	24.4	28.1	28.0	29.4	30.1	32.0	33.3
	Percent of live births to unmarried mothers										
All races and origins	10.7	14.3	18.4	22.0	28.0	32.2	33.2	35.8	36.9	38.5	39.7
White	5.5	7.1	11.2	14.7	20.4	25.3	27.1	30.5	31.7	33.3	34.8
Black or African American	37.5	49.5	56.1	61.2	66.5	69.9	68.5	68.8	69.3	70.2	71.2
American Indian or Alaska Native	22.4	32.7	39.2	46.8	53.6	57.2	58.4	62.3	63.5	64.6	65.3
Asian or Pacific Islander[4]	- - -	- - -	7.3	9.5	13.2	16.3	14.8	15.5	16.2	16.5	16.6
Hispanic or Latina[3]	- - -	- - -	23.6	29.5	36.7	40.8	42.7	46.4	48.0	49.9	51.3
Mexican	- - -	- - -	20.3	25.7	33.3	38.1	40.7	45.2	46.7	48.6	50.1
Puerto Rican	- - -	- - -	46.3	51.1	55.9	60.0	59.6	61.0	61.7	62.4	63.4
Cuban	- - -	- - -	10.0	16.1	18.2	23.8	27.3	33.2	36.4	39.4	41.8
Central and South American	- - -	- - -	27.1	34.9	41.2	44.1	44.7	47.6	49.2	51.5	52.7
Other and unknown Hispanic or Latina	- - -	- - -	22.4	31.1	37.2	44.0	46.2	46.6	48.6	49.2	51.3
Not Hispanic or Latina:[3]											
White	- - -	- - -	9.5	12.4	16.9	21.2	22.1	24.5	25.3	26.6	27.8
Black or African American	- - -	- - -	57.2	62.0	66.7	70.0	68.7	69.3	69.9	70.7	71.6
	Number of live births, in thousands										
Live births to unmarried mothers	399	448	666	828	1,165	1,254	1,347	1,470	1,527	1,642	1,715
Maternal age	Percent distribution of live births to unmarried mothers										
Under 20 years	50.1	52.1	40.8	33.8	30.9	30.9	28.0	23.7	23.1	22.7	22.5
20–24 years	31.8	29.9	35.6	36.3	34.7	34.5	37.4	38.5	38.3	38.1	37.6
25 years and over	18.1	18.0	23.5	29.9	34.4	34.7	34.6	37.8	38.7	39.2	39.9

- - - Data not available.

[1]Rates computed by relating births to unmarried mothers, regardless of age of mother, to unmarried women 15–44 years of age. Population data for unmarried American Indian or Alaska Native women are not available for rate calculations. Prior to 2000, population data for unmarried Asian or Pacific Islander women were not available for rate calculations.

[2]For 1970 and 1975, birth rates are by race of child.

[3]Prior to 1993, data from states lacking an Hispanic-origin item on the birth certificate were excluded. See Appendix II, Hispanic origin. Data for non-Hispanic white and non-Hispanic black women for years prior to 1989 are not nationally representative and are provided for comparison with Hispanic data.

[4]Starting with 2003 data, estimates are not available for Asian or Pacific Islander subgroups during the transition from single-race to multiple-race reporting. See Appendix II, Race, Birth file.

NOTES: National estimates for 1970 and 1975 for unmarried mothers are based on births occurring in states reporting marital status of mother. Changes in reporting procedures for marital status occurred in some states during the 1990s. Interpretation of trend data should also take into consideration expansion of reporting areas and immigration. See Appendix II, Marital status. The race groups white, black, American Indian or Alaska Native, and Asian or Pacific Islander include persons of Hispanic and non-Hispanic origin. Persons of Hispanic origin may be of any race. Starting with 2003 data, some states reported multiple-race data. The multiple-race data for these states were bridged to the single-race categories of the 1977 Office of Management and Budget standards for comparability with other states. See Appendix II, Race. Starting with *Health, United States, 2003*, rates for 1991–1999 were revised using intercensal population estimates based on the 2000 census. Rates for 2000 were computed using the 2000 census counts and starting with 2001, rates were computed using 2000-based postcensal estimates. Some data have been revised and differ from previous editions of *Health, United States*. Data for additional years are available. See Appendix III.

SOURCE: CDC/NCHS, National Vital Statistics System, Birth File. Martin JA, Hamilton BE, Sutton PD, Ventura SJ, Mathews TJ, Kirmeyer S, Osterman MJK. Births: Final data for 2007. National vital statistics reports; vol 58 no 24. Hyattsville, MD: NCHS. 2010; Hamilton BE, Sutton PD, Ventura SJ. Revised birth and fertility rates for the 1990s and new rates for Hispanic populations, 2000 and 2001: United States. National vital statistics reports; vol 51 no 12. Hyattsville, MD: NCHS. 2003; Births: Final data for each data year 1997–2006. National vital statistics reports. Hyattsville, MD; Final natality statistics for each data year 1993–1996. Monthly vital statistics report. Hyattsville, MD; Ventura SJ. Births to unmarried mothers: United States, 1980–1992. Vital Health Stat 21(53). 1995.

Table 8. Mothers who smoked cigarettes during pregnancy, by selected characteristics: United States, selected years 1990–2000 and selected states 2006–2007

[Data are based on birth certificates]

Characteristic of mother	1990[1]	2000[1]	28 reporting areas (1989 revision) 2006[1,2]	28 reporting areas (1989 revision) 2007[1,2]	17 reporting areas (2003 revision) 2006[1,3]	17 reporting areas (2003 revision) 2007[1,3]
Race of mother	Percent of mothers who smoked [1,4,5]					
All races	18.4	12.2	9.5	9.3	13.2	13.0
White.	19.4	13.2	10.4	10.2	14.0	13.8
Black or African American	15.9	9.1	7.5	7.4	10.4	10.4
American Indian or Alaska Native.	22.4	20.0	16.2	16.2	24.6	23.7
Asian or Pacific Islander[6,7]	5.5	2.8	2.1	2.0	2.4	2.3
Hispanic origin and race of mother[8]						
Hispanic or Latina[6]	6.7	3.5	2.6	2.4	2.8	2.7
Mexican	5.3	2.4	1.8	1.7	2.0	1.9
Puerto Rican.	13.6	10.3	7.8	7.4	14.3	14.1
Cuban	6.4	3.3	5.6	5.7	10.2	8.8
Central and South American	3.0	1.5	1.0	0.9	1.1	0.9
Other and unknown Hispanic or Latina	10.8	7.4	6.0	5.1	3.6	3.9
Not Hispanic or Latina:						
White.	21.0	15.6	12.8	12.7	18.1	18.0
Black or African American.	15.9	9.2	8.0	7.7	10.6	10.6
Age of mother[5]						
Under 15 years.	7.5	7.1	3.5	4.1	5.7	3.6
15–19 years.	20.8	17.8	13.1	12.5	17.5	17.1
15–17 years	17.6	15.0	10.0	9.3	12.7	12.0
18–19 years	22.5	19.2	14.6	14.0	19.7	19.4
20–24 years.	22.1	16.8	14.3	14.1	19.5	19.1
25–29 years.	18.0	10.5	9.2	9.2	12.6	12.6
30–34 years.	15.3	8.0	5.5	5.4	7.5	7.5
35–39 years.	13.3	9.1	5.3	5.1	7.3	7.1
40–54 years[9]	12.3	9.5	6.0	5.6	7.8	7.6
Education of mother[10]	Percent of mothers 20 years of age and over who smoked [1,5]					
0–8 years[2].	17.5	7.9	5.8	5.6	- - -	- - -
9–11 years[2].	40.5	28.2	23.4	22.8	- - -	- - -
12 years[2].	21.9	16.6	14.0	13.9	- - -	- - -
13–15 years[2].	12.8	9.1	8.0	8.0	- - -	- - -
16 years or more[2]	4.5	2.0	1.3	1.3	- - -	- - -
No high school diploma or GED[3]	- - -	- - -	- - -	- - -	18.4	18.5
High school diploma or GED[3]	- - -	- - -	- - -	- - -	20.7	20.3
Some college, no Bachelor's degree[3].	- - -	- - -	- - -	- - -	12.3	12.3
Bachelor's degree or more[3].	- - -	- - -	- - -	- - -	1.7	1.7

- - - Data not available.

[1]Maternal tobacco use during pregnancy was not reported on the birth certificates of California.

[2]Data are for the 28 reporting areas that used the 1989 Revision of the U.S. Standard Certificate of Live Birth for data on smoking in 2006 and 2007. Reporting areas that have implemented the 2003 revision of the U.S. Standard Certificate of Live Birth are excluded because maternal tobacco use and education data based on the 2003 revision are not comparable with data based on the 1989 revision. See Appendix II, Cigarette smoking.

[3]Data are for the 17 reporting areas that used the 2003 Revision of the U.S. Standard Certificate of Live Birth for data on smoking in 2006 and 2007. Reporting areas that used the 1989 Revision of the U.S. Standard Certificate of Live Birth are excluded because smoking and education data based on the 2003 revision are not comparable with data based on the 1989 revision.

[4]Data from states that did not require the reporting of mother's tobacco use during pregnancy on the birth certificate are not included. Reporting area for tobacco use increased from 43 states and the District of Columbia (D.C.) in 1989 to 49 states and D.C. in 2000–2002. See Appendix II, Cigarette smoking.

[5]Excludes live births for whom smoking status of mother is unknown.

[6]Data from California are excluded because mother's tobacco use is unknown. In 2007, California accounted for 29% of the births to Asian or Pacific Islander mothers and 28% of the births to Hispanic mothers.

[7]Starting with 2003 data, estimates are not available for Asian or Pacific Islander subgroups during the transition from single-race to multiple-race reporting. See Appendix II, Race, Birth file.

[8]Data from states that did not require the reporting of Hispanic origin of mother on the birth certificate are not included. Reporting of Hispanic origin increased from 47 states in 1989 to include all 50 states and D.C. by 1993. See Appendix II, Hispanic origin.

[9]Prior to 1997, data are for live births to mothers 40–49 years of age.

[10]Data from states that did not require the reporting of mother's education on the birth certificate are not included. See Appendix II, Education.

NOTES: Prior to 2003, all data are based on the 1989 Revision of the U.S. Standard Certificate of Live Birth. Starting in 2003 some states have implemented the 2003 Revision of the U.S. Standard Certificate of Live Birth on a voluntary basis. Data are not shown for 2006 and 2007 for the six states that implemented the 2003 revision mid-year 2006 or during 2007. See Appendix II, Cigarette smoking for a listing of states that used the 2003 revision in 2006 and 2007. The race groups white, black, American Indian or Alaska Native, and Asian or Pacific Islander include persons of Hispanic and non-Hispanic origin. Persons of Hispanic origin may be of any race. Starting with 2003 data, some states reported multiple-race data. The multiple-race data for these states were bridged to the single-race categories of the 1977 Office of Management and Budget standards for comparability with other states. See Appendix II, Race. Interpretation of trend data should take into consideration changes in reporting areas and immigration. Data for additional years are available. See Appendix III.

SOURCE: CDC/NCHS, National Vital Statistics System, Birth File.

Table 9. Low birthweight live births, by detailed race, Hispanic origin, and smoking status of mother: United States, selected years 1970–2007

[Data are based on birth certificates]

Birthweight, race and Hispanic origin of mother, and smoking status of mother	1970	1975	1980	1985	1990	1995	2000	2005	2006	2007
Low birthweight (less than 2,500 grams)					Percent of live births [1]					
All races	7.93	7.38	6.84	6.75	6.97	7.32	7.57	8.19	8.26	8.22
White	6.85	6.27	5.72	5.65	5.70	6.22	6.55	7.16	7.21	7.16
Black or African American	13.90	13.19	12.69	12.65	13.25	13.13	12.99	13.59	13.59	13.55
American Indian or Alaska Native	7.97	6.41	6.44	5.86	6.11	6.61	6.76	7.36	7.52	7.46
Asian or Pacific Islander [2]	- - -	- - -	6.68	6.16	6.45	6.90	7.31	7.98	8.12	8.10
Hispanic or Latina [3]	- - -	- - -	6.12	6.16	6.06	6.29	6.41	6.88	6.99	6.93
Mexican	- - -	- - -	5.62	5.77	5.55	5.81	6.01	6.49	6.58	6.50
Puerto Rican	- - -	- - -	8.95	8.69	8.99	9.41	9.30	9.92	10.14	9.83
Cuban	- - -	- - -	5.62	6.02	5.67	6.50	6.49	7.64	7.14	7.66
Central and South American	- - -	- - -	5.76	5.68	5.84	6.20	6.34	6.78	6.81	6.71
Other and unknown Hispanic or Latina	- - -	- - -	6.96	6.83	6.87	7.55	7.84	8.27	8.54	8.61
Not Hispanic or Latina: [3]										
White	- - -	- - -	5.69	5.61	5.61	6.20	6.60	7.29	7.32	7.28
Black or African American	- - -	- - -	12.71	12.62	13.32	13.21	13.13	14.02	13.97	13.90
									17 reporting areas	
Cigarette smoker [4]	- - -	- - -	- - -	- - -	A	A	A	A	12.02	12.08
Nonsmoker [4]	- - -	- - -	- - -	- - -	A	A	A	A	7.69	7.61
Very low birthweight (less than 1,500 grams)										
All races	1.17	1.16	1.15	1.21	1.27	1.35	1.43	1.49	1.49	1.49
White	0.95	0.92	0.90	0.94	0.95	1.06	1.14	1.20	1.20	1.19
Black or African American	2.40	2.40	2.48	2.71	2.92	2.97	3.07	3.15	3.05	3.11
American Indian or Alaska Native	0.98	0.95	0.92	1.01	1.01	1.10	1.16	1.17	1.28	1.27
Asian or Pacific Islander [2]	- - -	- - -	0.92	0.85	0.87	0.91	1.05	1.14	1.12	1.14
Hispanic or Latina [3]	- - -	- - -	0.98	1.01	1.03	1.11	1.14	1.20	1.19	1.21
Mexican	- - -	- - -	0.92	0.97	0.92	1.01	1.03	1.12	1.12	1.13
Puerto Rican	- - -	- - -	1.29	1.30	1.62	1.79	1.93	1.87	1.91	1.89
Cuban	- - -	- - -	1.02	1.18	1.20	1.19	1.21	1.50	1.28	1.27
Central and South American	- - -	- - -	0.99	1.01	1.05	1.13	1.20	1.19	1.13	1.15
Other and unknown Hispanic or Latina	- - -	- - -	1.01	0.96	1.09	1.28	1.42	1.36	1.36	1.44
Not Hispanic or Latina: [3]										
White	- - -	- - -	0.87	0.91	0.93	1.04	1.14	1.21	1.20	1.19
Black or African American	- - -	- - -	2.47	2.67	2.93	2.98	3.10	3.27	3.15	3.20
									17 reporting areas	
Cigarette smoker [4]	- - -	- - -	- - -	- - -	A	A	A	A	1.73	1.82
Nonsmoker [4]	- - -	- - -	- - -	- - -	A	A	A	A	1.41	1.40

- - - Data not available.

[A] Data not shown. Due to a change in reporting, data are not comparable to other years. See footnote 4.

[1] Excludes live births with unknown birthweight. Percent based on live births with known birthweight.

[2] Starting with 2003 data, estimates are not available for Asian or Pacific Islander subgroups during the transition from single-race to multiple-race reporting. See Appendix II, Race, Birth file.

[3] Prior to 1993, data from states lacking an Hispanic-origin item on the birth certificate were excluded. See Appendix II, Hispanic origin. Data for non-Hispanic white and non-Hispanic black women for years prior to 1989 are not nationally representative and are provided for comparison with Hispanic data.

[4] Percent based on live births with known smoking status of mother and known birthweight. Only reporting areas that have implemented the 2003 Revision of the U.S. Standard Certificate of Live Birth are shown because maternal tobacco use data based on the 2003 revision are not comparable with data based on the 1989 or earlier revisions to the U.S. Standard Certificate of Live Birth. In addition, California did not require reporting of tobacco use during pregnancy. Data are for the 17 reporting areas that used the 2003 Revision of the U.S. Standard Certificate of Live Birth for data on smoking in 2006 and 2007. See Appendix II, Cigarette smoking. For data for reporting areas that use the 1989 Revision of the U.S. Standard Certificate of Live Birth, see: Martin JA, Hamilton BE, Sutton PD, Ventura SJ, Menacker F, Kirmeyer S, Mathews TJ. Births: Final data for 2006. National vital statistics reports; vol 57 no 7. Hyattsville, MD: NCHS; 2009. Available from: http://www.cdc.gov/nchs/data/nvsr/nvsr57/nvsr57_07.pdf.

NOTES: The race groups, white, black, American Indian or Alaska Native, and Asian or Pacific Islander, include persons of Hispanic and non-Hispanic origin. Persons of Hispanic origin may be of any race. Starting with 2003 data, some states reported multiple-race data. The multiple-race data for these states were bridged to the single-race categories of the 1977 Office of Management and Budget standards for comparability with other states. See Appendix II, Race. Interpretation of trend data should take into consideration expansion of reporting areas and immigration. Data for additional years are available. See Appendix III.

SOURCE: CDC/NCHS, National Vital Statistics System, Birth File.

Table 10 (page 1 of 3). Low birthweight live births among mothers 20 years of age and over, by detailed race, Hispanic origin, and education of mother: United States, selected years and reporting areas 1989–2007

[Data are based on birth certificates]

Education, race, and Hispanic origin of mother	1989	1990	2000	2002	28 reporting areas (1989 revision)	
					2006[1]	2007[1]
Less than 12 years of education	Percent of live births weighing less than 2,500 grams[2]					
All races	9.0	8.6	8.2	8.2	9.2	9.1
White	7.3	7.0	7.1	7.1	7.9	7.7
Black or African American	17.0	16.5	14.9	15.0	15.0	15.6
American Indian or Alaska Native	7.3	7.4	7.2	8.4	7.6	8.1
Asian or Pacific Islander[3]	6.6	6.4	7.2	7.4	7.2	6.7
Hispanic or Latina[4]	6.0	5.7	6.0	6.0	6.6	6.4
Mexican	5.3	5.2	5.6	5.7	6.1	5.8
Puerto Rican	11.3	10.3	10.9	10.4	11.7	11.8
Cuban	9.4	7.9	8.4	7.5	*11.6	*
Central and South American	5.8	5.8	6.2	6.2	6.4	6.3
Other and unknown Hispanic or Latina	8.2	8.0	8.6	7.8	9.5	8.8
Not Hispanic or Latina:[4]						
White	8.4	8.3	9.0	9.3	10.1	10.2
Black or African American	17.6	16.7	15.2	15.3	16.3	16.5
12 years of education						
All races	7.1	7.1	7.9	8.2	9.1	9.0
White	5.7	5.8	6.8	7.0	7.7	7.6
Black or African American	13.4	13.1	13.0	13.4	13.9	13.9
American Indian or Alaska Native	5.6	6.1	6.7	7.1	7.5	7.3
Asian or Pacific Islander[3]	6.4	6.5	7.4	7.9	8.2	7.9
Hispanic or Latina[4]	5.9	6.0	6.2	6.5	7.1	7.0
Mexican	5.2	5.5	5.8	6.1	6.3	6.4
Puerto Rican	8.8	8.3	8.8	9.3	10.5	9.9
Cuban	5.3	5.2	6.5	6.0	8.1	8.2
Central and South American	5.7	5.8	6.0	6.4	6.5	6.3
Other and unknown Hispanic or Latina	6.1	6.6	7.3	7.7	8.7	8.5
Not Hispanic or Latina:[4]						
White	5.7	5.7	6.9	7.3	7.9	7.8
Black or African American	13.6	13.2	13.1	13.5	14.4	14.4
13 years or more of education						
All races	5.5	5.4	6.6	7.0	7.5	7.4
White	4.6	4.6	5.8	6.2	6.6	6.5
Black or African American	11.2	11.1	11.6	12.0	12.3	12.3
American Indian or Alaska Native	5.6	4.7	6.5	7.0	6.6	6.9
Asian or Pacific Islander[3]	6.1	6.0	7.0	7.6	8.4	8.3
Hispanic or Latina[4]	5.5	5.5	6.2	6.6	7.4	7.3
Mexican	5.1	5.2	5.8	6.2	6.8	6.1
Puerto Rican	7.4	7.4	7.9	8.9	9.5	9.3
Cuban	4.9	5.0	5.9	6.4	7.1	8.7
Central and South American	5.2	5.6	6.3	6.5	6.9	7.1
Other and unknown Hispanic or Latina	5.4	5.2	6.6	7.0	8.0	8.4
Not Hispanic or Latina:[4]						
White	4.6	4.5	5.8	6.2	6.5	6.4
Black or African American	11.2	11.1	11.7	12.1	12.6	12.5

See footnotes at end of table.

Table 10 (page 2 of 3). Low birthweight live births among mothers 20 years of age and over, by detailed race, Hispanic origin, and education of mother: United States, selected years and reporting areas 1989–2007

[Data are based on birth certificates]

Education, race, and Hispanic origin of mother	19 reporting areas (2003 revision)	
	2006[5]	2007[5]
No high school diploma or GED	Percent of live births weighing less than 2,500 grams[2]	
All races	7.9	8.0
White.	7.1	7.2
Black or African American	14.6	14.4
American Indian or Alaska Native	8.4	8.9
Asian or Pacific Islander[3]	7.5	7.0
Hispanic or Latina.	6.4	6.4
Mexican	6.1	6.2
Puerto Rican.	10.6	10.9
Cuban	9.5	8.3
Central and South American	6.8	6.3
Other and unknown Hispanic or Latina	8.5	8.7
Not Hispanic or Latina:		
White	9.4	9.6
Black or African American.	15.5	15.5
High school diploma or GED		
All races	8.5	8.3
White.	7.5	7.3
Black or African American	13.6	13.8
American Indian or Alaska Native	8.3	7.2
Asian or Pacific Islander[3]	8.1	7.5
Hispanic or Latina.	6.8	6.7
Mexican	6.6	6.4
Puerto Rican.	9.2	8.8
Cuban	6.6	7.3
Central and South American	6.6	6.4
Other and unknown Hispanic or Latina	8.0	8.3
Not Hispanic or Latina:		
White	7.9	7.8
Black or African American.	14.0	14.2
Some college, no Bachelor's degree		
All races	7.7	7.7
White.	6.8	6.8
Black or African American	12.5	12.5
American Indian or Alaska Native	7.3	6.8
Asian or Pacific Islander[3]	8.0	7.9
Hispanic or Latina.	7.0	7.1
Mexican	6.7	6.8
Puerto Rican.	8.9	8.6
Cuban	6.9	7.3
Central and South American	6.6	6.9
Other and unknown Hispanic or Latina	7.9	8.0
Not Hispanic or Latina:		
White	6.8	6.7
Black or African American.	12.7	12.8
Bachelor's degree or more		
All races	6.8	6.8
White.	6.3	6.3
Black or African American	11.2	11.2
American Indian or Alaska Native	7.1	6.5
Asian or Pacific Islander[3]	7.8	7.9
Hispanic or Latina.	6.8	6.7
Mexican	6.7	6.6
Puerto Rican.	7.1	8.3
Cuban	6.1	7.3
Central and South American	6.9	6.2
Other and unknown Hispanic or Latina	7.6	7.3
Not Hispanic or Latina:		
White	6.3	6.2
Black or African American.	11.4	11.4

See footnotes at end of table.

Table 10 (page 3 of 3). Low birthweight live births among mothers 20 years of age and over, by detailed race, Hispanic origin, and education of mother: United States, selected years and reporting areas 1989–2007

[Data are based on birth certificates]

* Percents preceded by an asterisk are based on fewer than 50 births in the numerator. Percents not shown are based on fewer than 20 births.
[1]Data are for the 28 reporting areas (26 states, District of Columbia (D.C.), and New York City) that used the 1989 Revision of the U.S. Standard Certificate of Live Birth in 2006 and 2007. Reporting areas that have implemented the 2003 Revision of the U.S. Standard Certificate of Live Birth are excluded because maternal education data based on the 2003 revision are not comparable with data based on the 1989 or earlier revisions See Appendix II, Education.
[2]Excludes live births with unknown birthweight. Percent based on live births with known birthweight.
[3]Starting with 2003 data, estimates are not available for Asian or Pacific Islander subgroups during the transition from single-race to multiple-race reporting. See Appendix II, Race, Birth file.
[4]Prior to 1993, data shown only for states with an Hispanic-origin item and education of mother item on the birth certificate. See Appendix II, Education; Hispanic origin.
[5]Data are for the 19 reporting areas that used the 2003 Revision of the U.S. Standard Certificate of Live Birth in 2006 and 2007. Reporting areas that used the 1989 Revision of the U.S. Standard Certificate of Live Birth are excluded because maternal education data based on the 2003 revision are not comparable with data based on the 1989 or earlier revisions See Appendix II, Education.

NOTES: Prior to 2003, all data are based on the 1989 or earlier revisions of the U.S. Standard Certificate of Live Birth. In 1992–2002, education of mother was reported on the birth certificate by all 50 states and D.C. Prior to 1992, data from states lacking an education of mother item were excluded. Starting in 2003 some states have implemented the 2003 Revision of the U.S. Standard Certificate of Live Birth on a voluntary basis. Data are not shown for 2006 and 2007 for the seven states that implemented the 2003 revision mid-year 2006 or during 2007. See Appendix II, Education, for a listing of states that used the 2003 revisions in 2006 and 2007. The race groups white, black, American Indian or Alaska Native, and Asian or Pacific Islander include persons of Hispanic and non-Hispanic origin. Persons of Hispanic origin may be of any race. Starting with 2003 data, some states reported multiple-race data. The multiple-race data for these states were bridged to the single-race categories of the 1977 Office of Management and Budget standards for comparability with other states. See Appendix II, Race. Interpretation of trend data should take into consideration changes in reporting areas and immigration. Some data have been revised and differ from previous editions of *Health, United States.* Data for additional years are available. See Appendix III.

SOURCE: CDC/NCHS, National Vital Statistics System, Birth File.

Table 11 (page 1 of 2). Low birthweight live births, by race and Hispanic origin of mother, and by state: United States, 1999–2001, 2002–2004, and 2005–2007

[Data are based on birth certificates]

| | All races | | | Not Hispanic or Latina | | | | | |
| | | | | White | | | Black or African American | | |
State	1999–2001	2002–2004	2005–2007	1999–2001	2002–2004	2005–2007	1999–2001	2002–2004	2005–2007
	Percent of live births weighing less than 2,500 grams [1]								
United States..........	7.62	7.94	8.22	6.67	7.05	7.30	13.14	13.56	13.96
Alabama	9.56	10.09	10.51	7.58	8.18	8.56	13.87	14.63	15.47
Alaska.............	5.70	5.93	5.90	5.03	4.98	5.78	10.64	9.52	12.08
Arizona	6.95	7.00	7.05	6.73	6.94	6.90	13.19	12.09	12.95
Arkansas	8.66	8.92	9.08	7.48	7.78	7.86	13.60	14.54	14.75
California	6.20	6.56	6.85	5.72	6.13	6.42	11.73	12.14	12.17
Colorado	8.43	8.94	9.04	8.02	8.71	8.78	14.39	14.98	15.26
Connecticut	7.47	7.68	8.05	6.33	6.60	6.94	12.53	12.60	12.73
Delaware	8.84	9.45	9.35	7.28	7.85	7.57	13.71	14.36	14.49
District of Columbia....	12.37	11.19	11.25	6.56	5.91	6.84	15.17	14.09	14.41
Florida.............	8.10	8.49	8.70	6.92	7.29	7.51	12.42	13.02	13.52
Georgia	8.72	9.08	9.54	6.85	7.29	7.49	12.82	13.42	14.37
Hawaii	7.74	8.26	8.08	5.60	6.47	6.01	10.77	11.47	10.45
Idaho.............	6.43	6.48	6.70	6.31	6.39	6.74	*	*8.87	*8.99
Illinois	7.99	8.28	8.55	6.59	7.13	7.32	14.03	14.45	14.65
Indiana	7.62	7.86	8.35	7.04	7.29	7.73	12.85	13.33	13.91
Iowa	6.23	6.74	6.97	5.97	6.57	6.80	12.58	11.50	11.65
Kansas	6.99	7.22	7.14	6.66	6.92	6.85	12.36	12.95	13.10
Kentucky	8.26	8.69	9.17	7.73	8.25	8.73	13.69	13.82	14.57
Louisiana	10.25	10.69	11.37	7.36	7.76	8.55	14.40	14.91	15.98
Maine	6.03	6.42	6.65	6.06	6.41	6.59	*9.97	*8.57	8.70
Maryland	8.88	9.13	9.21	6.70	7.14	7.25	13.12	13.16	13.13
Massachusetts	7.11	7.64	7.90	6.43	6.98	7.27	11.44	11.86	11.60
Michigan	7.95	8.17	8.35	6.43	6.90	7.11	14.47	14.21	14.15
Minnesota	6.17	6.34	6.59	5.79	5.86	6.07	10.61	10.51	10.82
Mississippi	10.55	11.40	12.17	7.72	8.50	8.88	14.03	15.31	16.40
Missouri...........	7.64	8.10	8.00	6.68	7.18	7.04	13.22	13.76	13.78
Montana	6.65	7.10	7.04	6.69	6.94	6.80	*	*15.63	*
Nebraska	6.73	7.04	7.03	6.37	6.86	6.52	12.81	12.32	13.59
Nevada	7.45	7.86	8.27	7.38	7.51	8.00	12.69	13.87	14.46
New Hampshire	6.36	6.44	6.72	6.04	6.51	6.62	11.88	10.19	10.30
New Jersey	7.94	8.13	8.43	6.54	7.03	7.32	13.45	13.42	13.65
New Mexico	7.87	8.21	8.74	7.85	8.01	8.72	13.37	14.99	14.76
New York	7.75	7.98	8.25	6.47	6.68	6.99	11.97	12.50	12.78
North Carolina	8.87	9.00	9.16	7.39	7.64	7.80	13.72	14.16	14.46
North Dakota	6.26	6.46	6.45	6.23	6.26	6.41	*	*10.25	*6.88
Ohio	7.93	8.38	8.74	6.95	7.36	7.67	13.36	13.83	14.19
Oklahoma	7.55	7.92	8.17	7.23	7.63	7.77	12.93	13.48	14.79
Oregon	5.52	5.99	6.08	5.32	5.92	5.94	10.64	10.67	9.82
Pennsylvania	7.84	8.14	8.42	6.68	6.97	7.26	13.87	13.86	13.78
Rhode Island	7.27	8.17	7.93	6.52	7.50	7.42	12.55	11.52	10.91
South Carolina	9.69	10.08	10.15	7.30	7.77	7.80	14.29	15.01	15.22
South Dakota	6.15	6.90	6.86	6.02	6.74	6.67	*11.42	*8.08	10.37
Tennessee	9.21	9.23	9.52	7.96	8.08	8.39	14.12	14.37	14.77
Texas	7.43	7.88	8.38	6.68	7.23	7.65	12.76	13.45	14.23
Utah	6.60	6.55	6.80	6.43	6.32	6.55	12.49	13.76	10.78
Vermont...........	5.90	6.63	6.43	5.79	6.67	6.31	*	*	*9.80
Virginia	7.85	8.13	8.35	6.52	6.80	7.15	12.39	12.82	13.11
Washington	5.74	6.04	6.31	5.40	5.61	5.84	10.30	10.83	10.10
West Virginia	8.28	8.96	9.58	8.11	8.80	9.44	13.20	13.52	14.80
Wisconsin	6.59	6.80	6.96	5.82	6.06	6.18	13.28	13.49	13.47
Wyoming	8.32	8.67	8.88	8.15	8.57	9.04	*14.29	*	*15.05

See footnotes at end of table.

Table 11 (page 2 of 2). Low birthweight live births, by race and Hispanic origin of mother, and by state: United States, 1999–2001, 2002–2004, and 2005–2007

[Data are based on birth certificates]

State	Hispanic or Latina[2]			American Indian or Alaska Native[3]			Asian or Pacific Islander[3]		
	1999–2001	2002–2004	2005–2007	1999–2001	2002–2004	2005–2007	1999–2001	2002–2004	2005–2007
	Percent of live births weighing less than 2,500 grams[1]								
United States.	6.42	6.68	6.94	7.08	7.35	7.45	7.42	7.82	8.07
Alabama	6.68	6.93	6.73	*8.25	11.50	*7.18	7.59	8.52	7.74
Alaska	6.09	5.62	5.51	5.83	6.08	5.13	7.05	6.79	6.54
Arizona	6.67	6.67	6.65	7.12	6.84	7.13	7.69	8.20	7.97
Arkansas	5.92	5.96	6.91	7.95	8.41	7.51	8.80	6.78	7.79
California	5.59	5.95	6.26	6.27	6.54	6.93	6.98	7.33	7.68
Colorado	8.23	8.46	8.54	8.60	9.82	10.08	10.10	10.14	10.21
Connecticut	8.60	8.41	8.46	*8.09	8.97	8.59	7.59	7.96	8.42
Delaware	6.62	7.06	7.22	*	*	*	8.98	9.61	8.49
District of Columbia. . . .	6.99	8.20	7.35	*	*	*	*8.79	7.36	8.96
Florida	6.49	6.90	7.05	7.08	7.68	6.96	8.51	8.57	8.38
Georgia	5.66	5.94	6.06	9.79	8.48	9.20	7.67	8.40	8.17
Hawaii	7.63	8.41	8.30	*6.11	*	*	8.29	8.79	8.81
Idaho	6.78	6.73	6.27	7.82	7.07	7.20	7.62	6.51	7.67
Illinois	6.38	6.41	6.90	9.05	8.63	8.89	8.37	8.23	8.57
Indiana	6.10	6.19	6.85	*6.89	*9.54	*6.94	7.42	7.59	8.02
Iowa	5.83	6.16	6.10	*7.36	8.72	8.48	7.72	7.11	8.25
Kansas	6.00	6.14	5.68	6.36	7.08	6.38	7.34	7.15	7.65
Kentucky	7.18	7.13	7.12	*	*9.93	*7.12	7.68	7.35	8.12
Louisiana	6.70	7.25	6.95	8.41	10.31	8.95	7.92	8.55	8.22
Maine	*4.91	*5.46	*7.40	*	*	*	*5.42	7.85	7.97
Maryland	6.80	7.09	7.07	9.95	11.07	*8.08	7.37	7.67	7.94
Massachusetts	8.28	8.46	8.27	*6.84	*6.13	11.21	7.38	7.66	8.15
Michigan	6.37	6.41	6.88	7.24	6.50	7.62	7.72	8.22	8.16
Minnesota	5.98	5.85	5.75	6.92	7.18	6.36	7.48	7.41	7.75
Mississippi	6.92	6.79	6.63	8.42	6.00	7.32	7.75	7.58	9.06
Missouri	5.98	6.39	5.92	8.95	6.53	7.10	6.89	7.83	7.30
Montana	7.02	8.11	7.89	6.77	7.71	7.97	*6.42	*8.76	*9.38
Nebraska	6.49	6.05	6.52	6.32	7.11	7.44	7.91	7.70	7.75
Nevada	6.21	6.61	6.71	7.80	6.73	7.59	7.88	9.41	10.62
New Hampshire	5.89	5.35	7.60	*	*	*	5.83	6.08	8.27
New Jersey	7.19	7.22	7.44	10.04	10.67	10.20	7.67	7.86	8.46
New Mexico	7.93	8.38	8.74	6.88	7.18	7.85	8.28	7.62	9.43
New York	7.41	7.48	7.82	8.44	6.84	7.10	7.24	7.84	7.91
North Carolina	6.21	6.22	6.32	10.33	11.16	10.64	8.05	7.79	8.52
North Dakota	*6.89	*6.42	7.22	6.21	7.15	6.31	*	*6.56	*6.32
Ohio	7.23	7.18	7.52	8.39	10.04	10.70	7.36	8.67	8.44
Oklahoma	6.03	6.55	6.46	6.34	6.53	7.19	7.19	7.13	7.15
Oregon	5.51	5.28	5.86	6.79	7.35	6.44	6.08	7.12	7.32
Pennsylvania	8.95	9.11	8.83	9.41	11.03	11.02	7.38	7.91	8.12
Rhode Island	7.07	8.24	8.11	*10.67	12.37	14.13	8.78	10.83	8.60
South Carolina	6.57	6.46	6.71	10.20	*9.11	9.67	7.10	8.97	8.01
South Dakota	*6.07	7.12	6.33	6.25	7.14	7.36	*9.37	*12.89	*7.23
Tennessee	6.57	5.97	6.34	*7.13	*7.43	6.55	8.03	8.22	8.26
Texas	6.76	7.08	7.54	6.76	7.54	8.16	7.74	8.19	8.69
Utah	7.33	7.06	7.31	6.58	7.64	7.57	7.18	7.94	8.45
Vermont	*	*	*	*	*	*	*	*6.52	*8.20
Virginia	5.96	6.31	6.18	*9.23	*10.13	*7.23	7.15	7.95	7.66
Washington	5.31	5.67	6.03	7.14	7.03	7.68	6.41	6.88	7.32
West Virginia	*	*8.26	*4.19	*	*	*	*7.94	*8.24	9.33
Wisconsin	6.29	6.10	6.36	5.97	6.29	6.44	7.02	7.45	7.27
Wyoming	7.86	8.60	7.36	8.93	10.62	8.37	*17.06	*	*11.11

* Percents preceded by an asterisk are based on fewer than 50 births. Percents not shown are based on fewer than 20 births.
[1]Excludes live births with unknown birthweight.
[2]Persons of Hispanic origin may be of any race. See Appendix II, Hispanic origin.
[3]Includes persons of Hispanic and non-Hispanic origin.

NOTES: For information on very low birthweight live births, see Table 37 in Martin JA, Hamilton BE, Sutton PD, Ventura SJ, Mathews TJ, Kirmeyer S, Osterman MJK. Births: Final data for 2007. National vital statistics reports; vol 58 no 24. Hyattsville, MD: NCHS; 2010. Available from: http://www.cdc.gov/nchs/data/nvsr/nvsr58/nvsr58_24.pdf; Starting with 2003 data, some states reported multiple-race data. The multiple-race data for these states were bridged to the single-race categories of the 1977 Office of Management and Budget standards for comparability with other states. See Appendix II, Race.

SOURCE: CDC/NCHS, National Vital Statistics System, Birth File.

Table 12 (page 1 of 2). Legal abortions and legal abortion ratios, by selected patient characteristics: United States, selected years 1973–2006

[Data are based on reporting by state health departments and by hospitals and other medical facilities]

Characteristic	1973	1975	1980	1985	1990	1995	1999[1]	2000[2]	2004[3]	2005[4]	2006[4]
	Number of legal abortions reported in thousands										
Centers for Disease Control and Prevention (CDC)	616	855	1,298	1,329	1,429	1,211	862	857	839	820	846
Guttmacher Institute[5]	745	1,034	1,554	1,589	1,609	1,359	1,315	1,313	1,222	1,206	- - -
	Abortions per 100 live births[6]										
Total CDC	19.6	27.2	35.9	35.4	34.4	31.1	25.6	24.5	23.8	23.3	23.3
Age											
Under 15 years	123.7	119.3	139.7	137.6	81.8	66.4	70.9	70.8	76.2	76.4	75.4
15–19 years	53.9	54.2	71.4	68.8	51.1	39.9	37.5	36.1	36.2	35.8	35.1
20–24 years	29.4	28.9	39.5	38.6	37.8	34.8	31.6	30.0	29.1	28.3	28.0
25–29 years	20.7	19.2	23.7	21.7	21.8	22.0	20.8	19.8	19.1	18.7	18.8
30–34 years	28.0	25.0	23.7	19.9	19.0	16.4	15.2	14.5	14.3	14.0	14.0
35–39 years	45.1	42.2	41.0	33.6	27.3	22.3	19.3	18.1	17.0	16.8	17.0
40 years and over	68.4	66.8	80.7	62.3	50.6	38.5	32.9	30.1	28.6	27.8	27.6
Race											
White[7]	32.6	27.7	33.2	27.7	25.8	20.3	17.7	16.7	16.1	15.8	16.2
Black or African American[8]	42.0	47.6	54.3	47.2	53.7	53.1	52.9	50.3	47.2	46.7	45.9
Hispanic origin[9]											
Hispanic or Latina	- - -	- - -	- - -	- - -	- - -	27.1	26.1	22.5	21.1	20.5	20.0
Not Hispanic or Latina	- - -	- - -	- - -	- - -	- - -	27.9	25.2	23.3	23.6	22.3	22.4
Marital status											
Married	7.6	9.6	10.5	8.0	8.7	7.6	7.0	6.5	6.1	5.8	- - -
Unmarried	139.8	161.0	147.6	117.4	86.3	64.5	60.4	57.0	51.0	48.5	- - -
Previous live births[10]											
0	43.7	38.4	45.7	45.1	36.0	28.6	24.3	22.6	23.0	22.6	- - -
1	23.5	22.0	20.2	21.6	22.7	22.0	20.6	19.4	19.0	18.2	- - -
2	36.8	36.8	29.5	29.9	31.5	30.6	29.0	27.4	26.4	25.4	- - -
3	46.9	47.7	29.8	18.2	30.1	30.7	29.8	28.5	27.4	26.4	- - -
4 or more[11]	44.7	43.5	24.3	21.5	26.6	23.7	24.2	23.7	22.9	21.9	- - -
	Percent distribution[12]										
Total	100.0	100.0	100.0	100.0	100.0	100.0	100.0	100.0	100.0	100.0	100.0
Period of gestation											
Under 9 weeks	36.1	44.6	51.7	50.3	51.6	54.0	57.6	58.1	61.4	62.1	62.0
9–10 weeks	29.4	28.4	26.2	26.6	25.3	23.1	20.2	19.8	17.6	17.1	17.1
11–12 weeks	17.9	14.9	12.2	12.5	11.7	10.9	10.2	10.2	9.3	9.3	9.3
13–15 weeks	6.9	5.0	5.1	5.9	6.4	6.3	6.2	6.2	6.3	6.3	6.3
16–20 weeks	8.0	6.1	3.9	3.9	4.0	4.3	4.3	4.3	4.0	3.8	3.8
21 weeks and over	1.7	1.0	0.9	0.8	1.0	1.4	1.5	1.4	1.4	1.4	1.4
Previous induced abortions											
0	- - -	81.9	67.6	60.1	57.1	55.1	53.7	54.7	55.0	54.9	55.2
1	- - -	14.9	23.5	25.7	26.9	26.9	27.1	26.4	25.8	25.8	25.5
2	- - -	2.5	6.6	9.8	10.1	10.9	11.5	11.3	11.3	11.4	11.2
3 or more	- - -	0.7	2.3	4.4	5.9	7.1	7.7	7.6	7.9	7.9	8.0

See footnotes at end of table.

Table 12 (page 2 of 2). Legal abortions and legal abortion ratios, by selected patient characteristics: United States, selected years 1973–2006

[Data are based on reporting by state health departments and by hospitals and other medical facilities]

- - - Data not available.

[1]In 1998 and 1999, Alaska, California, New Hampshire, and Oklahoma did not report abortion data to CDC. For comparison, in 1997, the 48 corresponding reporting areas reported about 900,000 legal abortions.

[2]In 2000, 2001, and 2002, Alaska, California, and New Hampshire did not report abortion data to CDC.

[3]In 2003 and 2004, California, New Hampshire, and West Virginia did not report abortion data to CDC.

[4]In 2005 and 2006, California, Louisiana, and New Hampshire did not report abortion data to CDC.

[5]No surveys were conducted in 1983, 1986, 1989, 1990, 1993, 1994, 1997, 1998, 2001, 2002, or 2003. Data for these years were estimated by interpolation. See Appendix I, Guttmacher Institute.

[6]For calculation of ratios by each characteristic, abortions with characteristic unknown were distributed in proportion to abortions with characteristic known.

[7]For 1989 and later years, white race includes women of Hispanic ethnicity.

[8]Before 1989, black race includes races other than white.

[9]Data from 20–22 states, the District of Columbia (DC), and New York City (NYC) were included in 1991–1993. The number of reporting areas increased to 25 states, DC, and NYC in 1994–2004. States were excluded either because they did not collect data on Hispanic origin or due to incomplete reporting of Hispanic data (greater than 15% unknown Hispanic origin). See Appendix I, Abortion Surveillance.

[10]For 1973–1975, data indicate number of living children.

[11]For 1975, data refer to four previous live births, not four or more. For five or more previous live births, the ratio is 47.3.

[12]For calculation of percent distribution by each characteristic, abortions with characteristic unknown were excluded.

NOTES: The number of areas reporting adequate data (less than or equal to 15% missing) for each characteristic varies from year to year. For methodological differences between these two data sources, see Appendix I, Abortion Surveillance; Guttmacher Institute Abortion Provider Survey. Data for additional years are available. See Appendix III.

SOURCE: CDC, National Center for Chronic Disease Prevention and Health Promotion: Abortion Surveillance, 1973, 1975, 1979–1980. Atlanta, GA: Public Health Service, 1975, 1977, 1983; CDC MMWR Surveillance Summaries. Abortion Surveillance, United States, 1984 and 1985, vol 38, no SS–2, 1989; 1990, vol 42, no SS–6, 1993; 1995, vol 47, no SS–2, 1998; 1997, vol 49, no SS–11, 2000; 1998, vol 51, no SS–3, 2002; 1999, vol 51, no SS–9, 2002; 2000, vol 52, no SS–12, 2003; 2001, vol 53, no SS–9, 2004; 2002, vol 54, no SS–7, 2005; 2003, vol 55, no SS–11, 2006; 2004, vol 56, no SS–09, 2007; 2005, vol 57, no SS–13, 2008; 2006, vol 58, no SS–08, 2009. Guttmacher Institute Abortion Provider Survey. Finer LB, Henshaw SK. Abortion incidence and services in the United States in 2000. Perspect Sex Reprod Health 2003;35(1)6–15. Finer LB, Henshaw SK. Estimates of U.S. abortion incidence, 2001–2003. Guttmacher Institute. August 2006. Jones RK, Zolna MRS, Henshaw SK, Finer LB. Abortion in the United States: Incidence and access to services, 2005. Perspect Sex Reprod Health 2008;40(1)6–16. Available from: http://www.guttmacher.org/journals/toc/psrh4001toc.html.

Table 13 (page 1 of 5). Contraceptive use in the past month among women 15–44 years of age, by age, race, Hispanic origin, and method of contraception: United States, selected years 1982–2008

[Data are based on household interviews of samples of women of childbearing age]

Race, Hispanic origin, and year[1]	Age in years				
	15–44	15–19	20–24	25–34	35–44
	Number of women in population in thousands				
All women:[2]					
1982	54,099	9,521	10,629	19,644	14,305
1995	60,201	8,961	9,041	20,758	21,440
2002	61,561	9,834	9,840	19,522	22,365
2006–2008	61,864	10,431	10,140	19,837	21,457
Not Hispanic or Latina:					
White only:					
1982	41,279	7,010	8,081	14,945	11,243
1995	42,154	5,865	6,020	14,471	15,798
2002	39,498	6,069	5,938	12,073	15,418
2006–2008	37,660	6,186	6,122	11,954	13,397
Black or African American only:					
1982	6,825	1,383	1,456	2,392	1,593
1995	8,060	1,334	1,305	2,780	2,641
2002	8,250	1,409	1,396	2,587	2,857
2006–2008	8,452	1,606	1,440	2,704	2,702
Hispanic or Latina:[3]					
1982	4,393	886	811	1,677	1,018
1995	6,702	1,150	1,163	2,450	1,940
2002	9,107	1,521	1,632	3,249	2,705
2006–2008	10,377	1,812	1,705	3,656	3,204
	Percent of women in population using contraception				
All women:[2]					
1982	55.7	24.2	55.8	66.7	61.6
1995	64.2	29.8	63.5	71.1	72.3
2002	61.9	31.5	60.7	68.6	69.9
2006–2008	61.8	28.2	54.7	67.2	76.5
Not Hispanic or Latina:					
White only:					
1982	57.3	23.6	58.7	67.8	63.5
1995	66.2	30.5	65.4	72.9	73.6
2002	64.6	35.0	66.3	69.9	71.4
2006–2008	64.7	31.7	57.6	69.6	78.8
Black or African American only:					
1982	51.6	29.8	52.3	63.5	52.0
1995	62.3	36.1	67.6	66.8	68.3
2002	57.6	32.9	50.8	67.9	63.8
2006–2008	54.5	25.3	46.4	62.5	68.2
Hispanic or Latina:[3]					
1982	50.6	*	*36.8	67.2	59.0
1995	59.0	26.1	50.6	69.2	70.8
2002	59.0	20.4	57.4	66.2	72.9
2006–2008	58.5	20.5	51.3	64.3	77.2

See footnotes at end of table.

Table 13 (page 2 of 5). Contraceptive use in the past month among women 15–44 years of age, by age, race, Hispanic origin, and method of contraception: United States, selected years 1982–2008

[Data are based on household interviews of samples of women of childbearing age]

Race, Hispanic origin, and year[1]	Age in years				
	15–44	15–19	20–24	25–34	35–44
	Number of sexually active women in population in thousands[4]				
All women:[2]					
1982	- - -	- - -	- - -	- - -	- - -
1995	41,796	3,341	6,272	15,687	16,495
2002	42,683	3,775	6,798	14,857	17,252
2006–2008	42,756	3,618	6,475	14,713	17,951
Not Hispanic or Latina:					
White only:					
1982	- - -	- - -	- - -	- - -	- - -
1995	29,994	2,202	4,276	11,194	12,322
2002	28,079	2,519	4,329	9,224	12,006
2006–2008	26,889	2,317	4,001	9,054	11,516
Black or African American only:					
1982	- - -	- - -	- - -	- - -	- - -
1995	5,579	598	967	2,039	1,975
2002	5,611	564	949	1,978	2,121
2006–2008	5,504	511	871	2,056	2,066
Hispanic or Latina:[3]					
1982	- - -	- - -	- - -	- - -	- - -
1995	4,330	409	685	1,794	1,442
2002	6,075	405	1,070	2,462	2,138
2006–2008	6,669	488	1,001	2,569	2,610
	Percent of sexually active women in population using contraception[4]				
All women:[2]					
1982	- - -	- - -	- - -	- - -	- - -
1995	92.5	80.2	91.7	94.0	93.9
2002	89.3	82.0	87.9	90.2	90.7
2006–2008	89.4	81.3	85.7	90.5	91.4
Not Hispanic or Latina:					
White only:					
1982	- - -	- - -	- - -	- - -	- - -
1995	93.0	81.7	93.0	93.9	94.2
2002	90.9	84.4	90.9	91.5	91.7
2006–2008	90.6	84.5	88.2	91.8	91.6
Black or African American only:					
1982	- - -	- - -	- - -	- - -	- - -
1995	90.0	80.0	91.3	91.6	90.9
2002	84.7	82.2	74.8	88.9	86.0
2006–2008	83.7	79.4	76.7	82.2	89.1
Hispanic or Latina:[3]					
1982	- - -	- - -	- - -	- - -	- - -
1995	91.4	75.5	82.5	95.4	95.2
2002	88.4	76.4	87.5	87.4	92.3
2006–2008	91.1	76.2	87.4	91.6	94.8

See footnotes at end of table.

Table 13 (page 3 of 5). Contraceptive use in the past month among women 15–44 years of age, by age, race, Hispanic origin, and method of contraception: United States, selected years 1982–2008

[Data are based on household interviews of samples of women of childbearing age]

Method of contraception and year	Age in years				
	15–44	15–19	20–24	25–34	35–44
Female sterilization	Percent of contracepting women				
1982	23.2	—	*4.5	22.1	43.5
1995	27.8	*	4.0	23.8	45.0
2002	27.0	—	3.6	21.7	45.8
2006–2008	27.1	*	*2.4	22.2	44.2
Male sterilization					
1982	10.9	*	*3.6	10.1	19.9
1995	10.9	—	*	7.8	19.5
2002	10.2	—	*	7.2	18.2
2006–2008	10.9	—	-	6.6	19.8
Implant and other hormonal contraceptives[5]					
1982	. . .	. . .	. . .	. . .	. . .
1995	1.3	*	3.7	*1.3	*
2002	1.2	*	*	*1.9	*
2006–2008	1.1	1.8	1.4	*1.7	0.5
Injectable[5]					
1982	. . .	. . .	. . .	. . .	. . .
1995	3.0	9.7	6.1	2.9	*0.8
2002	5.4	13.9	10.2	5.3	*1.8
2006–2008	3.2	9.4	*5.1	3.7	*1.1
Birth control pill					
1982	28.0	63.9	55.1	25.7	*3.7
1995	27.0	43.8	52.1	33.4	8.7
2002	31.0	53.8	52.5	34.8	15.0
2006–2008	29.1	54.6	48.1	31.4	16.3
Intrauterine device					
1982	7.1	*	*4.2	9.7	6.9
1995	0.8	—	*	*0.8	1.1
2002	2.2	*	1.8	3.7	*
2006–2008	5.6	3.6	5.9	6.5	5.0
Diaphragm					
1982	8.1	*6.0	10.2	10.3	4.0
1995	1.9	*	*	1.7	2.8
2002	—	-	*	*	*
2006–2008	—	-	—	*	*
Condom					
1982	12.0	20.8	10.7	11.4	11.3
1995	23.4	45.8	33.7	23.7	15.3
2002	23.8	44.6	36.0	23.1	15.6
2006–2008	22.5	37.6	37.2	26.3	11.7
Periodic abstinence–calendar rhythm					
1982	3.3	2.0	3.1	3.3	3.7
1995	3.3	*	*1.5	3.7	3.9
2002	2.0	*	*2.3	*1.7	*2.4
2006–2008	1.8	*	—	2.3	1.9
Periodic abstinence–natural family planning					
1982	0.6	—	*	0.9	*
1995	*0.5	—	*	*0.7	*
2002	*0.4	—	-	*	*
2006–2008	—	-	*	—	—
Withdrawal					
1982	2.0	2.9	3.0	1.8	1.3
1995	6.1	13.2	7.1	6.0	4.5
2002	8.8	15.0	11.9	10.7	4.7
2006–2008	10.1	11.0	14.0	12.6	6.6
Other methods[6]					
1982	4.9	2.6	5.4	4.8	5.3
1995	3.2	*	3.2	3.1	3.4
2002	1.7	*	*	*1.5	*1.8
2006–2008	2.9	—	*6.7	3.8	—

See footnotes at end of table.

Table 13 (page 4 of 5). **Contraceptive use in the past month among women 15–44 years of age, by age, race, Hispanic origin, and method of contraception: United States, selected years 1982–2008**

[Data are based on household interviews of samples of women of childbearing age]

Method of contraception and year	Not Hispanic or Latina[1]		Hispanic or Latina[3]
	White only	Black or African American only	
Female sterilization	*Percent of contracepting women*		
1982	22.0	30.0	23.0
1995	24.5	39.9	36.6
2002	23.9	39.2	33.8
2006–2008	23.0	39.9	33.5
Male sterilization			
1982	13.0	*1.5	*
1995	13.7	*1.8	*4.0
2002	12.9	*	4.7
2006–2008	14.1	2.4	6.1
Implant and other hormonal contraceptives[5]			
1982	. . .	. . .	. . .
1995	*1.0	*2.4	*2.0
2002	*0.8	*	*3.1
2006–2008	0.7	–	–
Injectable[5]			
1982	. . .	. . .	. . .
1995	2.4	5.4	4.7
2002	4.2	9.4	7.3
2006–2008	2.1	*7.5	*4.5
Birth control pill			
1982	26.4	37.9	30.2
1995	28.7	23.7	23.0
2002	34.9	23.1	22.1
2006–2008	34.1	21.9	20.3
Intrauterine device			
1982	5.8	9.3	19.2
1995	0.7	*	*
2002	1.7	*	5.3
2006–2008	5.1	–	8.3
Diaphragm			
1982	9.2	*3.2	*
1995	2.3	*	*
2002	*	*	–
2006–2008	–	–	*
Condom			
1982	13.1	6.3	*6.9
1995	22.5	24.9	21.2
2002	21.7	29.6	24.1
2006–2008	21.0	27.2	19.3
Periodic abstinence–calendar rhythm			
1982	3.2	2.9	3.9
1995	3.3	*1.7	3.2
2002	2.3	*	*
2006–2008	1.5	–	*2.5
Periodic abstinence–natural family planning			
1982	0.7	0.3	–
1995	0.7	*	*
2002	*	*	*
2006–2008	–	*	*
Withdrawal			
1982	2.1	1.3	2.6
1995	6.4	3.3	5.7
2002	9.5	4.9	6.3
2006–2008	10.3	6.3	9.8

See footnotes at end of table.

Table 13 (page 5 of 5). Contraceptive use in the past month among women 15–44 years of age, by age, race, Hispanic origin, and method of contraception: United States, selected years 1982–2008

[Data are based on household interviews of samples of women of childbearing age]

	Not Hispanic or Latina[1]		Hispanic or Latina[3]
Method of contraception and year	White only	Black or African American only	
Other methods[6]	Percent of contracepting women		
1982	4.6	7.3	5.0
1995	3.3	3.8	*2.2
2002	*1.7	*1.9	*1.2
2006–2008	3.2	3.2	2.3

- - - Data not available.
– Quantity zero.
. . . Data not applicable.
* Estimates are considered unreliable. Data preceded by an asterisk have a relative standard error (RSE) of 20%–30%. Data not shown have an RSE greater than 30%.
[1]Starting with 1995 data, race-specific estimates are tabulated according to 1997 Revisions to the Standards for the Classification of Federal Data on Race and Ethnicity and are not strictly comparable with estimates for earlier years. Starting with 1995 data, race-specific estimates are for persons who reported only one racial group. Prior to data year 1995, data were tabulated according to the 1977 Standards. Estimates for single-race categories prior to 1995 included persons who reported one race or, if they reported more than one race, identified one race as best representing their race. See Appendix II, Race.
[2]Includes women of other or unknown race not shown separately.
[3]Persons of Hispanic origin may be of any race. See Appendix II, Hispanic origin.
[4]Had sexual (vaginal) intercourse in the past 3 months.
[5]Data collected starting with the 1995 survey.
[6]In 2006–2008, includes contraceptive ring, female condom/vaginal pouch, foam, cervical cap, Today® sponge, suppository or insert, jelly or cream (without diaphragm), and other methods. See Appendix II, Contraception, for the list of other methods reported in previous surveys.

NOTES: Survey collects up to four methods of contraception used in the month of interview. Percents may not add to the total because more than one method could have been used in the month of interview. These data replace estimates of most effective method used and may differ from previous editions of *Health, United States*. Standard errors for selected years are available in the spreadsheet version of this table. Available from: http://www.cdc.gov/nchs/hus.htm. Data for additional years are available. See Appendix III.

SOURCE: CDC/NCHS, National Survey of Family Growth.

Table 14. Breastfeeding among mothers 15–44 years of age, by year of baby's birth and selected characteristics of mother: United States, average annual 1986–1988 through 2002–2004

[Data are based on household interviews of samples of women of childbearing age]

Selected characteristics of mother	1986–1988	1989–1991	1992–1994	1995–1998	1999–2001	2002–2004
			Percent of babies breastfed			
Total	54.1	53.3	57.6	64.4	66.5	73.3
Age at baby's birth						
Under 20 years.	28.4	34.7	41.0	49.5	47.3	73.2
20–24 years.	48.2	44.3	50.0	55.9	59.3	66.2
25–29 years.	58.2	56.4	57.4	68.1	63.5	72.5
30–44 years.	68.6	66.0	70.2	72.8	80.0	78.4
Race and Hispanic origin[1]						
Not Hispanic or Latina:						
White only.	59.1	58.4	61.7	66.5	68.7	79.1
Black or African American only	22.3	22.4	26.1	47.9	45.3	44.4
Hispanic or Latina	55.6	57.0	63.8	71.2	76.0	76.5
Education[2]						
No high school diploma or GED	31.8	36.5	44.6	50.6	46.6	61.0
High school diploma or GED	47.4	45.5	51.1	55.9	61.6	63.0
Some college, no bachelor's degree . . .	62.2	61.4	64.3	70.1	75.6	70.4
Bachelor's degree or higher	78.4	80.6	82.5	82.0	81.3	91.5
Geographic region[3]						
Northeast	51.3	53.5	56.5	61.6	66.9	75.5
Midwest	52.3	49.6	51.7	61.7	61.9	67.9
South.	44.6	43.6	48.6	58.1	60.9	70.2
West	71.4	69.5	77.3	78.1	78.9	84.0
			Percent of babies who were breastfed 3 months or more			
Total	34.6	31.8	33.6	45.8	48.4	53.2
Age at baby's birth						
Under 20 years.	18.5	*10.5	*11.7	30.0	30.0	48.8
20–24 years.	26.1	24.1	25.1	36.6	41.8	39.3
25–29 years.	36.9	32.3	35.6	46.3	43.7	50.5
30–44 years.	50.1	46.8	46.7	57.5	62.4	64.7
Race and Hispanic origin[1]						
Not Hispanic or Latina:						
White only.	37.7	35.2	36.6	47.8	49.7	57.1
Black or African American only	11.6	11.5	13.3	29.6	33.7	30.1
Hispanic or Latina	38.2	33.9	35.0	49.7	54.3	58.2
Education[2]						
No high school diploma or GED	21.8	17.6	25.2	33.9	37.0	45.8
High school diploma or GED	28.2	28.0	27.4	36.9	43.1	43.2
Some college, no bachelor's degree . . .	38.7	33.1	38.7	49.6	52.8	43.7
Bachelor's degree or higher	55.0	56.1	59.3	64.5	64.1	74.6
Geographic region[3]						
Northeast	29.9	37.2	36.4	48.2	48.8	61.1
Midwest	30.3	31.5	30.1	42.0	42.8	44.1
South.	27.7	20.1	26.2	38.9	44.4	50.1
West	52.4	42.9	45.3	58.2	59.2	64.5

* Estimates are considered unreliable. Data preceded by an asterisk have a relative standard error of 20%–30%.

[1]Starting with 1995 data, race-specific estimates are tabulated according to 1997 Revisions to the Standards for the Classification of Federal Data on Race and Ethnicity and are not strictly comparable with estimates for earlier years. Starting with 1995 data, race-specific estimates are for persons who reported only one racial group. Prior to data year 1995, data were tabulated according to the 1977 Standards. Estimates for single-race categories prior to 1995 included persons who reported one race or, if they reported more than one race, identified one race as best representing their race. See Appendix II, Race.

[2]Educational attainment is presented only for women 22–44 years of age. Education is as of year of interview. GED is General Educational Development high school equivalency diploma. See Appendix II, Education.

[3]See Appendix II, Geographic region.

NOTES: Data are based on single births to mothers 15–44 years of age at interview, including those births that occurred when the mothers were younger than 15 years of age. Data on breastfeeding during 1986–1994 are based on responses to questions in the National Survey of Family Growth (NSFG) Cycle 5, conducted in 1995. Data for 1995–2001 are based on the NSFG Cycle 6 conducted in 2002. Data for 2002–2004 are based on the NSFG Cycle 7 conducted in 2006–2008. See Appendix I, National Survey of Family Growth. Standard errors are available in the spreadsheet version of this table. Available from: http://www.cdc.gov/nchs/hus.htm.

SOURCE: CDC/NCHS, National Survey of Family Growth, Cycle 5 (1995), Cycle 6 (2002), and Cycle 7 (2006–2008).

Table 15. Infant, neonatal, and postneonatal mortality rates, by detailed race and Hispanic origin of mother: United States, selected years 1983–2006

[Data are based on linked birth and death certificates for infants]

Race and Hispanic origin of mother	1983[1]	1985[1]	1990[1]	1995[2]	2000[2]	2004[2]	2005[2]	2006[2]
Infant[3] deaths per 1,000 live births								
All mothers.	10.9	10.4	8.9	7.6	6.9	6.8	6.9	6.7
White.	9.3	8.9	7.3	6.3	5.7	5.7	5.7	5.6
Black or African American	19.2	18.6	16.9	14.6	13.5	13.2	13.3	12.9
American Indian or Alaska Native.	15.2	13.1	13.1	9.0	8.3	8.4	8.1	8.3
Asian or Pacific Islander[4]	8.3	7.8	6.6	5.3	4.9	4.7	4.9	4.5
Hispanic or Latina[5,6].	9.5	8.8	7.5	6.3	5.6	5.5	5.6	5.4
Mexican.	9.1	8.5	7.2	6.0	5.4	5.5	5.5	5.3
Puerto Rican.	12.9	11.2	9.9	8.9	8.2	7.8	8.3	8.0
Cuban	7.5	8.5	7.2	5.3	4.6	4.6	4.4	5.1
Central and South American	8.5	8.0	6.8	5.5	4.6	4.6	4.7	4.5
Other and unknown Hispanic or Latina	10.6	9.5	8.0	7.4	6.9	6.7	6.4	5.8
Not Hispanic or Latina:								
White[6]	9.2	8.6	7.2	6.3	5.7	5.7	5.8	5.6
Black or African American[6].	19.1	18.3	16.9	14.7	13.6	13.6	13.6	13.4
Neonatal[3] deaths per 1,000 live births								
All mothers.	7.1	6.8	5.7	4.9	4.6	4.5	4.5	4.5
White.	6.1	5.8	4.6	4.1	3.8	3.8	3.8	3.7
Black or African American	12.5	12.3	11.1	9.6	9.1	8.9	8.9	8.7
American Indian or Alaska Native.	7.5	6.1	6.1	4.0	4.4	4.3	4.0	4.3
Asian or Pacific Islander[4]	5.2	4.8	3.9	3.4	3.4	3.2	3.4	3.2
Hispanic or Latina[5,6].	6.2	5.7	4.8	4.1	3.8	3.8	3.9	3.7
Mexican.	5.9	5.4	4.5	3.9	3.6	3.7	3.8	3.7
Puerto Rican.	8.7	7.6	6.9	6.1	5.8	5.3	5.9	5.4
Cuban	*5.0	6.2	5.3	*3.6	*3.2	*2.8	*3.1	3.6
Central and South American.	5.8	5.6	4.4	3.7	3.3	3.4	3.2	3.1
Other and unknown Hispanic or Latina	6.4	5.6	5.0	4.8	4.6	4.7	4.3	3.7
Not Hispanic or Latina:								
White[6]	5.9	5.6	4.5	4.0	3.8	3.7	3.7	3.6
Black or African American[6].	12.0	11.9	11.0	9.6	9.2	9.1	9.1	9.0
Postneonatal[3] deaths per 1,000 live births								
All mothers.	3.8	3.6	3.2	2.6	2.3	2.3	2.3	2.2
White.	3.2	3.1	2.7	2.2	1.9	1.9	2.0	1.9
Black or African American	6.7	6.3	5.9	5.0	4.3	4.3	4.3	4.2
American Indian or Alaska Native.	7.7	7.0	7.0	5.1	3.9	4.2	4.0	4.0
Asian or Pacific Islander[4]	3.1	2.9	2.7	1.9	1.4	1.5	1.5	1.4
Hispanic or Latina[5,6].	3.3	3.2	2.7	2.1	1.8	1.7	1.8	1.7
Mexican.	3.2	3.2	2.7	2.1	1.8	1.7	1.7	1.6
Puerto Rican.	4.2	3.5	3.0	2.8	2.4	2.5	2.4	2.6
Cuban	*2.5	*2.3	*1.9	*1.7	*	*1.7	*1.4	*1.4
Central and South American.	2.6	2.4	2.4	1.9	1.4	1.2	1.5	1.4
Other and unknown Hispanic or Latina	4.2	3.9	3.0	2.6	2.3	2.0	2.1	2.1
Not Hispanic or Latina:								
White[6]	3.2	3.0	2.7	2.2	1.9	2.0	2.1	1.9
Black or African American[6].	7.0	6.4	5.9	5.0	4.4	4.5	4.5	4.4

* Estimates are considered unreliable. Rates preceded by an asterisk are based on fewer than 50 deaths in the numerator. Rates not shown are based on fewer than 20 deaths in the numerator.

[1]Rates based on unweighted birth cohort data.

[2]Rates based on a period file using weighted data. See Appendix I, National Vital Statistics System (NVSS), Linked Birth/Infant Death Data Set.

[3]Infant (under 1 year of age), neonatal (under 28 days), and postneonatal (28 days–11 months).

[4]Starting with 2003 data, estimates are not available for Asian or Pacific Islander subgroups during the transition from single-race to multiple-race reporting. See Appendix II, Race, Birth file.

[5]Persons of Hispanic origin may be of any race.

[6]Prior to 1995, data are shown only for states with an Hispanic-origin item on their birth certificates. See Appendix II, Hispanic origin.

NOTES: The race groups white, black, American Indian or Alaska Native, and Asian or Pacific Islander include persons of Hispanic and non-Hispanic origin. Starting with 2003 data, some states reported multiple-race data. The multiple-race data for these states were bridged to the single-race categories of the 1977 Office of Management and Budget standards for comparability with other states. See Appendix II, Race. National linked files do not exist for 1992–1994. Data for additional years are available. See Appendix III.

SOURCE: CDC/NCHS, National Vital Statistics System. Mathews TJ, MacDorman MF. Infant mortality statistics from the 2006 period: Linked birth/infant death data set. National vital statistics reports; vol 58 no 17. Hyattsville, MD: NCHS; 2010. Available from: http://www.cdc.gov/nchs/data/nvsr/nvsr58/nvsr58_17.pdf.

Table 16. Infant mortality rates, by birthweight: United States, selected years 1983–2006

[Data are based on linked birth and death certificates for infants]

Birthweight	1983[1]	1985[1]	1990[1]	1995[2]	2000[2]	2004[2]	2005[2]	2006[2]
	Infant deaths per 1,000 live births[3]							
All birthweights	10.9	10.4	8.9	7.6	6.9	6.8	6.9	6.7
Less than 2,500 grams	95.9	93.9	78.1	65.3	60.2	57.9	57.6	55.7
Less than 1,500 grams	400.6	387.7	317.6	270.7	246.9	245.2	245.7	241.4
Less than 500 grams	890.3	895.9	898.2	904.9	847.9	850.1	857.2	847.6
500–999 grams	584.2	559.2	440.1	351.0	313.8	314.6	305.1	303.8
1,000–1,499 grams	162.3	145.4	97.9	69.6	60.9	55.7	58.1	58.4
1,500–1,999 grams	58.4	54.0	43.8	33.5	28.7	27.4	27.0	26.2
2,000–2,499 grams	22.5	20.9	17.8	13.7	11.9	11.1	10.9	10.4
2,500 grams or more	4.7	4.3	3.7	3.0	2.5	2.3	2.3	2.3
2,500–2,999 grams	8.8	7.9	6.7	5.5	4.6	4.2	4.2	4.0
3,000–3,499 grams	4.4	4.3	3.7	2.9	2.4	2.1	2.2	2.1
3,500–3,999 grams	3.2	3.0	2.6	2.0	1.7	1.5	1.5	1.4
4,000 grams or more	3.3	3.2	2.4	2.0	1.6	1.5	1.6	1.5
4,000–4,499 grams	2.9	2.9	2.2	1.8	1.5	1.4	1.5	1.4
4,500–4,999 grams	3.9	3.8	2.5	2.2	2.1	1.5	2.2	1.9
5,000 grams or more[4]	14.4	14.7	9.8	8.5	*6.1	*4.9	*4.6	*5.4

* Estimates are considered unreliable. Rates preceded by an asterisk are based on fewer than 50 deaths in the numerator.
[1] Rates based on unweighted birth cohort data.
[2] Rates based on a period file using weighted data; unknown birthweight imputed when period of gestation is known and proportionately distributed when period of gestation is unknown. See Appendix I, National Vital Statistics System (NVSS), Linked Birth/Infant Death Data Set.
[3] For calculation of birthweight-specific infant mortality rates, unknown birthweight has been distributed in proportion to known birthweight separately for live births (denominator) and infant deaths (numerator).
[4] In 1989, a birthweight-gestational age consistency check instituted for the natality file resulted in a decrease in the number of deaths to infants coded with birthweights of 5,000 grams or more and a discontinuity in the mortality trend for infants weighing 5,000 grams or more at birth. Starting with 1989 data, the rates are believed to be more accurate.

NOTES: National linked files do not exist for 1992–1994. Data for additional years are available. See Appendix III.

SOURCE: CDC/NCHS, National Vital Statistics System, Linked Birth/Infant Death Data Set.

Table 17. Infant mortality rates, fetal mortality rates, and perinatal mortality rates, by race: United States, selected years 1950–2007

[Data are based on death certificates, fetal death records, and birth certificates]

Race and year	Infant[1]	Neonatal[1] Under 28 days	Neonatal[1] Under 7 days	Postneonatal[1]	Fetal mortality rate[2]	Late fetal mortality rate[3]	Perinatal mortality rate[4]
All races		Deaths per 1,000 live births					
1950[5]	29.2	20.5	17.8	8.7	18.4	14.9	32.5
1960[5]	26.0	18.7	16.7	7.3	15.8	12.1	28.6
1970	20.0	15.1	13.6	4.9	14.0	9.5	23.0
1980	12.6	8.5	7.1	4.1	9.1	6.2	13.2
1990	9.2	5.8	4.8	3.4	7.5	4.3	9.0
1995	7.6	4.9	4.0	2.7	7.0	3.6	7.6
2000	6.9	4.6	3.7	2.3	6.6	3.3	7.0
2002	7.0	4.7	3.7	2.3	6.4	3.2	6.9
2003	6.9	4.6	3.7	2.2	6.3	3.1	6.8
2004	6.8	4.5	3.6	2.3	6.3	3.1	6.7
2005	6.9	4.5	3.6	2.3	6.2	3.0	6.6
2006	6.7	4.5	3.5	2.2	- - -	- - -	- - -
2007	6.8	4.4	3.5	2.3	- - -	- - -	- - -
Race of child:[6] White							
1950[5]	26.8	19.4	17.1	7.4	16.6	13.3	30.1
1960[5]	22.9	17.2	15.6	5.7	13.9	10.8	26.2
1970	17.8	13.8	12.5	4.0	12.3	8.6	21.0
1980	11.0	7.5	6.2	3.5	8.1	5.7	11.9
Race of mother:[7] White							
1980	10.9	7.4	6.1	3.5	8.1	5.7	11.8
1990	7.6	4.8	3.9	2.8	6.4	3.8	7.7
1995	6.3	4.1	3.3	2.2	5.9	3.3	6.5
2000	5.7	3.8	3.0	1.9	5.6	2.9	5.9
2002	5.8	3.9	3.1	1.9	5.5	2.8	5.9
2003	5.7	3.9	3.1	1.8	5.3	2.7	5.8
2004	5.7	3.8	3.0	1.9	5.4	2.8	5.8
2005	5.7	3.8	3.0	1.9	5.3	2.7	5.7
2006	5.6	3.7	2.9	1.8	- - -	- - -	- - -
2007	5.6	3.7	2.9	1.9	- - -	- - -	- - -
Race of child:[6] Black or African American							
1950[5]	43.9	27.8	23.0	16.1	32.1	- - -	- - -
1960[5]	44.3	27.8	23.7	16.5	- - -	- - -	- - -
1970	32.6	22.8	20.3	9.9	23.2	- - -	34.5
1980	21.4	14.1	11.9	7.3	14.4	8.9	20.7
Race of mother:[7] Black or African American							
1980	22.2	14.6	12.3	7.6	14.7	9.1	21.3
1990	18.0	11.6	9.7	6.4	13.3	6.7	16.4
1995	15.1	9.8	8.2	5.3	12.7	5.7	13.8
2000	14.1	9.4	7.6	4.7	12.4	5.4	13.0
2001	14.0	9.2	7.6	4.8	12.1	5.3	12.8
2002	14.4	9.5	7.8	4.8	11.9	5.2	12.8
2003	14.0	9.4	7.5	4.6	12.1	5.1	12.5
2004	13.8	9.1	7.3	4.7	11.6	5.0	12.2
2005	13.7	9.1	7.3	4.7	11.4	4.9	12.1
2006	13.3	8.8	7.0	4.5	- - -	- - -	- - -
2007	13.2	8.6	6.9	4.6	- - -	- - -	- - -

- - - Data not available.

[1]Infant (under 1 year of age), neonatal (under 28 days), early neonatal (under 7 days), and postneonatal (28 days–11 months).
[2]Number of fetal deaths of 20 weeks or more gestation per 1,000 live births plus fetal deaths.
[3]Number of fetal deaths of 28 weeks or more gestation (late fetal deaths) per 1,000 live births plus late fetal deaths.
[4]Number of late fetal deaths plus infant deaths within 7 days of birth per 1,000 live births plus late fetal deaths.
[5]Includes births and deaths of persons who were not residents of the 50 states and the District of Columbia.
[6]Infant deaths, live births, and fetal deaths are tabulated by race of child. See Appendix II, Race.
[7]Infant deaths are tabulated by race of decedent; fetal deaths and live births are tabulated by race of mother. See Appendix II, Race.

NOTES: Infant mortality rates in this table are based on infant deaths from the mortality file (numerator) and live births from the natality file (denominator). Inconsistencies in reporting race for the same infant between the birth and death certificate can result in underestimated infant mortality rates for races other than white or black. Infant mortality rates for minority population groups are available from the Linked Birth/Infant Death Data Set and are presented in Table 18. Some numbers in this table have been revised and differ from previous editions of *Health, United States*. Data for additional years are available. See Appendix III.

SOURCE: CDC/NCHS, National Vital Statistics System; Xu JQ, Kochanek KD, Murphy SL, Tejada-Vera B. Deaths: Final data for 2007. National vital statistics reports; vol 58 no 19. Hyattsville, MD: NCHS; 2010. Available from: http://www.cdc.gov/nchs/data/nvsr/nvsr58/nvsr58_19.pdf and unpublished data.

Table 18 (page 1 of 2). Infant mortality rates, by race and Hispanic origin of mother, and state: United States, average annual 1989–1991, 2001–2003, and 2004–2006

[Data are based on linked birth and death certificates for infants]

State	All races			Not Hispanic or Latina White			Not Hispanic or Latina Black or African American		
	1989–1991[1]	2001–2003[2]	2004–2006[2]	1989–1991[1]	2001–2003[2]	2004–2006[2]	1989–1991[1]	2001–2003[2]	2004–2006[2]
	Infant[3] deaths per 1,000 live births								
United States.	9.0	6.9	6.8	7.3	5.7	5.7	17.2	13.6	13.5
Alabama	11.4	9.0	9.1	8.6	6.7	7.0	16.8	14.1	13.8
Alaska	9.2	6.8	6.5	7.2	5.1	5.0	*	*	*
Arizona	8.8	6.6	6.6	8.2	6.1	6.1	17.3	13.8	12.3
Arkansas	9.8	8.5	8.2	8.1	7.6	7.0	15.2	13.1	14.0
California	7.6	5.3	5.2	6.9	4.7	4.7	15.4	11.1	11.4
Colorado	8.7	6.0	6.1	8.0	5.2	5.2	16.7	14.2	14.0
Connecticut	7.9	6.0	5.8	5.9	4.6	4.0	17.0	13.6	13.4
Delaware	11.2	9.5	8.6	8.2	7.6	6.3	20.1	16.4	15.0
District of Columbia. . . .	20.3	10.9	12.6	*8.2	*3.8	*3.2	23.9	14.8	18.5
Florida.	9.4	7.4	7.2	7.2	5.9	5.9	16.2	13.3	12.8
Georgia	11.9	8.7	8.2	8.4	6.3	6.1	17.9	13.5	12.9
Hawaii	7.0	7.0	6.1	5.5	5.3	*3.7	*13.6	*	*21.1
Idaho.	8.9	6.2	6.3	8.9	6.0	6.0	*	*	*
Illinois	10.7	7.6	7.4	7.6	5.9	5.9	20.5	15.5	14.4
Indiana	9.4	7.7	7.9	8.4	7.0	7.0	17.3	13.8	16.1
Iowa	8.2	5.6	5.2	7.8	5.3	5.0	15.8	*12.3	*8.2
Kansas	8.5	7.1	7.3	7.8	6.3	6.8	15.4	15.8	14.4
Kentucky	8.7	6.6	7.0	8.1	6.3	6.5	14.4	10.1	12.5
Louisiana[4]	10.2	9.8	10.0	7.5	7.0	7.0	14.3	13.9	14.7
Maine	6.6	5.2	6.3	6.2	5.1	6.2	*	*	*
Maryland	9.1	8.0	7.9	6.3	5.4	5.5	15.0	13.2	12.9
Massachusetts	7.0	4.9	4.9	5.9	4.0	4.0	14.2	10.2	10.3
Michigan	10.5	8.2	7.6	7.7	6.3	5.7	20.7	16.7	15.7
Minnesota	7.3	5.1	5.0	6.4	4.5	4.4	18.5	8.4	9.6
Mississippi	11.5	10.5	10.6	7.9	7.1	6.8	15.2	14.7	15.4
Missouri.	9.7	7.9	7.5	8.0	6.5	6.5	18.0	15.7	13.8
Montana	9.0	7.3	6.0	8.0	6.9	5.0	*	*	*
Nebraska.	8.1	6.4	5.9	7.2	5.6	5.2	18.3	15.2	12.2
Nevada	8.6	5.8	6.2	7.8	5.4	5.5	16.9	12.8	14.4
New Hampshire[4]	7.1	4.3	5.6	7.2	4.2	5.3	*	*	*
New Jersey	8.4	5.9	5.4	6.1	3.9	3.7	17.8	13.1	11.8
New Mexico.	8.4	6.1	6.1	8.1	6.1	6.8	*17.2	*	*
New York.	9.5	6.0	5.9	6.3	4.6	4.6	18.4	11.2	11.5
North Carolina	10.7	8.3	8.5	8.0	6.2	6.4	16.9	15.1	15.7
North Dakota	8.0	7.5	5.9	7.3	6.8	5.4	*	*	*
Ohio	9.0	7.8	7.8	7.7	6.3	6.4	16.2	15.4	15.9
Oklahoma[4]	8.0	7.8	8.0	7.3	7.2	7.7	12.7	14.3	13.0
Oregon	8.0	5.6	5.6	7.4	5.6	5.5	21.3	*9.3	*9.6
Pennsylvania	9.2	7.4	7.4	7.2	6.0	5.8	19.1	14.1	13.8
Rhode Island	8.7	6.9	6.0	7.5	5.3	3.9	*13.6	*11.8	*11.5
South Carolina	11.8	8.9	9.0	8.4	6.1	6.3	17.2	14.5	14.3
South Dakota	9.5	6.9	7.3	7.5	5.7	6.2	*	*	*
Tennessee	10.2	9.1	8.7	7.8	7.1	6.9	18.2	16.9	15.9
Texas	7.9	6.2	6.3	6.9	5.7	5.8	14.1	11.9	12.1
Utah	7.0	5.2	5.0	6.8	4.8	4.7	*	*	*
Vermont.	6.6	5.1	5.5	6.3	5.0	5.6	*	*	*
Virginia	9.9	7.5	7.3	7.4	5.7	5.7	18.0	14.2	13.8
Washington	8.0	5.7	5.1	7.4	5.3	4.5	15.1	9.4	8.2
West Virginia	9.1	7.9	7.6	8.8	7.7	7.3	*15.7	*12.5	*15.1
Wisconsin	8.4	6.8	6.3	7.4	5.5	5.0	17.0	17.5	16.9
Wyoming	8.4	6.0	7.4	8.0	5.6	7.3	*	*	*

See footnotes at end of table.

[Data are based on linked birth and death certificates for infants]

State	Hispanic or Latina[5]			American Indian or Alaska Native[6]			Asian or Pacific Islander[6]		
	1989–1991[1]	2001–2003[2]	2004–2006[2]	1989–1991[1]	2001–2003[2]	2004–2006[2]	1989–1991[1]	2001–2003[2]	2004–2006[2]
	Infant[3] deaths per 1,000 live births								
United States..........	7.5	5.6	5.5	12.6	9.0	8.3	6.6	4.8	4.7
Alabama	*	7.0	7.4	*	*	*	*	*	*
Alaska..............	*	*	*	15.7	10.6	9.8	*	*	*
Arizona	8.0	6.2	6.7	11.4	9.7	7.2	*8.5	*6.2	5.9
Arkansas	*	*5.3	6.3	*	*	*	*	*	*
California	7.0	5.1	4.9	11.0	7.3	6.3	6.4	4.3	4.1
Colorado	8.5	6.3	7.0	*16.5	*	*	*7.8	*6.7	*5.6
Connecticut	7.9	6.3	7.8	*	*	*	*	*	*3.2
Delaware	*	*6.9	*5.5	*	*	*	*	*	*
District of Columbia....	*8.8	*7.2	*	*	*	*	*	*	*
Florida.............	7.1	5.3	5.1	*	*7.4	*	*6.2	5.1	5.5
Georgia	9.0	6.4	5.1	*	*	*	*8.2	6.5	5.9
Hawaii	10.7	*6.8	6.1	*	*	*	7.1	7.3	6.4
Idaho..............	*7.2	7.0	7.3	*	*	*	*	*	*
Illinois	9.2	5.9	6.2	*	*	*	6.0	5.4	5.1
Indiana	*7.2	6.4	6.7	*	*	*	*	*	*
Iowa	*11.9	*6.5	*5.0	*	*	*	*	*	*8.7
Kansas	8.7	7.3	6.5	*	*	*	*	*	*6.4
Kentucky	*	*4.9	7.3	*	*	*	*	*	*
Louisiana[7]	- - -	*4.5	*5.7	*	*	*	*	*9.9	*
Maine	*	*	*	*	*	*	*	*	*
Maryland	7.2	6.0	5.3	*	*	*	7.5	4.3	4.6
Massachusetts	8.3	6.3	6.4	*	*	*	5.7	3.4	3.6
Michigan	7.9	7.3	7.3	*10.7	*	*	*6.1	5.2	4.9
Minnesota	*8.4	5.7	4.3	17.3	*9.8	*9.5	*5.1	5.5	4.1
Mississippi	*	*	*5.8	*	*	*	*	*	*
Missouri............	*9.1	7.0	6.3	*	*	*	*9.1	*6.2	*5.5
Montana	*	*	*	16.7	*9.4	*10.0	*	*	*
Nebraska...........	*8.8	6.2	5.9	*18.2	*	*	*	*	*
Nevada	7.0	4.4	5.1	*	*	*	*	*4.3	*5.5
New Hampshire[7]	- - -	*	*	*	*	*	*	*	*
New Jersey	7.5	6.1	5.1	*	*	*	5.6	3.7	4.7
New Mexico.........	7.8	5.9	5.4	9.8	6.0	7.6	*	*	*
New York	9.4	5.5	5.3	*15.2	*11.9	*	6.4	3.4	3.8
North Carolina	*7.5	6.1	6.2	12.2	11.0	10.6	*6.3	*4.8	6.1
North Dakota	*	*	*	*13.8	*11.4	*9.8	*	*	*
Ohio	8.0	8.2	5.6	*	*	*	*4.8	*5.1	*4.3
Oklahoma[7]	- - -	5.6	5.4	7.8	7.4	8.3	*	*	*6.3
Oregon	8.5	4.7	5.4	*15.7	*8.9	*8.5	*8.4	*4.7	*5.1
Pennsylvania	10.9	8.0	7.7	*	*	*	7.8	4.0	5.6
Rhode Island	*7.2	8.8	8.0	*	*	*	*	*	*
South Carolina	*	5.3	7.4	*	*	*	*	*7.9	*6.1
South Dakota	*	*	*	19.9	12.6	12.4	*	*	*
Tennessee	*	6.6	6.5	*	*	*	*	*6.4	*7.5
Texas	7.0	5.4	5.5	*	*	*	6.8	4.4	4.2
Utah	*7.0	6.4	5.3	*10.0	*	*	*10.7	*7.9	*7.7
Vermont............	*	*	*	*	*	*	*	*	*
Virginia	7.6	4.9	5.3	*	*	*	6.0	5.0	4.0
Washington	7.6	5.2	4.8	19.6	10.6	9.3	6.2	4.7	4.5
West Virginia	*	*	*	*	*	*	*	*	*
Wisconsin	*7.3	6.9	5.7	*11.9	*12.7	*8.1	*6.7	*6.6	*5.7
Wyoming	*	*	*	*	*	*	*	*	*

* Estimates are considered unreliable. Rates preceded by an asterisk are based on fewer than 50 deaths in the numerator. Rates not shown are based on fewer than 20 deaths in the numerator.

- - - Data not available.

[1]Rates based on unweighted birth cohort data.

[2]Rates based on period file using weighted data. See Appendix I, National Vital Statistics System (NVSS), Linked Birth/Infant Death Data Set.

[3]Under 1 year of age.

[4]Rates for white and black are substituted for non-Hispanic white and non-Hispanic black for Louisiana for 1989, Oklahoma for 1989–1990, and New Hampshire for 1989–1991.

[5]Persons of Hispanic origin may be of any race. See Appendix II, Hispanic origin.

[6]Includes persons of Hispanic origin.

[7]Rates for Hispanic origin exclude data from states not reporting Hispanic origin on the birth certificate for 1 or more years in a 3-year period.

NOTES: Starting with 2003 data, some states reported multiple-race data. The multiple-race data for these states were bridged to the single-race categories of the 1977 Office of Management and Budget standards for comparability with other states. See Appendix II, Race. National linked files do not exist for 1992–1994.

SOURCE: CDC/NCHS, National Vital Statistics System, Linked Birth/Infant Death Data Set.

Table 19 (page 1 of 2). Neonatal mortality rates, by race and Hispanic origin of mother, and state: United States, average annual 1989–1991, 2001–2003, and 2004–2006

[Data are based on linked birth and death certificates for infants]

	All races			Not Hispanic or Latina White			Black or African American		
State	1989–1991[1]	2001–2003[2]	2004–2006[2]	1989–1991[1]	2001–2003[2]	2004–2006[2]	1989–1991[1]	2001–2003[2]	2004–2006[2]
	Neonatal[3] deaths per 1,000 live births								
United States.	5.7	4.6	4.5	4.6	3.8	3.7	11.1	9.2	9.1
Alabama	7.5	5.7	5.6	5.7	4.1	4.2	11.1	9.0	8.7
Alaska	4.1	3.0	3.4	3.7	*2.8	*2.6	*	*	*
Arizona	5.3	4.3	4.5	4.9	4.0	4.1	11.0	9.5	7.3
Arkansas	5.4	5.1	4.9	4.5	4.5	4.0	8.5	8.3	8.8
California	4.6	3.6	3.5	4.1	3.1	3.1	9.2	7.2	7.5
Colorado	5.0	4.3	4.5	4.7	3.5	3.8	10.9	11.0	9.7
Connecticut	5.7	4.4	4.4	4.2	3.5	3.0	12.5	9.2	9.7
Delaware	7.5	7.0	6.2	5.8	5.7	4.4	12.4	12.2	11.1
District of Columbia. . . .	14.1	7.7	8.7	*5.2	*	*	16.7	10.3	12.4
Florida	6.2	4.9	4.6	4.7	3.7	3.6	10.5	8.9	8.2
Georgia	7.9	5.8	5.5	5.5	4.1	3.8	12.0	9.2	8.9
Hawaii	4.3	4.8	4.4	3.5	*4.3	*2.9	*	*	*16.5
Idaho.	5.3	3.9	4.2	5.2	3.8	4.1	*	*	*
Illinois	7.0	5.2	5.0	5.1	4.3	4.0	12.7	9.9	9.0
Indiana	6.0	5.0	5.3	5.2	4.6	4.5	11.5	9.0	11.3
Iowa	4.8	3.5	3.3	4.5	3.2	3.2	*10.5	*9.1	*
Kansas	4.9	4.7	4.6	4.6	4.0	4.3	8.3	11.2	8.4
Kentucky	5.0	4.0	4.1	4.6	3.9	3.7	8.9	5.7	7.5
Louisiana[4]	6.3	6.2	5.9	4.8	4.3	3.8	8.5	9.0	9.1
Maine	4.5	4.0	4.5	4.2	3.9	4.4	*	*	*
Maryland	5.9	5.8	5.7	3.9	4.0	3.9	10.2	9.5	9.6
Massachusetts	4.9	3.7	3.7	4.1	3.0	3.1	10.4	7.8	7.8
Michigan	6.9	5.7	5.3	4.9	4.4	4.0	14.0	11.2	11.1
Minnesota	4.3	3.4	3.2	3.9	3.1	2.9	10.7	4.5	6.1
Mississippi	7.1	6.4	6.5	4.9	4.1	3.6	9.5	9.2	9.9
Missouri.	6.0	5.4	4.8	5.0	4.4	4.1	10.6	11.1	9.2
Montana	4.6	4.4	3.1	4.2	4.4	2.7	*	*	*
Nebraska.	4.5	4.4	3.7	4.2	4.0	3.3	*9.8	*11.2	*7.6
Nevada	4.3	3.4	4.0	3.8	3.0	3.7	*8.3	7.3	8.9
New Hampshire[4]	4.3	3.0	4.3	4.4	2.9	4.0	*	*	*
New Jersey	5.8	4.2	3.8	4.5	2.8	2.7	11.4	8.9	7.9
New Mexico.	5.0	3.9	3.7	4.8	3.8	4.2	*	*	*
New York.	6.5	4.2	4.1	4.3	3.3	3.3	12.6	7.7	7.6
North Carolina	7.3	5.8	5.9	5.3	4.1	4.1	11.9	10.9	11.2
North Dakota	5.0	5.2	4.1	4.7	4.8	3.9	*	*	*
Ohio	5.5	5.3	5.2	4.8	4.3	4.1	9.8	10.4	11.1
Oklahoma[4]	4.4	4.6	4.6	4.1	4.2	4.4	6.3	8.6	8.7
Oregon	4.4	3.7	3.8	4.0	3.7	3.8	*11.6	*	*
Pennsylvania	6.2	5.4	5.2	4.9	4.4	4.0	12.5	9.8	9.8
Rhode Island	6.4	5.1	4.8	5.3	3.7	3.3	*9.8	*9.6	*8.3
South Carolina	7.7	6.1	5.9	5.4	3.9	4.0	11.3	10.5	9.7
South Dakota	5.1	3.4	4.3	4.5	3.0	4.2	*	*	*
Tennessee	6.5	5.8	5.6	4.9	4.2	4.1	11.8	11.9	11.3
Texas	4.7	4.0	4.1	4.1	3.5	3.6	8.5	7.5	7.7
Utah	3.7	3.5	3.4	3.6	3.3	3.2	*	*	*
Vermont.	4.1	3.7	3.3	3.9	3.8	3.3	*	*	*
Virginia	6.8	5.1	5.0	4.8	3.7	3.8	13.0	10.1	9.6
Washington	4.3	3.7	3.1	3.8	3.5	2.5	9.7	6.1	5.6
West Virginia	5.8	5.1	4.6	5.6	4.8	4.4	*9.7	*9.6	*
Wisconsin	5.1	4.7	4.2	4.6	3.8	3.4	9.1	11.2	11.2
Wyoming	3.9	3.8	5.0	3.8	3.7	5.0	*	*	*

See footnotes at end of table.

[Data are based on linked birth and death certificates for infants]

State	Hispanic or Latina[5]			American Indian or Alaska Native[6]			Asian or Pacific Islander[6]		
	1989–1991[1]	2001–2003[2]	2004–2006[2]	1989–1991[1]	2001–2003[2]	2004–2006[2]	1989–1991[1]	2001–2003[2]	2004–2006[2]
	Neonatal[3] deaths per 1,000 live births								
United States.	4.8	3.8	3.8	5.9	4.5	4.2	3.9	3.3	3.2
Alabama	*	*4.3	4.1	*	*	*	*	*	*
Alaska	*	*	*	*5.7	*3.2	*4.4	*	*	*
Arizona	5.0	4.3	4.7	5.4	4.3	3.9	*	*	*
Arkansas	*	*3.5	4.2	*	*	*	*	*	*
California	4.4	3.5	3.4	6.3	*3.7	*3.5	3.6	2.9	2.8
Colorado	4.4	4.8	5.3	*	*	*	*	*4.7	*4.3
Connecticut	5.3	4.9	6.0	*	*	*	*	*	*
Delaware	*	*	*	*	*	*	*	*	*
District of Columbia. . . .	*	*	*	*	*	*	*4.4	3.7	3.7
Florida	5.1	3.6	3.5	*	*	*	*5.3	5.3	4.0
Georgia	*5.7	4.3	3.5	*	*	*	*5.3	5.3	4.0
Hawaii	*6.6	*4.4	*4.2	*	*	*	4.2	4.7	4.4
Idaho.	*	*5.1	*4.3	*	*	*	*	*	*
Illinois	6.4	4.1	4.4	*	*	*	3.9	3.9	3.9
Indiana	*4.7	4.3	4.6	*	*	*	*	*	*
Iowa	*	*4.6	*3.5	*	*	*	*	*	*
Kansas	*5.4	4.9	4.0	*	*	*	*	*	*
Kentucky	*	*	*6.0	*	*	*	*	*7.6	*
Louisiana[7]	- - -	*	*3.7	*	*	*	*	*	*
Maine	*	*	*	*	*	*	*	*	*
Maryland	*4.7	4.2	3.5	*	*	*	*4.5	*3.5	3.4
Massachusetts	5.8	4.7	4.7	*	*	*	*3.9	*2.6	*2.5
Michigan	5.2	5.1	4.8	*	*	*	*3.2	3.9	3.9
Minnesota	*	3.9	3.1	*4.9	*	*	*3.2	*3.4	*2.5
Mississippi	*	*	*	*	*	*	*	*	*
Missouri.	*	5.1	4.2	*	*	*	*	*4.5	*
Montana	*	*	*	*7.6	*	*4.8	*	*	*
Nebraska.	*	*3.9	*3.5	*	*	*	*	*	*4.1
Nevada	*4.1	2.7	3.1	*	*	*	*	*	*
New Hampshire[7]	- - -								
New Jersey	5.1	4.2	3.7	*	*	*	*3.4	2.7	3.0
New Mexico.	4.9	3.9	3.4	4.9	*3.4	*3.7	*	*	*
New York.	6.4	3.9	3.6	*	*	*	4.1	2.4	2.6
North Carolina	*5.5	4.1	4.5	*7.7	*8.0	*8.6	*	*3.4	*4.8
North Dakota	*	*	*	*	*	*	*	*4.2	*2.8
Ohio	*5.4	6.1	3.6	*	*	*	*	*	*
Oklahoma[7]	- - -	3.3	3.6	*3.7	3.8	4.0	*	*	*
Oregon	6.5	3.3	3.8	*	*	*	*5.3	*3.1	*3.4
Pennsylvania	7.3	5.4	5.6	*	*	*	*5.2	*3.2	4.0
Rhode Island	*4.9	*6.4	*6.2	*	*	*	*	*	*
South Carolina	*	*3.8	5.0	*	*	*	*	*	*
South Dakota	*	*	*	*8.2	*5.5	*5.3	*	*	*
Tennessee	*	4.4	4.5	*	*	*	*	*	*5.0
Texas	4.2	3.5	3.7	*	*	*	4.0	2.8	2.8
Utah	*3.6	4.3	3.9	*	*	*	*	*5.1	*4.9
Vermont.	*	*	*	*	*	*	*	*	*
Virginia	*4.8	3.6	3.8	*	*	*	*4.1	3.6	3.1
Washington	4.9	3.5	3.4	*8.5	*5.0	*4.5	*2.7	3.1	2.8
West Virginia	*	*	*	*	*	*	*	*	*
Wisconsin	*3.9	5.0	4.2	*	*6.5	*	*	*4.9	*4.2
Wyoming	*	*	*	*	*	*	*	*	*

* Estimates are considered unreliable. Rates preceded by an asterisk are based on fewer than 50 deaths in the numerator. Rates not shown are based on fewer than 20 deaths in the numerator.
- - - Data not available.
[1]Rates based on unweighted birth cohort data.
[2]Rates based on period file using weighted data. See Appendix I, National Vital Statistics System (NVSS), Linked Birth/Infant Death Data Set.
[3]Infants under 28 days of age.
[4]Rates for white and black are substituted for non-Hispanic white and non-Hispanic black for Louisiana for 1989, Oklahoma for 1989–1990, and New Hampshire for 1989–1991.
[5]Persons of Hispanic origin may be of any race. See Appendix II, Hispanic origin.
[6]Includes persons of Hispanic origin.
[7]Rates for Hispanic origin exclude data from states not reporting Hispanic origin on the birth certificate for 1 or more years in a 3-year period.

NOTES: Starting with 2003 data, some states reported multiple-race data. The multiple-race data for these states were bridged to the single-race categories of the 1977 Office of Management and Budget standards for comparability with other states. See Appendix II, Race. National linked files do not exist for 1992–1994.

SOURCE: CDC/NCHS, National Vital Statistics System, Linked Birth/Infant Death Data Set.

Table 20. Infant mortality rates and international rankings: Organisation for Economic Co-operation and Development (OECD) countries, selected years 1960–2007

[Data are based on reporting by OECD countries]

Country	1960	1970	1980	1990	2000	2006	2007	International rankings[1] 1960	International rankings[1] 2007
				Infant[2] deaths per 1,000 live births					
Australia	20.2	17.9	10.7	8.2	5.2	4.7	4.2	6	19
Austria	37.5	25.9	14.3	7.8	4.8	3.6	3.7	21	11
Belgium	23.9	21.1	12.1	8.0	4.8	4.0	4.0	12	16
Canada	27.3	18.8	10.4	6.8	5.3	5.0	- - -	14	- - -
Czech Republic	20.0	20.2	16.9	10.8	4.1	3.3	3.1	5	6
Denmark	21.5	14.2	8.4	7.5	5.3	3.8	4.0	9	16
Finland	21.0	13.2	7.6	5.6	3.8	2.8	2.7	7	5
France	27.7	18.2	10.0	7.3	4.5	3.8	- - -	15	- - -
Germany	35.0	22.5	12.4	7.0	4.4	3.8	3.9	20	14
Greece	40.1	29.6	17.9	9.7	5.4	3.7	3.6	22	10
Hungary	47.6	35.9	23.2	14.8	9.2	5.7	5.9	25	22
Iceland	13.1	13.3	7.8	5.8	3.0	1.4	2.0	1	2
Ireland	29.3	19.5	11.1	8.2	6.2	3.7	3.1	17	6
Italy	43.3	29.0	14.6	8.2	4.5	3.7	3.7	23	11
Japan	30.7	13.1	7.5	4.6	3.2	2.6	2.6	18	4
Luxembourg	31.5	24.9	11.5	7.3	5.1	2.5	1.8	19	1
Mexico	- - -	79.4	51.0	39.2	19.4	16.2	15.7	- - -	25
Netherlands	17.9	12.7	8.6	7.1	5.1	4.4	4.1	3	18
New Zealand	22.6	16.7	13.0	8.4	6.3	5.2	4.8	11	20
Norway	18.9	12.7	8.1	6.9	3.8	3.2	3.1	4	6
Poland	54.8	36.7	25.5	19.3	8.1	6.0	6.0	26	23
Portugal	77.5	55.5	24.2	11.0	5.5	3.3	3.4	27	9
Republic of Korea	- - -	45.0	- - -	- - -	- - -	4.1	- - -	- - -	- - -
Slovak Republic	28.6	25.7	20.9	12.0	8.6	6.6	6.1	16	24
Spain	43.7	28.1	12.3	7.6	4.4	3.8	3.7	24	11
Sweden	16.6	11.0	6.9	6.0	3.4	2.8	2.5	2	3
Switzerland	21.1	15.1	9.1	6.8	4.9	4.4	3.9	8	14
Turkey	189.5	145.0	117.5	55.4	28.9	22.3	20.7	28	26
United Kingdom	22.5	18.5	12.1	7.9	5.6	5.0	4.8	10	20
United States	26.0	20.0	12.6	9.2	6.9	6.7	- - -	13	- - -

- - - Data not available.

[1]Rankings are from lowest to highest infant mortality rates (IMR). Countries with the same IMR receive the same rank. The country with the next highest IMR is assigned the rank it would have received had the lower-ranked countries not been tied, i.e., skip a rank. Some of the variation in IMRs is due to variations among countries in registering practices of premature infants (whether they are reported as live births or not). In several countries, such as the United States, Canada, and the Nordic countries, very premature babies (with relatively low odds of survival) are registered as live births, which increases mortality rates compared with other countries that do not register them as live births.

[2]Under 1 year of age.

NOTES: Some rates for selected countries and selected years were revised and differ from previous editions of *Health, United States*. Data for additional years are available. See Appendix III.

SOURCE: The Organisation for Economic Co-operation and Development (OECD) Health Data 2009, incorporating revisions to the annual update. Available from: http://www.ecosante.org/oecd.htm.

Table 21 (page 1 of 2). Life expectancy at birth and at 65 years of age, by sex: Organisation for Economic Co-operation and Development (OECD) countries, selected years 1980–2007

[Data are based on reporting by OECD countries]

	Male						Female					
Country	1980	1990	1995	2000	2004	2007	1980	1990	1995	2000	2004	2007
At birth						Life expectancy in years						
Australia.................	71.0	73.9	75.0	76.6	78.1	79.0	78.1	80.1	80.8	82.0	83.0	83.7
Austria...................	69.0	72.2	73.3	75.1	76.4	77.3	76.1	78.8	79.9	81.1	82.1	82.9
Belgium.................	69.9	72.7	73.5	74.6	76.0	77.1	76.7	79.5	80.4	81.0	81.8	82.6
Canada	71.7	74.4	75.1	76.7	77.8	- - -	78.9	80.8	81.1	81.9	82.6	- - -
Czech Republic[1]	66.9	67.6	69.7	71.7	72.6	73.8	74.0	75.5	76.8	78.5	79.2	80.2
Denmark................	71.2	72.0	72.7	74.5	75.4	76.2	77.3	77.8	77.9	79.2	80.2	80.6
Finland.................	69.3	71.0	72.9	74.2	75.4	76.0	78.0	79.0	80.4	81.2	82.5	83.1
France..................	70.2	72.8	73.8	75.3	76.7	77.5	78.4	80.9	81.9	82.8	83.8	84.4
Germany[2]...............	69.6	72.0	73.3	75.1	76.5	77.4	76.2	78.5	79.9	81.2	81.9	82.7
Greece.................	72.2	74.6	75.0	75.5	76.6	77.0	76.8	79.5	80.3	80.5	81.5	82.0
Hungary................	65.5	65.1	65.3	67.4	68.6	69.2	72.7	73.7	74.5	75.9	76.9	77.3
Iceland................	73.7	75.4	75.9	78.4	79.2	79.4	79.7	80.5	80.0	81.8	82.7	82.9
Ireland	70.1	72.1	72.8	74.0	76.5	77.4	75.6	77.7	78.3	79.2	81.4	82.1
Italy	70.6	73.8	75.0	76.9	77.9	- - -	77.4	80.3	81.5	82.8	83.8	- - -
Japan..................	73.4	75.9	76.4	77.7	78.6	79.2	78.8	81.9	82.9	84.6	85.6	86.0
Luxembourg	70.0	72.4	73.0	74.6	76.0	76.7	75.6	78.7	80.6	81.3	82.4	82.2
Mexico.................	64.1	67.7	69.7	71.3	72.1	72.6	70.2	73.5	75.2	76.5	77.0	77.4
Netherlands	72.5	73.8	74.6	75.5	76.9	78.0	79.2	80.1	80.4	80.5	81.4	82.3
New Zealand.............	70.1	72.5	74.1	75.9	77.3	78.2	76.2	78.4	79.5	80.8	81.8	82.2
Norway.................	72.4	73.5	74.8	76.0	77.6	78.3	79.3	79.9	80.9	81.5	82.6	82.9
Poland	66.0	66.2	67.6	69.7	70.7	71.0	74.4	75.2	76.4	78.0	79.2	79.7
Portugal	67.9	70.6	71.7	73.2	75.0	75.9	74.9	77.5	79.0	80.2	81.5	82.2
Republic of Korea	61.8	67.3	69.6	72.3	74.5	76.1	70.0	75.5	77.4	79.6	81.4	82.7
Slovak Republic[1].........	66.8	66.6	68.4	69.1	70.3	70.5	74.3	75.4	76.3	77.4	77.8	78.1
Spain..................	72.3	73.4	74.4	75.8	76.9	77.8	78.5	80.6	81.8	82.9	83.7	84.3
Sweden	72.8	74.8	76.2	77.4	78.4	78.9	78.8	80.4	81.4	82.0	82.7	83.0
Switzerland..............	72.3	74.0	75.4	77.0	78.6	79.5	79.0	80.9	81.9	82.8	83.8	84.4
Turkey	55.8	65.4	67.2	69.0	70.5	71.1	60.3	69.5	71.3	73.1	74.6	75.6
United Kingdom...........	70.2	72.9	74.0	75.5	76.8	- - -	76.2	78.5	79.3	80.3	81.0	- - -
United States	70.0	71.8	72.5	74.1	74.9	75.4	77.4	78.8	78.9	79.3	79.9	80.4

See footnotes at end of table.

Table 21 (page 2 of 2). Life expectancy at birth and at 65 years of age, by sex: Organisation for Economic Co-operation and Development (OECD) countries, selected years 1980–2007

[Data are based on reporting by OECD countries]

Country	Male						Female					
	1980	1990	1995	2000	2004	2007	1980	1990	1995	2000	2004	2007
At 65 years	Life expectancy in years											
Australia	13.7	15.2	15.7	16.9	17.8	18.5	17.9	19.0	19.5	20.4	21.1	21.6
Austria	12.9	14.3	14.9	16.0	16.9	17.4	16.3	17.8	18.6	19.4	20.3	20.8
Belgium	12.9	14.3	14.8	15.6	16.4	17.3	16.8	18.8	19.3	19.8	20.2	21.0
Canada	14.5	15.7	16.0	16.8	17.7	- - -	18.9	19.9	20.0	20.4	21.0	- - -
Czech Republic[1]	11.2	11.7	12.7	13.8	14.2	15.1	14.4	15.3	16.2	17.3	17.6	18.5
Denmark	13.6	14.0	14.1	15.2	15.9	16.5	17.6	17.9	17.6	18.3	19.0	19.2
Finland	12.6	13.8	14.6	15.5	16.5	17.0	17.0	17.8	18.8	19.5	20.7	21.3
France	13.6	15.5	16.1	16.7	17.7	- - -	18.2	19.8	20.6	21.2	22.1	- - -
Germany[2]	12.8	14.0	14.8	15.8	16.7	17.4	16.3	17.7	18.7	19.6	20.1	20.7
Greece	14.6	15.7	16.1	16.2	17.0	17.4	16.8	18.0	18.4	18.3	19.2	19.6
Hungary	11.6	12.0	12.1	12.7	13.1	13.4	14.6	15.3	15.8	16.5	16.9	17.3
Iceland	15.8	16.2	16.2	18.1	17.9	18.3	19.1	19.5	19.0	19.7	20.5	20.6
Ireland	12.6	13.3	13.5	14.6	16.2	17.1	15.7	17.0	17.2	18.0	19.7	20.1
Italy	13.3	15.1	15.9	16.7	17.5	- - -	17.1	19.0	19.9	20.7	21.6	- - -
Japan	14.6	16.2	16.5	17.5	18.2	18.6	17.7	20.0	20.9	22.4	23.3	23.6
Luxembourg	12.6	14.3	14.8	15.5	16.5	16.4	16.5	18.5	19.7	20.1	20.5	20.3
Mexico	15.4	16.0	16.1	16.5	16.7	16.8	17.0	17.8	17.8	18.1	18.2	18.3
Netherlands	13.7	14.4	14.7	15.3	16.3	17.0	18.0	18.9	19.0	19.2	19.8	20.5
New Zealand	13.2	14.6	15.4	16.5	17.5	18.1	17.0	18.3	19.0	19.8	20.4	20.7
Norway	14.3	14.6	15.1	16.1	17.1	17.5	18.2	18.7	19.3	19.9	20.7	20.8
Poland	12.0	12.4	12.9	13.6	14.2	14.6	15.5	16.1	16.6	17.5	18.4	18.9
Portugal	13.1	14.0	14.7	15.4	16.3	16.8	16.1	17.1	18.1	18.9	19.7	20.2
Republic of Korea	10.5	12.4	13.3	14.3	15.5	16.3	15.1	16.3	17.0	18.2	19.4	20.5
Slovak Republic[1]	12.3	12.2	12.7	12.9	13.3	13.4	15.4	15.7	16.1	16.5	16.9	17.1
Spain	14.6	15.5	16.2	16.7	17.3	17.8	17.8	19.3	20.2	20.8	21.5	22.0
Sweden	14.3	15.3	16.0	16.7	17.4	17.8	17.9	19.0	19.6	20.0	20.6	20.7
Switzerland	14.3	15.3	16.2	17.0	18.2	18.6	18.2	19.7	20.4	20.9	21.6	22.2
Turkey	11.7	12.8	13.1	13.4	13.8	13.9	12.8	14.3	14.7	15.1	15.5	15.8
United Kingdom	12.6	14.0	14.6	15.8	16.8	- - -	16.6	17.9	18.2	19.0	19.4	- - -
United States	14.1	15.1	15.6	16.0	16.7	17.2	18.3	18.9	18.9	19.0	19.5	19.9

- - - Data not available.

[1]In 1993, Czechoslovakia was divided into two nations, the Czech Republic and Slovakia. Data for years prior to 1993 are from the Czech and Slovak regions of Czechoslovakia.
[2]Until 1990, estimates refer to the Federal Republic of Germany; from 1995 onwards, data refer to Germany after reunification.

NOTES: Since calculation of life expectancy (LE) estimates varies among countries, ranks are not presented; comparisons among countries and their interpretation should be made with caution. See Appendix II, Life expectancy. Some estimates for selected countries and selected years were revised and differ from the previous editions of *Health, United States*. Data for additional years are available. See Appendix III.

SOURCE: Organisation for Economic Co-operation and Development (OECD) Health Data 2009, A Comparative Analysis of 30 Countries, available from: http://www.oecd.org/els/health/; CDC/NCHS. Vital statistics of the United States (selected years). Public Health Service. Washington, DC.

Table 22. Life expectancy at birth, at 65 years of age, and at 75 years of age, by race and sex: United States, selected years 1900–2007

[Data are based on death certificates]

Specified age and year	All races Both sexes	All races Male	All races Female	White Both sexes	White Male	White Female	Black or African American[1] Both sexes	Black or African American[1] Male	Black or African American[1] Female
At birth				Remaining life expectancy in years					
1900[2,3]	47.3	46.3	48.3	47.6	46.6	48.7	33.0	32.5	33.5
1950[3]	68.2	65.6	71.1	69.1	66.5	72.2	60.8	59.1	62.9
1960[3]	69.7	66.6	73.1	70.6	67.4	74.1	63.6	61.1	66.3
1970	70.8	67.1	74.7	71.7	68.0	75.6	64.1	60.0	68.3
1980	73.7	70.0	77.4	74.4	70.7	78.1	68.1	63.8	72.5
1990	75.4	71.8	78.8	76.1	72.7	79.4	69.1	64.5	73.6
1995	75.8	72.5	78.9	76.5	73.4	79.6	69.6	65.2	73.9
1999	76.7	73.9	79.4	77.3	74.6	79.9	71.4	67.8	74.7
2000	76.8	74.1	79.3	77.3	74.7	79.9	71.8	68.2	75.1
2001	76.9	74.2	79.4	77.4	74.8	79.9	72.0	68.4	75.2
2002	76.9	74.3	79.5	77.4	74.9	79.9	72.1	68.6	75.4
2003	77.1	74.5	79.6	77.6	75.0	80.0	72.3	68.8	75.6
2004	77.5	74.9	79.9	77.9	75.4	80.4	72.8	69.3	76.0
2005	77.4	74.9	79.9	77.9	75.4	80.4	72.8	69.3	76.1
2006	77.7	75.1	80.2	78.2	75.7	80.6	73.2	69.7	76.5
2007	77.9	75.4	80.4	78.4	75.9	80.8	73.6	70.0	76.8
At 65 years									
1950[3]	13.9	12.8	15.0	- - -	12.8	15.1	13.9	12.9	14.9
1960[3]	14.3	12.8	15.8	14.4	12.9	15.9	13.9	12.7	15.1
1970	15.2	13.1	17.0	15.2	13.1	17.1	14.2	12.5	15.7
1980	16.4	14.1	18.3	16.5	14.2	18.4	15.1	13.0	16.8
1990	17.2	15.1	18.9	17.3	15.2	19.1	15.4	13.2	17.2
1995	17.4	15.6	18.9	17.6	15.7	19.1	15.6	13.6	17.1
1999	17.7	16.1	19.1	17.8	16.1	19.2	16.0	14.3	17.3
2000	17.6	16.0	19.0	17.7	16.1	19.1	16.1	14.1	17.5
2001	17.7	16.2	19.0	17.8	16.3	19.1	16.2	14.2	17.6
2002	17.8	16.2	19.1	17.9	16.3	19.2	16.3	14.4	17.7
2003	17.9	16.4	19.2	18.0	16.5	19.3	16.4	14.5	17.9
2004	18.2	16.7	19.5	18.3	16.8	19.5	16.7	14.8	18.2
2005	18.2	16.8	19.5	18.3	16.9	19.5	16.8	14.9	18.2
2006	18.5	17.0	19.7	18.6	17.1	19.8	17.1	15.1	18.6
2007	18.6	17.2	19.9	18.7	17.3	19.9	17.2	15.2	18.7
At 75 years									
1980	10.4	8.8	11.5	10.4	8.8	11.5	9.7	8.3	10.7
1990	10.9	9.4	12.0	11.0	9.4	12.0	10.2	8.6	11.2
1995	11.0	9.7	11.9	11.1	9.7	12.0	10.2	8.8	11.1
1999	11.2	10.0	12.1	11.2	10.0	12.1	10.4	9.2	11.1
2000	11.0	9.8	11.8	11.0	9.8	11.9	10.4	9.0	11.3
2001	11.1	9.9	11.9	11.1	9.9	11.9	10.5	9.1	11.4
2002	11.0	9.9	11.9	11.1	9.9	11.9	10.5	9.2	11.4
2003	11.1	10.0	11.9	11.1	10.0	11.9	10.6	9.3	11.5
2004	11.4	10.3	12.2	11.4	10.3	12.2	10.8	9.5	11.7
2005	11.3	10.2	12.1	11.4	10.3	12.1	10.8	9.5	11.7
2006	11.6	10.5	12.3	11.5	10.5	12.3	11.1	9.8	12.0
2007	11.7	10.6	12.5	11.7	10.6	12.4	11.2	9.9	12.1

- - - Data not available.

[1] Data shown for 1900–1960 are for the nonwhite population.

[2] Death registration area only. The death registration area increased from 10 states and the District of Columbia (D.C.) in 1900 to the coterminous United States in 1933. See Appendix II, Registration area.

[3] Includes deaths of persons who were not residents of the 50 states and D.C.

NOTES: Populations for computing life expectancy for 1991–1999 are 1990-based postcensal estimates of U.S. resident population. See Appendix I, Population Census and Population Estimates. In 1997, life table methodology was revised to construct complete life tables by single years of age that extend to age 100 (Anderson RN. Method for constructing complete annual U.S. life tables. NCHS. Vital Health Stat 2(129). 1999). Previously, abridged life tables were constructed for 5-year age groups ending with 85 years and over. Life table values for 2000 and later years were computed using a slight modification of the new life table method due to a change in the age detail of populations received from the U.S. Census Bureau. Values for data years 2000–2007 are based on a newly revised methodology that uses vital statistics death rates for ages under 66 and modeled probabilities of death for ages 66 to 100 based on blended vital statistics and Medicare probabilities of dying and may differ from figures previously published. The revised methodology is similar to that developed for the 1999–2001 decennial life tables. Starting with 2003 data, some states allowed the reporting of more than one race on the death certificate. The multiple-race data for these states were bridged to the single-race categories of the 1977 Office of Management and Budget Standards for comparability with other states. See Appendix II, Race. Some data have been revised and differ from previous editions of Health, United States. Data for additional years are available. See Appendix III.

SOURCE: CDC/NCHS, National Vital Statistics System; Grove RD, Hetzel AM. Vital statistics rates in the United States, 1940–1960. Washington, DC: U.S. Government Printing Office, 1968; Arias E, Rostron BL, Tejada-Vera B. United States life tables, 2005. National vital statistics reports; vol 58 no 10. Hyattsville, MD: NCHS. 2010. Xu J, Kochanek KD, Murphy SL, Tejada-Vera B. Deaths: Final Data for 2007. National vital statistics reports; vol 58 no 19. Hyattsville, MD: NCHS. 2010.

Table 23 (page 1 of 2). Age-adjusted death rates, by race, Hispanic origin, and state: United States, average annual 1979–1981, 1989–1991, and 2005–2007

[Data are based on death certificates]

State	All persons 1979–1981	All persons 1989–1991	All persons 2005–2007	White 2005–2007	Black or African American 2005–2007	American Indian or Alaska Native[1] 2005–2007	Asian or Pacific Islander 2005–2007	Hispanic or Latino[2] 2005–2007	White, not Hispanic or Latino 2005–2007
			Age-adjusted death rate per 100,000 population[3]						
United States	1,022.8	942.2	779.2	766.8	987.0	641.9	432.3	567.2	779.3
Alabama	1,091.2	1,037.9	952.9	916.4	1,105.5	306.5	351.9	315.4	921.2
Alaska	1,087.4	944.6	758.4	724.7	670.8	1,056.2	454.8	464.3	730.9
Arizona	951.5	873.5	714.3	711.6	807.6	807.9	347.5	647.0	715.3
Arkansas	1,017.0	996.3	894.3	869.6	1,113.9	356.8	468.1	346.4	878.4
California	975.5	911.0	699.2	719.5	977.2	405.9	448.2	564.8	749.6
Colorado	941.1	856.1	719.8	724.0	811.6	505.7	388.2	682.7	722.7
Connecticut	961.5	857.5	713.5	708.7	809.5	331.3	334.8	548.6	708.8
Delaware	1,069.7	1,001.9	800.9	780.7	943.5	*	314.5	497.9	781.3
District of Columbia	1,243.1	1,255.3	898.7	569.3	1,122.5	*	417.4	332.4	580.7
Florida	960.8	870.9	709.8	692.9	901.9	274.2	322.4	563.5	716.8
Georgia	1,094.3	1,037.9	859.4	826.2	988.5	511.3	407.7	283.4	839.5
Hawaii	801.2	752.2	626.8	665.9	430.3	*	619.5	952.5	685.6
Idaho	936.7	856.6	750.8	753.0	520.3	774.7	450.3	555.5	756.1
Illinois	1,063.7	973.8	783.4	755.5	1,050.1	263.1	363.7	453.3	769.5
Indiana	1,048.3	962.0	839.9	829.1	1,035.6	144.1	262.8	411.2	835.6
Iowa	919.9	848.2	735.1	733.4	966.5	623.6	330.6	350.8	736.7
Kansas	940.1	867.2	796.0	783.5	1,078.3	1,275.1	375.6	530.0	785.9
Kentucky	1,088.9	1,024.5	917.5	912.7	1,054.8	190.7	425.9	568.7	914.6
Louisiana	1,132.6	1,074.6	974.9	904.9	1,193.7	319.7	447.4	398.2	913.2
Maine	1,002.9	918.7	793.2	794.1	543.9	*	338.2	281.5	793.3
Maryland	1,063.3	985.2	796.6	758.6	952.7	318.7	373.8	342.4	770.0
Massachusetts	982.6	884.8	719.9	725.6	778.8	316.0	353.8	484.4	725.9
Michigan	1,050.2	966.0	816.1	785.3	1,060.2	947.1	366.6	684.0	784.8
Minnesota	892.9	825.2	676.6	668.5	861.7	1,025.4	492.8	408.9	669.3
Mississippi	1,108.7	1,071.4	970.4	908.7	1,119.8	827.4	457.3	265.5	913.3
Missouri	1,033.7	952.4	845.1	824.9	1,083.9	404.9	416.1	522.5	828.3
Montana	1,013.6	890.2	785.3	766.6	614.2	1,160.1	415.9	531.4	765.4
Nebraska	930.6	867.9	744.4	734.5	1,014.5	1,153.4	419.3	504.3	737.5
Nevada	1,077.4	1,017.4	844.1	865.3	908.2	630.2	454.6	436.7	910.7
New Hampshire	982.3	891.7	734.1	739.7	455.1	*	306.6	285.3	741.9
New Jersey	1,047.5	956.0	742.8	733.0	939.9	352.8	337.9	466.6	753.1
New Mexico	967.1	891.9	773.0	773.9	691.1	788.7	368.8	749.0	766.4
New York	1,051.8	973.7	699.6	704.1	760.5	249.5	367.4	545.6	705.6
North Carolina	1,050.4	986.0	850.4	813.0	1,030.7	855.5	368.6	275.9	821.8
North Dakota	922.4	818.4	708.7	688.4	*	1,338.4	*	*	668.9
Ohio	1,070.6	967.4	847.5	829.3	1,052.8	232.8	321.8	450.8	831.1
Oklahoma	1,025.6	961.4	933.8	924.4	1,112.1	929.1	416.9	490.5	935.3
Oregon	953.9	893.0	770.3	777.2	808.3	760.6	444.7	419.9	786.1
Pennsylvania	1,076.4	963.4	809.8	791.3	1,052.5	234.9	362.6	504.7	792.9
Rhode Island	990.8	889.6	761.7	763.5	797.5	*	408.9	398.7	768.7
South Carolina	1,104.6	1,030.0	869.3	819.4	1,041.6	416.0	348.4	451.6	823.5
South Dakota	941.9	846.4	726.1	689.8	745.6	1,329.7	*	375.8	691.1
Tennessee	1,045.5	1,011.8	907.1	882.3	1,103.8	300.7	406.9	287.2	887.7
Texas	1,014.9	947.6	789.0	778.5	1,001.2	202.0	390.4	651.3	809.5
Utah	924.9	823.2	701.5	703.0	765.2	729.8	551.1	529.9	709.4
Vermont	990.2	908.6	733.0	736.5	*	*	*	*	740.1
Virginia	1,054.0	963.1	787.2	761.8	977.9	271.3	401.1	366.4	769.5
Washington	947.7	869.4	731.7	739.5	873.0	894.5	456.7	473.8	745.9
West Virginia	1,100.3	1,031.5	950.7	952.0	1,071.7	*	*	173.8	956.5
Wisconsin	956.4	879.1	747.9	733.1	1,062.2	1,063.3	466.1	412.1	736.2
Wyoming	1,016.1	897.4	809.3	806.4	695.1	1,002.6	*	739.7	805.7

See footnotes at end of table.

Table 23 (page 2 of 2). Age-adjusted death rates, by race, Hispanic origin, and state: United States, average annual 1979–1981, 1989–1991, and 2005–2007

[Data are based on death certificates]

* Data for states with population under 10,000 in the middle year of a 3-year period or fewer than 50 deaths for the 3-year period are considered unreliable and are not shown.

[1] All data for the American Indian or Alaska Native (AIAN) category should be used with caution. Agreement between self-reported race and death certificate proxy reporting was found to be poor for the AIAN population. (Arias E, Schauman WS, Eschbach K, et al. The validity of race and Hispanic origin reporting on death certificates in the United States. National Center for Health Statistics. Vital Health Stat 2(148). 2008.) See Appendix II, Race, Mortality file.

[2] Caution should also be used when comparing death rates by Hispanic origin and race among states. Estimates of death rates may be affected by several factors, including possible misreporting of race and Hispanic origin on the death certificate, migration patterns between United States and country of origin for persons who were born outside the United States, and possible biases in population estimates. See Appendix I, National Vital Statistics System, Mortality file, and Appendix II, Hispanic origin; Race.

[3] Average annual death rates, age-adjusted using the year 2000 standard population. Prior to 2001, age-adjusted rates were calculated using standard million proportions based on rounded population numbers. Starting with 2001 data, unrounded population numbers are used to calculate age-adjusted rates. See Appendix II, Age adjustment. Denominators for rates are resident population estimates for the middle year of each 3-year period, multiplied by 3. See Appendix I, Population Census and Population Estimates.

NOTES: The race groups, white, black, American Indian or Alaska Native, and Asian or Pacific Islander, include persons of Hispanic and non-Hispanic origin. Persons of Hispanic origin may be of any race. Death rates for the American Indian or Alaska Native and Asian or Pacific Islander populations are known to be underestimated. See Appendix II, Race, for a discussion of sources of bias in death rates by race and Hispanic origin. Starting with 2003 data, some states allowed the reporting of more than one race on the death certificate. The multiple-race data for these states were bridged to the single-race categories of the 1977 Office of Management and Budget Standards, for comparability with other states. See Appendix II, Race.

SOURCE: CDC/NCHS, National Vital Statistics System; numerator data from annual mortality files; denominator data from state population estimates prepared by the U.S. Census Bureau 1980 from April 1, 1980 MARS Census File; 1990 from April 1, 1990 MARS Census File; 2006 from bridged-race Vintage 2008 file. Estimates of the July 1, 2006, resident populations of the United States by state and county, race, age, sex, and Hispanic origin, prepared under a collaborative arrangement with the U.S. Census Bureau. Available from: http://www.cdc.gov/nchs/nvss/bridged_race.htm.

Table 24 (page 1 of 4). Age-adjusted death rates for selected causes of death, by sex, race, and Hispanic origin: United States, selected years 1950–2007

[Data are based on death certificates]

Sex, race, Hispanic origin, and cause of death[1]	1950[2,3]	1960[2,3]	1970[3]	1980[3]	1990	2000[4]	2005[4]	2006[4]	2007[4]
All persons				Age-adjusted death rate per 100,000 population[5]					
All causes	1,446.0	1,339.2	1,222.6	1,039.1	938.7	869.0	798.8	776.5	760.2
Diseases of heart	588.8	559.0	492.7	412.1	321.8	257.6	211.1	200.2	190.9
Ischemic heart disease	- - -	- - -	- - -	345.2	249.6	186.8	144.4	134.9	126.0
Cerebrovascular diseases	180.7	177.9	147.7	96.2	65.3	60.9	46.6	43.6	42.2
Malignant neoplasms	193.9	193.9	198.6	207.9	216.0	199.6	183.8	180.7	178.4
Trachea, bronchus, and lung	15.0	24.1	37.1	49.9	59.3	56.1	52.6	51.5	50.6
Colon, rectum, and anus	- - -	30.3	28.9	27.4	24.5	20.8	17.5	17.2	16.9
Chronic lower respiratory diseases	- - -	- - -	- - -	28.3	37.2	44.2	43.2	40.5	40.8
Influenza and pneumonia	48.1	53.7	41.7	31.4	36.8	23.7	20.3	17.8	16.2
Chronic liver disease and cirrhosis	11.3	13.3	17.8	15.1	11.1	9.5	9.0	8.8	9.1
Diabetes mellitus	23.1	22.5	24.3	18.1	20.7	25.0	24.6	23.3	22.5
Human immunodeficiency virus (HIV) disease	- - -	- - -	- - -	- - -	10.2	5.2	4.2	4.0	3.7
Unintentional injuries	78.0	62.3	60.1	46.4	36.3	34.9	39.1	39.8	40.0
Motor vehicle-related injuries	24.6	23.1	27.6	22.3	18.5	15.4	15.2	15.0	14.4
Poisoning	2.5	1.7	2.8	1.9	2.3	4.5	7.9	9.1	9.8
Suicide[6]	13.2	12.5	13.1	12.2	12.5	10.4	10.9	10.9	11.3
Homicide[6]	5.1	5.0	8.8	10.4	9.4	5.9	6.1	6.2	6.1
Male									
All causes	1,674.2	1,609.0	1,542.1	1,348.1	1,202.8	1,053.8	951.1	924.8	905.6
Diseases of heart	699.0	687.6	634.0	538.9	412.4	320.0	260.9	248.5	237.7
Ischemic heart disease	- - -	- - -	- - -	459.7	328.2	241.4	187.4	176.5	165.4
Cerebrovascular diseases	186.4	186.1	157.4	102.2	68.5	62.4	46.9	43.9	42.5
Malignant neoplasms	208.1	225.1	247.6	271.2	280.4	248.9	225.1	220.1	217.5
Trachea, bronchus, and lung	24.6	43.6	67.5	85.2	91.1	76.7	69.0	67.0	65.1
Colon, rectum, and anus	- - -	31.8	32.3	32.8	30.4	25.1	20.9	20.5	20.1
Prostate	28.6	28.7	28.8	32.8	38.4	30.4	24.5	23.5	23.5
Chronic lower respiratory diseases	- - -	- - -	- - -	49.9	55.4	55.8	51.2	47.6	48.0
Influenza and pneumonia	55.0	65.8	54.0	42.1	47.8	28.9	23.9	21.2	19.3
Chronic liver disease and cirrhosis	15.0	18.5	24.8	21.3	15.9	13.4	12.4	12.1	12.7
Diabetes mellitus	18.8	19.9	23.0	18.1	21.7	27.8	28.4	27.4	26.4
Human immunodeficiency virus (HIV) disease	- - -	- - -	- - -	- - -	18.5	7.9	6.2	5.9	5.4
Unintentional injuries	101.8	85.5	87.4	69.0	52.9	49.3	54.2	55.2	55.2
Motor vehicle-related injuries	38.5	35.4	41.5	33.6	26.5	21.7	21.7	21.4	20.9
Poisoning	3.3	2.3	3.9	2.7	3.5	6.6	10.7	12.4	13.0
Suicide[6]	21.2	20.0	19.8	19.9	21.5	17.7	18.0	18.0	18.4
Homicide[6]	7.9	7.5	14.3	16.6	14.8	9.0	9.6	9.7	9.6
Female									
All causes	1,236.0	1,105.3	971.4	817.9	750.9	731.4	677.6	657.8	643.4
Diseases of heart	486.6	447.0	381.6	320.8	257.0	210.9	172.3	162.2	154.0
Ischemic heart disease	- - -	- - -	- - -	263.1	193.9	146.5	111.7	103.1	95.7
Cerebrovascular diseases	175.8	170.7	140.0	91.7	62.6	59.1	45.6	42.6	41.3
Malignant neoplasms	182.3	168.7	163.2	166.7	175.7	167.6	155.6	153.6	151.3
Trachea, bronchus, and lung	5.8	7.5	13.1	24.4	37.1	41.3	40.5	40.0	40.0
Colon, rectum, and anus	- - -	29.1	26.5	23.8	20.6	17.7	14.8	14.7	14.4
Breast	31.9	31.7	32.1	31.9	33.3	26.8	24.1	23.5	22.9
Chronic lower respiratory diseases	- - -	- - -	- - -	14.9	26.6	37.4	38.1	35.9	36.0
Influenza and pneumonia	41.9	43.8	32.7	25.1	30.5	20.7	17.9	15.5	14.2
Chronic liver disease and cirrhosis	7.8	8.7	11.9	9.9	7.1	6.2	5.8	5.8	5.9
Diabetes mellitus	27.0	24.7	25.1	18.0	19.9	23.0	21.6	20.1	19.5
Human immunodeficiency virus (HIV) disease	- - -	- - -	- - -	- - -	2.2	2.5	2.3	2.2	2.1
Unintentional injuries	54.0	40.0	35.1	26.1	21.5	22.0	25.0	25.5	25.8
Motor vehicle-related injuries	11.5	11.7	14.9	11.8	11.0	9.5	8.9	8.8	8.2
Poisoning	1.7	1.1	1.8	1.3	1.2	2.5	5.1	5.9	6.6
Suicide[6]	5.6	5.6	7.4	5.7	4.8	4.0	4.4	4.5	4.7
Homicide[6]	2.4	2.6	3.7	4.4	4.0	2.8	2.5	2.5	2.5

See footnotes at end of table.

Table 24 (page 2 of 4). Age-adjusted death rates for selected causes of death, by sex, race, and Hispanic origin: United States, selected years 1950–2007

[Data are based on death certificates]

Sex, race, Hispanic origin, and cause of death[1]	1950[2,3]	1960[2,3]	1970[3]	1980[3]	1990	2000[4]	2005[4]	2006[4]	2007[4]
White[7]	Age-adjusted death rate per 100,000 population[5]								
All causes	1,410.8	1,311.3	1,193.3	1,012.7	909.8	849.8	785.3	764.4	749.4
Diseases of heart	586.0	559.0	492.2	409.4	317.0	253.4	207.8	197.0	187.8
Ischemic heart disease	- - -	- - -	- - -	347.6	249.7	185.6	143.8	134.2	125.5
Cerebrovascular diseases	175.5	172.7	143.5	93.2	62.8	58.8	44.7	41.7	40.5
Malignant neoplasms	194.6	193.1	196.7	204.2	211.6	197.2	182.6	179.9	177.5
Trachea, bronchus, and lung	15.2	24.0	36.7	49.2	58.6	56.2	53.1	52.1	51.2
Colon, rectum, and anus	- - -	30.9	29.2	27.4	24.1	20.3	16.9	16.7	16.4
Chronic lower respiratory diseases	- - -	- - -	- - -	29.3	38.3	46.0	45.4	42.6	43.0
Influenza and pneumonia	44.8	50.4	39.8	30.9	36.4	23.5	20.2	17.7	16.0
Chronic liver disease and cirrhosis	11.5	13.2	16.6	13.9	10.5	9.6	9.2	9.1	9.4
Diabetes mellitus	22.9	21.7	22.9	16.7	18.8	22.8	22.5	21.2	20.5
Human immunodeficiency virus (HIV) disease	- - -	- - -	- - -	- - -	8.3	2.8	2.2	2.1	1.9
Unintentional injuries	77.0	60.4	57.8	45.3	35.5	35.1	40.1	41.0	41.5
Motor vehicle-related injuries	24.4	22.9	27.1	22.6	18.5	15.6	15.6	15.4	14.8
Poisoning	2.4	1.6	2.4	1.8	2.1	4.5	8.4	9.7	10.6
Suicide[6]	13.9	13.1	13.8	13.0	13.4	11.3	12.0	12.1	12.5
Homicide[6]	2.6	2.7	4.7	6.7	5.5	3.6	3.7	3.7	3.7
Black or African American[7]									
All causes	1,722.1	1,577.5	1,518.1	1,314.8	1,250.3	1,121.4	1,016.5	982.0	958.0
Diseases of heart	588.7	548.3	512.0	455.3	391.5	324.8	271.3	257.7	247.3
Ischemic heart disease	- - -	- - -	- - -	334.5	267.0	218.3	171.3	161.6	150.6
Cerebrovascular diseases	233.6	235.2	197.1	129.1	91.6	81.9	65.2	61.6	60.3
Malignant neoplasms	176.4	199.1	225.3	256.4	279.5	248.5	222.7	217.4	215.5
Trachea, bronchus, and lung	11.1	23.7	41.3	59.7	72.4	64.0	58.4	56.8	55.6
Colon, rectum, and anus	- - -	22.8	26.1	28.3	30.6	28.2	24.8	24.3	23.5
Chronic lower respiratory diseases	- - -	- - -	- - -	19.2	28.1	31.6	30.6	28.1	28.1
Influenza and pneumonia	76.7	81.1	57.2	34.4	39.4	25.6	21.7	19.6	18.4
Chronic liver disease and cirrhosis	9.0	13.6	28.1	25.0	16.5	9.4	7.7	7.0	7.4
Diabetes mellitus	23.5	30.9	38.8	32.7	40.5	49.5	46.9	45.1	42.8
Human immunodeficiency virus (HIV) disease	- - -	- - -	- - -	- - -	26.7	23.3	19.4	18.6	17.3
Unintentional injuries	79.9	74.0	78.3	57.6	43.8	37.7	38.7	38.3	36.6
Motor vehicle-related injuries	26.0	24.2	31.1	20.2	18.8	15.7	14.5	14.6	14.1
Poisoning	2.8	2.9	5.8	3.1	4.1	6.0	8.2	9.4	8.6
Suicide[6]	4.5	5.0	6.2	6.5	7.1	5.5	5.2	5.1	5.0
Homicide[6]	28.3	26.0	44.0	39.0	36.3	20.5	21.1	21.6	21.1
American Indian or Alaska Native[7]									
All causes	- - -	- - -	- - -	867.0	716.3	709.3	663.4	642.1	627.2
Diseases of heart	- - -	- - -	- - -	240.6	200.6	178.2	141.8	139.4	127.3
Ischemic heart disease	- - -	- - -	- - -	173.6	139.1	129.1	96.2	97.4	86.7
Cerebrovascular diseases	- - -	- - -	- - -	57.8	40.7	45.0	34.8	29.4	29.8
Malignant neoplasms	- - -	- - -	- - -	113.7	121.8	127.8	123.2	119.4	117.8
Trachea, bronchus, and lung	- - -	- - -	- - -	20.7	30.9	32.3	34.1	31.2	32.7
Colon, rectum, and anus	- - -	- - -	- - -	9.5	12.0	13.4	12.0	11.2	11.5
Chronic lower respiratory diseases	- - -	- - -	- - -	14.2	25.4	32.8	29.1	27.4	30.9
Influenza and pneumonia	- - -	- - -	- - -	44.4	36.1	22.3	20.4	14.2	13.8
Chronic liver disease and cirrhosis	- - -	- - -	- - -	45.3	24.1	24.3	22.6	22.1	24.8
Diabetes mellitus	- - -	- - -	- - -	29.6	34.1	41.5	41.5	39.6	37.2
Human immunodeficiency virus (HIV) disease	- - -	- - -	- - -	- - -	1.8	2.2	2.7	2.4	2.6
Unintentional injuries	- - -	- - -	- - -	99.0	62.6	51.3	54.7	56.7	55.7
Motor vehicle-related injuries	- - -	- - -	- - -	54.5	32.5	27.3	24.8	26.7	23.7
Poisoning	- - -	- - -	- - -	2.3	3.2	4.7	9.4	10.4	11.6
Suicide[6]	- - -	- - -	- - -	11.9	11.7	9.8	11.7	11.6	11.5
Homicide[6]	- - -	- - -	- - -	15.5	10.4	6.8	7.7	7.5	6.5

See footnotes at end of table.

Table 24 (page 3 of 4). Age-adjusted death rates for selected causes of death, by sex, race, and Hispanic origin: United States, selected years 1950–2007

[Data are based on death certificates]

Sex, race, Hispanic origin, and cause of death[1]	1950[2,3]	1960[2,3]	1970[3]	1980[3]	1990	2000[4]	2005[4]	2006[4]	2007[4]
Asian or Pacific Islander[7]				Age-adjusted death rate per 100,000 population[5]					
All causes............................	- - -	- - -	- - -	589.9	582.0	506.4	440.2	428.6	415.0
Diseases of heart	- - -	- - -	- - -	202.1	181.7	146.0	113.3	108.5	101.2
Ischemic heart disease.................	- - -	- - -	- - -	168.2	139.6	109.6	81.0	77.1	71.0
Cerebrovascular diseases	- - -	- - -	- - -	66.1	56.9	52.9	38.6	37.0	34.3
Malignant neoplasms...................	- - -	- - -	- - -	126.1	134.2	121.9	110.5	106.5	106.7
Trachea, bronchus, and lung...........	- - -	- - -	- - -	28.4	30.2	28.1	25.7	25.2	25.3
Colon, rectum, and anus..............	- - -	- - -	- - -	16.4	14.4	12.7	11.2	10.9	10.9
Chronic lower respiratory diseases	- - -	- - -	- - -	12.9	19.4	18.6	14.9	14.4	13.4
Influenza and pneumonia...............	- - -	- - -	- - -	24.0	31.4	19.7	15.5	14.7	13.6
Chronic liver disease and cirrhosis	- - -	- - -	- - -	6.1	5.2	3.5	3.6	3.5	3.3
Diabetes mellitus.....................	- - -	- - -	- - -	12.6	14.6	16.4	16.6	15.8	16.2
Human immunodeficiency virus (HIV) disease ...	- - -	- - -	- - -	- - -	2.2	0.6	0.6	0.6	0.5
Unintentional injuries	- - -	- - -	- - -	27.0	23.9	17.9	17.9	16.9	17.0
Motor vehicle-related injuries...........	- - -	- - -	- - -	13.9	14.0	8.6	7.6	7.5	7.2
Poisoning	- - -	- - -	- - -	0.5	0.7	0.7	1.3	1.4	1.5
Suicide[6]	- - -	- - -	- - -	7.8	6.7	5.5	5.2	5.6	6.1
Homicide[6]...........................	- - -	- - -	- - -	5.9	5.0	3.0	2.9	2.8	2.3
Hispanic or Latino[7,8]									
All causes............................	- - -	- - -	- - -	- - -	692.0	665.7	590.7	564.0	546.1
Diseases of heart	- - -	- - -	- - -	- - -	217.1	196.0	157.3	144.1	136.0
Ischemic heart disease.................	- - -	- - -	- - -	- - -	173.3	153.2	118.0	106.4	97.8
Cerebrovascular diseases	- - -	- - -	- - -	- - -	45.2	46.4	35.7	34.2	32.7
Malignant neoplasms...................	- - -	- - -	- - -	- - -	136.8	134.9	122.8	118.0	116.2
Trachea, bronchus, and lung...........	- - -	- - -	- - -	- - -	26.5	24.8	22.4	20.7	20.9
Colon, rectum, and anus..............	- - -	- - -	- - -	- - -	14.7	14.1	12.4	12.6	12.0
Chronic lower respiratory diseases	- - -	- - -	- - -	- - -	19.3	21.1	19.3	17.3	17.5
Influenza and pneumonia...............	- - -	- - -	- - -	- - -	29.7	20.6	16.8	15.0	13.1
Chronic liver disease and cirrhosis	- - -	- - -	- - -	- - -	18.3	16.5	13.9	13.3	13.8
Diabetes mellitus.....................	- - -	- - -	- - -	- - -	28.2	36.9	33.6	29.9	28.9
Human immunodeficiency virus (HIV) disease ...	- - -	- - -	- - -	- - -	16.3	6.7	4.7	4.5	4.1
Unintentional injuries	- - -	- - -	- - -	- - -	34.6	30.1	31.3	31.5	30.1
Motor vehicle-related injuries...........	- - -	- - -	- - -	- - -	19.5	14.7	14.7	14.6	13.3
Poisoning	- - -	- - -	- - -	- - -	3.2	4.1	5.2	5.7	5.8
Suicide[6]	- - -	- - -	- - -	- - -	7.8	5.9	5.6	5.3	6.0
Homicide[6]...........................	- - -	- - -	- - -	- - -	16.2	7.5	7.5	7.3	6.9

See footnotes at end of table.

Table 24 (page 4 of 4). Age-adjusted death rates for selected causes of death, by sex, race, and Hispanic origin: United States, selected years 1950–2007

[Data are based on death certificates]

Sex, race, Hispanic origin, and cause of death[1]	1950[2,3]	1960[2,3]	1970[3]	1980[3]	1990	2000[4]	2005[4]	2006[4]	2007[4]
White, not Hispanic or Latino[8]	Age-adjusted death rate per 100,000 population[5]								
All causes	- - -	- - -	- - -	- - -	914.5	855.5	796.6	777.0	763.3
Diseases of heart	- - -	- - -	- - -	- - -	319.7	255.5	210.7	200.3	191.4
Ischemic heart disease	- - -	- - -	- - -	- - -	251.9	186.6	145.2	136.0	127.4
Cerebrovascular diseases	- - -	- - -	- - -	- - -	63.5	59.0	45.0	41.9	40.7
Malignant neoplasms	- - -	- - -	- - -	- - -	215.4	200.6	187.0	184.6	182.3
Trachea, bronchus, and lung	- - -	- - -	- - -	- - -	60.3	58.2	55.5	54.7	53.9
Colon, rectum, and anus	- - -	- - -	- - -	- - -	24.6	20.5	17.2	17.0	16.7
Chronic lower respiratory diseases	- - -	- - -	- - -	- - -	39.2	47.2	47.2	44.4	44.9
Influenza and pneumonia	- - -	- - -	- - -	- - -	36.5	23.5	20.4	17.8	16.2
Chronic liver disease and cirrhosis	- - -	- - -	- - -	- - -	9.9	9.0	8.7	8.6	8.9
Diabetes mellitus	- - -	- - -	- - -	- - -	18.3	21.8	21.5	20.4	19.8
Human immunodeficiency virus (HIV) disease	- - -	- - -	- - -	- - -	7.4	2.2	1.8	1.7	1.5
Unintentional injuries	- - -	- - -	- - -	- - -	35.0	35.3	41.0	42.1	43.0
Motor vehicle-related injuries	- - -	- - -	- - -	- - -	18.2	15.6	15.5	15.3	14.9
Poisoning	- - -	- - -	- - -	- - -	2.0	4.6	9.0	10.5	11.6
Suicide[6]	- - -	- - -	- - -	- - -	13.8	12.0	12.9	13.2	13.5
Homicide[6]	- - -	- - -	- - -	- - -	4.0	2.8	2.7	2.7	2.8

- - - Data not available.

[1]Underlying cause of death code numbers are based on the applicable revision of the *International Classification of Diseases* (ICD) for data years shown. For the period 1980–1998, causes were coded using ICD–9 codes that are most nearly comparable with the 113 cause list for ICD–10. See Appendix II, Cause of death; Tables IV and V.

[2]Includes deaths of persons who were not residents of the 50 states and the District of Columbia (D.C.).

[3]Underlying cause of death was coded according to the 6th Revision of the *International Classification of Diseases* (ICD) in 1950, 7th Revision in 1960, 8th Revision in 1970, and 9th Revision in 1980–1998. See Appendix II, Cause of death; Tables IV and V.

[4]Starting with 1999 data, cause of death is coded according to ICD–10. See Appendix II, Cause of death, Table V; Comparability ratio, Table VI.

[5]Age-adjusted rates are calculated using the year 2000 standard population. Prior to 2003, age-adjusted rates were calculated using standard million proportions based on rounded population numbers. Starting with 2003 data, unrounded population numbers are used to calculate age-adjusted rates. See Appendix II, Age adjustment.

[6]Figures for 2001 (in Excel spreadsheet on the Web) include September 11-related deaths for which death certificates were filed as of October 24, 2002. See Appendix II, Cause of death; Table V for terrorism-related ICD–10 codes.

[7]The race groups, white, black, Asian or Pacific Islander, and American Indian or Alaska Native, include persons of Hispanic and non-Hispanic origin. Persons of Hispanic origin may be of any race. Death rates for the American Indian or Alaska Native and Asian or Pacific Islander populations are known to be underestimated. See Appendix II, Race, for a discussion of sources of bias in death rates by race and Hispanic origin.

[8]Prior to 1997, excludes data from states lacking an Hispanic-origin item on the death certificate. See Appendix II, Hispanic origin.

NOTES: Data for 1950 have been revised and differ from previous editions of *Health, United States*. Starting with *Health, United States, 2003*, rates for 1991–1999 were revised using intercensal population estimates based on the 2000 census. Rates for 2000 were revised based on 2000 census counts. Rates for 2001 and later years were computed using 2000-based postcensal estimates. See Appendix I, Population Census and Population Estimates. Starting with 2003 data, some states allowed the reporting of more than one race on the death certificate. The multiple-race data for these states were bridged to the single-race categories of the 1977 Office of Management and Budget Standards for comparability with other states. See Appendix II, Race. Data for additional years are available. See Appendix III.

SOURCE: CDC/NCHS, National Vital Statistics System; Grove RD, Hetzel AM. Vital statistics rates in the United States, 1940–1960. Washington, DC: U.S. Government Printing Office. 1968; numerator data from National Vital Statistics System, annual mortality files; denominator data from national population estimates for race groups from Table 1 and unpublished Hispanic population estimates for 1985–1996 prepared by the Housing and Household Economic Statistics Division, U.S. Census Bureau; additional mortality tables are available from: http://www.cdc.gov/nchs/nvss/mortality_tables.htm; Xu JQ, Kochanek KD, Murphy SL, Tejada-Vera B. Deaths: Final data for 2007. National vital statistics reports; vol 58 no 19. Hyattsville, MD: NCHS; 2010. Available from: http://www.cdc.gov/nchs/data/nvsr/nvsr58/nvsr58_19.pdf.

Table 25 (page 1 of 4). Years of potential life lost before age 75 for selected causes of death, by sex, race, and Hispanic origin: United States, selected years 1980–2007

[Data are based on death certificates]

Sex, race, Hispanic origin, and cause of death[2]	Crude 2007[3]	Age-adjusted[1]					
		1980	1990	2000[3]	2005[3]	2006[3]	2007[3]
		Years lost before age 75 per 100,000 population under 75 years of age					
All persons							
All causes	7,366.2	10,448.4	9,085.5	7,578.1	7,299.8	7,214.3	7,083.5
Diseases of heart	1,112.6	2,238.7	1,617.7	1,253.0	1,110.4	1,077.8	1,042.4
Ischemic heart disease.	694.0	1,729.3	1,153.6	841.8	701.8	675.5	642.1
Cerebrovascular diseases	195.4	357.5	259.6	223.3	193.3	190.2	184.5
Malignant neoplasms.	1,574.0	2,108.8	2,003.8	1,674.1	1,525.2	1,490.5	1,461.4
Trachea, bronchus, and lung.	402.9	548.5	561.4	443.1	392.9	378.7	366.8
Colorectal	136.8	190.0	164.7	141.9	124.7	126.1	126.7
Prostate[4]	55.4	84.9	96.8	63.6	55.1	54.8	53.5
Breast[5].	300.0	463.2	451.6	332.6	296.2	286.7	275.4
Chronic lower respiratory diseases	185.5	169.1	187.4	188.1	181.2	171.0	172.1
Influenza and pneumonia.	74.5	160.2	141.5	87.1	83.6	76.4	71.6
Chronic liver disease and cirrhosis	167.0	300.3	196.9	164.1	152.6	149.9	157.6
Diabetes mellitus.	181.9	134.4	155.9	178.4	179.9	176.5	170.1
Human immunodeficiency virus (HIV) disease	113.7	- - -	383.8	174.6	133.6	126.0	115.2
Unintentional injuries	1,155.5	1,543.5	1,162.1	1,026.5	1,132.7	1,167.5	1,159.5
Motor vehicle-related injuries.	536.4	912.9	716.4	574.3	564.4	561.2	538.4
Poisoning	351.2	68.0	81.2	163.6	287.3	332.5	354.3
Suicide[6]	357.2	392.0	393.1	334.5	347.3	348.7	357.5
Homicide[6]	276.0	425.5	417.4	266.5	276.8	281.8	278.3
Male							
All causes	9,171.1	13,777.2	11,973.5	9,572.2	9,206.1	9,092.6	8,919.9
Diseases of heart	1,528.7	3,352.1	2,356.0	1,766.0	1,561.6	1,517.5	1,468.2
Ischemic heart disease.	1,008.8	2,715.1	1,766.3	1,255.4	1,044.3	1,009.2	962.1
Cerebrovascular diseases	213.1	396.7	286.6	244.6	213.7	212.0	206.2
Malignant neoplasms.	1,642.2	2,360.8	2,214.6	1,810.8	1,639.7	1,595.2	1,565.1
Trachea, bronchus, and lung.	459.1	821.1	764.8	554.9	476.3	454.5	434.0
Colorectal	155.7	214.9	194.3	167.3	146.2	145.4	148.5
Prostate	55.4	84.9	96.8	63.6	55.1	54.8	53.5
Chronic lower respiratory diseases	194.0	235.1	224.8	206.0	195.8	182.4	187.5
Influenza and pneumonia.	85.6	202.5	180.0	102.8	97.8	88.9	83.5
Chronic liver disease and cirrhosis	231.9	415.0	283.9	236.9	216.1	210.9	222.4
Diabetes mellitus.	215.3	140.4	170.4	203.8	216.5	213.2	207.1
Human immunodeficiency virus (HIV) disease	158.5	- - -	686.2	258.9	192.0	178.3	161.0
Unintentional injuries	1,648.6	2,342.7	1,715.1	1,475.6	1,608.5	1,659.2	1,639.2
Motor vehicle-related injuries.	774.0	1,359.7	1,018.4	796.4	795.9	790.9	766.5
Poisoning	479.2	96.4	123.6	242.1	395.6	461.6	480.7
Suicide[6]	564.1	605.6	634.8	539.1	548.0	549.0	561.5
Homicide[6]	444.2	675.0	658.0	410.5	439.0	447.1	439.4
Female							
All causes	5,560.6	7,350.3	6,333.1	5,644.6	5,425.7	5,364.7	5,274.2
Diseases of heart	696.4	1,246.0	948.5	774.6	682.6	660.6	637.9
Ischemic heart disease.	379.2	852.1	600.3	457.6	379.0	360.6	339.7
Cerebrovascular diseases	177.7	324.0	235.9	203.9	174.4	169.8	164.3
Malignant neoplasms.	1,505.7	1,896.8	1,826.6	1,555.3	1,424.3	1,398.6	1,370.3
Trachea, bronchus, and lung.	346.8	310.4	382.2	342.1	316.9	309.7	305.6
Colorectal	117.9	168.7	138.7	118.7	104.9	108.4	106.6
Breast.	300.0	463.2	451.6	332.6	296.2	286.7	275.4
Chronic lower respiratory diseases	177.0	114.0	155.9	172.3	168.2	160.5	158.0
Influenza and pneumonia.	63.4	122.0	106.2	72.3	70.0	64.7	60.3
Chronic liver disease and cirrhosis	102.1	194.5	115.1	94.5	91.6	91.3	95.3
Diabetes mellitus.	148.4	128.5	142.3	154.4	145.1	141.7	135.0
Human immunodeficiency virus (HIV) disease	68.8	- - -	87.8	92.0	76.2	74.5	70.1
Unintentional injuries	662.1	755.3	607.4	573.2	648.0	666.1	670.2
Motor vehicle-related injuries.	298.8	470.4	411.6	348.5	327.1	325.4	304.5
Poisoning	223.1	40.2	39.1	85.0	177.2	201.0	225.3
Suicide[6]	150.4	184.2	153.3	129.1	144.1	145.7	150.8
Homicide[6]	107.7	181.3	174.3	118.9	108.7	110.4	111.2

See footnotes at end of table.

[Data are based on death certificates]

Sex, race, Hispanic origin, and cause of death[2]	Crude 2007[3]	Age-adjusted[1]					
		1980	1990	2000[3]	2005[3]	2006[3]	2007[3]
		Years lost before age 75 per 100,000 population under 75 years of age					
White[7]							
All causes	6,985.7	9,554.1	8,159.5	6,949.5	6,775.6	6,713.1	6,614.2
Diseases of heart	1,052.9	2,100.8	1,490.3	1,149.4	1,011.7	985.9	952.2
Ischemic heart disease	693.0	1,682.7	1,113.4	805.3	672.0	648.2	617.1
Cerebrovascular diseases	168.4	300.7	213.1	187.1	160.4	158.1	154.0
Malignant neoplasms	1,593.8	2,035.9	1,929.3	1,627.8	1,485.9	1,456.6	1,428.3
Trachea, bronchus, and lung	419.1	529.9	544.2	436.3	389.4	374.8	364.8
Colorectal	133.9	186.8	157.8	134.1	117.3	118.9	119.6
Prostate[4]	50.6	74.8	86.6	54.3	47.0	47.3	46.2
Breast[5]	289.1	460.2	441.7	315.6	275.1	269.0	256.9
Chronic lower respiratory diseases	197.2	165.4	182.3	185.3	182.2	172.0	174.0
Influenza and pneumonia	69.2	130.8	116.9	77.7	76.3	70.4	65.2
Chronic liver disease and cirrhosis	177.9	257.3	175.8	162.7	156.7	155.3	163.6
Diabetes mellitus	163.7	115.7	133.7	155.6	156.3	152.8	147.7
Human immunodeficiency virus (HIV) disease	57.5	- - -	309.0	94.7	69.8	64.6	58.1
Unintentional injuries	1,193.3	1,520.4	1,139.7	1,031.8	1,170.9	1,209.8	1,208.5
Motor vehicle-related injuries	548.5	939.9	726.7	586.1	585.7	580.5	557.5
Poisoning	385.7	64.9	74.4	167.2	310.6	360.6	391.9
Suicide[6]	392.6	414.5	417.7	362.0	381.2	383.5	393.8
Homicide[6]	158.2	271.7	234.9	156.6	159.7	160.1	162.4
Black or African American[7]							
All causes	11,005.6	17,873.4	16,593.0	12,897.1	11,890.7	11,646.3	11,259.8
Diseases of heart	1,728.1	3,619.9	2,891.8	2,275.2	2,046.0	1,969.3	1,906.3
Ischemic heart disease	864.8	2,305.1	1,676.1	1,300.1	1,080.2	1,034.5	972.4
Cerebrovascular diseases	375.0	883.2	656.4	507.0	441.7	431.8	416.5
Malignant neoplasms	1,768.4	2,946.1	2,894.8	2,294.7	2,069.7	2,003.1	1,966.9
Trachea, bronchus, and lung	415.8	776.0	811.3	593.0	511.8	496.4	470.9
Colorectal	178.4	232.3	241.8	222.4	199.6	198.9	199.5
Prostate[4]	103.3	200.3	223.5	171.0	144.8	140.0	138.8
Breast[5]	422.8	524.2	592.9	500.0	485.7	450.1	445.3
Chronic lower respiratory diseases	175.8	203.7	240.6	232.7	211.0	197.6	192.7
Influenza and pneumonia	117.4	384.9	330.8	161.2	145.3	127.6	123.7
Chronic liver disease and cirrhosis	119.9	644.0	371.8	185.6	138.4	127.0	130.4
Diabetes mellitus	321.7	305.3	361.5	383.4	379.9	375.4	358.6
Human immunodeficiency virus (HIV) disease	483.2	- - -	1,014.7	763.3	594.4	566.8	522.1
Unintentional injuries	1,139.3	1,751.5	1,392.7	1,152.8	1,134.6	1,170.7	1,116.5
Motor vehicle-related injuries	539.4	750.2	699.5	580.8	532.3	541.6	521.4
Poisoning	250.7	99.4	144.3	196.6	253.8	296.1	263.5
Suicide[6]	190.0	238.0	261.4	208.7	194.0	187.3	187.3
Homicide[6]	1,031.8	1,580.8	1,612.9	941.6	967.8	998.6	967.7
American Indian or Alaska Native[7]							
All causes	8,164.2	13,390.9	9,506.2	7,758.2	8,624.4	8,517.6	8,463.6
Diseases of heart	885.5	1,819.9	1,391.0	1,030.1	1,010.2	1,008.6	985.4
Ischemic heart disease	514.5	1,208.2	901.8	709.3	625.2	614.2	587.1
Cerebrovascular diseases	148.7	269.3	223.3	198.1	209.4	178.2	170.0
Malignant neoplasms	881.4	1,101.3	1,141.1	995.7	1,084.3	983.9	991.1
Trachea, bronchus, and lung	190.1	181.1	268.1	227.8	268.2	225.3	226.3
Colorectal	89.2	78.8	82.4	93.8	109.7	88.1	100.5
Prostate[4]	26.6	66.7	42.0	44.5	37.6	38.8	33.5
Breast[5]	153.8	205.5	213.4	174.1	149.2	172.9	163.8
Chronic lower respiratory diseases	147.3	89.3	129.0	151.8	155.3	144.6	171.4
Influenza and pneumonia	103.3	307.9	206.3	124.0	113.6	101.6	110.9
Chronic liver disease and cirrhosis	529.3	1,190.3	535.1	519.4	498.9	479.2	576.3
Diabetes mellitus	253.0	305.5	292.3	305.6	347.3	324.8	292.6
Human immunodeficiency virus (HIV) disease	72.0	- - -	70.1	68.4	89.9	76.1	79.7
Unintentional injuries	1,955.0	3,541.0	2,183.9	1,700.1	1,875.6	1,885.1	1,870.6
Motor vehicle-related injuries	1,009.1	2,102.4	1,301.5	1,032.2	1,004.9	1,021.7	930.5
Poisoning	421.9	92.9	119.5	180.1	333.8	358.5	416.7
Suicide[6]	514.3	515.0	495.9	403.1	498.6	487.8	470.6
Homicide[6]	305.3	628.9	434.2	278.5	337.5	328.3	283.3

See footnotes at end of table.

Table 25 (page 3 of 4). Years of potential life lost before age 75 for selected causes of death, by sex, race, and Hispanic origin: United States, selected years 1980–2007

[Data are based on death certificates]

Sex, race, Hispanic origin, and cause of death[2]	Crude 2007[3]	Age-adjusted[1]					
		1980	1990	2000[3]	2005[3]	2006[3]	2007[3]
Asian or Pacific Islander[7]		Years lost before age 75 per 100,000 population under 75 years of age					
All causes	3,388.3	5,378.4	4,705.2	3,811.1	3,533.2	3,450.6	3,404.9
Diseases of heart	445.5	952.8	702.2	567.9	513.8	471.8	454.5
Ischemic heart disease.	286.7	697.7	486.6	381.1	326.5	305.7	295.4
Cerebrovascular diseases	149.5	266.9	233.5	199.4	162.8	163.9	153.5
Malignant neoplasms.	882.2	1,218.6	1,166.4	1,033.8	945.3	912.7	895.8
Trachea, bronchus, and lung.	156.5	238.2	204.7	185.8	169.2	171.3	162.5
Colorectal	81.1	115.9	105.1	91.6	78.7	81.2	82.1
Prostate[4]	13.4	17.0	32.4	18.8	20.4	18.3	16.6
Breast[5].	163.3	222.2	216.5	200.8	178.4	173.3	156.3
Chronic lower respiratory diseases	34.0	56.4	72.8	56.5	36.0	37.4	35.9
Influenza and pneumonia.	35.4	79.3	74.0	48.6	40.3	36.8	37.1
Chronic liver disease and cirrhosis	41.8	85.6	72.4	44.8	43.6	44.3	41.3
Diabetes mellitus.	77.0	83.1	74.0	77.0	78.1	80.8	79.5
Human immunodeficiency virus (HIV) disease	16.1	- - -	77.0	19.9	16.6	15.4	15.0
Unintentional injuries	418.2	742.7	636.6	425.7	413.7	411.0	417.4
Motor vehicle-related injuries.	231.0	472.6	445.5	263.4	242.1	243.9	231.8
Poisoning	55.8	*	17.6	25.9	42.0	46.6	52.8
Suicide[6]	212.6	217.1	200.6	168.6	164.6	185.1	205.0
Homicide[6]	100.0	201.1	205.8	113.1	130.8	121.7	97.3
Hispanic or Latino[7,8]							
All causes	5,118.6	- - -	7,963.3	6,037.6	5,757.9	5,601.9	5,447.4
Diseases of heart	487.2	- - -	1,082.0	821.3	727.0	686.8	666.9
Ischemic heart disease.	280.7	- - -	756.6	564.6	483.2	446.2	418.0
Cerebrovascular diseases	131.4	- - -	238.0	207.8	184.9	184.5	176.0
Malignant neoplasms.	742.3	- - -	1,232.2	1,098.2	1,017.5	987.7	991.2
Trachea, bronchus, and lung.	80.9	- - -	193.7	152.1	138.1	125.0	126.0
Colorectal	65.2	- - -	100.2	101.4	86.4	91.5	92.7
Prostate[4]	22.6	- - -	47.7	42.9	41.7	43.8	43.5
Breast[5].	150.7	- - -	299.3	230.7	197.3	203.2	194.7
Chronic lower respiratory diseases	40.9	- - -	78.8	68.5	62.2	56.9	56.5
Influenza and pneumonia.	47.1	- - -	130.1	76.0	69.5	65.1	55.1
Chronic liver disease and cirrhosis	157.3	- - -	329.1	252.1	210.3	201.4	210.3
Diabetes mellitus.	122.3	- - -	177.8	215.6	202.2	181.1	178.6
Human immunodeficiency virus (HIV) disease	100.6	- - -	600.1	209.4	139.3	129.0	115.6
Unintentional injuries	977.1	- - -	1,190.6	920.1	980.1	993.0	929.0
Motor vehicle-related injuries.	551.1	- - -	740.8	540.2	569.2	564.7	509.1
Poisoning	196.7	- - -	121.9	145.9	179.5	195.6	202.1
Suicide[6]	205.4	- - -	256.2	188.5	193.2	185.1	200.3
Homicide[6]	362.2	- - -	720.8	335.1	343.0	335.3	322.6

See footnotes at end of table.

Table 25 (page 4 of 4). Years of potential life lost before age 75 for selected causes of death, by sex, race, and Hispanic origin: United States, selected years 1980–2007

[Data are based on death certificates]

Sex, race, Hispanic origin, and cause of death[2]	Crude 2007[3]	Age-adjusted[1]					
		1980	1990	2000[3]	2005[3]	2006[3]	2007[3]
White, not Hispanic or Latino[8]		Years lost before age 75 per 100,000 population under 75 years of age					
All causes	7,341.4	- - -	8,022.5	6,960.5	6,853.3	6,813.8	6,736.5
Diseases of heart	1,171.7	- - -	1,504.0	1,175.1	1,046.4	1,024.0	989.1
Ischemic heart disease	780.2	- - -	1,127.2	824.7	694.4	673.5	643.5
Cerebrovascular diseases	174.9	- - -	210.1	183.0	155.5	152.5	149.3
Malignant neoplasms	1,774.1	- - -	1,974.1	1,668.4	1,534.3	1,505.9	1,474.4
Trachea, bronchus, and lung	493.3	- - -	566.8	460.3	416.3	402.4	392.3
Colorectal	148.5	- - -	162.1	136.2	120.8	121.8	122.9
Prostate[4]	56.8	- - -	89.2	54.9	47.3	47.6	46.3
Breast[5]	316.8	- - -	451.5	322.3	283.6	275.5	263.1
Chronic lower respiratory diseases	231.3	- - -	188.1	193.8	194.0	183.4	186.5
Influenza and pneumonia	73.6	- - -	112.3	76.4	76.8	70.4	66.6
Chronic liver disease and cirrhosis	180.1	- - -	162.4	150.9	147.8	147.4	155.5
Diabetes mellitus	171.4	- - -	131.2	150.2	151.5	150.1	144.5
Human immunodeficiency virus (HIV) disease	46.6	- - -	271.2	76.0	56.6	51.5	45.8
Unintentional injuries	1,228.8	- - -	1,114.7	1,041.4	1,199.6	1,246.4	1,263.4
Motor vehicle-related injuries	541.1	- - -	715.7	588.8	579.9	575.4	561.1
Poisoning	424.8	- - -	68.3	169.4	338.2	397.9	435.8
Suicide[6]	431.7	- - -	433.0	389.2	416.6	422.7	433.8
Homicide[6]	109.0	- - -	162.0	113.2	109.1	109.9	115.4

- - - Data not available.

* Rates based on fewer than 20 deaths are considered unreliable and are not shown.

[1]Age-adjusted rates are calculated using the year 2000 standard population. Prior to 2003, age-adjusted rates were calculated using standard million proportions based on rounded population numbers. Starting with 2003 data, unrounded population numbers are used to calculate age-adjusted rates. See Appendix II, Age adjustment.

[2]Underlying cause of death was coded according to the 6th Revision of the *International Classification of Diseases* (ICD) in 1950, 7th Revision in 1960, 8th Revision in 1970, and 9th Revision in 1980–1998. See Appendix II, Cause of death; Tables IV and V.

[3]Starting with 1999 data, cause of death is coded according to ICD–10. See Appendix II, Cause of death, Table V; Comparability ratio, Table VI.

[4]Rate for male population only.

[5]Rate for female population only.

[6]Figures for 2001 (in Excel spreadsheet on the Web) include September 11-related deaths for which death certificates were filed as of October 24, 2002. See Appendix II, Cause of death; Table V for terrorism-related ICD–10 codes.

[7]The race groups, white, black, Asian or Pacific Islander, and American Indian or Alaska Native, include persons of Hispanic and non-Hispanic origin. Persons of Hispanic origin may be of any race. Death rates for the American Indian or Alaska Native and Asian or Pacific Islander populations are known to be underestimated. See Appendix II, Race, for a discussion of sources of bias in death rates by race and Hispanic origin.

[8]Prior to 1997, excludes data from states lacking an Hispanic-origin item on the death certificate. See Appendix II, Hispanic origin.

NOTES: Starting with *Health, United States, 2003*, rates for 1991–1999 were revised using intercensal population estimates based on the 2000 census. Rates for 2000 were revised based on 2000 census counts. Rates for 2001 and later years were computed using 2000-based postcensal estimates. See Appendix I, Population Census and Population Estimates. See Appendix II, Years of potential life lost (YPLL) for definition and method of calculation. Starting with 2003 data, some states allowed the reporting of more than one race on the death certificate. The multiple-race data for these states were bridged to the single-race categories of the 1977 Office of Management and Budget Standards for comparability with other states. See Appendix II, Race. Data for additional years are available. See Appendix III.

SOURCE: CDC/NCHS, National vital statistics system; numerator data from annual mortality files; denominator data from national population estimates for race groups from Table 1 and unpublished Hispanic population estimates for 1990–1996 prepared by the Housing and Household Economic Statistics Division, U.S. Census Bureau.

Table 26 (page 1 of 4). Leading causes of death and numbers of deaths, by sex, race, and Hispanic origin: United States, 1980 and 2007

[Data are based on death certificates]

Sex, race, Hispanic origin, and rank order	1980 Cause of death	Deaths	2007 Cause of death	Deaths
All persons				
Rank	All causes	1,989,841	All causes	2,423,712
1	Diseases of heart	761,085	Diseases of heart	616,067
2	Malignant neoplasms	416,509	Malignant neoplasms	562,875
3	Cerebrovascular diseases	170,225	Cerebrovascular diseases	135,952
4	Unintentional injuries	105,718	Chronic lower respiratory diseases	127,924
5	Chronic obstructive pulmonary diseases	56,050	Unintentional injuries	123,706
6	Pneumonia and influenza	54,619	Alzheimer's disease	74,632
7	Diabetes mellitus	34,851	Diabetes mellitus	71,382
8	Chronic liver disease and cirrhosis	30,583	Influenza and pneumonia	52,717
9	Atherosclerosis	29,449	Nephritis, nephrotic syndrome and nephrosis	46,448
10	Suicide	26,869	Septicemia	34,828
Male				
Rank	All causes	1,075,078	All causes	1,203,968
1	Diseases of heart	405,661	Diseases of heart	309,821
2	Malignant neoplasms	225,948	Malignant neoplasms	292,857
3	Unintentional injuries	74,180	Unintentional injuries	79,827
4	Cerebrovascular diseases	69,973	Chronic lower respiratory diseases	61,235
5	Chronic obstructive pulmonary diseases	38,625	Cerebrovascular diseases	54,111
6	Pneumonia and influenza	27,574	Diabetes mellitus	35,478
7	Suicide	20,505	Suicide	27,269
8	Chronic liver disease and cirrhosis	19,768	Influenza and pneumonia	24,071
9	Homicide	18,779	Nephritis, nephrotic syndrome and nephrosis	22,616
10	Diabetes mellitus	14,325	Alzheimer's disease	21,800
Female				
Rank	All causes	914,763	All causes	1,219,744
1	Diseases of heart	355,424	Diseases of heart	306,246
2	Malignant neoplasms	190,561	Malignant neoplasms	270,018
3	Cerebrovascular diseases	100,252	Cerebrovascular diseases	81,841
4	Unintentional injuries	31,538	Chronic lower respiratory diseases	66,689
5	Pneumonia and influenza	27,045	Alzheimer's disease	52,832
6	Diabetes mellitus	20,526	Unintentional injuries	43,879
7	Atherosclerosis	17,848	Diabetes mellitus	35,904
8	Chronic obstructive pulmonary diseases	17,425	Influenza and pneumonia	28,646
9	Chronic liver disease and cirrhosis	10,815	Nephritis, nephrotic syndrome and nephrosis	23,832
10	Certain conditions originating in the perinatal period	9,815	Septicemia	18,989
White				
Rank	All causes	1,738,607	All causes	2,074,151
1	Diseases of heart	683,347	Diseases of heart	531,636
2	Malignant neoplasms	368,162	Malignant neoplasms	483,939
3	Cerebrovascular diseases	148,734	Chronic lower respiratory diseases	118,081
4	Unintentional injuries	90,122	Cerebrovascular diseases	114,695
5	Chronic obstructive pulmonary diseases	52,375	Unintentional injuries	106,252
6	Pneumonia and influenza	48,369	Alzheimer's disease	68,933
7	Diabetes mellitus	28,868	Diabetes mellitus	56,390
8	Atherosclerosis	27,069	Influenza and pneumonia	45,947
9	Chronic liver disease and cirrhosis	25,240	Nephritis, nephrotic syndrome and nephrosis	36,871
10	Suicide	24,829	Suicide	31,348
Black or African American				
Rank	All causes	233,135	All causes	289,585
1	Diseases of heart	72,956	Diseases of heart	71,209
2	Malignant neoplasms	45,037	Malignant neoplasms	64,049
3	Cerebrovascular diseases	20,135	Cerebrovascular diseases	17,085
4	Unintentional injuries	13,480	Unintentional injuries	13,559
5	Homicide	10,172	Diabetes mellitus	12,459
6	Certain conditions originating in the perinatal period	6,961	Homicide	8,870
7	Pneumonia and influenza	5,648	Nephritis, nephrotic syndrome and nephrosis	8,392
8	Diabetes mellitus	5,544	Chronic lower respiratory diseases	7,901
9	Chronic liver disease and cirrhosis	4,790	Human immunodeficiency virus (HIV) disease	6,470
10	Nephritis, nephrotic syndrome, and nephrosis	3,416	Septicemia	6,297

See footnotes at end of table.

Table 26 (page 2 of 4). Leading causes of death and numbers of deaths, by sex, race, and Hispanic origin: United States, 1980 and 2007

[Data are based on death certificates]

Sex, race, Hispanic origin, and rank order	1980 Cause of death	1980 Deaths	2007 Cause of death	2007 Deaths
American Indian or Alaska Native				
Rank	All causes	6,923	All causes	14,367
1	Diseases of heart	1,494	Diseases of heart	2,648
2	Unintentional injuries	1,290	Malignant neoplasms	2,561
3	Malignant neoplasms	770	Unintentional injuries	1,701
4	Chronic liver disease and cirrhosis	410	Diabetes mellitus	790
5	Cerebrovascular diseases	322	Chronic liver disease and cirrhosis	709
6	Pneumonia and influenza	257	Chronic lower respiratory diseases	611
7	Homicide	217	Cerebrovascular diseases	586
8	Diabetes mellitus	210	Suicide	392
9	Certain conditions originating in the perinatal period .	199	Nephritis, nephrotic syndrome and nephrosis	292
10	Suicide	181	Influenza and pneumonia	280
Asian or Pacific Islander				
Rank	All causes	11,071	All causes	45,609
1	Diseases of heart	3,265	Malignant neoplasms	12,326
2	Malignant neoplasms	2,522	Diseases of heart	10,574
3	Cerebrovascular diseases	1,028	Cerebrovascular diseases	3,586
4	Unintentional injuries	810	Unintentional injuries	2,194
5	Pneumonia and influenza	342	Diabetes mellitus	1,743
6	Suicide	249	Influenza and pneumonia	1,335
7	Certain conditions originating in the perinatal period .	246	Chronic lower respiratory diseases	1,331
8	Diabetes mellitus	227	Suicide	900
9	Homicide	211	Nephritis, nephrotic syndrome and nephrosis	893
10	Chronic obstructive pulmonary diseases	207	Alzheimer's disease	748
Hispanic or Latino				
Rank		- - -	All causes	135,519
1		- - -	Diseases of heart	29,021
2		- - -	Malignant neoplasms	27,660
3		- - -	Unintentional injuries	11,723
4		- - -	Cerebrovascular diseases	7,078
5		- - -	Diabetes mellitus	6,417
6		- - -	Chronic liver disease and cirrhosis	3,913
7		- - -	Chronic lower respiratory diseases	3,531
8		- - -	Homicide	3,466
9		- - -	Certain conditions originating in the perinatal period .	2,946
10		- - -	Influenza and pneumonia	2,735
White male				
Rank	All causes	933,878	All causes	1,023,951
1	Diseases of heart	364,679	Diseases of heart	266,908
2	Malignant neoplasms	198,188	Malignant neoplasms	252,049
3	Unintentional injuries	62,963	Unintentional injuries	68,059
4	Cerebrovascular diseases	60,095	Chronic lower respiratory diseases	55,934
5	Chronic obstructive pulmonary diseases	35,977	Cerebrovascular diseases	44,714
6	Pneumonia and influenza	23,810	Diabetes mellitus	28,744
7	Suicide	18,901	Suicide	24,725
8	Chronic liver disease and cirrhosis	16,407	Influenza and pneumonia	20,720
9	Diabetes mellitus	12,125	Alzheimer's disease	20,185
10	Atherosclerosis	10,543	Nephritis, nephrotic syndrome and nephrosis . . .	18,242
Black or African American male				
Rank	All causes	130,138	All causes	148,309
1	Diseases of heart	37,877	Diseases of heart	35,669
2	Malignant neoplasms	25,861	Malignant neoplasms	33,069
3	Unintentional injuries	9,701	Unintentional injuries	9,268
4	Cerebrovascular diseases	9,194	Homicide	7,584
5	Homicide	8,274	Cerebrovascular diseases	7,549
6	Certain conditions originating in the perinatal period .	3,869	Diabetes mellitus	5,493
7	Pneumonia and influenza	3,386	Chronic lower respiratory diseases	4,207
8	Chronic liver disease and cirrhosis	3,020	Human immunodeficiency virus (HIV) disease	4,186
9	Chronic obstructive pulmonary diseases	2,429	Nephritis, nephrotic syndrome and nephrosis	3,772
10	Diabetes mellitus	2,010	Certain conditions originating in the perinatal period .	2,846

See footnotes at end of table.

Table 26 (page 3 of 4). **Leading causes of death and numbers of deaths, by sex, race, and Hispanic origin: United States, 1980 and 2007**

[Data are based on death certificates]

Sex, race, Hispanic origin, and rank order	1980		2007	
	Cause of death	Deaths	Cause of death	Deaths
American Indian or Alaska Native male				
Rank	All causes	4,193	All causes	7,885
1	Unintentional injuries	946	Diseases of heart	1,520
2	Diseases of heart	917	Malignant neoplasms	1,345
3	Malignant neoplasms	408	Unintentional injuries	1,129
4	Chronic liver disease and cirrhosis	239	Chronic liver disease and cirrhosis	415
5	Cerebrovascular diseases	163	Diabetes mellitus	381
6	Homicide	162	Suicide	310
7	Pneumonia and influenza	148	Chronic lower respiratory diseases	299
8	Suicide	147	Cerebrovascular diseases	267
9	Certain conditions originating in the perinatal period	107	Homicide	163
10	Diabetes mellitus	86	Influenza and pneumonia	150
Asian or Pacific Islander male				
Rank	All causes	6,809	All causes	23,823
1	Diseases of heart	2,174	Malignant neoplasms	6,394
2	Malignant neoplasms	1,485	Diseases of heart	5,724
3	Unintentional injuries	556	Cerebrovascular diseases	1,581
4	Cerebrovascular diseases	521	Unintentional injuries	1,371
5	Pneumonia and influenza	227	Diabetes mellitus	860
6	Suicide	159	Chronic lower respiratory diseases	795
7	Chronic obstructive pulmonary diseases	158	Influenza and pneumonia	703
8	Homicide	151	Suicide	628
9	Certain conditions originating in the perinatal period	128	Nephritis, nephrotic syndrome and nephrosis	476
10	Diabetes mellitus	103	Septicemia	302
Hispanic or Latino male				
Rank	---	---	All causes	75,708
1	---	---	Diseases of heart	15,657
2	---	---	Malignant neoplasms	14,493
3	---	---	Unintentional injuries	8,844
4	---	---	Cerebrovascular diseases	3,319
5	---	---	Diabetes mellitus	3,199
6	---	---	Homicide	2,926
7	---	---	Chronic liver disease and cirrhosis	2,799
8	---	---	Suicide	2,078
9	---	---	Chronic lower respiratory diseases	1,894
10	---	---	Certain conditions originating in the perinatal period	1,643
White female				
Rank	All causes	804,729	All causes	1,050,200
1	Diseases of heart	318,668	Diseases of heart	264,728
2	Malignant neoplasms	169,974	Malignant neoplasms	231,890
3	Cerebrovascular diseases	88,639	Cerebrovascular diseases	69,981
4	Unintentional injuries	27,159	Chronic lower respiratory diseases	62,147
5	Pneumonia and influenza	24,559	Alzheimer's disease	48,748
6	Diabetes mellitus	16,743	Unintentional injuries	38,193
7	Atherosclerosis	16,526	Diabetes mellitus	27,646
8	Chronic obstructive pulmonary diseases	16,398	Influenza and pneumonia	25,227
9	Chronic liver disease and cirrhosis	8,833	Nephritis, nephrotic syndrome and nephrosis	18,629
10	Certain conditions originating in the perinatal period	6,512	Septicemia	15,150
Black or African American female				
Rank	All causes	102,997	All causes	141,276
1	Diseases of heart	35,079	Diseases of heart	35,540
2	Malignant neoplasms	19,176	Malignant neoplasms	30,980
3	Cerebrovascular diseases	10,941	Cerebrovascular diseases	9,536
4	Unintentional injuries	3,779	Diabetes mellitus	6,966
5	Diabetes mellitus	3,534	Nephritis, nephrotic syndrome and nephrosis	4,620
6	Certain conditions originating in the perinatal period	3,092	Unintentional injuries	4,291
7	Pneumonia and influenza	2,262	Chronic lower respiratory diseases	3,694
8	Homicide	1,898	Septicemia	3,462
9	Chronic liver disease and cirrhosis	1,770	Alzheimer's disease	3,459
10	Nephritis, nephrotic syndrome, and nephrosis	1,722	Essential hypertension and hypertensive renal disease	2,661

See footnotes at end of table.

Table 26 (page 4 of 4). Leading causes of death and numbers of deaths, by sex, race, and Hispanic origin: United States, 1980 and 2007

[Data are based on death certificates]

Sex, race, Hispanic origin, and rank order	1980 Cause of death	1980 Deaths	2007 Cause of death	2007 Deaths
American Indian or Alaska Native female				
Rank	All causes	2,730	All causes	6,482
1	Diseases of heart	577	Malignant neoplasms	1,216
2	Malignant neoplasms	362	Diseases of heart	1,128
3	Unintentional injuries	344	Unintentional injuries	572
4	Chronic liver disease and cirrhosis	171	Diabetes mellitus	409
5	Cerebrovascular diseases	159	Cerebrovascular diseases	319
6	Diabetes mellitus	124	Chronic lower respiratory diseases	312
7	Pneumonia and influenza	109	Chronic liver disease and cirrhosis	294
8	Certain conditions originating in the perinatal period	92	Nephritis, nephrotic syndrome and nephrosis	166
9	Nephritis, nephrotic syndrome, and nephrosis	56	Influenza and pneumonia	130
10	Homicide	55	Septicemia	128
Asian or Pacific Islander female				
Rank	All causes	4,262	All causes	21,786
1	Diseases of heart	1,091	Malignant neoplasms	5,932
2	Malignant neoplasms	1,037	Diseases of heart	4,850
3	Cerebrovascular diseases	507	Cerebrovascular diseases	2,005
4	Unintentional injuries	254	Diabetes mellitus	883
5	Diabetes mellitus	124	Unintentional injuries	823
6	Certain conditions originating in the perinatal period	118	Influenza and pneumonia	632
7	Pneumonia and influenza	115	Chronic lower respiratory diseases	536
8	Congenital anomalies	104	Alzheimer's disease	503
9	Suicide	90	Nephritis, nephrotic syndrome and nephrosis	417
10	Homicide	60	Essential (primary) hypertension and hypertensive renal disease	348
Hispanic or Latina female				
Rank	- - -	- - -	All causes	59,811
1	- - -	- - -	Diseases of heart	13,364
2	- - -	- - -	Malignant neoplasms	13,167
3	- - -	- - -	Cerebrovascular diseases	3,759
4	- - -	- - -	Diabetes mellitus	3,218
5	- - -	- - -	Unintentional injuries	2,879
6	- - -	- - -	Alzheimer's disease	1,670
7	- - -	- - -	Chronic lower respiratory diseases	1,637
8	- - -	- - -	Influenza and pneumonia	1,374
9	- - -	- - -	Nephritis, nephrotic syndrome and nephrosis	1,328
10	- - -	- - -	Certain conditions originating in the perinatal period	1,303

- - - Data not available.

NOTES: For cause of death codes based on the *International Classification of Diseases*, 9th Revision (ICD–9) in 1980 and ICD–10 in 2007, see Appendix II, Cause of death; Tables IV and V. Starting in 2006, the category essential (primary) hypertension and hypertensive renal disease was changed to essential hypertension and hypertensive renal disease to reflect the addition of secondary hypertension. Starting with 2003 data, some states allowed the reporting of more than one race on the death certificate. The multiple-race data for these states were bridged to the single-race categories of the 1977 Office of Management and Budget standards for comparability with other states. The race groups, white, black, Asian or Pacific Islander, and American Indian or Alaska Native, include persons of Hispanic and non-Hispanic origin. Persons of Hispanic origin may be of any race. See Appendix II, Race; Hispanic origin.

SOURCE: CDC/NCHS, National Vital Statistics System; Vital statistics of the United States, vol II, mortality, part A, 1980. Washington, DC: Public Health Service. 1985; 2007 annual mortality file. Xu JQ, Kochanek KD, Murphy SL, Tejada-Vera B. Deaths: Final data for 2007. National vital statistics reports; vol 58 no 19. Hyattsville, MD: NCHS; 2010. Available from: http://www.cdc.gov/nchs/data/nvsr/nvsr58/nvsr58_19.pdf.

Table 27 (page 1 of 2). Leading causes of death and numbers of deaths, by age: United States, 1980 and 2007

[Data are based on death certificates]

Age and rank order	1980 Cause of death	Deaths	2007 Cause of death	Deaths
Under 1 year				
Rank	All causes	45,526	All causes	29,138
1	Congenital anomalies	9,220	Congenital malformations, deformations and chromosomal abnormalities	5,785
2	Sudden infant death syndrome	5,510	Disorders related to short gestation and low birth weight, not elsewhere classified	4,857
3	Respiratory distress syndrome	4,989	Sudden infant death syndrome	2,453
4	Disorders relating to short gestation and unspecified low birthweight	3,648	Newborn affected by maternal complications of pregnancy	1,769
5	Newborn affected by maternal complications of pregnancy	1,572	Unintentional injuries	1,285
6	Intrauterine hypoxia and birth asphyxia	1,497	Newborn affected by complications of placenta, cord and membranes	1,135
7	Unintentional injuries	1,166	Bacterial sepsis of newborn	820
8	Birth trauma	1,058	Respiratory distress of newborn	789
9	Pneumonia and influenza	1,012	Diseases of circulatory system	624
10	Newborn affected by complications of placenta, cord, and membranes	985	Neonatal hemorrhage	597
1–4 years				
Rank	All causes	8,187	All causes	4,703
1	Unintentional injuries	3,313	Unintentional injuries	1,588
2	Congenital anomalies	1,026	Congenital malformations, deformations and chromosomal abnormalities	546
3	Malignant neoplasms	573	Homicide	398
4	Diseases of heart	338	Malignant neoplasms	364
5	Homicide	319	Diseases of heart	173
6	Pneumonia and influenza	267	Influenza and pneumonia	109
7	Meningitis	223	Septicemia	78
8	Meningococcal infection	110	Certain conditions originating in the perinatal period	70
9	Certain conditions originating in the perinatal period	84	In situ neoplasms, benign neoplasms and neoplasms of uncertain or unknown behavior	59
10	Septicemia	71	Chronic lower respiratory diseases	57
5–14 years				
Rank	All causes	10,689	All causes	6,147
1	Unintentional injuries	5,224	Unintentional injuries	2,194
2	Malignant neoplasms	1,497	Malignant neoplasms	959
3	Congenital anomalies	561	Congenital malformations, deformations and chromosomal abnormalities	374
4	Homicide	415	Homicide	346
5	Diseases of heart	330	Diseases of heart	241
6	Pneumonia and influenza	194	Suicide	184
7	Suicide	142	Chronic lower respiratory diseases	118
8	Benign neoplasms	104	Influenza and pneumonia	103
9	Cerebrovascular diseases	95	In situ neoplasms, benign neoplasms and neoplasms of uncertain or unknown behavior	84
10	Chronic obstructive pulmonary diseases	85	Cerebrovascular diseases	83
15–24 years				
Rank	All causes	49,027	All causes	33,982
1	Unintentional injuries	26,206	Unintentional injuries	15,897
2	Homicide	6,537	Homicide	5,551
3	Suicide	5,239	Suicide	4,140
4	Malignant neoplasms	2,683	Malignant neoplasms	1,653
5	Diseases of heart	1,223	Diseases of heart	1,084
6	Congenital anomalies	600	Congenital malformations, deformations and chromosomal abnormalities	402
7	Cerebrovascular diseases	418	Cerebrovascular diseases	195
8	Pneumonia and influenza	348	Diabetes mellitus	168
9	Chronic obstructive pulmonary diseases	141	Influenza and pneumonia	163
10	Anemias	133	Septicemia	160

See footnotes at end of table.

Table 27 (page 2 of 2). Leading causes of death and numbers of deaths, by age: United States, 1980 and 2007

[Data are based on death certificates]

Age and rank order	1980		2007	
	Cause of death	Deaths	Cause of death	Deaths
25–44 years				
Rank	All causes	108,658	All causes	122,178
1	Unintentional injuries	26,722	Unintentional injuries	31,908
2	Malignant neoplasms	17,551	Malignant neoplasms	16,751
3	Diseases of heart.	14,513	Diseases of heart.	15,062
4	Homicide.	10,983	Suicide	12,000
5	Suicide	9,855	Homicide.	7,810
6	Chronic liver disease and cirrhosis.	4,782	Human immunodeficiency virus (HIV) disease. .	4,663
7	Cerebrovascular diseases.	3,154	Chronic liver disease and cirrhosis.	2,954
8	Diabetes mellitus	1,472	Cerebrovascular diseases.	2,638
9	Pneumonia and influenza	1,467	Diabetes mellitus	2,594
10	Congenital anomalies	817	Septicemia	1,207
45–64 years				
Rank	All causes	425,338	All causes	471,796
1	Diseases of heart.	148,322	Malignant neoplasms	153,338
2	Malignant neoplasms	135,675	Diseases of heart.	102,961
3	Cerebrovascular diseases.	19,909	Unintentional injuries	32,508
4	Unintentional injuries	18,140	Diabetes mellitus	17,057
5	Chronic liver disease and cirrhosis.	16,089	Chronic lower respiratory diseases	16,930
6	Chronic obstructive pulmonary diseases.	11,514	Cerebrovascular diseases.	16,885
7	Diabetes mellitus	7,977	Chronic liver disease and cirrhosis.	16,216
8	Suicide	7,079	Suicide	12,847
9	Pneumonia and influenza	5,804	Nephritis, nephrotic syndrome and nephrosis . .	6,673
10	Homicide.	4,019	Septicemia	6,662
65 years and over				
Rank	All causes	1,341,848	All causes	1,755,567
1	Diseases of heart.	595,406	Diseases of heart.	496,095
2	Malignant neoplasms	258,389	Malignant neoplasms	389,730
3	Cerebrovascular diseases.	146,417	Cerebrovascular diseases.	115,961
4	Pneumonia and influenza	45,512	Chronic lower respiratory diseases	109,562
5	Chronic obstructive pulmonary diseases.	43,587	Alzheimer's disease	73,797
6	Atherosclerosis	28,081	Diabetes mellitus	51,528
7	Diabetes mellitus	25,216	Influenza and pneumonia	45,941
8	Unintentional injuries	24,844	Nephritis, nephrotic syndrome and nephrosis . .	38,484
9	Nephritis, nephrotic syndrome, and nephrosis . .	12,968	Unintentional injuries	38,292
10	Chronic liver disease and cirrhosis.	9,519	Septicemia	26,362

NOTES: For cause of death codes based on the *International Classification of Diseases*, 9th Revision (ICD–9) in 1980 and ICD–10 in 2007, see Appendix II, Cause of death; Tables IV and V.

SOURCE: CDC/NCHS, National Vital Statistics System; Vital statistics of the United States, vol II, mortality, part A, 1980. Washington, DC: Public Health Service. 1985; 2007 annual mortality file; Xu JQ, Kochanek KD, Murphy SL, Tejada-Vera B. Deaths: Final data for 2007. National vital statistics reports; vol 58 no 19. Hyattsville, MD: NCHS; 2010. Available from: http://www.cdc.gov/nchs/data/nvsr/nvsr58/nvsr58_19.pdf.

Table 28 (page 1 of 3). Age-adjusted death rates, by race, sex, region, and urbanization level: United States, average annual, selected years 1996–1998 through 2005–2007

[Data are based on the National Vital Statistics System]

Sex, region, and urbanization level[1]	All races			White			Black or African American		
	1996–1998	1999–2001	2005–2007	1996–1998	1999–2001	2005–2007	1996–1998	1999–2001	2005–2007
Both sexes	Age-adjusted death rate per 100,000 standard population[2]								
All regions:									
Metropolitan counties:									
Large:									
Central.	894.5	869.0	753.3	858.8	836.7	729.7	1,164.2	1,133.6	994.2
Fringe	839.3	833.0	742.4	828.0	823.7	738.6	1,059.6	1,040.8	903.9
Medium.	865.6	859.0	779.5	846.5	842.2	767.3	1,152.4	1,137.3	1,005.6
Small	887.8	887.9	812.7	866.5	868.8	797.4	1,173.1	1,164.3	1,037.1
Nonmetropolitan counties:									
Micropolitan.	913.0	907.1	841.3	892.1	890.0	827.2	1,208.2	1,174.9	1,064.1
Nonmicropolitan.	933.0	923.2	863.3	909.6	902.8	845.6	1,191.6	1,162.8	1,062.6
Northeast:									
Metropolitan counties:									
Large:									
Central.	909.6	861.7	733.3	881.4	838.6	718.4	1,052.4	1,001.1	856.8
Fringe	827.8	814.0	718.4	823.3	810.8	721.5	1,000.0	986.6	836.4
Medium.	851.9	836.2	760.5	842.2	828.6	757.2	1,076.6	1,040.8	894.4
Small	852.0	849.5	776.5	847.8	846.5	773.7	1,106.9	1,072.4	975.5
Nonmetropolitan counties:									
Micropolitan.	878.4	854.4	783.8	877.9	855.7	787.0	*	*	*
Nonmicropolitan.	893.6	877.4	796.7	892.0	876.3	798.3	*	*	*
Midwest:									
Metropolitan counties:									
Large:									
Central.	951.7	939.6	826.7	880.7	868.9	762.0	1,213.7	1,205.9	1,069.3
Fringe	856.4	856.1	772.8	845.9	846.3	764.9	1,121.2	1,123.1	1,037.8
Medium.	876.1	873.5	796.6	857.0	856.1	781.5	1,168.9	1,151.6	1,038.3
Small	860.8	861.5	785.3	847.4	850.8	775.2	1,178.9	1,146.9	1,057.5
Nonmetropolitan counties:									
Micropolitan.	868.8	865.2	800.9	863.9	863.0	799.6	1,222.0	1,103.5	971.1
Nonmicropolitan.	867.6	852.7	795.3	858.2	845.9	788.5	1,388.1	1,058.9	924.4
South:									
Metropolitan counties:									
Large:									
Central.	938.1	926.8	804.1	864.9	859.1	746.3	1,241.9	1,212.8	1,068.9
Fringe	845.3	845.6	747.6	821.9	826.2	736.4	1,071.4	1,048.4	894.6
Medium.	891.8	892.4	805.7	852.1	855.8	775.6	1,172.6	1,164.4	1,031.2
Small	943.6	950.5	874.3	907.5	917.9	849.8	1,183.2	1,180.0	1,046.4
Nonmetropolitan counties:									
Micropolitan.	974.1	973.3	906.1	933.5	939.3	877.4	1,218.9	1,194.3	1,089.7
Nonmicropolitan.	1,005.3	1,003.0	944.2	975.9	978.5	925.7	1,188.4	1,171.2	1,074.9
West:									
Metropolitan counties:									
Large:									
Central.	819.2	792.4	690.7	829.4	804.1	708.3	1,107.9	1,077.7	956.7
Fringe	818.6	803.6	728.6	823.2	810.1	740.4	1,060.8	1,006.2	952.5
Medium.	814.7	800.5	728.9	826.9	815.8	747.6	1,045.4	996.3	877.0
Small	827.6	815.7	743.9	826.6	815.7	745.9	973.5	990.7	841.7
Nonmetropolitan counties:									
Micropolitan.	861.0	851.8	788.6	860.4	854.7	793.9	*	*	*
Nonmicropolitan.	867.1	847.4	780.1	845.9	828.6	761.3	*	*	*

See footnotes at end of table.

Table 28 (page 2 of 3). Age-adjusted death rates, by race, sex, region, and urbanization level: United States, average annual, selected years 1996–1998 through 2005–2007

[Data are based on the National Vital Statistics System]

Sex, region, and urbanization level[1]	All races			White			Black or African American		
	1996–1998	1999–2001	2005–2007	1996–1998	1999–2001	2005–2007	1996–1998	1999–2001	2005–2007
Male	Age-adjusted death rate per 100,000 standard population[2]								
All regions:									
Metropolitan counties:									
Large:									
Central.	1,108.6	1,057.6	905.2	1,060.6	1,015.2	873.3	1,503.8	1,436.1	1,246.6
Fringe	1,025.2	998.7	870.7	1,010.9	987.3	865.9	1,329.0	1,281.1	1,088.9
Medium.	1,069.9	1,038.5	928.1	1,045.4	1,017.7	911.5	1,469.0	1,409.2	1,234.7
Small	1,104.6	1,079.2	969.4	1,077.4	1,056.1	950.2	1,497.6	1,449.1	1,273.4
Nonmetropolitan counties:									
Micropolitan.	1,139.9	1,108.6	1,004.5	1,113.5	1,087.5	986.6	1,547.8	1,475.9	1,315.2
Nonmicropolitan.	1,172.3	1,132.9	1,036.7	1,143.3	1,108.3	1,015.3	1,529.0	1,457.3	1,313.5
Northeast:									
Metropolitan counties:									
Large:									
Central.	1,142.0	1,065.3	893.8	1,102.8	1,034.5	873.6	1,374.4	1,280.7	1,077.5
Fringe	1,018.1	985.3	852.3	1,012.6	982.3	857.6	1,263.0	1,219.0	997.7
Medium.	1,061.6	1,018.1	916.1	1,049.9	1,009.7	913.0	1,351.2	1,262.4	1,079.5
Small	1,062.7	1,034.1	936.2	1,057.9	1,032.3	934.6	1,376.8	1,280.7	1,136.6
Nonmetropolitan counties:									
Micropolitan.	1,093.5	1,042.5	941.9	1,093.7	1,045.6	947.9	*	*	*
Nonmicropolitan.	1,096.9	1,056.9	955.5	1,096.1	1,056.6	958.6	*	*	*
Midwest:									
Metropolitan counties:									
Large:									
Central.	1,192.6	1,155.5	1,003.5	1,101.0	1,064.6	918.9	1,559.8	1,525.5	1,353.8
Fringe	1,051.7	1,030.0	903.8	1,038.7	1,018.7	894.5	1,399.4	1,372.7	1,250.8
Medium.	1,089.0	1,063.2	956.9	1,065.3	1,043.8	938.1	1,470.0	1,394.4	1,283.0
Small	1,076.0	1,057.3	942.9	1,059.7	1,045.0	932.0	1,463.9	1,401.9	1,251.4
Nonmetropolitan counties:									
Micropolitan.	1,092.0	1,063.4	966.7	1,086.0	1,062.0	965.8	1,551.8	1,315.8	1,141.5
Nonmicropolitan.	1,094.7	1,050.5	960.2	1,083.0	1,043.3	953.1	1,788.2	1,225.3	1,046.9
South:									
Metropolitan counties:									
Large:									
Central.	1,172.0	1,130.9	968.7	1,074.6	1,042.9	894.9	1,616.0	1,542.6	1,344.2
Fringe	1,030.8	1,009.7	874.8	1,000.5	984.8	859.7	1,351.1	1,297.8	1,086.1
Medium.	1,106.6	1,081.2	957.7	1,053.0	1,033.8	918.8	1,517.1	1,466.2	1,278.6
Small	1,185.9	1,160.8	1,048.7	1,138.6	1,118.6	1,015.3	1,526.9	1,487.0	1,305.4
Nonmetropolitan counties:									
Micropolitan.	1,228.0	1,198.9	1,084.7	1,175.1	1,154.7	1,045.9	1,577.6	1,519.8	1,365.7
Nonmicropolitan.	1,275.7	1,240.6	1,139.6	1,239.3	1,210.2	1,115.2	1,530.4	1,478.0	1,338.5
West:									
Metropolitan counties:									
Large:									
Central.	996.3	949.8	819.8	1,006.7	962.4	837.3	1,383.8	1,323.2	1,157.5
Fringe	981.1	947.0	846.3	988.0	954.5	858.8	1,228.8	1,171.2	1,095.0
Medium.	987.4	952.8	860.5	1,003.1	969.3	876.8	1,230.6	1,165.1	1,011.5
Small	1,003.7	970.5	868.6	1,001.7	971.6	870.0	1,178.9	1,088.1	955.6
Nonmetropolitan counties:									
Micropolitan.	1,037.8	1,012.6	917.1	1,036.0	1,013.6	919.4	*	*	*
Nonmicropolitan.	1,048.7	1,010.9	909.5	1,023.0	986.8	884.7	*	*	*

See footnotes at end of table.

Table 28 (page 3 of 3). Age-adjusted death rates, by race, sex, region, and urbanization level: United States, average annual, selected years 1996–1998 through 2005–2007

[Data are based on the National Vital Statistics System]

Sex, region, and urbanization level[1]	All races			White			Black or African American		
	1996–1998	1999–2001	2005–2007	1996–1998	1999–2001	2005–2007	1996–1998	1999–2001	2005–2007
Female	Age-adjusted death rate per 100,000 standard population[2]								
All regions:									
Metropolitan counties:									
Large:									
Central.	738.9	730.1	635.1	711.3	703.8	616.4	934.4	929.3	816.1
Fringe	705.7	711.1	640.8	696.3	702.7	637.2	875.9	876.4	770.3
Medium.	716.8	724.6	660.3	701.9	710.6	650.8	932.0	945.4	836.1
Small	731.2	745.7	687.6	713.7	729.1	674.8	951.9	966.5	861.8
Nonmetropolitan counties:									
Micropolitan.	745.9	754.8	707.3	728.8	740.2	695.6	975.6	968.3	879.6
Nonmicropolitan.	750.6	759.5	715.7	731.4	741.9	700.8	951.5	953.0	870.5
Northeast:									
Metropolitan counties:									
Large:									
Central.	748.4	719.6	615.8	725.6	699.1	602.7	848.3	823.6	709.2
Fringe	696.3	692.6	617.6	692.4	689.3	618.8	827.2	828.1	718.6
Medium.	709.1	707.5	645.3	701.4	700.9	642.4	883.4	877.0	750.3
Small	706.7	717.3	655.5	703.2	713.8	652.6	919.9	930.0	843.6
Nonmetropolitan counties:									
Micropolitan.	725.0	717.5	660.7	724.3	718.1	662.3	*	*	*
Nonmicropolitan.	741.8	738.5	665.1	740.1	737.4	666.3	*	*	*
Midwest:									
Metropolitan counties:									
Large:									
Central.	784.1	786.2	695.7	729.7	730.9	646.2	974.4	984.5	869.1
Fringe	722.9	733.8	672.9	714.5	725.1	666.2	924.6	948.2	883.7
Medium.	728.9	739.6	676.6	713.6	724.3	664.5	955.1	972.7	857.1
Small	710.8	721.4	666.0	700.0	712.2	657.0	963.1	952.5	897.5
Nonmetropolitan counties:									
Micropolitan.	711.2	721.2	671.9	707.3	718.6	670.7	998.7	948.8	818.3
Nonmicropolitan.	696.1	700.0	658.0	688.9	693.9	651.9	1,123.8	955.4	805.4
South:									
Metropolitan counties:									
Large:									
Central.	768.6	776.3	675.7	712.1	721.7	628.3	988.2	989.8	875.8
Fringe	705.7	719.6	642.6	686.1	702.4	632.4	882.4	881.0	759.2
Medium.	731.2	746.6	678.6	700.1	716.0	653.3	938.9	958.2	853.7
Small	771.0	795.0	734.8	740.9	767.1	714.9	956.5	974.2	862.1
Nonmetropolitan counties:									
Micropolitan.	788.4	803.8	758.4	754.8	774.5	735.0	977.3	975.7	893.7
Nonmicropolitan.	803.4	821.3	780.1	778.3	799.5	764.4	946.7	955.0	876.8
West:									
Metropolitan counties:									
Large:									
Central.	682.6	670.1	584.8	691.8	679.9	600.9	906.0	899.3	796.8
Fringe	696.3	693.8	632.9	699.2	699.1	643.3	920.1	876.5	833.7
Medium.	680.5	681.3	620.1	691.6	696.1	639.7	890.3	855.7	751.7
Small	687.3	691.3	636.0	687.2	690.7	638.2	789.8	886.6	722.0
Nonmetropolitan counties:									
Micropolitan.	712.6	715.1	671.6	713.8	720.0	678.3	*	*	*
Nonmicropolitan.	710.4	704.0	655.8	694.2	690.7	642.9	*	*	*

* Estimates of death rates for the black population in nonmetropolitan counties in the Northeast and West may be unreliable, possibly due to anomalies in population estimates for the black population in nonmetropolitan counties in these regions.

[1]Urbanization levels are for county of residence of decedent. The levels were developed by NCHS using information from the Office of Management and Budget, Department of Agriculture, and Census Bureau. More information on this six-level urban-rural classification scheme is available from: http://www.cdc.gov/nchs/data_access/urban_rural.htm. See Appendix II, Urbanization.

[2]Average annual death rates are age-adjusted using the year 2000 standard population. In earlier editions of *Health, United States*, age-adjusted rates were calculated using standard million proportions based on rounded population numbers. Starting with *Health, United States 2006*, unrounded population numbers are used to calculate age-adjusted rates. See Appendix II, Age adjustment. Denominators for rates are population estimates for the middle year of each 3-year period multiplied by 3. The 1997 population estimates used to compute rates for 1996–1998 are intercensal population estimates based on the 2000 census. The 2000 population estimates used to compute rates for 1999–2001 are based on the 2000 census. The 2006 population estimates used to compute rates for 2005–2007 are postcensal population estimates based on the 2000 census. See Appendix I, Population Census and Population Estimates.

NOTES: The race groups, white and black, include persons of Hispanic and non-Hispanic origin. Starting with 2003 data, some states allowed the reporting of more than one race on the death certificate. The multiple-race data for these states were bridged to the single-race categories of the 1977 Office of Management and Budget standards for comparability with other states. See Appendix II, Race; Hispanic origin. Data have been revised and differ from previous editions of *Health, United States*. Data for additional years are available. See Appendix III.

SOURCE: CDC/NCHS, National Vital Statistics System, Compressed Mortality File.

Table 29 (page 1 of 4). Death rates for all causes, by sex, race, Hispanic origin, and age: United States, selected years 1950–2007

[Data are based on death certificates]

Sex, race, Hispanic origin, and age	1950[1]	1960[1]	1970	1980	1990	2000	2006	2007
All persons		Deaths per 100,000 resident population						
All ages, age-adjusted[2]	1,446.0	1,339.2	1,222.6	1,039.1	938.7	869.0	776.5	760.2
All ages, crude	963.8	954.7	945.3	878.3	863.8	854.0	810.4	803.6
Under 1 year	3,299.2	2,696.4	2,142.4	1,288.3	971.9	736.7	690.7	684.5
1–4 years	139.4	109.1	84.5	63.9	46.8	32.4	28.4	28.6
5–14 years	60.1	46.6	41.3	30.6	24.0	18.0	15.2	15.3
15–24 years	128.1	106.3	127.7	115.4	99.2	79.9	82.2	79.9
25–34 years	178.7	146.4	157.4	135.5	139.2	101.4	106.3	104.9
35–44 years	358.7	299.4	314.5	227.9	223.2	198.9	190.2	184.4
45–54 years	853.9	756.0	730.0	584.0	473.4	425.6	427.5	420.9
55–64 years	1,901.0	1,735.1	1,658.8	1,346.3	1,196.9	992.2	890.9	877.7
65–74 years	4,104.3	3,822.1	3,582.7	2,994.9	2,648.6	2,399.1	2,062.1	2,011.3
75–84 years	9,331.1	8,745.2	8,004.4	6,692.6	6,007.2	5,666.5	5,115.0	5,011.6
85 years and over	20,196.9	19,857.5	16,344.9	15,980.3	15,327.4	15,524.4	13,253.1	12,946.5
Male								
All ages, age-adjusted[2]	1,674.2	1,609.0	1,542.1	1,348.1	1,202.8	1,053.8	924.8	905.6
All ages, crude	1,106.1	1,104.5	1,090.3	976.9	918.4	853.0	814.8	809.9
Under 1 year	3,728.0	3,059.3	2,410.0	1,428.5	1,082.8	806.5	756.3	747.8
1–4 years	151.7	119.5	93.2	72.6	52.4	35.9	30.5	31.3
5–14 years	70.9	55.7	50.5	36.7	28.5	20.9	17.6	17.4
15–24 years	167.9	152.1	188.5	172.3	147.4	114.9	119.3	115.8
25–34 years	216.5	187.9	215.3	196.1	204.3	138.6	146.8	144.0
35–44 years	428.8	372.8	402.6	299.2	310.4	255.2	238.7	231.8
45–54 years	1,067.1	992.2	958.5	767.3	610.3	542.8	541.0	530.0
55–64 years	2,395.3	2,309.5	2,282.7	1,815.1	1,553.4	1,230.7	1,110.0	1,100.6
65–74 years	4,931.4	4,914.4	4,873.8	4,105.2	3,491.5	2,979.6	2,516.2	2,456.9
75–84 years	10,426.0	10,178.4	10,010.2	8,816.7	7,888.6	6,972.6	6,177.7	6,038.4
85 years and over	21,636.0	21,186.3	17,821.5	18,801.1	18,056.6	17,501.4	14,309.1	14,006.4
Female								
All ages, age-adjusted[2]	1,236.0	1,105.3	971.4	817.9	750.9	731.4	657.8	643.4
All ages, crude	823.5	809.2	807.8	785.3	812.0	855.0	806.1	797.4
Under 1 year	2,854.6	2,321.3	1,863.7	1,141.7	855.7	663.4	622.0	618.1
1–4 years	126.7	98.4	75.4	54.7	41.0	28.7	26.3	25.7
5–14 years	48.9	37.3	31.8	24.2	19.3	15.0	12.8	13.1
15–24 years	89.1	61.3	68.1	57.5	49.0	43.1	42.8	42.0
25–34 years	142.7	106.6	101.6	75.9	74.2	63.5	64.3	64.2
35–44 years	290.3	229.4	231.1	159.3	137.9	143.2	141.6	136.9
45–54 years	641.5	526.7	517.2	412.9	342.7	312.5	317.7	315.2
55–64 years	1,404.8	1,196.4	1,098.9	934.3	878.8	772.2	687.0	670.1
65–74 years	3,333.2	2,871.8	2,579.7	2,144.7	1,991.2	1,921.2	1,677.9	1,633.0
75–84 years	8,399.6	7,633.1	6,677.6	5,440.1	4,883.1	4,814.7	4,388.3	4,304.1
85 years and over	19,194.7	19,008.4	15,518.0	14,746.9	14,274.3	14,719.2	12,759.0	12,442.3
White male[3]								
All ages, age-adjusted[2]	1,642.5	1,586.0	1,513.7	1,317.6	1,165.9	1,029.4	908.2	890.5
All ages, crude	1,089.5	1,098.5	1,086.7	983.3	930.9	887.8	852.3	848.1
Under 1 year	3,400.5	2,694.1	2,113.2	1,230.3	896.1	667.6	632.7	627.8
1–4 years	135.5	104.9	83.6	66.1	45.9	32.6	27.5	28.3
5–14 years	67.2	52.7	48.0	35.0	26.4	19.8	16.4	16.2
15–24 years	152.4	143.7	170.8	167.0	131.3	105.8	111.8	108.1
25–34 years	185.3	163.2	176.6	171.3	176.1	124.1	135.4	134.2
35–44 years	380.9	332.6	343.5	257.4	268.2	233.6	224.4	218.2
45–54 years	984.5	932.2	882.9	698.9	548.7	496.9	505.2	498.4
55–64 years	2,304.4	2,225.2	2,202.6	1,728.5	1,467.2	1,163.3	1,050.6	1,042.7
65–74 years	4,864.9	4,848.4	4,810.1	4,035.7	3,397.7	2,905.7	2,455.8	2,396.7
75–84 years	10,526.3	10,299.6	10,098.8	8,829.8	7,844.9	6,933.1	6,182.2	6,049.2
85 years and over	22,116.3	21,750.0	18,551.7	19,097.3	18,268.3	17,716.4	14,576.8	14,286.4

See footnotes at end of table.

Table 29 (page 2 of 4). Death rates for all causes, by sex, race, Hispanic origin, and age: United States, selected years 1950–2007

[Data are based on death certificates]

Sex, race, Hispanic origin, and age	1950[1]	1960[1]	1970	1980	1990	2000	2006	2007
Black or African American male[3]			Deaths per 100,000 resident population					
All ages, age-adjusted[2]	1,909.1	1,811.1	1,873.9	1,697.8	1,644.5	1,403.5	1,215.6	1,184.4
All ages, crude	1,257.7	1,181.7	1,186.6	1,034.1	1,008.0	834.1	786.7	775.6
Under 1 year	- - -	5,306.8	4,298.9	2,586.7	2,112.4	1,567.6	1,407.1	1,363.2
1–4 years[4]	1,412.6	208.5	150.5	110.5	85.8	54.5	47.1	45.3
5–14 years	95.1	75.1	67.1	47.4	41.2	28.2	24.8	24.6
15–24 years	289.7	212.0	320.6	209.1	252.2	181.4	171.3	168.1
25–34 years	503.5	402.5	559.5	407.3	430.8	261.0	254.2	240.3
35–44 years	878.1	762.0	956.6	689.8	699.6	453.0	392.3	378.9
45–54 years	1,905.0	1,624.8	1,777.5	1,479.9	1,261.0	1,017.7	921.9	876.7
55–64 years	3,773.2	3,316.4	3,256.9	2,873.0	2,618.4	2,080.1	1,891.8	1,870.8
65–74 years	5,310.3	5,798.7	5,803.2	5,131.1	4,946.1	4,253.5	3,669.2	3,604.9
75–84 years[5]	10,101.9	8,605.1	9,454.9	9,231.6	9,129.5	8,486.0	7,393.2	7,169.0
85 years and over	- - -	14,844.8	12,222.3	16,098.8	16,954.9	16,791.0	13,206.0	12,964.7
American Indian or Alaska Native male[3]								
All ages, age-adjusted[2]	- - -	- - -	- - -	1,111.5	916.2	841.5	739.9	736.7
All ages, crude	- - -	- - -	- - -	597.1	476.4	415.6	477.1	488.2
Under 1 year	- - -	- - -	- - -	1,598.1	1,056.6	700.2	1,057.8	1,009.9
1–4 years	- - -	- - -	- - -	82.7	77.4	44.9	58.1	63.6
5–14 years	- - -	- - -	- - -	43.7	33.4	20.2	17.2	23.2
15–24 years	- - -	- - -	- - -	311.1	219.8	136.2	156.1	143.7
25–34 years	- - -	- - -	- - -	360.6	256.1	179.1	194.0	198.3
35–44 years	- - -	- - -	- - -	556.8	365.4	295.2	338.5	332.5
45–54 years	- - -	- - -	- - -	871.3	619.9	520.0	591.9	573.0
55–64 years	- - -	- - -	- - -	1,547.5	1,211.3	1,090.4	1,029.5	1,037.0
65–74 years	- - -	- - -	- - -	2,968.4	2,461.7	2,478.3	2,146.7	2,131.7
75–84 years	- - -	- - -	- - -	5,607.0	5,389.2	5,351.2	4,198.0	4,193.4
85 years and over	- - -	- - -	- - -	12,635.2	11,243.9	10,725.8	7,540.2	7,638.6
Asian or Pacific Islander male[3]								
All ages, age-adjusted[2]	- - -	- - -	- - -	786.5	716.4	624.2	516.0	499.2
All ages, crude	- - -	- - -	- - -	375.3	334.3	332.9	330.6	331.4
Under 1 year	- - -	- - -	- - -	816.5	605.3	529.4	469.7	483.5
1–4 years	- - -	- - -	- - -	50.9	45.0	23.3	18.1	25.3
5–14 years	- - -	- - -	- - -	23.4	20.7	12.9	11.3	12.2
15–24 years	- - -	- - -	- - -	80.8	76.0	55.2	61.7	61.0
25–34 years	- - -	- - -	- - -	83.5	79.6	55.0	54.2	50.1
35–44 years	- - -	- - -	- - -	128.3	130.8	104.9	88.5	88.9
45–54 years	- - -	- - -	- - -	342.3	287.1	249.7	232.5	229.1
55–64 years	- - -	- - -	- - -	881.1	789.1	642.4	550.7	523.1
65–74 years	- - -	- - -	- - -	2,236.1	2,041.4	1,661.0	1,329.2	1,304.7
75–84 years	- - -	- - -	- - -	5,389.5	5,008.6	4,328.2	3,606.4	3,538.4
85 years and over	- - -	- - -	- - -	13,753.6	12,446.3	12,125.3	9,524.7	8,918.0
Hispanic or Latino male[3,6]								
All ages, age-adjusted[2]	- - -	- - -	- - -	- - -	886.4	818.1	675.6	654.5
All ages, crude	- - -	- - -	- - -	- - -	411.6	331.3	323.9	321.8
Under 1 year	- - -	- - -	- - -	- - -	921.8	637.1	640.7	632.7
1–4 years	- - -	- - -	- - -	- - -	53.8	31.5	28.8	28.0
5–14 years	- - -	- - -	- - -	- - -	26.0	17.9	16.4	15.8
15–24 years	- - -	- - -	- - -	- - -	159.3	107.7	120.7	115.3
25–34 years	- - -	- - -	- - -	- - -	234.0	120.2	112.7	110.1
35–44 years	- - -	- - -	- - -	- - -	341.8	211.0	176.5	166.3
45–54 years	- - -	- - -	- - -	- - -	533.9	439.0	403.8	399.2
55–64 years	- - -	- - -	- - -	- - -	1,123.7	965.7	843.6	831.4
65–74 years	- - -	- - -	- - -	- - -	2,368.2	2,287.9	1,910.7	1,862.7
75–84 years	- - -	- - -	- - -	- - -	5,369.1	5,395.3	4,492.6	4,364.8
85 years and over	- - -	- - -	- - -	- - -	12,272.1	13,086.2	9,435.5	8,953.7

See footnotes at end of table.

Table 29 (page 3 of 4). Death rates for all causes, by sex, race, Hispanic origin, and age: United States, selected years 1950–2007

[Data are based on death certificates]

Sex, race, Hispanic origin, and age	1950[1]	1960[1]	1970	1980	1990	2000	2006	2007
White, not Hispanic or Latino male[6]			Deaths per 100,000 resident population					
All ages, age-adjusted[2]	- - -	- - -	- - -	- - -	1,170.9	1,035.4	922.8	906.8
All ages, crude	- - -	- - -	- - -	- - -	985.9	978.5	962.0	960.4
Under 1 year	- - -	- - -	- - -	- - -	865.4	658.7	621.9	616.8
1–4 years	- - -	- - -	- - -	- - -	43.8	32.4	26.7	28.1
5–14 years	- - -	- - -	- - -	- - -	25.7	20.0	16.2	16.1
15–24 years	- - -	- - -	- - -	- - -	123.4	103.5	107.6	104.6
25–34 years	- - -	- - -	- - -	- - -	165.3	123.0	141.1	140.8
35–44 years	- - -	- - -	- - -	- - -	257.1	233.9	233.1	228.4
45–54 years	- - -	- - -	- - -	- - -	544.5	497.7	515.1	508.7
55–64 years	- - -	- - -	- - -	- - -	1,479.7	1,170.9	1,064.0	1,057.5
65–74 years	- - -	- - -	- - -	- - -	3,434.5	2,930.5	2,490.3	2,432.7
75–84 years	- - -	- - -	- - -	- - -	7,920.4	6,977.8	6,278.3	6,152.7
85 years and over	- - -	- - -	- - -	- - -	18,505.4	17,853.2	14,841.1	14,588.3
White female[3]								
All ages, age-adjusted[2]	1,198.0	1,074.4	944.0	796.1	728.8	715.3	648.2	634.8
All ages, crude	803.3	800.9	812.6	806.1	846.9	912.3	863.9	854.9
Under 1 year	2,566.8	2,007.7	1,614.6	962.5	690.0	550.5	516.5	516.8
1–4 years	112.2	85.2	66.1	49.3	36.1	25.5	23.5	23.1
5–14 years	45.1	34.7	29.9	22.9	17.9	14.1	11.9	12.4
15–24 years	71.5	54.9	61.6	55.5	45.9	41.1	41.7	41.2
25–34 years	112.8	85.0	84.1	65.4	61.5	55.1	58.9	59.6
35–44 years	235.8	191.1	193.3	138.2	117.4	125.7	129.0	126.2
45–54 years	546.4	458.8	462.9	372.7	309.3	281.4	291.6	290.5
55–64 years	1,293.8	1,078.9	1,014.9	876.2	822.7	730.9	654.6	638.0
65–74 years	3,242.8	2,779.3	2,470.7	2,066.6	1,923.5	1,868.3	1,646.0	1,600.9
75–84 years	8,481.5	7,696.6	6,698.7	5,401.7	4,839.1	4,785.3	4,395.1	4,317.6
85 years and over	19,679.5	19,477.7	15,980.2	14,979.6	14,400.6	14,890.7	12,965.7	12,646.7
Black or African American female[3]								
All ages, age-adjusted[2]	1,545.5	1,369.7	1,228.7	1,033.3	975.1	927.6	813.0	793.8
All ages, crude	1,002.0	905.0	829.2	733.3	747.9	733.0	684.0	675.7
Under 1 year	- - -	4,162.2	3,368.8	2,123.7	1,735.5	1,279.8	1,194.6	1,132.2
1–4 years[4]	1,139.3	173.3	129.4	84.4	67.6	45.3	39.4	39.0
5–14 years	72.8	53.8	43.8	30.5	27.5	20.0	17.4	17.0
15–24 years	213.1	107.5	111.9	70.5	68.7	58.3	51.3	48.9
25–34 years	393.3	273.2	231.0	150.0	159.5	121.8	106.6	102.1
35–44 years	758.1	568.5	533.0	323.9	298.6	271.9	245.0	229.1
45–54 years	1,576.4	1,177.0	1,043.9	768.2	639.4	588.3	548.1	537.2
55–64 years	3,089.4	2,510.9	1,986.2	1,561.0	1,452.6	1,227.2	1,076.3	1,047.4
65–74 years	4,000.2	4,064.2	3,860.9	3,057.4	2,865.7	2,689.6	2,239.7	2,209.5
75–84 years[5]	8,347.0	6,730.0	6,691.5	6,212.1	5,688.3	5,696.5	5,028.9	4,902.9
85 years and over	- - -	13,052.6	10,706.6	12,367.2	13,309.5	13,941.3	12,196.7	11,997.4
American Indian or Alaska Native female[3]								
All ages, age-adjusted[2]	- - -	- - -	- - -	662.4	561.8	604.5	555.7	533.2
All ages, crude	- - -	- - -	- - -	380.1	330.4	346.1	399.9	400.0
Under 1 year	- - -	- - -	- - -	1,352.6	688.7	492.2	689.9	830.3
1–4 years	- - -	- - -	- - -	87.5	37.8	39.8	50.5	46.0
5–14 years	- - -	- - -	- - -	33.5	25.5	17.7	16.6	13.0
15–24 years	- - -	- - -	- - -	90.3	69.0	58.9	63.5	61.3
25–34 years	- - -	- - -	- - -	178.5	102.3	84.8	92.1	90.6
35–44 years	- - -	- - -	- - -	286.0	156.4	171.9	204.6	196.0
45–54 years	- - -	- - -	- - -	491.4	380.9	284.9	342.4	346.4
55–64 years	- - -	- - -	- - -	837.1	805.9	772.1	686.6	693.5
65–74 years	- - -	- - -	- - -	1,765.5	1,679.4	1,899.8	1,657.3	1,611.9
75–84 years	- - -	- - -	- - -	3,612.9	3,073.2	3,850.0	3,746.4	3,436.8
85 years and over	- - -	- - -	- - -	8,567.4	8,201.1	9,118.2	6,633.7	6,248.2

See footnotes at end of table.

[Data are based on death certificates]

Sex, race, Hispanic origin, and age	1950[1]	1960[1]	1970	1980	1990	2000	2006	2007
Asian or Pacific Islander female[3]				Deaths per 100,000 resident population				
All ages, age-adjusted[2]	- - -	- - -	- - -	425.9	469.3	416.8	362.6	350.6
All ages, crude	- - -	- - -	- - -	222.5	234.3	262.3	285.6	287.2
Under 1 year	- - -	- - -	- - -	755.8	518.2	434.3	356.9	397.6
1–4 years	- - -	- - -	- - -	35.4	32.0	20.0	21.1	17.9
5–14 years	- - -	- - -	- - -	21.5	13.0	11.7	10.3	9.8
15–24 years	- - -	- - -	- - -	32.3	28.8	22.4	25.4	24.4
25–34 years	- - -	- - -	- - -	45.4	37.5	27.6	28.5	28.1
35–44 years	- - -	- - -	- - -	89.7	69.9	65.6	56.8	54.9
45–54 years	- - -	- - -	- - -	214.1	182.7	155.5	145.2	136.2
55–64 years	- - -	- - -	- - -	440.8	483.4	390.9	332.7	329.2
65–74 years	- - -	- - -	- - -	1,027.7	1,089.2	996.4	897.9	832.7
75–84 years	- - -	- - -	- - -	2,833.6	3,127.9	2,882.4	2,525.5	2,470.6
85 years and over	- - -	- - -	- - -	7,923.3	10,254.0	9,052.2	7,560.2	7,334.0
Hispanic or Latina female[3,6]								
All ages, age-adjusted[2]	- - -	- - -	- - -	- - -	537.1	546.0	468.6	452.7
All ages, crude	- - -	- - -	- - -	- - -	285.4	274.6	274.6	272.1
Under 1 year	- - -	- - -	- - -	- - -	746.6	553.6	538.3	539.9
1–4 years	- - -	- - -	- - -	- - -	42.1	27.5	24.0	23.8
5–14 years	- - -	- - -	- - -	- - -	17.3	13.4	11.8	12.3
15–24 years	- - -	- - -	- - -	- - -	40.6	31.7	35.2	33.5
25–34 years	- - -	- - -	- - -	- - -	62.9	43.4	43.1	43.4
35–44 years	- - -	- - -	- - -	- - -	109.3	100.5	87.1	82.7
45–54 years	- - -	- - -	- - -	- - -	253.3	223.8	215.3	204.0
55–64 years	- - -	- - -	- - -	- - -	607.5	548.4	486.5	476.9
65–74 years	- - -	- - -	- - -	- - -	1,453.8	1,423.2	1,222.7	1,162.1
75–84 years	- - -	- - -	- - -	- - -	3,351.3	3,624.5	3,222.9	3,196.2
85 years and over	- - -	- - -	- - -	- - -	10,098.7	11,202.8	8,803.5	8,318.9
White, not Hispanic or Latina female[6]								
All ages, age-adjusted[2]	- - -	- - -	- - -	- - -	734.6	721.5	660.0	647.7
All ages, crude	- - -	- - -	- - -	- - -	903.6	1,007.3	974.7	967.6
Under 1 year	- - -	- - -	- - -	- - -	655.3	530.9	503.7	499.6
1–4 years	- - -	- - -	- - -	- - -	34.0	24.4	23.2	22.7
5–14 years	- - -	- - -	- - -	- - -	17.6	13.9	11.8	12.3
15–24 years	- - -	- - -	- - -	- - -	46.0	42.6	42.9	42.7
25–34 years	- - -	- - -	- - -	- - -	60.6	56.8	62.5	63.4
35–44 years	- - -	- - -	- - -	- - -	116.8	128.1	136.3	134.4
45–54 years	- - -	- - -	- - -	- - -	312.1	285.0	299.8	300.5
55–64 years	- - -	- - -	- - -	- - -	834.5	742.1	668.0	651.3
65–74 years	- - -	- - -	- - -	- - -	1,940.2	1,891.0	1,677.4	1,634.9
75–84 years	- - -	- - -	- - -	- - -	4,887.3	4,819.3	4,460.7	4,385.4
85 years and over	- - -	- - -	- - -	- - -	14,533.1	14,971.7	13,150.7	12,856.7

- - - Data not available.

[1] Includes deaths of persons who were not residents of the 50 states and the District of Columbia (D.C.).

[2] Age-adjusted rates are calculated using the year 2000 standard population. Prior to 2003, age-adjusted rates were calculated using standard million proportions based on rounded population numbers. Starting with 2003 data, unrounded population numbers are used to calculate age-adjusted rates. See Appendix II, Age adjustment.

[3] The race groups, white, black, Asian or Pacific Islander, and American Indian or Alaska Native, include persons of Hispanic and non-Hispanic origin. Persons of Hispanic origin may be of any race. Death rates for the American Indian or Alaska Native and Asian or Pacific Islander populations are known to be underestimated. See Appendix II, Race, for a discussion of sources of bias in death rates by race and Hispanic origin.

[4] In 1950, rate is for the age group under 5 years.

[5] In 1950, rate is for the age group 75 years and over.

[6] Prior to 1997, excludes data from states lacking an Hispanic-origin item on the death certificate. See Appendix II, Hispanic origin.

NOTES: Starting with *Health, United States, 2003*, rates for 1991–1999 were revised using intercensal population estimates based on the 2000 census. Rates for 2000 were revised based on 2000 census counts. Rates for 2001 and later years were computed using 2000-based postcensal estimates. See Appendix I, Population Census and Population Estimates. Starting with 2003 data, some states allowed the reporting of more than one race on the death certificate. The multiple-race data for these states were bridged to the single-race categories of the 1977 Office of Management and Budget standards for comparability with other states. See Appendix II, Race. Data for additional years are available. See Appendix III.

SOURCE: CDC/NCHS, National Vital Statistics System; Grove RD, Hetzel AM. Vital statistics rates in the United States, 1940–1960. Washington, DC: U.S. Government Printing Office, 1968; numerator data from National Vital Statistics System, annual mortality files; denominator data from national population estimates for race groups from Table 1 and unpublished Hispanic population estimates for 1985–1996 prepared by the Housing and Household Economic Statistics Division, U.S. Census Bureau; additional mortality tables are available from: http://www.cdc.gov/nchs/nvss/mortality_tables.htm; Xu JQ, Kochanek KD, Murphy SL, Tejada-Vera B. Deaths: Final data for 2007. National vital statistics reports; vol 58 no 19. Hyattsville, MD: NCHS; 2010. Available from: http://www.cdc.gov/nchs/data/nvsr/nvsr58/nvsr58_19.pdf.

Table 30 (page 1 of 3). Death rates for diseases of heart, by sex, race, Hispanic origin, and age: United States, selected years 1950–2007

[Data are based on death certificates]

Sex, race, Hispanic origin, and age	1950[1,2]	1960[1,2]	1970[2]	1980[2]	1990[2]	2000[3]	2006[3]	2007[3]
All persons				Deaths per 100,000 resident population				
All ages, age-adjusted[4]	588.8	559.0	492.7	412.1	321.8	257.6	200.2	190.9
All ages, crude	356.8	369.0	362.0	336.0	289.5	252.6	211.0	204.3
Under 1 year	4.1	6.6	13.1	22.8	20.1	13.0	8.4	10.0
1–4 years	1.6	1.3	1.7	2.6	1.9	1.2	1.0	1.1
5–14 years	3.9	1.3	0.8	0.9	0.9	0.7	0.6	0.6
15–24 years	8.2	4.0	3.0	2.9	2.5	2.6	2.5	2.6
25–34 years	20.9	15.6	11.4	8.3	7.6	7.4	8.2	7.9
35–44 years	88.3	74.6	66.7	44.6	31.4	29.2	28.3	27.4
45–54 years	309.2	271.8	238.4	180.2	120.5	94.2	88.0	85.3
55–64 years	804.3	737.9	652.3	494.1	367.3	261.2	207.3	200.3
65–74 years	1,857.2	1,740.5	1,558.2	1,218.6	894.3	665.6	490.3	462.9
75–84 years	4,311.0	4,089.4	3,683.8	2,993.1	2,295.7	1,780.3	1,383.1	1,315.0
85 years and over	9,152.5	9,317.8	7,891.3	7,777.1	6,739.9	5,926.1	4,480.8	4,267.7
Male								
All ages, age-adjusted[4]	699.0	687.6	634.0	538.9	412.4	320.0	248.5	237.7
All ages, crude	424.7	439.5	422.5	368.6	297.6	249.8	214.0	208.4
Under 1 year	4.7	7.8	15.1	25.5	21.9	13.3	8.8	10.9
1–4 years	1.7	1.4	1.9	2.8	1.9	1.4	1.1	1.0
5–14 years	3.5	1.4	0.9	1.0	0.9	0.8	0.7	0.6
15–24 years	8.3	4.2	3.7	3.7	3.1	3.2	3.3	3.2
25–34 years	24.4	20.1	15.2	11.4	10.3	9.6	11.2	10.5
35–44 years	120.4	112.7	103.2	68.7	48.1	41.4	39.5	38.6
45–54 years	441.2	420.4	376.4	282.6	183.0	140.2	128.9	124.6
55–64 years	1,100.5	1,066.9	987.2	746.8	537.3	371.7	296.8	288.8
65–74 years	2,310.2	2,291.3	2,170.3	1,728.0	1,250.0	898.3	660.5	624.9
75–84 years	4,825.8	4,742.4	4,534.8	3,834.3	2,968.2	2,248.1	1,743.5	1,656.5
85 years and over	9,661.4	9,788.9	8,426.2	8,752.7	7,418.4	6,430.0	4,819.9	4,621.8
Female								
All ages, age-adjusted[4]	486.6	447.0	381.6	320.8	257.0	210.9	162.2	154.0
All ages, crude	289.7	300.6	304.5	305.1	281.8	255.3	208.0	200.2
Under 1 year	3.4	5.4	10.9	20.0	18.3	12.5	7.9	9.0
1–4 years	1.6	1.1	1.6	2.5	1.9	1.0	0.9	1.1
5–14 years	4.3	1.2	0.8	0.9	0.8	0.5	0.6	0.6
15–24 years	8.2	3.7	2.3	2.1	1.8	2.1	1.8	1.9
25–34 years	17.6	11.3	7.7	5.3	5.0	5.2	5.1	5.3
35–44 years	57.0	38.2	32.2	21.4	15.1	17.2	17.0	16.2
45–54 years	177.8	127.5	109.9	84.5	61.0	49.8	48.5	47.2
55–64 years	507.0	429.4	351.6	272.1	215.7	159.3	124.1	117.9
65–74 years	1,434.9	1,261.3	1,082.7	828.6	616.8	474.0	346.3	325.4
75–84 years	3,873.0	3,582.7	3,120.8	2,497.0	1,893.8	1,475.1	1,136.7	1,079.7
85 years and over	8,798.1	9,016.8	7,591.8	7,350.5	6,478.1	5,720.9	4,322.1	4,099.3
White male[5]								
All ages, age-adjusted[4]	701.4	694.5	640.2	539.6	409.2	316.7	245.2	234.8
All ages, crude	434.2	454.6	438.3	384.0	312.7	265.8	226.9	221.1
45–54 years	424.1	413.2	365.7	269.8	170.6	130.7	119.2	116.2
55–64 years	1,082.6	1,056.0	979.3	730.6	516.7	351.8	278.9	271.4
65–74 years	2,309.4	2,297.9	2,177.2	1,729.7	1,230.5	877.8	636.6	603.0
75–84 years	4,908.0	4,839.9	4,617.6	3,883.2	2,983.4	2,247.0	1,743.3	1,659.3
85 years and over	9,952.3	10,135.8	8,818.0	8,958.0	7,558.7	6,560.8	4,947.1	4,756.1
Black or African American male[5]								
All ages, age-adjusted[4]	641.5	615.2	607.3	561.4	485.4	392.5	320.6	305.9
All ages, crude	348.4	330.6	330.3	301.0	256.8	211.1	191.8	186.5
45–54 years	624.1	514.0	512.8	433.4	328.9	247.2	229.8	216.3
55–64 years	1,434.0	1,236.8	1,135.4	987.2	824.0	631.2	526.4	516.3
65–74 years	2,140.1	2,281.4	2,237.8	1,847.2	1,632.9	1,268.8	1,044.6	989.4
75–84 years[6]	4,107.9	3,533.6	3,783.4	3,578.8	3,107.1	2,597.6	2,129.9	1,999.2
85 years and over	- - -	6,037.9	5,367.6	6,819.5	6,479.6	5,633.5	4,073.1	3,879.6

See footnotes at end of table.

Table 30 (page 2 of 3). Death rates for diseases of heart, by sex, race, Hispanic origin, and age: United States, selected years 1950–2007

[Data are based on death certificates]

Sex, race, Hispanic origin, and age	1950[1,2]	1960[1,2]	1970[2]	1980[2]	1990[2]	2000[3]	2006[3]	2007[3]
American Indian or Alaska Native male[5]				Deaths per 100,000 resident population				
All ages, age-adjusted[4]	- - -	- - -	- - -	320.5	264.1	222.2	170.2	159.8
All ages, crude	- - -	- - -	- - -	130.6	108.0	90.1	95.8	94.1
45–54 years	- - -	- - -	- - -	238.1	173.8	108.5	119.5	112.4
55–64 years	- - -	- - -	- - -	496.3	411.0	285.0	256.2	235.8
65–74 years	- - -	- - -	- - -	1,009.4	839.1	748.2	573.6	521.5
75–84 years	- - -	- - -	- - -	2,062.2	1,788.8	1,655.7	1,176.6	1,129.5
85 years and over	- - -	- - -	- - -	4,413.7	3,860.3	3,318.3	2,066.9	1,901.1
Asian or Pacific Islander male[5]								
All ages, age-adjusted[4]	- - -	- - -	- - -	286.9	220.7	185.5	136.3	126.0
All ages, crude	- - -	- - -	- - -	119.8	88.7	90.6	82.4	79.6
45–54 years	- - -	- - -	- - -	112.0	70.4	61.1	55.7	51.5
55–64 years	- - -	- - -	- - -	306.7	226.1	182.6	145.4	131.5
65–74 years	- - -	- - -	- - -	852.4	623.5	482.5	344.3	321.3
75–84 years	- - -	- - -	- - -	2,010.9	1,642.2	1,354.7	963.3	906.3
85 years and over	- - -	- - -	- - -	5,923.0	4,617.8	4,154.2	2,985.9	2,665.8
Hispanic or Latino male[5,7]								
All ages, age-adjusted[4]	- - -	- - -	- - -	- - -	270.0	238.2	175.2	165.0
All ages, crude	- - -	- - -	- - -	- - -	91.0	74.7	67.7	66.6
45–54 years	- - -	- - -	- - -	- - -	116.4	84.3	75.6	73.3
55–64 years	- - -	- - -	- - -	- - -	363.0	264.8	202.3	201.9
65–74 years	- - -	- - -	- - -	- - -	829.9	684.8	505.6	477.0
75–84 years	- - -	- - -	- - -	- - -	1,971.3	1,733.2	1,308.4	1,233.4
85 years and over	- - -	- - -	- - -	- - -	4,711.9	4,897.5	3,257.9	2,960.8
White, not Hispanic or Latino male[7]								
All ages, age-adjusted[4]	- - -	- - -	- - -	- - -	413.6	319.9	250.0	239.8
All ages, crude	- - -	- - -	- - -	- - -	336.5	297.5	260.3	254.3
45–54 years	- - -	- - -	- - -	- - -	172.8	134.3	124.5	121.6
55–64 years	- - -	- - -	- - -	- - -	521.3	356.3	284.5	276.6
65–74 years	- - -	- - -	- - -	- - -	1,243.4	885.1	644.3	610.9
75–84 years	- - -	- - -	- - -	- - -	3,007.7	2,261.9	1,767.4	1,685.0
85 years and over	- - -	- - -	- - -	- - -	7,663.4	6,606.6	5,032.8	4,858.5
White female[5]								
All ages, age-adjusted[4]	479.2	441.7	376.7	315.9	250.9	205.6	158.6	150.5
All ages, crude	290.5	306.5	313.8	319.2	298.4	274.5	224.2	215.5
45–54 years	142.4	103.4	91.4	71.2	50.2	40.9	40.7	40.0
55–64 years	460.7	383.0	317.7	248.1	192.4	141.3	111.4	105.3
65–74 years	1,401.6	1,229.8	1,044.0	796.7	583.6	445.2	325.8	304.4
75–84 years	3,926.2	3,629.7	3,143.5	2,493.6	1,874.3	1,452.4	1,123.9	1,068.9
85 years and over	9,086.9	9,280.8	7,839.9	7,501.6	6,563.4	5,801.4	4,402.6	4,169.6
Black or African American female[5]								
All ages, age-adjusted[4]	538.9	488.9	435.6	378.6	327.5	277.6	212.5	204.5
All ages, crude	289.9	268.5	261.0	249.7	237.0	212.6	174.3	170.0
45–54 years	526.8	360.7	290.9	202.4	155.3	125.0	111.0	107.1
55–64 years	1,210.7	952.3	710.5	530.1	442.0	332.8	251.3	242.5
65–74 years	1,659.4	1,680.5	1,553.2	1,210.3	1,017.5	815.2	578.3	563.5
75–84 years[6]	3,499.3	2,926.9	2,964.1	2,707.2	2,250.9	1,913.1	1,461.7	1,384.0
85 years and over	- - -	5,650.0	5,003.8	5,796.5	5,766.1	5,298.7	4,049.4	3,962.0

See footnotes at end of table.

Table 30 (page 3 of 3)

Table 30 (page 3 of 3). Death rates for diseases of heart, by sex, race, Hispanic origin, and age: United States, selected years 1950–2007

[Data are based on death certificates]

Sex, race, Hispanic origin, and age	1950[1,2]	1960[1,2]	1970[2]	1980[2]	1990[2]	2000[3]	2006[3]	2007[3]
American Indian or Alaska Native female[5]				Deaths per 100,000 resident population				
All ages, age-adjusted[4]	- - -	- - -	- - -	175.4	153.1	143.6	113.2	99.8
All ages, crude	- - -	- - -	- - -	80.3	77.5	71.9	75.1	69.6
45–54 years	- - -	- - -	- - -	65.2	62.0	40.2	41.8	36.7
55–64 years	- - -	- - -	- - -	193.5	197.0	149.4	125.2	108.7
65–74 years	- - -	- - -	- - -	577.2	492.8	391.8	322.3	288.5
75–84 years	- - -	- - -	- - -	1,364.3	1,050.3	1,044.1	937.9	779.2
85 years and over	- - -	- - -	- - -	2,893.3	2,868.7	3,146.3	1,883.1	1,697.9
Asian or Pacific Islander female[5]								
All ages, age-adjusted[4]	- - -	- - -	- - -	132.3	149.2	115.7	87.3	82.0
All ages, crude	- - -	- - -	- - -	57.0	62.0	65.0	64.9	63.9
45–54 years	- - -	- - -	- - -	28.6	17.5	15.9	15.9	12.1
55–64 years	- - -	- - -	- - -	92.9	99.0	68.8	48.4	46.8
65–74 years	- - -	- - -	- - -	313.3	323.9	229.6	187.4	168.5
75–84 years	- - -	- - -	- - -	1,053.2	1,130.9	866.2	639.8	611.4
85 years and over	- - -	- - -	- - -	3,211.0	4,161.2	3,367.2	2,492.6	2,345.6
Hispanic or Latina female[5,7]								
All ages, age-adjusted[4]	- - -	- - -	- - -	- - -	177.2	163.7	118.9	111.8
All ages, crude	- - -	- - -	- - -	- - -	79.4	71.5	62.6	60.8
45–54 years	- - -	- - -	- - -	- - -	43.5	28.2	27.3	23.4
55–64 years	- - -	- - -	- - -	- - -	153.2	111.2	86.9	81.4
65–74 years	- - -	- - -	- - -	- - -	460.4	366.3	273.0	249.7
75–84 years	- - -	- - -	- - -	- - -	1,259.7	1,169.4	894.5	856.6
85 years and over	- - -	- - -	- - -	- - -	4,440.3	4,605.8	3,078.3	2,888.2
White, not Hispanic or Latina female[7]								
All ages, age-adjusted[4]	- - -	- - -	- - -	- - -	252.6	206.8	160.9	153.0
All ages, crude	- - -	- - -	- - -	- - -	320.0	304.9	254.7	245.5
45–54 years	- - -	- - -	- - -	- - -	50.2	41.9	42.2	42.1
55–64 years	- - -	- - -	- - -	- - -	193.6	142.9	113.2	107.1
65–74 years	- - -	- - -	- - -	- - -	584.7	448.5	329.1	308.1
75–84 years	- - -	- - -	- - -	- - -	1,890.2	1,458.9	1,135.8	1,081.0
85 years and over	- - -	- - -	- - -	- - -	6,615.2	5,822.7	4,460.8	4,230.8

- - - Data not available.

[1]Includes deaths of persons who were not residents of the 50 states and the District of Columbia (D.C.).

[2]Underlying cause of death was coded according to the 6th Revision of the *International Classification of Diseases* (ICD) in 1950, 7th Revision in 1960, 8th Revision in 1970, and 9th Revision in 1980–1998. See Appendix II, Cause of death; Tables IV and V.

[3]Starting with 1999 data, cause of death is coded according to ICD–10. See Appendix II, Cause of death, Table V; Comparability ratio, Table VI.

[4]Age-adjusted rates are calculated using the year 2000 standard population. Prior to 2003, age-adjusted rates were calculated using standard million proportions based on rounded population numbers. Starting with 2003 data, unrounded population numbers are used to calculate age-adjusted rates. See Appendix II, Age adjustment.

[5]The race groups, white, black, Asian or Pacific Islander, and American Indian or Alaska Native, include persons of Hispanic and non-Hispanic origin. Persons of Hispanic origin may be of any race. Death rates for the American Indian or Alaska Native and Asian or Pacific Islander populations are known to be underestimated. See Appendix II, Race, for a discussion of sources of bias in death rates by race and Hispanic origin.

[6]In 1950, rate is for the age group 75 years and over.

[7]Prior to 1997, excludes data from states lacking an Hispanic-origin item on the death certificate. See Appendix II, Hispanic origin.

NOTES: Starting with *Health, United States, 2003*, rates for 1991–1999 were revised using intercensal population estimates based on the 2000 census. Rates for 2000 were revised based on 2000 census counts. Rates for 2001 and later years were computed using 2000-based postcensal estimates. See Appendix I, Population Census and Population Estimates. For the period 1980–1998, diseases of heart was coded using ICD–9 codes that are most nearly comparable with diseases of heart codes in the 113 cause list for ICD–10. See Appendix II, Cause of death; Table V. Age groups were selected to minimize the presentation of unstable age-specific death rates based on small numbers of deaths and for consistency among comparison groups. Starting with 2003 data, some states allowed the reporting of more than one race on the death certificate. The multiple-race data for these states were bridged to the single-race categories of the 1977 Office of Management and Budget standards for comparability with other states. See Appendix II, Race. Data for additional years are available. See Appendix III.

SOURCE: CDC/NCHS, National Vital Statistics System; numerator data from National Vital Statistics System, annual mortality files; denominator data from national population estimates for race groups from Table 1 and unpublished Hispanic population estimates for 1985–1996 prepared by the Housing and Household Economic Statistics Division, U.S. Census Bureau; additional mortality tables are available from: http://www.cdc.gov/nchs/nvss/mortality_tables.htm; Xu JQ, Kochanek KD, Murphy SL, Tejada-Vera B. Deaths: Final data for 2007. National vital statistics reports; vol 58 no 19. Hyattsville, MD: NCHS; 2010. Available from: http://www.cdc.gov/nchs/data/nvsr/nvsr58/nvsr58_19.pdf.

Table 31 (page 1 of 3). Death rates for cerebrovascular diseases, by sex, race, Hispanic origin, and age: United States, selected years 1950–2007

[Data are based on death certificates]

Sex, race, Hispanic origin, and age	1950[1,2]	1960[1,2]	1970[2]	1980[2]	1990[2]	2000[3]	2006[3]	2007[3]
All persons	Deaths per 100,000 resident population							
All ages, age-adjusted[4]	180.7	177.9	147.7	96.2	65.3	60.9	43.6	42.2
All ages, crude	104.0	108.0	101.9	75.0	57.8	59.6	45.8	45.1
Under 1 year	5.1	4.1	5.0	4.4	3.8	3.3	3.4	3.1
1–4 years	0.9	0.8	1.0	0.5	0.3	0.3	0.3	0.3
5–14 years	0.5	0.7	0.7	0.3	0.2	0.2	0.2	0.2
15–24 years	1.6	1.8	1.6	1.0	0.6	0.5	0.5	0.5
25–34 years	4.2	4.7	4.5	2.6	2.2	1.5	1.3	1.2
35–44 years	18.7	14.7	15.6	8.5	6.4	5.8	5.1	4.9
45–54 years	70.4	49.2	41.6	25.2	18.7	16.0	14.7	14.6
55–64 years	194.2	147.3	115.8	65.1	47.9	41.0	33.3	32.1
65–74 years	554.7	469.2	384.1	219.0	144.2	128.6	96.3	93.0
75–84 years	1,499.6	1,491.3	1,254.2	786.9	498.0	461.3	335.1	322.3
85 years and over	2,990.1	3,680.5	3,014.3	2,283.7	1,628.9	1,589.2	1,039.6	1,015.5
Male								
All ages, age-adjusted[4]	186.4	186.1	157.4	102.2	68.5	62.4	43.9	42.5
All ages, crude	102.5	104.5	94.5	63.4	46.7	46.9	37.0	36.4
Under 1 year	6.4	5.0	5.8	5.0	4.4	3.8	3.9	3.5
1–4 years	1.1	0.9	1.2	0.4	0.3	*	0.3	0.2
5–14 years	0.5	0.7	0.8	0.3	0.2	0.2	0.3	0.2
15–24 years	1.8	1.9	1.8	1.1	0.7	0.5	0.5	0.5
25–34 years	4.2	4.5	4.4	2.6	2.1	1.5	1.4	1.2
35–44 years	17.5	14.6	15.7	8.7	6.8	5.8	5.3	5.3
45–54 years	67.9	52.2	44.4	27.2	20.5	17.5	16.4	16.2
55–64 years	205.2	163.8	138.7	74.6	54.3	47.2	38.7	38.0
65–74 years	589.6	530.7	449.5	258.6	166.6	145.0	108.0	105.2
75–84 years	1,543.6	1,555.9	1,361.6	866.3	551.1	490.8	345.5	333.2
85 years and over	3,048.6	3,643.1	2,895.2	2,193.6	1,528.5	1,484.3	932.4	895.7
Female								
All ages, age-adjusted[4]	175.8	170.7	140.0	91.7	62.6	59.1	42.6	41.3
All ages, crude	105.6	111.4	109.0	85.9	68.4	71.8	54.4	53.5
Under 1 year	3.7	3.2	4.0	3.8	3.1	2.7	2.9	2.6
1–4 years	0.7	0.7	0.7	0.5	0.3	0.4	0.4	0.4
5–14 years	0.4	0.6	0.6	0.3	0.2	0.2	0.2	0.2
15–24 years	1.5	1.6	1.4	0.8	0.6	0.5	0.5	0.4
25–34 years	4.3	4.9	4.7	2.6	2.2	1.5	1.2	1.3
35–44 years	19.9	14.8	15.6	8.4	6.1	5.7	4.8	4.6
45–54 years	72.9	46.3	39.0	23.3	17.0	14.5	13.0	12.9
55–64 years	183.1	131.8	95.3	56.8	42.2	35.3	28.2	26.6
65–74 years	522.1	415.7	333.3	188.7	126.7	115.1	86.5	82.7
75–84 years	1,462.2	1,441.1	1,183.1	740.1	466.2	442.1	328.0	314.9
85 years and over	2,949.4	3,704.4	3,081.0	2,323.1	1,667.6	1,632.0	1,089.8	1,072.4
White male[5]								
All ages, age-adjusted[4]	182.1	181.6	153.7	98.7	65.5	59.8	41.7	40.2
All ages, crude	100.5	102.7	93.5	63.1	46.9	48.4	37.7	37.0
45–54 years	53.7	40.9	35.6	21.7	15.4	13.6	12.8	13.0
55–64 years	182.2	139.0	119.9	64.0	45.7	39.7	31.5	31.4
65–74 years	569.7	501.0	420.0	239.8	152.9	133.8	97.1	94.3
75–84 years	1,556.3	1,564.8	1,361.6	852.7	539.2	480.0	338.5	323.1
85 years and over	3,127.1	3,734.8	3,018.1	2,230.8	1,545.4	1,490.7	941.3	905.0
Black or African American male[5]								
All ages, age-adjusted[4]	228.8	238.5	206.4	142.0	102.2	89.6	67.1	67.1
All ages, crude	122.0	122.9	108.8	73.0	53.0	46.1	39.3	39.5
45–54 years	211.9	166.1	136.1	82.1	68.4	49.5	43.5	41.0
55–64 years	522.8	439.9	343.4	189.7	141.7	115.4	105.9	99.8
65–74 years	783.6	899.2	780.1	472.3	326.9	268.5	218.7	223.3
75–84 years[6]	1,504.9	1,475.2	1,445.7	1,066.3	721.5	659.2	471.1	491.9
85 years and over	- - -	2,700.0	1,963.1	1,873.2	1,421.5	1,458.8	882.0	866.9

See footnotes at end of table.

Table 31 (page 2 of 3). Death rates for cerebrovascular diseases, by sex, race, Hispanic origin, and age: United States, selected years 1950–2007

[Data are based on death certificates]

Sex, race, Hispanic origin, and age	1950[1,2]	1960[1,2]	1970[2]	1980[2]	1990[2]	2000[3]	2006[3]	2007[3]
American Indian or Alaska Native male[5]				Deaths per 100,000 resident population				
All ages, age-adjusted[4]	- - -	- - -	- - -	66.4	44.3	46.1	25.8	31.1
All ages, crude	- - -	- - -	- - -	23.1	16.0	16.8	14.4	16.5
45–54 years	- - -	- - -	- - -	*	*	13.3	16.3	13.9
55–64 years	- - -	- - -	- - -	72.0	39.8	48.6	35.0	37.0
65–74 years	- - -	- - -	- - -	170.5	120.3	144.7	82.9	83.3
75–84 years	- - -	- - -	- - -	523.9	325.9	373.3	174.3	266.0
85 years and over	- - -	- - -	- - -	1,384.7	949.8	834.9	344.5	481.0
Asian or Pacific Islander male[5]								
All ages, age-adjusted[4]	- - -	- - -	- - -	71.4	59.1	58.0	39.8	35.5
All ages, crude	- - -	- - -	- - -	28.7	23.3	27.2	23.6	22.0
45–54 years	- - -	- - -	- - -	17.0	15.6	15.0	13.4	14.7
55–64 years	- - -	- - -	- - -	59.9	51.8	49.3	36.3	31.5
65–74 years	- - -	- - -	- - -	197.9	167.9	135.6	108.9	90.7
75–84 years	- - -	- - -	- - -	619.5	483.9	438.7	294.9	274.2
85 years and over	- - -	- - -	- - -	1,399.0	1,196.6	1,415.6	865.9	748.7
Hispanic or Latino male[5,7]								
All ages, age-adjusted[4]	- - -	- - -	- - -	- - -	46.5	50.5	35.9	34.4
All ages, crude	- - -	- - -	- - -	- - -	15.6	15.8	14.3	14.1
45–54 years	- - -	- - -	- - -	- - -	20.0	18.1	17.0	16.5
55–64 years	- - -	- - -	- - -	- - -	49.2	48.8	41.1	42.9
65–74 years	- - -	- - -	- - -	- - -	126.4	136.1	100.1	94.6
75–84 years	- - -	- - -	- - -	- - -	356.6	392.9	292.8	263.6
85 years and over	- - -	- - -	- - -	- - -	866.3	1,029.9	581.9	594.6
White, not Hispanic or Latino male[7]								
All ages, age-adjusted[4]	- - -	- - -	- - -	- - -	66.3	59.9	41.7	40.3
All ages, crude	- - -	- - -	- - -	- - -	50.6	53.9	42.6	41.9
45–54 years	- - -	- - -	- - -	- - -	14.9	13.0	12.1	12.3
55–64 years	- - -	- - -	- - -	- - -	45.1	38.7	30.3	30.0
65–74 years	- - -	- - -	- - -	- - -	154.5	133.1	96.5	93.8
75–84 years	- - -	- - -	- - -	- - -	547.3	482.3	340.5	326.3
85 years and over	- - -	- - -	- - -	- - -	1,578.7	1,505.9	960.2	922.4
White female[5]								
All ages, age-adjusted[4]	169.7	165.0	135.5	89.0	60.3	57.3	41.1	39.9
All ages, crude	103.3	110.1	109.8	88.6	71.6	76.9	57.9	57.0
45–54 years	55.0	33.8	30.5	18.6	13.5	11.2	10.4	10.0
55–64 years	156.9	103.0	78.1	48.6	35.8	30.2	24.1	22.5
65–74 years	498.1	383.3	303.2	172.5	116.1	107.3	79.3	75.8
75–84 years	1,471.3	1,444.7	1,176.8	728.8	456.5	434.2	321.5	310.5
85 years and over	3,017.9	3,795.7	3,167.6	2,362.7	1,685.9	1,646.7	1,102.2	1,083.8
Black or African American female[5]								
All ages, age-adjusted[4]	238.4	232.5	189.3	119.6	84.0	76.2	57.0	55.0
All ages, crude	128.3	127.7	112.2	77.8	60.7	58.3	46.5	45.6
45–54 years	248.9	166.2	119.4	61.8	44.1	38.1	31.3	33.0
55–64 years	567.7	452.0	272.4	138.4	96.9	76.4	61.1	58.4
65–74 years	754.4	830.5	673.5	361.7	236.7	190.9	148.9	143.8
75–84 years[6]	1,496.7	1,413.1	1,338.3	917.5	595.0	549.2	415.6	387.9
85 years and over	- - -	2,578.9	2,210.5	1,891.6	1,495.2	1,556.5	1,060.5	1,050.6

See footnotes at end of table.

Table 31 (page 3 of 3). Death rates for cerebrovascular diseases, by sex, race, Hispanic origin, and age: United States, selected years 1950–2007

[Data are based on death certificates]

Sex, race, Hispanic origin, and age	1950[1,2]	1960[1,2]	1970[2]	1980[2]	1990[2]	2000[3]	2006[3]	2007[3]
American Indian or Alaska Native female[5]				Deaths per 100,000 resident population				
All ages, age-adjusted[4]	- - -	- - -	- - -	51.2	38.4	43.7	30.9	28.4
All ages, crude	- - -	- - -	- - -	22.0	19.3	21.5	19.8	19.7
45–54 years	- - -	- - -	- - -	*	*	14.4	*	10.0
55–64 years	- - -	- - -	- - -	*	40.7	37.9	16.2	23.7
65–74 years	- - -	- - -	- - -	128.3	100.5	79.5	78.8	83.4
75–84 years	- - -	- - -	- - -	404.2	282.0	391.1	267.6	198.7
85 years and over	- - -	- - -	- - -	1,095.5	776.2	931.5	648.1	599.9
Asian or Pacific Islander female[5]								
All ages, age-adjusted[4]	- - -	- - -	- - -	60.8	54.9	49.1	34.9	33.2
All ages, crude	- - -	- - -	- - -	26.4	24.3	28.7	26.7	26.4
45–54 years	- - -	- - -	- - -	20.3	19.7	13.3	10.4	9.9
55–64 years	- - -	- - -	- - -	43.7	42.1	33.3	28.8	25.2
65–74 years	- - -	- - -	- - -	136.1	124.0	102.8	80.8	72.6
75–84 years	- - -	- - -	- - -	446.6	396.6	386.0	284.2	259.7
85 years and over	- - -	- - -	- - -	1,545.2	1,395.0	1,246.6	777.0	802.4
Hispanic or Latina female[5,7]								
All ages, age-adjusted[4]	- - -	- - -	- - -	- - -	43.7	43.0	32.3	30.8
All ages, crude	- - -	- - -	- - -	- - -	20.1	19.4	17.5	17.1
45–54 years	- - -	- - -	- - -	- - -	15.2	12.4	11.8	11.0
55–64 years	- - -	- - -	- - -	- - -	38.5	31.9	27.8	25.4
65–74 years	- - -	- - -	- - -	- - -	102.6	95.2	76.9	71.6
75–84 years	- - -	- - -	- - -	- - -	308.5	311.3	240.6	244.2
85 years and over	- - -	- - -	- - -	- - -	1,055.3	1,108.9	742.9	684.5
White, not Hispanic or Latina female[7]								
All ages, age-adjusted[4]	- - -	- - -	- - -	- - -	61.0	57.6	41.5	40.3
All ages, crude	- - -	- - -	- - -	- - -	77.2	85.5	65.5	64.7
45–54 years	- - -	- - -	- - -	- - -	13.2	10.9	10.1	9.8
55–64 years	- - -	- - -	- - -	- - -	35.7	29.9	23.5	22.1
65–74 years	- - -	- - -	- - -	- - -	116.9	107.6	79.0	75.9
75–84 years	- - -	- - -	- - -	- - -	461.9	438.3	325.9	314.4
85 years and over	- - -	- - -	- - -	- - -	1,714.7	1,661.6	1,118.7	1,103.7

* Rates based on fewer than 20 deaths are considered unreliable and are not shown.

- - - Data not available.

[1]Includes deaths of persons who were not residents of the 50 states and the District of Columbia (D.C.).

[2]Underlying cause of death was coded according to the 6th Revision of the *International Classification of Diseases* (ICD) in 1950, 7th Revision in 1960, 8th Revision in 1970, and 9th Revision in 1980–1998. See Appendix II, Cause of death; Tables IV and V.

[3]Starting with 1999 data, cause of death is coded according to ICD–10. See Appendix II, Cause of death, Table V; Comparability ratio, Table VI.

[4]Age-adjusted rates are calculated using the year 2000 standard population. Prior to 2003, age-adjusted rates were calculated using standard million proportions based on rounded population numbers. Starting with 2003 data, unrounded population numbers are used to calculate age-adjusted rates. See Appendix II, Age adjustment.

[5]The race groups, white, black, Asian or Pacific Islander, and American Indian or Alaska Native, include persons of Hispanic and non-Hispanic origin. Persons of Hispanic origin may be of any race. Death rates for the American Indian or Alaska Native and Asian or Pacific Islander populations are known to be underestimated. See Appendix II, Race, for a discussion of sources of bias in death rates by race and Hispanic origin.

[6]In 1950, rate is for the age group 75 years and over.

[7]Prior to 1997, excludes data from states lacking an Hispanic-origin item on the death certificate. See Appendix II, Hispanic origin.

NOTES: Starting with *Health, United States, 2003*, rates for 1991–1999 were revised using intercensal population estimates based on the 2000 census. Rates for 2000 were revised based on 2000 census counts. Rates for 2001 and later years were computed using 2000-based postcensal estimates. See Appendix I, Population Census and Population Estimates. For the period 1980–1998, cerebrovascular diseases was coded using ICD–9 codes that are most nearly comparable with cerebrovascular diseases codes in the 113 cause list for ICD–10. See Appendix II, Cause of death; Table V. Age groups were selected to minimize the presentation of unstable age-specific death rates based on small numbers of deaths and for consistency among comparison groups. Starting with 2003 data, some states allowed the reporting of more than one race on the death certificate. The multiple-race data for these states were bridged to the single-race categories of the 1977 Office of Management and Budget standards for comparability with other states. See Appendix II, Race. Data for additional years are available. See Appendix III.

SOURCE: CDC/NCHS, National Vital Statistics System; Grove RD, Hetzel AM. Vital statistics rates in the United States, 1940–1960. Washington, DC: U.S. Government Printing Office. 1968; numerator data from National Vital Statistics System, annual mortality files; denominator data from national population estimates for race groups from Table 1 and unpublished Hispanic population estimates for 1985–1996 prepared by the Housing and Household Economic Statistics Division, U.S. Census Bureau; additional mortality tables are available from: http://www.cdc.gov/nchs/nvss/mortality_tables.htm; Xu JQ, Kochanek KD, Murphy SL, Tejada-Vera B. Deaths: Final data for 2007. National vital statistics reports; vol 58 no 19. Hyattsville, MD: NCHS; 2010. Available from: http://www.cdc.gov/nchs/data/nvsr/nvsr58/nvsr58_19.pdf.

Table 32 (page 1 of 4). **Death rates for malignant neoplasms, by sex, race, Hispanic origin, and age: United States, selected years 1950–2007**

[Data are based on death certificates]

Sex, race, Hispanic origin, and age	1950[1,2]	1960[1,2]	1970[2]	1980[2]	1990[2]	2000[3]	2006[3]	2007[3]
All persons				Deaths per 100,000 resident population				
All ages, age-adjusted[4]	193.9	193.9	198.6	207.9	216.0	199.6	180.7	178.4
All ages, crude	139.8	149.2	162.8	183.9	203.2	196.5	187.0	186.6
Under 1 year	8.7	7.2	4.7	3.2	2.3	2.4	1.8	1.7
1–4 years	11.7	10.9	7.5	4.5	3.5	2.7	2.3	2.2
5–14 years	6.7	6.8	6.0	4.3	3.1	2.5	2.2	2.4
15–24 years	8.6	8.3	8.3	6.3	4.9	4.4	3.9	3.9
25–34 years	20.0	19.5	16.5	13.7	12.6	9.8	9.0	8.5
35–44 years	62.7	59.7	59.5	48.6	43.3	36.6	31.9	30.8
45–54 years	175.1	177.0	182.5	180.0	158.9	127.5	116.3	114.3
55–64 years	390.7	396.8	423.0	436.1	449.6	366.7	321.2	315.4
65–74 years	698.8	713.9	754.2	817.9	872.3	816.3	727.2	715.5
75–84 years	1,153.3	1,127.4	1,169.2	1,232.3	1,348.5	1,335.6	1,263.8	1,256.3
85 years and over	1,451.0	1,450.0	1,320.7	1,594.6	1,752.9	1,819.4	1,606.1	1,590.2
Male								
All ages, age-adjusted[4]	208.1	225.1	247.6	271.2	280.4	248.9	220.1	217.5
All ages, crude	142.9	162.5	182.1	205.3	221.3	207.2	196.6	197.0
Under 1 year	9.7	7.7	4.4	3.7	2.4	2.6	1.8	1.8
1–4 years	12.5	12.4	8.3	5.2	3.7	3.0	2.5	2.3
5–14 years	7.4	7.6	6.7	4.9	3.5	2.7	2.5	2.4
15–24 years	9.7	10.2	10.4	7.8	5.7	5.1	4.6	4.5
25–34 years	17.7	18.8	16.3	13.4	12.6	9.2	8.6	8.2
35–44 years	45.6	48.9	53.0	44.0	38.5	32.7	27.4	26.4
45–54 years	156.2	170.8	183.5	188.7	162.5	130.9	119.0	117.5
55–64 years	413.1	459.9	511.8	520.8	532.9	415.8	363.6	358.5
65–74 years	791.5	890.5	1,006.8	1,093.2	1,122.2	1,001.9	870.4	854.3
75–84 years	1,332.6	1,389.4	1,588.3	1,790.5	1,914.4	1,760.6	1,631.3	1,617.4
85 years and over	1,668.3	1,741.2	1,720.8	2,369.5	2,739.9	2,710.7	2,248.7	2,249.2
Female								
All ages, age-adjusted[4]	182.3	168.7	163.2	166.7	175.7	167.6	153.6	151.3
All ages, crude	136.8	136.4	144.4	163.6	186.0	186.2	177.6	176.5
Under 1 year	7.6	6.8	5.0	2.7	2.2	2.3	1.8	1.6
1–4 years	10.8	9.3	6.7	3.7	3.2	2.5	2.1	2.2
5–14 years	6.0	6.0	5.2	3.6	2.8	2.2	2.0	2.3
15–24 years	7.6	6.5	6.2	4.8	4.1	3.6	3.1	3.2
25–34 years	22.2	20.1	16.7	14.0	12.6	10.4	9.5	8.9
35–44 years	79.3	70.0	65.6	53.1	48.1	40.4	36.4	35.2
45–54 years	194.0	183.0	181.5	171.8	155.5	124.2	113.7	111.3
55–64 years	368.2	337.7	343.2	361.7	375.2	321.3	281.8	275.2
65–74 years	612.3	560.2	557.9	607.1	677.4	663.6	605.9	597.6
75–84 years	1,000.7	924.1	891.9	903.1	1,010.3	1,058.5	1,012.5	1,007.4
85 years and over	1,299.7	1,263.9	1,096.7	1,255.7	1,372.1	1,456.4	1,305.5	1,276.7
White male[5]								
All ages, age-adjusted[4]	210.0	224.7	244.8	265.1	272.2	243.9	217.9	215.1
All ages, crude	147.2	166.1	185.1	208.7	227.7	218.1	208.7	208.8
25–34 years	17.7	18.8	16.2	13.6	12.3	9.2	8.6	8.1
35–44 years	44.5	46.3	50.1	41.1	35.8	30.9	26.7	25.9
45–54 years	150.8	164.1	172.0	175.4	149.9	123.5	113.6	112.0
55–64 years	409.4	450.9	498.1	497.4	508.2	401.9	352.9	346.7
65–74 years	798.7	887.3	997.0	1,070.7	1,090.7	984.3	862.0	845.4
75–84 years	1,367.6	1,413.7	1,592.7	1,779.7	1,883.2	1,736.0	1,631.3	1,617.4
85 years and over	1,732.7	1,791.4	1,772.2	2,375.6	2,715.1	2,693.7	2,258.3	2,253.2
Black or African American male[5]								
All ages, age-adjusted[4]	178.9	227.6	291.9	353.4	397.9	340.3	284.9	282.3
All ages, crude	106.6	136.7	171.6	205.5	221.9	188.5	172.3	172.9
25–34 years	18.0	18.4	18.8	14.1	15.7	10.1	10.0	9.5
35–44 years	55.7	72.9	81.3	73.8	64.3	48.4	36.5	34.0
45–54 years	211.7	244.7	311.2	333.0	302.6	214.2	182.2	178.0
55–64 years	490.8	579.7	689.2	812.5	859.2	626.4	542.9	544.1
65–74 years	636.5	938.5	1,168.9	1,417.2	1,613.9	1,363.8	1,156.5	1,139.5
75–84 years[6]	853.5	1,053.3	1,624.8	2,029.6	2,478.3	2,351.8	1,979.1	1,936.9
85 years and over	- - -	1,155.2	1,387.0	2,393.9	3,238.3	3,264.8	2,543.3	2,637.1

See footnotes at end of table.

Table 32 (page 2 of 4). **Death rates for malignant neoplasms, by sex, race, Hispanic origin, and age: United States, selected years 1950–2007**

[Data are based on death certificates]

Sex, race, Hispanic origin, and age	1950[1,2]	1960[1,2]	1970[2]	1980[2]	1990[2]	2000[3]	2006[3]	2007[3]
American Indian or Alaska Native male[5]				Deaths per 100,000 resident population				
All ages, age-adjusted[4]	- - -	- - -	- - -	140.5	145.8	155.8	135.5	139.4
All ages, crude	- - -	- - -	- - -	58.1	61.4	67.0	76.1	83.3
25–34 years	- - -	- - -	- - -	*	*	*	*	0.0
35–44 years	- - -	- - -	- - -	*	22.8	21.4	15.1	16.0
45–54 years	- - -	- - -	- - -	86.9	86.9	70.3	74.5	78.3
55–64 years	- - -	- - -	- - -	213.4	246.2	255.6	222.8	264.5
65–74 years	- - -	- - -	- - -	613.0	530.6	648.0	583.5	565.5
75–84 years	- - -	- - -	- - -	936.4	1,038.4	1,152.5	1,016.8	984.5
85 years and over	- - -	- - -	- - -	1,471.2	1,654.4	1,584.2	1,161.0	1,271.2
Asian or Pacific Islander male[5]								
All ages, age-adjusted[4]	- - -	- - -	- - -	165.2	172.5	150.8	126.7	130.2
All ages, crude	- - -	- - -	- - -	81.9	82.7	85.2	84.5	89.0
25–34 years	- - -	- - -	- - -	6.3	9.2	7.4	6.9	6.5
35–44 years	- - -	- - -	- - -	29.4	27.7	26.1	19.6	18.8
45–54 years	- - -	- - -	- - -	108.2	92.6	78.5	70.2	73.4
55–64 years	- - -	- - -	- - -	298.5	274.6	229.2	197.2	190.0
65–74 years	- - -	- - -	- - -	581.2	687.2	559.4	459.9	470.7
75–84 years	- - -	- - -	- - -	1,147.6	1,229.9	1,086.1	942.3	1,014.5
85 years and over	- - -	- - -	- - -	1,798.7	1,837.0	1,823.2	1,439.0	1,427.4
Hispanic or Latino male[5,7]								
All ages, age-adjusted[4]	- - -	- - -	- - -	- - -	174.7	171.7	143.4	141.4
All ages, crude	- - -	- - -	- - -	- - -	65.5	61.3	60.4	61.6
25–34 years	- - -	- - -	- - -	- - -	8.0	6.9	6.1	6.3
35–44 years	- - -	- - -	- - -	- - -	22.5	20.1	16.0	17.4
45–54 years	- - -	- - -	- - -	- - -	96.6	79.4	71.4	74.2
55–64 years	- - -	- - -	- - -	- - -	294.0	253.1	224.8	221.9
65–74 years	- - -	- - -	- - -	- - -	655.5	651.2	574.8	560.3
75–84 years	- - -	- - -	- - -	- - -	1,233.4	1,306.4	1,098.4	1,072.6
85 years and over	- - -	- - -	- - -	- - -	2,019.4	2,049.7	1,440.1	1,417.9
White, not Hispanic or Latino male[7]								
All ages, age-adjusted[4]	- - -	- - -	- - -	- - -	276.7	247.7	223.4	220.8
All ages, crude	- - -	- - -	- - -	- - -	246.2	244.4	239.9	240.6
25–34 years	- - -	- - -	- - -	- - -	12.8	9.7	9.3	8.6
35–44 years	- - -	- - -	- - -	- - -	36.8	32.3	28.9	27.7
45–54 years	- - -	- - -	- - -	- - -	153.9	127.2	118.7	116.8
55–64 years	- - -	- - -	- - -	- - -	520.6	412.0	363.4	357.6
65–74 years	- - -	- - -	- - -	- - -	1,109.0	1,002.1	883.0	867.3
75–84 years	- - -	- - -	- - -	- - -	1,906.6	1,750.2	1,662.9	1,652.8
85 years and over	- - -	- - -	- - -	- - -	2,744.4	2,714.1	2,300.2	2,300.4
White female[5]								
All ages, age-adjusted[4]	182.0	167.7	162.5	165.2	174.0	166.9	153.6	151.2
All ages, crude	139.9	139.8	149.4	170.3	196.1	199.4	190.1	188.8
25–34 years	20.9	18.8	16.3	13.5	11.9	10.1	9.1	8.6
35–44 years	74.5	66.6	62.4	50.9	46.2	38.2	34.9	33.9
45–54 years	185.8	175.7	177.3	166.4	150.9	120.1	109.5	107.1
55–64 years	362.5	329.0	338.6	355.5	368.5	319.7	279.1	271.8
65–74 years	616.5	562.1	554.7	605.2	675.1	665.6	611.5	602.3
75–84 years	1,026.6	939.3	903.5	905.4	1,011.8	1,063.4	1,023.0	1,017.7
85 years and over	1,348.3	1,304.9	1,126.6	1,266.8	1,372.3	1,459.1	1,317.5	1,291.6

See footnotes at end of table.

Table 32 (page 3 of 4). Death rates for malignant neoplasms, by sex, race, Hispanic origin, and age: United States, selected years 1950–2007

[Data are based on death certificates]

Sex, race, Hispanic origin, and age	1950[1,2]	1960[1,2]	1970[2]	1980[2]	1990[2]	2000[3]	2006[3]	2007[3]
Black or African American female[5]				Deaths per 100,000 resident population				
All ages, age-adjusted[4]	174.1	174.3	173.4	189.5	205.9	193.8	176.1	174.9
All ages, crude	111.8	113.8	117.3	136.5	156.1	151.8	147.7	148.2
25–34 years	34.3	31.0	20.9	18.3	18.7	13.5	12.5	12.0
35–44 years	119.8	102.4	94.6	73.5	67.4	58.9	50.8	48.5
45–54 years	277.0	254.8	228.6	230.2	209.9	173.9	158.7	156.1
55–64 years	484.6	442.7	404.8	450.4	482.4	391.0	356.9	352.5
65–74 years	477.3	541.6	615.8	662.4	773.2	753.1	672.9	681.0
75–84 years[6]	605.3	696.3	763.3	923.9	1,059.9	1,124.0	1,065.3	1,071.7
85 years and over	- - -	728.9	791.5	1,159.9	1,431.3	1,527.7	1,324.4	1,265.2
American Indian or Alaska Native female[5]								
All ages, age-adjusted[4]	- - -	- - -	- - -	94.0	106.9	108.3	108.3	102.1
All ages, crude	- - -	- - -	- - -	50.4	62.1	61.3	76.8	75.0
25–34 years	- - -	- - -	- - -	*	*	*	*	0.0
35–44 years	- - -	- - -	- - -	36.9	31.0	23.7	25.4	20.3
45–54 years	- - -	- - -	- - -	96.9	104.5	59.7	72.8	75.6
55–64 years	- - -	- - -	- - -	198.4	213.3	200.9	193.8	190.3
65–74 years	- - -	- - -	- - -	350.8	438.9	458.3	469.8	444.3
75–84 years	- - -	- - -	- - -	446.4	554.3	714.0	756.8	712.1
85 years and over	- - -	- - -	- - -	786.5	843.7	983.2	684.8	639.5
Asian or Pacific Islander female[5]								
All ages, age-adjusted[4]	- - -	- - -	- - -	93.0	103.0	100.7	92.2	90.0
All ages, crude	- - -	- - -	- - -	54.1	60.5	72.1	77.8	78.2
25–34 years	- - -	- - -	- - -	9.5	7.3	8.1	7.3	6.0
35–44 years	- - -	- - -	- - -	38.7	29.8	28.9	24.7	24.0
45–54 years	- - -	- - -	- - -	99.8	93.9	78.2	73.5	70.0
55–64 years	- - -	- - -	- - -	174.7	196.2	176.5	160.2	162.2
65–74 years	- - -	- - -	- - -	301.9	346.2	357.4	330.9	308.8
75–84 years	- - -	- - -	- - -	522.1	641.4	650.1	602.4	601.2
85 years and over	- - -	- - -	- - -	800.0	971.7	988.5	878.4	875.2
Hispanic or Latina female[5,7]								
All ages, age-adjusted[4]	- - -	- - -	- - -	- - -	111.9	110.8	100.4	98.6
All ages, crude	- - -	- - -	- - -	- - -	60.7	58.5	59.7	59.9
25–34 years	- - -	- - -	- - -	- - -	9.7	7.8	8.5	8.9
35–44 years	- - -	- - -	- - -	- - -	34.8	30.7	27.9	26.5
45–54 years	- - -	- - -	- - -	- - -	100.5	84.7	78.1	75.5
55–64 years	- - -	- - -	- - -	- - -	205.4	192.5	174.4	175.6
65–74 years	- - -	- - -	- - -	- - -	404.8	410.0	370.2	364.4
75–84 years	- - -	- - -	- - -	- - -	663.0	716.5	665.9	665.7
85 years and over	- - -	- - -	- - -	- - -	1,022.7	1,056.5	884.9	814.2

See footnotes at end of table.

Table 32 (page 4 of 4). Death rates for malignant neoplasms, by sex, race, Hispanic origin, and age: United States, selected years 1950–2007

[Data are based on death certificates]

Sex, race, Hispanic origin, and age	1950[1,2]	1960[1,2]	1970[2]	1980[2]	1990[2]	2000[3]	2006[3]	2007[3]
White, not Hispanic or Latina female[7]				Deaths per 100,000 resident population				
All ages, age-adjusted[4]	- - -	- - -	- - -	- - -	177.5	170.0	157.6	155.3
All ages, crude	- - -	- - -	- - -	- - -	210.6	220.6	214.7	213.7
25–34 years	- - -	- - -	- - -	- - -	11.9	10.5	9.2	8.4
35–44 years	- - -	- - -	- - -	- - -	47.0	38.9	35.9	35.2
45–54 years	- - -	- - -	- - -	- - -	154.9	123.0	113.0	110.9
55–64 years	- - -	- - -	- - -	- - -	379.5	328.9	288.5	280.6
65–74 years	- - -	- - -	- - -	- - -	688.5	681.0	631.3	622.2
75–84 years	- - -	- - -	- - -	- - -	1,027.2	1,075.3	1,044.4	1,040.1
85 years and over	- - -	- - -	- - -	- - -	1,385.7	1,468.7	1,336.7	1,315.2

- - - Data not available.
* Rates based on fewer than 20 deaths are considered unreliable and are not shown.
0.0 Quantity more than zero but less than 0.05.
[1]Includes deaths of persons who were not residents of the 50 states and the District of Columbia (D.C.).
[2]Underlying cause of death was coded according to the 6th Revision of the *International Classification of Diseases* (ICD) in 1950, 7th Revision in 1960, 8th Revision in 1970, and 9th Revision in 1980–1998. See Appendix II, Cause of death; Tables IV and V.
[3]Starting with 1999 data, cause of death is coded according to ICD–10. See Appendix II, Cause of death, Table V; Comparability ratio, Table VI.
[4]Age-adjusted rates are calculated using the year 2000 standard population. Prior to 2003, age-adjusted rates were calculated using standard million proportions based on rounded population numbers. Starting with 2003 data, unrounded population numbers are used to calculate age-adjusted rates. See Appendix II, Age adjustment.
[5]The race groups, white, black, Asian or Pacific Islander, and American Indian or Alaska Native, include persons of Hispanic and non-Hispanic origin. Persons of Hispanic origin may be of any race. Death rates for the American Indian or Alaska Native and Asian or Pacific Islander populations are known to be underestimated. See Appendix II, Race, for a discussion of sources of bias in death rates by race and Hispanic origin.
[6]In 1950, rate is for the age group 75 years and over.
[7]Prior to 1997, excludes data from states lacking an Hispanic-origin item on the death certificate. See Appendix II, Hispanic origin.

NOTES: Starting with *Health, United States, 2003*, rates for 1991–1999 were revised using intercensal population estimates based on the 2000 census. Rates for 2000 were revised based on 2000 census counts. Rates for 2001 and later years were computed using 2000-based postcensal estimates. See Appendix I, Population Census and Population Estimates. See Appendix II, Cause of death; Tables IV and V. Age groups were selected to minimize the presentation of unstable age-specific death rates based on small numbers of deaths and for consistency among comparison groups. Starting with 2003 data, some states allowed the reporting of more than one race on the death certificate. The multiple-race data for these states were bridged to the single-race categories of the 1977 Office of Management and Budget standards for comparability with other states. See Appendix II, Race. Data for additional years are available. See Appendix III.

SOURCE: CDC/NCHS, National Vital Statistics System; Grove RD, Hetzel AM. Vital statistics rates in the United States, 1940–1960. Washington, DC: U.S. Government Printing Office. 1968; numerator data from National Vital Statistics System, annual mortality files; denominator data from national population estimates for race groups from Table 1 and unpublished Hispanic population estimates for 1985–1996 prepared by the Housing and Household Economic Statistics Division, U.S. Census Bureau; additional mortality tables are available from: http://www.cdc.gov/nchs/nvss/mortality_tables.htm; Xu JQ, Kochanek KD, Murphy SL, Tejada-Vera B. Deaths: Final data for 2007. National vital statistics reports; vol 58 no 19. Hyattsville, MD: NCHS; 2010. Available from: http://www.cdc.gov/nchs/data/nvsr/nvsr58/nvsr58_19.pdf.

Table 33 (page 1 of 3). Death rates for malignant neoplasms of trachea, bronchus, and lung, by sex, race, Hispanic origin, and age: United States, selected years 1950–2007

[Data are based on death certificates]

Sex, race, Hispanic origin, and age	1950[1,2]	1960[1,2]	1970[2]	1980[2]	1990[2]	2000[3]	2006[3]	2007[3]
All persons			Deaths per 100,000 resident population					
All ages, age-adjusted[4]	15.0	24.1	37.1	49.9	59.3	56.1	51.5	50.6
All ages, crude	12.2	20.3	32.1	45.8	56.8	55.3	53.0	52.6
Under 25 years	0.1	0.0	0.1	0.0	0.0	0.0	0.0	0.0
25–34 years	0.8	1.0	0.9	0.6	0.7	0.5	0.4	0.3
35–44 years	4.5	6.8	11.0	9.2	6.8	6.1	4.6	4.3
45–54 years	20.4	29.6	43.4	54.1	46.8	31.6	29.1	28.4
55–64 years	48.7	75.3	109.1	138.2	160.6	122.4	99.1	95.4
65–74 years	59.7	108.1	164.5	233.3	288.4	284.2	253.1	248.8
75–84 years	55.8	91.5	163.2	240.5	333.3	370.8	373.5	371.3
85 years and over	42.3	65.6	101.7	176.0	242.5	302.1	300.5	299.8
Male								
All ages, age-adjusted[4]	24.6	43.6	67.5	85.2	91.1	76.7	67.0	65.1
All ages, crude	19.9	35.4	53.4	68.6	75.1	65.5	60.5	59.4
Under 25 years	0.0	0.0	0.1	0.1	0.0	*	*	0.0
25–34 years	1.1	1.4	1.3	0.8	0.9	0.5	0.4	0.4
35–44 years	7.1	10.5	16.1	11.9	8.5	6.9	4.7	4.2
45–54 years	35.0	50.6	67.5	76.0	59.7	38.5	33.8	32.1
55–64 years	83.8	139.3	189.7	213.6	222.9	154.0	121.6	116.2
65–74 years	98.7	204.3	320.8	403.9	430.4	377.9	319.4	310.2
75–84 years	82.6	167.1	330.8	488.8	572.9	532.2	509.9	498.3
85 years and over	62.5	107.7	194.0	368.1	513.2	521.2	457.7	453.0
Female								
All ages, age-adjusted[4]	5.8	7.5	13.1	24.4	37.1	41.3	40.0	40.0
All ages, crude	4.5	6.4	11.9	24.3	39.4	45.4	45.7	46.0
Under 25 years	0.1	0.0	0.0	*	*	*	*	*
25–34 years	0.5	0.5	0.5	0.5	0.5	0.5	0.4	0.3
35–44 years	1.9	3.2	6.1	6.5	5.2	5.3	4.5	4.4
45–54 years	5.8	9.2	21.0	33.7	34.5	25.0	24.6	24.9
55–64 years	13.6	15.4	36.8	72.0	105.0	93.3	78.2	76.1
65–74 years	23.3	24.4	43.1	102.7	177.6	206.9	197.0	196.7
75–84 years	32.9	32.8	52.4	94.1	190.1	265.6	280.3	283.8
85 years and over	28.2	38.8	50.0	91.9	138.1	212.8	226.9	227.0
White male[5]								
All ages, age-adjusted[4]	25.1	43.6	67.1	83.8	89.0	75.7	66.8	64.8
All ages, crude	20.8	36.4	54.6	70.2	77.8	69.4	64.6	63.4
45–54 years	35.1	49.2	63.3	70.9	55.2	35.7	31.7	30.2
55–64 years	85.4	139.2	186.8	205.6	213.7	150.8	118.3	113.1
65–74 years	101.5	207.5	325.0	401.0	422.1	374.9	319.8	310.4
75–84 years	85.5	170.4	336.7	493.5	572.2	529.9	514.6	502.7
85 years and over	67.4	109.4	199.6	374.1	516.3	522.4	464.0	453.3
Black or African American male[5]								
All ages, age-adjusted[4]	17.8	42.6	75.4	107.6	125.4	101.1	83.7	82.2
All ages, crude	12.1	28.1	47.7	66.6	73.7	58.3	52.0	51.5
45–54 years	34.4	68.4	115.4	133.8	114.9	70.7	56.9	54.1
55–64 years	68.3	146.8	234.3	321.1	358.6	223.5	184.3	177.7
65–74 years	53.8	168.3	300.5	472.3	585.4	488.8	402.7	395.6
75–84 years[6]	36.2	107.3	271.6	472.9	645.4	642.5	563.9	546.2
85 years and over	- - -	82.8	137.0	311.3	499.5	562.8	442.3	504.8
American Indian or Alaska Native male[5]								
All ages, age-adjusted[4]	- - -	- - -	- - -	31.7	47.5	42.9	37.6	40.7
All ages, crude	- - -	- - -	- - -	14.2	20.0	18.1	21.2	23.8
45–54 years	- - -	- - -	- - -	*	26.6	14.5	18.3	14.4
55–64 years	- - -	- - -	- - -	72.0	97.8	86.0	64.4	82.4
65–74 years	- - -	- - -	- - -	202.8	194.3	184.8	202.2	202.6
75–84 years	- - -	- - -	- - -	*	356.2	367.9	294.1	300.5
85 years and over	- - -	- - -	- - -	*	*	*	*	286.3

See footnotes at end of table.

Table 33 (page 2 of 3). Death rates for malignant neoplasms of trachea, bronchus, and lung, by sex, race, Hispanic origin, and age: United States, selected years 1950–2007

[Data are based on death certificates]

Sex, race, Hispanic origin, and age	1950[1,2]	1960[1,2]	1970[2]	1980[2]	1990[2]	2000[3]	2006[3]	2007[3]
Asian or Pacific Islander male[5]				Deaths per 100,000 resident population				
All ages, age-adjusted[4]	- - -	- - -	- - -	43.3	44.2	40.9	35.3	34.7
All ages, crude	- - -	- - -	- - -	22.1	20.7	22.7	23.2	22.9
45–54 years	- - -	- - -	- - -	33.3	18.8	17.2	18.0	17.1
55–64 years	- - -	- - -	- - -	94.4	74.4	61.4	56.2	44.1
65–74 years	- - -	- - -	- - -	174.3	215.8	183.2	141.2	135.2
75–84 years	- - -	- - -	- - -	301.3	307.5	323.2	285.6	301.5
85 years and over	- - -	- - -	- - -	*	421.3	378.0	342.6	357.3
Hispanic or Latino male[5,7]								
All ages, age-adjusted[4]	- - -	- - -	- - -	- - -	44.1	39.0	30.3	29.6
All ages, crude	- - -	- - -	- - -	- - -	16.2	13.3	12.0	12.0
45–54 years	- - -	- - -	- - -	- - -	21.5	14.8	10.5	10.3
55–64 years	- - -	- - -	- - -	- - -	80.7	58.6	44.8	42.1
65–74 years	- - -	- - -	- - -	- - -	195.5	167.3	140.1	140.7
75–84 years	- - -	- - -	- - -	- - -	313.4	327.5	254.2	246.1
85 years and over	- - -	- - -	- - -	- - -	420.7	368.8	263.9	256.1
White, not Hispanic or Latino male[7]								
All ages, age-adjusted[4]	- - -	- - -	- - -	- - -	91.1	77.9	69.7	67.7
All ages, crude	- - -	- - -	- - -	- - -	84.7	78.9	75.8	74.6
45–54 years	- - -	- - -	- - -	- - -	57.8	37.7	34.5	33.0
55–64 years	- - -	- - -	- - -	- - -	221.0	157.7	124.8	119.8
65–74 years	- - -	- - -	- - -	- - -	431.4	387.3	334.0	324.2
75–84 years	- - -	- - -	- - -	- - -	580.4	537.7	531.2	520.4
85 years and over	- - -	- - -	- - -	- - -	520.9	527.3	474.2	464.7
White female[5]								
All ages, age-adjusted[4]	5.9	6.8	13.1	24.5	37.6	42.3	41.1	41.2
All ages, crude	4.7	5.9	12.3	25.6	42.4	49.9	50.2	50.7
45–54 years	5.7	9.0	20.9	33.0	34.6	24.8	24.0	24.7
55–64 years	13.7	15.1	37.2	71.9	105.7	96.1	80.5	78.3
65–74 years	23.7	24.8	42.9	104.6	181.3	213.2	205.2	204.7
75–84 years	34.0	32.7	52.6	95.2	194.6	272.7	288.8	293.0
85 years and over	29.3	39.1	50.6	92.4	138.3	215.9	231.9	232.3
Black or African American female[5]								
All ages, age-adjusted[4]	4.5	6.8	13.7	24.8	36.8	39.8	39.0	38.1
All ages, crude	2.8	4.3	9.4	18.3	28.1	30.8	32.3	31.8
45–54 years	7.5	11.3	23.9	43.4	41.3	32.9	34.7	32.5
55–64 years	12.9	17.9	33.5	79.9	117.9	95.3	82.6	78.6
65–74 years	14.0	18.1	46.1	88.0	164.3	194.1	179.1	180.4
75–84 years[6]	*	31.3	49.1	79.4	148.1	224.3	251.3	249.3
85 years and over	- - -	34.2	44.8	85.8	134.9	185.9	191.9	190.9
American Indian or Alaska Native female[5]								
All ages, age-adjusted[4]	- - -	- - -	- - -	11.7	19.3	24.8	26.3	26.8
All ages, crude	- - -	- - -	- - -	6.0	11.2	14.0	18.5	19.2
45–54 years	- - -	- - -	- - -	*	22.9	12.1	12.1	10.9
55–64 years	- - -	- - -	- - -	*	53.7	52.6	59.7	52.3
65–74 years	- - -	- - -	- - -	*	78.5	151.5	144.7	160.0
75–84 years	- - -	- - -	- - -	*	111.8	136.3	173.0	180.6
85 years and over	- - -	- - -	- - -	*	*	*	*	*

See footnotes at end of table.

[Data are based on death certificates]

Sex, race, Hispanic origin, and age	1950[1,2]	1960[1,2]	1970[2]	1980[2]	1990[2]	2000[3]	2006[3]	2007[3]
Asian or Pacific Islander female[5]				Deaths per 100,000 resident population				
All ages, age-adjusted[4]	- - -	- - -	- - -	15.4	18.9	18.4	17.7	18.5
All ages, crude	- - -	- - -	- - -	8.4	10.5	12.6	14.5	15.7
45–54 years	- - -	- - -	- - -	13.5	11.3	9.9	10.2	10.6
55–64 years	- - -	- - -	- - -	24.6	38.3	30.4	27.5	33.2
65–74 years	- - -	- - -	- - -	62.4	71.6	77.0	75.0	74.7
75–84 years	- - -	- - -	- - -	117.7	137.9	135.0	130.0	139.8
85 years and over	- - -	- - -	- - -	*	172.9	175.3	166.4	166.2
Hispanic or Latina female[5,7]								
All ages, age-adjusted[4]	- - -	- - -	- - -	- - -	14.1	14.7	13.6	14.4
All ages, crude	- - -	- - -	- - -	- - -	7.2	7.2	7.5	8.2
45–54 years	- - -	- - -	- - -	- - -	8.7	7.1	6.3	6.7
55–64 years	- - -	- - -	- - -	- - -	25.1	22.2	19.0	22.2
65–74 years	- - -	- - -	- - -	- - -	66.8	66.0	65.2	66.7
75–84 years	- - -	- - -	- - -	- - -	94.3	112.3	107.6	111.7
85 years and over	- - -	- - -	- - -	- - -	118.2	137.5	106.0	123.0
White, not Hispanic or Latina female[7]								
All ages, age-adjusted[4]	- - -	- - -	- - -	- - -	39.0	44.1	43.5	43.5
All ages, crude	- - -	- - -	- - -	- - -	46.2	56.4	58.4	59.0
45–54 years	- - -	- - -	- - -	- - -	36.6	26.4	26.3	27.1
55–64 years	- - -	- - -	- - -	- - -	111.3	102.2	86.4	83.8
65–74 years	- - -	- - -	- - -	- - -	186.4	222.9	217.3	216.7
75–84 years	- - -	- - -	- - -	- - -	199.1	279.2	300.5	305.2
85 years and over	- - -	- - -	- - -	- - -	139.0	218.0	237.8	237.7

0.0 Quantity more than zero but less than 0.05.

* Rates based on fewer than 20 deaths are considered unreliable and are not shown.

- - - Data not available.

[1]Includes deaths of persons who were not residents of the 50 states and the District of Columbia (D.C.).

[2]Underlying cause of death was coded according to the 6th Revision of the *International Classification of Diseases* (ICD) in 1950, 7th Revision in 1960, 8th Revision in 1970, and 9th Revision in 1980–1998. See Appendix II, Cause of death; Tables IV and V.

[3]Starting with 1999 data, cause of death is coded according to ICD–10. See Appendix II, Cause of death, Table V; Comparability ratio, Table VI.

[4]Age-adjusted rates are calculated using the year 2000 standard population. Prior to 2003, age-adjusted rates were calculated using standard million proportions based on rounded population numbers. Starting with 2003 data, unrounded population numbers are used to calculate age-adjusted rates. See Appendix II, Age adjustment.

[5]The race groups, white, black, Asian or Pacific Islander, and American Indian or Alaska Native, include persons of Hispanic and non-Hispanic origin. Persons of Hispanic origin may be of any race. Death rates for the American Indian or Alaska Native and Asian or Pacific Islander populations are known to be underestimated. See Appendix II, Race, for a discussion of sources of bias in death rates by race and Hispanic origin.

[6]In 1950, rate is for the age group 75 years and over.

[7]Prior to 1997, excludes data from states lacking an Hispanic-origin item on the death certificate. See Appendix II, Hispanic origin.

NOTES: Starting with *Health, United States, 2003*, rates for 1991–1999 were revised using intercensal population estimates based on the 2000 census. Rates for 2000 were revised based on 2000 census counts. Rates for 2001 and later years were computed using 2000-based postcensal estimates. See Appendix I, Population Census and Population Estimates. For the period 1980–1998, lung cancer was coded using ICD–9 codes that are most comparable with lung cancer codes in the 113 cause list for ICD–10. See Appendix II, Cause of death; Table V. Age groups were selected to minimize the presentation of unstable age-specific death rates based on small numbers of deaths and for consistency among comparison groups. Starting with 2003 data, some states allowed the reporting of more than one race on the death certificate. The multiple-race data for these states were bridged to the single-race categories of the 1977 Office of Management and Budget standards for comparability with other states. See Appendix II, Race. Data for additional years are available. See Appendix III.

SOURCE: CDC/NCHS, National Vital Statistics System; Grove RD, Hetzel AM. Vital statistics rates in the United States, 1940–1960. Washington, DC: U.S. Government Printing Office. 1968; numerator data from National Vital Statistics System, annual mortality files; denominator data from national population estimates for race groups from Table 1 and unpublished Hispanic population estimates for 1985–1996 prepared by the Housing and Household Economic Statistics Division, U.S. Census Bureau; additional mortality tables are available from: http://www.cdc.gov/nchs/nvss/mortality_tables.htm; Xu JQ, Kochanek KD, Murphy SL, Tejada-Vera B. Deaths: Final data for 2007. National vital statistics reports; vol 58 no 19. Hyattsville, MD: NCHS; 2010. Available from: http://www.cdc.gov/nchs/data/nvsr/nvsr58/nvsr58_19.pdf.

Table 34 (page 1 of 2). Death rates for malignant neoplasm of breast among females, by race, Hispanic origin, and age: United States, selected years 1950–2007

[Data are based on death certificates]

Race, Hispanic origin, and age	1950[1,2]	1960[1,2]	1970[2]	1980[2]	1990[2]	2000[3]	2006[3]	2007[3]
All females			Deaths per 100,000 resident population					
All ages, age-adjusted[4]	31.9	31.7	32.1	31.9	33.3	26.8	23.5	22.9
All ages, crude	24.7	26.1	28.4	30.6	34.0	29.2	26.9	26.5
Under 25 years	*	*	*	*	*	*	*	*
25–34 years	3.8	3.8	3.9	3.3	2.9	2.3	1.8	1.7
35–44 years	20.8	20.2	20.4	17.9	17.8	12.4	10.8	10.1
45–54 years	46.9	51.4	52.6	48.1	45.4	33.0	27.6	26.7
55–64 years	69.9	70.8	77.6	80.5	78.6	59.3	53.7	51.3
65–74 years	95.0	90.0	93.8	101.1	111.7	88.3	76.9	77.3
75–84 years	139.8	129.9	127.4	126.4	146.3	128.9	119.2	116.3
85 years and over	195.5	191.9	157.1	169.3	196.8	205.7	169.9	170.4
White[5]								
All ages, age-adjusted[4]	32.4	32.0	32.5	32.1	33.2	26.3	22.9	22.3
All ages, crude	25.7	27.2	29.9	32.3	35.9	30.7	27.9	27.6
35–44 years	20.8	19.7	20.2	17.3	17.1	11.3	9.8	9.1
45–54 years	47.1	51.2	53.0	48.1	44.3	31.2	25.6	24.7
55–64 years	70.9	71.8	79.3	81.3	78.5	57.9	52.0	49.4
65–74 years	96.3	91.6	95.9	103.7	113.3	89.3	77.1	77.3
75–84 years	143.6	132.8	129.6	128.4	148.2	130.2	120.4	117.3
85 years and over	204.2	199.7	161.9	171.7	198.0	205.5	170.3	172.1
Black or African American[5]								
All ages, age-adjusted[4]	25.3	27.9	28.9	31.7	38.1	34.5	31.6	31.4
All ages, crude	16.4	18.7	19.7	22.9	29.0	27.9	27.5	27.7
35–44 years	21.0	24.8	24.4	24.1	25.8	20.9	19.0	18.2
45–54 years	46.5	54.4	52.0	52.7	60.5	51.5	44.5	44.3
55–64 years	64.3	63.2	64.7	79.9	93.1	80.9	76.3	75.7
65–74 years	67.0	72.3	77.3	84.3	112.2	98.6	91.2	96.0
75–84 years[6]	81.0	87.5	101.8	114.1	140.5	139.8	138.2	135.2
85 years and over	- - -	92.1	112.1	149.9	201.5	238.7	199.2	191.9
American Indian or Alaska Native[5]								
All ages, age-adjusted[4]	- - -	- - -	- - -	10.8	13.7	13.6	12.8	12.7
All ages, crude	- - -	- - -	- - -	6.1	8.6	8.7	10.0	10.4
35–44 years	- - -	- - -	- - -	*	*	*	*	*
45–54 years	- - -	- - -	- - -	*	23.9	14.4	15.8	18.1
55–64 years	- - -	- - -	- - -	*	*	40.0	30.9	34.8
65–74 years	- - -	- - -	- - -	*	*	42.5	43.0	38.3
75–84 years	- - -	- - -	- - -	*	*	71.8	54.1	51.6
85 years and over	- - -	- - -	- - -	*	*	*	*	*
Asian or Pacific Islander[5]								
All ages, age-adjusted[4]	- - -	- - -	- - -	11.9	13.7	12.3	12.1	11.1
All ages, crude	- - -	- - -	- - -	8.2	9.3	10.2	11.1	10.4
35–44 years	- - -	- - -	- - -	10.4	8.4	8.1	5.2	5.8
45–54 years	- - -	- - -	- - -	23.4	26.4	22.3	19.6	15.4
55–64 years	- - -	- - -	- - -	35.7	33.8	31.3	33.0	28.9
65–74 years	- - -	- - -	- - -	*	38.5	34.7	39.1	35.7
75–84 years	- - -	- - -	- - -	*	48.0	37.5	42.5	48.8
85 years and over	- - -	- - -	- - -	*	*	68.2	68.8	52.4
Hispanic or Latina[5,7]								
All ages, age-adjusted[4]	- - -	- - -	- - -	- - -	19.5	16.9	15.0	14.5
All ages, crude	- - -	- - -	- - -	- - -	11.5	9.7	9.6	9.4
35–44 years	- - -	- - -	- - -	- - -	11.7	8.7	7.9	7.4
45–54 years	- - -	- - -	- - -	- - -	32.8	23.9	19.6	19.4
55–64 years	- - -	- - -	- - -	- - -	45.8	39.1	36.4	33.9
65–74 years	- - -	- - -	- - -	- - -	64.8	54.9	47.3	48.3
75–84 years	- - -	- - -	- - -	- - -	67.2	74.9	68.8	66.5
85 years and over	- - -	- - -	- - -	- - -	102.8	105.8	89.9	88.3

See footnotes at end of table.

Table 34 (page 2 of 2). Death rates for malignant neoplasm of breast among females, by race, Hispanic origin, and age: United States, selected years 1950–2007

[Data are based on death certificates]

Race, Hispanic origin, and age	1950[1,2]	1960[1,2]	1970[2]	1980[2]	1990[2]	2000[3]	2006[3]	2007[3]
White, not Hispanic or Latina[7]				Deaths per 100,000 resident population				
All ages, age-adjusted[4]	- - -	- - -	- - -	- - -	33.9	26.8	23.5	23.0
All ages, crude	- - -	- - -	- - -	- - -	38.5	33.8	31.4	31.1
35–44 years	- - -	- - -	- - -	- - -	17.5	11.6	10.0	9.3
45–54 years	- - -	- - -	- - -	- - -	45.2	31.7	26.3	25.3
55–64 years	- - -	- - -	- - -	- - -	80.6	59.2	53.4	50.8
65–74 years	- - -	- - -	- - -	- - -	115.7	91.4	79.6	79.8
75–84 years	- - -	- - -	- - -	- - -	151.4	132.2	123.6	120.7
85 years and over	- - -	- - -	- - -	- - -	201.5	208.3	174.1	176.3

* Rates based on fewer than 20 deaths are considered unreliable and are not shown.
- - - Data not available.
[1]Includes deaths of persons who were not residents of the 50 states and the District of Columbia (D.C.).
[2]Underlying cause of death was coded according to the 6th Revision of the *International Classification of Diseases* (ICD) in 1950, 7th Revision in 1960, 8th Revision in 1970, and 9th Revision in 1980–1998. See Appendix II, Cause of death; Tables IV and V.
[3]Starting with 1999 data, cause of death is coded according to ICD–10. See Appendix II, Cause of death, Table V; Comparability ratio, Table VI.
[4]Age-adjusted rates are calculated using the year 2000 standard population. Prior to 2003, age-adjusted rates were calculated using standard million proportions based on rounded population numbers. Starting with 2003 data, unrounded population numbers are used to calculate age-adjusted rates. See Appendix II, Age adjustment.
[5]The race groups, white, black, Asian or Pacific Islander, and American Indian or Alaska Native, include persons of Hispanic and non-Hispanic origin. Persons of Hispanic origin may be of any race. Death rates for the American Indian or Alaska Native and Asian or Pacific Islander populations are known to be underestimated. See Appendix II, Race, for a discussion of sources of bias in death rates by race and Hispanic origin.
[6]In 1950, rate is for the age group 75 years and over.
[7]Prior to 1997, excludes data from states lacking an Hispanic-origin item on the death certificate. See Appendix II, Hispanic origin.

NOTES: Starting with *Health, United States, 2003*, rates for 1991–1999 were revised using intercensal population estimates based on the 2000 census. Rates for 2000 were revised based on 2000 census counts. Rates for 2001 and beyond were computed using 2000-based postcensal estimates. See Appendix I, Population Census and Population Estimates. Age groups were selected to minimize the presentation of unstable age-specific death rates based on small numbers of deaths and for consistency among comparison groups. Starting with 2003 data, some states allowed the reporting of more than one race on the death certificate. The multiple-race data for these states were bridged to the single-race categories of the 1977 Office of Management and Budget standards for comparability with other states. See Appendix II, Race. Data for additional years are available. See Appendix III.

SOURCE: CDC/NCHS, National Vital Statistics System; numerator data from National Vital Statistics System, annual mortality files; denominator data from national population estimates for race groups from Table 1 and unpublished Hispanic population estimates for 1985–1996 prepared by the Housing and Household Economic Statistics Division, U.S. Census Bureau; additional mortality tables are available from: http://www.cdc.gov/nchs/nvss/mortality_tables.htm; Xu JQ, Kochanek KD, Murphy SL, Tejada-Vera B. Deaths: Final data for 2007. National vital statistics reports; vol 58 no 19. Hyattsville, MD: NCHS; 2010. Available from: http://www.cdc.gov/nchs/data/nvsr/nvsr58/nvsr58_19.pdf.

Table 35 (page 1 of 2). Death rates for human immunodeficiency virus (HIV) disease, by sex, race, Hispanic origin, and age: United States, selected years 1987–2007

[Data are based on death certificates]

Sex, race, Hispanic origin, and age[1]	1987[2]	1990[2]	1995[2]	1996	1997	1998	1999[3]	2000[3]	2005[3]	2006[3]	2007[3]
All persons				Deaths per 100,000 resident population							
All ages, age-adjusted[4]	5.6	10.2	16.2	11.5	6.0	4.9	5.3	5.2	4.2	4.0	3.7
All ages, crude	5.6	10.1	16.2	11.6	6.1	4.9	5.3	5.1	4.2	4.0	3.7
Under 1 year	2.3	2.7	1.5	1.1	*	*	*	*	*	*	*
1–4 years	0.7	0.8	1.3	0.9	0.3	0.2	0.2	*	*	*	*
5–14 years	0.1	0.2	0.5	0.5	0.3	0.1	0.2	0.1	*	*	*
15–24 years	1.3	1.5	1.7	1.1	0.7	0.5	0.5	0.5	0.4	0.5	0.4
25–34 years	11.7	19.7	28.3	19.2	9.7	7.1	6.8	6.1	3.3	2.9	2.7
35–44 years	14.0	27.4	44.2	31.3	16.0	12.8	13.8	13.1	9.9	9.2	8.3
45–54 years	8.0	15.2	26.0	19.1	10.3	8.9	10.7	11.0	10.6	10.1	9.5
55–64 years	3.5	6.2	10.9	8.3	4.8	4.3	4.8	5.1	5.3	5.5	5.3
65–74 years	1.3	2.0	3.6	2.7	1.8	1.6	2.2	2.2	2.3	2.5	2.3
75–84 years	0.8	0.7	0.7	0.8	0.6	0.5	0.6	0.7	0.8	0.8	0.8
85 years and over	*	*	*	*	*	*	*	*	*	*	*
Male											
All ages, age-adjusted[4]	10.4	18.5	27.3	19.0	9.6	7.6	8.2	7.9	6.2	5.9	5.4
All ages, crude	10.2	18.5	27.6	19.2	9.7	7.6	8.2	7.9	6.3	5.9	5.4
Under 1 year	2.2	2.4	1.7	1.1	*	*	*	*	*	*	*
1–4 years	0.7	0.8	1.2	0.9	0.3	*	*	*	*	*	*
5–14 years	0.2	0.3	0.5	0.5	0.3	0.1	0.2	0.1	*	*	*
15–24 years	2.2	2.2	2.0	1.3	0.8	0.5	0.5	0.5	0.4	0.6	0.4
25–34 years	20.7	34.5	45.5	30.2	14.4	10.0	9.5	8.0	4.0	3.5	3.2
35–44 years	26.3	50.2	75.5	51.7	25.4	20.0	21.0	19.8	14.3	12.9	11.6
45–54 years	15.5	29.1	46.2	33.1	17.1	14.8	17.5	17.8	16.4	15.3	14.0
55–64 years	6.8	12.0	19.7	14.7	8.3	7.2	8.3	8.7	8.8	8.9	8.5
65–74 years	2.4	3.7	6.4	5.0	3.4	2.9	3.8	3.8	4.1	4.2	4.2
75–84 years	1.2	1.1	1.3	1.5	1.0	0.9	1.0	1.3	1.4	1.6	1.6
85 years and over	*	*	*	*	*	*	*	*	*	*	*
Female											
All ages, age-adjusted[4]	1.1	2.2	5.3	4.2	2.6	2.2	2.5	2.5	2.3	2.2	2.1
All ages, crude	1.1	2.2	5.3	4.3	2.6	2.2	2.5	2.5	2.2	2.2	2.1
Under 1 year	2.5	3.0	1.2	*	*	*	*	*	*	*	*
1–4 years	0.7	0.8	1.5	1.0	0.4	*	*	*	*	*	*
5–14 years	*	0.2	0.5	0.4	0.2	0.2	0.2	0.1	*	*	*
15–24 years	0.3	0.7	1.4	0.9	0.7	0.5	0.5	0.4	0.3	0.4	0.3
25–34 years	2.8	4.9	10.9	8.2	4.9	4.2	4.1	4.2	2.6	2.3	2.2
35–44 years	2.1	5.2	13.3	11.2	6.7	5.7	6.7	6.5	5.6	5.4	4.9
45–54 years	0.8	1.9	6.6	5.6	3.7	3.1	4.1	4.4	5.1	5.1	5.1
55–64 years	0.5	1.1	2.8	2.5	1.6	1.6	1.6	1.8	2.0	2.3	2.2
65–74 years	0.5	0.8	1.4	0.8	0.5	0.6	0.8	0.8	0.9	1.1	0.8
75–84 years	0.5	0.4	0.3	0.3	0.4	0.3	0.3	0.3	0.4	0.3	0.3
85 years and over	*	*	*	*	*	*	*	*	*	*	*
All ages, age-adjusted[4]											
White male	8.7	15.7	20.4	13.1	5.9	4.5	4.9	4.6	3.6	3.4	3.1
Black or African American male	26.2	46.3	89.0	70.3	40.9	33.2	36.1	35.1	28.2	26.3	24.5
American Indian or Alaska Native male	*	3.3	10.5	6.4	3.3	3.5	4.2	3.5	4.0	3.3	3.6
Asian or Pacific Islander male	2.5	4.3	6.0	4.4	1.6	1.3	1.4	1.2	1.0	1.1	0.8
Hispanic or Latino male[5]	18.8	28.8	40.8	28.0	14.0	10.2	10.9	10.6	7.5	7.0	6.3
White, not Hispanic or Latino male[5]	10.7	14.1	17.9	11.2	4.8	3.7	4.0	3.8	3.0	2.8	2.5
White female	0.6	1.1	2.5	1.9	1.0	0.8	1.0	1.0	0.8	0.7	0.7
Black or African American female	4.6	10.1	24.4	20.8	13.7	12.0	13.1	13.2	12.0	12.2	11.3
American Indian or Alaska Native female	*	*	2.5	1.4	1.0	0.6	1.0	1.0	1.5	1.5	1.7
Asian or Pacific Islander female	*	*	0.6	0.5	0.2	0.3	0.2	0.2	*	*	*
Hispanic or Latina female[5]	2.1	3.8	8.8	6.3	3.3	2.8	3.0	2.9	1.9	1.9	1.8
White, not Hispanic or Latina female[5]	0.5	0.7	1.7	1.3	0.7	0.5	0.7	0.7	0.6	0.6	0.5

See footnotes at end of table.

Table 35 (page 2 of 2). Death rates for human immunodeficiency virus (HIV) disease, by sex, race, Hispanic origin, and age: United States, selected years 1987–2007

[Data are based on death certificates]

Sex, race, Hispanic origin, and age[1]	1987[2]	1990[2]	1995[2]	1996	1997	1998	1999[3]	2000[3]	2005[3]	2006[3]	2007[3]
Age 25–44 years	Deaths per 100,000 resident population										
All persons	12.7	23.2	36.3	25.4	12.9	10.1	10.5	9.8	6.8	6.2	5.6
White male	19.2	35.0	46.1	29.1	12.9	9.6	9.7	8.8	5.7	5.1	4.5
Black or African American male	60.2	102.0	179.4	136.8	75.2	58.1	59.3	55.4	36.2	32.9	29.4
American Indian or Alaska Native male	*	7.7	28.5	16.6	9.5	7.5	9.1	5.5	6.1	5.4	5.1
Asian or Pacific Islander male	4.1	8.1	12.1	7.7	3.3	2.4	2.4	1.9	1.4	1.0	0.9
Hispanic or Latino male[5]	36.8	59.3	73.9	48.0	23.3	16.6	16.5	14.3	8.3	7.6	6.5
White, not Hispanic or Latino male[5]	23.3	31.6	41.2	25.6	10.9	8.1	8.2	7.4	4.9	4.3	3.7
White female	1.2	2.3	5.9	4.3	2.3	1.8	2.2	2.1	1.5	1.3	1.2
Black or African American female	11.6	23.6	53.6	45.7	28.6	25.5	26.6	26.7	20.7	19.9	18.6
American Indian or Alaska Native female	*	*	*	*	*	*	*	*	*	*	*
Asian or Pacific Islander female	*	*	1.2	*	*	*	*	*	*	*	*
Hispanic or Latina female[5]	4.9	8.9	17.2	12.0	6.2	4.6	5.3	4.6	2.6	2.5	2.3
White, not Hispanic or Latina female[5]	1.0	1.5	4.2	3.1	1.7	1.3	1.6	1.6	1.2	1.0	0.9
Age 45–64 years											
All persons	5.8	11.1	19.9	14.8	8.1	7.0	8.4	8.7	8.4	8.1	7.7
White male	9.9	18.6	26.0	17.3	7.9	6.6	7.8	8.1	7.3	7.2	6.4
Black or African American male	27.3	53.0	133.2	110.7	69.3	60.9	70.7	71.6	66.2	61.4	58.3
American Indian or Alaska Native male	*	*	*	*	*	*	*	*	8.9	6.4	7.6
Asian or Pacific Islander male	*	6.5	9.1	7.9	2.3	2.4	2.3	2.1	2.0	2.3	2.2
Hispanic or Latino male[5]	25.8	37.9	67.1	49.7	25.1	18.3	21.2	23.3	18.0	16.6	14.9
White, not Hispanic or Latino male[5]	12.6	16.9	22.4	14.2	6.3	5.4	6.4	6.5	6.0	5.9	5.2
White female	0.5	0.9	2.4	1.9	1.1	0.9	1.2	1.3	1.4	1.3	1.4
Black or African American female	2.6	7.5	27.0	24.3	17.5	15.4	18.6	19.6	22.0	23.4	22.1
American Indian or Alaska Native female	*	*	*	*	*	*	*	*	*	*	*
Asian or Pacific Islander female	*	*	*	*	*	*	*	*	*	*	*
Hispanic or Latina female[5]	*	3.1	12.6	9.8	5.4	4.9	5.1	5.8	4.1	3.9	4.1
White, not Hispanic or Latina female[5]	0.5	0.7	1.5	1.2	0.7	0.5	0.8	0.9	1.1	0.9	1.0

* Rates based on fewer than 20 deaths are considered unreliable and are not shown.

[1] The race groups, white, black, Asian or Pacific Islander, and American Indian or Alaska Native, include persons of Hispanic and non-Hispanic origin. Persons of Hispanic origin may be of any race. Death rates for the American Indian or Alaska Native and Asian or Pacific Islander populations are known to be underestimated. See Appendix II, Race, for a discussion of sources of bias in death rates by race and Hispanic origin.

[2] Categories for the coding and classification of human immunodeficiency virus (HIV) disease were introduced in the United States in 1987. For the period 1987–1998, underlying cause of death was coded according to the 9th Revision of the *International Classification of Diseases* (ICD). See Appendix II, Cause of death; Human immunodeficiency virus (HIV) disease; Tables IV and V.

[3] Starting with 1999 data, cause of death is coded according to ICD–10. To estimate change between 1998 and 1999, compare the 1999 rate with the comparability-modified rate for 1998. Additional years of data available in spreadsheet version of this table. Available from: http://www.cdc.gov/nchs/hus.htm; See Appendix II, Cause of death, Table V; Comparability ratio, Table VI.

[4] Age-adjusted rates are calculated using the year 2000 standard population. Prior to 2003, age-adjusted rates were calculated using standard million proportions based on rounded population numbers. Starting with 2003 data, unrounded population numbers are used to calculate age-adjusted rates. See Appendix II, Age adjustment.

[5] Prior to 1997, excludes data from states lacking an Hispanic-origin item on the death certificate. See Appendix II, Hispanic origin.

NOTES: Starting with *Health, United States, 2003*, rates for 1991–1999 were revised using intercensal population estimates based on the 2000 census. Rates for 2000 were revised based on 2000 census counts. Rates for 2001 and beyond were computed using 2000-based postcensal estimates. See Appendix I, Population Census and Population Estimates. Starting with 2003 data, some states allowed the reporting of more than one race on the death certificate. The multiple-race data for these states were bridged to the single-race categories of the 1977 Office of Management and Budget standards for comparability with other states. See Appendix II, Race. Data for additional years are available. See Appendix III.

SOURCE: CDC/NCHS, National Vital Statistics System; numerator data from annual mortality files; denominator data from national population estimates for race groups from Table 1 and unpublished Hispanic population estimates for 1987–1996 prepared by the Housing and Household Economic Statistics Division, U.S. Census Bureau; additional mortality tables are available from: http://www.cdc.gov/nchs/nvss/mortality_tables.htm; Xu JQ, Kochanek KD, Murphy SL, Tejada-Vera B. Deaths: Final data for 2007. National vital statistics reports; vol 58 no 19. Hyattsville, MD: NCHS; 2010. Available from: http://www.cdc.gov/nchs/data/nvsr/nvsr58/nvsr58_19.pdf.

Table 36. Maternal mortality for complications of pregnancy, childbirth, and the puerperium, by race, Hispanic origin, and age: United States, selected years 1950–2007

[Data are based on death certificates]

Race, Hispanic origin, and age	1950[1,2]	1960[1,2]	1970[2]	1980[2]	1990[2]	2000[3]	2005[3,4]	2006[3,4]	2007[3,4]
	Number of deaths								
All persons	2,960	1,579	803	334	343	396	623	569	548
White	1,873	936	445	193	177	240	360	313	335
Black or African American	1,041	624	342	127	153	137	231	218	179
American Indian or Alaska Native	- - -	- - -	- - -	3	4	6	5	9	10
Asian or Pacific Islander	- - -	- - -	- - -	11	9	13	27	29	24
Hispanic or Latina[5]	- - -	- - -	- - -	- - -	47	81	95	106	95
White, not Hispanic or Latina[5]	- - -	- - -	- - -	- - -	125	160	267	210	242
All persons	Deaths per 100,000 live births								
All ages, age-adjusted[6]	73.7	32.1	21.5	9.4	7.6	8.2	12.4	11.2	10.2
All ages, crude	83.3	37.1	21.5	9.2	8.2	9.8	15.1	13.3	12.7
Under 20 years	70.7	22.7	18.9	7.6	7.5	*	7.4	5.0	7.1
20–24 years	47.6	20.7	13.0	5.8	6.1	7.4	10.7	10.2	8.1
25–29 years	63.5	29.8	17.0	7.7	6.0	7.9	11.8	11.7	9.4
30–34 years	107.7	50.3	31.6	13.6	9.5	10.0	12.8	12.6	12.1
35 years and over[7]	222.0	104.3	81.9	36.3	20.7	22.7	38.0	29.3	32.3
White									
All ages, age-adjusted[6]	53.1	22.4	14.4	6.7	5.1	6.2	9.1	8.1	7.7
All ages, crude	61.1	26.0	14.3	6.6	5.4	7.5	11.1	9.5	10.0
Under 20 years	44.9	14.8	13.8	5.8	*	*	*	*	*
20–24 years	35.7	15.3	8.4	4.2	3.9	5.6	9.0	8.3	5.9
25–29 years	45.0	20.3	11.1	5.4	4.8	5.9	7.2	7.4	6.7
30–34 years	75.9	34.3	18.7	9.3	5.0	7.1	9.3	8.2	9.7
35 years and over[7]	174.1	73.9	59.3	25.5	12.6	18.0	28.9	20.5	27.5
Black or African American									
All ages, age-adjusted[6]	- - -	92.0	65.5	24.9	21.7	20.1	31.7	28.7	23.8
All ages, crude	- - -	103.6	60.9	22.4	22.4	22.0	36.5	32.7	26.5
Under 20 years	- - -	54.8	32.3	13.1	*	*	*	*	*
20–24 years	- - -	56.9	41.9	13.9	14.7	15.3	18.2	17.8	18.6
25–29 years	- - -	92.8	65.2	22.4	14.9	21.8	37.1	36.0	24.7
30–34 years	- - -	150.6	117.8	44.0	44.2	34.8	46.6	45.1	31.3
35 years and over[7]	- - -	299.5	207.5	100.6	79.7	62.8	112.8	97.0	74.0
Hispanic or Latina[5,8]									
All ages, age-adjusted[6]	- - -	- - -	- - -	- - -	7.4	9.0	8.2	8.8	7.2
All ages, crude	- - -	- - -	- - -	- - -	7.9	9.9	9.6	10.2	8.9
White, not Hispanic or Latina[5]									
All ages, age-adjusted[6]	- - -	- - -	- - -	- - -	4.4	5.5	9.6	8.0	8.1
All ages, crude	- - -	- - -	- - -	- - -	4.8	6.8	11.7	9.1	10.5

- - - Data not available.
– Quantity zero.
* Rates based on fewer than 20 deaths are considered unreliable and are not shown.
[1]Includes deaths of persons who were not residents of the 50 states and the District of Columbia (D.C.).
[2]Underlying cause of death was coded according to the 6th Revision of the *International Classification of Diseases* (ICD) in 1950, 7th Revision in 1960, 8th Revision in 1970, and 9th Revision in 1980–1998. See Appendix II, Cause of death; Tables IV and V.
[3]Starting with 1999 data, cause of death is coded according to ICD–10. Major changes in the classification and coding of maternal deaths account for an increase in the number of maternal deaths under ICD–10. See Appendix II, Cause of death, Table V; Comparability ratio, Table VI; *International Classification of Diseases* (ICD); Maternal death.
[4]In 2003, states began adopting the 2003 revision of the U.S. Standard Certificate of death that introduced a standard question format for maternal deaths. Increases are due to methodological changes in reporting and data processing. See Appendix II, Maternal death.
[5]Prior to 1997, excludes data from states lacking an Hispanic-origin item on the death certificate. See Appendix II, Hispanic origin.
[6]Rates are age-adjusted to the 1970 distribution of live births by mother's age in the United States. See Appendix II, Age adjustment; Table III.
[7]Rates computed by relating deaths of women 35 years of age and over to live births to women 35–49 years of age. See Appendix II, Rate: Death and related rates.
[8]Age-specific maternal mortality rates are not calculated because rates based on fewer than 20 deaths are considered unreliable.

NOTES: The race groups, white, black, Asian or Pacific Islander, and American Indian or Alaska Native, include persons of Hispanic and non-Hispanic origin. Persons of Hispanic origin may be of any race. For 1950 and 1960, rates were based on live births by race of child; for all other years, rates are based on live births by race of mother. Starting with 2003 data, some states allowed the reporting of more than one race on the death certificate. The multiple-race data for these states were bridged to the single-race categories of the 1977 Office of Management and Budget standards for comparability with other states. See Appendix II, Race. Rates are not calculated for American Indian or Alaska Native and Asian or Pacific Islander mothers because rates based on fewer than 20 deaths are considered unreliable. Data for additional years are available. See Appendix III.

SOURCE: CDC/NCHS, National Vital Statistics System; numerator data from annual mortality files; denominator data from annual natality files; Xu JQ, Kochanek KD, Murphy SL, Tejada-Vera B. Deaths: Final data for 2007. National vital statistics reports; vol 58 no 19. Hyattsville, MD: NCHS. 2010. Available from: http://www.cdc.gov/nchs/data/nvsr/nvsr58/nvsr58_19.pdf.

Table 37 (page 1 of 4). Death rates for motor vehicle-related injuries, by sex, race, Hispanic origin, and age: United States, selected years 1950–2007

[Data are based on death certificates]

Sex, race, Hispanic origin, and age	1950[1,2]	1960[1,2]	1970[2]	1980[2]	1990[2]	2000[3]	2006[3]	2007[3]
All persons	\multicolumn{8}{c}{Deaths per 100,000 resident population}
All ages, age-adjusted[4]	24.6	23.1	27.6	22.3	18.5	15.4	15.0	14.4
All ages, crude	23.1	21.3	26.9	23.5	18.8	15.4	15.1	14.6
Under 1 year	8.4	8.1	9.8	7.0	4.9	4.4	3.4	2.9
1–14 years	9.8	8.6	10.5	8.2	6.0	4.3	3.4	3.2
1–4 years	11.5	10.0	11.5	9.2	6.3	4.2	3.6	3.3
5–14 years	8.8	7.9	10.2	7.9	5.9	4.3	3.3	3.2
15–24 years	34.4	38.0	47.2	44.8	34.1	26.9	26.0	24.9
15–19 years	29.6	33.9	43.6	43.0	33.1	26.0	23.2	22.0
20–24 years	38.8	42.9	51.3	46.6	35.0	28.0	28.8	27.8
25–34 years	24.6	24.3	30.9	29.1	23.6	17.3	18.2	17.5
35–44 years	20.3	19.3	24.9	20.9	16.9	15.3	15.3	14.8
45–64 years	25.2	23.0	26.5	18.0	15.7	14.3	14.9	14.2
45–54 years	22.2	21.4	25.5	18.6	15.6	14.2	15.3	14.9
55–64 years	29.0	25.1	27.9	17.4	15.9	14.4	14.3	13.3
65 years and over	43.1	34.7	36.2	22.5	23.1	21.4	19.0	18.6
65–74 years	39.1	31.4	32.8	19.2	18.6	16.5	15.4	15.2
75–84 years	52.7	41.8	43.5	28.1	29.1	25.7	22.3	21.8
85 years and over	45.1	37.9	34.2	27.6	31.2	30.4	23.4	23.2
Male								
All ages, age-adjusted[4]	38.5	35.4	41.5	33.6	26.5	21.7	21.4	20.9
All ages, crude	35.4	31.8	39.7	35.3	26.7	21.3	21.4	20.9
Under 1 year	9.1	8.6	9.3	7.3	5.0	4.6	3.3	2.6
1–14 years	12.3	10.7	13.0	10.0	7.0	4.9	3.7	3.7
1–4 years	13.0	11.5	12.9	10.2	6.9	4.7	3.8	3.7
5–14 years	11.9	10.4	13.1	9.9	7.0	5.0	3.7	3.7
15–24 years	56.7	61.2	73.2	68.4	49.5	37.4	36.6	35.1
15–19 years	46.3	51.7	64.1	62.6	45.5	33.9	30.2	28.5
20–24 years	66.7	73.2	84.4	74.3	53.3	41.2	42.9	41.7
25–34 years	40.8	40.1	49.4	46.3	35.7	25.5	27.4	26.2
35–44 years	32.5	29.9	37.7	31.7	24.7	22.0	21.8	21.7
45–64 years	37.7	33.3	38.9	26.5	21.9	20.2	21.7	21.0
45–54 years	33.6	31.6	37.2	27.6	22.0	20.4	22.6	22.2
55–64 years	43.1	35.6	40.9	25.4	21.7	19.8	20.5	19.4
65 years and over	66.6	52.1	54.4	33.9	32.1	29.5	26.5	27.1
65–74 years	59.1	45.8	47.3	27.3	24.2	21.7	21.1	21.6
75–84 years	85.0	66.0	68.2	44.3	41.2	35.6	30.8	31.9
85 years and over	78.1	62.7	63.1	56.1	64.5	57.5	41.0	39.8
Female								
All ages, age-adjusted[4]	11.5	11.7	14.9	11.8	11.0	9.5	8.8	8.2
All ages, crude	10.9	11.0	14.7	12.3	11.3	9.7	9.0	8.4
Under 1 year	7.6	7.5	10.4	6.7	4.9	4.2	3.5	3.2
1–14 years	7.2	6.3	7.9	6.3	4.9	3.7	3.1	2.8
1–4 years	10.0	8.4	10.0	8.1	5.6	3.8	3.4	3.0
5–14 years	5.7	5.4	7.2	5.7	4.7	3.6	2.9	2.7
15–24 years	12.6	15.1	21.6	20.8	17.9	15.9	14.7	14.1
15–19 years	12.9	16.0	22.7	22.8	20.0	17.5	15.7	15.2
20–24 years	12.2	14.0	20.4	18.9	16.0	14.2	13.7	12.9
25–34 years	9.3	9.2	13.0	12.2	11.5	8.8	8.7	8.4
35–44 years	8.5	9.1	12.9	10.4	9.2	8.8	8.8	7.7
45–64 years	12.6	13.1	15.3	10.3	10.1	8.7	8.3	7.7
45–54 years	10.9	11.6	14.5	10.2	9.6	8.2	8.2	7.8
55–64 years	14.9	15.2	16.2	10.5	10.8	9.5	8.5	7.6
65 years and over	21.9	20.3	23.1	15.0	17.2	15.8	13.5	12.5
65–74 years	20.6	19.0	21.6	13.0	14.1	12.3	10.6	9.7
75–84 years	25.2	23.0	27.2	18.5	21.9	19.2	16.5	14.9
85 years and over	22.1	22.0	18.0	15.2	18.3	19.3	15.2	15.2
White male[5]								
All ages, age-adjusted[4]	37.9	34.8	40.4	33.8	26.3	21.8	21.8	21.3
All ages, crude	35.1	31.5	39.1	35.9	26.7	21.6	22.0	21.5
Under 1 year	9.1	8.8	9.1	7.0	4.8	4.2	3.2	2.7
1–14 years	12.4	10.6	12.5	9.8	6.6	4.8	3.5	3.7
15–24 years	58.3	62.7	75.2	73.8	52.5	39.6	39.2	37.4
25–34 years	39.1	38.6	47.0	46.6	35.4	25.1	27.6	26.5
35–44 years	30.9	28.4	35.2	30.7	23.7	21.8	22.2	21.8
45–64 years	36.2	31.7	36.5	25.2	20.6	19.7	21.6	21.1
65 years and over	67.1	52.1	54.2	32.7	31.4	29.4	26.8	27.2

See footnotes at end of table.

Table 37 (page 2 of 4). **Death rates for motor vehicle-related injuries, by sex, race, Hispanic origin, and age: United States, selected years 1950–2007**

[Data are based on death certificates]

Sex, race, Hispanic origin, and age	1950[1,2]	1960[1,2]	1970[2]	1980[2]	1990[2]	2000[3]	2006[3]	2007[3]
Black or African American male[5]			Deaths per 100,000 resident population					
All ages, age-adjusted[4]	34.8	39.6	51.0	34.2	29.9	24.4	22.6	22.5
All ages, crude	37.2	33.1	44.3	31.1	28.1	22.5	21.5	21.2
Under 1 year	---	*	10.6	7.8	*	6.7	*	*
1–14 years[6]	10.4	11.2	16.3	11.4	8.9	5.5	4.8	4.1
15–24 years	42.5	46.4	58.1	34.9	36.1	30.2	27.2	27.3
25–34 years	54.4	51.0	70.4	44.9	39.5	32.6	33.0	30.6
35–44 years	46.7	43.6	59.5	41.2	33.5	27.2	25.3	27.6
45–64 years	54.6	47.8	61.7	39.5	33.3	27.1	26.2	25.1
65 years and over	52.6	48.2	53.4	42.4	36.3	32.1	26.4	27.8
American Indian or Alaska Native male[5]								
All ages, age-adjusted[4]	---	---	---	78.9	48.3	35.8	36.8	32.0
All ages, crude	---	---	---	74.6	47.6	33.6	37.1	32.4
1–14 years	---	---	---	15.1	11.6	7.8	5.8	6.0
15–24 years	---	---	---	126.1	75.2	56.8	56.2	48.2
25–34 years	---	---	---	107.0	78.2	49.8	49.7	48.2
35–44 years	---	---	---	82.8	57.0	36.3	38.9	37.2
45–64 years	---	---	---	77.4	45.9	32.0	45.1	30.8
65 years and over	---	---	---	97.0	43.0	48.5	35.5	36.5
Asian or Pacific Islander male[5]								
All ages, age-adjusted[4]	---	---	---	19.0	17.9	10.6	9.5	9.4
All ages, crude	---	---	---	17.1	15.8	9.8	8.8	8.6
1–14 years	---	---	---	8.2	6.3	2.5	2.7	1.9
15–24 years	---	---	---	27.2	25.7	17.0	16.8	18.4
25–34 years	---	---	---	18.8	17.0	10.4	8.5	7.3
35–44 years	---	---	---	13.1	12.2	6.9	5.8	5.9
45–64 years	---	---	---	13.7	15.1	10.1	8.6	7.7
65 years and over	---	---	---	37.3	33.6	21.1	19.3	20.7
Hispanic or Latino male[5,7]								
All ages, age-adjusted[4]	---	---	---	---	29.5	21.3	21.2	19.3
All ages, crude	---	---	---	---	29.2	20.1	20.7	18.7
1–14 years	---	---	---	---	7.2	4.4	4.4	4.1
15–24 years	---	---	---	---	48.2	34.7	41.1	36.3
25–34 years	---	---	---	---	41.0	24.9	25.6	24.3
35–44 years	---	---	---	---	28.0	21.6	20.6	17.8
45–64 years	---	---	---	---	28.9	21.7	21.4	18.6
65 years and over	---	---	---	---	35.3	28.9	23.7	24.4
White, not Hispanic or Latino male[7]								
All ages, age-adjusted[4]	---	---	---	---	25.7	21.7	21.6	21.4
All ages, crude	---	---	---	---	26.0	21.5	22.0	21.8
1–14 years	---	---	---	---	6.4	4.9	3.2	3.5
15–24 years	---	---	---	---	52.3	40.3	38.1	37.2
25–34 years	---	---	---	---	34.0	24.7	27.8	26.8
35–44 years	---	---	---	---	23.1	21.6	22.2	22.5
45–64 years	---	---	---	---	19.8	19.3	21.4	21.2
65 years and over	---	---	---	---	31.1	29.3	26.9	27.3
White female[5]								
All ages, age-adjusted[4]	11.4	11.7	14.9	12.2	11.2	9.8	9.1	8.5
All ages, crude	10.9	11.2	14.8	12.8	11.6	10.0	9.4	8.8
Under 1 year	7.8	7.5	10.2	7.1	4.7	3.5	3.0	2.8
1–14 years	7.2	6.2	7.5	6.2	4.8	3.7	3.0	2.7
15–24 years	12.6	15.6	22.7	23.0	19.5	17.1	15.9	15.1
25–34 years	9.0	9.0	12.7	12.2	11.6	8.9	8.9	8.8
35–44 years	8.1	8.9	12.3	10.6	9.2	8.9	9.1	8.0
45–64 years	12.7	13.1	15.1	10.4	9.9	8.7	8.3	7.8
65 years and over	22.2	20.8	23.7	15.3	17.4	16.2	13.9	12.9

See footnotes at end of table.

Table 37 (page 3 of 4). **Death rates for motor vehicle-related injuries, by sex, race, Hispanic origin, and age: United States, selected years 1950–2007**

[Data are based on death certificates]

Sex, race, Hispanic origin, and age	1950[1,2]	1960[1,2]	1970[2]	1980[2]	1990[2]	2000[3]	2006[3]	2007[3]
Black or African American female[5]				Deaths per 100,000 resident population				
All ages, age-adjusted[4]	9.3	10.4	14.1	8.5	9.6	8.4	7.8	7.0
All ages, crude	10.2	9.7	13.4	8.3	9.4	8.2	7.7	7.0
Under 1 year	- - -	8.1	11.9	*	7.0	*	*	*
1–14 years[6]	7.2	6.9	10.2	6.3	5.3	3.9	3.4	3.3
15–24 years	11.6	9.9	13.4	8.0	9.9	11.7	10.0	9.8
25–34 years	10.8	9.8	13.3	10.6	11.1	9.4	8.7	7.5
35–44 years	11.1	11.0	16.1	8.3	9.4	8.2	8.1	7.1
45–64 years	11.8	12.7	16.7	9.2	10.7	9.0	8.9	7.6
65 years and over	14.3	13.2	15.7	9.5	13.5	10.4	9.4	8.7
American Indian or Alaska Native female[5]								
All ages, age-adjusted[4]	- - -	- - -	- - -	32.0	17.5	19.5	16.9	15.6
All ages, crude	- - -	- - -	- - -	32.0	17.3	18.6	17.1	15.9
1–14 years	- - -	- - -	- - -	15.0	8.1	6.5	*	*
15–24 years	- - -	- - -	- - -	42.3	31.4	30.3	27.7	24.7
25–34 years	- - -	- - -	- - -	52.5	18.8	22.3	21.8	22.5
35–44 years	- - -	- - -	- - -	38.1	18.2	22.0	20.6	22.5
45–64 years	- - -	- - -	- - -	32.6	17.6	17.8	14.5	11.8
65 years and over	- - -	- - -	- - -	*	*	24.0	16.2	*
Asian or Pacific Islander female[5]								
All ages, age-adjusted[4]	- - -	- - -	- - -	9.3	10.4	6.7	5.6	5.2
All ages, crude	- - -	- - -	- - -	8.2	9.0	5.9	5.3	4.9
1–14 years	- - -	- - -	- - -	7.4	3.6	2.3	1.8	*
15–24 years	- - -	- - -	- - -	7.4	11.4	6.0	7.3	8.0
25–34 years	- - -	- - -	- - -	7.3	7.3	4.5	3.4	3.2
35–44 years	- - -	- - -	- - -	8.6	7.5	4.9	4.1	2.7
45–64 years	- - -	- - -	- - -	8.5	11.8	6.4	6.2	5.6
65 years and over	- - -	- - -	- - -	18.6	24.3	18.5	13.3	13.2
Hispanic or Latina female[5,7]								
All ages, age-adjusted[4]	- - -	- - -	- - -	- - -	9.6	7.9	7.7	6.9
All ages, crude	- - -	- - -	- - -	- - -	8.9	7.2	7.2	6.5
1–14 years	- - -	- - -	- - -	- - -	4.8	3.9	3.2	2.8
15–24 years	- - -	- - -	- - -	- - -	11.6	10.6	11.6	10.9
25–34 years	- - -	- - -	- - -	- - -	9.4	6.5	6.8	6.8
35–44 years	- - -	- - -	- - -	- - -	8.0	7.3	7.2	6.8
45–64 years	- - -	- - -	- - -	- - -	11.4	8.3	8.0	6.8
65 years and over	- - -	- - -	- - -	- - -	14.9	13.4	11.7	10.2

See footnotes at end of table.

Table 37 (page 4 of 4). Death rates for motor vehicle-related injuries, by sex, race, Hispanic origin, and age: United States, selected years 1950–2007

[Data are based on death certificates]

Sex, race, Hispanic origin, and age	1950[1,2]	1960[1,2]	1970[2]	1980[2]	1990[2]	2000[3]	2006[3]	2007[3]
White, not Hispanic or Latina female[7]				Deaths per 100,000 resident population				
All ages, age-adjusted[4]	- - -	- - -	- - -	- - -	11.3	10.0	9.3	8.7
All ages, crude	- - -	- - -	- - -	- - -	11.7	10.3	9.7	9.1
1–14 years	- - -	- - -	- - -	- - -	4.7	3.5	2.9	2.6
15–24 years	- - -	- - -	- - -	- - -	20.4	18.4	16.7	16.0
25–34 years	- - -	- - -	- - -	- - -	11.7	9.3	9.4	9.3
35–44 years	- - -	- - -	- - -	- - -	9.3	9.0	9.3	8.2
45–64 years	- - -	- - -	- - -	- - -	9.7	8.7	8.3	7.9
65 years and over	- - -	- - -	- - -	- - -	17.5	16.3	14.0	13.0

- - - Data not available.

* Rates based on fewer than 20 deaths are considered unreliable and are not shown.

[1]Includes deaths of persons who were not residents of the 50 states and the District of Columbia (D.C.).

[2]Underlying cause of death was coded according to the 6th Revision of the *International Classification of Diseases* (ICD) in 1950, 7th Revision in 1960, 8th Revision in 1970, and 9th Revision in 1980–1998. See Appendix II, Cause of death; Tables IV and V.

[3]Starting with 1999 data, cause of death is coded according to ICD–10. See Appendix II, Cause of death, Table V; Comparability ratio, Table VI.

[4]Age-adjusted rates are calculated using the year 2000 standard population. Prior to 2003, age-adjusted rates were calculated using standard million proportions based on rounded population numbers. Starting with 2003 data, unrounded population numbers are used to calculate age-adjusted rates. See Appendix II, Age adjustment.

[5]The race groups, white, black, Asian or Pacific Islander, and American Indian or Alaska Native, include persons of Hispanic and non-Hispanic origin. Persons of Hispanic origin may be of any race. Death rates for the American Indian or Alaska Native and Asian or Pacific Islander populations are known to be underestimated. See Appendix II, Race, for a discussion of sources of bias in death rates by race and Hispanic origin.

[6]In 1950, rate is for the age group under 15 years.

[7]Prior to 1997, excludes data from states lacking an Hispanic-origin item on the death certificate. See Appendix II, Hispanic origin.

NOTES: Starting with *Health, United States, 2003*, rates for 1991–1999 were revised using intercensal population estimates based on the 2000 census. Rates for 2000 were revised based on 2000 census counts. Rates for 2001 and later years were computed using 2000-based postcensal estimates. See Appendix I, Population Census and Population Estimates. Age groups were selected to minimize the presentation of unstable age-specific death rates based on small numbers of deaths and for consistency among comparison groups. For additional injury-related statistics, see Web-based Injury Statistics Query and Reporting System, available from: http://www.cdc.gov/injury/wisqars/index.html. Starting with 2003 data, some states allowed the reporting of more than one race on the death certificate. The multiple-race data for these states were bridged to the single-race categories of the 1977 Office of Management and Budget standards for comparability with other states. See Appendix II, Race. Data for additional years are available. See Appendix III.

SOURCE: CDC/NCHS, National Vital Statistics System; Grove RD, Hetzel AM. Vital statistics rates in the United States, 1940–1960. Washington, DC: U.S. Government Printing Office, 1968; numerator data from National Vital Statistics System, annual mortality files; denominator data from national population estimates for race groups from Table 1 and unpublished Hispanic population estimates for 1985–1996 prepared by the Housing and Household Economic Statistics Division, U.S. Census Bureau; additional mortality tables are available from: http://www.cdc.gov/nchs/nvss/mortality_tables.htm; Xu JQ, Kochanek KD, Murphy SL, Tejada-Vera B. Deaths: Final data for 2007. National vital statistics reports; vol 58 no 19. Hyattsville, MD: NCHS; 2010. Available from: http://www.cdc.gov/nchs/data/nvsr/nvsr58/nvsr58_19.pdf.

Table 38 (page 1 of 4). Death rates for homicide, by sex, race, Hispanic origin, and age: United States, selected years 1950–2007

[Data are based on death certificates]

Sex, race, Hispanic origin, and age	1950[1,2]	1960[1,2]	1970[2]	1980[2]	1990[2]	2000[3]	2006[3]	2007[3]
All persons	\multicolumn{8}{c}{Deaths per 100,000 resident population}							
All ages, age-adjusted[4]	5.1	5.0	8.8	10.4	9.4	5.9	6.2	6.1
All ages, crude	5.0	4.6	8.1	10.6	9.9	6.0	6.2	6.1
Under 1 year	4.4	4.8	4.3	5.9	8.4	9.2	8.1	8.3
1–14 years	0.6	0.6	1.1	1.5	1.8	1.3	1.3	1.3
1–4 years	0.6	0.7	1.9	2.5	2.5	2.3	2.2	2.4
5–14 years	0.5	0.5	0.9	1.2	1.5	0.9	1.0	0.9
15–24 years	5.8	5.6	11.3	15.4	19.7	12.6	13.5	13.1
15–19 years	3.9	3.9	7.7	10.5	16.9	9.5	10.7	10.4
20–24 years	8.5	7.7	15.6	20.2	22.2	16.0	16.2	15.8
25–44 years	8.9	8.5	14.9	17.5	14.7	8.7	9.2	9.3
25–34 years	9.3	9.2	16.2	19.3	17.4	10.4	11.7	11.7
35–44 years	8.4	7.8	13.5	14.9	11.6	7.1	6.9	7.1
45–64 years	5.0	5.3	8.7	9.0	6.3	4.0	4.3	4.1
45–54 years	5.9	6.1	10.0	11.0	7.5	4.7	5.1	4.9
55–64 years	3.9	4.1	7.1	7.0	5.0	3.0	3.2	3.0
65 years and over	3.0	2.7	4.6	5.5	4.0	2.4	2.1	2.0
65–74 years	3.2	2.8	4.9	5.7	3.8	2.4	2.1	2.1
75–84 years	2.5	2.3	4.0	5.2	4.3	2.4	2.1	2.1
85 years and over	2.3	2.4	4.2	5.3	4.6	2.4	1.9	1.5
Male								
All ages, age-adjusted[4]	7.9	7.5	14.3	16.6	14.8	9.0	9.7	9.6
All ages, crude	7.7	6.8	13.1	17.1	15.9	9.3	10.0	9.8
Under 1 year	4.5	4.7	4.5	6.3	8.8	10.4	9.4	9.5
1–14 years	0.6	0.6	1.2	1.6	2.0	1.5	1.6	1.5
1–4 years	0.5	0.7	1.9	2.7	2.7	2.5	2.5	2.5
5–14 years	0.6	0.5	1.0	1.2	1.7	1.1	1.2	1.0
15–24 years	8.6	8.4	18.2	24.0	32.5	20.9	22.8	22.1
15–19 years	5.5	5.7	12.1	15.9	27.8	15.5	18.2	17.6
20–24 years	13.5	11.8	25.6	32.2	36.9	26.7	27.5	26.7
25–44 years	13.8	12.8	24.4	28.9	23.5	13.3	14.7	14.9
25–34 years	14.4	13.9	26.8	31.9	27.7	16.7	19.4	19.4
35–44 years	13.2	11.7	21.7	24.5	18.6	10.3	10.4	10.6
45–64 years	8.1	8.1	14.8	15.2	10.2	6.0	6.5	6.2
45–54 years	9.5	9.4	16.8	18.4	11.9	6.9	7.6	7.3
55–64 years	6.3	6.4	12.1	11.8	8.0	4.6	4.8	4.6
65 years and over	4.8	4.3	7.7	8.8	5.8	3.3	2.8	2.8
65–74 years	5.2	4.6	8.5	9.2	5.8	3.4	3.0	3.1
75–84 years	3.9	3.7	5.9	8.1	5.7	3.2	2.7	2.8
85 years and over	2.5	3.6	7.4	7.5	6.7	3.3	2.3	1.5
Female								
All ages, age-adjusted[4]	2.4	2.6	3.7	4.4	4.0	2.8	2.5	2.5
All ages, crude	2.4	2.4	3.4	4.5	4.2	2.8	2.5	2.5
Under 1 year	4.2	4.9	4.1	5.6	8.0	7.9	6.8	7.0
1–14 years	0.6	0.5	1.0	1.4	1.6	1.1	1.1	1.2
1–4 years	0.7	0.7	1.9	2.2	2.3	2.1	2.0	2.3
5–14 years	0.5	0.4	0.7	1.1	1.2	0.7	0.7	0.7
15–24 years	3.0	2.8	4.6	6.6	6.2	3.9	3.5	3.5
15–19 years	2.4	1.9	3.2	4.9	5.4	3.1	2.9	2.8
20–24 years	3.7	3.8	6.2	8.2	7.0	4.7	4.2	4.2
25–44 years	4.2	4.3	5.8	6.4	6.0	4.0	3.6	3.6
25–34 years	4.5	4.6	6.0	6.9	7.1	4.1	3.7	3.7
35–44 years	3.8	4.0	5.7	5.7	4.8	4.0	3.4	3.5
45–64 years	1.9	2.5	3.1	3.4	2.8	2.1	2.2	2.1
45–54 years	2.3	2.9	3.7	4.1	3.2	2.5	2.6	2.5
55–64 years	1.4	2.0	2.5	2.8	2.3	1.6	1.7	1.5
65 years and over	1.4	1.3	2.3	3.3	2.8	1.8	1.6	1.4
65–74 years	1.3	1.3	2.2	3.0	2.2	1.6	1.3	1.3
75–84 years	1.4	1.3	2.7	3.5	3.4	2.0	1.8	1.5
85 years and over	2.1	1.6	2.5	4.3	3.8	2.0	1.8	1.4

See footnotes at end of table.

Table 38 (page 2 of 4). Death rates for homicide, by sex, race, Hispanic origin, and age: United States, selected years 1950–2007

[Data are based on death certificates]

Sex, race, Hispanic origin, and age	1950[1,2]	1960[1,2]	1970[2]	1980[2]	1990[2]	2000[3]	2006[3]	2007[3]
White male[5]			Deaths per 100,000 resident population					
All ages, age-adjusted[4]	3.8	3.9	7.2	10.4	8.3	5.2	5.4	5.4
All ages, crude	3.6	3.6	6.6	10.7	8.8	5.2	5.4	5.4
Under 1 year	4.3	3.8	2.9	4.3	6.4	8.2	7.4	7.7
1–14 years	0.4	0.5	0.7	1.2	1.3	1.2	1.1	1.0
15–24 years	3.2	5.0	7.6	15.1	15.2	9.9	10.6	10.5
25–44 years	5.4	5.5	11.6	17.2	13.0	7.4	7.8	8.1
25–34 years	4.9	5.7	12.5	18.5	14.7	8.4	9.3	9.9
35–44 years	6.1	5.2	10.8	15.2	11.1	6.5	6.4	6.4
45–64 years	4.8	4.6	8.3	9.8	6.9	4.1	4.4	4.2
65 years and over	3.8	3.1	5.4	6.7	4.1	2.5	2.2	2.2
Black or African American male[5]								
All ages, age-adjusted[4]	47.0	42.3	78.2	69.4	63.1	35.4	37.8	37.1
All ages, crude	44.7	35.0	66.0	65.7	68.5	37.2	40.6	39.7
Under 1 year	- - -	10.3	14.3	18.6	21.4	23.3	20.7	19.2
1–14 years[6]	1.8	1.5	4.4	4.1	5.8	3.1	4.0	3.9
15–24 years	53.8	43.2	98.3	82.6	137.1	85.3	88.2	85.3
25–44 years	92.8	80.5	140.2	130.0	105.4	55.8	63.2	62.3
25–34 years	104.3	86.4	154.5	142.9	123.7	73.9	86.2	82.5
35–44 years	80.0	74.4	124.0	109.3	81.2	38.5	39.8	41.2
45–64 years	46.0	44.6	82.3	70.6	41.4	21.9	23.3	22.5
65 years and over	16.5	17.3	33.3	30.9	25.7	12.8	10.0	10.8
American Indian or Alaska Native male[5]								
All ages, age-adjusted[4]	- - -	- - -	- - -	23.3	16.7	10.7	11.9	9.2
All ages, crude	- - -	- - -	- - -	23.1	16.6	10.7	12.9	10.1
15–24 years	- - -	- - -	- - -	35.4	25.1	17.0	22.5	14.7
25–44 years	- - -	- - -	- - -	39.2	25.7	17.0	17.9	17.1
45–64 years	- - -	- - -	- - -	22.1	14.8	*	9.1	6.5
Asian or Pacific Islander male[5]								
All ages, age-adjusted[4]	- - -	- - -	- - -	9.1	7.3	4.3	4.4	3.3
All ages, crude	- - -	- - -	- - -	8.3	7.9	4.4	4.5	3.5
15–24 years	- - -	- - -	- - -	9.3	14.9	7.8	11.5	7.4
25–44 years	- - -	- - -	- - -	11.3	9.6	4.6	4.0	3.9
45–64 years	- - -	- - -	- - -	10.4	7.0	6.1	4.7	3.3
Hispanic or Latino male[5,7]								
All ages, age-adjusted[4]	- - -	- - -	- - -	- - -	27.4	11.8	11.7	11.2
All ages, crude	- - -	- - -	- - -	- - -	31.0	13.4	13.1	12.4
Under 1 year	- - -	- - -	- - -	- - -	8.7	6.6	10.1	8.3
1–14 years	- - -	- - -	- - -	- - -	3.1	1.7	1.6	1.3
15–24 years	- - -	- - -	- - -	- - -	55.4	28.5	31.0	30.0
25–44 years	- - -	- - -	- - -	- - -	46.4	17.2	16.5	16.0
25–34 years	- - -	- - -	- - -	- - -	50.9	19.9	19.7	19.9
35–44 years	- - -	- - -	- - -	- - -	39.3	13.5	12.5	11.2
45–64 years	- - -	- - -	- - -	- - -	20.5	9.1	8.3	7.7
65 years and over	- - -	- - -	- - -	- - -	9.4	4.4	3.1	3.7
White, not Hispanic or Latino male[7]								
All ages, age-adjusted[4]	- - -	- - -	- - -	- - -	5.6	3.6	3.6	3.7
All ages, crude	- - -	- - -	- - -	- - -	5.8	3.6	3.6	3.7
Under 1 year	- - -	- - -	- - -	- - -	5.4	8.3	6.5	7.2
1–14 years	- - -	- - -	- - -	- - -	0.9	1.0	0.9	0.9
15–24 years	- - -	- - -	- - -	- - -	7.5	4.7	4.7	4.9
25–44 years	- - -	- - -	- - -	- - -	8.7	5.2	5.1	5.6
25–34 years	- - -	- - -	- - -	- - -	9.3	5.2	5.5	6.2
35–44 years	- - -	- - -	- - -	- - -	8.0	5.2	4.9	5.1
45–64 years	- - -	- - -	- - -	- - -	5.7	3.6	3.9	3.7
65 years and over	- - -	- - -	- - -	- - -	3.7	2.3	2.1	2.0

See footnotes at end of table.

Table 38 (page 3 of 4). Death rates for homicide, by sex, race, Hispanic origin, and age: United States, selected years 1950–2007

[Data are based on death certificates]

Sex, race, Hispanic origin, and age	1950[1,2]	1960[1,2]	1970[2]	1980[2]	1990[2]	2000[3]	2006[3]	2007[3]
White female[5]				Deaths per 100,000 resident population				
All ages, age-adjusted[4]	1.4	1.5	2.3	3.2	2.7	2.1	1.9	2.0
All ages, crude	1.4	1.4	2.1	3.2	2.8	2.1	1.9	1.9
Under 1 year	3.9	3.5	2.9	4.3	5.1	5.0	6.3	6.1
1–14 years	0.4	0.4	0.7	1.1	1.0	0.8	0.8	0.9
15–24 years	1.3	1.5	2.7	4.7	4.0	2.7	2.4	2.5
25–44 years	2.0	2.1	3.3	4.2	3.8	2.9	2.5	2.7
45–64 years	1.5	1.7	2.1	2.6	2.3	1.8	1.8	1.7
65 years and over	1.2	1.2	1.9	2.9	2.2	1.6	1.5	1.3
Black or African American female[5]								
All ages, age-adjusted[4]	11.1	11.4	14.7	13.2	12.5	7.1	6.4	6.1
All ages, crude	11.5	10.4	13.2	13.5	13.4	7.2	6.6	6.2
Under 1 year	- - -	13.8	10.7	12.8	22.8	22.2	11.1	11.4
1–14 years[6]	1.8	1.2	3.1	3.3	4.7	2.7	2.5	2.7
15–24 years	16.5	11.9	17.7	18.4	18.9	10.7	9.5	8.9
25–44 years	22.5	22.7	25.3	22.6	21.0	11.0	10.1	9.1
45–64 years	6.8	10.3	13.4	10.8	6.5	4.5	5.2	4.9
65 years and over	3.6	3.0	7.4	8.0	9.4	3.5	2.5	2.6
American Indian or Alaska Native female[5]								
All ages, age-adjusted[4]	- - -	- - -	- - -	8.1	4.6	3.0	2.9	3.6
All ages, crude	- - -	- - -	- - -	7.7	4.8	2.9	3.0	3.5
15–24 years	- - -	- - -	- - -	*	*	*	*	*
25–44 years	- - -	- - -	- - -	13.7	6.9	5.9	6.0	5.1
45–64 years	- - -	- - -	- - -	*	*	*	*	*
Asian or Pacific Islander female[5]								
All ages, age-adjusted[4]	- - -	- - -	- - -	3.1	2.8	1.7	1.4	1.3
All ages, crude	- - -	- - -	- - -	3.1	2.8	1.7	1.4	1.4
15–24 years	- - -	- - -	- - -	*	*	*	*	*
25–44 years	- - -	- - -	- - -	4.6	3.8	2.2	1.6	1.9
45–64 years	- - -	- - -	- - -	*	*	2.0	2.0	1.5
Hispanic or Latina female[5,7]								
All ages, age-adjusted[4]	- - -	- - -	- - -	- - -	4.3	2.8	2.3	2.3
All ages, crude	- - -	- - -	- - -	- - -	4.7	2.8	2.4	2.5
Under 1 year	- - -	- - -	- - -	- - -	*	7.4	6.5	7.3
1–14 years	- - -	- - -	- - -	- - -	1.9	1.0	1.0	1.3
15–24 years	- - -	- - -	- - -	- - -	8.1	3.7	3.8	3.5
25–44 years	- - -	- - -	- - -	- - -	6.1	3.7	3.1	3.3
45–64 years	- - -	- - -	- - -	- - -	3.3	2.9	1.9	1.7
65 years and over	- - -	- - -	- - -	- - -	*	2.4	*	*
White, not Hispanic or Latina female[7]								
All ages, age-adjusted[4]	- - -	- - -	- - -	- - -	2.5	1.9	1.8	1.8
All ages, crude	- - -	- - -	- - -	- - -	2.5	1.9	1.8	1.8
Under 1 year	- - -	- - -	- - -	- - -	4.4	4.1	6.2	5.7
1–14 years	- - -	- - -	- - -	- - -	0.8	0.8	0.8	0.8
15–24 years	- - -	- - -	- - -	- - -	3.3	2.3	2.0	2.2
25–44 years	- - -	- - -	- - -	- - -	3.5	2.7	2.3	2.5
45–64 years	- - -	- - -	- - -	- - -	2.2	1.6	1.8	1.7
65 years and over	- - -	- - -	- - -	- - -	2.2	1.6	1.5	1.3

See footnotes at end of table.

Table 38 (page 4 of 4). Death rates for homicide, by sex, race, Hispanic origin, and age: United States, selected years 1950–2007

[Data are based on death certificates]

- - - Data not available.

* Rates based on fewer than 20 deaths are considered unreliable and are not shown.

[1]Includes deaths of persons who were not residents of the 50 states and the District of Columbia (D.C.).

[2]Underlying cause of death was coded according to the 6th Revision of the *International Classification of Diseases* (ICD) in 1950, 7th Revision in 1960, 8th Revision in 1970, and 9th Revision in 1980–1998. See Appendix II, Cause of death; Tables IV and V.

[3]Starting with 1999 data, cause of death is coded according to ICD–10. See Appendix II, Cause of death, Table V; Comparability ratio, Table VI.

[4]Age-adjusted rates are calculated using the year 2000 standard population. Prior to 2003, age-adjusted rates were calculated using standard million proportions based on rounded population numbers. Starting with 2003 data, unrounded population numbers are used to calculate age-adjusted rates. See Appendix II, Age adjustment.

[5]The race groups, white, black, Asian or Pacific Islander, and American Indian or Alaska Native, include persons of Hispanic and non-Hispanic origin. Persons of Hispanic origin may be of any race. Death rates for the American Indian or Alaska Native and Asian or Pacific Islander populations are known to be underestimated. See Appendix II, Race, for a discussion of sources of bias in death rates by race and Hispanic origin.

[6]In 1950, rate is for the age group under 15 years.

[7]Prior to 1997, excludes data from states lacking an Hispanic-origin item on the death certificate. See Appendix II, Hispanic origin.

NOTES: Starting with *Health, United States, 2003*, rates for 1991–1999 were revised using intercensal population estimates based on the 2000 census. Rates for 2000 were revised based on 2000 census counts. Rates for 2001 and later years were computed using 2000-based postcensal estimates. See Appendix I, Population Census and Population Estimates. Figures for 2001 include September 11-related deaths for which death certificates were filed as of October 24, 2002. For the period 1980–1998, homicide was coded using ICD–9 codes that are most nearly comparable with homicide codes in the 113 cause list for ICD–10. See Appendix II, Cause of death; Table V for terrorism-related ICD–10 codes. Age groups were selected to minimize the presentation of unstable age-specific death rates based on small numbers of deaths and for consistency among comparison groups. For additional injury-related statistics, see Web-based Injury Statistics Query and Reporting System, available from: http://www.cdc.gov/injury/wisqars/index.html. Starting with 2003 data, some states allowed the reporting of more than one race on the death certificate. The multiple-race data for these states were bridged to the single-race categories of the 1977 Office of Management and Budget standards for comparability with other states. See Appendix II, Race. Data for additional years are available. See Appendix III.

SOURCE: CDC/NCHS, National Vital Statistics System; Grove RD, Hetzel AM. Vital statistics rates in the United States, 1940–1960. Washington, DC: U.S. Government Printing Office, 1968; numerator data from National Vital Statistics System, annual mortality files; denominator data from national population estimates for race groups from Table 1 and unpublished Hispanic population estimates for 1985–1996 prepared by the Housing and Household Economic Statistics Division, U.S. Census Bureau; additional mortality tables are available from: http://www.cdc.gov/nchs/nvss/mortality_tables.htm; Xu JQ, Kochanek KD, Murphy SL, Tejada-Vera B. Deaths: Final data for 2007. National vital statistics reports; vol 58 no 19. Hyattsville, MD: NCHS; 2010. Available from: http://www.cdc.gov/nchs/data/nvsr58/nvsr58_19.pdf.

Table 39 (page 1 of 3). Death rates for suicide, by sex, race, Hispanic origin, and age: United States, selected years 1950–2007

[Data are based on death certificates]

Sex, race, Hispanic origin, and age	1950[1,2]	1960[1,2]	1970[2]	1980[2]	1990[2]	2000[3]	2006[3]	2007[3]
All persons	\multicolumn{8}{c}{Deaths per 100,000 resident population}							
All ages, age-adjusted[4]	13.2	12.5	13.1	12.2	12.5	10.4	10.9	11.3
All ages, crude	11.4	10.6	11.6	11.9	12.4	10.4	11.1	11.5
Under 1 year	. . .	. . .	. . .	. . .	. . .	. . .	. . .	. . .
1–4 years	. . .	. . .	. . .	. . .	. . .	. . .	. . .	. . .
5–14 years	0.2	0.3	0.3	0.4	0.8	0.7	0.5	0.5
15–24 years	4.5	5.2	8.8	12.3	13.2	10.2	9.9	9.7
15–19 years	2.7	3.6	5.9	8.5	11.1	8.0	7.3	6.9
20–24 years	6.2	7.1	12.2	16.1	15.1	12.5	12.5	12.6
25–44 years	11.6	12.2	15.4	15.6	15.2	13.4	13.8	14.3
25–34 years	9.1	10.0	14.1	16.0	15.2	12.0	12.3	13.0
35–44 years	14.3	14.2	16.9	15.4	15.3	14.5	15.1	15.6
45–64 years	23.5	22.0	20.6	15.9	15.3	13.5	16.0	16.8
45–54 years	20.9	20.7	20.0	15.9	14.8	14.4	17.2	17.7
55–64 years	26.8	23.7	21.4	15.9	16.0	12.1	14.5	15.5
65 years and over	30.0	24.5	20.8	17.6	20.5	15.2	14.2	14.3
65–74 years	29.6	23.0	20.8	16.9	17.9	12.5	12.6	12.6
75–84 years	31.1	27.9	21.2	19.1	24.9	17.6	15.9	16.3
85 years and over	28.8	26.0	19.0	19.2	22.2	19.6	15.9	15.6
Male								
All ages, age-adjusted[4]	21.2	20.0	19.8	19.9	21.5	17.7	18.0	18.4
All ages, crude	17.8	16.5	16.8	18.6	20.4	17.1	17.8	18.3
Under 1 year	. . .	. . .	. . .	. . .	. . .	. . .	. . .	. . .
1–4 years	. . .	. . .	. . .	. . .	. . .	. . .	. . .	. . .
5–14 years	0.3	0.4	0.5	0.6	1.1	1.2	0.7	0.6
15–24 years	6.5	8.2	13.5	20.2	22.0	17.1	16.2	15.9
15–19 years	3.5	5.6	8.8	13.8	18.1	13.0	11.5	11.1
20–24 years	9.3	11.5	19.3	26.8	25.7	21.4	20.8	20.8
25–44 years	17.2	17.9	20.9	24.0	24.4	21.3	21.5	22.3
25–34 years	13.4	14.7	19.8	25.0	24.8	19.6	19.7	20.7
35–44 years	21.3	21.0	22.1	22.5	23.9	22.8	23.2	23.8
45–64 years	37.1	34.4	30.0	23.7	24.3	21.3	24.8	25.8
45–54 years	32.0	31.6	27.9	22.9	23.2	22.4	26.2	27.0
55–64 years	43.6	38.1	32.7	24.5	25.7	19.4	22.7	24.3
65 years and over	52.8	44.0	38.4	35.0	41.6	31.1	28.5	28.6
65–74 years	50.5	39.6	36.0	30.4	32.2	22.7	22.7	22.5
75–84 years	58.3	52.5	42.8	42.3	56.1	38.6	33.3	34.3
85 years and over	58.3	57.4	42.4	50.6	65.9	57.5	43.2	41.8
Female								
All ages, age-adjusted[4]	5.6	5.6	7.4	5.7	4.8	4.0	4.5	4.7
All ages, crude	5.1	4.9	6.6	5.5	4.8	4.0	4.6	4.8
Under 1 year	. . .	. . .	. . .	. . .	. . .	. . .	. . .	. . .
1–4 years	. . .	. . .	. . .	. . .	. . .	. . .	. . .	. . .
5–14 years	0.1	0.1	0.2	0.2	0.4	0.3	0.3	0.3
15–24 years	2.6	2.2	4.2	4.3	3.9	3.0	3.2	3.2
15–19 years	1.8	1.6	2.9	3.0	3.7	2.7	2.8	2.5
20–24 years	3.3	2.9	5.7	5.5	4.1	3.2	3.6	3.9
25–44 years	6.2	6.6	10.2	7.7	6.2	5.4	5.9	6.2
25–34 years	4.9	5.5	8.6	7.1	5.6	4.3	4.7	5.0
35–44 years	7.5	7.7	11.9	8.5	6.8	6.4	7.0	7.3
45–64 years	9.9	10.2	12.0	8.9	7.1	6.2	7.7	8.2
45–54 years	9.9	10.2	12.6	9.4	6.9	6.7	8.4	8.8
55–64 years	9.9	10.2	11.4	8.4	7.3	5.4	6.8	7.3
65 years and over	9.4	8.4	8.1	6.1	6.4	4.0	3.9	3.9
65–74 years	10.1	8.4	9.0	6.5	6.7	4.0	4.1	4.2
75–84 years	8.1	8.9	7.0	5.5	6.3	4.0	4.0	3.8
85 years and over	8.2	6.0	5.9	5.5	5.4	4.2	3.1	3.1
White male[5]								
All ages, age-adjusted[4]	22.3	21.1	20.8	20.9	22.8	19.1	19.6	20.2
All ages, crude	19.0	17.6	18.0	19.9	22.0	18.8	19.8	20.5
15–24 years	6.6	8.6	13.9	21.4	23.2	17.9	17.1	16.9
25–44 years	17.9	18.5	21.5	24.6	25.4	22.9	23.5	24.5
45–64 years	39.3	36.5	31.9	25.0	26.0	23.2	27.4	28.8
65 years and over	55.8	46.7	41.1	37.2	44.2	33.3	30.9	31.1
65–74 years	53.2	42.0	38.7	32.5	34.2	24.3	24.7	24.7
75–84 years	61.9	55.7	45.5	45.5	60.2	41.1	36.0	36.9
85 years and over	61.9	61.3	45.8	52.8	70.3	61.6	46.1	45.4

See footnotes at end of table.

Table 39 (page 2 of 3). Death rates for suicide, by sex, race, Hispanic origin, and age: United States, selected years 1950–2007

[Data are based on death certificates]

Sex, race, Hispanic origin, and age	1950[1,2]	1960[1,2]	1970[2]	1980[2]	1990[2]	2000[3]	2006[3]	2007[3]
Black or African American male[5]			Deaths per 100,000 resident population					
All ages, age-adjusted[4]	7.5	8.4	10.0	11.4	12.8	10.0	9.4	8.8
All ages, crude	6.3	6.4	8.0	10.3	12.0	9.4	8.8	8.4
15–24 years	4.9	4.1	10.5	12.3	15.1	14.2	10.6	10.3
25–44 years	9.8	12.6	16.1	19.2	19.6	14.3	14.3	13.7
45–64 years	12.7	13.0	12.4	11.8	13.1	9.9	9.9	9.4
65 years and over	9.0	9.9	8.7	11.4	14.9	11.5	10.4	8.7
65–74 years	10.0	11.3	8.7	11.1	14.7	11.1	8.8	8.3
75–84 years[6]	*	*	*	10.5	14.4	12.1	11.6	11.2
85 years and over	- - -	*	*	*	*	*	*	*
American Indian or Alaska Native male[5]								
All ages, age-adjusted[4]	- - -	- - -	- - -	19.3	20.1	16.0	18.3	18.1
All ages, crude	- - -	- - -	- - -	20.9	20.9	15.9	19.3	19.2
15–24 years	- - -	- - -	- - -	45.3	49.1	26.2	35.9	32.3
25–44 years	- - -	- - -	- - -	31.2	27.8	24.5	26.0	28.6
45–64 years	- - -	- - -	- - -	*	*	15.4	18.0	15.9
65 years and over	- - -	- - -	- - -	*	*	*	*	*
Asian or Pacific Islander male[5]								
All ages, age-adjusted[4]	- - -	- - -	- - -	10.7	9.6	8.6	7.9	9.0
All ages, crude	- - -	- - -	- - -	8.8	8.7	7.9	8.0	8.7
15–24 years	- - -	- - -	- - -	10.8	13.5	9.1	12.0	13.4
25–44 years	- - -	- - -	- - -	11.0	10.6	9.9	9.2	9.8
45–64 years	- - -	- - -	- - -	13.0	9.7	9.7	9.7	10.7
65 years and over	- - -	- - -	- - -	18.6	16.8	15.4	10.6	12.9
Hispanic or Latino male[5,7]								
All ages, age-adjusted[4]	- - -	- - -	- - -	- - -	13.7	10.3	8.8	10.1
All ages, crude	- - -	- - -	- - -	- - -	11.4	8.4	7.9	8.8
15–24 years	- - -	- - -	- - -	- - -	14.7	10.9	11.6	11.5
25–44 years	- - -	- - -	- - -	- - -	16.2	11.2	10.8	11.9
45–64 years	- - -	- - -	- - -	- - -	16.1	12.0	10.3	12.9
65 years and over	- - -	- - -	- - -	- - -	23.4	19.5	12.1	15.9
White, not Hispanic or Latino male[7]								
All ages, age-adjusted[4]	- - -	- - -	- - -	- - -	23.5	20.2	21.4	21.9
All ages, crude	- - -	- - -	- - -	- - -	23.1	20.4	22.3	22.9
15–24 years	- - -	- - -	- - -	- - -	24.4	19.5	18.5	18.2
25–44 years	- - -	- - -	- - -	- - -	26.4	25.1	26.9	28.0
45–64 years	- - -	- - -	- - -	- - -	26.8	24.0	29.3	30.6
65 years and over	- - -	- - -	- - -	- - -	45.4	33.9	32.3	32.2
White female[5]								
All ages, age-adjusted[4]	6.0	5.9	7.9	6.1	5.2	4.3	5.1	5.2
All ages, crude	5.5	5.3	7.1	5.9	5.3	4.4	5.2	5.4
15–24 years	2.7	2.3	4.2	4.6	4.2	3.1	3.4	3.4
25–44 years	6.6	7.0	11.0	8.1	6.6	6.0	6.8	7.0
45–64 years	10.6	10.9	13.0	9.6	7.7	6.9	8.8	9.3
65 years and over	9.9	8.8	8.5	6.4	6.8	4.3	4.1	4.2
Black or African American female[5]								
All ages, age-adjusted[4]	1.8	2.0	2.9	2.4	2.4	1.8	1.4	1.7
All ages, crude	1.5	1.6	2.6	2.2	2.3	1.7	1.4	1.7
15–24 years	1.8	*	3.8	2.3	2.3	2.2	1.8	1.6
25–44 years	2.3	3.0	4.8	4.3	3.8	2.6	2.0	2.7
45–64 years	2.7	3.1	2.9	2.5	2.9	2.1	1.9	2.3
65 years and over	*	*	2.6	*	1.9	1.3	*	*

See footnotes at end of table.

[Data are based on death certificates]

Sex, race, Hispanic origin, and age	1950[1,2]	1960[1,2]	1970[2]	1980[2]	1990[2]	2000[3]	2006[3]	2007[3]
American Indian or Alaska Native female[5]				Deaths per 100,000 resident population				
All ages, age-adjusted[4]	- - -	- - -	- - -	4.7	3.6	3.8	5.1	4.9
All ages, crude	- - -	- - -	- - -	4.7	3.7	4.0	5.4	5.1
15–24 years	- - -	- - -	- - -	*	*	*	8.9	7.8
25–44 years	- - -	- - -	- - -	10.7	*	7.2	8.0	6.9
45–64 years	- - -	- - -	- - -	*	*	*	*	*
65 years and over	- - -	- - -	- - -	*	*	*	*	*
Asian or Pacific Islander female[5]								
All ages, age-adjusted[4]	- - -	- - -	- - -	5.5	4.1	2.8	3.4	3.5
All ages, crude	- - -	- - -	- - -	4.7	3.4	2.7	3.3	3.6
15–24 years	- - -	- - -	- - -	*	3.9	2.7	4.0	3.8
25–44 years	- - -	- - -	- - -	5.4	3.8	3.3	3.3	4.6
45–64 years	- - -	- - -	- - -	7.9	5.0	3.2	4.2	4.0
65 years and over	- - -	- - -	- - -	*	8.5	5.2	6.9	5.2
Hispanic or Latina female[5,7]								
All ages, age-adjusted[4]	- - -	- - -	- - -	- - -	2.3	1.7	1.8	1.9
All ages, crude	- - -	- - -	- - -	- - -	2.2	1.5	1.7	1.8
15–24 years	- - -	- - -	- - -	- - -	3.1	2.0	2.6	2.2
25–44 years	- - -	- - -	- - -	- - -	3.1	2.1	2.3	2.7
45–64 years	- - -	- - -	- - -	- - -	2.5	2.5	2.4	2.8
65 years and over	- - -	- - -	- - -	- - -	*	*	1.7	*
White, not Hispanic or Latina female[7]								
All ages, age-adjusted[4]	- - -	- - -	- - -	- - -	5.4	4.7	5.6	5.7
All ages, crude	- - -	- - -	- - -	- - -	5.6	4.9	5.9	6.1
15–24 years	- - -	- - -	- - -	- - -	4.3	3.3	3.5	3.7
25–44 years	- - -	- - -	- - -	- - -	7.0	6.7	7.8	8.0
45–64 years	- - -	- - -	- - -	- - -	8.0	7.3	9.5	10.0
65 years and over	- - -	- - -	- - -	- - -	7.0	4.4	4.3	4.4

. . . Category not applicable.
* Rates based on fewer than 20 deaths are considered unreliable and are not shown.
- - - Data not available.
[1]Includes deaths of persons who were not residents of the 50 states and the District of Columbia (D.C.).
[2]Underlying cause of death was coded according to the 6th Revision of the International Classification of Diseases (ICD) in 1950, 7th Revision in 1960, 8th Revision in 1970, and 9th Revision in 1980–1998. See Appendix II, Cause of death; Tables IV and V.
[3]Starting with 1999 data, cause of death is coded according to ICD–10. See Appendix II, Cause of death, Table V; Comparability ratio, Table VI.
[4]Age-adjusted rates are calculated using the year 2000 standard population. Prior to 2003, age-adjusted rates were calculated using standard million proportions based on rounded population numbers. Starting with 2003 data, unrounded population numbers are used to calculate age-adjusted rates. See Appendix II, Age adjustment.
[5]The race groups, white, black, Asian or Pacific Islander, and American Indian or Alaska Native, include persons of Hispanic and non-Hispanic origin. Persons of Hispanic origin may be of any race. Death rates for the American Indian or Alaska Native and Asian or Pacific Islander populations are known to be underestimated. See Appendix II, Race, for a discussion of sources of bias in death rates by race and Hispanic origin.
[6]In 1950, rate is for the age group 75 years and over.
[7]Prior to 1997, excludes data from states lacking an Hispanic-origin item on the death certificate. See Appendix II, Hispanic origin.

NOTES: Starting with Health, United States, 2003, rates for 1991–1999 were revised using intercensal population estimates based on the 2000 census. Rates for 2000 were revised based on 2000 census counts. Rates for 2001 and later years were computed using 2000-based postcensal estimates. See Appendix I, Population Census and Population Estimates. Figures for 2001 include September 11-related deaths for which death certificates were filed as of October 24, 2002. See Appendix II, Cause of death; Table V for terrorism-related ICD–10 codes. Age groups were selected to minimize the presentation of unstable age-specific death rates based on small numbers of deaths and for consistency among comparison groups. For additional injury-related statistics, see Web-based Injury Statistics Query and Reporting System, available from: http://www.cdc.gov/injury/wisqars/index.html. Starting with 2003 data, some states allowed the reporting of more than one race on the death certificate. The multiple-race data for these states were bridged to the single-race categories of the 1977 Office of Management and Budget standards for comparability with other states. See Appendix II, Race. Data for additional years are available. See Appendix III.

SOURCE: CDC/NCHS, National Vital Statistics System; Grove RD, Hetzel AM. Vital statistics rates in the United States, 1940–1960. Washington, DC: U.S. Government Printing Office, 1968; numerator data from National Vital Statistics System, annual mortality files; denominator data from national population estimates for race groups from Table 1 and unpublished Hispanic population estimates for 1985–1996 prepared by the Housing and Household Economic Statistics Division, U.S. Census Bureau; additional mortality tables are available from: http://www.cdc.gov/nchs/nvss/mortality_tables.htm; Xu JQ, Kochanek KD, Murphy SL, Tejada-Vera B. Deaths: Final data for 2007. National vital statistics reports; vol 58 no 19. Hyattsville, MD: NCHS; 2010. Available from: http://www.cdc.gov/nchs/data/nvsr/nvsr58/nvsr58_19.pdf.

Table 40 (page 1 of 3). Death rates for firearm-related injuries, by sex, race, Hispanic origin, and age: United States, selected years 1970–2007

[Data are based on death certificates]

Sex, race, Hispanic origin, and age	1970[1]	1980[1]	1990[1]	1995[1]	2000[2]	2005[2]	2006[2]	2007[2]
All persons			Deaths per 100,000 resident population					
All ages, age-adjusted[3]	14.3	14.8	14.6	13.4	10.2	10.2	10.2	10.2
All ages, crude	13.1	14.9	14.9	13.5	10.2	10.4	10.3	10.4
Under 1 year	*	*	*	*	*	*	*	*
1–14 years	1.6	1.4	1.5	1.6	0.7	0.7	0.7	0.7
1–4 years	1.0	0.7	0.6	0.6	0.3	0.4	0.3	0.4
5–14 years	1.7	1.6	1.9	1.9	0.9	0.8	0.9	0.8
15–24 years	15.5	20.6	25.8	26.7	16.8	16.2	16.9	16.2
15–19 years	11.4	14.7	23.3	24.1	12.9	12.5	13.2	12.4
20–24 years	20.3	26.4	28.1	29.2	20.9	20.0	20.6	20.1
25–44 years	20.9	22.5	19.3	16.9	13.1	13.6	13.3	13.6
25–34 years	22.2	24.3	21.8	19.6	14.5	15.7	15.3	15.5
35–44 years	19.6	20.0	16.3	14.3	11.9	11.6	11.5	11.9
45–64 years	17.6	15.2	13.6	11.7	10.0	10.6	10.6	10.7
45–54 years	18.1	16.4	13.9	12.0	10.5	11.2	11.2	11.1
55–64 years	17.0	13.9	13.3	11.3	9.4	9.8	9.8	10.2
65 years and over	13.8	13.5	16.0	14.1	12.2	11.8	11.2	11.3
65–74 years	14.5	13.8	14.4	12.8	10.6	10.3	10.0	10.0
75–84 years	13.4	13.4	19.4	16.3	13.9	13.7	12.9	13.2
85 years and over	10.2	11.6	14.7	14.4	14.2	12.0	11.5	11.6
Male								
All ages, age-adjusted[3]	24.8	25.9	26.1	23.8	18.1	18.3	18.1	18.2
All ages, crude	22.2	25.7	26.2	23.6	17.8	18.3	18.1	18.2
Under 1 year	*	*	*	*	*	*	*	*
1–14 years	2.3	2.0	2.2	2.3	1.1	1.0	1.0	1.0
1–4 years	1.2	0.9	0.7	0.8	0.4	0.5	0.5	0.5
5–14 years	2.7	2.5	2.9	2.9	1.4	1.2	1.2	1.2
15–24 years	26.4	34.8	44.7	46.5	29.4	28.7	29.8	28.5
15–19 years	19.2	24.5	40.1	41.6	22.4	22.0	23.3	21.8
20–24 years	35.1	45.2	49.1	51.5	37.0	35.3	36.2	35.3
25–44 years	34.1	38.1	32.6	28.4	22.0	23.1	22.6	23.2
25–34 years	36.5	41.4	37.0	33.2	24.9	27.2	26.6	27.0
35–44 years	31.6	33.2	27.4	23.6	19.4	19.2	18.9	19.5
45–64 years	31.0	25.9	23.4	20.0	17.1	18.3	17.9	18.3
45–54 years	30.7	27.3	23.2	20.1	17.6	18.9	18.5	18.6
55–64 years	31.3	24.5	23.7	19.8	16.3	17.4	17.0	17.9
65 years and over	29.7	29.7	35.3	30.7	26.4	25.1	24.1	24.2
65–74 years	29.5	27.8	28.2	25.1	20.3	19.7	19.2	19.1
75–84 years	31.0	33.0	46.9	37.8	32.2	30.8	29.1	29.5
85 years and over	26.2	34.9	49.3	47.1	44.7	35.4	33.6	33.5
Female								
All ages, age-adjusted[3]	4.8	4.7	4.2	3.8	2.8	2.7	2.7	2.7
All ages, crude	4.4	4.7	4.3	3.8	2.8	2.7	2.8	2.7
Under 1 year	*	*	*	*	*	*	*	*
1–14 years	0.8	0.7	0.8	0.8	0.3	0.4	0.4	0.4
1–4 years	0.9	0.5	0.5	0.5	*	0.3	*	0.4
5–14 years	0.8	0.7	1.0	0.9	0.4	0.4	0.4	0.4
15–24 years	4.8	6.1	6.0	5.9	3.5	3.0	3.2	3.2
15–19 years	3.5	4.6	5.7	5.6	2.9	2.4	2.5	2.6
20–24 years	6.4	7.7	6.3	6.1	4.2	3.6	3.8	3.9
25–44 years	8.3	7.4	6.1	5.5	4.2	3.9	3.9	3.9
25–34 years	8.4	7.5	6.7	5.8	4.0	3.8	3.7	3.6
35–44 years	8.2	7.2	5.4	5.2	4.4	4.0	4.1	4.2
45–64 years	5.4	5.4	4.5	3.9	3.4	3.3	3.6	3.4
45–54 years	6.4	6.2	4.9	4.2	3.6	3.7	4.0	3.7
55–64 years	4.2	4.6	4.0	3.5	3.0	2.8	3.2	3.0
65 years and over	2.4	2.5	3.1	2.8	2.2	2.1	1.9	2.0
65–74 years	2.8	3.1	3.6	3.0	2.5	2.5	2.2	2.3
75–84 years	1.7	1.7	2.9	2.8	2.0	2.1	1.8	2.0
85 years and over	*	1.3	1.3	1.8	1.7	1.3	1.1	1.1
White male[4]								
All ages, age-adjusted[3]	19.7	22.1	22.0	20.1	15.9	15.7	15.3	15.6
All ages, crude	17.6	21.8	21.8	19.9	15.6	15.8	15.4	15.8
1–14 years	1.8	1.9	1.9	1.9	1.0	0.8	0.8	0.7
15–24 years	16.9	28.4	29.5	30.8	19.6	18.2	18.4	17.5
25–44 years	24.2	29.5	25.7	23.2	18.0	17.9	17.3	18.3
25–34 years	24.3	31.1	27.8	25.2	18.1	18.6	17.7	18.9
35–44 years	24.1	27.1	23.3	21.2	17.9	17.2	17.0	17.6
45–64 years	27.4	23.3	22.8	19.5	17.4	19.0	18.4	19.0
65 years and over	29.9	30.1	36.8	32.2	28.2	27.1	26.0	26.2

See footnotes at end of table.

Table 40 (page 2 of 3). Death rates for firearm-related injuries, by sex, race, Hispanic origin, and age: United States, selected years 1970–2007

[Data are based on death certificates]

Sex, race, Hispanic origin, and age	1970[1]	1980[1]	1990[1]	1995[1]	2000[2]	2005[2]	2006[2]	2007[2]
Black or African American male[4]			Deaths per 100,000 resident population					
All ages, age-adjusted[3]	70.8	60.1	56.3	49.2	34.2	36.4	37.4	36.2
All ages, crude	60.8	57.7	61.9	52.9	36.1	38.7	40.0	38.9
1–14 years	5.3	3.0	4.4	4.4	1.8	2.1	2.2	2.2
15–24 years	97.3	77.9	138.0	138.7	89.3	86.8	91.8	89.1
25–44 years	126.2	114.1	90.3	70.2	54.1	63.6	63.8	62.3
25–34 years	145.6	128.4	108.6	92.3	74.8	88.4	89.0	84.8
35–44 years	104.2	92.3	66.1	46.3	34.3	38.7	38.1	38.9
45–64 years	71.1	55.6	34.5	28.3	18.4	17.8	19.3	19.0
65 years and over	30.6	29.7	23.9	21.8	13.8	13.6	13.4	11.1
American Indian or Alaska Native male[4]								
All ages, age-adjusted[3]	- - -	24.0	19.4	19.4	13.1	15.7	14.7	12.4
All ages, crude	- - -	27.5	20.5	20.9	13.2	16.7	15.8	13.2
15–24 years	- - -	55.3	49.1	40.9	26.9	32.7	32.7	25.1
25–44 years	- - -	43.9	25.4	31.2	16.6	23.2	21.2	16.3
45–64 years	- - -	*	*	14.2	12.2	13.0	11.0	11.7
65 years and over	- - -	*	*	*	*	*	*	*
Asian or Pacific Islander male[4]								
All ages, age-adjusted[3]	- - -	7.8	8.8	9.2	6.0	5.3	5.4	5.2
All ages, crude	- - -	8.2	9.4	10.0	6.2	5.5	5.7	5.3
15–24 years	- - -	10.8	21.0	24.3	9.3	12.1	14.5	11.4
25–44 years	- - -	12.8	10.9	10.6	8.1	6.4	5.7	5.9
45–64 years	- - -	10.4	8.1	8.2	7.4	5.7	5.6	5.7
65 years and over	- - -	*	*	*	*	*	*	4.4
Hispanic or Latino male[4,5]								
All ages, age-adjusted[3]	- - -	- - -	27.6	23.8	13.6	13.3	12.7	12.9
All ages, crude	- - -	- - -	29.9	26.2	14.2	14.2	13.7	13.4
1–14 years	- - -	- - -	2.6	2.8	1.0	0.7	1.1	0.8
15–24 years	- - -	- - -	55.5	61.7	30.8	33.0	33.6	31.4
25–44 years	- - -	- - -	42.7	31.4	17.3	18.8	17.4	17.2
25–34 years	- - -	- - -	47.3	36.4	20.3	22.9	20.9	21.1
35–44 years	- - -	- - -	35.4	24.2	13.2	13.4	12.9	12.4
45–64 years	- - -	- - -	21.4	17.2	12.0	9.1	8.5	9.6
65 years and over	- - -	- - -	19.1	16.5	12.2	9.8	7.6	10.7
White, not Hispanic or Latino male[5]								
All ages, age-adjusted[3]	- - -	- - -	20.6	18.6	15.5	15.3	15.0	15.4
All ages, crude	- - -	- - -	20.4	18.5	15.7	15.9	15.6	16.1
1–14 years	- - -	- - -	1.6	1.6	1.0	0.8	0.7	0.7
15–24 years	- - -	- - -	24.1	23.5	16.2	13.9	13.9	13.4
25–44 years	- - -	- - -	23.3	21.4	17.9	17.4	17.1	18.3
25–34 years	- - -	- - -	24.7	22.5	17.2	16.9	16.3	18.0
35–44 years	- - -	- - -	21.6	20.4	18.4	17.8	17.8	18.6
45–64 years	- - -	- - -	22.7	19.5	17.8	20.0	19.5	20.1
65 years and over	- - -	- - -	37.4	32.5	29.0	28.2	27.3	27.4
White female[4]								
All ages, age-adjusted[3]	4.0	4.2	3.8	3.5	2.7	2.6	2.6	2.6
All ages, crude	3.7	4.1	3.8	3.5	2.7	2.6	2.6	2.7
15–24 years	3.4	5.1	4.8	4.5	2.8	2.3	2.3	2.6
25–44 years	6.9	6.2	5.3	4.9	3.9	3.7	3.5	3.7
45–64 years	5.0	5.1	4.5	4.0	3.5	3.6	3.9	3.7
65 years and over	2.2	2.5	3.1	2.8	2.4	2.3	2.0	2.1

See footnotes at end of table.

Table 40 (page 3 of 3). Death rates for firearm-related injuries, by sex, race, Hispanic origin, and age: United States, selected years 1970–2007

[Data are based on death certificates]

Sex, race, Hispanic origin, and age	1970[1]	1980[1]	1990[1]	1995[1]	2000[2]	2005[2]	2006[2]	2007[2]
Black or African American female[4]			Deaths per 100,000 resident population					
All ages, age-adjusted[3]	11.1	8.7	7.3	6.2	3.9	3.6	4.0	3.8
All ages, crude	10.0	8.8	7.8	6.5	4.0	3.7	4.1	3.9
15–24 years	15.2	12.3	13.3	13.2	7.6	6.7	7.7	7.1
25–44 years	19.4	16.1	12.4	9.8	6.5	6.0	7.0	6.4
45–64 years	10.2	8.2	4.8	4.1	3.1	2.7	2.6	2.8
65 years and over	4.3	3.1	3.1	2.6	1.3	1.3	1.0	1.2
American Indian or Alaska Native female[4]								
All ages, age-adjusted[3]	- - -	5.8	3.3	3.8	2.9	2.4	2.4	2.0
All ages, crude	- - -	5.8	3.4	4.1	2.9	2.6	2.4	2.0
15–24 years	- - -	*	*	*	*	*	*	*
25–44 years	- - -	10.2	*	7.0	5.5	*	*	*
45–64 years	- - -	*	*	*	*	*	*	*
65 years and over	- - -	*	*	*	*	*	*	*
Asian or Pacific Islander female[4]								
All ages, age-adjusted[3]	- - -	2.0	1.9	2.0	1.1	0.9	1.0	0.7
All ages, crude	- - -	2.1	2.1	2.1	1.2	0.9	1.0	0.7
15–24 years	- - -	*	*	3.9	*	2.3	*	*
25–44 years	- - -	3.2	2.7	2.7	1.5	1.0	1.2	1.0
45–64 years	- - -	*	*	*	*	*	1.3	*
65 years and over	- - -	*	*	*	*	*	*	*
Hispanic or Latina female[4,5]								
All ages, age-adjusted[3]	- - -	- - -	3.3	3.1	1.8	1.6	1.5	1.5
All ages, crude	- - -	- - -	3.6	3.3	1.8	1.6	1.5	1.5
15–24 years	- - -	- - -	6.9	6.1	2.9	2.6	2.7	2.9
25–44 years	- - -	- - -	5.1	4.7	2.5	2.7	2.3	2.3
45–64 years	- - -	- - -	2.4	2.4	2.2	1.2	1.4	1.5
65 years and over	- - -	- - -	*	*	*	*	*	*
White, not Hispanic or Latina female[5]								
All ages, age-adjusted[3]	- - -	- - -	3.7	3.4	2.8	2.7	2.7	2.8
All ages, crude	- - -	- - -	3.7	3.5	2.9	2.8	2.8	2.9
15–24 years	- - -	- - -	4.3	4.1	2.7	2.2	2.2	2.5
25–44 years	- - -	- - -	5.1	4.8	4.2	4.0	3.8	4.1
45–64 years	- - -	- - -	4.6	4.1	3.6	3.8	4.2	3.9
65 years and over	- - -	- - -	3.2	2.8	2.4	2.4	2.2	2.2

* Rates based on fewer than 20 deaths are considered unreliable and are not shown.

- - - Data not available.

[1]Underlying cause of death was coded according to the 8th Revision of the *International Classification of Diseases* (ICD) in 1970 and 9th Revision in 1980–1998. See Appendix II, Cause of death; Tables IV and V.

[2]Starting with 1999 data, cause of death is coded according to ICD–10. See Appendix II, Cause of death, Table V; Comparability ratio, Table VI.

[3]Age-adjusted rates are calculated using the year 2000 standard population. Prior to 2003, age-adjusted rates were calculated using standard million proportions based on rounded population numbers. Starting with 2003 data, unrounded population numbers are used to calculate age-adjusted rates. See Appendix II, Age adjustment.

[4]The race groups, white, black, Asian or Pacific Islander, and American Indian or Alaska Native, include persons of Hispanic and non-Hispanic origin. Persons of Hispanic origin may be of any race. Death rates for the American Indian or Alaska Native and Asian or Pacific Islander populations are known to be underestimated. See Appendix II, Race, for a discussion of sources of bias in death rates by race and Hispanic origin.

[5]Prior to 1997, excludes data from states lacking an Hispanic-origin item on the death certificate. See Appendix II, Hispanic origin.

NOTES: Starting with *Health, United States, 2003*, rates for 1991–1999 were revised using intercensal population estimates based on the 2000 census. Rates for 2000 were revised based on 2000 census counts. Rates for 2001 and later years were computed using 2000-based postcensal estimates. See Appendix I, Population Census and Population Estimates. Age groups were selected to minimize the presentation of unstable age-specific death rates based on small numbers of deaths and for consistency among comparison groups. For additional injury-related statistics, see Web-based Injury Statistics Query and Reporting System, available from: http://www.cdc.gov/injury/wisqars/index.html. Starting with 2003 data, some states allowed the reporting of more than one race on the death certificate. The multiple-race data for these states were bridged to the single-race categories of the 1977 Office of Management and Budget standards for comparability with other states. See Appendix II, Race. Data for additional years are available. See Appendix III.

SOURCE: CDC/NCHS, National Vital Statistics System; numerator data from National Vital Statistics System, annual mortality files; denominator data from national population estimates for race groups from Table 1 and unpublished Hispanic population estimates for 1985–1996 prepared by the Housing and Household Economic Statistics Division, U.S. Census Bureau; additional mortality tables are available from: http://www.cdc.gov/nchs/nvss/mortality_tables.htm; Xu JQ, Kochanek KD, Murphy SL, Tejada-Vera B. Deaths: Final data for 2007. National vital statistics reports; vol 58 no 19. Hyattsville, MD: NCHS; 2010. Available from: http://www.cdc.gov/nchs/data/nvsr/nvsr58/nvsr58_19.pdf.

Table 41. Deaths from selected occupational diseases among persons 15 years of age and over: United States, selected years 1980–2007

[Data are based on death certificates]

Cause of death	1980[1]	1985[1]	1990[1]	1995[1]	2000[2]	2005[2]	2006[2]	2007[2]
Underlying and nonunderlying cause of death	Number of death certificates with cause of death code(s) mentioned							
Angiosarcoma of liver[3]	- - -	- - -	- - -	- - -	16	26	23	22
Malignant mesothelioma[4]	699	715	874	897	2,531	2,704	2,588	2,606
Pneumoconiosis[5]	4,151	3,783	3,644	3,151	2,859	2,425	2,308	2,189
Coal workers' pneumoconiosis	2,576	2,615	1,990	1,413	949	652	654	524
Asbestosis	339	534	948	1,169	1,486	1,416	1,340	1,393
Silicosis	448	334	308	242	151	160	126	122
Other (including unspecified)	814	321	413	343	290	222	206	163
Underlying cause of death	Number of deaths							
Angiosarcoma of liver[3]	- - -	- - -	- - -	- - -	15	23	21	20
Malignant mesothelioma[4]	531	573	725	780	2,384	2,553	2,452	2,432
Pneumoconiosis	1,581	1,355	1,335	1,117	1,142	983	907	898
Coal workers' pneumoconiosis	982	958	734	533	389	270	266	209
Asbestosis	101	139	302	355	558	532	485	538
Silicosis	207	143	150	114	71	74	67	72
Other (including unspecified)	291	115	149	115	124	107	89	79

- - - Data not available.

[1]For the period 1980–1998, underlying cause of death was coded according to the 9th Revision of the *International Classification of Diseases* (ICD). See Appendix II, Cause of death; Tables IV and V.

[2]Starting with 1999 data, ICD–10 was introduced for coding cause of death. Discontinuities exist between 1998 and 1999 due to ICD–10 coding and classification changes. Caution should be exercised in interpreting trends for the causes of death in this table, especially for those with major ICD–10 changes (e.g., malignant mesothelioma). See Appendix II, *International Classification of Diseases* (ICD) and Table V.

[3]Prior to 1999, there was no discrete code for this condition.

[4]Prior to 1999, the combined ICD–9 categories of malignant neoplasm of peritoneum and malignant neoplasm of pleura served as a crude surrogate for malignant mesothelioma category under ICD–10.

[5]For underlying and nonunderlying cause of death, counts for pneumoconiosis subgroups may sum to slightly more than total pneumoconiosis due to the reporting of more than one type of pneumoconiosis on some death certificates.

NOTES: Cause-of-death titles for selected occupational diseases and corresponding code numbers according to the *International Classification of Diseases*, 9th and 10th Revisions. See Appendix II, Cause of death; Table V. See Appendix I, National Vital Statistics System, Multiple Cause of Death File, for information about tabulating cause-of-death data in this table. Selection of occupational diseases is based on definitions in Mullan RJ, Murthy LI. Occupational sentinel health events: An updated list for physician recognition and public health surveillance. 1991; Am J Ind Med 19(6):775–99. For more detailed information about pneumoconiosis deaths, see *Work-Related Lung Disease Surveillance Report 2007*, DHHS (NIOSH) Publication Number 2008–143 available from: http://www2a.cdc.gov/drds/WorldReportData. Data for additional years are available. See Appendix III.

SOURCE: CDC/NCHS, National Vital Statistics System; annual mortality files for underlying and multiple cause of death.

Table 42 (page 1 of 2). Occupational injury deaths and rates, by industry, sex, age, race, and Hispanic origin: United States, selected years 1995–2008

[Data are compiled from various federal, state, and local administrative sources]

Characteristic	1995	2000	2001[1]	2004	2005	2006	2007	2008[2]
	Deaths per 100,000 employed workers[3]							
Total workforce	4.9	4.3	4.3	4.1	4.0	4.0	3.8	3.7
Sex								
Male	8.3	7.4	7.4	7.1	6.9	6.9	6.6	6.1
Female	0.9	0.7	0.7	0.6	0.6	0.7	0.6	0.6
Age								
16–17 years	1.6	1.6	1.3	1.1	1.4	0.9	0.9	2.5
18–19 years	3.3	2.7	2.8	2.7	2.9	2.8	2.6	2.4
20–24 years	3.8	3.2	3.2	3.0	2.8	2.7	3.0	2.8
25–34 years	4.3	3.8	3.8	3.2	3.3	3.3	3.1	2.8
35–44 years	4.6	4.0	4.0	3.9	3.6	3.7	3.4	3.3
45–54 years	5.2	4.4	4.5	4.3	4.2	4.2	4.1	3.8
55–64 years	7.2	6.1	5.5	5.2	5.1	5.0	4.6	4.7
65 years and over	14.0	12.0	12.7	11.8	11.3	11.2	10.2	12.7
Race and Hispanic origin[4]								
Hispanic or Latino	5.5	5.6	6.0	5.0	4.9	5.0	4.6	4.2
Not Hispanic or Latino	- - -	- - -	- - -	- - -	- - -	- - -	- - -	- - -
White	- - -	4.2	4.2	4.1	3.9	4.0	3.8	3.8
Black or African American	- - -	3.8	3.8	3.7	3.9	3.7	3.9	3.7
Industry[5]								
Private sector	- - -	- - -	- - -	4.4	4.3	4.3	4.1	4.0
Agriculture, forestry, fishing, and hunting	- - -	- - -	- - -	30.5	32.5	30.0	27.9	30.4
Mining	- - -	- - -	- - -	28.3	25.6	28.1	25.1	18.1
Utilities	- - -	- - -	- - -	6.1	3.6	6.3	4.0	3.9
Construction	- - -	- - -	- - -	12.0	11.1	10.9	10.5	9.7
Manufacturing	- - -	- - -	- - -	2.8	2.4	2.8	2.5	2.5
Wholesale trade	- - -	- - -	- - -	4.5	4.6	4.9	4.7	4.4
Retail trade	- - -	- - -	- - -	2.3	2.4	2.2	2.1	2.0
Transportation and warehousing	- - -	- - -	- - -	18.0	17.7	16.8	16.9	14.9
Information	- - -	- - -	- - -	1.7	2.0	2.0	2.3	1.5
Finance and insurance	- - -	- - -	- - -	0.7	0.6	0.6	0.6	0.3
Real estate and rental and leasing	- - -	- - -	- - -	2.4	1.9	2.6	2.4	3.1
Professional, scientific, and technical services	- - -	- - -	- - -	0.9	1.0	0.9	0.9	0.8
Management of companies and enterprises	- - -	- - -	- - -	*	*	*	*	*
Administrative and support and waste management and remediation services	- - -	- - -	- - -	6.7	7.2	6.6	6.3	6.1
Educational services	- - -	- - -	- - -	1.3	1.3	1.3	0.9	0.9
Health care and social assistance	- - -	- - -	- - -	0.8	0.7	0.8	0.7	0.7
Arts, entertainment, and recreation	- - -	- - -	- - -	4.3	3.2	3.5	3.9	4.0
Accommodation and food services	- - -	- - -	- - -	1.6	1.5	2.0	1.7	1.8
Other services (except public administration)	- - -	- - -	- - -	3.0	3.0	2.6	2.5	2.6
Government[6]	- - -	- - -	- - -	2.5	2.4	2.4	2.5	2.4
	Number of deaths[7]							
Total workforce	6,275	5,920	5,915	5,764	5,734	5,840	5,657	5,214
Sex								
Male	5,736	5,471	5,442	5,349	5,328	5,396	5,228	4,827
Female	539	449	473	415	406	444	429	387
Age								
Under 16 years	26	29	20	13	23	11	18	11
16–17 years	42	44	33	25	31	21	20	23
18–19 years	130	127	122	103	111	106	97	66
20–24 years	486	446	441	421	403	390	424	353
25–34 years	1,409	1,163	1,142	996	1,017	1,041	991	850
35–44 years	1,571	1,473	1,478	1,342	1,243	1,288	1,168	1,113
45–54 years	1,256	1,313	1,368	1,384	1,389	1,417	1,425	1,292
55–64 years	827	831	775	907	933	963	934	920
65 years and over	515	488	530	569	578	599	574	580
Unspecified	13	6	6	4	6	4	6	6

See footnotes at end of table.

Table 42 (page 2 of 2). Occupational injury deaths and rates, by industry, sex, age, race, and Hispanic origin: United States, selected years 1995–2008

[Data are compiled from various federal, state, and local administrative sources]

Characteristic	1995	2000	2001[1]	2004	2005	2006	2007	2008[2]
Race and Hispanic origin	\multicolumn{8}{c}{Number of deaths[7]}							
White.	5,120	- - -	- - -	- - -	- - -	- - -	- - -	- - -
Black or African American	697	- - -	- - -	- - -	- - -	- - -	- - -	- - -
Hispanic or Latino.	619	815	895	902	923	990	937	804
Not Hispanic or Latino.	5,656	5,105	5,020	4,862	4,809	4,850	4,734	4,410
White.	4,599	4,244	4,175	4,066	3,977	4,019	3,867	3,663
Black or African American.	684	575	565	546	584	565	609	533
American Indian or Alaska Native	27	33	48	28	50	46	29	32
Asian[8]	188	171	173	168	154	148	166	145
Native Hawaiian or Other Pacific Islander . .	- - -	14	9	12	9	11	6	7
Multiple races	- - -	- - -	6	4	- - -	11	10	6
Other races or not reported	158	68	44	38	35	50	33	24
Industry[5]								
Private sector.	- - -	- - -	- - -	5,229	5,214	5,320	5,112	4,670
Agriculture, forestry, fishing, and hunting.	- - -	- - -	- - -	669	715	655	585	672
Mining	- - -	- - -	- - -	152	159	192	183	176
Utilities	- - -	- - -	- - -	51	30	53	34	37
Construction	- - -	- - -	- - -	1,234	1,192	1,239	1,204	975
Manufacturing.	- - -	- - -	- - -	463	393	456	400	411
Wholesale trade	- - -	- - -	- - -	205	209	222	207	180
Retail trade.	- - -	- - -	- - -	377	400	359	348	301
Transportation and warehousing	- - -	- - -	- - -	840	885	860	890	796
Information	- - -	- - -	- - -	55	65	66	79	47
Finance and insurance.	- - -	- - -	- - -	46	42	44	46	24
Real estate and rental and leasing	- - -	- - -	- - -	70	57	82	73	82
Professional, scientific, and technical services	- - -	- - -	- - -	77	83	78	77	69
Management of companies and enterprises	- - -	- - -	- - -	*	*	*	4	*
Administrative and support and waste management and remediation services . . .	- - -	- - -	- - -	373	398	381	395	332
Educational services	- - -	- - -	- - -	44	46	49	34	28
Health care and social assistance	- - -	- - -	- - -	113	104	129	115	113
Arts, entertainment, and recreation	- - -	- - -	- - -	99	77	80	96	92
Accommodation and food services	- - -	- - -	- - -	148	136	185	164	146
Other services (except public administration).	- - -	- - -	- - -	207	210	183	175	178
Government[6]	- - -	- - -	- - -	535	520	520	545	544

- - - Data not available.

* Estimates are unreliable or data do not meet publication criteria.

[1]2,886 fatalities due to the September 11 terrorist attacks are not included.

[2]Starting with 2008 data, fatal injury rates are based on hours, rather than employment, and consequently are not directly comparable with earlier data. Hours-based rates standardize the amount of exposure and are considered more accurate than employment-based rates. Employment- and hours-based rates will be similar for groups of workers who usually work full-time. Differences in these rates are more likely for groups of workers who have a high percentage of part-time workers, like younger workers. Hours worked data are provided by the Current Population Survey (CPS). For more information see http://www.bls.gov/iif/oshnotice10.htm.

[3]Numerator excludes deaths to workers under the age of 16 years. For data prior to 2008, employment data in denominators are average annual estimates of employed civilians 16 years of age and over from the CPS, regardless of the number of hours worked. These data are supplemented by data for the resident military, which was supplied by the U.S. Census Bureau (1995–1998) and the Department of Defense (1999–2008). Starting with 2004 data, rates are taken directly from the U.S. Department of Labor, Bureau of Labor Statistics, Census of Fatal Occupational Injuries. Revised annual data. Starting with 2008 data, employment data in denominators are based on hours. See Appendix I, Census of Fatal Occupational Injuries.

[4]Employment data for American Indian or Alaska Native workers and, prior to 2003, Asian or Pacific Islander workers, were not available for the calculation of rates. Employment data for non-Hispanic white and non-Hispanic black workers were not available before the year 2000. In 1999 and earlier years, the race groups white and black included persons of Hispanic and non-Hispanic origin.

[5]Starting with 2003 data, establishments were classified by industry according to the North American Industry Classification System (NAICS). Prior to 2003, the Standard Industrial Classification (SIC) system was used. Because of substantial differences between these systems, industry data classified by these two systems are not comparable. Industry data for 1995–2002 classified by SIC are available in Health, United States, 2004, Table 49 available from: http://www.cdc.gov/nchs/hus.htm. See Appendix II, Industry of employment.

[6]Includes fatalities to workers employed by governmental organizations, regardless of industry.

[7]Includes fatalities to all workers, regardless of age.

[8]In 1999 and earlier years, category also included Native Hawaiian or Other Pacific Islander.

NOTES: Fatalities and rates are based on revised data and may differ from originally published data from the Census of Fatal Occupational Injuries (CFOI). See Appendix I, Census of Fatal Occupational Injuries. CFOI began collecting fatality data in 1992. For data for prior years, see CDC. Fatal Occupational Injuries—United States, 1980–1997. MMWR 2001;50(16):317–20, Available from: http://www.cdc.gov/mmwr/preview/mmwrhtml/mm5016a4.htm. which reports trend data from the National Traumatic Occupational Fatalities (NTOF) surveillance system. NTOF was established at the National Institute of Occupational Safety and Health (NIOSH) to monitor occupational injury deaths through death certificates. Because of methodological differences between CFOI and NTOF, the data are not directly comparable. Industry categories presented in this table differ from those shown in some previous editions of Health, United States.

SOURCE: Department of Labor, Bureau of Labor Statistics, Census of Fatal Occupational Injuries. Revised annual data.

Table 43. Nonfatal occupational injuries and illnesses with days away from work, job transfer, or restriction, by industry: United States, selected years 2003–2008

[Data are based on employer records from a sample of business establishments]

| | Injuries and illnesses with days away from work, job transfer, or restriction | | | | | | | |
| | Cases per 100 full-time workers[1] | | | | Number of cases in thousands[2] | | | |
Industry	2003	2006	2007	2008	2003	2006	2007	2008
Total private sector[3]	2.6	2.3	2.1	2.0	2,301.9	2,114.6	2,036.0	1,900.8
Agriculture, forestry, fishing, and hunting[4]	3.3	3.2	2.8	2.9	29.3	27.6	26.6	26.0
Mining[5]	2.0	2.1	2.0	2.0	11.2	14.0	14.1	16.4
Utilities	2.2	2.2	2.1	1.9	12.2	11.8	11.4	10.6
Construction	3.6	3.2	2.8	2.5	218.0	223.7	197.5	171.6
Manufacturing	3.8	3.3	3.0	2.7	538.0	473.4	427.1	372.9
Wholesale trade	2.8	2.5	2.4	2.2	147.4	140.6	139.3	130.9
Retail trade	2.7	2.6	2.5	2.3	319.6	308.6	309.1	283.4
Transportation and warehousing[6]	5.4	4.3	4.3	3.9	204.0	176.3	179.4	164.3
Information	1.1	1.0	1.1	1.1	30.8	28.3	29.1	28.0
Finance and insurance	0.4	0.3	0.4	0.3	21.3	17.7	20.7	18.7
Real estate and rental and leasing	2.1	1.8	1.6	1.8	35.6	33.0	29.0	32.1
Professional, scientific, and technical services	0.6	0.5	0.5	0.5	36.0	34.5	31.8	33.5
Management of companies and enterprises	1.6	1.1	0.9	0.7	25.1	17.9	15.1	12.7
Administrative and support and waste management and remediation services	2.4	1.9	1.8	1.8	96.7	87.0	89.2	87.0
Educational services	1.2	0.9	1.0	1.0	17.9	14.5	15.8	16.0
Health care and social assistance	3.1	2.7	2.5	2.5	337.9	310.0	303.7	302.6
Arts, entertainment, and recreation	2.9	2.5	2.5	2.4	34.1	28.7	31.9	31.9
Accommodation and food services	2.0	1.7	1.6	1.5	135.2	124.6	119.6	116.0
Other services, except public administration	1.7	1.4	1.5	1.5	51.7	42.4	45.7	46.2

[1]Incidence rate calculated as (N/EH) x 200,000, where N = total number of injuries and illnesses, EH = total hours worked by all employees during the calendar year, and 200,000 = base for 100 full-time equivalent employees working 40 hours per week, 50 weeks per year.

[2]Because of rounding, components may not add to total number of cases in private sector.

[3]Totals include data for industries not shown separately. Excludes self-employed, private households, and employees in federal, state, and local government agencies.

[4]Excludes farms with fewer than 11 employees.

[5]Data for Mining include establishments not governed by the Mine Safety and Health Administration rules and reporting, such as those in Oil and Gas Extraction and related support activities. Data for mining operators in coal, metal, and nonmetal mining are provided to BLS by the Mine Safety and Health Administration, U.S. Department of Labor. Independent mining contractors are excluded from the coal, metal, and nonmetal mining industries. These data do not reflect the changes the Occupational Safety and Health Administration made to its recordkeeping requirements effective January 1, 2002. Therefore, estimates for these industries are not comparable to estimates in other industries. For more information, see http://www.bls.gov/news.release/pdf/osh.pdf.

[6]Data for railroad transportation are provided to BLS by the Federal Railroad Administration, U.S. Department of Transportation.

NOTES: Starting with 2003 data, the Survey of Occupational Injuries and Illnesses began using the North American Industry Classification System (NAICS) to classify establishments by industry. Prior to 2003, the survey used the Standard Industrial Classification (SIC) system. Because of substantial differences between these systems, the data measured by these surveys are not directly comparable. See Appendix II, Industry of employment. Data for previous years are presented in *Health, United States, 2004*, Table 50. Available from: http://www.cdc.gov/nchs/hus.htm. See Appendix I, Survey of Occupational Injuries and Illnesses (SOII). Data for additional years are available. See Appendix III.

SOURCE: U.S. Department of Labor, Bureau of Labor Statistics (BLS), Survey of Occupational Injuries and Illnesses: Workplace injuries and illnesses, 2003–2008 editions. Summary News Release. 2004–2009. Available from: http://www.bls.gov/iif/home.htm.

Table 44 (page 1 of 2). Selected notifiable disease rates and number new of cases: United States, selected years 1950–2008

[Data are based on reporting by state health departments]

Disease	1950	1960	1970	1980	1990	2000	2006	2007	2008
	New cases per 100,000 population								
Diphtheria	3.83	0.51	0.21	0.00	0.00	0.00	–	–	–
Haemophilus influenzae, invasive	- - -	- - -	- - -	- - -	- - -	0.51	0.82	0.85	0.96
Hepatitis A	- - -	- - -	27.87	12.84	12.64	4.91	1.21	1.00	0.86
Hepatitis B	- - -	- - -	4.08	8.39	8.48	2.95	1.62	1.51	1.34
Lyme disease	- - -	- - -	- - -	- - -	- - -	6.53	6.75	9.21	11.67
Meningococcal disease	- - -	- - -	1.23	1.25	0.99	0.83	0.40	0.36	0.39
Mumps	- - -	- - -	55.55	3.86	2.17	0.13	2.22	0.27	0.15
Pertussis (whooping cough)	79.82	8.23	2.08	0.76	1.84	2.88	5.27	3.49	4.40
Poliomyelitis, total	22.02	1.77	0.02	0.00	0.00	–	–	–	–
Paralytic[1]	- - -	1.40	0.02	0.00	0.00	–	–	–	–
Rocky Mountain spotted fever	- - -	- - -	0.19	0.52	0.26	0.18	0.80	0.77	0.85
Rubella (German measles)	- - -	- - -	27.75	1.72	0.45	0.06	–	–	0.01
Rubeola (measles)	211.01	245.42	23.23	5.96	11.17	0.03	0.02	0.01	0.05
Salmonellosis, excluding typhoid fever	- - -	3.85	10.84	14.88	19.54	14.51	15.45	16.03	16.92
Shigellosis	15.45	6.94	6.79	8.41	10.89	8.41	5.23	6.60	7.50
Tuberculosis[2]	- - -	30.83	18.28	12.25	10.33	6.01	4.65	4.44	4.28
Sexually transmitted diseases:[3]									
Syphilis[4]	146.02	68.78	44.80	30.30	54.32	11.20	12.34	13.57	15.34
Primary and secondary	16.73	9.06	10.80	12.00	20.26	2.12	3.26	3.80	4.48
Early latent	39.71	10.11	8.00	8.90	22.19	3.35	3.07	3.57	4.11
Late and late latent[5]	70.22	45.91	24.70	9.20	10.32	5.53	5.89	6.05	6.61
Congenital[6]	368.30	103.70	52.30	7.70	92.95	14.29	8.72	10.10	10.10
Chlamydia[7]	- - -	- - -	- - -	- - -	160.19	251.38	344.33	367.47	401.34
Gonorrhea[8]	192.50	145.40	294.20	442.10	276.43	128.67	119.70	118.03	111.64
Chancroid	3.34	0.94	0.70	0.30	1.69	0.03	0.01	0.01	0.01
	Number of new cases								
Diphtheria	5,796	918	435	3	4	1	–	–	–
Haemophilus influenzae, invasive	- - -	- - -	- - -	- - -	- - -	1,398	2,496	2,541	2,886
Hepatitis A	- - -	- - -	56,797	29,087	31,441	13,397	3,579	2,979	2,585
Hepatitis B	- - -	- - -	8,310	19,015	21,102	8,036	4,713	4,519	4,033
Lyme disease	- - -	- - -	- - -	- - -	- - -	17,730	19,931	27,444	35,198
Meningococcal disease	- - -	- - -	2,505	2,840	2,451	2,256	1,194	1,077	1,172
Mumps	- - -	- - -	104,953	8,576	5,292	338	6,584	800	454
Pertussis (whooping cough)	120,718	14,809	4,249	1,730	4,570	7,867	15,632	10,454	13,278
Poliomyelitis, total	33,300	3,190	33	9	6	–	–	–	–
Paralytic[1]	- - -	2,525	31	9	6	–	–	–	–
Rocky Mountain spotted fever	- - -	- - -	380	1,163	651	495	2,288	2,221	2,563
Rubella (German measles)	- - -	- - -	56,552	3,904	1,125	176	11	12	16
Rubeola (measles)	319,124	441,703	47,351	13,506	27,786	86	55	43	140
Salmonellosis, excluding typhoid fever	- - -	6,929	22,096	33,715	48,603	39,574	45,808	47,995	51,040
Shigellosis	23,367	12,487	13,845	19,041	27,077	22,922	15,503	19,758	22,625
Tuberculosis[2]	- - -	55,494	37,137	27,749	25,701	16,377	13,779	13,299	12,904
Sexually transmitted diseases:[3]									
Syphilis[4]	217,558	122,538	91,382	68,832	135,590	31,618	36,958	40,921	46,277
Primary and secondary	23,939	16,145	21,982	27,204	50,578	5,979	9,756	11,466	13,500
Early latent	59,256	18,017	16,311	20,297	55,397	9,465	9,186	10,768	12,401
Late and late latent[5]	113,569	81,798	50,348	20,979	25,750	15,594	17,644	18,256	19,945
Congenital[6]	13,377	4,416	1,953	277	3,865	580	372	431	431
Chlamydia[7]	- - -	- - -	- - -	- - -	323,663	709,452	1,030,911	1,108,374	1,210,523
Gonorrhea[8]	286,746	258,933	600,072	1,004,029	690,042	363,136	358,366	355,991	336,742
Chancroid	4,977	1,680	1,416	788	4,212	78	19	23	25

See footnotes at end of table.

[Data are based on reporting by state health departments]

0.00 Rate greater than zero but less than 0.005.
– Quantity zero.
- - - Data not available.

[1]Cases of vaccine-associated parylytic poliomyelitis caused by polio vaccine virus.

[2]Case reporting for tuberculosis began in 1953. Data prior to 1975 are not comparable with subsequent years because of changes in reporting criteria effective in 1975. Data from 1993 to 2008 were updated through the Division of Tuberculosis Elimination, National Center for HIV/AIDS, Viral Hepatitis, STD, and TB Prevention (NCHHSTP), as of May 15, 2009.

[3]Starting with 1991, data include both civilian and military cases. Adjustments to the number of cases reported from state health departments were made for hardcopy forms and for electronic data submissions through June 10, 2009. For 1950, data for Alaska and Hawaii were not included. Cases and rates shown, do not include outlying areas of Guam, Puerto Rico, and the Virgin Islands.

[4]Includes stage of syphilis not stated.

[5]Includes cases of unknown duration.

[6]Rates include all cases of congenitally acquired syphilis per 100,000 live births. Cases of congenitally acquired syphilis were reported through 1994; starting with 1995 data, only congenital syphilis for cases less than 1 year of age were reported. See STD Surveillance Report for congenital syphilis rates per 100,000 live births.

[7]Prior to 1994, chlamydia was not notifiable. In 1994–1999, cases for New York were exclusively reported by New York City. Starting with 2000 data, includes cases for the entire state.

[8]Data for 1994 do not include cases from Georgia.

NOTES: The total resident population was used to calculate all rates except sexually transmitted diseases (STDs), which used the civilian resident population prior to 1991. STD rates for 1990–2002 have been revised and may differ from previous editions of *Health, United States*. Revised rates are due to revision of population estimates to incorporate bridged single-race estimates. 2007 population estimates were used to calculate 2008 rates. See Appendix I, Population Census and Population Estimates. Population data from those states where diseases were not notifiable or not available were excluded from the rate calculation; see Appendix II, Notifiable Disease. See Appendix I, National Notifiable Disease Surveillance System (NNDSS), for information on underreporting of notifiable diseases. Data for additional years are available. See Appendix III.

SOURCE: CDC, National Center for Public Health Informatics, Division of Integrated Surveillance Systems and Services; Summary of notifiable diseases, United States, 2008. MMWR 2010;57(54):1–94 and CDC. http://www.cdc.gov/mmwr/preview/mmwrhtml/mm5754a1.htm. Sexually transmitted disease surveillance, 2008. Atlanta, GA: U.S. Department of Health and Human Services, 2008. http://www.cdc.gov/std/stats08/default.htm.

Table 45 (page 1 of 3). Acquired immunodeficiency syndrome (AIDS) diagnoses, by year of diagnosis and selected characteristics: United States, 2005–2008

[Data are based on reporting by 50 states and the District of Columbia]

Sex, race and Hispanic origin, age at diagnosis, and region of residence	Year of diagnosis				
	All years[1]	2005	2006	2007	2008
	Estimated number of AIDS diagnoses[2]				
All persons[3]	1,073,128	37,290	36,442	36,333	37,151
Male, 13 years and over	851,974	27,436	26,741	26,619	27,543
Female, 13 years and over	211,804	9,799	9,661	9,683	9,567
Children, under 13 years	9,349	55	40	30	41
Male, 13 years and over					
Hispanic origin and race:					
Not Hispanic or Latino:					
White	376,372	9,338	9,101	8,809	8,980
Black or African American	315,145	11,763	11,296	11,391	11,968
Asian[4]	7,016	316	365	397	427
Native Hawaiian or Other Pacific Islander	691	39	39	47	44
American Indian or Alaska Native	2,922	135	121	108	155
Hispanic or Latino[5]	144,438	5,539	5,490	5,533	5,660
Multiple Race	5,080	306	329	334	310
Age at diagnosis:					
13–14 years	663	32	26	27	20
15–24 years	32,831	1,480	1,454	1,769	1,891
25–34 years	266,130	5,645	5,441	5,513	5,888
35–44 years	338,443	10,609	10,157	9,452	9,233
45–54 years	154,898	7,035	6,802	7,072	7,352
55–64 years	45,942	2,082	2,233	2,202	2,505
65 years and over	13,067	553	627	584	655
Female, 13 years and over					
Hispanic origin and race:					
Not Hispanic or Latina:					
White	41,920	1,543	1,584	1,599	1,583
Black or African American	131,988	6,458	6,267	6,303	6,336
Asian[4]	1,189	82	77	92	97
Native Hawaiian or Other Pacific Islander	133	11	15	11	7
American Indian or Alaska Native	785	38	35	48	44
Hispanic or Latina[5]	33,824	1,519	1,549	1,487	1,379
Multiple Race	1,908	148	133	143	121
Age at diagnosis:					
13–14 years	557	41	49	46	29
15–24 years	14,589	660	590	613	582
25–34 years	69,179	2,310	2,246	2,125	2,189
35–44 years	78,089	3,519	3,363	3,304	3,169
45–54 years	34,772	2,386	2,442	2,490	2,514
55–64 years	10,713	702	759	871	877
65 years and over	3,905	182	212	235	206
Children, under 13 years					
Hispanic origin and race:					
Not Hispanic or Latino:					
White	1,612	4	3	4	7
Black or African American	5,782	40	30	22	25
Asian[4]	49	1	1	0	1
Native Hawaiian or Other Pacific Islander	7	0	0	0	0
American Indian or Alaska Native	33	0	0	0	0
Hispanic or Latino[5]	1,798	8	4	3	4
Multiple Race	66	1	1	0	3
Region of residence					
Northeast	328,748	9,323	9,168	9,011	8,386
Midwest	111,137	4,427	4,126	3,993	4,251
South	414,914	17,204	16,711	16,781	17,471
West	218,331	6,336	6,436	6,548	7,042

See footnotes at end of table.

Table 45 (page 2 of 3). Acquired immunodeficiency syndrome (AIDS) diagnoses, by year of diagnosis and selected characteristics: United States, 2005–2008

[Data are based on reporting by 50 states and the District of Columbia]

Sex, race and Hispanic origin, age at diagnosis, and region of residence	All years[1]	Year of diagnosis			
		2005	2006	2007	2008
	Percent distribution[6]				
All persons[3]	100.0	100.0	100.0	100.0	100.0
Male, 13 years and over.	79.4	73.6	73.4	73.3	74.1
Female, 13 years and over.	19.7	26.3	26.5	26.7	25.8
Children, under 13 years	0.9	0.1	0.1	0.1	0.1
Male, 13 years and over					
Hispanic origin and race:					
Not Hispanic or Latino:					
White.	44.2	34.0	34.0	33.1	32.6
Black or African American	37.0	42.9	42.2	42.8	43.4
Asian[4]	0.8	1.2	1.4	1.5	1.6
Native Hawaiian or Other Pacific Islander . . .	0.3	0.5	0.5	0.4	0.6
American Indian or Alaska Native	0.1	0.1	0.1	0.2	0.2
Hispanic or Latino[5].	17.0	20.2	20.5	20.8	20.5
Multiple Race.	0.6	1.1	1.2	1.3	1.1
Age at diagnosis:					
13–14 years.	0.1	0.1	0.1	0.1	0.1
15–24 years.	3.9	5.4	5.4	6.6	6.9
25–34 years.	31.2	20.6	20.3	20.7	21.4
35–44 years.	39.7	38.7	38.0	35.5	33.5
45–54 years.	18.2	25.6	25.4	26.6	26.7
55–64 years.	5.4	7.6	8.4	8.3	9.1
65 years and over	1.5	2.0	2.3	2.2	2.4
Female, 13 years and over					
Hispanic origin and race:					
Not Hispanic or Latina:					
White.	19.8	15.8	16.4	16.5	16.5
Black or African American	62.3	65.9	64.9	65.1	66.2
Asian[4]	0.6	0.8	0.8	0.9	1.0
Native Hawaiian or Other Pacific Islander . . .	0.1	0.1	0.2	0.1	0.1
American Indian or Alaska Native	0.4	0.4	0.4	0.5	0.5
Hispanic or Latina[5].	16.0	15.5	16.0	15.4	14.4
Multiple Race.	0.9	1.5	1.4	1.5	1.3
Age at diagnosis:					
13–14 years.	0.3	0.4	0.5	0.5	0.3
15–24 years.	6.9	6.7	6.1	6.3	6.1
25–34 years.	32.7	23.6	23.2	21.9	22.9
35–44 years.	36.9	35.9	34.8	34.1	33.1
45–54 years.	16.4	24.3	25.3	25.7	26.3
55–64 years.	5.1	7.2	7.9	9.0	9.2
65 years and over	1.8	1.9	2.2	2.4	2.2
Children, under 13 years					
Hispanic origin and race:					
Not Hispanic or Latino:					
White.	17.2	7.5	8.2	14.5	17.2
Black or African American	61.8	73.2	75.8	74.8	61.1
Asian[4]	0.5	2.0	2.6	–	2.8
Native Hawaiian or Other Pacific Islander . . .	0.1	–	–	–	–
American Indian or Alaska Native	0.4	–	–	–	–
Hispanic or Latino[5].	19.2	15.4	10.7	10.7	10.3
Multiple Race.	0.7	1.9	2.6	2.6	8.6
Region of residence					
Northeast	30.6	25.0	25.2	24.8	22.6
Midwest	10.4	11.9	11.3	11.0	11.4
South.	38.7	46.1	45.9	46.2	47.0
West	20.3	17.0	17.7	18.0	19.0

See footnotes at end of table.

Table 45 (page 3 of 3). Acquired immunodeficiency syndrome (AIDS) diagnoses, by year of diagnosis and selected characteristics: United States, 2005–2008

[Data are based on reporting by 50 states and the District of Columbia]

– Quantity zero.

[1]Based on diagnoses reported to CDC from the beginning of the epidemic (1981) through June 30, 2009.

[2]Numbers are point estimates that result from statisitcal adjustments for reporting delays and missing risk factor information. The estimates do not include adjustments for incomplete reporting. See Appendix I, AIDS Surveillance.

[3]Total for all years includes 368 persons of unknown races and 1 person of unknown sex. All persons totals were calculated independent of values for subpopulations. Consequently, sums of subpopulations may not equal totals for all persons.

[4]Includes Asian and Pacific Islander legacy cases.

[5]Persons of Hispanic origin may be of any race. See Appendix II, Hispanic origin.

[6]Percents may not sum to 100% due to rounding and because persons of unknown race and Hispanic origin are included in totals.

NOTES: See Appendix II, Acquired immunodeficiency syndrome (AIDS), for discussion of AIDS diagnoses reporting definitions and other issues affecting interpretation of trends. Data are for the 50 states and the District of Columbia. This table replaces surveillance data by year of report in previous editions of *Health, United States*. Starting with HUS 2010, the title of this table was changed from AIDS cases to AIDS diagnoses to be consistent with language used by CDC.

SOURCE: CDC, National Center for HIV, STD, and TB Prevention, Division of HIV/AIDS Prevention—Surveillance and Epidemiology; Diagnoses of HIV infection and AIDS in the United States and Dependent Areas, 2008 (vol 20). Atlanta, GA: U.S. Department of Health and Human Services, CDC. 2010. Available from: http://www.cdc.gov/hiv/surveillance/resources/reports/2008report/index.htm.

Table 46 (page 1 of 5). Health conditions among children under 18 years of age, by selected characteristics: United States, average annual, selected years 1997–1999 through 2007–2009

[Data are based on household interviews of a sample of the civilian noninstitutionalized population]

Characteristic	Current asthma[1]				Asthma attack in the past 12 months[2]			
	1997–1999	2000–2002	2003–2005	2007–2009	1997–1999	2000–2002	2003–2005	2007–2009
	Percent of children							
Under 18 years[3].	- - -	- - -	8.7	9.4	5.4	5.7	5.4	5.4
Age								
0–4 years.	- - -	- - -	6.1	6.4	4.3	4.7	4.2	4.3
5–17 years.	- - -	- - -	9.6	10.6	5.7	6.1	5.8	5.9
5–9 years	- - -	- - -	9.1	10.2	5.6	6.3	6.1	6.2
10–17 years	- - -	- - -	9.9	10.8	5.8	5.9	5.7	5.7
Sex								
Male	- - -	- - -	9.9	10.8	6.2	6.6	6.3	6.2
Female	- - -	- - -	7.3	7.9	4.5	4.7	4.4	4.6
Race[4]								
White only	- - -	- - -	7.7	8.0	5.0	5.2	4.9	4.7
Black or African American only.	- - -	- - -	13.0	16.0	7.0	8.0	7.6	8.6
American Indian or Alaska Native only . . .	- - -	- - -	12.2	*10.8	6.4	*8.7	*6.1	*
Asian only	- - -	- - -	4.8	6.3	4.3	4.7	3.3	4.1
Native Hawaiian or Other Pacific Islander only.	- - -	- - -	*	*	- - -	*	*	*
2 or more races	- - -	- - -	13.5	13.9	- - -	7.3	8.8	9.3
Hispanic origin and race[4]								
Hispanic or Latino.	- - -	- - -	7.6	7.9	4.8	4.2	4.6	4.6
Not Hispanic or Latino.	- - -	- - -	8.9	9.8	5.5	6.0	5.6	5.7
White only.	- - -	- - -	7.9	8.2	5.1	5.5	5.0	4.8
Black or African American only	- - -	- - -	13.0	16.0	7.0	7.9	7.5	8.5
Percent of poverty level[5]								
Below 100%.	- - -	- - -	10.4	12.2	6.1	7.1	6.5	6.9
100%–199%.	- - -	- - -	8.6	9.8	5.3	5.4	5.2	5.7
200%–399%.	- - -	- - -	8.3	8.2	5.0	5.3	5.2	4.7
400% or more	- - -	- - -	7.9	8.4	5.2	5.5	4.9	5.0
Health insurance status at the time of interview[6]								
Insured	- - -	- - -	9.0	9.7	5.6	5.9	5.6	5.6
Private	- - -	- - -	8.0	8.4	5.0	5.3	5.0	5.1
Medicaid.	- - -	- - -	11.4	12.1	7.7	7.7	7.1	6.7
Uninsured	- - -	- - -	5.6	6.3	3.9	4.3	3.3	3.5

See footnotes at end of table.

Table 46 (page 2 of 5). **Health conditions among children under 18 years of age, by selected characteristics: United States, average annual, selected years 1997–1999 through 2007–2009**

[Data are based on household interviews of a sample of the civilian noninstitutionalized population]

Characteristic	Attention deficit hyperactivity disorder[7]				Serious emotional or behavioral difficulties[8]			
	1997–1999	2000–2002	2003–2005	2007–2009	1997–1999	2000–2002	2003–2005	2007–2009
Age	Percent of children							
5–17 years	6.5	7.5	7.6	9.0	- - -	- - -	5.1	5.5
5–9 years	4.8	5.2	5.6	5.8	- - -	- - -	4.3	4.7
10–17 years	7.6	9.0	8.9	10.9	- - -	- - -	5.6	6.0
Sex								
Male	9.6	10.8	10.7	12.3	- - -	- - -	6.1	6.9
Female	3.2	4.2	4.4	5.5	- - -	- - -	4.1	4.0
Race[4]								
White only	7.1	8.1	7.8	9.2	- - -	- - -	5.1	5.2
Black or African American only	5.0	7.0	7.7	9.3	- - -	- - -	5.3	6.6
American Indian or Alaska Native only	*8.5	*	*9.4	*	- - -	- - -	*	*
Asian only	*1.7	*	*1.6	*1.8	- - -	- - -	*1.7	*
Native Hawaiian or Other Pacific Islander only	- - -	*	*	*	- - -	- - -	*	*3.3
2 or more races	- - -	7.4	9.7	13.1	- - -	- - -	8.2	10.3
Hispanic origin and race[4]								
Hispanic or Latino	3.6	4.2	4.6	4.9	- - -	- - -	3.8	3.6
Not Hispanic or Latino	7.0	8.2	8.3	10.0	- - -	- - -	5.4	5.9
White only	7.7	9.0	8.8	10.6	- - -	- - -	5.6	5.8
Black or African American only	5.0	6.8	7.5	9.5	- - -	- - -	5.2	6.5
Percent of poverty level[5]								
Below 100%	7.2	8.2	8.4	10.3	- - -	- - -	7.4	8.7
100%–199%	6.7	7.5	7.8	10.6	- - -	- - -	5.4	6.9
200%–399%	6.2	7.7	7.8	8.1	- - -	- - -	4.9	4.6
400% or more	6.1	7.1	6.9	7.8	- - -	- - -	3.7	3.3
Health insurance status at the time of interview[6]								
Insured	6.7	7.8	7.8	9.3	- - -	- - -	5.2	5.6
Private	5.9	7.0	7.0	7.6	- - -	- - -	4.1	3.9
Medicaid	10.5	10.7	10.3	12.7	- - -	- - -	8.5	9.1
Uninsured	4.8	5.4	6.1	6.1	- - -	- - -	4.6	4.2

See footnotes at end of table.

Table 46 (page 3 of 5). Health conditions among children under 18 years of age, by selected characteristics: United States, average annual, selected years 1997–1999 through 2007–2009

[Data are based on household interviews of a sample of the civilian noninstitutionalized population]

Characteristic	Food allergy[9]				Skin allergy[10]			
	1997–1999	2000–2002	2003–2005	2007–2009	1997–1999	2000–2002	2003–2005	2007–2009
	Percent of children							
Under 18 years.	3.4	3.6	3.8	4.6	7.4	8.1	9.6	10.7
Age								
0–4 years.	3.8	4.0	4.3	5.0	8.1	8.7	11.0	12.4
5–17 years.	3.3	3.4	3.6	4.4	7.2	7.9	9.1	10.1
5–9 years.	3.1	3.6	3.5	4.6	7.5	8.6	10.0	11.4
10–17 years	3.4	3.3	3.6	4.3	7.1	7.5	8.6	9.3
Sex								
Male	3.4	3.7	3.8	4.6	7.3	7.9	9.5	10.6
Female	3.5	3.4	3.8	4.5	7.6	8.4	9.8	10.8
Race[4]								
White only	3.5	3.6	3.8	4.4	7.1	7.6	9.0	9.7
Black or African American only.	3.1	3.0	3.7	4.4	9.0	10.4	12.4	14.5
American Indian or Alaska Native only . . .	*	*4.8	*	*7.9	*4.1	*9.1	11.3	*9.8
Asian only	3.9	4.4	4.3	4.3	8.0	8.4	7.5	10.6
Native Hawaiian or Other Pacific								
Islander only.	- - -	*	*	*	- - -	*	*	*
2 or more races	- - -	5.2	4.6	5.7	- - -	10.9	14.0	15.7
Hispanic origin and race[4]								
Hispanic or Latino.	2.1	2.5	2.8	3.7	5.5	5.6	7.2	8.6
Not Hispanic or Latino.	3.7	3.8	4.0	4.8	7.8	8.7	10.2	11.3
White only.	3.8	3.9	4.1	4.7	7.5	8.2	9.7	10.2
Black or African American only	3.1	3.1	3.7	4.5	9.0	10.4	12.4	14.6
Percent of poverty level[5]								
Below 100%.	3.3	3.2	3.3	3.9	7.3	7.1	9.0	11.4
100%–199%.	3.0	3.4	3.8	4.4	7.2	7.6	8.7	10.1
200%–399%.	3.2	3.4	3.8	4.8	7.3	8.5	10.0	10.2
400% or more	4.2	4.0	4.1	5.0	7.9	8.8	10.5	11.4
Health insurance status at the time of interview[6]								
Insured	3.5	3.7	3.9	4.6	7.7	8.5	10.0	11.0
Private	3.5	3.7	4.0	4.8	7.4	8.5	10.1	10.7
Medicaid.	3.6	3.7	3.6	4.2	8.4	8.4	9.5	11.0
Uninsured	2.6	2.4	3.0	3.9	5.9	5.3	6.8	7.9

See footnotes at end of table.

Table 46 (page 4 of 5). Health conditions among children under 18 years of age, by selected characteristics: United States, average annual, selected years 1997–1999 through 2007–2009

[Data are based on household interviews of a sample of the civilian noninstitutionalized population]

Characteristic	Hay fever or respiratory allergy[11]				Three or more ear infections[12]			
	1997–1999	2000–2002	2003–2005	2007–2009	1997–1999	2000–2002	2003–2005	2007–2009
	Percent of children							
Under 18 years..................	17.5	17.7	17.3	16.6	7.1	6.7	5.8	5.5
Age								
0–4 years.......................	10.7	10.4	10.1	10.1	13.7	12.8	11.0	10.5
5–17 years......................	19.9	20.3	20.0	19.2	4.8	4.5	3.8	3.5
5–9 years.....................	17.3	18.1	17.9	17.3	7.1	6.9	5.7	5.6
10–17 years	21.6	21.7	21.2	20.4	3.2	2.9	2.7	2.2
Sex								
Male	18.6	18.8	18.9	18.1	7.3	6.9	5.9	5.6
Female	16.3	16.5	15.6	15.1	6.9	6.5	5.6	5.4
Race[4]								
White only....................	17.9	18.5	17.8	17.2	7.4	7.2	6.3	5.9
Black or African American only.........	16.2	15.6	15.2	14.2	5.9	5.0	4.1	3.8
American Indian or Alaska Native only ...	15.2	16.4	16.5	*13.0	*10.8	*6.3	*5.1	*7.6
Asian only	15.3	12.6	11.3	13.2	3.7	2.6	3.3	2.7
Native Hawaiian or Other Pacific Islander only..................	- - -	*	*	*	- - -	*	*	*
2 or more races	- - -	20.9	20.8	20.5	- - -	7.4	5.0	6.1
Hispanic origin and race[4]								
Hispanic or Latino..................	12.4	12.4	12.8	11.8	6.1	6.7	6.2	6.3
Not Hispanic or Latino..............	18.4	18.8	18.3	18.0	7.3	6.7	5.7	5.3
White only....................	19.1	19.9	19.4	19.1	7.7	7.3	6.3	5.8
Black or African American only	16.3	15.5	15.1	14.2	5.9	4.9	4.0	3.8
Percent of poverty level[5]								
Below 100%....................	14.3	14.0	14.2	13.7	8.3	7.9	6.7	7.1
100%–199%....................	15.4	15.6	16.0	14.6	7.1	6.8	5.7	5.9
200%–399%....................	18.5	18.1	17.7	16.8	6.8	6.5	5.6	4.9
400% or more	20.3	21.1	19.7	20.3	6.6	6.1	5.5	4.7
Health insurance status at the time of interview[6]								
Insured	18.0	18.3	17.7	16.9	7.3	6.9	5.8	5.7
Private	18.8	19.2	18.5	18.6	6.6	6.4	5.2	4.7
Medicaid.....................	15.0	16.0	16.1	13.9	10.2	8.7	7.4	7.4
Uninsured	14.3	12.6	13.5	13.9	5.9	4.9	5.4	3.8

See footnotes at end of table.

Table 46 (page 5 of 5). Health conditions among children under 18 years of age, by selected characteristics: United States, average annual, selected years 1997–1999 through 2007–2009

[Data are based on household interviews of a sample of the civilian noninstitutionalized population]

- - - Data not available.

*Estimates are considered unreliable. Data preceded by an asterisk have a relative standard error (RSE) of 20%–30%. Data not shown have an RSE greater than 30%.

[1]Based on parents responding "yes" to both of the questions, "Has a doctor or other health professional ever told you that your child had asthma?" and "Does your child still have asthma?"

[2]Based on parents responding "yes" to both questions, "Has a doctor or other health professional ever told you that your child had asthma?" and "During the past 12 months, did your child have an episode of asthma or an asthma attack?"

[3]Includes all other races not shown separately and unknown health insurance status.

[4]The race groups white, black, American Indian or Alaska Native, Asian, Native Hawaiian or Other Pacific Islander, and 2 or more races include persons of Hispanic and non-Hispanic origin. Persons of Hispanic origin may be of any race. Starting with 1999 data, race-specific estimates are tabulated according to the 1997 Revisions to the Standards for the Classification of Federal Data on Race and Ethnicity and are not strictly comparable with estimates for earlier years. The five single-race categories plus multiple-race categories shown in the table conform to the 1997 Standards. Starting with 1999 data, race-specific estimates are for persons who reported only one racial group; the category 2 or more races includes persons who reported more than one racial group. Prior to 1999, data were tabulated according to the 1977 Standards with four racial groups, and the Asian only category included Native Hawaiian or Other Pacific Islander. Estimates for single-race categories prior to 1999 included persons who reported one race or, if they reported more than one race, identified one race as best representing their race. Starting with 2003 data, race responses of other race and unspecified multiple race were treated as missing, and then race was imputed if these were the only race responses. Almost all persons with a race response of other race were of Hispanic origin. See Appendix II, Hispanic origin; Race.

[5]Percent of poverty level is based on family income and family size and composition using U.S. Census Bureau poverty thresholds. Missing family income data were imputed for 1997 and beyond. See Appendix II, Family income; Poverty; Table VII.

[6]Health insurance categories are mutually exclusive. Persons who reported both Medicaid and private coverage are classified as having private coverage. Starting with 1997 data, state-sponsored health plan coverage is included as Medicaid coverage. Starting with 1999 data, coverage by the Children's Health Insurance Program (CHIP) is included as Medicaid coverage. In addition to private and Medicaid, the insured category also includes military, other government, and Medicare coverage. Persons not covered by private insurance, Medicaid, CHIP, state-sponsored or other government-sponsored health plans, Medicare, or military plans are considered to have no health insurance coverage. Persons with only Indian Health Service coverage are considered to have no health insurance coverage. See Appendix II, Health insurance coverage.

[7]Based on parents responding "yes" to the question: "Has a doctor or health professional ever told you that your child had attention deficit hyperactivity disorder (ADHD) or attention deficit disorder (ADD)?"

[8]Based on parents responding "yes, definite" or "yes, severe" to the question, "Overall, do you think that [child] has difficulties in any of the following areas: emotions, concentration, behavior, or being able to get along with other people?"

[9]Based on parents responding "yes" to the question, "During the past 12 months, has your child had any kind of food or digestive allergy?"

[10]Based on parents responding "yes" to the question, "During the past 12 months, has your child had any eczema or any kind of skin allergy?"

[11]Based on parents responding "yes" to the question "During the past 12 months, has your child had hay fever?" or "yes" to the question, "During the past 12 months, has your child had any kind of respiratory allergy?"

[12]Based on parents responding "yes" to the question "During the past 12 months, has your child had three or more ear infections?"

NOTES: Answers to questions are supplied by the parents or knowledgable adult in the family. Standard errors are available in the spreadsheet version of this table. Available from: http://www.cdc.gov/nchs/hus.htm. Data for additional years are available. See Appendix III.

SOURCE: CDC/NCHS, National Health Interview Survey, sample child and family core questionnaire.

Table 47 (page 1 of 3). Age-adjusted cancer incidence rates for selected cancer sites, by sex, race, and Hispanic origin: United States, selected geographic areas, selected years 1990–2007

[Data are based on the Surveillance, Epidemiology, and End Results (SEER) Program's 13 population-based cancer registries]

Site, sex, race, and Hispanic origin	1990	1995	2000	2002	2003	2004	2005	2006	2007	1990–2007 APC[1]
All sites	Number of new cases per 100,000 population[2]									
All persons	475.5	470.6	473.3	470.0	457.9	457.7	450.3	446.3	446.7	⌃0.5
White	483.1	477.2	484.7	480.5	468.2	467.5	461.5	456.8	455.4	⌃0.5
Black or African American	512.5	534.2	518.1	516.1	502.7	504.3	483.6	474.6	470.0	⌃0.8
American Indian or Alaska Native[3]	346.2	367.6	357.5	346.1	366.5	392.2	387.8	371.1	332.0	0.1
Asian or Pacific Islander	333.9	336.2	335.1	340.0	328.2	331.0	323.6	317.0	322.2	⌃0.4
Hispanic or Latino[4]	354.4	356.0	354.5	357.7	342.1	349.9	344.2	327.9	326.5	⌃0.6
White, not Hispanic or Latino[4]	495.3	491.5	503.6	499.8	488.5	487.1	482.0	479.7	479.4	⌃0.3
Male	583.7	563.5	562.8	552.8	538.5	536.8	520.4	515.9	518.3	⌃1.0
White	590.8	563.0	567.6	558.0	543.0	542.3	528.1	521.8	523.1	⌃1.0
Black or African American	685.6	734.1	696.4	678.2	653.8	649.4	604.1	589.2	584.6	⌃1.5
American Indian or Alaska Native[3]	393.2	420.6	367.5	371.0	423.8	389.2	406.8	368.6	352.0	−0.7
Asian or Pacific Islander	384.9	394.1	392.1	381.1	378.1	374.3	359.7	356.2	355.4	⌃0.8
Hispanic or Latino[4]	414.9	435.5	424.9	422.6	399.8	410.7	394.5	373.7	373.8	⌃1.0
White, not Hispanic or Latino[4]	606.7	577.5	588.0	578.0	564.4	562.9	549.8	546.4	549.6	⌃0.9
Female	411.2	410.1	412.8	413.7	402.8	403.2	402.3	398.1	396.5	−0.2
White	421.2	423.2	429.7	428.4	417.8	416.4	416.5	412.2	408.4	−0.1
Black or African American	403.8	400.7	397.9	407.2	400.2	407.0	402.2	396.0	391.8	−0.1
American Indian or Alaska Native[3]	314.7	334.0	356.8	327.0	328.0	399.8	374.9	377.0	321.5	⌃0.8
Asian or Pacific Islander	293.9	293.8	295.8	314.5	295.6	303.8	301.5	292.9	302.3	0.1
Hispanic or Latina[4]	321.6	307.3	313.2	317.6	306.9	312.5	313.2	300.2	297.9	⌃0.3
White, not Hispanic or Latina[4]	430.8	437.2	446.6	446.6	436.7	434.5	435.5	433.3	429.5	0.1
Lung and bronchus										
Male	95.0	86.9	77.7	75.2	74.8	71.0	70.3	68.0	65.4	⌃2.1
White	94.2	85.0	76.3	74.6	73.8	69.8	69.7	66.8	64.9	⌃2.1
Black or African American	133.9	136.7	110.5	108.3	110.3	100.6	95.1	95.4	87.2	⌃2.6
Asian or Pacific Islander	64.2	60.0	63.2	57.1	57.6	58.5	56.5	55.5	52.4	⌃1.1
Hispanic or Latino[4]	59.4	52.5	44.8	48.0	44.5	38.9	41.2	36.2	38.0	⌃2.3
White, not Hispanic or Latino[4]	97.4	88.4	80.3	78.1	77.6	74.2	73.8	71.5	69.1	⌃1.9
Female	47.2	49.3	48.5	49.1	49.4	48.6	49.3	48.2	47.4	0.0
White	48.4	51.8	50.8	51.3	52.0	50.2	51.1	50.1	49.9	0.0
Black or African American	52.8	49.7	54.4	54.9	54.1	56.6	57.0	56.0	51.2	0.3
Asian or Pacific Islander	28.3	27.2	27.2	29.1	28.8	30.6	30.5	29.4	27.0	0.3
Hispanic or Latina[4]	26.3	24.9	24.0	24.5	24.3	25.5	22.9	22.1	22.5	⌃1.0
White, not Hispanic or Latina[4]	50.8	54.9	54.4	55.3	56.2	54.0	55.6	54.7	54.5	⌃0.3
Colon and rectum										
Male	72.2	63.2	62.5	59.6	57.7	55.9	53.4	51.7	50.7	⌃1.9
White	73.0	62.5	62.1	58.5	56.5	55.1	53.0	50.5	49.6	⌃2.0
Black or African American	72.7	74.3	72.7	70.9	74.4	72.3	63.8	62.3	61.2	⌃1.0
Asian or Pacific Islander	60.9	58.1	57.2	57.6	52.1	49.2	46.5	49.8	46.5	⌃1.4
Hispanic or Latino[4]	47.5	45.1	49.4	43.9	44.9	45.6	43.2	42.0	41.5	⌃0.9
White, not Hispanic or Latino[4]	75.1	64.1	63.6	60.1	57.9	56.2	54.2	51.7	50.7	⌃2.0
Female	50.2	45.9	46.0	44.9	43.1	41.7	40.7	40.4	39.0	⌃1.2
White	49.8	45.5	45.6	43.9	42.6	40.5	39.7	39.5	37.9	⌃1.3
Black or African American	61.0	54.8	57.6	55.5	54.3	53.1	52.3	52.2	50.1	⌃0.7
Asian or Pacific Islander	37.7	38.4	37.1	41.0	36.1	36.9	36.4	34.6	34.5	⌃0.8
Hispanic or Latina[4]	34.4	31.7	33.6	31.2	33.2	31.7	31.8	30.4	31.5	⌃0.4
White, not Hispanic or Latina[4]	50.9	46.8	46.9	45.5	43.7	41.7	40.9	40.8	38.8	⌃1.3
Prostate										
Male	166.7	166.0	178.0	176.2	163.5	162.8	149.7	157.6	158.3	⌃1.5
White	168.3	161.1	174.0	172.6	159.3	159.3	145.2	153.3	152.0	⌃1.7
Black or African American	218.3	274.8	286.4	276.1	247.3	244.0	228.1	224.5	227.4	⌃1.6
American Indian or Alaska Native[3]	98.4	92.6	66.8	88.1	105.3	84.4	83.0	82.7	77.9	⌃2.1
Asian or Pacific Islander	88.3	102.8	105.1	100.9	101.7	99.2	92.3	92.6	93.3	⌃1.0
Hispanic or Latino[4]	118.2	137.9	144.8	143.1	129.9	140.2	123.0	118.8	116.2	⌃1.1
White, not Hispanic or Latino[4]	172.2	163.8	178.4	176.8	163.8	162.3	148.7	159.0	158.7	⌃1.6
Breast										
Female	129.3	130.8	133.9	131.7	122.8	123.1	122.3	120.2	122.5	⌃0.4
White	134.2	136.4	140.8	137.8	127.7	127.4	127.4	124.3	125.5	−0.4
Black or African American	116.6	122.2	120.3	121.1	120.8	120.2	115.5	119.6	120.5	0.0
American Indian or Alaska Native[3]	68.0	94.5	95.8	79.4	91.1	100.2	102.3	81.3	83.4	0.2
Asian or Pacific Islander	87.3	86.5	92.9	99.3	90.3	95.6	93.0	91.8	98.0	⌃0.7
Hispanic or Latina[4]	89.8	87.7	94.3	88.3	83.4	86.5	88.1	85.5	83.8	−0.3
White, not Hispanic or Latina[4]	138.8	142.2	147.6	145.7	135.0	134.6	134.7	131.3	133.5	−0.3

See footnotes at end of table.

[Data are based on the Surveillance, Epidemiology, and End Results (SEER) Program's 13 population-based cancer registries]

Site, sex, race, and Hispanic origin	1990	1995	2000	2002	2003	2004	2005	2006	2007	1990–2007 APC[1]
Cervix uteri	Number of new cases per 100,000 population[2]									
Female	11.9	9.9	8.9	8.3	8.1	7.8	7.8	7.4	7.2	^−2.7
White	11.3	9.2	8.9	8.3	7.8	7.7	7.6	7.4	7.1	^−2.4
Black or African American	16.4	14.7	10.6	9.9	10.6	9.7	8.9	8.0	8.1	^−4.0
Asian or Pacific Islander	12.0	11.0	7.9	8.1	8.0	7.1	7.8	6.9	6.9	^−4.0
Hispanic or Latina[4]	21.4	17.7	16.9	14.3	13.7	12.7	13.5	11.3	10.1	^−3.8
White, not Hispanic or Latina[4]	9.7	7.8	7.1	7.0	6.5	6.6	6.3	6.6	6.4	^−2.3
Corpus uteri[5]										
Female	24.2	24.4	23.4	23.4	22.8	23.2	23.3	23.1	23.4	^−0.3
White	26.0	26.0	25.2	24.3	24.2	24.4	24.6	24.5	24.2	^−0.4
Black or African American	16.2	16.9	16.3	21.2	18.6	19.0	20.0	17.6	21.1	^1.4
Asian or Pacific Islander	12.9	17.1	16.2	18.5	16.3	18.7	18.5	17.7	18.8	^1.5
Hispanic or Latina[4]	17.3	15.9	15.2	16.8	16.7	18.1	18.1	16.6	16.8	0.3
White, not Hispanic or Latina[4]	26.7	27.1	26.5	25.3	25.3	25.2	25.5	25.7	25.4	^−0.3
Ovary										
Female	15.5	14.5	14.2	13.8	13.4	12.9	12.9	12.5	12.6	^−1.1
White	16.4	15.4	15.1	14.6	14.1	13.6	13.6	13.3	13.2	^−1.2
Black or African American	11.3	10.8	10.7	9.8	11.3	10.7	10.3	8.6	11.0	−0.5
Asian or Pacific Islander	11.2	10.4	10.1	12.0	10.0	9.9	10.7	10.4	10.1	−0.1
Hispanic or Latina[4]	12.3	11.7	10.7	13.6	11.3	11.7	11.4	10.4	10.2	−0.6
White, not Hispanic or Latina[4]	16.7	15.9	15.6	14.6	14.6	13.9	13.9	13.9	13.7	^−1.1
Oral cavity and pharynx										
Male	18.5	16.5	15.7	15.6	15.0	15.1	14.7	14.2	14.5	^−1.5
White	17.9	16.3	15.6	15.7	15.1	15.4	15.0	14.3	14.8	^−1.2
Black or African American	25.4	22.3	19.2	17.9	17.1	15.9	15.2	15.2	14.4	^−3.1
Asian or Pacific Islander	14.8	11.7	13.2	12.8	11.6	11.3	11.1	11.2	10.6	^−1.5
Hispanic or Latino[4]	10.8	12.1	8.9	9.1	8.4	9.9	9.3	7.1	8.1	^−2.2
White, not Hispanic or Latino[4]	18.7	16.9	16.6	16.8	16.2	16.4	16.0	15.6	16.2	^−0.9
Female	7.3	7.0	6.2	6.5	5.9	6.1	6.0	6.1	5.9	^−1.3
White	7.4	7.1	6.2	6.5	5.8	6.0	5.9	6.1	5.9	^−1.3
Black or African American	6.4	6.7	5.3	6.3	6.7	5.8	6.8	5.4	5.3	^−1.1
Asian or Pacific Islander	6.1	5.2	6.1	5.9	5.1	5.7	5.8	5.2	5.0	^−0.9
Hispanic or Latina[4]	4.1	3.7	3.7	3.7	3.6	3.6	3.4	3.7	3.8	^−1.3
White, not Hispanic or Latina[4]	7.8	7.6	6.6	7.1	6.2	6.5	6.4	6.5	6.4	^−1.1
Stomach										
Male	14.6	13.5	12.5	11.9	11.6	11.8	11.2	11.0	10.9	^−1.9
White	12.8	11.9	10.7	10.4	10.0	10.2	9.4	9.5	9.4	^−1.9
Black or African American	21.4	18.6	18.4	15.7	18.1	15.9	16.8	15.4	16.1	^−2.3
Asian or Pacific Islander	26.8	24.3	22.4	20.2	18.8	19.8	19.6	17.6	17.2	^−2.8
Hispanic or Latino[4]	20.2	19.5	16.0	15.9	15.5	16.1	14.7	14.0	15.9	^−2.2
White, not Hispanic or Latino[4]	12.1	11.0	10.0	9.6	9.1	9.3	8.6	8.6	8.3	^−2.2
Female	6.7	6.2	6.1	6.2	5.9	5.9	5.6	5.8	5.4	^−1.0
White	5.7	5.1	5.0	5.0	4.9	5.0	4.6	4.9	4.4	^−1.1
Black or African American	9.9	9.8	8.6	9.8	9.3	7.4	7.8	9.2	7.5	^−1.4
Asian or Pacific Islander	15.4	13.0	12.9	11.2	11.1	11.0	10.3	9.0	10.1	^−2.8
Hispanic or Latina[4]	10.8	11.1	10.8	10.6	9.9	10.1	10.1	9.6	9.2	^−0.7
White, not Hispanic or Latina[4]	5.1	4.5	4.2	4.2	4.1	4.1	3.7	4.1	3.5	^−1.9
Pancreas										
Male	13.0	12.7	12.8	12.7	12.4	13.3	13.4	13.3	13.1	0.2
White	12.7	12.4	12.6	12.9	12.2	13.1	13.2	13.4	13.1	^0.4
Black or African American	19.3	19.1	18.1	13.7	17.0	17.6	17.6	16.6	15.6	^−1.0
Asian or Pacific Islander	11.0	10.3	10.7	9.7	10.1	11.7	11.5	10.0	11.3	−0.4
Hispanic or Latino[4]	10.7	12.1	12.1	10.6	9.7	10.9	11.6	11.6	10.2	0.1
White, not Hispanic or Latino[4]	12.8	12.4	12.7	13.2	12.6	13.3	13.3	13.7	13.5	^0.5
Female	10.0	9.9	9.9	10.4	10.3	10.3	10.6	10.7	10.3	^0.3
White	9.8	9.6	9.6	10.1	10.1	10.1	10.4	10.3	10.1	^0.3
Black or African American	12.9	15.5	12.6	15.7	14.2	14.2	15.8	14.9	13.8	−0.3
Asian or Pacific Islander	9.9	8.1	9.2	8.8	8.1	8.9	7.8	9.5	8.2	0.4
Hispanic or Latina[4]	9.9	8.9	9.3	10.8	8.7	9.0	11.1	9.2	9.9	0.0
White, not Hispanic or Latina[4]	9.7	9.7	9.6	10.0	10.4	10.2	10.4	10.5	10.1	^0.4

See footnotes at end of table.

Table 47 (page 3 of 3). **Age-adjusted cancer incidence rates for selected cancer sites, by sex, race, and Hispanic origin: United States, selected geographic areas, selected years 1990–2007**

[Data are based on the Surveillance, Epidemiology, and End Results (SEER) Program's 13 population-based cancer registries]

Site, sex, race, and Hispanic origin	1990	1995	2000	2002	2003	2004	2005	2006	2007	1990–2007 APC[1]
Urinary bladder	Number of new cases per 100,000 population[2]									
Male	37.2	35.3	36.8	35.4	36.5	36.5	36.1	34.8	35.3	^−0.2
White	40.7	38.9	40.7	39.0	40.3	40.5	39.9	38.3	39.0	−0.2
Black or African American	19.6	19.2	20.1	20.4	22.4	22.0	21.6	18.5	20.1	0.1
Asian or Pacific Islander	15.4	16.4	16.5	19.0	17.3	16.8	16.5	17.9	16.8	^0.9
Hispanic or Latino[4]	21.9	17.4	19.7	19.7	18.9	17.9	18.2	18.3	17.3	^−0.7
White, not Hispanic or Latino[4]	42.4	41.1	43.2	41.5	43.1	43.5	42.8	41.1	42.3	0.0
Female	9.5	9.3	9.1	9.1	9.1	9.1	8.8	8.7	8.3	^−0.5
White	10.0	10.1	9.9	10.0	9.9	10.0	9.5	9.3	9.1	^−0.3
Black or African American	8.6	7.2	7.7	8.3	7.6	8.1	7.7	8.4	7.4	0.1
Asian or Pacific Islander	5.3	4.4	4.2	3.2	4.9	3.8	5.1	3.7	3.5	−0.8
Hispanic or Latina[4]	5.6	5.1	5.7	6.1	4.2	5.4	5.8	4.9	4.8	−0.6
White, not Hispanic or Latina[4]	10.4	10.6	10.4	10.6	10.8	10.6	10.1	10.0	9.7	−0.1
Non-Hodgkin's lymphoma										
Male	22.6	25.0	23.4	23.6	23.8	24.6	24.0	23.0	23.7	0.1
White	23.6	26.2	24.8	24.8	25.2	25.9	25.2	24.4	25.3	0.1
Black or African American	17.4	21.3	17.4	17.9	18.8	21.4	18.8	18.9	16.0	−0.1
Asian or Pacific Islander	16.7	16.4	15.9	16.1	16.1	16.1	17.5	14.7	15.5	−0.3
Hispanic or Latino[4]	17.3	20.9	20.0	19.7	18.5	20.6	18.3	17.4	18.8	−0.2
White, not Hispanic or Latino[4]	24.3	26.7	25.3	25.5	26.1	26.7	26.3	25.5	26.5	^0.3
Female	14.5	15.2	15.9	16.3	17.0	17.1	16.2	16.4	16.1	^0.9
White	15.4	15.9	16.8	17.3	17.8	18.0	17.3	17.5	17.0	^0.9
Black or African American	10.2	10.1	11.8	11.7	13.1	13.2	12.9	12.0	12.7	^1.8
Asian or Pacific Islander	9.1	11.9	11.3	12.2	12.6	12.0	9.5	10.7	11.1	0.6
Hispanic or Latina[4]	13.5	12.9	13.3	13.2	14.6	14.9	14.5	14.4	13.7	^0.7
White, not Hispanic or Latina[4]	15.6	16.2	17.3	17.9	18.3	18.5	17.7	18.1	17.7	^1.0
Leukemia										
Male	17.1	17.5	16.7	16.6	16.5	16.5	16.3	15.0	15.6	^−0.5
White	17.9	18.8	17.7	17.9	17.6	17.3	17.5	16.0	16.8	^−0.4
Black or African American	16.0	13.1	13.4	12.2	13.7	15.6	11.8	12.7	11.2	−0.7
Asian or Pacific Islander	8.5	10.0	10.3	9.2	10.2	10.0	8.9	8.3	8.8	−0.6
Hispanic or Latino[4]	12.1	14.5	12.4	12.0	11.2	12.0	12.3	11.8	10.3	−0.4
White, not Hispanic or Latino[4]	18.2	19.2	18.3	18.5	18.3	17.8	17.9	16.3	17.6	−0.3
Female	9.8	10.1	10.2	9.7	9.7	10.0	9.4	10.0	9.1	−0.2
White	10.3	10.8	10.8	10.5	10.2	10.5	9.9	10.7	9.7	−0.1
Black or African American	8.4	8.2	9.5	7.3	8.7	9.1	8.6	7.7	6.8	−0.5
Asian or Pacific Islander	5.8	6.3	6.3	6.3	6.3	6.4	6.2	6.3	5.8	−0.4
Hispanic or Latina[4]	8.5	8.1	7.5	8.4	6.8	8.7	7.8	8.4	7.2	−0.3
White, not Hispanic or Latina[4]	10.2	10.9	10.9	10.5	10.7	10.7	10.0	10.9	10.1	0.1

^ Annual percent change (APC) is significantly different from 0 (p < 0.05).
0.0 APC is greater than −0.05 but less than 0.05.
[1]APC has been calculated by fitting a linear regression model to the natural logarithm of the yearly rates from 1990–2007.
[2]Age-adjusted by 5-year age groups to the year 2000 U.S. standard population. Age-adjusted rates are based on at least 25 cases. See Appendix II, Age adjustment.
[3]Starting with *Health, United States, 2007*, estimates for American Indian or Alaska Native population are based on the Contract Health Service Delivery Area (CHSDA) counties within SEER areas. Estimates for American Indian or Alaska Native are not shown for some sites because of the small number of annual cases.
[4]Starting with *Health, United States, 2007*, Hispanic data exclude cases from Alaska. The race groups, white, black, Asian or Pacific Islander, and American Indian or Alaska Native, include persons of Hispanic and non-Hispanic origin. Persons of Hispanic origin may be of any race. The North American Association of Central Cancer Registries (NAACCR) Hispanic Identification Algorithm was used on a combination of variables to classify cases as Hispanic for analytic purposes. See the report, NAACCR Guideline for Enhancing Hispanic-Latino Identification, for more information; available from: http://seer.cancer.gov/seerstat/variables/seer/yr1973_2006/race_ethnicity/. See Appendix II, Hispanic origin.
[5]Includes corpus uteri only cases and not uterus, not elsewhere specified cases.

NOTES: See Appendix II, Incidence. Estimates are based on 13 SEER areas November 2009 submission and differ from published estimates based on 9 SEER areas or other submission dates. See Appendix I,Surveillance, Epidemiology, and End Results Program (SEER). The site variable distinguishes Kaposi Sarcoma and Mesothelioma as individual cancer sites. As a result, Kaposi Sarcoma and Mesothelioma cases do not contribute to other cancer sites. Data have been revised and differ from previous editions of *Health, United States*. Data for additional years are available. See Appendix III.

SOURCE: National Institutes of Health, National Cancer Institute, Surveillance, Epidemiology, and End Results (SEER) Program. Available from: http://www.seer.cancer.gov.

Table 48. Five-year relative cancer survival rates for selected cancer sites, by race and sex: United States, selected geographic areas, selected years 1975–1977 through 1999–2006

[Data are based on the Surveillance, Epidemiology, and End Results (SEER) Program's nine population-based cancer registries]

Sex and site	White					Black or African American				
	1975–1977	1981–1983	1987–1989	1996–1998	1999–2006	1975–1977	1981–1983	1987–1989	1996–1998	1999–2006
Both sexes					Percent of patients					
All sites	51.2	52.6	57.8	65.8	69.1	39.9	39.6	43.6	55.7	59.2
Oral cavity and pharynx.	54.8	54.9	56.6	61.1	64.7	36.3	31.9	34.3	36.6	45.4
Esophagus.	5.7	7.6	11.1	15.0	20.0	3.1	4.3	6.7	10.4	12.5
Stomach	14.8	16.9	19.2	21.1	25.6	16.3	17.2	20.0	23.6	26.2
Colon	51.9	56.6	61.8	64.1	67.2	46.6	49.7	53.2	54.7	55.4
Rectum	49.6	53.5	59.6	64.9	69.5	45.1	40.7	53.6	56.3	60.4
Pancreas.	2.6	2.8	3.4	4.4	5.8	2.3	3.7	5.9	3.6	4.9
Lung and bronchus.	12.8	13.9	13.8	15.5	16.8	11.6	11.7	11.2	12.7	13.2
Urinary bladder.	74.8	79.1	81.4	81.3	82.0	50.8	60.1	63.4	62.8	66.2
Non-Hodgkin's lymphoma . . .	48.5	52.7	52.8	61.2	70.5	49.1	50.6	47.4	54.5	60.0
Leukemia.	36.1	40.1	45.6	51.3	56.2	33.6	34.1	36.8	39.4	47.2
Male										
All sites	43.5	47.4	53.3	65.1	69.2	32.8	34.3	38.8	57.7	62.1
Oral cavity and pharynx.	54.3	53.6	54.4	60.1	64.4	29.8	26.3	30.0	31.7	40.1
Esophagus.	5.0	6.8	11.4	14.6	19.8	1.6	3.6	5.3	8.9	10.2
Stomach	13.8	16.0	16.1	19.1	23.5	16.4	16.8	17.2	20.9	24.1
Colon	51.3	57.3	62.5	64.2	67.8	45.6	46.0	51.5	56.0	54.4
Rectum	48.6	52.1	59.7	63.9	69.6	42.0	38.6	49.4	54.8	59.3
Pancreas.	2.7	2.3	3.2	5.0	5.8	2.7	4.0	5.5	3.3	3.5
Lung and bronchus.	11.5	12.2	12.5	13.6	14.5	10.8	10.5	11.0	11.1	11.8
Prostate gland	70.2	74.6	85.3	98.6	99.9	61.4	63.7	72.1	95.2	97.3
Urinary bladder.	75.9	80.1	83.4	82.4	82.8	57.0	65.4	68.1	66.0	70.3
Non-Hodgkin's lymphoma . . .	47.9	52.4	49.1	59.0	68.9	42.7	49.8	42.4	52.4	54.5
Leukemia.	35.2	39.9	47.6	51.1	56.5	30.5	33.4	35.0	40.2	48.3
Female										
All sites	58.0	57.5	62.1	66.4	69.0	47.3	45.6	48.9	53.4	55.9
Colon	52.4	55.9	61.1	64.0	66.6	47.0	52.3	54.5	53.6	56.2
Rectum	50.8	55.2	59.5	66.3	69.4	47.6	42.9	57.8	57.6	61.5
Pancreas.	2.3	3.2	3.5	3.8	5.8	2.0	3.3	6.1	3.7	6.0
Lung and bronchus.	16.0	17.0	15.8	17.7	19.4	14.1	15.1	11.5	15.2	15.0
Melanoma of skin	86.9	87.7	91.5	93.3	95.1	*	*	89.5	78.5	73.6
Breast	76.1	77.6	85.4	89.7	91.2	62.4	64.1	71.3	76.4	78.4
Cervix uteri	70.8	68.9	73.6	74.7	72.5	65.2	61.6	58.1	65.2	63.5
Corpus uteri[1]	89.4	83.9	85.7	87.0	87.0	62.0	54.3	59.1	64.0	62.8
Ovary	36.6	40.3	40.0	45.2	45.0	43.2	39.2	35.2	41.0	36.7
Non-Hodgkin's lymphoma . . .	49.1	53.0	57.3	63.9	72.3	56.3	51.5	53.5	57.5	66.4

* Data for population groups with fewer than 25 cases are not shown because estimates are considered unreliable.
[1]Includes corpus uteri only cases and not uterus, not elsewhere specified cases.

NOTES: Rates are based on followup of patients through 2007. The rate is the ratio of the observed survival rate for the patient group to the expected survival rate for persons in the general population similar to the patient group with respect to age, sex, race, and calendar year of observation. It estimates the chance of surviving the effects of cancer. The site variable distinguishes Kaposi Sarcoma and Mesothelioma as individual cancer sites. As a result, Kaposi Sarcoma and Mesothelioma cases are excluded from each of the sites shown except all sites combined. The race groups, white and black, include persons of Hispanic and non-Hispanic origin. Due to death certificate race-ethnicity classification and other methodological issues related to developing life tables, survival rates for race-ethnicity groups other than white and black are not calculated. Data have been revised and differ from previous editions of *Health, United States*. Data for additional years are available. See Appendix III.

SOURCE: National Institutes of Health, National Cancer Institute, Surveillance, Epidemiology, and End Results (SEER) Program. Available from: http://www.seer.cancer.gov.

Table 49 (page 1 of 2). Respondent-reported prevalence of heart disease, cancer, and stroke among adults 18 years of age and over, by selected characteristics: United States, average annual, selected years 1997–1998 through 2008–2009

[Data are based on household interviews of a sample of the civilian noninstitutionalized population]

Characteristic	Heart disease[1]				Cancer[2]				Stroke[3]			
	1997–1998	1999–2000	2005–2006	2008–2009	1997–1998	1999–2000	2005–2006	2008–2009	1997–1998	1999–2000	2005–2006	2008–2009
	Percent of persons											
18 years and over, age-adjusted[4,5]	12.0	11.1	11.2	11.5	4.9	5.1	5.7	5.9	2.3	2.2	2.5	2.7
18 years and over, crude[5]	11.6	10.9	11.4	11.8	4.8	4.9	5.7	6.1	2.2	2.1	2.5	2.8
Age												
18–44 years	4.6	4.3	4.0	4.5	1.7	1.7	1.8	1.6	0.4	0.4	0.4	0.6
18–24 years.	3.2	3.3	3.2	3.3	0.8	1.0	0.9	0.8	*	*	*	*
25–44 years.	5.0	4.6	4.2	4.9	2.0	1.9	2.2	1.9	0.4	0.5	0.5	0.7
45–64 years	13.5	12.6	12.9	12.7	5.4	5.2	6.0	6.7	2.3	2.0	2.3	2.7
45–54 years.	10.9	10.0	9.4	9.5	4.0	4.0	4.4	4.9	1.4	1.3	1.5	1.8
55–64 years.	17.4	16.6	17.8	16.8	7.4	7.2	8.2	9.2	3.8	3.1	3.5	3.8
65 years and over	31.8	29.6	31.2	31.7	14.1	15.2	17.1	17.7	8.1	8.1	9.2	9.2
65–74 years.	27.8	25.8	26.5	26.2	12.4	13.1	14.3	15.8	6.7	6.2	6.9	6.3
75 years and over	37.0	34.3	36.6	38.0	16.2	17.7	20.2	20.0	9.8	10.3	11.8	12.5
Sex[4]												
Male.	12.3	11.9	12.2	12.8	4.1	4.4	5.1	5.0	2.6	2.4	2.6	2.7
Female.	11.8	10.5	10.5	10.5	5.8	5.8	6.4	6.8	2.1	2.1	2.4	2.7
Sex and age												
Male:												
18–44 years.	3.7	3.6	3.3	4.4	0.8	0.8	0.8	0.7	0.3	0.3	0.4	0.5
45–54 years.	11.0	10.0	9.8	10.0	2.0	2.0	2.6	2.9	1.2	1.3	1.5	1.6
55–64 years.	18.7	19.7	20.5	18.8	5.8	5.9	6.8	7.0	4.6	3.7	3.9	4.4
65–74 years.	32.0	30.4	31.6	30.5	12.8	13.9	15.5	16.2	8.1	6.7	7.7	6.7
75 years and over	40.8	39.2	43.1	46.6	18.3	20.3	24.3	22.2	11.2	11.3	12.5	12.8
Female:												
18–44 years.	5.5	4.9	4.7	4.7	2.6	2.5	2.9	2.5	0.4	0.4	0.5	0.8
45–54 years.	10.8	9.9	9.1	9.0	6.0	5.9	6.2	6.8	1.5	1.4	1.4	2.1
55–64 years.	16.2	13.8	15.4	14.9	8.8	8.4	9.5	11.2	3.2	2.6	3.1	3.3
65–74 years.	24.5	22.0	22.2	22.6	12.1	12.5	13.3	15.6	5.5	5.8	6.3	6.0
75 years and over	34.6	31.2	32.4	32.3	14.9	16.1	17.6	18.5	9.0	9.6	11.5	12.3
Race[4,6]												
White only.	12.2	11.3	11.5	11.9	5.2	5.4	6.0	6.2	2.2	2.1	2.3	2.6
Black or African American only	11.4	10.6	10.1	10.7	3.5	3.5	3.9	4.3	3.3	3.5	4.0	3.7
American Indian or Alaska Native only. . .	18.6	14.7	15.9	10.2	*6.5	*5.7	*7.4	*5.4	*5.0	*5.4	*	*
Asian only.	6.9	6.3	6.8	5.7	2.4	*2.3	2.9	3.0	*1.2	*1.2	1.9	1.5
Native Hawaiian or Other Pacific Islander only	- - -	*	*	*	- - -	*	*	*	- - -	*	*	*
2 or more races.	- - -	17.0	14.2	16.4	- - -	*4.7	8.6	9.9	- - -	*4.0	*3.2	*3.4
Hispanic origin and race[4,6]												
Hispanic or Latino	8.7	8.0	8.0	8.4	2.9	3.0	3.5	3.6	2.1	1.9	2.1	2.3
Mexican.	7.5	7.4	7.5	8.4	3.0	2.8	3.1	3.3	2.5	2.0	2.5	2.5
Not Hispanic or Latino	12.2	11.4	11.6	11.9	5.1	5.2	5.9	6.1	2.3	2.2	2.5	2.7
White only	12.5	11.6	12.0	12.4	5.4	5.5	6.3	6.5	2.2	2.1	2.3	2.7
Black or African American only.	11.4	10.5	10.2	10.8	3.6	3.6	3.9	4.2	3.3	3.5	4.1	3.7
Education[7,8]												
No high school diploma or GED	15.1	13.8	14.2	14.5	5.3	5.5	5.7	6.1	3.9	3.8	4.1	4.5
High school diploma or GED.	12.8	11.9	12.6	12.7	5.5	5.8	6.4	6.4	2.5	2.5	2.9	3.3
Some college or more	12.7	12.0	11.9	12.4	6.0	5.9	6.9	7.1	2.1	1.9	2.3	2.5

See footnotes at end of table.

Table 49 (page 2 of 2). Respondent-reported prevalence of heart disease, cancer, and stroke among adults 18 years of age and over, by selected characteristics: United States, average annual, selected years 1997–1998 through 2008–2009

[Data are based on household interviews of a sample of the civilian noninstitutionalized population]

Characteristic	Heart disease[1]				Cancer[2]				Stroke[3]			
	1997–1998	1999–2000	2005–2006	2008–2009	1997–1998	1999–2000	2005–2006	2008–2009	1997–1998	1999–2000	2005–2006	2008–2009
Percent of poverty level[4,9]					Percent of persons							
Below 100%	15.3	13.6	14.6	14.1	4.9	4.9	5.3	6.2	4.3	3.7	4.1	4.4
100%–199%	13.2	12.0	12.5	13.2	4.8	5.3	5.7	6.0	3.1	3.2	3.2	3.6
200%–399%	11.5	11.0	11.0	11.6	4.9	5.1	5.5	5.5	2.1	2.1	2.4	2.7
400% or more	11.0	10.2	10.1	10.1	5.2	5.1	6.1	6.0	1.6	1.5	1.8	1.8
Hispanic origin and race and percent of poverty level[4,6,9]												
Hispanic or Latino:												
Below 100%	9.7	9.7	11.0	10.3	2.2	2.3	3.5	3.8	3.0	2.0	3.1	2.6
100%–199%	8.7	8.4	8.1	8.8	2.8	3.2	3.3	3.2	2.2	2.2	1.8	2.6
200%–399%	8.4	8.2	6.9	7.7	2.7	2.7	3.6	3.3	*1.8	*2.3	*2.0	2.4
400% or more	8.4	5.6	5.1	7.1	*5.5	*4.5	*3.4	4.2	*	*	*	*
Not Hispanic or Latino:												
White only:												
Below 100%	17.8	15.2	16.9	15.9	6.3	6.2	6.9	8.1	4.4	3.8	4.1	4.4
100%–199%	14.1	12.8	14.3	15.6	5.6	6.2	6.7	7.4	3.2	3.0	3.2	4.0
200%–399%	12.2	11.6	11.9	12.8	5.2	5.5	6.0	6.1	2.1	2.1	2.3	2.8
400% or more	11.3	10.6	10.6	10.6	5.4	5.3	6.5	6.2	1.6	1.5	1.8	1.8
Black or African American only:												
Below 100%	14.6	13.0	13.2	15.2	4.4	4.0	3.6	4.9	5.0	4.5	5.3	6.4
100%–199%	12.9	11.2	10.7	10.9	3.3	3.2	4.3	3.6	4.2	5.1	4.6	4.0
200%–399%	9.2	10.2	9.1	9.3	3.2	3.7	4.2	4.0	2.5	2.7	4.1	2.8
400% or more	9.5	8.9	8.5	8.9	4.0	4.3	3.6	5.0	*	*	*2.6	*2.5
Geographic region[4]												
Northeast	11.6	10.6	11.0	11.1	4.5	5.0	5.6	6.2	1.8	1.8	1.9	2.3
Midwest	12.1	11.4	12.3	12.4	5.1	5.2	5.7	5.8	2.3	2.2	2.5	2.6
South	12.5	11.5	11.5	12.3	5.0	5.0	5.6	5.9	2.6	2.5	2.9	3.2
West	11.1	10.4	9.8	9.7	5.1	5.0	5.7	5.6	2.1	2.0	2.1	2.2
Location of residence[4,10]												
Within MSA	11.7	10.7	10.9	11.2	4.9	5.0	5.6	5.7	2.2	2.1	2.4	2.6
Outside MSA	12.8	12.5	13.0	13.1	5.1	5.5	6.0	7.0	2.7	2.5	2.9	3.0

* Estimates are considered unreliable. Data preceded by an asterisk have a relative standard error (RSE) of 20%–30%. Data not shown have an RSE greater than 30%.

- - - Data not available.

[1]Heart disease is based on self-reported responses to questions about whether respondents had ever been told by a doctor or other health professional that they had coronary heart disease, angina (angina pectoris), a heart attack (myocardial infarction), or any other kind or heart disease or heart condition.

[2]Cancer is based on self-reported responses to a question about whether respondents had ever been told by a doctor or other health professional that they had cancer or a malignancy of any kind. Excludes squamous cell and basal cell carcinomas.

[3]Stroke is based on self-reported responses to a question about whether respondents had ever been told by a doctor or other health professional that they had a stroke.

[4]Estimates are age-adjusted to the year 2000 standard population using five age groups: 18–44 years, 45–54 years, 55–64 years, 65–74 years, and 75 years and over. Age-adjusted estimates in this table may differ from other age-adjusted estimates based on the same data and presented elsewhere if different age groups are used in the adjustment procedure. See Appendix II, Age adjustment.

[5]Includes all other races not shown separately and unknown education level.

[6]The race groups white, black, American Indian or Alaska Native, Asian, Native Hawaiian or Other Pacific Islander, and 2 or more races include persons of Hispanic and non-Hispanic origin. Persons of Hispanic origin may be of any race. Starting with 1999 data, race-specific estimates are tabulated according to the 1997 Revisions to the Standards for the Classification of Federal Data on Race and Ethnicity and are not strictly comparable with estimates for earlier years. The five single-race categories plus multiple-race categories shown in the table conform to the 1997 Standards. Starting with 1999 data, race-specific estimates are for persons who reported only one racial group; the category 2 or more races includes persons who reported more than one racial group. Prior to 1999, data were tabulated according to the 1977 Standards with four racial groups and the Asian only category included Native Hawaiian or Other Pacific Islander. Estimates for single-race categories prior to 1999 included persons who reported one race or, if they reported more than one race, identified one race as best representing their race. Starting with 2003 data, race responses of other race and unspecified multiple race were treated as missing, and then race was imputed if these were the only race responses. Almost all persons with a race response of other race were of Hispanic origin. See Appendix II, Hispanic origin; Race.

[7]Estimates are for persons 25 years of age and over and are age-adjusted to the year 2000 standard population using five age groups: 25–44 years, 45–54 years, 55–64 years, 65–74 years, and 75 years and over. See Appendix II, Age adjustment.

[8]GED is General Educational Development high school equivalency diploma. See Appendix II, Education.

[9]Percent of poverty level is based on family income and family size and composition using U.S. Census Bureau poverty thresholds. Missing family income data were imputed for 1997–1998 and beyond. See Appendix II, Family income; Poverty; Table VII.

[10]MSA is metropolitan statistical area. Starting with 2006 data, MSA status is determined using 2000 census data and the 2000 standards for defining MSAs. For data prior to 2006, see Appendix II, Metropolitan statistical area (MSA) for the applicable standards.

NOTES: Standard errors are available in the spreadsheet version of this table. Available from: http://www.cdc.gov/nchs/hus.htm. Data for additional years are available. See Appendix III.

SOURCE: CDC/NCHS, National Health Interview Survey, family core and sample adult questionnaires.

Table 50. Diabetes among adults 20 years of age and over, by sex, age, and race and Hispanic origin: United States, selected years 1988–1994 through 2005–2008

[Data are based on interviews and physical examinations of a sample of the civilian noninstitutionalized population]

Sex, age, and race and Hispanic origin[3]	Physician-diagnosed and undiagnosed diabetes[1,2]			Physician-diagnosed diabetes[1]			Undiagnosed diabetes[2]		
	1988–1994	1999–2002	2005–2008	1988–1994	1999–2002	2005–2008	1988–1994	1999–2002	2005–2008
20 years and over, age-adjusted[4]	Percent of population								
All persons[5]	9.1	9.8	10.9	5.5	6.6	7.9	3.6	3.2	3.0
Male	9.6	10.8	11.7	5.5	7.0	7.7	4.1	3.8	4.0
Female	8.7	8.8	10.2	5.6	6.2	8.0	3.1	2.6	2.2
Not Hispanic or Latino:									
White only	8.0	8.3	9.2	5.1	5.3	6.5	2.9	3.0	2.6
Black or African American only	16.0	16.3	19.9	8.8	11.9	14.4	7.2	4.4	5.5
Mexican	14.9	13.2	16.9	9.8	10.1	11.8	5.0	*3.1	5.1
Percent of poverty level:[6]									
Below 100%	14.2	14.5	15.7	8.8	9.1	12.1	5.4	5.4	*3.7
100%–199%	10.9	12.6	14.9	6.6	9.0	10.3	4.3	*3.6	4.6
200%–399%	8.4	10.0	10.2	4.8	6.8	7.3	3.6	3.2	*2.9
400% or more	6.8	5.9	7.7	4.3	3.6	5.5	2.6	2.3	*2.2
20 years and over, crude									
All persons[5]	8.4	9.7	11.3	5.1	6.5	8.2	3.3	3.2	3.1
Male	8.6	10.4	11.7	4.8	6.7	7.8	3.7	3.7	3.9
Female	8.3	9.0	10.8	5.4	6.3	8.5	3.0	2.7	2.3
Not Hispanic or Latino:									
White only	7.8	8.7	10.2	5.0	5.5	7.2	2.8	3.2	2.9
Black or African American only	12.9	14.1	18.6	6.9	10.1	13.6	6.0	4.0	5.0
Mexican	9.7	8.5	11.9	5.6	6.5	8.1	4.1	1.9	3.7
Percent of poverty level:[6]									
Below 100%	11.3	13.0	13.6	7.0	8.1	10.3	4.3	4.9	*3.4
100%–199%	10.1	12.6	16.3	6.4	9.1	11.3	3.8	*3.5	5.0
200%–399%	7.3	9.6	10.6	4.3	6.5	7.5	3.1	*3.1	*3.1
400% or more	6.5	6.0	7.9	4.1	3.7	5.6	*2.4	2.2	2.2
Age									
20–44 years	2.6	3.4	3.7	1.6	2.3	2.7	*1.0	*	*1.0
45–64 years	13.9	13.0	13.7	7.9	8.5	10.5	6.0	4.5	3.2
65 years and over	19.6	22.4	26.9	12.9	15.8	18.4	6.7	6.6	8.6

* Estimates are considered unreliable. Data preceded by an asterisk have a relative standard error (RSE) of 20%–30%. Data not shown have an RSE greater than 30%.

[1]Physician-diagnosed diabetes was obtained by self-report and excludes women who reported having diabetes only during pregnancy.

[2]Undiagnosed diabetes is defined as a fasting blood glucose (FBG) of at least 126 mg/dL or a hemoglobin A1c of at least 6.5% and no reported physician diagnosis. Respondents had fasted for at least 8 hours and less than 24 hours. Estimates in some prior editions of Health, United States included data from respondents who had fasted for at least 9 hours and less than 24 hours. In 2005–2006 and 2007–2008, testing was performed at a different laboratory and using different instruments than testing in earlier years. National Health and Nutrition Examination Survey (NHANES) conducted a crossover study to evaluate the impact of these changes on FBG and A1c measurements. As a result of that study, NHANES recommended that 2005–2008 data on FBG and A1c measurements be adjusted to be compatible with earlier years. Undiagnosed diabetes estimates in Health, United States were produced after adjusting the 2005–2008 laboratory data as recommended. For more information, see http://www.cdc.gov/nchs/nhanes/nhanes2007-2008/Glu_E.htm. The definition of undiagnosed diabetes in previous editions of Health, United States did not consider hemoglobin A1c. The revised definition of undiagnosed diabetes was based on recommendations from the American Diabetes Association. For more information, see Standards of medical care in diabetes—2010. Diabetes Care 2010;33(suppl 1):S11-S61. Also see Appendix II, Diabetes.

[3]Persons of Mexican origin may be of any race. Starting with 1999 data, race-specific estimates are tabulated according to the 1997 Revisions to the Standards for the Classification of Federal Data on Race and Ethnicity and are not strictly comparable with estimates for earlier years. The two non-Hispanic race categories shown in the table conform to the 1997 Standards. Starting with 1999 data, race-specific estimates are for persons who reported only one racial group. Prior to data year 1999, estimates were tabulated according to the 1977 Standards. Estimates for single-race categories prior to 1999 included persons who reported one race or, if they reported more than one race, identified one race as best representing their race. See Appendix II, Hispanic origin; Race.

[4]Estimates are age-adjusted to the year 2000 standard population using three age groups: 20–44 years, 45–64 years, and 65 years and over. Age-adjusted estimates in this table may differ from other age-adjusted estimates based on the same data and presented elsewhere if different age groups are used in the adjustment procedure. See Appendix II, Age adjustment.

[5]Includes all other races and Hispanic origins not shown separately.

[6]Percent of poverty level is based on family income and family size. Persons with unknown percent of poverty level are excluded (5% in 2005–2008). See Appendix II, Family income; Poverty.

NOTES: Standard errors are available in the spreadsheet version of this table. Available from: http://www.cdc.gov/nchs/hus.htm. Starting with Health, United States, 2007, data use a revised weighting scheme. The definition of undiagnosed diabetes has been revised and differs from that used in previous editions of Health, United States. Data for additional years are available. See Appendix III.

SOURCE: CDC/NCHS, National Health and Nutrition Examination Survey.

Table 51 (page 1 of 2). Incidence and prevalence of end-stage renal disease, by selected characteristics: United States, selected years 1980–2007

[Data are based on the Centers for Medicare & Medicaid Services' Renal Beneficiary and Utilization System]

Characteristic	Incidence					Prevalence				
	1980	1990	2000	2006	2007	1980	1990	2000	2006	2007
	Number of new patients					Number of patients alive on December 31				
Total	17,335	49,758	92,036	108,967	108,891	58,220	182,541	383,605	494,695	514,642
Age										
Under 20 years	736	1,049	1,173	1,240	1,245	2,365	4,482	6,288	7,089	7,209
20–44 years.	4,701	10,348	12,802	13,671	13,504	20,189	57,118	87,795	93,804	94,938
45–64 years.	6,949	17,154	32,116	40,888	41,239	23,670	67,065	156,609	217,987	228,434
65–74 years.	3,644	13,338	23,335	25,110	24,986	9,206	35,572	76,178	97,350	102,627
75 years and over	1,305	7,869	22,610	28,058	27,917	2,790	18,304	56,735	78,465	81,434
Sex										
Male	9,658	26,670	49,148	60,825	61,001	32,161	98,400	209,379	276,717	288,933
Female	7,677	23,088	42,888	48,142	47,890	26,059	84,141	174,226	217,978	225,709
Race[1]										
White	12,293	33,134	61,033	71,961	71,453	41,015	118,483	236,899	305,150	316,576
Black or African American	4,814	14,829	26,660	31,220	31,357	16,431	57,356	126,116	159,688	166,076
American Indian or Alaska Native. . .	124	599	1,201	1,203	1,235	374	2,175	5,390	6,742	7,012
Asian or Pacific Islander	104	1,196	3,142	4,583	4,846	400	4,527	15,200	23,115	24,978
Hispanic origin[1,2]										
Hispanic	- - -	- - -	10,721	13,418	13,678	- - -	- - -	42,390	64,663	69,719
Not Hispanic[3].	- - -	- - -	81,315	95,549	95,213	- - -	- - -	341,215	430,032	444,923
Primary diagnosis										
Diabetes	2,590	17,707	41,097	48,284	47,778	5,580	46,938	135,939	184,034	192,388
Hypertension	3,093	15,195	24,669	29,533	30,402	9,422	47,221	94,598	120,828	125,953
Glomerulonephritis	2,724	6,909	8,425	7,871	7,436	13,343	39,672	67,601	78,266	79,592
Cystic kidney	757	1,551	2,135	2,629	2,601	3,624	9,967	17,855	23,345	24,447
Other urologic	460	1,261	2,671	1,638	1,519	1,587	6,094	11,671	13,096	12,844
Other cause.	1,783	4,796	8,910	13,635	13,993	6,549	21,378	39,221	52,452	55,601
Unknown cause	1,513	1,863	3,678	4,809	4,600	5,856	8,236	13,984	19,132	20,097
Missing disease	4,415	476	451	568	562	12,259	3,035	2,736	3,542	3,720

See footnotes at end of table.

Table 51 (page 2 of 2). Incidence and prevalence of end-stage renal disease, by selected characteristics: United States, selected years 1980–2007

[Data are based on the Centers for Medicare & Medicaid Services' Renal Beneficiary and Utilization System]

Characteristic	Incidence					Prevalence				
	1980	1990	2000	2006	2007	1980	1990	2000	2006	2007
	New patients per million population					Patients alive on December 31 per million population				
Total	76.3	199.3	326.1	364.7	361.0	254.9	726.4	1,352.4	1,648.0	1,698.2
Age										
Under 20 years	10.2	14.6	14.6	15.1	15.1	32.7	62.1	78.0	86.3	87.3
20–44 years.	55.6	103.3	122.9	130.5	128.9	236.3	565.7	841.2	895.4	905.8
45–64 years.	156.2	370.4	514.6	546.8	538.5	530.6	1,439.6	2,469.8	2,880.2	2,948.0
65–74 years.	232.8	736.7	1,270.3	1,327.9	1,291.1	583.4	1,954.6	4,152.3	5,088.6	5,243.2
75 years and over	129.8	598.7	1,353.2	1,529.6	1,506.1	273.4	1,373.1	3,365.5	4,255.3	4,370.6
Sex										
Male	87.5	219.1	354.9	413.3	410.3	289.7	802.8	1,503.7	1,870.9	1,933.9
Female	65.7	180.5	298.4	317.6	313.1	221.9	653.6	1,206.5	1,431.4	1,469.0
Race[1]										
White	63.0	158.3	264.7	297.8	293.3	209.3	562.9	1,022.9	1,257.7	1,294.6
Black or African American	179.7	483.8	725.9	789.9	783.4	608.9	1,852.0	3,411.3	4,014.7	4,122.8
American Indian or Alaska Native. . .	86.7	291.0	404.6	376.4	381.7	255.7	1,039.3	1,804.1	2,096.6	2,153.8
Asian or Pacific Islander	27.1	158.4	264.5	319.1	328.0	99.6	583.9	1,256.4	1,586.7	1,667.5
Hispanic origin[1,2]										
Hispanic	- - -	- - -	300.7	304.6	300.6	- - -	- - -	1,165.9	1,444.0	1,508.1
Not Hispanic[3].	- - -	- - -	329.8	375.1	371.8	- - -	- - -	1,379.8	1,683.7	1,732.4
Primary diagnosis										
Diabetes	11.4	70.9	145.6	161.6	158.4	24.4	186.8	479.2	613.1	634.8
Hypertension	13.6	60.9	87.4	98.9	100.8	41.3	187.9	333.5	402.5	415.6
Glomerulonephritis	12.0	27.7	29.9	26.4	24.7	58.4	157.9	238.3	260.7	262.6
Cystic kidney	3.3	6.2	7.6	8.8	8.6	15.9	39.7	63.0	77.8	80.7
Other urologic	2.0	5.1	9.5	5.5	5.0	7.0	24.3	41.2	43.6	42.4
Other cause.	7.9	19.2	31.6	45.6	46.4	28.7	85.1	138.3	174.7	183.5
Unknown cause	6.7	7.5	13.0	16.1	15.3	25.6	32.8	49.3	63.7	66.3
Missing disease	19.4	1.9	1.6	1.9	1.9	53.7	12.1	9.7	11.8	12.3

- - - Data not available.

[1]The race groups, white, black or African American, American Indian or Alaska Native, and Asian or Pacific Islander, include persons of Hispanic and non-Hispanic origin. Persons of Hispanic origin may be of any race. See Appendix II, Hispanic origin; Race.
[2]Centers for Medicare & Medicaid Services began collecting Hispanic ethnicity data in April 1995.
[3]Not Hispanic includes unknown ethnicity.

NOTES: Persons with unknown age, gender, or race are excluded. For incidence estimates, age is determined as of the date of diagnosis with end-stage renal disease (ESRD). For prevalence estimates, age is calculated as of December 31 of each year. Prevalence estimates include patients with a functioning transplant. See Appendix I, United States Renal Data System (USRDS). See Appendix II, End-stage renal disease; Incidence; Prevalence. Data for additional years are available. See Appendix III.

SOURCE: United States Renal Data System, USRDS 2009 Annual data report: Atlas of chronic kidney disease and end-stage renal disease in the United States, National Institutes of Health, National Institute of Diabetes and Digestive and Kidney Diseases, Bethesda, MD, 2009. Available from: http://www.usrds.org/reference.htm.

Table 52 (page 1 of 3). Severe headache or migraine, low back pain, and neck pain among adults 18 years of age and over, by selected characteristics: United States, selected years 1997–2009

[Data are based on household interviews of a sample of the civilian noninstitutionalized population]

Characteristic	Severe headache or migraine[1]			Low back pain[1]			Neck pain[1]		
	1997	2008	2009	1997	2008	2009	1997	2008	2009
	Percent of adults with pain during past 3 months								
18 years and over, age-adjusted[2,3]	15.8	13.6	16.1	28.2	27.2	28.1	14.7	13.8	15.1
18 years and over, crude[3]	16.0	13.4	15.8	28.1	27.4	28.5	14.6	14.0	15.4
Age									
18–44 years	18.7	16.6	19.7	26.1	24.5	24.5	13.3	12.7	13.0
18–24 years	18.7	16.3	17.0	21.9	20.7	18.1	9.8	8.8	8.4
25–44 years	18.7	16.7	20.6	27.3	25.9	26.7	14.3	14.1	14.6
45–64 years	15.8	13.3	15.0	31.3	29.5	32.6	17.0	16.5	19.1
45–54 years	17.8	15.4	17.2	31.3	29.3	31.9	17.3	16.7	19.6
55–64 years	12.7	10.5	12.2	31.2	29.7	33.4	16.6	16.3	18.6
65 years and over	7.0	4.4	6.3	29.5	31.7	31.8	15.0	12.6	14.6
65–74 years	8.2	5.7	6.9	30.2	32.1	30.1	15.0	13.2	15.2
75 years and over	5.4	3.0	5.6	28.6	31.3	33.9	15.0	11.9	13.7
Sex[2]									
Male	9.9	8.1	10.1	26.5	25.0	26.0	12.6	11.2	12.6
Female	21.4	18.9	21.9	29.6	29.3	30.1	16.6	16.2	17.5
Sex and age									
Male:									
18–44 years	11.9	9.5	11.8	24.8	22.3	22.2	11.6	10.0	10.5
45–54 years	10.3	9.7	11.5	29.4	28.8	31.8	13.9	13.9	17.1
55–64 years	8.8	6.9	8.4	30.7	27.5	30.9	14.6	13.5	15.5
65–74 years	5.0	3.4	4.8	29.0	28.3	26.3	13.6	11.2	11.8
75 years and over	*2.4	*2.0	3.4	22.5	27.4	30.6	12.6	9.8	13.6
Female:									
18–44 years	25.4	23.6	27.5	27.3	26.8	26.7	14.9	15.3	15.5
45–54 years	24.9	20.8	22.8	33.1	29.8	32.1	20.6	19.3	22.0
55–64 years	16.3	14.0	15.7	31.7	31.8	35.8	18.4	18.9	21.4
65–74 years	10.7	7.6	8.6	31.1	35.3	33.3	16.1	14.9	18.2
75 years and over	7.4	3.7	7.0	32.4	33.8	36.2	16.5	13.3	13.9
Race[2,4]									
White only	15.9	14.0	16.3	28.7	28.1	28.8	15.1	14.5	15.7
Black or African American only	16.7	12.7	17.0	26.9	23.6	26.6	13.3	10.4	12.9
American Indian or Alaska Native only	18.9	16.0	21.8	33.3	31.5	30.5	16.2	16.8	19.0
Asian only	11.7	7.7	8.4	21.0	17.7	17.8	9.2	9.0	8.5
Native Hawaiian or Other Pacific Islander only	- - -	*	*	- - -	*	*	- - -	*	*
2 or more races	- - -	20.3	21.0	- - -	39.4	36.2	- - -	23.5	19.7
Hispanic origin and race[2,4]									
Hispanic or Latino	15.5	12.5	16.4	26.4	25.3	26.3	13.9	14.4	15.1
Mexican	14.6	12.6	15.9	25.2	22.8	22.9	12.9	13.0	14.1
Not Hispanic or Latino	15.9	13.9	16.2	28.4	27.6	28.5	14.9	13.9	15.3
White only	16.1	14.5	16.6	29.1	28.9	29.4	15.4	14.8	16.1
Black or African American only	16.8	12.3	16.9	26.9	23.3	26.6	13.3	10.2	12.9
Education[5,6]									
25 years and over:									
No high school diploma or GED	19.2	16.5	19.9	33.6	32.0	35.0	16.5	16.4	18.4
High school diploma or GED	16.0	13.5	16.2	30.2	30.5	32.2	15.5	14.9	16.9
Some college or more	13.8	12.4	14.9	26.9	26.4	27.4	14.6	14.0	15.3

See footnotes at end of table.

Table 52 (page 2 of 3). Severe headache or migraine, low back pain, and neck pain among adults 18 years of age and over, by selected characteristics: United States, selected years 1997–2009

[Data are based on household interviews of a sample of the civilian noninstitutionalized population]

Characteristic	Severe headache or migraine[1]			Low back pain[1]			Neck pain[1]		
	1997	2008	2009	1997	2008	2009	1997	2008	2009
Percent of poverty level[2,7]	Percent of adults with pain during the past 3 months								
Below 100%	23.3	19.5	22.0	35.4	32.4	35.4	18.6	17.6	20.8
100%–199%	18.9	16.5	19.5	30.8	32.1	32.7	16.1	15.8	17.0
200%–399%	15.5	12.7	16.3	27.9	26.4	28.4	14.8	13.7	14.7
400% or more	12.4	11.4	12.5	24.8	24.8	23.9	12.8	12.3	13.1
Hispanic origin and race and percent of poverty level[2,4,7]									
Hispanic or Latino:									
Below 100%	18.9	16.9	19.4	29.5	32.9	31.3	16.4	18.3	19.4
100%–199%	15.7	13.3	17.6	26.8	26.3	25.3	12.9	15.1	15.0
200%–399%	14.0	11.4	16.1	25.0	21.1	26.1	13.8	13.5	14.3
400% or more	13.0	9.8	11.0	21.6	24.6	23.9	12.1	12.6	11.2
Not Hispanic or Latino:									
White only:									
Below 100%	26.1	23.3	23.2	38.9	36.3	39.1	20.5	20.2	23.4
100%–199%	20.4	19.0	21.9	33.3	36.9	36.3	18.0	18.2	19.0
200%–399%	16.3	13.6	17.4	29.1	29.0	30.4	15.9	15.1	16.4
400% or more	12.5	12.1	13.0	25.4	25.5	24.9	13.1	12.9	13.7
Black or African American only:									
Below 100%	22.7	16.7	23.0	34.5	26.2	33.3	17.9	13.0	17.7
100%–199%	17.6	15.4	18.8	27.7	26.8	32.4	14.0	11.2	14.7
200%–399%	14.0	11.0	13.9	24.3	21.4	22.6	10.2	8.4	9.8
400% or more	12.9	7.5	13.1	21.5	20.9	19.9	11.9	9.8	10.7
Disability measure[2,8]									
Any basic actions difficulty or complex activity limitation	29.3	26.5	30.0	48.0	46.3	50.1	27.2	25.0	29.4
Any basic actions difficulty	30.0	27.6	31.0	49.3	47.6	51.6	27.9	25.8	30.2
Any complex activity limitation	34.6	30.6	33.5	55.1	52.9	55.0	33.1	29.5	34.4
No disability	11.0	9.2	11.3	19.4	19.1	18.6	9.1	9.2	9.2
Geographic region[2]									
Northeast	14.5	13.4	14.7	27.1	27.4	27.7	14.0	13.8	14.6
Midwest	15.6	14.1	16.3	28.7	27.4	29.2	15.3	12.9	15.5
South	17.1	14.0	17.0	27.5	26.8	28.1	13.9	13.5	14.2
West	15.3	12.6	15.4	30.0	27.5	27.4	16.1	15.3	16.5
Location of residence[2,9]									
Within MSA	15.2	13.1	15.5	27.0	26.8	27.1	14.2	13.6	14.6
Outside MSA	18.1	16.3	19.3	32.5	29.6	33.3	16.4	14.9	17.7

See footnotes at end of table.

Table 52 (page 3 of 3). Severe headache or migraine, low back pain, and neck pain among adults 18 years of age and over, by selected characteristics: United States, selected years 1997–2009

[Data are based on household interviews of a sample of the civilian noninstitutionalized population]

* Estimates are considered unreliable. Data preceded by an asterisk have a relative standard error (RSE) of 20%–30%. Data not shown have an RSE greater than 30%.

- - - Data not available.

[1]In three separate questions, respondents were asked, "During the past 3 months, did you have a severe headache or migraine? ...low back pain? ...neck pain?" Respondents were instructed to report pain that had lasted a whole day or more, and not to report fleeting or minor aches or pains. Persons may be represented in more than one column.

[2]Estimates are age-adjusted to the year 2000 standard population using five age groups: 18–44 years, 45–54 years, 55–64 years, 65–74 years, and 75 years and over. Age-adjusted estimates in this table may differ from other age-adjusted estimates based on the same data and presented elsewhere if different age groups are used in the adjustment procedure. See Appendix II, Age adjustment.

[3]Includes all other races not shown separately, unknown education level, and unknown disability status.

[4]The race groups white, black, American Indian or Alaska Native, Asian, Native Hawaiian or Other Pacific Islander, and 2 or more races include persons of Hispanic and non-Hispanic origin. Persons of Hispanic origin may be of any race. Starting with 1999 data, race-specific estimates are tabulated according to the 1997 Revisions to the Standards for the Classification of Federal Data on Race and Ethnicity and are not strictly comparable with estimates for earlier years. The five single-race categories plus multiple-race categories shown in the table conform to the 1997 Standards. Starting with 1999 data, race-specific estimates are for persons who reported only one racial group; the category 2 or more races includes persons who reported more than one racial group. Prior to 1999, data were tabulated according to the 1977 Standards with four racial groups and the Asian only category included Native Hawaiian or Other Pacific Islander. Estimates for single-race categories prior to 1999 included persons who reported one race or, if they reported more than one race, identified one race as best representing their race. Starting with 2003 data, race responses of other race and unspecified multiple race were treated as missing, and then race was imputed if these were the only race responses. Almost all persons with a race response of other race were of Hispanic origin. See Appendix II, Hispanic origin; Race.

[5]Estimates are for persons 25 years of age and over and are age-adjusted to the year 2000 standard population using five age groups: 25–44 years, 45–54 years, 55–64 years, 65–74 years, and 75 years and over. See Appendix II, Age adjustment.

[6]GED is General Educational Development high school equivalency diploma. See Appendix II, Education.

[7]Percent of poverty level is based on family income and family size and composition using U.S. Census Bureau poverty thresholds. Missing family income data were imputed for 1997 and beyond. See Appendix II, Family income; Poverty; Table VII.

[8]Any basic actions difficulty or complex activity limitation is defined as having one or more of the following limitations or difficulties: movement difficulty, emotional difficulty, sensory (seeing or hearing) difficulty, cognitive difficulty, self-care (ADL or IADL) limitation, social limitation, or work limitation. For more information, see Appendix II, Basic actions difficulty; Complex activity limitation. Starting with 2007 data, the hearing question, a component of the basic actions difficulty measure, was revised. Consequently, data prior to 2007 are not comparable with data for 2007 and beyond. For more information on the impact of the revised hearing question, see Appendix II, Hearing trouble.

[9]MSA is metropolitan statistical area. Starting with 2006 data, MSA status is determined using 2000 census data and the 2000 standards for defining MSAs. For data prior to 2006, see Appendix II, Metropolitan statistical area (MSA) for the applicable standards.

NOTES: Standard errors are available in the spreadsheet version of this table. Available from: http://www.cdc.gov/nchs/hus.htm. Data for additional years are available. See Appendix III.

SOURCE: CDC/NCHS, National Health Interview Survey, sample adult questionnaire.

Table 53 (page 1 of 5). Joint pain among adults 18 years of age and over, by selected characteristics: United States, selected years 2002–2009

[Data are based on household interviews of a sample of the civilian noninstitutionalized population]

Characteristic	Any joint pain[1]			Knee pain[1]			Shoulder pain[1]		
	2002	2008	2009	2002	2008	2009	2002	2008	2009
	Percent of adults reporting joint pain in past 30 days								
18 years and over, age-adjusted[2,3]	29.5	30.5	32.0	16.5	18.5	19.5	8.6	9.0	9.0
18 years and over, crude[3]	29.5	31.3	33.0	16.5	19.0	20.2	8.7	9.3	9.3
Age									
18–44 years	19.3	20.3	20.7	10.5	12.1	12.4	4.9	5.2	5.3
18–24 years	14.2	15.6	14.8	8.3	9.3	8.8	3.4	3.0	3.0
25–44 years	21.0	22.0	22.8	11.2	13.1	13.7	5.4	5.9	6.1
45–64 years	37.5	39.3	41.8	20.4	24.6	26.2	12.3	12.3	12.4
45–54 years	34.3	36.2	37.5	18.4	22.5	23.8	10.5	10.8	11.0
55–64 years	42.3	43.3	47.3	23.4	27.4	29.4	15.1	14.1	14.2
65 years and over	47.2	47.4	50.6	28.6	28.0	30.3	14.1	15.5	14.9
65–74 years	46.0	46.8	47.9	27.6	28.2	28.9	14.0	15.5	14.2
75 years and over	48.7	48.1	53.8	29.7	27.7	31.9	14.1	15.6	15.7
Sex[2]									
Male	28.0	28.8	30.8	15.2	17.4	18.3	8.4	9.3	9.2
Female	30.7	32.0	32.9	17.6	19.4	20.5	8.8	8.7	8.7
Sex and age									
Male:									
18–44 years	20.1	20.5	21.8	10.7	12.3	12.9	5.5	5.8	6.0
45–54 years	31.1	34.8	37.1	16.2	21.8	23.0	9.5	10.9	10.9
55–64 years	37.3	37.8	41.7	20.1	23.8	24.4	13.7	15.0	14.5
65–74 years	41.7	40.8	42.0	24.1	24.4	23.6	13.3	14.1	14.6
75 years and over	43.9	43.6	47.5	25.7	24.1	28.3	11.4	15.0	13.5
Female:									
18–44 years	18.4	20.1	19.7	10.2	12.0	11.9	4.2	4.5	4.6
45–54 years	37.3	37.6	38.0	20.5	23.2	24.5	11.4	10.7	11.1
55–64 years	46.8	48.4	52.4	26.4	30.7	33.9	16.3	13.3	13.9
65–74 years	49.6	52.1	52.9	30.5	31.5	33.5	14.7	16.7	13.9
75 years and over	51.6	51.0	58.1	32.1	30.1	34.3	15.7	15.9	17.1
Race[2,4]									
White only	29.8	31.5	32.8	16.3	18.9	19.7	8.8	9.3	9.1
Black or African American only	30.8	29.0	30.8	20.2	19.8	20.7	8.3	7.8	9.0
American Indian or Alaska Native only	36.7	29.4	35.8	24.5	15.1	22.5	*11.3	13.2	*8.3
Asian only	18.1	16.1	18.3	8.5	9.2	11.0	3.9	5.2	5.4
Native Hawaiian or Other Pacific Islander only	*	*	*	*	*	*	*	*	*
2 or more races	42.7	43.7	46.4	28.1	28.1	29.7	15.4	15.0	15.0
Hispanic origin and race[2,4]									
Hispanic or Latino	23.4	23.7	25.0	13.6	13.9	15.7	7.6	7.6	8.0
Mexican	24.6	23.2	25.6	14.1	13.8	16.6	8.3	7.3	8.2
Not Hispanic or Latino	30.4	31.5	33.1	17.0	19.2	20.2	8.9	9.3	9.2
White only	30.8	33.0	34.4	16.9	19.9	20.6	9.1	9.8	9.4
Black or African American only	30.8	29.1	31.0	20.1	19.9	21.0	8.3	7.8	9.1
Education[5,6]									
25 years of age and over:									
No high school diploma or GED	33.0	33.2	36.1	19.5	20.7	23.4	10.8	11.4	11.4
High school diploma or GED	32.9	34.0	35.6	18.6	21.5	21.7	10.2	11.1	10.6
Some college or more	31.1	32.0	33.8	16.9	18.8	20.3	8.8	8.9	9.2

See footnotes at end of table.

Table 53 (page 2 of 5). Joint pain among adults 18 years of age and over, by selected characteristics: United States, selected years 2002–2009

[Data are based on household interviews of a sample of the civilian noninstitutionalized population]

Characteristic	Any joint pain[1]			Knee pain[1]			Shoulder pain[1]		
	2002	2008	2009	2002	2008	2009	2002	2008	2009
Percent of poverty level[2,7]	Percent of adults reporting joint pain in past 30 days								
Below 100%.	31.7	33.2	35.5	19.9	21.3	23.2	11.2	11.4	12.3
100%–199%.	31.7	33.0	35.4	19.0	21.2	22.0	10.4	10.1	10.2
200%–399%.	30.1	30.2	32.0	16.4	18.0	20.4	8.8	9.4	9.2
400% or more.	27.6	29.1	29.5	14.9	17.3	16.8	7.3	7.6	7.5
Hispanic origin and race and percent of poverty level[2,4,7]									
Hispanic or Latino:									
Below 100%.	26.8	23.1	26.8	16.1	14.1	18.3	11.5	7.4	11.3
100%–199%.	24.5	24.2	24.9	14.4	16.0	15.8	8.2	8.0	6.7
200%–399%.	21.6	24.4	25.6	11.7	12.3	15.6	5.7	8.2	8.3
400% or more.	21.9	22.5	22.6	12.3	13.5	13.4	4.9	*6.7	6.2
Not Hispanic or Latino:									
White only:									
Below 100%.	34.2	38.9	38.5	21.3	25.1	24.9	12.4	13.7	12.8
100%–199%.	34.9	38.9	41.6	20.3	24.4	24.9	11.6	12.0	11.8
200%–399%.	32.0	32.8	34.8	17.0	19.7	22.5	9.6	10.4	9.8
400% or more.	28.2	30.4	30.9	15.1	17.8	17.2	7.6	8.0	7.8
Black or African American only:									
Below 100%.	31.6	34.3	39.1	20.8	23.0	25.1	9.1	11.2	13.2
100%–199%.	34.0	29.8	31.1	23.2	21.4	22.7	10.9	8.4	8.5
200%–399%.	29.1	27.0	27.3	19.1	17.7	17.1	7.4	6.7	8.3
400% or more.	29.8	28.6	28.7	18.2	19.6	20.7	*8.0	6.1	6.6
Disability measure[2,8]									
Any basic actions difficulty or complex activity limitation	52.5	50.2	54.5	32.1	33.0	35.8	17.8	16.2	17.0
Any basic actions difficulty.	54.0	51.8	56.2	33.4	34.3	37.3	18.3	16.6	17.7
Any complex activity limitation	56.4	54.9	57.4	35.2	36.0	38.6	22.0	21.3	21.4
No disability	19.6	20.9	21.6	9.4	11.1	11.7	4.6	5.1	4.9
Geographic region[2]									
Northeast.	27.5	28.2	28.6	15.8	17.2	17.6	7.9	8.7	7.5
Midwest.	32.1	33.2	35.6	18.4	20.5	22.5	8.6	9.2	10.2
South.	29.3	30.7	32.2	16.7	19.0	19.6	9.1	9.0	9.1
West.	28.4	29.0	30.5	14.6	16.6	17.7	8.6	9.1	8.7
Location of residence[2,9]									
Within MSA.	28.3	29.5	31.1	16.0	17.8	18.8	8.1	8.7	8.6
Outside MSA.	33.9	35.2	36.1	18.7	21.6	23.0	10.8	10.7	10.7

See footnotes at end of table.

Table 53 (page 3 of 5). Joint pain among adults 18 years of age and over, by selected characteristics: United States, selected years 2002–2009

[Data are based on household interviews of a sample of the civilian noninstitutionalized population]

Characteristic	Finger pain[1]			Hip pain[1]		
	2002	2008	2009	2002	2008	2009
	Percent of adults reporting joint pain in past 30 days					
18 years and over, age-adjusted[2,3]	7.5	7.2	7.6	6.6	6.9	7.1
18 years and over, crude[3]	7.5	7.5	8.0	6.6	7.1	7.4
Age						
18–44 years	3.4	3.3	3.4	3.2	3.5	3.7
18–24 years	2.0	2.1	2.4	1.6	*1.6	2.0
25–44 years	3.9	3.7	3.7	3.8	4.2	4.2
45–64 years	11.0	9.9	10.8	9.1	9.2	9.9
45–54 years	9.1	7.9	8.6	7.8	7.6	7.8
55–64 years	13.9	12.5	13.5	11.0	11.3	12.5
65 years and over	13.9	15.2	15.8	12.9	13.6	13.0
65–74 years	14.4	15.2	15.3	12.6	13.9	11.3
75 years and over	13.3	15.1	16.3	13.3	13.3	14.9
Sex[2]						
Male	5.8	5.6	5.9	5.1	5.1	5.3
Female	8.9	8.7	9.2	8.0	8.5	8.7
Sex and age						
Male:						
18–44 years	3.0	2.7	3.1	2.5	2.7	2.5
45–54 years	6.6	6.5	6.6	5.6	5.3	5.3
55–64 years	10.5	10.0	10.2	8.0	6.9	9.7
65–74 years	11.2	10.5	10.2	10.5	9.9	8.0
75 years and over	10.0	10.8	11.1	10.1	12.7	14.2
Female:						
18–44 years	3.8	3.9	3.7	3.9	4.3	4.8
45–54 years	11.5	9.3	10.6	9.9	9.8	10.2
55–64 years	17.0	14.9	16.5	13.7	15.4	15.1
65–74 years	17.1	19.3	19.7	14.2	17.3	14.1
75 years and over	15.3	17.9	19.8	15.2	13.6	15.4
Race[2,4]						
White only	7.6	7.6	8.0	6.9	7.4	7.3
Black or African American only	6.5	5.0	6.0	5.6	5.0	7.0
American Indian or Alaska Native only	*12.9	12.4	*7.7	*10.4	*8.1	*6.0
Asian only	*3.2	3.2	4.0	*2.3	*1.8	*1.8
Native Hawaiian or Other Pacific Islander only	*	*	*	*	*	*
2 or more races	12.8	16.2	16.3	10.0	11.0	11.8
Hispanic origin and race[2,4]						
Hispanic or Latino	6.8	5.6	6.9	3.8	4.6	4.1
Mexican	7.8	6.5	7.0	4.0	4.2	3.8
Not Hispanic or Latino	7.6	7.4	7.7	6.9	7.2	7.5
White only	7.8	8.0	8.1	7.3	7.9	7.8
Black or African American only	6.5	5.0	5.9	5.7	5.0	7.0
Education[5,6]						
25 years of age and over:						
No high school diploma or GED	9.5	8.8	10.2	7.3	7.8	9.0
High school diploma or GED	8.3	9.2	9.2	7.3	8.2	8.6
Some college or more	8.2	7.3	7.7	7.5	7.4	7.3

See footnotes at end of table.

[Data are based on household interviews of a sample of the civilian noninstitutionalized population]

Characteristic	Finger pain[1]			Hip pain[1]		
	2002	2008	2009	2002	2008	2009
Percent of poverty level[2,7]	Percent of adults reporting joint pain in past 30 days					
Below 100%	9.8	9.2	9.5	8.5	8.7	9.5
100%–199%	8.9	8.7	9.4	7.5	8.4	7.8
200%–399%	7.9	7.1	7.9	6.8	6.8	7.2
400% or more	6.2	6.2	6.4	5.8	5.9	5.9
Hispanic origin and race and percent of poverty level[2,4,7]						
Hispanic or Latino:						
Below 100%	8.6	7.4	8.3	5.9	*5.2	6.5
100%–199%	8.2	5.5	5.6	3.9	4.5	*2.6
200%–399%	6.2	5.6	7.8	3.2	*4.7	4.8
400% or more	*5.3	*4.4	6.2	*1.8	*4.3	*3.0
Not Hispanic or Latino:						
White only:						
Below 100%	10.9	11.5	10.5	9.9	11.3	10.7
100%–199%	9.9	10.6	11.9	9.1	11.3	9.7
200%–399%	8.5	7.8	8.5	7.5	7.8	8.3
400% or more	6.5	6.7	6.4	6.2	6.3	6.3
Black or African American only:						
Below 100%	7.9	5.4	7.8	8.1	7.3	10.3
100%–199%	7.4	6.5	4.9	6.4	4.6	6.9
200%–399%	6.0	5.4	4.9	4.7	4.8	5.5
400% or more	*4.8	*2.7	*6.6	*4.5	*5.0	*6.3
Disability measure[2,8]						
Any basic actions difficulty or complex activity limitation	14.5	12.8	13.7	13.8	13.5	14.6
Any basic actions difficulty	14.9	13.4	14.3	14.4	14.1	15.0
Any complex activity limitation	17.8	15.5	16.3	17.8	17.7	18.4
No disability	4.0	4.5	4.5	3.1	3.3	3.3
Geographic region[2]						
Northeast	6.6	5.4	6.2	5.7	6.7	5.8
Midwest	7.5	7.4	8.2	6.9	7.4	7.9
South	7.6	8.0	7.9	7.0	6.8	7.6
West	8.0	7.2	7.7	6.4	6.7	6.3
Location of residence[2,9]						
Within MSA	7.2	6.9	7.4	6.2	6.4	6.6
Outside MSA	8.4	8.8	8.9	8.0	9.0	9.1

See footnotes at end of table.

Table 53 (page 5 of 5). Joint pain among adults 18 years of age and over, by selected characteristics: United States, selected years 2002–2009

[Data are based on household interviews of a sample of the civilian noninstitutionalized population]

* Estimates are considered unreliable. Data preceded by an asterisk have a relative standard error (RSE) of 20%–30%. Data not shown have an RSE greater than 30%.

[1]Starting with 2002 data, respondents were asked, "During the past 30 days, have you had any symptoms of pain, aching, or stiffness in or around a joint?" Respondents were instructed not to include the back or neck. To facilitate their response, respondents were shown a card illustrating the body joints. Respondents reporting more than one type of joint pain were included in each response category. This table shows the most commonly reported joints.

[2]Estimates are age-adjusted to the year 2000 standard population using five age groups: 18–44 years, 45–54 years, 55–64 years, 65–74 years, and 75 years and over. See Appendix II, Age adjustment.

[3]Includes all other races not shown separately, unknown education level, and unknown disability status.

[4]The race groups white, black, American Indian or Alaska Native, Asian, Native Hawaiian or Other Pacific Islander, and 2 or more races include persons of Hispanic and non-Hispanic origin. Persons of Hispanic origin may be of any race. The five single-race categories plus multiple-race categories shown in the table conform to the 1997 Revisions to the Standards for the Classification of Federal Data on Race and Ethnicity. Starting with 2003 data, race responses of other race and unspecified multiple race were treated as missing, and then race was imputed if these were the only race responses. Almost all persons with a race response of other race were of Hispanic origin. See Appendix II, Hispanic origin; Race.

[5]Estimates are for persons 25 years of age and over and are age-adjusted to the year 2000 standard population using five age groups: 25–44 years, 45–54 years, 55–64 years, 65–74 years, and 75 years and over. See Appendix II, Age adjustment.

[6]GED is General Educational Development high school equivalency diploma. See Appendix II, Education.

[7]Percent of poverty level is based on family income and family size and composition using U.S. Census Bureau poverty thresholds. Missing family income data were imputed for 2002 and beyond. See Appendix II, Family income; Poverty; Table VII.

[8]Any basic actions difficulty or complex activity limitation is defined as having one or more of the following limitations or difficulties: movement difficulty, emotional difficulty, sensory (seeing or hearing) difficulty, cognitive difficulty, self-care (ADL or IADL) limitation, social limitation, or work limitation. For more information, see Appendix II, Basic actions difficulty; Complex activity limitation. Starting with 2007 data, the hearing question, a component of the basic actions difficulty measure, was revised. Consequently, data prior to 2007 are not comparable with data for 2007 and beyond. For more information on the impact of the revised hearing question, see Appendix II, Hearing trouble.

[9]MSA is metropolitan statistical area. Starting with 2006 data, MSA status is determined using 2000 census data and the 2000 standards for defining MSAs. For data prior to 2006, see Appendix II, Metropolitan statistical area (MSA) for the applicable standards.

NOTES: Standard errors are available in the spreadsheet version of this table. Available from: http://www.cdc.gov/nchs/hus.htm. Data for additional years are available. See Appendix III.

SOURCE: CDC/NCHS, National Health Interview Survey, sample adult questionnaire.

Table 54 (page 1 of 2). Basic actions difficulty and complex activity limitation among adults 18 years of age and over, by selected characteristics: United States, selected years 1997–2009

[Data are based on household interviews of a sample of the civilian noninstitutionalized population]

Characteristic	18 years and over				18–64 years				65 years and over			
	1997	2000	2008[1]	2009[1]	1997	2000	2008[1]	2009[1]	1997	2000	2008[1]	2009[1]
	Number in millions											
At least one basic actions difficulty or complex activity limitation[2,3]	60.9	59.0	71.7	71.4	41.3	39.3	49.5	49.2	19.6	19.7	22.2	22.1
At least one basic actions difficulty[3]	56.7	55.2	66.6	66.7	38.1	36.4	45.6	45.6	18.6	18.7	21.0	21.1
At least one complex activity limitation[4]	29.0	27.2	33.5	34.3	18.1	16.7	21.4	22.7	11.0	10.5	12.0	11.7
	At least one basic actions difficulty or complex activity limitation[2,3]											
	Percent											
Total, age-adjusted[4,5]	32.5	29.9	32.0	31.3	. . .	. . .	. . .	. . .	. . .	. . .	. . .	. . .
Total, crude[4]	31.8	29.5	32.5	32.0	25.8	23.5	26.8	26.4	62.2	60.8	62.2	60.8
	At least one basic actions difficulty[2]											
	Percent											
Total, age-adjusted[4,5]	30.1	27.9	29.8	29.3	. . .	. . .	. . .	. . .	. . .	. . .	. . .	. . .
Total, crude[4]	29.4	27.5	30.3	29.9	23.6	21.7	24.7	24.4	58.8	58.1	59.2	58.2
Sex												
Male	25.6	23.8	25.7	26.0	20.7	18.9	21.3	21.3	54.5	53.4	51.7	53.2
Female	32.9	31.0	34.5	33.7	26.4	24.3	28.0	27.5	61.9	61.5	64.9	62.1
Race[6]												
White only	29.6	28.1	30.8	30.4	23.5	21.8	25.0	24.4	58.5	58.0	59.1	58.9
Black or African American only	31.4	27.2	30.3	31.0	26.9	22.7	25.9	27.5	64.4	60.6	64.2	57.7
American Indian or Alaska Native only	43.8	36.8	27.5	33.5	41.9	34.1	24.7	31.1	66.0	70.2	*52.1	*61.7
Asian only	15.5	15.5	18.5	16.3	13.0	12.6	14.1	12.5	46.4	44.7	48.2	43.2
Native Hawaiian or Other Pacific Islander only	- - -	*	*	*22.2	- - -	*	*	*	- - -	*	*	*
2 or more races	- - -	38.0	39.4	39.3	- - -	34.4	35.6	37.2	- - -	70.7	71.0	56.2
Hispanic origin and race[6]												
Hispanic or Latino	23.8	19.6	23.4	22.7	21.0	16.6	20.2	19.8	54.6	57.5	59.3	56.2
Not Hispanic or Latino	30.0	28.5	31.4	31.1	23.9	22.4	25.5	25.3	59.0	58.2	59.2	58.4
White only	30.3	29.1	32.3	31.8	23.8	22.5	26.0	25.4	58.7	58.2	59.2	59.0
Black or African American only	31.5	27.3	30.4	31.5	27.0	22.9	26.0	28.0	64.4	60.4	64.4	58.5
Percent of poverty level[7]												
Below 100%	41.9	38.4	42.1	39.0	36.2	31.9	38.0	34.5	74.1	71.6	73.1	72.3
100%–199%	38.2	37.1	40.7	38.5	29.2	26.5	32.0	31.2	66.6	69.4	70.4	66.4
200%–399%	28.4	28.2	31.2	31.5	22.0	22.1	24.2	24.3	56.1	53.9	61.1	61.5
400% or more	21.0	19.4	21.3	21.7	18.2	16.8	18.2	18.3	45.5	44.7	43.3	44.1
Location of residence[8]												
Within MSA	27.7	25.9	28.7	28.5	22.3	20.3	23.4	23.3	56.6	56.7	58.7	57.1
Outside MSA	35.6	33.6	37.9	37.0	28.6	26.8	31.7	30.4	65.8	62.6	60.7	62.6

See footnotes at end of table.

Table 54 (page 2 of 2). Basic actions difficulty and complex activity limitation among adults 18 years of age and over, by selected characteristics: United States, selected years 1997–2009

[Data are based on household interviews of a sample of the civilian noninstitutionalized population]

Characteristic	18 years and over				18–64 years				65 years and over			
	1997	2000	2008	2009	1997	2000	2008	2009	1997	2000	2008	2009
	At least one complex activity limitation[3]											
	Percent											
Total, age-adjusted[4,5]	15.6	13.7	14.7	14.8	. . .	. . .	. . .	. . .	. . .	. . .	. . .	. . .
Total, crude[4]	15.1	13.4	15.1	15.2	11.2	9.8	11.5	12.0	35.1	32.0	33.3	31.5
Sex												
Male	13.7	12.0	13.5	14.0	10.6	9.4	10.9	11.4	31.9	28.1	29.1	29.1
Female	16.5	14.7	16.5	16.4	11.9	10.3	12.1	12.7	37.4	34.9	36.5	33.4
Race[6]												
White only	15.0	13.6	15.2	15.0	10.9	9.8	11.5	11.6	34.3	31.5	32.7	30.9
Black or African American only	19.0	15.0	17.0	18.9	15.2	11.7	13.7	16.1	47.1	40.4	42.3	39.3
American Indian or Alaska Native only	23.7	20.6	17.5	15.3	22.1	17.8	14.5	14.9	*42.6	*54.9	*44.6	*
Asian only	5.7	4.7	6.3	7.4	4.9	3.6	3.8	5.1	*14.8	*15.5	22.9	23.3
Native Hawaiian or Other Pacific Islander only	- - -	*	*	*	- - -	*	*	*	- - -	*	*	*
2 or more races	- - -	22.5	21.9	27.6	- - -	20.3	18.3	25.0	- - -	*42.2	50.6	*49.9
Hispanic origin and race[6]												
Hispanic or Latino	11.9	9.1	10.6	10.7	9.8	7.3	8.5	9.1	33.9	32.4	33.3	28.2
Not Hispanic or Latino	15.5	14.0	15.8	16.0	11.4	10.2	12.0	12.6	35.1	32.0	33.3	31.8
White only	15.4	14.1	16.0	15.8	11.1	10.1	12.1	12.2	34.4	31.5	32.7	31.1
Black or African American only	18.8	15.1	17.2	19.1	15.0	11.7	13.9	16.2	46.8	40.3	42.4	39.9
Percent of poverty level[7]												
Below 100%	30.0	26.0	29.6	29.3	25.2	22.0	26.4	26.0	56.9	46.7	53.8	53.4
100%–199%	23.3	22.0	23.9	22.6	16.7	15.1	17.8	17.7	43.9	42.8	44.9	40.8
200%–399%	13.3	12.8	14.5	15.0	9.3	9.2	10.1	10.9	30.6	27.5	33.0	32.0
400% or more	7.3	6.4	7.2	7.3	5.8	5.0	5.6	5.8	20.2	19.6	18.5	17.6
Location of residence[8]												
Within MSA	14.1	12.1	13.9	14.2	10.6	8.9	10.6	11.2	32.7	29.8	31.9	30.4
Outside MSA	19.0	18.2	21.0	20.5	13.6	13.4	16.3	16.5	42.8	38.8	38.0	36.0

. . . Category not applicable.

* Estimates are considered unreliable. Data preceded by an asterisk have a relative standard error (RSE) of 20%–30%. Data not shown have an RSE greater than 30%.

- - - Data not available.

[1]Starting with 2007 data, the hearing question, a component of the basic actions difficulty measure, was revised. Consequently, data for basic actions difficulty prior to 2007 are not comparable with 2007 data and beyond. For more information on the impact of the revised hearing question, see Appendix II, Hearing trouble.

[2]A basic actions difficulty is defined as having one or more of the following difficulties: movement, emotional, sensory (seeing or hearing), or cognitive. For more information, see Appendix II, Basic actions difficulty. Starting with 2007 data, the hearing question, a component of basic actions difficulty, was revised. Consequently, data prior to 2007 are not comparable with data for 2007 and beyond. For more information on the impact of the revised hearing question, see Appendix II, Hearing trouble.

[3]A complex activity limitation is defined as having one or more of the following limitations: self-care (activities of daily living or instrumental activities of daily living), social, or work. For more information, see Appendix II, Complex activity limitation.

[4]Includes all other races not shown separately.

[5]Estimates are age-adjusted to the year 2000 standard population using five age groups: 18–44 years, 45–54 years, 55–64 years, 65–74 years, and 75 years and over. See Appendix II, Age adjustment.

[6]The race groups, white, black, American Indian or Alaska Native, Asian, Native Hawaiian or Other Pacific Islander, and 2 or more races, include persons of Hispanic and non-Hispanic origin. Persons of Hispanic origin may be of any race. Starting with 1999 data, race-specific estimates are tabulated according to the 1997 Revisions to the Standards for the Classification of Federal Data on Race and Ethnicity and are not strictly comparable with estimates for earlier years. The five single-race categories plus multiple-race categories shown in the table conform to the 1997 Standards. Starting with 1999 data, race-specific estimates are for persons who reported only one racial group; the category 2 or more races includes persons who reported more than one racial group. Prior to 1999, data were tabulated according to the 1977 Standards with four racial groups and the Asian only category included Native Hawaiian or Other Pacific Islander. Estimates for single-race categories prior to 1999 included persons who reported one race or, if they reported more than one race, identified one race as best representing their race. Starting with 2003 data, race responses of other race and unspecified multiple race were treated as missing, and then race was imputed if these were the only race responses. Almost all persons with a race response of other race were of Hispanic origin. See Appendix II, Hispanic origin; Race.

[7]Percent of poverty level is based on family income and family size and composition using U.S. Census Bureau poverty thresholds. Missing family income data were imputed for 1997 and beyond. See Appendix II, Family income; Poverty; Table VII.

[8]MSA is metropolitan statistical area. Starting with 2006 data, MSA status is determined using 2000 census data and the 2000 standards for defining MSAs. For data prior to 2006, see Appendix II, Metropolitan statistical area (MSA) for the applicable standards.

NOTES: Standard errors are available in the spreadsheet version of this table. Available from: http://www.cdc.gov/nchs/hus.htm. Data have been revised and differ from previous editions of *Health, United States*. Data for additional years are available. See Appendix III.

SOURCE: CDC/NCHS, National Health Interview Survey, sample adult questionnaire.

Table 55 (page 1 of 2). Vision and hearing limitations among adults 18 years of age and over, by selected characteristics: United States, selected years 1997–2009

[Data are based on household interviews of a sample of the civilian noninstitutionalized population]

Characteristic	Any trouble seeing, even with glasses or contacts[1]				A lot of trouble hearing or deaf[2]			
	1997	2000	2008	2009	1997	2000	2008	2009
	Percent of adults							
18 years and over, age-adjusted[3,4]	10.0	9.0	10.9	8.3	3.2	3.2	1.9	2.0
18 years and over, crude[4]	9.8	8.9	11.2	8.6	3.1	3.1	1.9	2.1
Age								
18–44 years	6.2	5.3	7.2	5.3	1.0	0.9	0.5	0.4
18–24 years...................	5.4	4.2	7.8	4.8	*0.5	*0.7	*	*
25–44 years...................	6.5	5.7	7.0	5.6	1.2	1.0	0.6	*0.4
45–64 years	12.0	10.7	13.8	10.8	3.1	3.0	1.6	1.9
45–54 years...................	12.2	10.9	13.3	10.5	2.6	2.3	1.3	*1.4
55–64 years...................	11.6	10.5	14.4	11.2	3.9	4.0	2.0	2.5
65 years and over	18.1	17.4	17.5	13.1	9.8	10.5	6.5	7.4
65–74 years..................	14.2	13.6	14.3	10.3	6.6	7.4	3.7	4.1
75 years and over...............	23.1	21.9	21.1	16.5	14.1	14.3	9.7	11.4
Sex[3]								
Male........................	8.8	7.9	9.3	7.2	4.2	4.3	2.5	2.5
Female......................	11.1	10.1	12.5	9.3	2.4	2.3	1.4	1.6
Sex and age								
Male:								
18–44 years..................	5.3	4.4	6.1	4.5	1.2	1.1	*0.6	*0.2
45–54 years..................	10.1	8.8	11.3	9.1	3.6	2.9	*1.6	*1.4
55–64 years..................	10.5	9.5	11.9	9.7	5.4	6.2	3.0	3.9
65–74 years..................	13.2	12.8	11.3	9.3	9.4	10.8	5.7	5.2
75 years and over...............	21.4	20.7	19.8	15.1	17.7	18.0	12.4	15.3
Female:								
18–44 years..................	7.1	6.2	8.4	6.2	0.9	0.8	*0.5	*0.5
45–54 years..................	14.2	12.8	15.2	11.9	1.7	1.8	*1.1	*
55–64 years..................	12.6	11.5	16.7	12.6	2.6	1.9	*1.0	*1.2
65–74 years..................	15.0	14.4	16.9	11.2	4.4	4.5	*2.0	*3.2
75 years and over...............	24.2	22.7	22.0	17.4	11.7	12.1	7.9	8.8
Race[3,5]								
White only....................	9.7	8.8	10.9	8.1	3.4	3.4	2.0	2.1
Black or African American only	12.8	10.6	11.7	10.4	2.0	1.6	*0.8	*
American Indian or Alaska Native only	19.2	16.6	14.2	*12.3	14.1	*	*	*
Asian only....................	6.2	6.3	8.9	5.5	*	*2.4	*1.1	*2.0
Native Hawaiian or Other Pacific Islander only	- - -	*	*	*	- - -	*	*	*
2 or more races....................	- - -	16.2	16.1	14.8	- - -	*5.7	*4.1	*
Hispanic origin and race[3,5]								
Hispanic or Latino	10.0	9.7	10.4	8.7	1.5	2.3	*1.2	1.1
Mexican........................	10.2	8.3	10.4	8.7	1.8	3.0	*	*1.2
Not Hispanic or Latino	10.0	9.1	11.0	8.3	3.3	3.3	2.0	2.1
White only......................	9.8	8.9	11.1	8.1	3.5	3.5	2.2	2.2
Black or African American only........	12.8	10.6	11.7	10.5	2.0	1.6	*0.8	*
Education[6,7]								
25 years of age and over:								
No high school diploma or GED	15.0	12.2	15.9	12.6	4.8	4.6	3.0	3.1
High school diploma or GED	10.6	9.5	11.2	9.2	3.7	3.9	2.1	2.4
Some college or more..............	8.9	8.9	10.4	7.6	2.9	2.8	1.9	2.0

See footnotes at end of table.

Table 55 (page 2 of 2). Vision and hearing limitations among adults 18 years of age and over, by selected characteristics: United States, selected years 1997–2009

[Data are based on household interviews of a sample of the civilian noninstitutionalized population]

Characteristic	Any trouble seeing, even with glasses or contacts[1]				A lot of trouble hearing or deaf[2]			
	1997	2000	2008	2009	1997	2000	2008[2]	2009[2]
Percent of poverty level[3,8]				Percent of adults				
Below 100%	17.0	12.9	16.7	14.3	4.5	3.7	2.4	2.8
100%–199%	12.9	11.6	14.2	11.1	3.6	4.2	2.5	2.4
200%–399%	9.1	8.8	11.3	8.0	3.3	3.3	1.9	2.0
400% or more	7.3	7.1	7.8	5.7	2.7	2.5	1.4	1.7
Hispanic origin and race and percent of poverty level[3,5,8]								
Hispanic or Latino:								
Below 100%	12.8	11.0	12.9	12.2	*1.9	3.3	*	*
100%–199%	11.2	9.4	11.3	8.1	*1.5	*2.3	*	*
200%–399%	8.1	9.2	10.2	9.0	*	*	*	*
400% or more	*8.1	10.5	7.5	*4.6	*	*	*	*
Not Hispanic or Latino:								
White only:								
Below 100%	17.9	13.1	19.5	13.4	5.8	4.5	3.7	2.7
100%–199%	13.1	12.0	15.6	12.1	4.3	5.0	3.2	2.9
200%–399%	9.2	9.2	11.5	8.3	3.7	3.7	2.2	2.3
400% or more	7.3	7.0	7.9	5.8	2.7	2.6	1.5	1.8
Black or African American only:								
Below 100%	17.9	13.6	16.9	17.8	3.3	*1.6	*	*
100%–199%	16.0	12.9	14.5	11.7	*2.0	*2.0	*	*
200%–399%	9.3	7.7	9.8	8.1	*	*	*	*
400% or more	7.7	8.3	7.4	5.6	*	*	*	*
Geographic region[3]								
Northeast	8.6	7.4	9.3	7.3	2.2	2.4	1.7	1.7
Midwest	9.5	9.6	10.7	8.2	3.5	3.5	2.1	2.3
South	11.4	9.2	12.4	8.7	3.5	3.3	1.7	2.1
West	9.7	9.9	10.2	8.6	3.4	3.5	2.0	1.8
Location of residence[3]								
Within MSA[9]	9.5	8.5	10.6	8.2	2.9	3.0	1.7	1.9
Outside MSA[9]	12.0	11.1	12.5	9.0	4.5	3.9	2.8	2.5

* Estimates are considered unreliable. Data preceded by an asterisk have a relative standard error (RSE) of 20%–30%. Data not shown have an RSE greater than 30%.

- - - Data not available.

[1]Respondents were asked, "Do you have any trouble seeing, even when wearing glasses or contact lenses?" Respondents were also asked, "Are you blind or unable to see at all?" In this analysis, any trouble seeing and blind are combined into one category. In 2009, 0.4% of adults 18 years of age and over identified themselves as blind.

[2]Prior to 2007 data, respondents were asked, "Which statement best describes your hearing without a hearing aid: good, a little trouble, a lot of trouble, or deaf?" In this analysis, a lot of trouble and deaf are combined into one category. Starting with 2007 data, the question was revised to expand the response categories. Respondents were asked, "Which statement best describes your hearing without a hearing aid: excellent, good, a little trouble, moderate trouble, a lot of trouble, or deaf?" For 2007 and beyond, a lot of trouble and deaf are combined into one category. The decline from 2006 to 2007 in the estimate of those with hearing trouble is likely due to the addition of the "moderate trouble" response category. Data prior to 2007 are not comparable with 2007 and later data due to the revised question. For more information on the impact of this revised question, see Appendix II, Hearing trouble. In 2006, 0.3% of adults 18 years of age and over identified themselves as deaf; in 2007, 2008, and 2009, this estimate was 0.2%.

[3]Estimates are age-adjusted to the year 2000 standard population using five age groups: 18–44 years, 45–54 years, 55–64 years, 65–74 years, and 75 years and over. Age-adjusted estimates in this table may differ from other age-adjusted estimates based on the same data and presented elsewhere if different age groups are used in the adjustment procedure. See Appendix II, Age adjustment.

[4]Includes all other races not shown separately and unknown education level.

[5]The race groups, white, black, American Indian or Alaska Native, Asian, Native Hawaiian or Other Pacific Islander, and 2 or more races, include persons of Hispanic and non-Hispanic origin. Persons of Hispanic origin may be of any race. Starting with 1999 data, race-specific estimates are tabulated according to the 1997 Revisions to the Standards for the Classification of Federal Data on Race and Ethnicity and are not strictly comparable with estimates for earlier years. The five single-race categories plus multiple-race categories shown in the table conform to the 1997 Standards. Starting with 1999 data, race-specific estimates are for persons who reported only one racial group; the category 2 or more races includes persons who reported more than one racial group. Prior to 1999, data were tabulated according to the 1977 Standards with four racial groups and the Asian only category included Native Hawaiian or Other Pacific Islander. Estimates for single-race categories prior to 1999 included persons who reported one race or, if they reported more than one race, identified one race as best representing their race. Starting with 2003 data, race responses of other race and unspecified multiple race were treated as missing, and then race was imputed if these were the only race responses. Almost all persons with a race response of other race were of Hispanic origin. See Appendix II, Hispanic origin; Race.

[6]Estimates are for persons 25 years of age and over and are age-adjusted to the year 2000 standard population using five age groups: 25–44 years, 45–54 years, 55–64 years, 65–74 years, and 75 years and over. See Appendix II, Age adjustment.

[7]GED is General Educational Development high school equivalency diploma. See Appendix II, Education.

[8]Percent of poverty level is based on family income and family size and composition using U.S. Census Bureau poverty thresholds. Missing family income data were imputed for 1997 and beyond. See Appendix II, Family Income; Poverty; Table VII.

[9]MSA is metropolitan statistical area. Starting with 2006 data, MSA status is determined using 2000 census data and the 2000 standards for defining MSAs. For data prior to 2006, see Appendix II, Metropolitan statistical area (MSA) for the applicable standards.

NOTES: Standard errors are available in the spreadsheet version of this table. Available from: http://www.cdc.gov/nchs/hus.htm. Data for additional years are available. See Appendix III.

SOURCE: CDC/NCHS, National Health Interview Survey, sample adult questionnaire.

Table 56 (page 1 of 2). Respondent-assessed health status, by selected characteristics: United States, selected years 1991–2009

[Data are based on household interviews of a sample of the civilian noninstitutionalized population]

Characteristic	1991[1]	1995[1]	1997	2000	2005	2007	2008	2009
	Percent of persons with fair or poor health[2]							
All ages, age-adjusted[3,4]	10.4	10.6	9.2	9.0	9.2	9.5	9.5	9.4
All ages, crude[4].	10.0	10.1	8.9	8.9	9.3	9.8	9.9	9.9
Age								
Under 18 years	2.6	2.6	2.1	1.7	1.8	1.7	1.8	1.8
Under 6 years	2.7	2.7	1.9	1.5	1.6	1.5	1.2	1.3
6–17 years.	2.6	2.5	2.1	1.8	1.9	1.7	2.1	2.0
18–44 years	6.1	6.6	5.3	5.1	5.5	5.9	6.3	6.3
18–24 years	4.8	4.5	3.4	3.3	3.3	3.3	4.0	3.6
25–44 years.	6.4	7.2	5.9	5.7	6.3	6.8	7.2	7.2
45–54 years.	13.4	13.4	11.7	11.9	11.6	13.3	12.9	13.1
55–64 years.	20.7	21.4	18.2	17.9	18.3	17.9	18.8	19.1
65 years and over	29.0	28.3	26.7	26.9	26.6	26.8	24.9	24.0
65–74 years.	26.0	25.6	23.1	22.5	23.4	23.4	21.8	19.9
75 years and over.	33.6	32.2	31.5	32.1	30.2	30.7	28.4	28.9
Sex[3]								
Male.	10.0	10.1	8.8	8.8	8.8	9.1	9.1	9.1
Female	10.8	11.1	9.7	9.3	9.5	9.9	9.8	9.7
Race[3,5]								
White only.	9.6	9.7	8.3	8.2	8.6	8.8	8.9	8.7
Black or African American only	16.8	17.2	15.8	14.6	14.3	14.2	14.6	14.2
American Indian or Alaska Native only	18.3	18.7	17.3	17.2	13.2	17.1	14.5	16.3
Asian only.	7.8	9.3	7.8	7.4	6.8	7.1	6.7	8.4
Native Hawaiian or Other Pacific Islander only	- - -	- - -	- - -	*	*	*	*	*
2 or more races.	- - -	- - -	- - -	16.2	14.5	16.8	12.9	15.3
Black or African American; White	- - -	- - -	- - -	*14.5	8.3	*16.6	20.2	18.0
American Indian or Alaska Native; White.	- - -	- - -	- - -	18.7	17.2	19.2	14.6	15.2
Hispanic origin and race[3,5]								
Hispanic or Latino	15.6	15.1	13.0	12.8	13.3	13.0	12.8	13.3
Mexican	17.0	16.7	13.1	12.8	14.3	13.2	13.4	13.7
Not Hispanic or Latino	10.0	10.1	8.9	8.7	8.7	9.1	9.1	8.9
White only	9.1	9.1	8.0	7.9	8.0	8.3	8.4	8.0
Black or African American only.	16.8	17.3	15.8	14.6	14.4	14.1	14.6	14.2
Percent of poverty level[3,6]								
Below 100%	22.8	23.7	20.8	19.6	20.4	21.0	21.8	21.8
100%–199%	14.7	15.5	13.9	14.1	14.4	15.3	15.4	14.9
200%–399%	7.9	7.9	8.2	8.4	8.3	9.0	8.7	8.6
400% or more	4.9	4.7	4.1	4.5	4.7	4.7	4.4	4.3
Hispanic origin and race and percent of poverty level[3,5,6]								
Hispanic or Latino:								
Below 100%.	23.6	22.7	19.9	18.7	20.2	21.0	21.0	22.1
100%–199%.	18.0	16.9	13.5	15.3	15.3	15.1	14.6	16.2
200%–399%.	10.3	10.1	10.0	10.3	10.3	10.5	10.7	9.7
400% or more	6.6	4.0	5.7	5.5	7.6	7.2	5.6	5.6
Not Hispanic or Latino:								
White only:								
Below 100%	21.9	22.8	19.7	18.8	20.1	20.9	22.1	20.5
100%–199%	14.0	14.8	13.3	13.4	13.8	15.2	15.7	14.6
200%–399%	7.5	7.3	7.7	7.9	7.9	8.4	8.3	8.1
400% or more	4.7	4.6	3.9	4.2	4.3	4.3	4.1	4.0
Black or African American only:								
Below 100%	25.8	27.7	25.3	23.8	23.3	22.6	25.1	25.2
100%–199%	17.0	19.3	19.2	18.2	17.6	17.7	18.1	16.6
200%–399%	12.0	11.4	12.2	11.7	11.2	11.3	11.2	11.0
400% or more	5.9	6.5	6.1	7.3	7.1	7.2	6.9	5.9

See footnotes at end of table.

Table 56 (page 2 of 2). Respondent-assessed health status, by selected characteristics: United States, selected years 1991–2009

[Data are based on household interviews of a sample of the civilian noninstitutionalized population]

Characteristic	1991[1]	1995[1]	1997	2000	2005	2007	2008	2009
Disability measure among adults 18 years and over[3,7]	Percent of persons with fair or poor health[2]							
Any basic actions difficulty or complex activity limitation.............	- - -	- - -	27.0	27.6	28.5	31.2	28.5	30.3
Any basic actions difficulty...........	- - -	- - -	27.3	27.7	29.1	31.6	28.7	30.9
Any complex activity limitation........	- - -	- - -	42.9	45.6	46.3	50.8	47.9	48.8
No disability.......................	- - -	- - -	3.4	3.8	3.6	4.0	4.2	3.6
Geographic region[3]								
Northeast........................	8.3	9.1	8.0	7.6	7.5	8.4	8.0	8.4
Midwest..........................	9.1	9.7	8.1	8.0	8.3	8.6	8.8	8.6
South............................	13.1	12.3	10.8	10.7	11.0	11.0	11.0	10.9
West.............................	9.7	10.1	8.8	8.8	8.6	9.0	9.0	8.8
Location of residence[3,8]								
Within MSA.......................	9.9	10.1	8.7	8.5	8.7	9.0	9.1	9.1
Outside MSA......................	11.9	12.6	11.1	11.1	11.2	12.0	11.7	11.2

- - - Data not available.

*Estimates are considered unreliable. Data preceded by an asterisk have a relative standard error (RSE) of 20%–30%. Data not shown have an RSE greater than 30%.

[1]Data prior to 1997 are not strictly comparable with data for later years due to the 1997 questionnaire redesign. See Appendix I, National Health Interview Survey.

[2]See Appendix II, Health status, respondent-assessed.

[3]Estimates are age-adjusted to the year 2000 standard population using six age groups: under 18 years, 18–44 years, 45–54 years, 55–64 years, 65–74 years, and 75 years and over. The disability measure is age-adjusted using the five adult age groups. See Appendix II, Age adjustment.

[4]Includes all other races not shown separately and unknown disability status.

[5]The race groups white, black, American Indian or Alaska Native, Asian, Native Hawaiian or Other Pacific Islander, and 2 or more races include persons of Hispanic and non-Hispanic origin. Persons of Hispanic origin may be of any race. Starting with 1999 data, race-specific estimates are tabulated according to the 1997 Revisions to the Standards for the Classification of Federal Data on Race and Ethnicity and are not strictly comparable with estimates for earlier years. The five single-race categories plus multiple-race categories shown in the table conform to the 1997 Standards. Starting with 1999 data, race-specific estimates are for persons who reported only one racial group; the category 2 or more races includes persons who reported more than one racial group. Prior to 1999, data were tabulated according to the 1977 Standards with four racial groups and the Asian only category included Native Hawaiian or Other Pacific Islander. Estimates for single-race categories prior to 1999 included persons who reported one race or, if they reported more than one race, identified one race as best representing their race. Starting with 2003 data, race responses of other race and unspecified multiple race were treated as missing, and then race was imputed if these were the only race responses. Almost all persons with a race response of other race were of Hispanic origin. See Appendix II, Hispanic origin; Race.

[6]Percent of poverty level is based on family income and family size and composition using U.S. Census Bureau poverty thresholds. Missing family income data were imputed for starting in 1991. See Appendix II, Family income; Poverty; Table VII.

[7]Any basic actions difficulty or complex activity limitation is defined as having one or more of the following limitations or difficulties: movement difficulty, emotional difficulty, sensory (seeing or hearing) difficulty, cognitive difficulty, self-care (ADL or IADL) limitation, social limitation, or work limitation. For more information, see Appendix II, Basic actions difficulty; Complex activity limitation. Starting with 2007 data, the hearing question, a component of the basic actions difficulty measure, was revised. Consequently, data prior to 2007 are not comparable with data for 2007 and beyond. For more information on the impact of the revised hearing question, see Appendix II, Hearing trouble.

[8]MSA is metropolitan statistical area. Starting with 2006 data, MSA status is determined using 2000 census data and the 2000 standards for defining MSAs. For data prior to 2006, see Appendix II, Metropolitan statistical area (MSA) for the applicable standards.

NOTES: Standard errors for selected years are available in the spreadsheet version of this table. Available from: http://www.cdc.gov/nchs/hus.htm. Data for additional years are available. See Appendix III.

SOURCE: CDC/NCHS, National Health Interview Survey, family core and sample adult questionnaire.

Table 57 (page 1 of 2). Serious psychological distress in the past 30 days among adults 18 years of age and over, by selected characteristics: United States, average annual, selected years 1997–1998 through 2008–2009

[Data are based on household interviews of a sample of the civilian noninstitutionalized population]

Characteristic	1997–1998	1999–2000	2001–2002	2004–2005	2007–2008	2008–2009
	Percent of persons with serious psychological distress [1]					
18 years and over, age-adjusted [2,3]	3.2	2.6	3.1	3.0	2.9	3.2
18 years and over, crude [3]	3.2	2.6	3.1	3.0	2.9	3.2
Age						
18–44 years	2.9	2.3	2.9	2.8	2.7	3.1
18–24 years	2.7	2.2	2.8	2.5	2.3	2.5
25–44 years	3.0	2.4	3.0	2.9	2.8	3.3
45–64 years	3.7	3.2	3.9	3.7	3.6	3.7
45–54 years	3.9	3.5	4.2	3.9	3.6	3.9
55–64 years	3.4	2.6	3.4	3.4	3.6	3.6
65 years and over	3.1	2.4	2.4	2.5	2.4	2.4
65–74 years	2.5	2.3	2.4	2.2	2.4	2.2
75 years and over	3.8	2.5	2.4	2.9	2.4	2.6
Sex [2]						
Male	2.5	2.0	2.4	2.3	2.2	2.7
Female	3.8	3.1	3.8	3.7	3.5	3.6
Race [2,4]						
White only	3.1	2.5	3.0	2.9	2.9	3.2
Black or African American only	4.0	2.9	3.5	3.6	3.2	3.7
American Indian or Alaska Native only	7.8	*7.2	8.1	*3.5	*	*3.8
Asian only	2.0	*1.4	*1.8	1.7	*1.0	*1.1
Native Hawaiian or Other Pacific Islander only	- - -	*	*	*	*	*
2 or more races	- - -	4.8	5.0	7.9	5.9	*4.9
Hispanic origin and race [2,4]						
Hispanic or Latino	5.0	3.5	4.0	3.7	3.6	3.4
Mexican	5.2	2.9	3.8	3.6	3.3	2.9
Not Hispanic or Latino	3.0	2.5	3.1	3.0	2.8	3.1
White only	2.9	2.4	3.0	2.9	2.9	3.2
Black or African American only	3.9	2.9	3.5	3.6	3.1	3.7
Percent of poverty level [2,5]						
Below 100%	9.1	6.8	8.4	8.6	8.3	9.0
100%–199%	5.0	4.4	5.2	5.0	4.7	4.9
200%–399%	2.5	2.3	2.8	2.5	2.4	2.7
400% or more	1.3	1.2	1.3	1.1	1.1	1.1
Hispanic origin and race and percent of poverty level [2,4,5]						
Hispanic or Latino:						
Below 100%	8.6	6.1	7.5	6.6	7.0	6.7
100%–199%	5.4	3.8	4.1	3.9	4.5	4.5
200%–399%	3.4	2.1	3.5	2.6	2.2	1.8
400% or more	*	2.3	*	*1.9	*1.6	*1.0
Not Hispanic or Latino:						
White only:						
Below 100%	9.6	7.8	9.2	10.2	10.7	11.2
100%–199%	5.2	4.9	5.9	5.6	5.4	5.7
200%–399%	2.5	2.3	2.9	2.6	2.6	3.1
400% or more	1.3	1.1	1.3	1.1	1.0	1.0
Black or African American only:						
Below 100%	8.7	6.0	7.2	7.6	6.2	8.0
100%–199%	4.3	3.6	4.9	4.8	3.6	3.1
200%–399%	2.2	*1.7	2.3	2.1	2.4	2.9
400% or more	*	*1.0	*	*	*	*

See footnotes at end of table.

Table 57 (page 2 of 2). Serious psychological distress in the past 30 days among adults 18 years of age and over, by selected characteristics: United States, average annual, selected years 1997–1998 through 2008–2009

[Data are based on household interviews of a sample of the civilian noninstitutionalized population]

Characteristic	1997–1998	1999–2000	2001–2002	2004–2005	2007–2008	2008–2009
Geographic region[2]	Percent of persons with serious psychological distress[1]					
Northeast	2.7	1.9	2.8	2.5	2.6	2.9
Midwest	2.6	2.5	2.9	2.7	2.7	3.2
South	3.8	2.9	3.5	3.7	3.3	3.5
West.	3.3	2.8	3.0	2.8	2.7	2.8
Location of residence[2]						
Within MSA[6]	3.0	2.3	3.0	2.8	2.7	3.0
Outside MSA[6]	3.9	3.5	3.8	4.0	3.7	4.0

* Estimates are considered unreliable. Data preceded by an asterisk have a relative standard error (RSE) of 20%–30%. Data not shown have an RSE greater than 30%.

- - - Data not available.

[1]Serious psychological distress is measured by a six-question scale that asks respondents how often they experienced each of six symptoms of psychological distress in the past 30 days. See Appendix II, Serious psychological distress.

[2]Estimates are age-adjusted to the year 2000 standard population using five age groups: 18–44 years, 45–54 years, 55–64 years, 65–74 years, and 75 years and over. See Appendix II, Age adjustment.

[3]Includes all other races not shown separately.

[4]The race groups, white, black, American Indian or Alaska Native, Asian, Native Hawaiian or Other Pacific Islander, and 2 or more races, include persons of Hispanic and non-Hispanic origin. Persons of Hispanic origin may be of any race. Starting with 1999 data, race-specific estimates are tabulated according to the 1997 Revisions to the Standards for the Classification of Federal Data on Race and Ethnicity and are not strictly comparable with estimates for earlier years. The five single-race categories plus multiple-race categories shown in the table conform to the 1997 Standards. Starting with 1999 data, race-specific estimates are for persons who reported only one racial group; the category 2 or more races includes persons who reported more than one racial group. Prior to 1999, data were tabulated according to the 1977 Standards with four racial groups and the Asian only category included Native Hawaiian or Other Pacific Islander. Estimates for single-race categories prior to 1999 included persons who reported one race or, if they reported more than one race, identified one race as best representing their race. Starting with 2003 data, race responses of other race and unspecified multiple race were treated as missing, and then race was imputed if these were the only race responses. Almost all persons with a race response of other race were of Hispanic origin. See Appendix II, Hispanic origin; Race.

[5]Percent of poverty level is based on family income and family size and composition using U.S. Census Bureau poverty thresholds. Missing family income data were imputed for 1997 and beyond. See Appendix II, Family income; Poverty; Table VII.

[6]MSA is metropolitan statistical area. Starting with 2006–2007 data (shown in spreadsheet), MSA status is determined using 2000 census data and the 2000 standards for defining MSAs. For data prior to 2006, see Appendix II, Metropolitan statistical area (MSA) for the applicable standards.

NOTES: Standard errors for selected years are available in the spreadsheet version of this table. Available from: http://www.cdc.gov/nchs/hus.htm. Data for additional years are available. See Appendix III.

SOURCE: CDC/NCHS, National Health Interview Survey, family core questionnaire.

Table 58 (page 1 of 2). Current cigarette smoking among adults 18 years of age and over, by sex, race, and age: United States, selected years 1965–2009

[Data are based on household interviews of a sample of the civilian noninstitutionalized population]

Sex, race, and age	1965[1]	1974[1]	1979[1]	1985[1]	1990[1]	1995[1]	2000	2005	2007	2008	2009
18 years and over, age-adjusted[2]	Percent of persons who were current cigarette smokers[3]										
All persons	41.9	37.0	33.3	29.9	25.3	24.6	23.1	20.8	19.7	20.6	20.6
Male	51.2	42.8	37.0	32.2	28.0	26.5	25.2	23.4	22.0	22.8	23.2
Female	33.7	32.2	30.1	27.9	22.9	22.7	21.1	18.3	17.5	18.5	18.1
White male[4]	50.4	41.7	36.4	31.3	27.6	26.2	25.4	23.3	22.2	23.0	23.6
Black or African American male[4]	58.8	53.6	43.9	40.2	32.8	29.4	25.7	25.9	23.4	24.7	23.1
White female[4]	33.9	32.0	30.3	27.9	23.5	23.4	22.0	19.1	18.5	19.5	18.7
Black or African American female[4]	31.8	35.6	30.5	30.9	20.8	23.5	20.7	17.1	15.6	17.4	18.5
18 years and over, crude											
All persons	42.4	37.1	33.5	30.1	25.5	24.7	23.2	20.9	19.8	20.6	20.6
Male	51.9	43.1	37.5	32.6	28.4	27.0	25.6	23.9	22.3	23.1	23.5
Female	33.9	32.1	29.9	27.9	22.8	22.6	20.9	18.1	17.4	18.3	17.9
White male[4]	51.1	41.9	36.8	31.7	28.0	26.6	25.7	23.6	22.3	23.1	23.6
Black or African American male[4]	60.4	54.3	44.1	39.9	32.5	28.5	26.2	26.5	24.6	25.3	23.7
White female[4]	34.0	31.7	30.1	27.7	23.4	23.1	21.4	18.7	18.1	19.1	18.3
Black or African American female[4]	33.7	36.4	31.1	31.0	21.2	23.5	20.8	17.3	15.9	17.8	18.8
All males											
18–24 years	54.1	42.1	35.0	28.0	26.6	27.8	28.1	28.0	25.4	23.6	28.0
25–34 years	60.7	50.5	43.9	38.2	31.6	29.5	28.9	27.7	28.8	28.5	27.6
35–44 years	58.2	51.0	41.8	37.6	34.5	31.5	30.2	26.0	23.2	24.3	25.4
45–64 years	51.9	42.6	39.3	33.4	29.3	27.1	26.4	25.2	22.6	24.8	24.5
65 years and over	28.5	24.8	20.9	19.6	14.6	14.9	10.2	8.9	9.3	10.5	9.5
White male[4]											
18–24 years	53.0	40.8	34.3	28.4	27.4	28.4	30.4	29.7	26.5	25.2	30.0
25–34 years	60.1	49.5	43.6	37.3	31.6	29.9	29.7	27.7	29.0	29.5	28.4
35–44 years	57.3	50.1	41.3	36.6	33.5	31.2	30.6	26.3	24.4	24.9	26.3
45–64 years	51.3	41.2	38.3	32.1	28.7	26.3	25.8	24.5	22.1	24.0	24.0
65 years and over	27.7	24.3	20.5	18.9	13.7	14.1	9.8	7.9	8.9	9.9	9.3
Black or African American male[4]											
18–24 years	62.8	54.9	40.2	27.2	21.3	*14.6	20.9	21.6	21.4	*17.0	18.9
25–34 years	68.4	58.5	47.5	45.6	33.8	25.1	23.2	29.8	32.3	25.9	24.1
35–44 years	67.3	61.5	48.6	45.0	42.0	36.3	30.7	23.3	17.4	21.8	24.0
45–64 years	57.9	57.8	50.0	46.1	36.7	33.9	32.2	32.4	28.3	33.6	28.9
65 years and over	36.4	29.7	26.2	27.7	21.5	28.5	14.2	16.8	14.3	17.5	14.0
All females											
18–24 years	38.1	34.1	33.8	30.4	22.5	21.8	24.9	20.7	19.1	19.0	15.6
25–34 years	43.7	38.8	33.7	32.0	28.2	26.4	22.3	21.5	19.6	21.4	21.8
35–44 years	43.7	39.8	37.0	31.5	24.8	27.1	26.2	21.3	19.6	20.9	21.2
45–64 years	32.0	33.4	30.7	29.9	24.8	24.0	21.7	18.8	19.5	20.5	19.5
65 years and over	9.6	12.0	13.2	13.5	11.5	11.5	9.3	8.3	7.6	8.3	9.5
White female[4]											
18–24 years	38.4	34.0	34.5	31.8	25.4	24.9	28.5	22.6	21.6	20.1	16.7
25–34 years	43.4	38.6	34.1	32.0	28.5	27.3	24.9	23.1	21.4	23.1	22.7
35–44 years	43.9	39.3	37.2	31.0	25.0	27.0	26.6	22.2	20.7	22.6	22.9
45–64 years	32.7	33.0	30.6	29.7	25.4	24.3	21.4	18.9	19.6	20.9	19.4
65 years and over	9.8	12.3	13.8	13.3	11.5	11.7	9.1	8.4	8.0	8.6	9.6
Black or African American female[4]											
18–24 years	37.1	35.6	31.8	23.7	10.0	*8.8	14.2	14.2	*8.7	16.6	13.3
25–34 years	47.8	42.2	35.2	36.2	29.1	26.7	15.5	16.9	14.9	17.6	20.1
35–44 years	42.8	46.4	37.7	40.2	25.5	31.9	30.2	19.0	17.7	19.6	20.0
45–64 years	25.7	38.9	34.2	33.4	22.6	27.5	25.6	21.0	22.6	21.3	22.7
65 years and over	7.1	*8.9	*8.5	14.5	11.1	13.3	10.2	10.0	6.4	8.1	11.5

See footnotes at end of table.

Table 58 (page 2 of 2). Current cigarette smoking among adults 18 years of age and over, by sex, race, and age: United States, selected years 1965–2009

[Data are based on household interviews of a sample of the civilian noninstitutionalized population]

* Estimates are considered unreliable. Data preceded by an asterisk have a relative standard error of 20%–30%.

[1]Data prior to 1997 are not strictly comparable with data for later years due to the 1997 questionnaire redesign. See Appendix I, National Health Interview Survey.

[2]Estimates are age-adjusted to the year 2000 standard population using five age groups: 18–24 years, 25–34 years, 35–44 years, 45–64 years, 65 years and over. Age-adjusted estimates in this table may differ from other age-adjusted estimates based on the same data and presented elsewhere if different age groups are used in the adjustment procedure. See Appendix II, Age adjustment.

[3]Starting with 1993 data (shown in spreadsheet version), current cigarette smokers were defined as ever smoking 100 cigarettes in their lifetime and smoking now every day or some days. For previous definition, see Appendix II, Cigarette smoking.

[4]The race groups, white and black, include persons of Hispanic and non-Hispanic origin. Starting with 1999 data, race-specific estimates are tabulated according to the *1997 Revisions to the Standards for the Classification of Federal Data on Race and Ethnicity* and are not strictly comparable with estimates for earlier years. The single-race categories shown in the table conform to the 1997 Standards. Starting with 1999 data, race-specific estimates are for persons who reported only one racial group. Prior to 1999, data were tabulated according to the 1977 Standards. Estimates for single-race categories prior to 1999 included persons who reported one race or, if they reported more than one race, identified one race as best representing their race. Starting with 2003 data, race responses of other race and unspecified multiple race were treated as missing, and then race was imputed if these were the only race responses. Almost all persons with a race response of other race were of Hispanic origin. See Appendix II, Hispanic origin; Race. For additional data on cigarette smoking by racial groups, see Table 60.

NOTES: Standard errors for selected years are available in the spreadsheet version of this table. Available from: http://www.cdc.gov/nchs/hus.htm. Data for additional years are available. See Appendix III.

SOURCE: CDC/NCHS, National Health Interview Survey. Data are from the core questionnaire (1965) and the following questionnaire supplements: hypertension (1974), smoking (1979), alcohol and health practices (1983), health promotion and disease prevention (1985, 1990–1991), cancer control and cancer epidemiology (1992), and year 2000 objectives (1993–1995). Starting with 1997, data are from the family core and sample adult questionnaires.

Table 59. Age-adjusted prevalence of current cigarette smoking among adults 25 years of age and over, by sex, race, and education level: United States, selected years 1974–2009

[Data are based on household interviews of a sample of the civilian noninstitutionalized population]

Sex, race, and education level	1974[1]	1979[1]	1985[1]	1990[1]	1995[1]	2000	2005	2007	2008	2009
25 years and over, age-adjusted[2]	Percent of persons who were current cigarette smokers[3]									
All persons[4]	36.9	33.1	30.0	25.4	24.5	22.6	20.3	19.3	20.5	20.4
No high school diploma or GED	43.7	40.7	40.8	36.7	35.6	31.6	28.2	26.9	29.8	28.9
High school diploma or GED	36.2	33.6	32.0	29.1	29.1	29.2	27.0	26.6	28.1	28.7
Some college, no bachelor's degree	35.9	33.2	29.5	23.4	22.6	21.7	21.8	20.1	22.1	21.4
Bachelor's degree or higher	27.2	22.6	18.5	13.9	13.6	10.9	9.1	9.0	8.5	9.0
All males[4]	42.9	37.3	32.8	28.2	26.4	24.7	22.7	21.4	22.6	22.4
No high school diploma or GED	52.3	47.6	45.7	42.0	39.7	36.0	31.7	30.8	32.5	32.3
High school diploma or GED	42.4	38.9	35.5	33.1	32.7	32.1	29.9	29.4	31.4	31.4
Some college, no bachelor's degree	41.8	36.5	32.9	25.9	23.7	23.3	24.9	21.6	24.3	23.0
Bachelor's degree or higher	28.3	22.7	19.6	14.5	13.8	11.6	9.7	10.4	9.1	9.6
White males[4,5]	41.9	36.7	31.7	27.6	25.9	24.7	22.4	21.6	22.6	22.7
No high school diploma or GED	51.5	47.6	45.0	41.8	38.7	38.2	31.6	30.8	33.1	32.2
High school diploma or GED	42.0	38.5	34.8	32.9	32.9	32.4	30.0	29.9	31.9	32.4
Some college, no bachelor's degree	41.6	36.4	32.2	25.4	23.3	23.5	24.5	21.8	23.7	22.4
Bachelor's degree or higher	27.8	22.5	19.1	14.4	13.4	11.3	9.3	10.5	9.1	9.6
Black or African American males[4,5]	53.4	44.4	42.1	34.5	31.6	26.4	26.5	23.7	25.9	23.7
No high school diploma or GED	58.1	49.7	50.5	41.6	41.9	38.2	35.9	30.4	35.0	39.1
High school diploma or GED	*50.7	48.6	41.8	37.4	36.6	29.0	30.1	29.6	28.3	26.0
Some college, no bachelor's degree	*45.3	39.2	41.8	28.1	26.4	19.9	27.4	23.6	29.5	26.5
Bachelor's degree or higher	*41.4	*36.8	*32.0	*20.8	*17.3	14.6	10.0	*13.5	*10.0	9.9
All females[4]	32.0	29.5	27.5	22.9	22.9	20.5	18.0	17.2	18.4	18.5
No high school diploma or GED	36.6	34.8	36.5	31.8	31.7	27.1	24.6	22.7	27.0	24.8
High school diploma or GED	32.2	29.8	29.5	26.1	26.4	26.6	24.1	23.8	25.0	26.1
Some college, no bachelor's degree	30.1	30.0	26.3	21.0	21.6	20.4	19.1	18.9	20.1	20.0
Bachelor's degree or higher	25.9	22.5	17.1	13.3	13.3	10.1	8.5	7.7	8.1	8.4
White females[4,5]	31.7	29.7	27.3	23.3	23.1	21.0	18.6	18.0	19.4	19.0
No high school diploma or GED	36.8	35.8	36.7	33.4	32.4	28.4	24.6	23.8	28.4	24.4
High school diploma or GED	31.9	29.9	29.4	26.5	26.8	27.8	25.9	25.2	27.1	26.5
Some college, no bachelor's degree	30.4	30.7	26.7	21.2	22.2	21.1	19.5	19.6	21.6	21.2
Bachelor's degree or higher	25.5	21.9	16.5	13.4	13.5	10.2	9.1	8.2	8.5	9.1
Black or African American females[4,5]	35.6	30.3	32.0	22.4	25.7	21.6	17.5	16.6	17.5	19.3
No high school diploma or GED	36.1	31.6	39.4	26.3	32.3	31.1	27.8	23.1	28.9	31.0
High school diploma or GED	40.9	32.6	32.1	24.1	27.8	25.4	18.2	19.8	20.0	27.3
Some college, no bachelor's degree	32.3	*28.9	23.9	22.7	20.8	20.4	17.5	17.2	15.9	16.2
Bachelor's degree or higher	*36.3	*43.3	26.6	17.0	17.3	10.8	*6.6	*6.0	*9.3	*7.3

* Estimates are considered unreliable. Data preceded by an asterisk have a relative standard error of 20%–30%.

[1]Data prior to 1997 are not strictly comparable with data for later years due to the 1997 questionnaire redesign. See Appendix I, National Health Interview Survey.

[2]Estimates are age-adjusted to the year 2000 standard population using four age groups: 25–34 years, 35–44 years, 45–64 years, and 65 years and over. See Appendix II, Age adjustment. For age groups where smoking was 0% or 100%, the age-adjustment procedure was modified to substitute the percentage smoking from the next lower education group.

[3]Starting with 1993 data (shown in spreadsheet version), current cigarette smokers were defined as ever smoking 100 cigarettes in their lifetime and smoking now every day or some days. For previous definition, see Appendix II, Cigarette smoking.

[4]Includes unknown education level. Education categories shown are for 1997 and subsequent years. GED stands for General Educational Development high school equivalency diploma. In 1974–1995 the following categories based on number of years of school completed were used: less than 12 years, 12 years, 13–15 years, 16 years or more. See Appendix II, Education.

[5]The race groups, white and black, include persons of Hispanic and non-Hispanic origin. Starting with 1999 data, race-specific estimates are tabulated according to the 1997 Revisions to the Standards for the Classification of Federal Data on Race and Ethnicity and are not strictly comparable with estimates for earlier years. The single-race categories shown in the table conform to the 1997 Standards. Starting with 1999 data, race-specific estimates are for persons who reported only one racial group. Prior to 1999, data were tabulated according to the 1977 Standards. Estimates for single-race categories prior to 1999 included persons who reported one race or, if they reported more than one race, identified one race as best representing their race. Starting with 2003 data, race responses of other race and unspecified multiple race were treated as missing, and then race was imputed if these were the only race responses. Almost all persons with a race response of other race were of Hispanic origin. See Appendix II, Hispanic origin; Race. For additional data on cigarette smoking by racial groups, see Table 60.

NOTES: Standard errors for selected years are available in the spreadsheet version of this table. Available from: http://www.cdc.gov/nchs/hus.htm. Data for additional years are available. See Appendix III.

SOURCE: CDC/NCHS, National Health Interview Survey. Data are from the following questionnaire supplements: hypertension (1974), smoking (1979), alcohol and health practices (1983), health promotion and disease prevention (1985, 1990–1991), cancer control and cancer epidemiology (1992), and year 2000 objectives (1993–1995). Starting with 1997, data are from the family core and sample adult questionnaires.

Table 60 (page 1 of 3). Current cigarette smoking among adults, by sex, race, Hispanic origin, age, and education level: United States, average annual, selected years 1990–1992 through 2007–2009

[Data are based on household interviews of a sample of the civilian noninstitutionalized population]

Characteristic	Male			Female		
	1990–1992[1]	1999–2001	2007–2009	1990–1992[1]	1999–2001	2007–2009
18 years and over, age-adjusted[2]	Percent of persons who were current cigarette smokers[3]					
All persons[4]	27.9	25.0	22.6	23.7	21.1	18.0
Race[5]						
White only.	27.4	25.1	22.9	24.3	22.2	18.9
Black or African American only	33.9	27.2	23.7	23.1	19.7	17.2
American Indian or Alaska Native only	34.2	30.3	28.3	36.7	34.7	20.0
Asian only.	24.8	20.3	15.4	6.3	6.7	5.4
Native Hawaiian or Other Pacific Islander only	- - -	*30.2	18.9	- - -	*27.1	*20.7
2 or more races.	- - -	34.4	25.4	- - -	30.7	22.8
American Indian or Alaska Native; White.	- - -	38.7	36.0	- - -	38.9	26.4
Hispanic origin and race[5]						
Hispanic or Latino	25.7	22.2	18.0	15.8	12.1	9.4
Mexican.	26.2	21.9	18.1	14.8	10.6	8.3
Not Hispanic or Latino	28.1	25.5	23.6	24.4	22.3	19.5
White only	27.7	25.5	24.1	25.2	23.5	20.9
Black or African American only	33.9	27.2	24.0	23.2	19.7	17.3
18 years and over, crude						
All persons[4]	28.4	25.5	23.0	23.6	21.0	17.9
Race[5]						
White only.	27.8	25.4	23.0	24.1	21.7	18.5
Black or African American only	33.2	27.5	24.5	23.3	19.8	17.5
American Indian or Alaska Native only	35.5	31.8	28.5	37.3	36.9	21.2
Asian only.	24.9	21.4	16.1	6.3	6.9	5.6
Native Hawaiian or Other Pacific Islander only	- - -	*36.3	*20.3	- - -	*	*
2 or more races.	- - -	35.9	27.4	- - -	31.5	24.0
American Indian or Alaska Native; White.	- - -	41.1	33.6	- - -	40.1	27.8
Hispanic origin and race[5]						
Hispanic or Latino	26.5	23.2	19.2	16.6	12.6	9.6
Mexican.	27.1	22.8	19.2	15.0	11.0	8.5
Not Hispanic or Latino	28.5	25.8	23.6	24.2	21.9	19.1
White only	28.0	25.5	23.7	24.8	22.7	20.1
Black or African American only	33.3	27.5	24.7	23.3	19.8	17.6
Age and Hispanic origin and race[5]						
18–24 years:						
Hispanic or Latino.	19.3	22.6	19.5	12.8	12.9	7.7
Not Hispanic or Latino:						
White only.	28.9	32.7	29.3	28.7	30.8	22.5
Black or African American only	17.7	21.9	19.2	10.8	13.0	13.1
25–34 years:						
Hispanic or Latino.	29.9	23.2	20.6	19.2	12.5	9.6
Not Hispanic or Latino:						
White only.	32.7	30.8	31.8	30.9	27.4	26.3
Black or African American only	34.6	23.3	27.6	29.2	16.9	17.7
35–44 years:						
Hispanic or Latino.	32.1	25.3	20.0	19.9	14.1	10.3
Not Hispanic or Latino:						
White only.	32.3	29.6	26.5	27.3	28.3	24.7
Black or African American only	44.1	32.0	21.5	31.3	27.5	19.1
45–64 years:						
Hispanic or Latino.	26.6	24.7	19.7	17.1	13.5	12.1
Not Hispanic or Latino:						
White only.	28.4	25.1	23.9	26.1	22.1	21.0
Black or African American only	38.0	34.0	30.4	26.1	23.6	22.4
65 years and over:						
Hispanic or Latino.	16.1	12.6	8.6	6.6	5.9	4.5
Not Hispanic or Latino:						
White only.	14.2	10.0	9.5	12.3	9.8	9.1
Black or African American only	25.2	17.6	15.4	10.7	11.0	8.8

See footnotes at end of table.

Table 60 (page 2 of 3). Current cigarette smoking among adults, by sex, race, Hispanic origin, age, and education level: United States, average annual, selected years 1990–1992 through 2007–2009

[Data are based on household interviews of a sample of the civilian noninstitutionalized population]

Characteristic	Male			Female		
	1990–1992[1]	1999–2001	2007–2009	1990–1992[1]	1999–2001	2007–2009
Percent of poverty level[2,6]	Percent of persons who were current cigarette smokers[3]					
Below 100%	40.5	36.5	31.1	30.7	29.1	28.4
100%–199%	35.0	32.8	29.1	26.9	25.6	22.7
200%–399%	26.5	27.3	25.0	22.6	22.3	18.2
400% or more	22.5	18.8	16.5	19.0	15.9	12.5
Hispanic origin and race and percent of poverty level[2,4,6]						
Hispanic or Latino:						
Below 100%	29.2	25.3	19.6	16.3	14.4	12.0
100%–199%	29.5	22.0	18.6	16.0	11.8	8.4
200%–399%	23.7	23.6	18.9	15.9	12.0	9.4
400% or more	19.7	18.1	16.4	13.6	9.4	7.7
Not Hispanic or Latino:						
White only:						
Below 100%	44.2	40.7	37.8	37.8	38.3	38.9
100%–199%	36.3	37.5	34.5	31.1	32.0	31.6
200%–399%	26.4	28.5	27.8	23.7	24.8	21.9
400% or more	22.5	19.1	16.9	19.5	17.1	13.8
Black or African American only:						
Below 100%	43.5	40.6	37.9	28.9	27.7	26.6
100%–199%	36.0	33.9	31.1	20.3	21.3	19.1
200%–399%	31.4	24.9	21.1	21.4	17.3	11.9
400% or more	24.3	17.9	15.8	19.2	12.6	9.2
Disability measure[7]						
Any basic actions difficulty or complex activity limitation	- - -	33.1	31.0	- - -	28.1	26.9
Any basic actions difficulty	- - -	33.2	31.3	- - -	28.2	27.1
Any complex activity limitation	- - -	37.6	33.8	- - -	30.6	32.5
No disability	- - -	22.8	20.1	- - -	18.8	14.8
Education, Hispanic origin, and race[5,8]						
25 years and over, age-adjusted[9]						
No high school diploma or GED:						
Hispanic or Latino	30.2	24.3	18.8	15.8	12.1	8.3
Not Hispanic or Latino:						
White only	46.1	43.5	44.0	40.4	39.3	44.5
Black or African American only	45.4	40.0	36.5	31.3	29.4	28.1
High school diploma or GED:						
Hispanic or Latino	29.6	24.1	20.4	18.4	12.5	10.6
Not Hispanic or Latino:						
White only	32.9	31.8	34.4	28.4	29.2	29.8
Black or African American only	38.2	31.4	27.8	25.4	23.0	22.6
Some college or more:						
Hispanic or Latino	20.4	17.1	15.0	14.3	11.1	10.5
Not Hispanic or Latino:						
White only	19.3	17.6	15.8	18.1	16.7	15.1
Black or African American only	25.6	19.2	20.0	22.8	16.9	13.2

See footnotes at end of table.

Table 60 (page 3 of 3). Current cigarette smoking among adults, by sex, race, Hispanic origin, age, and education level: United States, average annual, selected years 1990–1992 through 2007–2009

[Data are based on household interviews of a sample of the civilian noninstitutionalized population]

- - - Data not available.
* Estimates are considered unreliable. Data preceded by an asterisk have a relative standard error (RSE) of 20%–30%. Data not shown have an RSE greater than 30%.

[1]Data prior to 1997 are not strictly comparable with data for later years due to the 1997 questionnaire redesign. See Appendix I, National Health Interview Survey.

[2]Estimates are age-adjusted to the year 2000 standard population using five age groups: 18–24 years, 25–34 years, 35–44 years, 45–64 years, and 65 years and over. See Appendix II, Age adjustment. For age groups where smoking is 0% or 100%, the age-adjustment procedure was modified to substitute the percentage smoking from the previous 3-year period.

[3]Starting with 1993 data, current cigarette smokers were defined as ever smoking 100 cigarettes in their lifetime and smoking now every day or some days. For previous definition, see Appendix II, Cigarette smoking.

[4]Includes all other races not shown separately, unknown education level, and unknown disability measure.

[5]The race groups white, black, American Indian or Alaska Native (AI/AN), Asian, Native Hawaiian or Other Pacific Islander, and 2 or more races include persons of Hispanic and non-Hispanic origin. Persons of Hispanic origin may be of any race. Starting with 1999 data, race-specific estimates are tabulated according to the 1997 Revisions to the Standards for the Classification of Federal Data on Race and Ethnicity and are not strictly comparable with estimates for earlier years. The five single-race categories plus multiple-race categories shown in the table conform to the 1997 Standards. Starting with 1999–2001 data, race-specific estimates are for persons who reported only one racial group; the category 2 or more races includes persons who reported more than one racial group. Prior to 1999, data were tabulated according to the 1977 Standards with four racial groups and the Asian only category included Native Hawaiian or Other Pacific Islander. Estimates for single-race categories prior to 1999 included persons who reported one race or, if they reported more than one race, identified one race as best representing their race. Starting with 2003 data, race responses of other race and unspecified multiple race were treated as missing, and then race was imputed if these were the only race responses. Almost all persons with a race response of other race were of Hispanic origin. See Appendix II, Hispanic origin; Race.

[6]Percent of poverty level is based on family income and family size and composition using U.S. Census Bureau poverty thresholds. Missing family income data were imputed for 1990 and beyond. See Appendix II, Family income; Poverty; Table VII.

[7]Any basic actions difficulty or complex activity limitation is defined as having one or more of the following limitations or difficulties: movement difficulty, emotional difficulty, sensory (seeing or hearing) difficulty, cognitive difficulty, self-care (ADL or IADL) limitation, social limitation, or work limitation. For more information, see Appendix II, Basic actions difficulty; Complex activity limitation. Starting with 2007 data, the hearing question, a component of the basic actions difficulty measure, was revised. Consequently, data prior to 2007 are not comparable with data for 2007 and beyond. For more information on the impact of the revised hearing question, see Appendix II, Hearing trouble.

[8]Education categories shown are for 1997 and subsequent years. GED is General Educational Development high school equivalency diploma. In years prior to 1997, the following categories based on number of years of school completed were used: less than 12 years, 12 years, 13 years or more. See Appendix II, Education.

[9]Estimates are age-adjusted to the year 2000 standard using four age groups: 25–34 years, 35–44 years, 45–64 years, and 65 years and over. See Appendix II, Age adjustment.

NOTES: Standard errors for selected years are available in the spreadsheet version of this table. Available from: http://www.cdc.gov/nchs/hus.htm. Data for additional years are available. See Appendix III.

SOURCE: CDC/NCHS, National Health Interview Survey. Data are from the following questionnaire supplements: health promotion and disease prevention (1990–1991), cancer control and cancer epidemiology (1992), and year 2000 objectives (1993–1995). Starting with 1997, data are from the family core and sample adult questionnaires.

Table 61 (page 1 of 2). Use of selected substances in the past month among persons 12 years of age and over, by age, sex, race, and Hispanic origin: United States, selected years 2002–2008

[Data are based on household interviews of a sample of the civilian noninstitutionalized population 12 years of age and over]

Age, sex, race, and Hispanic origin	Any illicit drug[1]			Marijuana			Nonmedical use of any psychotherapeutic drug[2]		
	2002	2007	2008	2002	2007	2008	2002	2007	2008
	Percent of population								
12 years and over	8.3	8.0	8.0	6.2	5.8	6.1	2.7	2.8	2.5
Age									
12–13 years	4.2	3.3	3.3	1.4	0.9	1.0	1.7	1.4	1.5
14–15 years	11.2	8.9	8.6	7.6	5.7	5.7	4.0	3.4	3.0
16–17 years	19.8	16.0	15.2	15.7	13.1	12.7	6.3	4.9	4.0
18–25 years	20.2	19.7	19.6	17.3	16.4	16.5	5.5	6.0	5.9
26–34 years	10.5	10.9	11.2	7.7	7.9	8.8	3.7	3.5	3.2
35 years and over	4.6	4.6	4.7	3.1	3.0	3.2	1.6	1.9	1.6
Sex									
Male	10.3	10.4	9.9	8.1	8.0	7.9	2.8	3.2	2.6
Female	6.4	5.8	6.3	4.4	3.8	4.4	2.6	2.3	2.4
Age and sex									
12–17 years	11.6	9.5	9.3	8.2	6.7	6.7	4.0	3.3	2.9
Male	12.3	10.0	9.5	9.1	7.5	7.3	3.6	3.0	2.5
Female	10.9	9.1	9.1	7.2	5.8	6.0	4.4	3.5	3.3
Hispanic origin and race[3]									
Not Hispanic or Latino:									
White only	8.5	8.2	8.2	6.5	6.0	6.2	2.8	3.0	2.8
Black or African American only	9.7	9.5	10.1	7.4	7.2	8.3	2.0	2.2	1.8
American Indian or Alaska Native only	10.1	12.6	9.5	6.7	7.9	8.2	3.2	4.5	3.0
Native Hawaiian or Other Pacific Islander only	7.9	*	7.3	4.4	2.8	5.5	3.8	*	1.7
Asian only	3.5	4.2	3.6	1.8	2.6	2.0	0.7	1.5	1.0
2 or more races	11.4	11.8	14.7	9.0	10.4	13.1	3.5	4.1	2.7
Hispanic or Latino	7.2	6.6	6.2	4.3	4.5	4.2	2.9	2.3	1.8

Age, sex, race, and Hispanic origin	Alcohol use			Binge alcohol use[4]			Heavy alcohol use[5]		
	2002	2007	2008	2002	2007	2008	2002	2007	2008
	Percent of population								
12 years and over	51.0	51.1	51.6	22.9	23.3	23.3	6.7	6.9	6.9
Age									
12–13 years	4.3	3.5	3.4	1.8	1.5	1.5	0.3	0.1	0.2
14–15 years	16.6	14.7	13.1	9.2	7.8	6.9	1.9	1.4	1.1
16–17 years	32.6	29.0	26.2	21.4	19.4	17.2	5.6	5.4	4.4
18–25 years	60.5	61.2	61.2	40.9	41.8	41.0	14.9	14.7	14.5
26–34 years	61.4	62.6	63.5	33.1	35.1	36.4	9.0	9.7	10.6
35 years and over	52.1	52.2	52.8	18.6	18.9	18.8	5.2	5.3	5.3
Sex									
Male	57.4	56.6	57.7	31.2	31.7	31.6	10.8	10.6	10.6
Female	44.9	46.0	45.9	15.1	15.4	15.4	3.0	3.3	3.4
Age and sex									
12–17 years	17.6	15.9	14.6	10.7	9.7	8.8	2.5	2.3	2.0
Male	17.4	15.9	14.2	11.4	10.6	8.9	3.1	2.8	2.3
Female	17.9	16.0	15.0	9.9	8.8	8.7	1.9	1.8	1.6
Hispanic origin and race[3]									
Not Hispanic or Latino:									
White only	55.0	56.1	56.2	23.4	24.6	24.0	7.5	7.8	7.7
Black or African American only	39.9	39.3	41.9	21.0	19.1	20.4	4.4	4.1	5.6
American Indian or Alaska Native only	44.7	44.7	43.3	27.9	28.2	24.4	8.7	11.6	5.7
Native Hawaiian or Other Pacific Islander only	*	*	*	25.2	*	*	8.3	*	3.5
Asian only	37.1	35.2	37.0	12.4	12.6	11.9	2.6	2.6	2.4
2 or more races	49.9	47.5	47.5	19.8	23.2	22.0	7.5	7.3	7.4
Hispanic or Latino	42.8	42.1	43.2	24.8	23.4	25.6	5.9	5.5	5.7

See footnotes at end of table.

Table 61 (page 2 of 2). Use of selected substances in the past month among persons 12 years of age and over, by age, sex, race, and Hispanic origin: United States, selected years 2002–2008

[Data are based on household interviews of a sample of the civilian noninstitutionalized population 12 years of age and over]

Age, sex, race, and Hispanic origin	Any tobacco[6]			Cigarettes			Cigars		
	2002	2007	2008	2002	2007	2008	2002	2007	2008
	Percent of population								
12 years and over	30.4	28.6	28.4	26.0	24.2	23.9	5.4	5.4	5.3
Age									
12–13 years	3.8	2.4	2.5	3.2	1.8	2.1	0.7	0.7	0.6
14–15 years	13.4	10.8	9.7	11.2	8.4	7.6	3.8	3.4	3.1
16–17 years	29.0	23.4	21.1	24.9	18.9	16.8	9.3	8.4	7.3
18–25 years	45.3	41.8	41.4	40.8	36.2	35.7	11.0	11.8	11.3
26–34 years	38.2	38.6	38.3	32.7	33.4	33.6	6.6	7.1	7.2
35 years and over	27.9	26.2	26.1	23.4	22.0	21.6	4.1	3.8	3.8
Sex									
Male.	37.0	35.2	34.5	28.7	27.1	26.3	9.4	9.1	9.0
Female.	24.3	22.4	22.5	23.4	21.5	21.7	1.7	1.8	1.7
Age and sex									
12–17 years	15.2	12.4	11.4	13.0	9.8	9.1	4.5	4.2	3.8
Male.	16.0	14.1	12.6	12.3	10.0	9.0	6.2	6.0	5.3
Female	14.4	10.6	10.2	13.6	9.7	9.2	2.7	2.4	2.2
Hispanic origin and race[3]									
Not Hispanic or Latino:									
White only.	32.0	30.7	30.4	26.9	25.6	25.2	5.5	5.5	5.3
Black or African American only.	28.8	26.8	28.6	25.3	23.2	24.8	6.8	6.7	7.0
American Indian or Alaska Native only . .	44.3	41.8	48.7	37.1	34.4	44.1	5.2	8.4	5.6
Native Hawaiian or Other Pacific									
Islander only.	28.8	*	*	*	*	*	4.1	*	2.2
Asian only	18.6	15.4	13.9	17.7	14.2	11.9	1.1	1.5	1.2
2 or more races	38.1	35.2	37.3	35.0	29.9	32.2	5.5	7.9	7.2
Hispanic or Latino	25.2	22.7	21.3	23.0	20.5	19.4	5.0	4.2	4.5

* Estimates are considered unreliable. Data not shown if the relative standard error is greater than 17.5% of the log transformation of the proportion, the minimum effective sample size is less than 68, the minimum nominal sample size is less than 100, or the prevalence is close to 0% or 100%.
[1]Any illicit drug includes marijuana/hashish, cocaine (including crack), heroin, hallucinogens (including LSD and PCP), inhalants, or any prescription-type psychotherapeutic drug used nonmedically.
[2]Nonmedical use of prescription-type psychotherapeutic drugs includes the nonmedical use of pain relievers, tranquilizers, stimulants, or sedatives and does not include over-the-counter drugs. Special questions on methamphetamine were added in 2005 and 2006. Data for years prior to 2007 have been adjusted for comparability.
[3]Persons of Hispanic origin may be of any race. Race and Hispanic origin were collected using the *1997 Revisions to the Standards for the Classification of Federal Data on Race and Ethnicity*. Single-race categories shown include persons who reported only one racial group. The category 2 or more races includes persons who reported more than one racial group. See Appendix II, Hispanic origin; Race.
[4]Binge alcohol use is defined as drinking five or more drinks on the same occasion on at least 1 day in the past 30 days. Occasion is defined as at the same time or within a couple of hours of each other. See Appendix II, Binge drinking.
[5]Heavy alcohol use is defined as drinking five or more drinks on the same occasion on each of 5 or more days in the past 30 days. By definition, all heavy alcohol users are also binge alcohol users.
[6]Any tobacco product includes cigarettes, smokeless tobacco (i.e., chewing tobacco or snuff), cigars, or pipe tobacco.

NOTES: The National Survey on Drug Use & Health (NSDUH), formerly called the National Household Survey on Drug Abuse (NHSDA), began a new baseline in 2002 and cannot be compared with previous years. Because of methodological differences among the National Survey on Drug Use & Health, the Monitoring the Future Study (MTF), and the Youth Risk Behavior Survey (YRBS), rates of substance use measured by these surveys are not directly comparable. See Appendix I, MTF, NSDUH, and YRBS. Data for additional years are available. See Appendix III.

SOURCE: Substance Abuse and Mental Health Services Administration, Office of Applied Studies, National Survey on Drug Use & Health. Available from: http://www.oas.samhsa.gov/nsduh.htm.

[Data are based on a survey of high school seniors, 10th graders, and 8th graders in the coterminous United States]

Substance, grade in school, sex, and race	1980	1985	1990	1991	1995	2000	2006	2007	2008	2009
Cigarettes				Percent using substance in the past month						
All high school seniors	30.5	30.1	29.4	28.3	33.5	31.4	21.6	21.6	20.4	20.1
Male	26.8	28.2	29.1	29.0	34.5	32.8	22.4	23.1	21.5	22.1
Female	33.4	31.4	29.2	27.5	32.0	29.7	20.1	19.6	19.1	17.6
White	31.0	31.7	32.5	31.8	37.3	36.6	24.7	25.2	24.1	23.7
Black or African American	25.2	18.7	12.0	9.4	15.0	13.6	11.0	10.6	10.1	9.3
All 10th graders	- - -	- - -	- - -	20.8	27.9	23.9	14.5	14.0	12.3	13.1
Male	- - -	- - -	- - -	20.8	27.7	23.8	13.4	14.6	12.7	13.7
Female	- - -	- - -	- - -	20.7	27.9	23.6	15.5	13.3	11.9	12.5
White	- - -	- - -	- - -	23.9	31.2	27.3	16.3	16.1	14.1	14.6
Black or African American	- - -	- - -	- - -	6.4	12.2	11.3	8.5	5.8	7.1	6.4
All 8th graders	- - -	- - -	- - -	14.3	19.1	14.6	8.7	7.1	6.8	6.5
Male	- - -	- - -	- - -	15.5	18.8	14.3	8.1	7.5	6.7	6.7
Female	- - -	- - -	- - -	13.1	19.0	14.7	8.9	6.4	6.7	6.0
White	- - -	- - -	- - -	15.0	21.7	16.4	9.1	7.1	7.3	7.3
Black or African American	- - -	- - -	- - -	5.3	8.2	8.4	5.4	4.8	4.4	4.5
Marijuana										
All high school seniors	33.7	25.7	14.0	13.8	21.2	21.6	18.3	18.8	19.4	20.6
Male	37.8	28.7	16.1	16.1	24.6	24.7	19.7	22.3	22.2	24.3
Female	29.1	22.4	11.5	11.2	17.2	18.3	16.4	15.0	16.2	16.8
White	34.2	26.4	15.6	15.0	21.5	22.0	19.2	19.9	20.4	21.2
Black or African American	26.5	21.7	5.2	6.5	17.8	17.5	16.7	15.4	17.1	20.6
All 10th graders	- - -	- - -	- - -	8.7	17.2	19.7	14.2	14.2	13.8	15.9
Male	- - -	- - -	- - -	10.1	19.2	23.3	15.7	15.8	15.2	18.7
Female	- - -	- - -	- - -	7.3	15.0	16.2	12.6	12.5	12.3	13.2
White	- - -	- - -	- - -	9.4	17.7	20.1	14.7	14.8	13.5	15.6
Black or African American	- - -	- - -	- - -	3.8	15.1	17.0	14.2	11.0	12.3	15.1
All 8th graders	- - -	- - -	- - -	3.2	9.1	9.1	6.5	5.7	5.8	6.5
Male	- - -	- - -	- - -	3.8	9.8	10.2	6.7	6.2	6.6	7.5
Female	- - -	- - -	- - -	2.6	8.2	7.8	6.0	4.9	4.8	5.3
White	- - -	- - -	- - -	3.0	9.0	8.3	5.7	5.1	4.9	5.9
Black or African American	- - -	- - -	- - -	2.1	7.0	8.5	6.7	6.0	6.2	7.2
Cocaine										
All high school seniors	5.2	6.7	1.9	1.4	1.8	2.1	2.5	2.0	1.9	1.3
Male	6.0	7.7	2.3	1.7	2.2	2.7	3.0	2.4	2.3	1.5
Female	4.3	5.6	1.3	0.9	1.3	1.6	2.1	1.5	1.3	0.9
White	5.4	7.0	1.8	1.3	1.7	2.2	2.6	2.3	2.0	1.2
Black or African American	2.0	2.7	0.5	0.8	0.4	1.0	1.0	0.5	0.5	0.2
All 10th graders	- - -	- - -	- - -	0.7	1.7	1.8	1.5	1.3	1.2	0.9
Male	- - -	- - -	- - -	0.7	1.8	2.1	1.6	1.4	1.4	1.0
Female	- - -	- - -	- - -	0.6	1.5	1.4	1.3	1.1	1.0	0.8
White	- - -	- - -	- - -	0.6	1.7	1.7	1.5	1.2	1.0	0.7
Black or African American	- - -	- - -	- - -	0.2	0.4	0.4	0.7	0.4	0.7	0.5
All 8th graders	- - -	- - -	- - -	0.5	1.2	1.2	1.0	0.9	0.8	0.8
Male	- - -	- - -	- - -	0.7	1.1	1.3	1.0	0.7	0.9	0.8
Female	- - -	- - -	- - -	0.4	1.2	1.1	0.9	1.0	0.7	0.7
White	- - -	- - -	- - -	0.4	1.0	1.1	0.8	0.6	0.6	0.6
Black or African American	- - -	- - -	- - -	0.4	0.4	0.5	0.4	0.6	0.4	0.7

See footnotes at end of table.

[Data are based on a survey of high school seniors, 10th graders, and 8th graders in the coterminous United States]

Substance, grade in school, sex, and race	1980	1985	1990	1991	1995	2000	2006	2007	2008	2009
Inhalants				Percent using substance in the past month						
All high school seniors	1.4	2.2	2.7	2.4	3.2	2.2	1.5	1.2	1.4	1.2
Male	1.8	2.8	3.5	3.3	3.9	2.9	1.5	1.5	1.6	1.2
Female.	1.0	1.7	2.0	1.6	2.5	1.7	1.4	0.9	1.2	1.0
White.	1.4	2.4	3.0	2.4	3.7	2.1	1.5	1.2	1.5	1.1
Black or African American	1.0	0.8	1.5	1.5	1.1	2.1	1.2	0.9	1.0	1.1
All 10th graders	- - -	- - -	- - -	2.7	3.5	2.6	2.3	2.5	2.1	2.2
Male	- - -	- - -	- - -	2.9	3.8	3.0	2.2	2.7	1.9	1.8
Female.	- - -	- - -	- - -	2.6	3.2	2.2	2.4	2.4	2.3	2.6
White.	- - -	- - -	- - -	2.9	3.9	2.8	2.4	2.6	1.6	1.9
Black or African American	- - -	- - -	- - -	2.0	1.2	1.5	1.8	1.5	1.9	1.3
All 8th graders	- - -	- - -	- - -	4.4	6.1	4.5	4.1	3.9	4.1	3.8
Male	- - -	- - -	- - -	4.1	5.6	4.1	3.6	3.4	2.9	3.3
Female.	- - -	- - -	- - -	4.7	6.6	4.8	4.7	4.3	5.3	4.3
White.	- - -	- - -	- - -	4.5	7.0	4.8	4.2	3.6	3.8	3.7
Black or African American	- - -	- - -	- - -	2.3	2.3	2.3	2.7	2.8	2.8	3.4
MDMA (Ecstasy)										
All high school seniors	- - -	- - -	- - -	- - -	- - -	3.6	1.3	1.6	1.8	1.8
Male	- - -	- - -	- - -	- - -	- - -	4.1	1.5	1.5	2.3	2.4
Female.	- - -	- - -	- - -	- - -	- - -	3.1	1.1	1.6	1.2	1.2
White.	- - -	- - -	- - -	- - -	- - -	3.9	1.4	1.7	1.7	1.7
Black or African American	- - -	- - -	- - -	- - -	- - -	1.9	0.6	0.8	1.1	1.8
All 10th graders	- - -	- - -	- - -	- - -	- - -	2.6	1.2	1.2	1.1	1.3
Male	- - -	- - -	- - -	- - -	- - -	2.5	1.5	1.3	1.6	1.6
Female.	- - -	- - -	- - -	- - -	- - -	2.5	0.8	1.1	0.7	1.0
White.	- - -	- - -	- - -	- - -	- - -	2.5	1.3	1.4	1.0	1.0
Black or African American	- - -	- - -	- - -	- - -	- - -	1.8	1.0	0.4	0.1	0.6
All 8th graders	- - -	- - -	- - -	- - -	- - -	1.4	0.7	0.6	0.8	0.6
Male	- - -	- - -	- - -	- - -	- - -	1.6	0.5	0.7	0.7	0.5
Female.	- - -	- - -	- - -	- - -	- - -	1.2	0.8	0.6	0.9	0.6
White.	- - -	- - -	- - -	- - -	- - -	1.4	0.5	0.5	0.7	0.6
Black or African American	- - -	- - -	- - -	- - -	- - -	0.8	0.7	0.8	0.3	0.1
Alcohol [1]										
All high school seniors	72.0	65.9	57.1	54.0	51.3	50.0	45.3	44.4	43.1	43.5
Male	77.4	69.8	61.3	58.4	55.7	54.0	47.3	47.1	45.8	47.8
Female.	66.8	62.1	52.3	49.0	47.0	46.1	43.0	41.4	40.9	38.9
White.	75.8	70.2	62.2	57.7	54.8	55.3	49.1	49.4	47.8	46.6
Black or African American	47.7	43.6	32.9	34.4	37.4	29.3	29.5	27.9	29.3	32.2
All 10th graders	- - -	- - -	- - -	42.8	38.8	41.0	33.8	33.4	28.8	30.4
Male	- - -	- - -	- - -	45.5	39.7	43.3	33.8	33.4	28.6	31.0
Female.	- - -	- - -	- - -	40.3	37.8	38.6	33.8	33.3	29.0	29.8
White.	- - -	- - -	- - -	45.7	41.3	44.3	36.0	35.7	30.5	32.4
Black or African American	- - -	- - -	- - -	30.2	24.9	24.7	22.4	21.0	20.4	20.1
All 8th graders	- - -	- - -	- - -	25.1	24.6	22.4	17.2	15.9	15.9	14.9
Male	- - -	- - -	- - -	26.3	25.0	22.5	16.3	15.6	15.4	14.7
Female.	- - -	- - -	- - -	23.8	24.0	22.0	17.6	16.0	16.4	14.9
White.	- - -	- - -	- - -	26.0	25.4	23.9	16.5	14.7	15.8	15.1
Black or African American	- - -	- - -	- - -	17.8	17.3	15.1	12.4	12.3	13.5	11.1

See footnotes at end of table.

Table 62 (page 3 of 3). Use of selected substances among high school seniors, 10th graders, and 8th graders, by sex and race: United States, selected years 1980–2009

[Data are based on a survey of high school seniors, 10th graders, and 8th graders in the coterminous United States]

Substance, grade in school, sex, and race	1980	1985	1990	1991	1995	2000	2006	2007	2008	2009
Binge drinking[2]				Percent in the last 2 weeks						
All high school seniors	41.2	36.7	32.2	29.8	29.8	30.0	25.4	25.9	24.6	25.2
Male	52.1	45.3	39.1	37.8	36.9	36.7	28.9	30.7	28.4	30.5
Female.	30.5	28.2	24.4	21.2	23.0	23.5	21.5	21.5	21.3	20.2
White.	44.6	40.1	36.2	32.9	32.9	34.4	28.9	30.5	29.3	28.7
Black or African American	17.0	16.7	11.6	11.8	15.5	11.0	11.9	11.0	10.8	13.7
All 10th graders	- - -	- - -	- - -	21.0	22.0	24.1	19.9	19.6	16.0	17.5
Male	- - -	- - -	- - -	24.1	24.1	27.6	21.0	20.9	16.6	18.8
Female.	- - -	- - -	- - -	18.1	19.7	20.6	18.9	18.3	15.4	16.1
White.	- - -	- - -	- - -	22.8	24.1	26.6	21.8	21.7	17.4	18.4
Black or African American	- - -	- - -	- - -	11.8	9.6	10.6	9.9	10.0	9.6	10.0
All 8th graders	- - -	- - -	- - -	10.9	12.3	11.7	8.7	8.3	8.1	7.8
Male	- - -	- - -	- - -	12.1	12.5	11.7	8.6	8.2	8.1	7.8
Female.	- - -	- - -	- - -	9.6	12.1	11.3	8.5	8.2	8.0	7.7
White.	- - -	- - -	- - -	11.0	12.6	12.5	8.4	7.7	8.0	7.4
Black or African American	- - -	- - -	- - -	6.7	7.8	6.2	5.5	5.7	5.7	4.8

- - - Data not available.

[1]In 1993, the alcohol question was changed to indicate that a drink meant more than a few sips. Data for 1993, available in the spreadsheet version of this table, are based on a half sample. See Appendix II, Alcohol consumption.

[2]Five or more alcoholic drinks in a row at least once in the prior 2-week period. See Appendix II, Binge drinking. For 8th and 10th graders only: The 1991–2007 data have been revised and differ from previous editions of *Health, United States*. As a result of the revisions, the 1991–2007 data are on average 2 percentage points lower than those previously reported.

NOTES: Estimates for Hispanic students are not shown due to small sample size. For 2-year estimates for Hispanic students, see Johnston LD, O'Malley PM, Bachman JG, Schulenberg JE. Monitoring the Future National Survey results on drug use: 1975–2009. Volume I: Secondary school students. NIH pub no. 10–7584, 2010. Bethesda, MD: National Institute on Drug Abuse, available from http://www.monitoringthefuture.org/pubs/monographs/vol1_2009.pdf. Because of methodological differences among the National Survey on Drug Use & Health (NSDUH), the Monitoring the Future Study (MTF), and the Youth Risk Behavior Survey (YRBS), rates of substance use measured by these surveys are not directly comparable. See Appendix I, National Survey on Drug Use & Health (NSDUH); Monitoring the Future Study (MTF); Youth Risk Behavior Survey (YRBS). Data for additional years are available. See Appendix III.

SOURCE: National Institutes of Health, National Institute on Drug Abuse (NIDA), Monitoring the Future Study, annual surveys.

Table 63 (page 1 of 2). Health risk behaviors among students in grades 9–12, by sex, grade level, race, and Hispanic origin: United States, selected years 1991–2009

[Data are based on a national sample of high school students, grades 9–12]

Sex, grade level, race, and Hispanic origin	Seriously considered suicide			In a physical fight[1]			Carried a weapon[2,3]		
	1991	2007	2009	1991	2007	2009	1991	2007	2009
	Percent of students								
Total	29.0	14.5	13.8	42.5	35.5	31.5	26.1	18.0	17.5
Male									
Total	20.8	10.3	10.5	50.2	44.4	39.3	40.6	28.5	27.1
9th grade	17.6	10.8	10.0	57.8	49.6	45.1	44.4	31.0	27.3
10th grade	19.5	9.3	10.0	50.2	45.1	41.2	41.5	29.3	28.5
11th grade	25.3	10.7	11.4	51.0	46.3	36.2	44.0	27.7	25.6
12th grade	20.7	10.2	10.5	42.3	34.3	32.5	33.1	25.0	26.5
Not Hispanic or Latino:									
White	21.7	10.2	10.5	49.1	41.9	36.0	41.2	30.3	29.3
Black or African American	13.3	8.5	7.8	58.4	50.3	48.3	43.4	24.6	21.0
Hispanic or Latino	18.0	10.7	10.7	48.5	47.3	43.8	40.0	28.2	26.5
Female									
Total	37.2	18.7	17.4	34.4	26.5	22.9	10.9	7.5	7.1
9th grade	40.3	19.0	20.3	42.9	31.8	27.8	10.4	8.9	7.6
10th grade	39.7	22.0	17.2	35.4	27.2	24.8	11.2	8.1	7.2
11th grade	38.4	16.3	17.8	34.5	23.5	20.5	12.9	6.0	6.3
12th grade	30.7	16.7	13.6	25.4	21.8	17.0	9.5	6.2	6.4
Not Hispanic or Latina:									
White	38.6	17.8	16.1	32.2	21.5	18.2	7.5	6.1	6.5
Black or African American	29.4	18.0	18.1	43.8	39.4	33.9	23.6	10.0	7.8
Hispanic or Latina	34.6	21.1	20.2	34.8	33.5	28.5	12.9	9.0	7.9

Sex, grade level, race, and Hispanic origin	Rarely or never wore a seatbelt[4]			Rode with a driver who had been drinking alcohol[2,5]			Drove while drinking alcohol[2,5]		
	1991	2007	2009	1991	2007	2009	1991	2007	2009
	Percent of students								
Total	25.9	11.1	9.7	39.9	29.1	28.3	16.7	10.5	9.7
Male									
Total	30.0	13.6	11.5	40.0	29.5	27.8	21.5	12.8	11.6
9th grade	30.0	15.1	11.2	40.0	27.6	25.3	8.6	6.8	5.1
10th grade	25.5	13.2	11.7	33.9	27.1	28.3	16.1	10.0	11.0
11th grade	29.5	12.2	11.2	36.6	31.4	29.2	26.4	13.7	13.0
12th grade	34.7	13.8	12.0	45.0	32.5	28.6	34.5	23.6	19.3
Not Hispanic or Latino:									
White	28.6	13.0	11.2	40.2	27.8	25.5	23.3	13.9	12.7
Black or African American	37.5	14.7	14.8	37.4	28.1	31.2	14.0	7.5	8.7
Hispanic or Latino	37.1	14.3	9.8	47.2	36.0	33.5	25.1	13.0	11.0
Female									
Total	21.6	8.5	7.7	39.8	28.8	28.8	11.7	8.1	7.6
9th grade	25.0	9.2	9.8	36.0	27.6	30.0	3.3	4.1	4.8
10th grade	20.4	8.3	6.8	38.8	30.4	27.6	7.3	7.3	5.3
11th grade	20.8	8.9	6.0	39.7	26.8	29.6	14.2	9.1	9.6
12th grade	20.2	7.3	8.0	44.8	30.5	27.9	21.7	13.1	11.4
Not Hispanic or Latina:									
White	18.7	7.3	7.6	40.9	28.0	26.9	13.6	9.3	8.7
Black or African American	31.9	10.0	8.3	33.8	26.9	28.7	6.2	3.9	4.1
Hispanic or Latina	25.9	11.4	7.8	46.7	35.1	34.9	9.5	7.7	7.9

See footnotes at end of table.

Table 63 (page 2 of 2). Health risk behaviors among students in grades 9–12, by sex, grade level, race, and Hispanic origin: United States, selected years 1991–2009

[Data are based on a national sample of high school students, grades 9–12]

Sex, grade level, race, and Hispanic origin	Ever had sexual intercourse			Used a condom at last sex[6]			Physically forced to have sex		
	1991	2007	2009	1991	2007	2009	1991	2007	2009
	Percent of students								
Total	54.1	47.8	46.0	46.2	61.5	61.1	- - -	7.8	7.4
Male									
Total	57.4	49.8	46.1	54.5	68.5	68.6	- - -	4.5	4.5
9th grade	45.6	38.1	33.6	56.0	75.8	69.9	- - -	4.1	4.1
10th grade	50.9	45.6	41.9	56.9	73.2	71.9	- - -	3.4	4.0
11th grade	64.5	57.3	53.4	56.8	69.3	68.9	- - -	5.0	5.4
12th grade	68.3	62.8	59.6	50.7	59.6	65.0	- - -	5.7	4.9
Not Hispanic or Latino:									
White	52.7	43.6	39.6	55.2	66.4	71.0	- - -	3.2	3.2
Black or African American	88.1	72.6	72.1	57.0	74.0	72.5	- - -	7.8	7.9
Hispanic or Latino	64.1	58.2	52.8	47.0	69.9	61.7	- - -	6.2	5.7
Female									
Total	50.8	45.9	45.7	38.0	54.9	53.9	- - -	11.3	10.5
9th grade	32.2	27.4	29.3	50.3	61.0	57.7	- - -	9.2	9.4
10th grade	45.3	41.9	39.6	36.4	59.5	63.5	- - -	13.1	10.6
11th grade	60.2	53.6	52.5	40.7	55.1	54.0	- - -	12.0	11.2
12th grade	65.2	66.2	65.0	32.6	49.9	46.3	- - -	10.9	10.8
Not Hispanic or Latina:									
White	47.1	43.7	44.7	38.0	53.9	56.1	- - -	11.0	10.0
Black or African American	75.9	60.9	58.3	39.4	60.1	51.8	- - -	13.3	12.0
Hispanic or Latina	43.3	45.8	45.4	26.9	52.1	48.0	- - -	11.4	11.2

- - - Data not available.
[1]During the last 12 months.
[2]During the last 30 days.
[3]Weapon refers to gun, knife, or club.
[4]When riding in a car driven by someone else.
[5]In car or other vehicle.
[6]Among students who had sexual intercourse in the last 3 months.

NOTES: Only youths attending school participated in the survey. Persons of Hispanic origin may be of any race. See Appendix II, Hispanic origin; Race; Suicidal ideation. Standard errors for selected years are available in the spreadsheet version of this table. Available from: http://www.cdc.gov/nchs/hus.htm. See Appendix III.

SOURCE: CDC/National Center for Chronic Disease Prevention and Health Promotion, National Youth Risk Behavior Survey (YRBS).

Table 64 (page 1 of 3). **Lifetime alcohol drinking status among adults 18 years of age and over, by selected characteristics: United States, selected years 1997–2009**

[Data are based on household interviews of a sample of the civilian noninstitutionalized population]

	Lifetime alcohol drinking status[1]											
	Current drinker				Former drinker				Lifetime abstainer			
Characteristic	1997	2000	2008	2009	1997	2000	2008	2009	1997	2000	2008	2009
	Percent of adults											
18 years and over, age-adjusted[2]	63.1	61.4	64.6	65.3	15.7	14.4	14.3	14.6	21.2	24.2	21.1	20.0
18 years and over, crude	63.4	61.6	64.4	65.1	15.5	14.3	14.5	15.0	21.1	24.1	21.0	19.9
Both sexes												
Age												
All persons:												
18–44 years	69.4	67.3	70.1	70.5	10.6	9.7	8.3	8.7	19.9	23.1	21.6	20.8
18–24 years	62.2	59.1	63.6	62.0	5.9	5.2	3.6	5.6	31.8	35.7	32.8	32.5
25–44 years	71.6	69.9	72.4	73.5	12.0	11.1	9.9	9.9	16.4	19.1	17.7	16.6
45–64 years	63.3	62.0	66.0	66.2	18.5	16.8	17.1	18.2	18.3	21.1	16.9	15.6
45–54 years	67.1	65.1	70.0	68.8	16.8	15.0	14.6	16.1	16.1	20.0	15.3	15.1
55–64 years	57.3	57.3	60.8	62.8	21.1	19.7	20.3	21.0	21.6	22.9	18.9	16.1
65 years and over	43.4	42.1	44.3	47.0	26.7	25.0	27.8	26.4	29.9	33.0	27.9	26.6
65–74 years	48.6	47.0	50.0	53.6	24.8	23.8	25.2	23.9	26.6	29.3	24.7	22.5
75 years and over	36.6	36.2	37.7	39.1	29.1	26.4	30.7	29.5	34.3	37.4	31.5	31.4
Race[2,3]												
White only	66.0	64.5	67.4	68.4	15.2	14.2	14.1	14.3	18.7	21.3	18.5	17.3
Black or African American only	47.8	46.7	51.4	53.2	21.0	17.1	18.3	18.0	31.1	36.1	30.3	28.8
American Indian or Alaska Native only	53.9	54.2	59.0	57.2	22.9	21.7	15.6	18.5	23.2	*24.1	25.3	24.3
Asian only	45.8	43.0	49.8	45.7	8.8	9.2	7.8	11.2	45.3	47.8	42.4	43.1
Native Hawaiian or Other Pacific Islander only	- - -	*	*	*	- - -	*	*	*	- - -	*	*	*
2 or more races	- - -	61.4	64.5	63.8	- - -	19.5	15.5	21.6	- - -	19.1	20.1	14.6
Hispanic origin and race[2,3]												
Hispanic or Latino	53.4	52.4	55.3	54.9	14.7	12.4	13.1	15.0	32.0	35.2	31.6	30.1
Mexican	53.0	51.0	54.8	53.8	14.4	14.4	12.5	16.5	32.6	35.6	32.7	29.7
Not Hispanic or Latino	64.1	62.6	66.1	67.0	15.8	14.6	14.4	14.6	20.1	22.8	19.5	18.4
White only	67.5	65.9	69.8	71.1	15.4	14.4	14.2	14.2	17.1	19.7	16.0	14.8
Black or African American only	47.8	46.7	51.5	53.3	21.0	17.1	18.3	17.9	31.2	36.2	30.2	28.8
Percent of poverty level[2,4]												
Below 100%	46.1	45.3	48.1	49.7	20.2	18.8	20.6	19.7	33.6	35.9	31.3	30.6
100%–199%	52.8	50.6	54.2	53.1	20.1	17.9	18.9	19.8	27.1	31.5	27.0	27.1
200%–399%	62.1	60.1	62.9	63.9	16.5	15.0	15.1	15.7	21.3	24.9	22.1	20.4
400% or more	74.6	71.3	74.3	76.8	11.5	11.3	10.3	9.9	13.9	17.4	15.4	13.3
Disability measure[2,5]												
Any basic actions difficulty or complex activity limitation	58.4	57.0	60.2	59.8	20.8	19.3	19.0	19.5	20.9	23.6	20.9	20.8
Any basic actions difficulty	58.9	57.3	61.1	60.5	20.5	19.4	18.6	19.5	20.7	23.4	20.3	20.0
Any complex activity limitation	50.3	49.4	49.1	50.8	25.3	24.0	24.6	23.7	24.4	26.6	26.3	25.5
No disability	67.0	64.5	68.2	69.1	12.5	11.8	11.2	11.7	20.5	23.7	20.6	19.2
Male												
18 years and over, age-adjusted[2]	69.8	67.6	70.9	71.6	16.2	14.8	14.6	14.8	14.0	17.5	14.6	13.6
18 years and over, crude	70.5	68.2	71.1	71.6	15.6	14.3	14.5	14.9	14.0	17.5	14.5	13.5
Age												
18–44 years	74.8	73.0	76.2	75.5	9.8	8.5	7.4	7.8	15.4	18.5	16.5	16.7
18–24 years	66.7	63.6	69.0	65.9	5.3	3.5	*2.9	4.5	28.0	32.8	28.1	29.6
25–44 years	77.2	76.0	78.7	79.0	11.1	10.2	8.9	9.0	11.6	13.9	12.3	12.0
45–64 years	70.8	68.1	71.2	71.9	19.2	17.2	18.1	19.3	10.1	14.7	10.7	8.8
45–54 years	73.8	70.3	75.7	73.6	17.2	15.5	14.7	17.5	9.0	14.2	9.6	8.9
55–64 years	65.8	64.5	65.2	69.7	22.3	20.0	22.6	21.7	11.8	15.4	12.2	8.6
65 years and over	52.7	50.2	53.1	58.0	31.4	30.2	30.4	28.4	15.8	19.6	16.4	13.6
65–74 years	56.7	52.7	57.9	65.4	29.7	28.2	26.6	23.3	13.5	19.1	15.5	11.3
75 years and over	46.7	46.7	46.7	47.8	34.0	33.1	35.5	35.4	19.3	20.3	17.7	16.8

See footnotes at end of table.

Table 64 (page 2 of 3). Lifetime alcohol drinking status among adults 18 years of age and over, by selected characteristics: United States, selected years 1997–2009

[Data are based on household interviews of a sample of the civilian noninstitutionalized population]

Characteristic	Current drinker 1997	2000	2008	2009	Former drinker 1997	2000	2008	2009	Lifetime abstainer 1997	2000	2008	2009
Race[2,3]					Percent of adults							
White only	71.8	69.7	72.7	74.0	15.8	14.7	14.3	14.5	12.4	15.7	13.0	11.5
Black or African American only	56.9	56.2	61.3	60.2	22.6	17.2	18.5	18.0	20.5	26.6	20.2	21.8
American Indian or Alaska Native only	66.1	62.4	62.5	64.9	*17.8	*23.3	21.7	21.8	*16.1	*	*15.8	*13.3
Asian only	60.2	55.9	62.1	58.2	10.1	10.3	10.1	12.8	29.8	33.8	27.8	29.0
Native Hawaiian or Other Pacific Islander only	- - -	*	*	*	- - -	*	*	*	- - -	*	*	*
2 or more races	- - -	70.5	65.6	74.2	- - -	*19.4	*17.3	*14.0	- - -	*10.1	*17.1	*11.9
Hispanic origin and race[2,3]												
Hispanic or Latino	64.6	63.8	67.6	65.7	17.5	14.2	14.8	16.9	17.9	22.0	17.6	17.4
Mexican	66.9	64.5	67.3	65.6	17.3	15.1	14.2	17.7	15.9	20.5	18.5	16.7
Not Hispanic or Latino	70.2	68.2	71.4	72.5	16.2	14.9	14.5	14.6	13.6	16.9	14.1	12.9
White only	72.7	70.4	73.8	75.5	15.7	14.7	14.2	14.3	11.6	14.9	12.0	10.2
Black or African American only	57.1	56.4	61.2	60.5	22.3	17.1	18.5	17.8	20.5	26.5	20.3	21.7
Percent of poverty level[2,4]												
Below 100%	57.2	55.3	55.7	58.9	21.8	18.7	22.7	21.6	21.1	26.0	21.6	19.5
100%–199%	60.6	59.0	62.5	59.9	21.5	20.2	19.3	20.8	17.9	20.8	18.2	19.3
200%–399%	68.6	66.2	69.0	68.8	17.4	15.5	15.4	16.4	14.0	18.3	15.7	14.8
400% or more	78.1	74.8	78.6	81.2	11.6	11.2	10.5	9.7	10.3	14.0	10.9	9.2
Disability measure[2,5]												
Any basic actions difficulty or complex activity limitation	63.8	62.9	67.0	64.6	22.5	21.1	19.5	20.3	13.7	16.0	13.5	15.1
Any basic actions difficulty	64.5	63.5	68.7	65.5	22.3	21.0	18.7	20.2	13.2	15.5	12.6	14.4
Any complex activity limitation	55.8	52.7	54.5	54.4	27.3	28.3	25.5	24.5	16.9	19.0	20.0	21.1
No disability	73.3	70.1	73.7	75.0	12.8	11.9	11.3	11.8	13.9	18.1	14.9	13.2
Female												
18 years and over, age-adjusted[2]	57.0	55.8	58.8	59.6	15.3	14.2	14.2	14.6	27.6	30.0	27.1	25.8
18 years and over, crude	57.0	55.5	58.3	59.0	15.4	14.4	14.6	15.1	27.7	30.1	27.1	25.9
Age												
18–44 years	64.2	61.7	64.1	65.5	11.5	10.7	9.2	9.7	24.3	27.5	26.7	24.8
18–24 years	57.7	54.6	58.3	58.1	6.6	6.8	4.3	6.6	35.7	38.5	37.4	35.3
25–44 years	66.1	64.0	66.2	68.1	12.9	12.0	10.9	10.8	21.0	24.1	23.0	21.1
45–64 years	56.2	56.4	61.2	60.8	17.9	16.5	16.2	17.2	25.9	27.2	22.6	22.0
45–54 years	60.7	60.1	64.7	64.3	16.4	14.5	14.6	14.7	22.9	25.4	20.7	21.0
55–64 years	49.4	50.7	56.7	56.5	20.0	19.5	18.2	20.4	30.5	29.8	25.1	23.1
65 years and over	36.6	36.2	37.6	38.5	23.2	21.2	25.8	25.0	40.2	42.5	36.6	36.5
65–74 years	42.0	42.3	43.3	43.4	20.9	20.2	24.1	24.5	37.1	37.5	32.7	32.1
75 years and over	30.2	29.8	31.8	33.2	25.9	22.3	27.6	25.5	43.8	47.9	40.6	41.3
Race[2,3]												
White only	60.7	59.8	62.4	63.2	15.0	14.0	14.1	14.1	24.3	26.2	23.5	22.7
Black or African American only	40.9	39.5	43.8	47.7	19.9	17.2	18.2	18.1	39.3	43.3	38.0	34.2
American Indian or Alaska Native only	45.2	47.0	54.0	49.0	26.1	*20.3	*12.1	*17.1	28.7	32.7	33.9	34.0
Asian only	31.6	29.3	38.3	34.6	8.1	8.0	5.6	9.9	60.3	62.7	56.1	55.5
Native Hawaiian or Other Pacific Islander only	- - -	*	*	*	- - -	*	*	*	- - -	*	*	*
2 or more races	- - -	52.5	63.6	54.8	- - -	19.1	*13.8	29.4	- - -	28.4	22.6	15.7

See footnotes at end of table.

Table 64 (page 3 of 3). Lifetime alcohol drinking status among adults 18 years of age and over, by selected characteristics: United States, selected years 1997–2009

[Data are based on household interviews of a sample of the civilian noninstitutionalized population]

| | Lifetime alcohol drinking status[1] | | | | | | | | | | | |
| | Current drinker | | | | Former drinker | | | | Lifetime abstainer | | | |
Characteristic	1997	2000	2008	2009	1997	2000	2008	2009	1997	2000	2008	2009
Hispanic origin and race[2,3]					Percent of adults							
Hispanic or Latina	42.1	41.2	42.9	43.8	12.5	11.2	11.8	13.6	45.4	47.6	45.4	42.6
Mexican	38.9	36.9	41.5	40.4	11.6	12.2	11.1	15.4	49.4	50.8	47.3	44.2
Not Hispanic or Latina	58.7	57.6	61.3	62.2	15.6	14.5	14.4	14.6	25.7	27.9	24.3	23.3
White only	62.9	61.9	66.2	67.1	15.2	14.3	14.3	14.1	21.9	23.8	19.4	18.8
Black or African American only	40.7	39.3	43.9	47.7	20.0	17.2	18.3	18.0	39.3	43.5	37.8	34.3
Percent of poverty level[2,4]												
Below 100%	39.1	38.5	42.7	43.3	19.9	19.2	19.3	18.8	41.1	42.2	38.0	37.9
100%–199%	46.0	43.4	47.0	47.6	19.5	16.4	18.8	19.3	34.5	40.1	34.2	33.1
200%–399%	56.3	54.5	57.2	59.3	15.9	14.6	15.0	15.2	27.9	30.9	27.9	25.5
400% or more	71.0	67.7	70.0	72.2	11.3	11.5	10.0	10.2	17.8	20.8	20.0	17.6
Disability measure[2,5]												
Any basic actions difficulty or complex activity limitation	54.3	52.7	55.1	56.2	19.6	18.1	18.6	18.9	26.1	29.2	26.3	24.9
Any basic actions difficulty	54.8	52.9	55.7	56.9	19.2	18.2	18.6	19.1	26.0	28.9	25.7	24.0
Any complex activity limitation	46.1	47.1	44.8	48.1	23.8	21.1	24.2	23.2	30.1	31.8	31.0	28.7
No disability	60.6	59.1	62.5	63.1	12.4	11.8	11.0	11.6	27.0	29.2	26.5	25.4

* Estimates are considered unreliable. Data preceded by an asterisk have a relative standard error (RSE) of 20%–30%. Data not shown have an RSE of greater than 30%.

- - - Data not available.

[1]Lifetime alcohol drinking status categories are based on self-reported responses to questions about alcohol consumption. Current drinkers had at least 12 drinks in their lifetime and at least one drink in the past year. Former drinkers had at least 12 drinks in their lifetime and none in the past year. Lifetime abstainers had fewer than 12 drinks in their lifetime. See Appendix II, Alcohol consumption.

[2]Estimates are age-adjusted to the year 2000 standard population using four age groups: 18–24 years, 25–44 years, 45–64 years, and 65 years and over. Age-adjusted estimates in this table may differ from other age-adjusted estimates based on the same data and presented elsewhere if different age groups are used in the adjustment procedure. See Appendix II, Age adjustment.

[3]The race groups, white, black, American Indian or Alaska Native, Asian, Native Hawaiian or Other Pacific Islander, and 2 or more races, include persons of Hispanic and non-Hispanic origin. Persons of Hispanic origin may be of any race. Starting with 1999 data, race-specific estimates are tabulated according to the 1997 Revisions to the Standards for the Classification of Federal Data on Race and Ethnicity and are not strictly comparable with estimates for earlier years. The five single-race categories plus multiple-race categories shown in the table conform to the 1997 Standards. Starting with 1999 data, race-specific estimates are for persons who reported only one racial group; the category 2 or more races includes persons who reported more than one racial group. Prior to 1999, data were tabulated according to the 1977 Standards with four racial groups and the Asian only category included Native Hawaiian or Other Pacific Islander. Estimates for single-race categories prior to 1999 included persons who reported one race or, if they reported more than one race, identified one race as best representing their race. Starting with 2003 data, race responses of other race and unspecified multiple race were treated as missing, and then race was imputed if these were the only race responses. Almost all persons with a race response of other race were of Hispanic origin. See Appendix II, Hispanic origin; Race.

[4]Percent of poverty level is based on family income and family size and composition using U.S. Census Bureau poverty thresholds. Missing family income data were imputed for 1997 and beyond. See Appendix II, Family income; Poverty; Table VII.

[5]Any basic actions difficulty or complex activity limitation is defined as having one or more of the following limitations or difficulties: movement difficulty, emotional difficulty, sensory (seeing or hearing) difficulty, cognitive difficulty, self-care (ADL or IADL) limitation, social limitation, or work limitation. For more information, see Appendix II, Basic actions difficulty; Complex activity limitation. Starting with 2007 data, the hearing question, a component of the basic actions difficulty measure, was revised. Consequently, data prior to 2007 are not comparable with data for 2007 and beyond. For more information on the impact of the revised hearing question, see Appendix II, Hearing trouble.

NOTES: Standard errors are available in the spreadsheet version of this table. Available from: http://www.cdc.gov/nchs/hus.htm. Data for additional years are available. See Appendix III.

SOURCE: CDC/NCHS, National Health Interview Survey, family core and sample adult questionnaires.

Table 65 (page 1 of 3). Heavier drinking and drinking five or more drinks in a day among adults 18 years of age and over, by selected characteristics: United States, selected years 1997–2009

[Data are based on household interviews of a sample of the civilian noninstitutionalized population]

Characteristic	Heavier drinker[1]				Five or more drinks in a day on at least 1 day in the past year[1]				Five or more drinks in a day on at least 12 days in the past year[1]			
	1997	2000	2008	2009	1997	2000	2008	2009	1997	2000	2008	2009
	Percent of adults											
18 years and over, age-adjusted[2]	4.9	4.3	5.7	5.3	21.1	19.2	23.2	23.6	9.7	8.7	10.5	10.0
18 years and over, crude	5.0	4.3	5.7	5.3	21.5	19.3	22.7	23.0	9.8	8.7	10.3	9.7
Both sexes												
Age												
All persons:												
18–44 years	5.2	4.7	6.3	5.6	29.2	26.9	32.0	32.3	13.2	12.2	14.9	13.7
18–24 years	5.3	5.8	8.2	6.2	31.8	30.3	35.7	35.5	15.2	15.5	18.4	16.7
25–44 years	5.2	4.3	5.6	5.4	28.5	25.8	30.8	31.2	12.6	11.1	13.6	12.6
45–64 years	5.5	4.6	5.9	5.8	15.9	14.4	17.7	18.7	7.6	6.4	7.7	7.8
45–54 years	5.5	4.4	6.7	6.0	19.0	16.4	21.8	22.2	8.7	7.0	9.3	9.6
55–64 years	5.4	5.0	4.8	5.5	11.1	11.3	12.3	14.4	5.8	5.4	5.5	5.5
65 years and over	3.1	2.6	3.5	3.5	4.9	3.8	5.4	5.2	2.2	1.8	2.2	2.4
65–74 years	3.9	3.1	4.4	4.5	6.7	5.2	8.3	7.9	3.0	2.5	3.5	3.4
75 years and over	2.1	2.0	2.4	2.3	2.4	2.1	2.1	1.9	1.1	*0.9	*0.7	*1.1
Race[2,3]												
White only	5.2	4.5	6.3	5.9	22.9	20.8	25.5	26.0	10.3	9.2	11.6	11.0
Black or African American only	4.0	3.5	3.4	3.3	11.7	11.6	13.8	14.2	6.5	6.5	6.1	5.8
American Indian or Alaska Native only	*	*	*	*4.4	29.2	23.7	23.2	24.5	17.4	*12.1	*10.8	*15.3
Asian only	*1.9	*2.3	*1.6	*1.7	11.4	8.8	11.0	10.8	*4.8	3.6	4.4	4.3
Native Hawaiian or Other Pacific Islander only	- - -	*	*	*	- - -	*	*	*	- - -	*	*	*
2 or more races	- - -	*7.5	*7.0	*6.2	- - -	28.0	23.8	26.3	- - -	15.9	11.3	11.7
Hispanic origin and race[2,3]												
Hispanic or Latino	3.9	3.2	3.7	3.1	20.4	17.3	19.4	19.9	11.2	9.0	9.9	9.6
Mexican	4.4	3.8	5.0	3.3	21.2	19.9	21.3	21.0	12.6	10.8	11.7	10.4
Not Hispanic or Latino	5.1	4.5	6.0	5.7	21.3	19.7	23.9	24.4	9.5	8.8	10.6	10.0
White only	5.4	4.7	6.7	6.3	23.5	21.5	27.0	27.5	10.3	9.3	12.0	11.2
Black or African American only	3.9	3.4	3.4	3.4	11.6	11.5	13.8	14.3	6.5	6.5	6.2	5.8
Percent of poverty level[2,4]												
Below 100%	4.8	4.3	6.0	5.2	17.3	15.0	19.5	18.4	9.7	8.6	10.3	9.1
100%–199%	4.9	4.2	4.6	5.2	18.4	15.7	19.0	20.6	9.8	8.0	9.4	10.3
200%–399%	4.9	4.2	5.7	5.1	21.0	18.7	22.7	23.1	9.8	8.9	10.7	9.6
400% or more	5.1	4.4	6.1	5.5	24.3	22.1	26.3	27.2	9.7	8.9	11.0	10.2
Disability measure[2,5]												
Any basic actions difficulty or complex activity limitation	5.7	5.2	6.7	6.1	20.2	18.8	22.5	22.6	10.2	9.3	10.7	9.2
Any basic actions difficulty	5.8	5.3	6.9	5.9	20.6	19.1	22.9	23.0	10.5	9.4	10.8	9.2
Any complex activity limitation	4.5	4.3	5.0	5.3	16.4	14.3	17.3	16.8	8.8	7.3	8.3	7.2
No disability	4.9	4.1	5.3	5.1	21.8	19.7	23.7	24.1	9.6	8.7	10.5	10.1
Male												
18 years and over, age-adjusted[2]	6.1	5.1	6.4	6.2	30.7	28.3	31.9	33.0	15.8	14.4	16.6	15.8
18 years and over, crude	6.1	5.2	6.4	6.2	31.7	29.0	31.9	32.9	16.3	14.7	16.5	15.7
Age												
All persons:												
18–44 years	6.5	5.6	7.0	6.9	40.6	37.8	42.0	43.4	21.1	19.6	22.6	21.4
18–24 years	6.0	6.3	8.3	7.6	40.6	38.0	43.1	43.7	22.9	22.9	25.6	24.1
25–44 years	6.6	5.3	6.5	6.6	40.6	37.7	41.7	43.2	20.6	18.5	21.6	20.4
45–64 years	6.6	5.5	6.8	6.2	25.3	23.5	26.7	27.9	12.7	11.3	12.8	12.5
45–54 years	6.6	5.7	7.9	5.7	29.4	26.3	32.0	31.5	14.5	12.3	15.3	14.2
55–64 years	6.6	5.4	5.3	6.7	18.9	19.0	19.7	23.2	10.0	9.8	9.6	10.2
65 years and over	3.7	3.1	3.8	4.1	9.3	7.4	9.7	9.8	4.7	3.7	4.5	4.7
65–74 years	4.8	3.9	5.2	5.1	12.2	9.5	13.8	14.2	6.1	4.9	6.5	6.6
75 years and over	*2.1	*2.0	*2.0	*2.8	5.1	4.4	4.3	3.9	*2.5	*2.0	*1.9	*2.1

See footnotes at end of table.

Table 65 (page 2 of 3).
Heavier drinking and drinking five or more drinks in a day among adults 18 years of age and over, by selected characteristics: United States, selected years 1997–2009

[Data are based on household interviews of a sample of the civilian noninstitutionalized population]

Characteristic	Heavier drinker[1]				Five or more drinks in a day on at least 1 day in the past year[1]				Five or more drinks in a day on at least 12 days in the past year[1]			
	1997	2000	2008	2009	1997	2000	2008	2009	1997	2000	2008	2009
Race[2,3]							Percent of adults					
White only	6.3	5.1	6.9	6.8	32.8	29.9	34.1	35.9	16.7	14.9	18.0	17.4
Black or African American only	5.3	5.4	4.5	4.0	18.4	19.8	22.8	21.5	11.0	12.4	10.8	9.5
American Indian or Alaska Native only	*	*	*	*	45.7	29.2	30.7	33.5	30.4	*14.0	*14.7	*20.7
Asian only	*2.3	*3.5	*	*2.6	17.8	14.1	17.8	16.7	*7.5	*5.9	7.8	7.1
Native Hawaiian or Other Pacific Islander only	- - -	*	*	*	- - -	*	*	*	- - -	*	*	*
2 or more races	- - -	*12.1	*10.3	*	- - -	39.2	39.1	33.6	- - -	23.7	*19.0	*16.2
Hispanic origin and race[2,3]												
Hispanic or Latino	5.7	5.2	5.0	4.7	30.9	27.9	29.1	30.4	18.8	15.9	16.3	15.8
Mexican	6.9	6.6	6.8	5.0	34.2	32.2	31.8	32.1	21.9	19.1	18.9	17.0
Not Hispanic or Latino	6.1	5.2	6.6	6.5	30.7	28.6	32.5	33.7	15.5	14.3	16.6	15.8
White only	6.4	5.2	7.3	7.2	33.3	30.6	35.5	37.3	16.6	15.0	18.4	17.6
Black or African American only	5.3	5.4	4.4	4.1	18.4	19.7	22.8	21.6	11.1	12.3	11.0	9.6
Percent of poverty level[2,4]												
Below 100%	6.8	6.4	8.3	7.6	26.9	24.8	28.5	28.6	16.5	15.7	16.7	15.9
100%–199%	7.1	5.8	6.1	7.0	27.3	23.6	27.0	29.5	16.4	13.3	16.0	16.4
200%–399%	6.6	5.3	6.9	6.0	30.4	27.4	31.3	32.3	16.0	14.7	16.6	15.2
400% or more	5.0	4.4	5.9	5.5	33.6	31.3	35.2	36.1	15.4	14.4	17.0	15.7
Disability measure[2,5]												
Any basic actions difficulty or complex activity limitation	7.2	6.8	7.9	7.3	29.4	28.9	32.4	30.8	17.0	16.5	17.9	14.3
Any basic actions difficulty	7.5	6.8	8.5	7.2	30.4	29.8	33.6	31.7	17.7	16.8	18.5	14.5
Any complex activity limitation	5.4	5.8	5.8	6.5	23.1	20.5	23.8	23.0	14.2	11.9	13.3	11.0
No disability	5.8	4.8	5.9	5.8	31.5	28.5	32.0	33.5	15.6	14.1	16.1	15.9
Female												
18 years and over, age-adjusted[2]	3.9	3.5	5.0	4.5	12.2	10.8	15.0	14.7	3.9	3.4	4.8	4.4
18 years and over, crude	3.9	3.5	5.0	4.5	12.1	10.6	14.2	14.0	3.9	3.3	4.6	4.2
Age												
All persons:												
18–44 years	4.0	3.8	5.6	4.4	18.3	16.5	22.3	21.6	5.5	5.2	7.4	6.2
18–24 years	4.5	5.2	8.1	4.8	23.0	22.8	28.4	27.4	7.6	8.3	11.4	9.4
25–44 years	3.9	3.4	4.7	4.3	16.9	14.5	20.2	19.5	4.9	4.2	5.9	5.1
45–64 years	4.4	3.8	5.1	5.5	7.2	6.0	9.3	10.2	2.9	1.9	2.9	3.4
45–54 years	4.5	3.2	5.6	6.3	9.2	7.1	12.3	13.4	3.3	2.1	3.7	5.2
55–64 years	4.4	4.6	4.4	4.4	4.1	4.4	5.4	6.3	2.1	1.5	1.8	1.2
65 years and over	2.6	2.2	3.2	3.0	1.6	1.2	2.2	1.6	*0.4	*0.4	*	*0.6
65–74 years	3.1	2.5	3.8	4.0	2.3	1.7	3.7	2.5	*	*	*	*
75 years and over	2.0	1.9	*2.7	*2.0	*0.7	*	*	*	*	*	*	*
Race[2,3]												
White only	4.2	4.0	5.7	4.9	13.5	12.1	17.2	16.5	4.2	3.7	5.4	4.8
Black or African American only	2.9	2.0	2.5	2.7	6.5	5.2	6.8	8.4	2.9	1.9	2.5	2.8
American Indian or Alaska Native only	*	*	*	*	18.1	*19.0	*16.1	*14.9	*	*	*	*
Asian only	*	*	*	*	*5.2	*3.7	*4.6	5.4	*	*	*	*
Native Hawaiian or Other Pacific Islander only	- - -	*	*	*	- - -	*	*	*	- - -	*	*	*
2 or more races	- - -	*	*	*	- - -	17.0	*11.8	18.9	- - -	*8.2	*6.2	*

See footnotes at end of table.

Table 65 (page 3 of 3). Heavier drinking and drinking five or more drinks in a day among adults 18 years of age and over, by selected characteristics: United States, selected years 1997–2009

[Data are based on household interviews of a sample of the civilian noninstitutionalized population]

Characteristic	Heavier drinker[1]				Five or more drinks in a day on at least 1 day in the past year[1]				Five or more drinks in a day on at least 12 days in the past year[1]			
	1997	2000	2008	2009	1997	2000	2008	2009	1997	2000	2008	2009
Hispanic origin and race[2,3]					Percent of adults							
Hispanic or Latina	2.2	1.2	2.5	1.5	9.7	6.8	9.4	9.2	3.5	2.1	3.2	3.1
Mexican.	*1.9	*1.1	*2.9	*1.4	8.2	7.1	10.0	8.6	3.2	*2.2	3.8	*3.1
Not Hispanic or Latina	4.1	3.8	5.4	4.9	12.6	11.5	16.0	15.7	4.0	3.6	5.1	4.6
White only	4.4	4.3	6.2	5.5	14.2	13.0	19.0	18.2	4.3	4.0	6.0	5.1
Black or African American only	2.9	2.0	2.6	2.8	6.2	5.2	6.6	8.4	2.9	1.9	2.5	2.8
Percent of poverty level[2,4]												
Below 100%	3.6	2.8	4.5	3.5	10.8	8.2	12.7	11.2	5.1	3.6	5.6	4.2
100%–199%	3.1	2.9	3.4	3.7	10.5	9.0	11.8	12.9	4.0	3.5	3.6	5.1
200%–399%	3.3	3.2	4.5	4.1	12.1	10.7	14.6	13.9	4.0	3.5	5.0	3.9
400% or more	5.2	4.5	6.3	5.4	14.2	12.6	17.3	18.1	3.4	3.3	5.0	4.4
Disability measure[2,5]												
Any basic actions difficulty or complex activity limitation.	4.5	4.1	5.7	5.1	13.1	11.3	15.0	16.2	5.0	4.1	5.2	5.3
Any basic actions difficulty	4.5	4.2	5.7	4.9	13.2	11.6	15.2	16.4	5.1	4.1	5.2	5.3
Any complex activity limitation	3.7	*3.2	4.3	4.3	10.8	9.1	11.9	11.6	4.2	*3.1	4.1	3.9
No disability.	3.9	3.5	4.7	4.4	12.0	10.9	15.0	14.5	3.6	3.3	4.7	4.1

* Estimates are considered unreliable. Data preceded by an asterisk have a relative standard error (RSE) of 20%–30%. Data not shown have an RSE of greater than 30%.

- - - Data not available.

[1]Heavier drinking is based on self-reported responses to questions about average alcohol consumption and is defined as more than 14 drinks per week for men and more than seven drinks per week for women on average. U.S. Department of Agriculture: Dietary Guidelines for Americans, 2005. Available from: http://www.health.gov/Dietaryguidelines/. Respondents were also asked, "In the past year, on how many days did you have five or more drinks of any alcoholic beverage?" See Appendix II, Alcohol consumption.

[2]Estimates are age-adjusted to the year 2000 standard population using four age groups: 18–24 years, 25–44 years, 45–64 years, and 65 years and over. Age-adjusted estimates in this table may differ from other age-adjusted estimates based on the same data and presented elsewhere if different age groups are used in the adjustment procedure. See Appendix II, Age adjustment.

[3]The race groups, white, black, American Indian or Alaska Native, Asian, Native Hawaiian or Other Pacific Islander, and 2 or more races, include persons of Hispanic and non-Hispanic origin. Persons of Hispanic origin may be of any race. Starting with 1999 data, race-specific estimates are tabulated according to the 1997 Revisions to the Standards for the Classification of Federal Data on Race and Ethnicity and are not strictly comparable with estimates for earlier years. The five single-race categories plus multiple-race categories shown in the table conform to the 1997 Standards. Starting with 1999 data, race-specific estimates are for persons who reported only one racial group; the category 2 or more races includes persons who reported more than one racial group. Prior to 1999, data were tabulated according to the 1977 Standards with four racial groups and the Asian only category included Native Hawaiian or Other Pacific Islander. Estimates for single-race categories prior to 1999 included persons who reported one race or, if they reported more than one race, identified one race as best representing their race. Starting with 2003 data, race responses of other race and unspecified multiple race were treated as missing, and then race was imputed if these were the only race responses. Almost all persons with a race response of other race were of Hispanic origin. See Appendix II, Hispanic origin; Race.

[4]Percent of poverty level is based on family income and family size and composition using U.S. Census Bureau poverty thresholds. Missing family income data were imputed for 1997 and beyond. See Appendix II, Family income; Poverty; Table VII.

[5]Any basic actions difficulty or complex activity limitation is defined as having one or more of the following limitations or difficulties: movement difficulty, emotional difficulty, sensory (seeing or hearing) difficulty, cognitive difficulty, self-care (ADL or IADL) limitation, social limitation, or work limitation. For more information, see Appendix II, Basic actions difficulty; Complex activity limitation. Starting with 2007 data, the hearing question, a component of the basic actions difficulty measure, was revised. Consequently, data prior to 2007 are not comparable with data for 2007 and beyond. For more information on the impact of the revised hearing question, see Appendix II, Hearing trouble.

NOTES: Standard errors are available in the spreadsheet version of this table. Available from: http://www.cdc.gov/nchs/hus.htm. For more data on alcohol consumption, see the Early Release reports on the National Health Interview Survey home page: http://www.cdc.gov/nchs/nhis.htm. Data for additional years are available. See Appendix III.

SOURCE: CDC/NCHS, National Health Interview Survey, family core and sample adult questionnaires.

Table 66 (page 1 of 2). Selected health conditions and risk factors: United States, selected years 1988–1994 through 2007–2008

[Data are based on interviews and physical examinations of a sample of the civilian noninstitutionalized population]

Health condition	1988–1994	1999–2000	2001–2002	2003–2004	2005–2006	2007–2008
Diabetes[1]	Percent of persons 20 years of age and over					
Total, age-adjusted[2]	9.1	9.0	10.5	10.8	10.4	11.5
Total, crude.	8.4	8.5	10.1	10.8	10.7	11.9
High cholesterol[3]						
Total, age-adjusted[4]	22.8	25.0	24.4	27.5	27.0	27.2
Total, crude.	21.5	24.0	23.9	27.5	27.6	28.3
High serum total cholesterol[5]						
Total, age-adjusted[4]	20.8	18.3	16.5	16.9	15.6	14.2
Total, crude.	19.6	17.7	16.4	17.0	15.9	14.6
Hypertension[6]						
Total, age-adjusted[4]	25.5	30.0	29.7	32.1	30.5	31.2
Total, crude.	24.1	28.9	28.9	32.5	31.7	32.6
Uncontrolled high blood pressure among persons with hypertension[7]						
Total, age-adjusted[4]	77.2	71.9	68.3	63.8	63.0	56.2
Total, crude.	73.9	69.1	65.4	60.8	56.6	51.8
Overweight (includes obesity)[8]						
Total, age-adjusted[4]	56.0	64.0	65.3	66.0	66.6	67.9
Total, crude.	54.9	63.6	65.2	66.2	67.0	68.1
Obesity[9]						
Total, age-adjusted[4].	22.9	30.1	29.9	32.0	33.9	33.5
Total, crude	22.3	29.9	30.0	32.0	34.2	33.7
Untreated dental caries[10]						
Total, age-adjusted[4]	27.7	24.3	21.3	30.0	23.6	21.2
Total, crude.	28.2	25.0	21.6	30.3	23.7	21.2
Obesity[11]	Percent of persons under 20 years of age					
2–5 years	7.2	10.3	10.6	14.0	11.0	10.4
6–11 years	11.3	15.1	16.3	18.8	15.1	19.6
12–19 years	10.5	14.8	16.7	17.4	17.8	18.1
Untreated dental caries[10,12]						
6–19 years	23.6	22.7	20.6	25.2	- - -	16.1

See footnotes at end of table.

Table 66 (page 2 of 2). Selected health conditions and risk factors: United States, selected years 1988–1994 through 2007–2008

[Data are based on interviews and physical examinations of a sample of the civilian noninstitutionalized population]

- - - Data not available.

[1]Includes physician-diagnosed and undiagnosed diabetes. Physician-diagnosed diabetes was obtained by self-report and excludes women who reported having diabetes only during pregnancy. Undiagnosed diabetes is defined as a fasting blood glucose (FBG) of at least 126 mg/dL or a hemoglobin A1c of at least 6.5% and no reported physician diagnosis. Respondents had fasted for at least 8 hours and less than 24 hours. Estimates in some prior editions of *Health, United States* included data from respondents who had fasted for at least 9 hours and less than 24 hours. In 2005–2006 and 2007–2008, testing was performed at a different laboratory and using different instruments than testing in earlier years. NHANES conducted a crossover study to evaluate the impact of these changes on FBG and A1c measurements. As a result of that study, NHANES recommended that 2005–2008 data on FBG and A1c measurements be adjusted to be compatible with earlier years. Undiagnosed diabetes estimates in *Health, United States* were produced after adjusting the 2005–2008 lab data as recommended. For more information, see: http://www.cdc.gov/nchs/nhanes/nhanes2007-2008/GLU_E.htm. The definition of undiagnosed diabetes in previous editions of *Health, United States* did not consider hemoglobin A1c. The revised definition of undiagnosed diabetes was based on recommendations from the American Diabetes Association. For more information, see: Standards of medical care in diabetes—2010. Diabetes Care 2010;33(suppl 1):S11-S61. Also see Appendix II, Diabetes. See related Table 50.

[2]Age-adjusted to the 2000 standard population using three age groups: 20–44 years, 45–64 years, and 65 years and over. Age-adjusted estimates may differ from other age-adjusted estimates based on the same data and presented elsewhere if different age groups are used in the adjustment procedure. See Appendix II, Age adjustment.

[3]High cholesterol is defined as measured serum total cholesterol greater than or equal to 240 mg/dL or reporting taking cholesterol-lowering medication. Respondents were asked, "Are you now following this advice [from a doctor of health professional] to take prescribed medicine [to lower your cholesterol]?" Risk levels for serum total cholesterol have been defined by the Third Report of the National Cholesterol Education Program Expert Panel on Detection, Evaluation, and Treatment of High Blood Cholesterol in Adults. National Heart, Lung, and Blood Institute, National Institutes of Health. September 2002. (Available from: http://www.nhlbi.nih.gov/guidelines/cholesterol/index.htm and summarized in JAMA 2001;285(19):2486–97.) See Appendix II, Cholesterol. See related Table 68.

[4]Age-adjusted to the 2000 standard population using five age groups: 20–34 years, 35–44 years, 45–54 years, 55–64 years, and 65 years and over. Age-adjusted estimates may differ from other age-adjusted estimates based on the same data and presented elsewhere if different age groups are used in the adjustment procedure. See Appendix II, Age adjustment.

[5]High serum total cholesterol is defined as greater than or equal to 240 mg/dL (6.20 mmol/L). This second measure of cholesterol presented in *Health, United States*, is based solely on measured high serum total cholesterol. See Appendix II, Cholesterol. See related Table 68.

[6]Hypertension is defined as having elevated blood pressure and/or taking antihypertensive medication. Elevated blood pressure is defined as having systolic pressure of at least 140 mmHg or diastolic pressure of at least 90 mmHg. Those with elevated blood pressure may be taking prescribed medicine for high blood pressure. Respondents were asked, "Are you now taking prescribed medicine for your high blood pressure?" See Appendix II, Blood pressure, high. See related Table 67.

[7]Uncontrolled high blood pressure among persons with hypertension is defined as measured systolic pressure of at least 140 mmHg or diastolic pressure of at least 90 mmHg, among those with measured high blood pressure or reporting taking antihypertensive medication. See Appendix II, Blood pressure, high. See related Table 67.

[8]Excludes pregnant women. Overweight is defined as body mass index (BMI) greater than or equal to 25 kg/m[2]. See Appendix II, Body mass index. See related Table 71.

[9]Excludes pregnant women. Obesity is defined as body mass index (BMI) greater than or equal to 30 kg/m[2]. See Appendix II, Body mass index. See related Table 71.

[10]Untreated dental caries refers to untreated coronal caries. Starting with 2005–2006 NHANES data, dental caries data were collected using a simplified examination process. Because of this change in data collection and because estimates from 2003–2004 and earlier years considered whether the teeth were primary or permanent, 2005–2006 estimates and beyond are not comparable with earlier data. In addition, dental caries data are no longer collected on children younger than 5 years of age. For more information on the methodology changes, see Appendix II, Dental caries and http://www.cdc.gov/nchs/data/nhanes/nhanes_05_06/ohx_d.pdf. See related Table 73.

[11]Obesity is defined as body mass index (BMI) at or above the sex- and age-specific 95th percentile BMI cutoff points from the 2000 CDC Growth Charts: United States. Advance data from vital and health statistics; no 314. Hyattsville, MD: NCHS. 2000. Starting with *Health United States, 2010*, the terminology describing height for weight among children changed from previous editions. The term obesity now refers to children who were formerly labeled as overweight. This is a change in terminology only and not in measurement; the previous definition of overweight is now the definition of obesity. For more information, see: Ogden CL, Flegal KM. Changes in terminology for childhood overweight and obesity. National health statistics report; no. 25. Hyattsville, MD: NCHS; 2010. Available from: http://www.cdc.gov/nchs/data/nhsr/nhsr025.pdf. Excludes pregnant girls. See related Table 72.

[12]Estimate is for 2005–2008. The 4-year estimate is shown for children because it is more reliable than the 2-year estimates.

NOTES: See related Tables 50, 67, 68, 71, 72, and 73. Standard errors for selected years are available in the spreadsheet version of this table. Available from: http://www.cdc.gov/nchs/hus.htm.

SOURCE: CDC/NCHS, National Health and Nutrition Examination Survey.

Table 67 (page 1 of 2). Hypertension and high blood pressure among persons 20 years of age and over, by selected characteristics: United States, selected years 1988–1994 through 2005–2008

[Data are based on interviews and physical examinations of a sample of the civilian noninstitutionalized population]

Sex, age, race and Hispanic origin[1], and percent of poverty level	Hypertension[2,3] (high blood pressure and/or taking antihypertensive medication)			Uncontrolled high blood pressure among persons with hypertension[4]		
	1988–1994	1999–2002	2005–2008	1988–1994	1999–2002	2005–2008
20 years and over, age-adjusted[5]		Percent of population				
Both sexes[6]	25.5	30.0	30.9	77.2	70.6	59.4
Male	26.4	28.8	31.6	83.2	73.3	63.8
Female	24.4	30.6	29.8	68.5	61.8	48.5
Not Hispanic or Latino:						
White only, male	25.6	27.6	31.5	82.6	70.3	60.8
White only, female	23.0	28.5	28.1	67.0	63.6	47.4
Black or African American only, male	37.5	40.6	41.4	84.0	74.3	70.6
Black or African American only, female	38.3	43.5	44.4	71.1	67.2	51.5
Mexican male	26.9	26.8	26.3	87.9	89.5	68.8
Mexican female	25.0	27.9	26.2	77.6	71.5	65.3
Percent of poverty level:[7]						
Below 100%	31.7	33.9	33.8	75.0	71.2	57.7
100%–199%	26.6	33.5	33.7	76.0	73.4	65.7
200%–399%	24.7	30.1	31.8	76.2	67.8	58.8
400% or more	22.6	26.4	28.7	81.5	70.3	56.7
20 years and over, crude						
Both sexes[6]	24.1	30.2	32.1	73.9	67.3	54.1
Male	23.8	27.6	31.4	79.3	67.1	56.3
Female	24.4	32.7	32.8	68.8	67.4	52.1
Not Hispanic or Latino:						
White only, male	24.3	28.3	33.2	78.0	64.0	53.6
White only, female	24.6	32.8	33.4	67.8	66.9	51.1
Black or African American only, male	31.1	35.9	38.9	83.3	71.3	64.2
Black or African American only, female	32.5	41.9	44.0	70.0	67.5	51.8
Mexican male	16.4	16.5	17.7	86.5	86.9	64.0
Mexican female	15.9	18.8	19.2	80.6	74.5	62.8
Percent of poverty level:[7]						
Below 100%	25.7	30.3	28.5	74.0	71.3	58.8
100%–199%	26.7	34.8	37.0	75.1	70.7	61.9
200%–399%	22.4	29.9	33.7	73.4	64.4	52.0
400% or more	22.0	26.8	29.0	74.3	63.8	49.5
Male						
20–34 years	7.1	*8.1	9.1	92.6	89.9	81.4
35–44 years	17.1	17.1	21.1	89.0	73.3	66.9
45–54 years	29.2	31.0	33.6	76.2	66.4	55.4
55–64 years	40.6	45.0	51.3	70.3	55.9	50.0
65–74 years	54.4	59.6	64.0	74.3	59.1	47.7
75 years and over	60.4	69.0	67.2	82.5	74.3	53.5
Female						
20–34 years	2.9	*2.7	3.2	82.2	56.9	49.1
35–44 years	11.2	15.1	13.8	56.8	58.6	40.9
45–54 years	23.9	31.8	33.0	58.5	61.1	46.3
55–64 years	42.6	53.9	52.7	64.3	60.0	52.4
65–74 years	56.2	72.7	68.4	68.7	73.5	51.2
75 years and over	73.6	83.1	80.4	81.9	78.1	62.9

See footnotes at end of table.

Table 67 (page 2 of 2). Hypertension and high blood pressure among persons 20 years of age and over, by selected characteristics: United States, selected years 1988–1994 through 2005–2008

[Data are based on interviews and physical examinations of a sample of the civilian noninstitutionalized population]

* Estimates are considered unreliable. Data preceded by an asterisk have a relative standard error (RSE) of 20%–30%.

[1]Persons of Mexican origin may be of any race. Starting with 1999 data, race-specific estimates are tabulated according to the 1997 Revisions to the Standards for the Classification of Federal Data on Race and Ethnicity and are not strictly comparable with estimates for earlier years. The two non-Hispanic race categories shown in the table conform to the 1997 Standards. Starting with 1999 data, race-specific estimates are for persons who reported only one racial group. Prior to data year 1999, estimates were tabulated according to the 1977 Standards. Estimates for single-race categories prior to 1999 included persons who reported one race or, if they reported more than one race, identified one race as best representing their race. See Appendix II, Hispanic origin; Race.

[2]Hypertension is defined as having measured high blood pressure and/or taking antihypertensive medication. High blood pressure is defined as having a measured systolic pressure of at least 140 mmHg or diastolic pressure of at least 90 mmHg. Those with high blood pressure also may be taking prescribed medicine for high blood pressure. Those taking antihypertensive medication may not have measured high blood pressure but are still classified as having hypertension. See Appendix II, Blood pressure, high.

[3]Respondents were asked, "Are you now taking prescribed medicine for your high blood pressure?"

[4]Uncontrolled high blood pressure among hypertensives is defined as measured systolic pressure of at least 140 mmHg or diastolic pressure of at least 90 mmHg, among those with measured high blood pressure or reporting taking antihypertensive medication.

[5]Age-adjusted to the 2000 standard population using five age groups: 20–34 years, 35–44 years, 45–54 years, 55–64 years, and 65 years and over. Age-adjusted estimates may differ from other age-adjusted estimates based on the same data and presented elsewhere if different age groups are used in the adjustment procedure. See Appendix II, Age adjustment.

[6]Includes persons of all races and Hispanic origins, not just those shown separately.

[7]Percent of poverty level is based on family income and family size. Persons with unknown percent of poverty level are excluded (5% in 2005–2008). See Appendix II, Family income; Poverty.

NOTES: Percentages are based on the average of blood pressure measurements taken. In 2005–2008, 81% of participants had three blood pressure readings. See *Health, United States, 2003*, Table 66, for a longer trend based on a single blood pressure measurement, which provides comparable data across five time periods (1960–1962 through 1999–2000). Excludes pregnant women. Estimates for persons 20 years of age and over are used for setting and tracking *Healthy People 2010* objectives. Standard errors are available in the spreadsheet version of this table. Available from: http://www.cdc.gov/nchs/hus.htm. Data for additional years are available. See Appendix III.

SOURCE: CDC/NCHS, National Health and Nutrition Examination Survey.

[Data are based on interviews and laboratory data of a sample of the civilian noninstitutionalized population]

Sex, age, race and Hispanic origin[1], and percent of poverty level	1988–1994	1999–2002	2005–2008
20 years and over, age-adjusted[2]	Percent of population with high cholesterol (serum total cholesterol greater than or equal to 240 mg/dL or taking cholesterol-lowering medications)[3]		
Both sexes[4]	22.8	25.0	27.5
Male	21.1	25.3	27.3
Female	24.0	24.3	27.5
Not Hispanic or Latino:			
White only, male	21.1	26.0	27.9
White only, female	24.2	25.1	28.1
Black or African American only, male	18.6	20.1	24.1
Black or African American only, female	23.1	22.0	25.3
Mexican male	19.9	21.6	26.2
Mexican female	19.8	19.3	25.0
Percent of poverty level:[5]			
Below 100%	23.0	25.0	27.1
100%–199%	22.1	25.9	26.3
200%–399%	23.1	26.5	28.7
400% or more	21.7	23.1	27.5
20 years and over, crude			
Both sexes[4]	21.5	25.0	28.4
Male	19.6	25.1	27.7
Female	23.2	24.8	29.1
Not Hispanic or Latino:			
White only, male	20.0	26.8	29.7
White only, female	24.5	27.0	31.2
Black or African American only, male	16.0	18.5	22.7
Black or African American only, female	19.7	19.9	24.5
Mexican male	16.2	17.0	21.1
Mexican female	14.9	13.8	20.6
Percent of poverty level:[5]			
Below 100%	19.4	21.6	23.1
100%–199%	21.3	25.4	27.8
200%–399%	21.3	26.2	29.8
400% or more	21.9	24.2	28.9
Male			
20–34 years	8.2	10.4	10.1
35–44 years	21.0	23.1	21.5
45–54 years	29.6	34.1	33.2
55–64 years	30.8	39.1	43.4
65–74 years	27.4	36.3	49.5
75 years and over	24.4	29.0	39.4
Female			
20–34 years	7.3	9.1	9.5
35–44 years	13.5	14.4	17.0
45–54 years	28.2	27.2	29.9
55–64 years	45.8	39.2	50.0
65–74 years	46.9	51.9	51.8
75 years and over	41.2	44.0	51.7

See footnotes at end of table.

[Data are based on interviews and laboratory data of a sample of the civilian noninstitutionalized population]

Sex, age, race and Hispanic origin[1], and percent of poverty level	1988–1994	1999–2002	2005–2008
20 years and over, age-adjusted[2]	Percent of population with high serum total cholesterol (greater than or equal to 240 mg/dL)[6]		
Both sexes[4]	20.8	17.3	14.9
Male	19.0	16.4	13.4
Female	22.0	17.8	16.0
Not Hispanic or Latino:			
White only, male	18.8	16.5	13.5
White only, female	22.2	18.1	16.8
Black or African American only, male	16.9	12.4	9.5
Black or African American only, female	21.4	17.7	13.2
Mexican male	18.5	17.4	16.8
Mexican female	18.7	13.8	13.9
Percent of poverty level:[5]			
Below 100%	20.6	18.3	15.6
100%–199%	20.6	19.1	15.0
200%–399%	20.8	18.9	16.1
400% or more	19.5	14.4	14.0
20 years and over, crude			
Both sexes[4]	19.6	17.3	15.2
Male	17.7	16.5	13.8
Female	21.3	18.0	16.6
Not Hispanic or Latino:			
White only, male	18.0	16.9	14.0
White only, female	22.5	19.1	17.8
Black or African American only, male	14.7	12.2	9.6
Black or African American only, female	18.2	16.1	12.8
Mexican male	15.4	15.0	15.5
Mexican female	14.3	10.7	13.0
Percent of poverty level:[5]			
Below 100%	17.6	16.4	14.0
100%–199%	19.8	18.2	14.8
200%–399%	19.3	18.7	16.0
400% or more	19.9	15.5	15.3
Male			
20–34 years	8.2	9.8	9.1
35–44 years	19.4	19.7	16.0
45–54 years	26.6	23.6	19.8
55–64 years	28.0	19.9	16.2
65–74 years	21.9	13.7	7.9
75 years and over	20.4	10.2	8.6
Female			
20–34 years	7.3	8.9	8.4
35–44 years	12.3	12.4	13.7
45–54 years	26.7	21.4	18.6
55–64 years	40.9	25.6	27.1
65–74 years	41.3	32.3	21.8
75 years and over	38.2	26.5	19.4

Table 68 (page 3 of 4). Cholesterol among persons 20 years of age and over, by selected characteristics: United States, selected years 1988–1994 through 2005–2008

[Data are based on interviews and laboratory data of a sample of the civilian noninstitutionalized population]

Sex, age, race and Hispanic origin[1], and percent of poverty level	1988–1994	1999–2002	2005–2008
20 years and over, age-adjusted[2]	Mean serum total cholesterol level, mg/dL[7]		
Both sexes[4]	206	203	198
Male	204	202	195
Female	207	204	200
Not Hispanic or Latino:			
White only, male	205	202	194
White only, female	208	205	201
Black or African American only, male	202	195	190
Black or African American only, female	207	202	193
Mexican male	206	204	202
Mexican female	206	199	198
Percent of poverty level:[5]			
Below 100%	205	201	198
100%–199%	205	204	199
200%–399%	207	205	197
400% or more	205	202	197
20 years and over, crude			
Both sexes[4]	204	203	198
Male	202	202	195
Female	206	204	201
Not Hispanic or Latino:			
White only, male	203	203	195
White only, female	208	206	203
Black or African American only, male	198	194	190
Black or African American only, female	201	199	193
Mexican male	199	200	201
Mexican female	198	194	196
Percent of poverty level:[5]			
Below 100%	200	198	196
100%–199%	202	202	198
200%–399%	205	204	197
400% or more	206	204	200
Male			
20–34 years	186	188	186
35–44 years	206	207	205
45–54 years	216	215	205
55–64 years	216	212	199
65–74 years	212	202	184
75 years and over	205	195	179
Female			
20–34 years	184	185	186
35–44 years	195	198	196
45–54 years	217	211	209
55–64 years	235	221	216
65–74 years	233	224	209
75 years and over	229	217	203

See footnotes at end of table.

Table 68 (page 4 of 4). Cholesterol among persons 20 years of age and over, by selected characteristics: United States, selected years 1988–1994 through 2005–2008

[Data are based on interviews and laboratory data of a sample of the civilian noninstitutionalized population]

[1]Persons of Mexican origin may be of any race. Starting with 1999 data, race-specific estimates are tabulated according to the 1997 Revisions to the Standards for the Classification of Federal Data on Race and Ethnicity and are not strictly comparable with estimates for earlier years. The two non-Hispanic race categories shown in the table conform to the 1997 Standards. Starting with 1999 data, race-specific estimates are for persons who reported only one racial group. Prior to data year 1999, estimates were tabulated according to the 1977 Standards. Estimates for single-race categories prior to 1999 included persons who reported one race or, if they reported more than one race, identified one race as best representing their race. See Appendix II, Hispanic origin; Race.

[2]Age-adjusted to the 2000 standard population using five age groups: 20–34 years, 35–44 years, 45–54 years, 55–64 years, and 65 years and over. Age-adjusted estimates may differ from other age-adjusted estimates based on the same data and presented elsewhere if different age groups are used in the adjustment procedure. See Appendix II, Age adjustment.

[3]High cholesterol is defined as measured serum total cholesterol greater than or equal to 240 mg/dL or reporting taking cholesterol-lowering medications. Respondents were asked, "Are you now following this advice [from a doctor of health professional] to take prescribed medicine [to lower your cholesterol]?"

[4]Includes persons of all races and Hispanic origins, not just those shown separately.

[5]Percent of poverty level is based on family income and family size. Persons with unknown percent of poverty level are excluded (4% in 2005–2008). See Appendix II, Family income; Poverty.

[6]High serum total cholesterol is defined as greater than or equal to 240 mg/dL (6.20 mmol/L), regardless of whether the respondent reported taking cholesterol-lowering medications.

[7]Risk levels for cholesterol have been defined by the Third Report of the National Cholesterol Education Program Expert Panel on Detection, Evaluation, and Treatment of High Blood Cholesterol in Adults. National Heart, Lung, and Blood Institute, National Institutes of Health. September 2002. (Available from: http://www.nhlbi.nih.gov/guidelines/cholesterol/index.htm and summarized in JAMA 2001;285(19):2486–97). Serum total cholesterol greater than or equal to 240 mg/dL (6.20 mmol/L) is considered high. Serum total cholesterol greater than or equal to 200 mg/dL and less than 240 mg/dL is considered borderline high.

NOTES: See Appendix II, Cholesterol. Standard errors for selected years are available in the spreadsheet version of this table. Available from: http://www.cdc.gov/nchs/hus.htm. Data for additional years are available. See Appendix III.

SOURCE: CDC/NCHS, National Health and Nutrition Examination Survey.

Table 69 (page 1 of 2). Mean energy and macronutrient intake among persons 20 years of age and over, by sex and age: United States, selected years 1971–1974 through 2005–2008

[Data are based on dietary recall interviews of a sample of the civilian noninstitutionalized population]

Sex and age	1971–1974	1976–1980	1988–1994	1999–2002	2005–2008
	Mean energy intake in kilocalories (kcals)				
Male, age-adjusted[1]	2,450	2,439	2,592	2,570	2,656
Male, crude	2,461	2,459	2,648	2,593	2,672
20–39 years	2,784	2,753	2,964	2,854	2,946
40–59 years	2,303	2,315	2,567	2,601	2,702
60–74 years	1,918	1,906	2,104	2,124	2,170
75 years and over	- - -	- - -	1,814	1,876	1,941
Female, age-adjusted[1]	1,542	1,522	1,762	1,837	1,811
Female, crude.	1,540	1,525	1,772	1,832	1,803
20–39 years	1,652	1,643	1,956	2,031	1,973
40–59 years	1,510	1,473	1,734	1,823	1,798
60–74 years	1,325	1,322	1,520	1,582	1,605
75 years and over	- - -	- - -	1,401	1,435	1,466
	Percent kcals from carbohydrates				
Male, age-adjusted[1]	42.4	42.6	48.5	49.1	47.4
Male, crude	42.4	42.7	48.4	49.0	47.4
20–39 years	42.2	43.1	48.1	50.1	48.0
40–59 years	41.6	41.5	47.8	47.7	46.5
60–74 years	44.8	44.1	49.7	48.9	47.3
75 years and over	- - -	- - -	50.9	50.8	49.0
Female, age-adjusted[1]	45.4	46.0	51.0	51.7	49.5
Female, crude.	45.5	46.1	51.0	51.7	49.4
20–39 years	45.8	46.0	50.6	52.6	50.0
40–59 years	44.4	45.0	50.0	50.4	48.0
60–74 years	46.8	48.6	52.6	51.4	49.9
75 years and over	- - -	- - -	54.2	53.5	52.6
	Percent kcals from protein				
Male, age-adjusted[1]	16.5	16.1	15.5	15.3	15.6
Male, crude	16.4	16.0	15.4	15.3	15.6
20–39 years	16.1	15.8	15.0	14.8	15.5
40–59 years	16.9	16.3	15.7	15.5	15.5
60–74 years	16.5	16.3	15.9	16.2	16.2
75 years and over	- - -	- - -	16.3	15.7	15.7
Female, age-adjusted[1]	16.9	16.0	15.4	15.1	15.8
Female, crude.	16.8	16.0	15.4	15.1	15.9
20–39 years	16.4	15.8	14.8	14.6	15.4
40–59 years	17.3	16.3	15.6	15.3	16.4
60–74 years	17.0	16.1	16.4	16.0	15.9
75 years and over	- - -	- - -	15.9	15.3	15.6
	Percent kcals from total fat				
Male, age-adjusted[1]	36.9	36.7	33.8	33.0	33.6
Male, crude	36.9	36.7	33.9	33.0	33.6
20–39 years	37.0	36.2	34.0	32.1	32.7
40–59 years	36.9	37.2	34.2	33.7	34.1
60–74 years	36.4	36.8	32.9	33.8	34.2
75 years and over	- - -	- - -	32.9	33.5	34.1
Female, age-adjusted[1]	36.1	36.0	33.2	33.2	33.8
Female, crude.	36.0	35.9	33.2	33.2	33.8
20–39 years	36.3	36.0	33.6	32.5	33.6
40–59 years	36.3	36.4	34.0	33.9	34.2
60–74 years	34.9	34.7	31.6	33.4	34.2
75 years and over	- - -	- - -	31.5	32.8	32.5
	Percent kcals from saturated fat				
Male, age-adjusted[1]	13.5	13.2	11.3	10.8	11.1
Male, crude	13.5	13.2	11.4	10.8	11.1
20–39 years	13.6	13.1	11.5	10.7	11.0
40–59 years	13.5	13.4	11.3	10.8	11.2
60–74 years	13.3	13.1	10.9	10.7	11.2
75 years and over	- - -	- - -	11.2	10.8	11.5
Female, age-adjusted[1]	13.0	12.5	11.1	10.7	11.3
Female, crude.	12.9	12.5	11.1	10.7	11.3
20–39 years	13.0	12.6	11.4	10.8	11.2
40–59 years	13.1	12.6	11.3	10.9	11.5
60–74 years	12.4	11.8	10.4	10.5	11.3
75 years and over	- - -	- - -	10.5	10.2	10.9

See footnotes at end of table.

Table 69 (page 2 of 2). Mean energy and macronutrient intake among persons 20 years of age and over, by sex and age: United States, selected years 1971–1974 through 2005–2008

[Data are based on dietary recall interviews of a sample of the civilian noninstitutionalized population]

- - - Data not available.

[1]Age-adjusted to the 2000 standard population using four age groups: 20–39 years, 40–59 years, 60–74 years, and 75 years and over. Age-adjusted estimates in this table may differ from other age-adjusted estimates based on the same data and presented elsewhere if different age groups are used in the adjustment procedure. See Appendix II, Age adjustment.

NOTES: Estimates of energy intake include kilocalories (kcals) from all foods and beverages, including alcoholic beverages, consumed during the preceding 24 hours. Individuals who reported no energy intake were excluded. Starting in 2001, data collection method also included a second-day recall that was conducted by telephone (Day 2 file). This table includes only data collected in Day 1 file in the Mobile Examination Center (MEC) to calculate dietary intake. Standard errors are available in the spreadsheet version of this table. Available from: http://www.cdc.gov/nchs/hus.htm. Data for additional years are available. See Appendix III.

SOURCE: CDC/NCHS, National Health and Nutrition Examination Survey. U.S. Department of Agriculture, Agriculture Research Service. Beltsville Human Nutrition Research Center, Food Surveys Research Group, What We Eat in America.

Table 70 (page 1 of 5). Participation in leisure-time aerobic and muscle-strengthening activities that meet the 2008 federal physical activity guidelines for adults 18 years of age and over, by selected characteristics: United States, selected years 1998–2009

[Data are based on household interviews of a sample of the civilian noninstitutionalized population]

Characteristic	2008 Physical Activity Guidelines for Adults[1]							
	Aerobic activity and muscle-strengthening				Inactive			
	1998	2000	2008	2009	1998	2000	2008	2009
	Percent of adults that meet both the aerobic activity and muscle-strengthening guidelines				Percent of adults that meet neither the aerobic activity nor the muscle-strengthening guidelines			
18 years and over, age-adjusted[2,3]	14.3	15.0	18.4	19.1	56.6	54.7	52.7	49.3
18 years and over, crude[3]	14.5	15.1	18.1	18.8	56.3	54.6	52.9	49.5
Age								
18–44 years	18.9	18.9	22.3	23.3	50.7	49.1	47.6	43.6
18–24 years.	23.8	23.8	26.1	25.2	46.5	44.5	44.3	40.0
25–44 years.	17.4	17.3	21.0	22.6	51.9	50.6	48.7	44.9
45–64 years	11.4	12.8	16.3	16.8	58.8	57.6	54.7	51.8
45–54 years.	13.2	14.5	17.9	18.0	56.9	55.4	53.1	50.5
55–64 years.	8.6	10.1	14.2	15.4	61.8	61.0	56.9	53.5
65 years and over	5.5	6.8	9.5	10.0	71.0	67.0	65.1	62.2
65–74 years.	7.0	8.4	11.3	12.8	65.6	60.3	60.8	54.6
75 years and over.	3.5	4.9	7.5	6.6	77.8	75.0	69.9	71.3
Sex[2]								
Male.	17.5	17.9	21.9	22.2	50.8	49.6	48.4	45.0
Female	11.4	12.3	15.0	16.2	61.9	59.4	56.6	53.2
Sex and age								
Male:								
18–44 years.	23.0	23.0	27.3	27.7	44.3	43.0	43.1	38.9
45–54 years.	16.1	16.0	20.0	18.9	52.9	52.7	50.0	48.1
55–64 years.	9.4	11.3	15.5	18.0	58.2	58.7	54.1	50.0
65–74 years.	9.5	9.4	11.6	13.8	58.9	55.3	56.4	50.1
75 years and over.	4.9	7.1	11.4	9.1	69.5	66.7	62.3	65.4
Female:								
18–44 years.	14.9	15.0	17.4	19.0	56.9	55.0	52.0	48.2
45–54 years.	10.5	13.1	15.8	17.1	60.8	57.9	56.2	52.8
55–64 years.	7.8	9.0	13.1	13.1	65.0	63.1	59.4	56.6
65–74 years.	5.1	7.7	11.0	12.0	70.9	64.3	64.5	58.5
75 years and over.	2.6	3.6	4.9	4.9	83.0	80.0	74.9	75.2
Race[2,4]								
White only.	14.8	15.7	19.1	19.8	55.2	53.1	51.2	47.9
Black or African American only	11.7	12.2	15.2	17.5	65.7	64.6	61.5	56.8
American Indian or Alaska Native only	16.0	*10.6	*9.7	*14.8	57.6	67.1	66.2	52.4
Asian only	13.5	14.1	14.6	13.9	59.1	55.0	52.5	54.7
Native Hawaiian or Other Pacific								
Islander only	- - -	*	*	*	- - -	*	54.5	47.7
2 or more races.	- - -	19.0	20.7	16.6	- - -	52.8	52.2	44.8
Hispanic origin and race[2,4]								
Hispanic or Latino	9.4	9.2	11.3	12.5	67.7	66.5	62.7	59.0
Mexican.	8.7	8.1	11.0	11.8	69.5	67.0	61.6	58.3
Not Hispanic or Latino	14.9	15.8	19.6	20.3	55.3	53.2	50.8	47.6
White only	15.5	16.5	20.8	21.3	53.6	51.4	48.7	45.6
Black or African American only.	11.7	12.2	14.9	17.8	65.8	64.6	61.6	56.5
Education[5,6]								
No high school diploma or GED	4.6	4.3	5.3	5.9	76.3	74.0	73.8	69.1
High school diploma or GED.	8.6	9.5	11.0	10.4	64.6	61.7	62.5	59.6
Some college or more	18.2	18.9	22.9	24.5	48.0	47.1	44.8	42.1

See footnotes at end of table.

Table 70 (page 2 of 5). Participation in leisure-time aerobic and muscle-strengthening activities that meet the 2008 federal physical activity guidelines for adults 18 years of age and over, by selected characteristics: United States, selected years 1998–2009

[Data are based on household interviews of a sample of the civilian noninstitutionalized population]

| | 2008 Physical Activity Guidelines for Adults[1] | | | | | | | |
| | Aerobic activity and muscle-strengthening | | | | Inactive | | | |
Characteristic	1998	2000	2008	2009	1998	2000	2008	2009
	Percent of adults that meet both the aerobic activity and muscle-strengthening guidelines				Percent of adults that meet neither the aerobic activity nor the muscle-strengthening guidelines			
Percent of poverty level[2,7]								
Below 100%	8.0	9.3	11.2	11.9	71.3	68.0	66.7	62.2
100%–199%	9.0	9.0	10.5	10.9	67.1	65.5	64.8	59.3
200%–399%	12.6	13.2	15.2	16.8	58.0	56.8	55.6	52.1
400% or more	20.2	20.5	26.5	27.1	46.2	45.0	40.7	38.3
Hispanic origin and race and percent of poverty level[2,4,7]								
Hispanic or Latino:								
Below 100%	4.6	4.4	8.9	6.5	78.0	75.2	71.0	65.4
100%–199%	7.0	5.0	6.1	7.8	71.2	72.2	70.9	67.9
200%–399%	11.1	10.2	10.8	15.2	63.8	63.1	59.4	55.1
400% or more	17.4	19.6	21.3	22.7	55.6	52.8	48.9	44.1
Not Hispanic or Latino:								
White only:								
Below 100%	9.9	11.7	13.4	15.8	66.9	63.5	71.0	58.0
100%–199%	9.6	10.3	13.0	12.8	65.1	62.6	70.9	55.2
200%–399%	13.1	13.9	16.4	16.7	56.1	54.7	59.4	51.2
400% or more	20.2	21.0	27.6	28.2	45.2	43.7	48.9	36.5
Black or African American only:								
Below 100%	7.1	9.5	9.7	11.5	74.6	72.1	70.8	66.2
100%–199%	8.8	9.5	10.4	10.3	69.8	69.2	70.7	59.9
200%–399%	10.6	11.8	13.1	20.1	64.5	64.3	60.4	55.1
400% or more	21.2	17.6	25.6	27.8	54.2	54.9	46.5	45.3
Disability measure[2,8]								
Any basic actions difficulty or complex activity limitation	10.2	10.3	12.5	13.0	64.4	62.2	63.0	59.3
Any basic actions difficulty	9.8	10.3	12.4	13.1	64.8	62.1	63.3	59.4
Any complex activity limitation	7.7	7.2	8.2	9.2	71.9	71.2	72.2	67.4
No disability	16.0	17.0	21.3	22.1	52.5	50.6	46.9	43.4
Geographic region[2]								
Northeast	14.2	17.0	18.2	18.6	57.0	51.8	53.6	51.3
Midwest	15.0	16.4	20.1	19.9	54.9	53.4	50.1	48.9
South	11.8	12.1	16.7	18.3	61.4	59.7	56.4	51.9
West	18.5	16.7	19.2	20.0	49.5	50.1	48.8	43.8
Location of residence[2]								
Within MSA[9]	14.9	15.7	19.4	20.2	55.8	54.1	51.5	47.6
Outside MSA[9]	12.2	12.3	12.5	13.5	59.7	56.9	59.3	57.9

See footnotes at end of table.

Table 70 (page 3 of 5). Participation in leisure-time aerobic and muscle-strengthening activities that meet the 2008 federal physical activity guidelines for adults 18 years of age and over, by selected characteristics: United States, selected years 1998–2009

[Data are based on household interviews of a sample of the civilian noninstitutionalized population]

| | 2008 Physical Activity Guidelines for Adults[1] | | | | | | | |
| | Met aerobic guidelines | | | | Met muscle-strengthening guidelines | | | |
Characteristic	1998	2000	2008	2009	1998	2000	2008	2009
	Percent of adults that met the respective guideline							
18 years and over, age-adjusted[2,3]	40.0	42.2	43.6	47.3	17.7	18.0	22.1	22.7
18 years and over, crude[3]	40.3	42.4	43.4	47.0	17.9	18.1	21.8	22.4
Age								
18–44 years	45.7	47.7	49.0	53.4	22.5	22.1	25.8	26.5
18–24 years..........................	49.3	52.2	52.4	56.5	28.0	27.2	29.3	29.1
25–44 years..........................	44.6	46.3	47.8	52.3	20.8	20.5	24.6	25.6
45–64 years	38.2	39.7	41.6	44.8	14.4	15.5	19.9	20.2
45–54 years..........................	40.1	42.1	43.3	46.2	16.2	17.0	21.4	21.2
55–64 years..........................	35.3	36.1	39.3	43.0	11.5	13.1	17.9	19.0
65 years and over	26.0	30.1	30.4	32.8	8.6	9.8	14.1	15.0
65–74 years..........................	31.7	36.8	34.2	41.1	9.7	11.3	16.3	17.1
75 years and over	18.7	22.1	26.0	22.9	7.2	8.0	11.6	12.5
Sex[2]								
Male.................................	45.4	47.4	47.6	51.2	21.2	20.8	25.9	26.0
Female...............................	35.1	37.6	40.1	43.7	14.4	15.4	18.4	19.4
Sex and age								
Male:								
18–44 years..........................	51.5	53.6	52.6	57.6	27.2	26.3	31.8	31.3
45–54 years..........................	44.3	45.2	46.3	48.3	18.8	18.0	23.5	22.5
55–64 years..........................	38.3	38.9	42.7	46.7	12.9	13.8	18.5	21.2
65–74 years..........................	38.5	41.8	38.5	45.6	12.0	12.2	16.5	18.1
75 years and over	26.1	30.7	34.8	29.1	9.5	10.1	14.3	14.7
Female:								
18–44 years..........................	40.0	42.0	45.5	49.3	17.9	17.9	20.0	21.7
45–54 years..........................	36.1	39.1	40.4	44.2	13.7	16.1	19.3	19.9
55–64 years..........................	32.5	33.5	36.3	39.5	10.3	12.4	17.4	16.9
65–74 years..........................	26.2	32.6	30.6	37.4	7.8	10.5	16.0	16.2
75 years and over	14.0	16.8	20.3	18.7	5.7	6.7	9.8	11.0
Race[2,4]								
White only............................	41.5	44.1	45.2	48.8	18.0	18.5	22.7	23.1
Black or African American only	30.4	31.7	34.3	39.1	15.6	16.0	19.5	21.8
American Indian or Alaska Native only.........	39.7	29.7	32.9	44.2	18.2	13.9	*10.7	18.7
Asian only............................	37.1	41.7	42.5	41.9	17.2	17.2	19.7	17.2
Native Hawaiian or Other Pacific Islander only	- - -	*	*	50.2	- - -	*	*	*
2 or more races........................	- - -	43.9	44.2	48.9	- - -	22.2	24.1	23.7
Hispanic origin and race[2,4]								
Hispanic or Latino	29.1	30.8	33.4	37.5	12.7	11.9	15.1	16.3
Mexican.............................	27.4	30.0	34.3	37.6	11.9	11.3	15.1	16.1
Not Hispanic or Latino	41.3	43.7	45.4	49.0	18.3	18.8	23.3	23.8
White only	43.1	45.7	47.8	51.1	18.7	19.3	24.3	24.6
Black or African American only.	30.4	31.7	34.1	39.4	15.6	16.0	19.3	22.1
Education[5,6]								
No high school diploma or GED	21.4	23.9	23.5	27.7	7.0	6.6	8.1	9.2
High school diploma or GED.	32.6	35.7	34.1	37.0	11.4	12.1	14.5	14.0
Some college or more	48.1	49.4	50.9	54.3	22.1	22.4	27.2	28.1

See footnotes at end of table.

Table 70 (page 4 of 5). Participation in leisure-time aerobic and muscle-strengthening activities that meet the 2008 federal physical activity guidelines for adults 18 years of age and over, by selected characteristics: United States, selected years 1998–2009

[Data are based on household interviews of a sample of the civilian noninstitutionalized population]

| | 2008 Physical Activity Guidelines for Adults[1] | | | | | | | |
| | Met aerobic guidelines | | | | Met muscle-strengthening guidelines | | | |
Characteristic	1998	2000	2008	2009	1998	2000	2008	2009
Percent of poverty level[2,7]	Percent of adults that met the respective guideline							
Below 100%	25.9	29.3	30.5	34.4	10.8	12.3	14.0	15.5
100%–199%	29.9	32.0	31.8	37.4	12.0	11.5	14.2	14.5
200%–399%	38.8	39.9	40.6	44.5	15.9	16.5	18.9	20.4
400% or more	50.0	52.0	55.3	58.2	24.0	23.4	30.5	30.6
Hispanic origin and race and percent of poverty level[2,4,7]								
Hispanic or Latino:								
Below 100%	19.5	22.1	27.3	30.8	7.1	7.2	10.5	10.7
100%–199%	25.6	25.8	25.0	29.2	10.2	7.1	10.3	11.4
200%–399%	33.1	33.0	35.7	40.7	14.6	14.0	15.6	19.6
400% or more	40.6	45.1	46.5	53.6	21.1	21.7	25.6	24.9
Not Hispanic or Latino:								
White only:								
Below 100%	30.2	34.0	35.2	39.1	12.8	14.7	16.3	18.7
100%–199%	32.2	34.8	36.6	41.9	12.5	12.9	16.8	15.8
200%–399%	40.8	42.3	42.6	45.7	16.2	16.9	19.6	20.0
400% or more	51.0	53.4	57.2	60.0	24.0	23.8	31.5	31.6
Black or African American only:								
Below 100%	22.7	25.4	24.8	29.5	10.0	12.1	14.0	15.8
100%–199%	26.9	28.0	26.8	34.7	12.1	12.3	12.8	15.7
200%–399%	30.6	31.4	34.3	41.3	15.5	16.2	18.6	23.7
400% or more	41.7	40.3	48.8	51.1	25.4	22.4	30.4	31.8
Disability measure[2,8]								
Any basic actions difficulty or complex activity limitation	31.8	34.2	32.6	36.5	13.9	14.0	16.9	17.4
Any basic actions difficulty	31.3	34.0	32.5	36.4	13.6	14.2	16.6	17.5
Any complex activity limitation	24.4	24.9	23.2	28.3	11.5	11.3	13.0	13.8
No disability	44.3	46.6	49.7	53.5	19.3	19.8	24.7	25.3
Geographic region[2]								
Northeast	39.6	45.3	42.3	45.3	17.5	20.0	22.4	22.3
Midwest	42.0	43.5	45.6	47.5	18.2	19.3	24.3	23.5
South	35.3	37.3	40.4	44.7	15.0	15.1	20.0	21.7
West	46.7	46.9	47.5	52.6	22.3	19.7	22.8	23.6
Location of residence[2]								
Within MSA[9]	40.8	42.9	44.8	48.8	18.3	18.6	23.2	23.9
Outside MSA[9]	37.1	39.9	37.3	39.3	15.4	15.5	16.1	16.5

See footnotes at end of table.

Table 70 (page 5 of 5). Participation in leisure-time aerobic and muscle-strengthening activities that meet the 2008 federal physical activity guidelines for adults 18 years of age and over, by selected characteristics: United States, selected years 1998–2009

[Data are based on household interviews of a sample of the civilian noninstitutionalized population]

---

* Estimates are considered unreliable. Data preceded by an asterisk have a relative standard error (RSE) of 20%–30%. Data not shown have an RSE of greater than 30%.

- - - Data not available.

[1]Starting with *Health, United States, 2010*, measures of physical activity shown in this table changed to reflect the 2008 Federal Physical Activity Guidelines for Americans (available from: http://www.health.gov/PAGuidelines/). This new table presents four measures of physical activity: the percentage of adults that fully met the 2008 federal guidelines for both aerobic activity and muscle strengthening; the percentage of adults that did not meet the aerobic activity guideline and did not meet the muscle-strengthening guideline (inactive); the percentage of adults who met the aerobic activity component; and the percentage of adults who met the muscle-strengthening component of the 2008 guidelines. The inactive category contains persons who were completely inactive in addition to those who had some activity but amounts were insufficient to meet the guidelines. The 2008 federal guidelines recommend that for substantial health benefits, adults perform at least 150 minutes (2 hours and 30 minutes) a week of moderate-intensity, or 75 minutes (1 hour and 15 minutes) a week of vigorous-intensity aerobic physical activity, or an equivalent combination of moderate- and vigorous-intensity aerobic activity. Aerobic activity should be performed in episodes of at least 10 minutes, and preferably, it should be spread throughout the week. The 2008 guidelines also recommend that adults perform muscle-strengthening activities that are moderate or high intensity and involve all major muscle groups on 2 or more days a week, because these activities provide additional health benefits. See Appendix II, Physical activity, leisure-time.

[2]Estimates are age-adjusted to the year 2000 standard population using five age groups: 18–44 years, 45–54 years, 55–64 years, 65–74 years, and 75 years and over. Age-adjusted estimates in this table may differ from other age-adjusted estimates based on the same data and presented elsewhere if different age groups are used in the adjustment procedure. See Appendix II, Age adjustment.

[3]Includes all other races not shown separately, unknown education level, and unknown disability status.

[4]The race groups, white, black, American Indian or Alaska Native, Asian, Native Hawaiian or Other Pacific Islander, and 2 or more races, include persons of Hispanic and non-Hispanic origin. Persons of Hispanic origin may be of any race. Starting with 1999 data, race-specific estimates are tabulated according to the 1997 Revisions to the Standards for the Classification of Federal Data on Race and Ethnicity and are not strictly comparable with estimates for earlier years. The five single-race categories plus multiple-race categories shown in the table conform to the 1997 Standards. Starting with 1999 data, race-specific estimates are for persons who reported only one racial group; the category 2 or more races includes persons who reported more than one racial group. Prior to 1999, data were tabulated according to the 1977 Standards with four racial groups and the Asian only category included Native Hawaiian or Other Pacific Islander. Estimates for single-race categories prior to 1999 included persons who reported one race or, if they reported more than one race, identified one race as best representing their race. Starting with 2003 data, race responses of other race and unspecified multiple race were treated as missing, and then race was imputed if these were the only race responses. Almost all persons with a race response of other race were of Hispanic origin. See Appendix II, Hispanic origin; Race.

[5]Estimates are for persons 25 years of age and over and are age-adjusted to the year 2000 standard population using five age groups: 25–44 years, 45–54 years, 55–64 years, 65–74 years, and 75 years and over. See Appendix II, Age adjustment.

[6]GED is General Educational Development high school equivalency diploma. See Appendix II, Education.

[7]Percent of poverty level is based on family income and family size and composition using U.S. Census Bureau poverty thresholds. Missing family income data were imputed for 1997 and beyond. See Appendix II, Family income; Poverty; Table VII.

[8]Any basic actions difficulty or complex activity limitation is defined as having one or more of the following limitations or difficulties: movement difficulty, emotional difficulty, sensory (seeing or hearing) difficulty, cognitive difficulty, self-care (ADL or IADL) limitation, social limitation, or work limitation. For more information, see Appendix II, Basic actions difficulty; Complex activity limitation. Starting with 2007 data, the hearing question, a component of the basic actions difficulty measure, was revised. Consequently, data prior to 2007 are not comparable with data for 2007 and beyond. For more information on the impact of the revised hearing question, see Appendix II, Hearing trouble.

[9]MSA is metropolitan statistical area. Starting with 2006 data, MSA status is determined using 2000 census data and the 2000 standards for defining MSAs. For data prior to 2006, see Appendix II, Metropolitan statistical area (MSA) for the applicable standards.

NOTES: Standard errors are available in the spreadsheet version of this table. Available from: http://www.cdc.gov/nchs/hus.htm. Data for additional years are available. See Appendix III.

SOURCE: CDC/NCHS, National Health Interview Survey, family core and sample adult questionnaires.

Table 71 (page 1 of 4). Overweight, obesity, and healthy weight among persons 20 years of age and over, by selected characteristics: United States, selected years 1960–1962 through 2005–2008

[Data are based on measured height and weight of a sample of the civilian noninstitutionalized population]

Sex, age, race and Hispanic origin[1], and percent of poverty level	Overweight (includes obesity)[2]					
	1960–1962	1971–1974	1976–1980[3]	1988–1994	1999–2002	2005–2008
20–74 years, age-adjusted[4]			Percent of population			
Both sexes[5]	44.8	47.7	47.4	56.0	65.2	67.7
Male.	49.5	54.7	52.9	61.0	68.8	73.0
Female.	40.2	41.1	42.0	51.2	61.7	62.6
Not Hispanic or Latino:						
White only, male.	- - -	- - -	53.8	61.6	69.5	72.9
White only, female	- - -	- - -	38.7	47.2	57.0	59.4
Black or African American only, male . . .	- - -	- - -	51.3	58.2	62.0	71.8
Black or African American only, female . .	- - -	- - -	62.6	68.5	77.6	79.1
Mexican male	- - -	- - -	61.6	69.4	74.1	79.2
Mexican female	- - -	- - -	61.7	69.6	71.4	75.6
Percent of poverty level:[6]						
Below 100%.	- - -	49.3	50.0	59.8	65.2	67.6
100%–199%.	- - -	50.9	49.0	58.2	68.0	70.3
200% or more	- - -	46.7	46.6	54.5	64.9	67.0
200%–399%.	- - -	48.4	- - -	56.0	68.7	69.0
400% or more.	- - -	43.4	- - -	51.8	61.8	65.1
20 years and over, age-adjusted[4]						
Both sexes[5]	- - -	- - -	- - -	56.0	65.1	67.5
Male.	- - -	- - -	- - -	60.9	68.8	72.9
Female.	- - -	- - -	- - -	51.4	61.6	62.5
Not Hispanic or Latino:						
White only, male.	- - -	- - -	- - -	61.6	69.4	72.9
White only, female	- - -	- - -	- - -	47.5	57.2	59.6
Black or African American only, male . . .	- - -	- - -	- - -	57.8	62.6	71.7
Black or African American only, female . .	- - -	- - -	- - -	68.2	77.2	78.0
Mexican male	- - -	- - -	- - -	68.9	73.2	77.7
Mexican female	- - -	- - -	- - -	68.9	71.2	74.8
Percent of poverty level:[6]						
Below 100%.	- - -	- - -	- - -	59.6	64.7	67.7
100%–199%.	- - -	- - -	- - -	58.0	67.3	69.6
200% or more	- - -	- - -	- - -	54.8	65.1	67.0
200%–399%.	- - -	- - -	- - -	56.0	68.6	68.7
400% or more.	- - -	- - -	- - -	52.4	62.2	65.3
20 years and over, crude						
Both sexes[5]	- - -	- - -	- - -	54.9	65.2	67.8
Male.	- - -	- - -	- - -	59.4	68.6	72.8
Female.	- - -	- - -	- - -	50.7	62.0	63.0
Not Hispanic or Latino:						
White only, male.	- - -	- - -	- - -	60.6	69.9	73.4
White only, female	- - -	- - -	- - -	47.4	58.2	60.7
Black or African American only, male . . .	- - -	- - -	- - -	56.7	61.7	71.1
Black or African American only, female . .	- - -	- - -	- - -	66.0	76.9	78.1
Mexican male	- - -	- - -	- - -	63.9	70.1	76.8
Mexican female	- - -	- - -	- - -	65.9	69.3	73.9
Percent of poverty level:[6]						
Below 100%.	- - -	- - -	- - -	56.8	62.5	65.9
100%–199%.	- - -	- - -	- - -	55.7	66.2	69.1
200% or more	- - -	- - -	- - -	54.2	65.8	67.9
200%–399%.	- - -	- - -	- - -	54.9	68.5	68.7
400% or more.	- - -	- - -	- - -	53.3	63.7	67.2
Male						
20–34 years	42.7	42.8	41.2	47.5	57.4	60.5
35–44 years	53.5	63.2	57.2	65.5	70.5	78.9
45–54 years	53.9	59.7	60.2	66.1	75.7	76.8
55–64 years	52.2	58.5	60.2	70.5	75.4	80.5
65–74 years	47.8	54.6	54.2	68.5	76.2	79.1
75 years and over	- - -	- - -	- - -	56.5	67.4	70.8
Female						
20–34 years	21.2	25.8	27.9	37.0	52.9	55.6
35–44 years	37.2	40.5	40.7	49.6	60.6	62.1
45–54 years	49.3	49.0	48.7	60.3	65.1	65.8
55–64 years	59.9	54.5	53.7	66.3	72.2	69.4
65–74 years	60.9	55.9	59.5	60.3	70.9	69.6
75 years and over	- - -	- - -	- - -	52.3	59.9	61.3

See footnotes at end of table.

Table 71 (page 2 of 4). **Overweight, obesity, and healthy weight among persons 20 years of age and over, by selected characteristics: United States, selected years 1960–1962 through 2005–2008**

[Data are based on measured height and weight of a sample of the civilian noninstitutionalized population]

Sex, age, race and Hispanic origin[1], and percent of poverty level	Obesity[7]					
	1960–1962	1971–1974	1976–1980[3]	1988–1994	1999–2002	2005–2008
20–74 years, age-adjusted[4]	Percent of population					
Both sexes[5]	13.3	14.6	15.1	23.3	31.1	34.7
Male	10.7	12.2	12.8	20.6	28.1	33.3
Female	15.7	16.8	17.1	26.0	34.0	36.2
Not Hispanic or Latino:						
White only, male	- - -	- - -	12.4	20.7	28.7	33.2
White only, female	- - -	- - -	15.4	23.3	31.3	33.8
Black or African American only, male	- - -	- - -	16.5	21.3	27.9	37.7
Black or African American only, female	- - -	- - -	31.0	39.1	49.4	51.8
Mexican male	- - -	- - -	15.7	24.4	29.0	32.2
Mexican female	- - -	- - -	26.6	36.1	38.9	44.0
Percent of poverty level:[6]						
Below 100%	- - -	20.7	21.9	29.2	36.0	36.4
100%–199%	- - -	18.4	18.7	26.6	35.4	39.2
200% or more	- - -	12.4	12.9	21.4	29.2	33.2
200%–399%	- - -	13.7	- - -	23.2	33.0	36.7
400% or more	- - -	10.1	- - -	18.9	25.8	29.9
20 years and over, age-adjusted[4]						
Both sexes[5]	- - -	- - -	- - -	22.9	30.4	34.0
Male	- - -	- - -	- - -	20.2	27.5	32.7
Female	- - -	- - -	- - -	25.5	33.2	35.4
Not Hispanic or Latino:						
White only, male	- - -	- - -	- - -	20.3	28.0	32.6
White only, female	- - -	- - -	- - -	22.9	30.7	33.1
Black or African American only, male	- - -	- - -	- - -	20.9	27.8	37.6
Black or African American only, female	- - -	- - -	- - -	38.3	48.6	51.0
Mexican male	- - -	- - -	- - -	23.8	27.8	32.0
Mexican female	- - -	- - -	- - -	35.2	38.0	43.3
Percent of poverty level:[6]						
Below 100%	- - -	- - -	- - -	28.1	34.7	35.9
100%–199%	- - -	- - -	- - -	26.1	34.1	38.0
200% or more	- - -	- - -	- - -	21.1	28.7	32.5
200%–399%	- - -	- - -	- - -	22.7	32.1	35.8
400% or more	- - -	- - -	- - -	18.7	25.5	29.4
20 years and over, crude						
Both sexes[5]	- - -	- - -	- - -	22.3	30.5	34.3
Male	- - -	- - -	- - -	19.5	27.5	32.9
Female	- - -	- - -	- - -	25.0	33.4	35.6
Not Hispanic or Latino:						
White only, male	- - -	- - -	- - -	19.9	28.4	33.1
White only, female	- - -	- - -	- - -	22.7	31.3	33.3
Black or African American only, male	- - -	- - -	- - -	20.7	27.5	37.3
Black or African American only, female	- - -	- - -	- - -	36.7	48.7	51.1
Mexican male	- - -	- - -	- - -	20.6	26.0	30.9
Mexican female	- - -	- - -	- - -	33.3	37.0	42.9
Percent of poverty level:[6]						
Below 100%	- - -	- - -	- - -	25.9	33.0	35.4
100%–199%	- - -	- - -	- - -	24.3	32.8	37.0
200% or more	- - -	- - -	- - -	20.9	29.3	33.4
200%–399%	- - -	- - -	- - -	22.1	31.8	35.6
400% or more	- - -	- - -	- - -	19.3	27.2	31.7
Male						
20–34 years	9.2	9.7	8.9	14.1	21.7	25.4
35–44 years	12.1	13.5	13.5	21.5	28.5	35.9
45–54 years	12.5	13.7	16.7	23.2	30.6	35.9
55–64 years	9.2	14.1	14.1	27.2	35.5	40.4
65–74 years	10.4	10.9	13.2	24.1	31.9	36.6
75 years and over	- - -	- - -	- - -	13.2	18.0	25.6
Female						
20–34 years	7.2	9.7	11.0	18.5	28.3	31.4
35–44 years	14.7	17.7	17.8	25.5	32.1	36.7
45–54 years	20.3	18.9	19.6	32.4	36.9	39.1
55–64 years	24.4	24.1	22.9	33.7	42.1	42.4
65–74 years	23.2	22.0	21.5	26.9	39.3	35.6
75 years and over	- - -	- - -	- - -	19.2	23.6	25.9

See footnotes at end of table.

Table 71 (page 3 of 4). Overweight, obesity, and healthy weight among persons 20 years of age and over, by selected characteristics: United States, selected years 1960–1962 through 2005–2008

[Data are based on measured height and weight of a sample of the civilian noninstitutionalized population]

Sex, age, race and Hispanic origin[1], and percent of poverty level	Healthy weight[8]					
	1960–1962	1971–1974	1976–1980[3]	1988–1994	1999–2002	2005–2008
20–74 years, age-adjusted[4]	Percent of population					
Both sexes[5]	51.2	48.8	49.6	41.7	32.9	30.6
Male	48.3	43.0	45.4	37.9	30.2	26.0
Female	54.1	54.3	53.7	45.3	35.6	35.1
Not Hispanic or Latino:						
White only, male	- - -	- - -	45.3	37.4	29.5	26.0
White only, female	- - -	- - -	56.7	49.2	39.7	38.0
Black or African American only, male	- - -	- - -	46.6	40.0	35.5	26.6
Black or African American only, female	- - -	- - -	35.0	28.9	21.2	19.3
Mexican male	- - -	- - -	37.1	29.8	25.6	20.3
Mexican female	- - -	- - -	36.4	29.0	27.6	23.1
Percent of poverty level:[6]						
Below 100%	- - -	45.8	45.1	37.3	32.4	29.3
100%–199%	- - -	45.1	47.6	39.2	29.7	27.7
200% or more	- - -	50.2	51.0	43.4	33.5	31.8
200%–399%	- - -	48.3	- - -	41.9	29.5	29.7
400% or more	- - -	53.9	- - -	46.0	36.9	33.9
20 years and over, age-adjusted[4]						
Both sexes[5]	- - -	- - -	- - -	41.6	33.0	30.8
Male	- - -	- - -	- - -	37.9	30.2	26.1
Female	- - -	- - -	- - -	45.0	35.7	35.2
Not Hispanic or Latino:						
White only, male	- - -	- - -	- - -	37.3	29.6	26.0
White only, female	- - -	- - -	- - -	48.7	39.5	37.8
Black or African American only, male	- - -	- - -	- - -	40.1	34.7	26.6
Black or African American only, female	- - -	- - -	- - -	29.2	21.6	20.4
Mexican male	- - -	- - -	- - -	30.2	26.5	21.8
Mexican female	- - -	- - -	- - -	29.7	27.5	24.1
Percent of poverty level:[6]						
Below 100%	- - -	- - -	- - -	37.5	32.7	29.1
100%–199%	- - -	- - -	- - -	39.3	30.5	28.3
200% or more	- - -	- - -	- - -	43.1	33.4	31.8
200%–399%	- - -	- - -	- - -	41.8	29.6	30.0
400% or more	- - -	- - -	- - -	45.5	36.5	33.5
20 years and over, crude						
Both sexes[5]	- - -	- - -	- - -	42.6	32.9	30.5
Male	- - -	- - -	- - -	39.4	30.4	26.1
Female	- - -	- - -	- - -	45.7	35.4	34.8
Not Hispanic or Latino:						
White only, male	- - -	- - -	- - -	38.2	29.2	25.4
White only, female	- - -	- - -	- - -	48.8	38.7	36.9
Black or African American only, male	- - -	- - -	- - -	41.5	35.9	27.4
Black or African American only, female	- - -	- - -	- - -	31.2	21.8	20.3
Mexican male	- - -	- - -	- - -	35.2	29.4	22.8
Mexican female	- - -	- - -	- - -	32.4	29.5	24.7
Percent of poverty level:[6]						
Below 100%	- - -	- - -	- - -	39.8	34.5	30.9
100%–199%	- - -	- - -	- - -	41.5	31.5	28.8
200% or more	- - -	- - -	- - -	43.6	32.8	31.0
200%–399%	- - -	- - -	- - -	42.9	29.7	30.0
400% or more	- - -	- - -	- - -	44.6	35.3	31.8
Male						
20–34 years	55.3	54.7	57.1	51.1	40.3	38.0
35–44 years	45.2	35.2	41.3	33.4	29.0	20.9
45–54 years	44.8	38.5	38.7	33.6	24.0	21.7
55–64 years	44.9	38.3	38.7	28.6	23.8	18.5
65–74 years	46.2	42.1	42.3	30.1	22.8	20.2
75 years and over	- - -	- - -	- - -	40.9	32.0	28.1
Female						
20–34 years	67.6	65.8	65.0	57.9	42.5	40.5
35–44 years	58.4	56.7	55.6	47.1	37.1	36.2
45–54 years	47.6	49.3	48.7	37.2	33.1	32.1
55–64 years	38.1	41.1	43.5	31.5	27.6	29.9
65–74 years	36.4	40.6	37.8	37.0	26.4	28.8
75 years and over	- - -	- - -	- - -	43.0	36.9	36.3

See footnotes at end of table.

Table 71 (page 4 of 4). Overweight, obesity, and healthy weight among persons 20 years of age and over, by selected characteristics: United States, selected years 1960–1962 through 2005–2008

[Data are based on measured height and weight of a sample of the civilian noninstitutionalized population]

- - - Data not available.

[1]Persons of Mexican origin may be of any race. Starting with 1999 data, race-specific estimates are tabulated according to the 1997 Revisions to the Standards for the Classification of Federal Data on Race and Ethnicity and are not strictly comparable with estimates for earlier years. The two non-Hispanic race categories shown in the table conform to the 1997 Standards. Starting with 1999 data, race-specific estimates are for persons who reported only one racial group. Prior to data year 1999, estimates were tabulated according to the 1977 Standards. Estimates for single-race categories prior to 1999 included persons who reported one race or, if they reported more than one race, identified one race as best representing their race. See Appendix II, Hispanic origin; Race.

[2]Body mass index (BMI) greater than or equal to 25 kilograms/meter^2. See Appendix II, Body mass index.

[3]Data for Mexicans are for 1982–1984. See Appendix I, National Health and Nutrition Examination Survey (NHANES).

[4]Age-adjusted to the 2000 standard population using five age groups: 20–34 years, 35–44 years, 45–54 years, 55–64 years, and 65 years and over (65–74 years for estimates for 20–74 years). Age-adjusted estimates in this table may differ from other age-adjusted estimates based on the same data and presented elsewhere if different age groups are used in the adjustment procedure. See Appendix II, Age adjustment.

[5]Includes persons of all races and Hispanic origins, not just those shown separately.

[6]Percent of poverty level is based on family income and family size. Persons with unknown percent of poverty level are excluded (7% in 2005–2008). See Appendix II, Family income; Poverty.

[7]Body mass index (BMI) greater than or equal to 30 kilograms/meter^2.

[8]BMI of 18.5 to less than 25 kilograms/meter^2.

NOTES: Percents do not sum to 100 because the percentage of persons with BMI less than 18.5 kilograms/meter^2 is not shown and the percentage of persons with obesity is a subset of the percentage with overweight. Height was measured without shoes; 2 pounds were deducted from data for 1960–1962 to allow for weight of clothing. Excludes pregnant women. Standard errors for selected years are available in the spreadsheet version of this table. Available from: http://www.cdc.gov/nchs/hus.htm. Data for additional years are available. See Appendix III.

SOURCE: CDC/NCHS, National Health and Nutrition Examination Survey, Hispanic Health and Nutrition Examination Survey (1982–1984), and National Health Examination Survey (1960–1962).

Table 72 (page 1 of 2). Obesity among children and adolescents 2–19 years of age, by selected characteristics: United States, selected years 1963–1965 through 2005–2008

[Data are based on physical examinations of a sample of the civilian noninstitutionalized population]

Sex, age, race and Hispanic origin[1], and percent of poverty level	1963–1965 1966–1970[2]	1971–1974	1976–1980[3]	1988–1994	1999–2002	2005–2008
2–5 years of age			Percent of population			
Both sexes[4]	- - -	- - -	- - -	7.2	10.3	10.7
Not Hispanic or Latino:						
White only	- - -	- - -	- - -	5.2	8.7	9.4
Black or African American only	- - -	- - -	- - -	7.7	8.8	14.0
Mexican	- - -	- - -	- - -	12.3	13.1	14.1
Boys	- - -	- - -	- - -	6.1	10.0	10.2
Not Hispanic or Latino:						
White only	- - -	- - -	- - -	*4.5	*8.2	*7.8
Black or African American only	- - -	- - -	- - -	7.7	*8.0	13.8
Mexican	- - -	- - -	- - -	12.4	14.1	17.3
Girls	- - -	- - -	- - -	8.2	10.6	11.1
Not Hispanic or Latina:						
White only	- - -	- - -	- - -	5.9	*9.0	11.3
Black or African American only	- - -	- - -	- - -	7.6	9.6	14.2
Mexican	- - -	- - -	- - -	12.3	*12.2	10.7
Percent of poverty level:[5]						
Below 100%	- - -	- - -	- - -	9.7	10.9	12.5
100%–199%	- - -	- - -	- - -	7.2	*13.8	10.8
200%–399%	- - -	- - -	- - -	5.6	*7.6	11.5
400% or more	- - -	- - -	- - -	*	*	*
6–11 years of age			Percent of population			
Both sexes[4]	4.2	4.0	6.5	11.3	15.9	17.4
Boys	4.0	*4.3	6.6	11.6	16.9	18.7
Not Hispanic or Latino:						
White only	- - -	- - -	6.1	10.7	14.0	16.5
Black or African American only	- - -	- - -	6.8	12.3	17.0	18.7
Mexican	- - -	- - -	13.3	17.5	26.5	28.4
Girls	4.5	*3.6	6.4	11.0	14.7	16.0
Not Hispanic or Latina:						
White only	- - -	- - -	5.2	*9.8	13.1	14.5
Black or African American only	- - -	- - -	11.2	17.0	22.8	21.3
Mexican	- - -	- - -	9.8	15.3	17.1	21.2
Percent of poverty level:[5]						
Below 100%	- - -	- - -	- - -	11.4	19.1	21.5
100%–199%	- - -	- - -	- - -	11.1	16.4	22.2
200%–399%	- - -	- - -	- - -	11.7	15.3	16.8
400% or more	- - -	- - -	- - -	*8.3	12.9	*9.5
12–19 years of age						
Both sexes[4]	4.6	6.1	5.0	10.5	16.0	17.9
Boys	4.5	6.1	4.8	11.3	16.7	18.7
Not Hispanic or Latino:						
White only	- - -	- - -	3.8	11.6	14.6	16.1
Black or African American only	- - -	- - -	6.1	10.7	18.8	19.1
Mexican	- - -	- - -	7.7	14.1	24.7	26.2
Girls	4.7	6.2	5.3	9.7	15.3	17.0
Not Hispanic or Latina:						
White only	- - -	- - -	4.6	8.9	12.6	14.0
Black or African American only	- - -	- - -	10.7	16.3	23.5	29.5
Mexican	- - -	- - -	8.8	*13.4	19.6	21.3
Percent of poverty level:[5]						
Below 100%	- - -	- - -	- - -	15.8	19.8	23.1
100%–199%	- - -	- - -	- - -	11.2	15.1	19.8
200%–399%	- - -	- - -	- - -	9.4	15.7	17.2
400% or more	- - -	- - -	- - -	2.7	13.9	14.0

See footnotes at end of table.

Table 72 (page 2 of 2). Obesity among children and adolescents 2–19 years of age, by selected characteristics: United States, selected years 1963–1965 through 2005–2008

[Data are based on physical examinations of a sample of the civilian noninstitutionalized population]

- - - Data not available.

* Estimates are considered unreliable. Data preceded by an asterisk have a relative standard error of 20%–30%. Data not shown have an RSE greater than 30%.

[1]Persons of Mexican origin may be of any race. Starting with 1999 data, race-specific estimates are tabulated according to the 1997 Revisions to the Standards for the Classification of Federal Data on Race and Ethnicity and are not strictly comparable with estimates for earlier years. The two non-Hispanic race categories shown in the table conform to the 1997 Standards. Starting with 1999 data, race-specific estimates are for persons who reported only one racial group. Prior to data year 1999, estimates were tabulated according to the 1977 Standards. Estimates for single-race categories prior to 1999 included persons who reported one race or, if they reported more than one race, identified one race as best representing their race. See Appendix II, Hispanic origin; Race.

[2]Data for 1963–1965 are for children 6–11 years of age; data for 1966–1970 are for adolescents 12–17 years of age, not 12–19 years.

[3]Data for Mexicans are for 1982–1984. See Appendix I, National Health and Nutrition Examination Survey (NHANES).

[4]Includes persons of all races and Hispanic origins, not just those shown separately.

[5]Percent of poverty level is based on family income and family size. Persons with unknown percent of poverty level are excluded (5% in 2005–2008). See Appendix II, Family income; Poverty.

NOTES: Obesity is defined as body mass index (BMI) at or above the sex- and age-specific 95th percentile BMI cutoff points from the 2000 CDC Growth Charts: United States. Kuczmarski RJ, Ogden CL, Guo SS, Grummer-Strawn LM, Flegal KM, Mei Z, Wei R, Curtin LR, Roche AF, Johnson CL. 2000 CDC Growth Charts for the United States: methods and development. Vital Health Stat 11. 2002 May;(246):1–190. Available at: http://www.cdc.gov/nchs/data/series/sr_11/sr11_246.pdf. Starting with *Health United States, 2010*, the terminology describing weight for height among children changed from prior editions. The term "obesity" now refers to children who were formerly labeled as overweight. This is a change in terminology only and not measurement; the previous definition of overweight is now the definition of obesity. Ogden CL, Flegal KM. Changes in terminology for childhood overweight and obesity. National health statistics report; no. 25. Hyattsville, MD: NCHS; 2010. Available from: http://www.cdc.gov/nchs/data/nhsr/nhsr025.pdf. Age is at time of examination at the mobile examination center. Crude rates, not age-adjusted rates, are shown. Excludes pregnant females starting with 1971–1974. Pregnancy status not available for 1963–1965 and 1966–1970. Standard errors for selected years are available in the spreadsheet version of this table. Available from: http://www.cdc.gov/nchs/hus.htm. Data for additional years are available. See Appendix III.

SOURCE: CDC/NCHS, National Health and Nutrition Examination Survey, Hispanic Health and Nutrition Examination Survey (1982–1984), and National Health Examination Survey (1963–1965 and 1966–1970). Available from: http://www.cdc.gov/nchs/data/nhsr/nhsr025.pdf.

Table 73 (page 1 of 2). Untreated dental caries, by selected characteristics: United States, selected years 1971–1974 through 2005–2008

[Data are based on dental examinations of a sample of the civilian noninstitutionalized population]

Sex, race and Hispanic origin[1], and percent of poverty level	Age 2–5 years			Age 6–19 years		
	1971–1974	1988–1994	2005–2008	1971–1974	1988–1994	2005–2008
	Percent of persons with untreated dental caries					
Total[2]	25.0	19.1	. . .	54.7	23.6	16.1
Sex						
Male	26.4	19.3	. . .	54.9	22.8	17.0
Female	23.6	18.9	. . .	54.5	24.5	15.3
Race and Hispanic origin						
Not Hispanic or Latino:						
White only	23.7	13.8	. . .	51.6	18.8	12.8
Black or African American only	29.0	24.7	. . .	71.0	33.7	22.1
Mexican	- - -	34.9	. . .	- - -	36.5	22.2
Percent of poverty level:[3]						
Below 100%	32.0	30.2	. . .	68.0	38.3	25.3
100%–199%	29.9	24.3	. . .	60.3	28.2	18.3
200% or more	17.8	9.4	. . .	46.2	15.1	11.9
200%–399%	- - -	10.7	. . .	- - -	16.3	14.2
400% or more	- - -	*	. . .	- - -	*10.2	9.3
Race, Hispanic origin, and percent of poverty level[3]						
Not Hispanic or Latino:						
White only:						
Below 100% of poverty level	32.1	25.7	. . .	65.9	33.5	25.2
100% or more of poverty level	22.0	11.7	. . .	49.9	16.7	11.0
Black or African American only:						
Below 100% of poverty level	29.1	27.2	. . .	73.9	37.0	26.9
100% or more of poverty level	27.9	22.5	. . .	67.3	31.0	19.1
Mexican:						
Below 100% of poverty level	- - -	38.8	. . .	- - -	46.4	25.3
100% or more of poverty level	- - -	30.3	. . .	- - -	26.4	20.4

Sex, race and Hispanic origin[1], and percent of poverty level	Age 20–64 years			Age 65–74 years		
	1971–1974	1988–1994	2005–2008	1971–1974	1988–1994	2005–2008
	Percent of persons with untreated dental caries					
Total[2]	48.0	28.3	23.2	29.7	25.4	18.3
Sex						
Male	50.5	31.5	26.6	32.6	29.8	22.9
Female	45.6	25.3	19.9	27.4	21.5	14.6
Race and Hispanic origin						
Not Hispanic or Latino:						
White only	45.3	23.9	18.8	28.3	22.7	16.6
Black or African American only	67.3	48.5	39.0	41.5	46.7	31.3
Mexican	- - -	40.2	34.6	- - -	43.8	31.9
Percent of poverty level:[3]						
Below 100%	63.5	48.1	41.2	34.3	46.6	41.7
100%–199%	56.2	43.5	36.7	35.6	40.1	22.2
200% or more	42.7	19.6	16.3	26.2	19.2	14.2
200%–399%	- - -	24.6	23.9	- - -	24.1	*16.2
400% or more	- - -	12.7	10.9	- - -	13.5	11.5
Race, Hispanic origin, and percent of poverty level[3]						
Not Hispanic or Latino:						
White only:						
Below 100% of poverty level	60.2	43.7	39.4	33.3	*39.0	*38.5
100% or more of poverty level	44.2	21.8	16.7	28.3	22.7	15.1
Black or African American only:						
Below 100% of poverty level	71.9	60.4	50.7	39.8	49.7	54.0
100% or more of poverty level	65.3	43.9	36.4	41.1	43.8	27.6
Mexican:						
Below 100% of poverty level	- - -	52.7	43.6	- - -	55.5	47.8
100% or more of poverty level	- - -	31.8	30.2	- - -	35.6	*23.2

See footnotes at end of table.

Table 73 (page 2 of 2). Untreated dental caries, by selected characteristics: United States, selected years 1971–1974 through 2005–2008

[Data are based on dental examinations of a sample of the civilian noninstitutionalized population]

Sex, race and Hispanic origin[1], and percent of poverty level	Age 75 years and over		
	1971–1974	1988–1994	2005–2008
	Percent of persons with untreated dental caries		
Total[2]	- - -	30.3	17.7
Sex			
Male	- - -	34.4	22.1
Female	- - -	28.1	14.3
Race and Hispanic origin			
Not Hispanic or Latino:			
White only.	- - -	27.8	15.4
Black or African American only	- - -	62.6	40.5
Mexican.	- - -	55.6	41.1
Percent of poverty level:[3]			
Below 100%	- - -	47.1	36.0
100%–199%	- - -	34.5	20.2
200% or more	- - -	23.2	11.9
200%–399%	- - -	24.3	11.5
400% or more	- - -	21.6	*
Race, Hispanic origin, and percent of poverty level[3]			
Not Hispanic or Latino:			
White only:			
Below 100% of poverty level	- - -	38.0	*
100% or more of poverty level.	- - -	26.1	13.7
Black or African American only:			
Below 100% of poverty level	- - -	68.6	*55.1
100% or more of poverty level.	- - -	60.2	33.0
Mexican:			
Below 100% of poverty level.	- - -	79.4	71.4
100% or more of poverty level	- - -	*	*28.0

. . . Category not applicable.

- - - Data not available.

* Estimates are considered unreliable. Data preceded by an asterisk have a relative standard error (RSE) of 20%–30%. Data not shown have an RSE greater than 30%.

[1]Persons of Mexican origin may be of any race. Starting with 1999 data, race-specific estimates are tabulated according to the 1997 Revisions to the Standards for the Classification of Federal Data on Race and Ethnicity and are not strictly comparable with estimates for earlier years. The two non-Hispanic race categories shown in the table conform to the 1997 Standards. Starting with 1999 data, race-specific estimates are for persons who reported only one racial group. Prior to data year 1999, estimates were tabulated according to the 1977 Standards. Estimates for single-race categories prior to 1999 included persons who reported one race or, if they reported more than one race, identified one race as best representing their race. See Appendix II, Hispanic origin; Race.

[2]Includes persons of all races and Hispanic origins, not just those shown separately, and those with unknown percent of poverty level.

[3]Percent of poverty level is based on family income and family size. Persons with unknown percent of poverty level are excluded (5% in 2005–2008). See Appendix II, Family income; Poverty.

NOTES: Root caries are not included. Persons without at least one primary or one permanent tooth or one root tip were classified as edentulous and were excluded from this analysis. The majority of edentulous persons are 65 years of age and over. Estimates of edentulism among persons 65 years of age and over are 46% in 1971–1974, 33% in 1988–1994, and 23% in 2005–2008. For estimates prior to 2005–2008, only dental caries in primary teeth was evaluated for children 2–5 years of age. Caries in both permanent and primary teeth was evaluated for children 6–11 years of age. For children 12–19 years of age and adults, only dental caries in permanent teeth was evaluated. Starting with 2005–2006 data, dental caries data were collected using a simplified examination process that used health technologists to screen for caries instead of using dentists to conduct a comprehensive caries exam. In addition, dental caries data were not collected on children younger than 5 years of age. Because of this change in the examination process and because 2005–2008 dental caries data are based on both primary and permanent teeth, regardless of age, data for 2005–2008 need to be interpreted with caution, especially when comparing with earlier data. For more information on the methodology changes, see Appendix II, Dental caries; http://www.cdc.gov/nchs/data/nhanes/nhanes_05_06/ohx_d.pdf and Dye BA, Barker LK, Li X, Lewis BG, Beltran-Aguilar ED. Overview and quality assurance for the Oral Health Component of the National Health and Nutrition Examination Survey (NHANES), 2005–08. J Public Health Dent, in press. Standard errors are available in the spreadsheet version of this table. Available from: http://www.cdc.gov/nchs/hus.htm. Data for additional years are available. See Appendix III.

SOURCE: CDC/NCHS, National Health and Nutrition Examination Survey.

Table 74 (page 1 of 2). No usual source of health care among children under 18 years of age, by selected characteristics: United States, average annual, selected years 1993–1994 through 2008–2009

[Data are based on household interviews of a sample of the civilian noninstitutionalized population]

Characteristic	Under 18 years			Under 6 years			6–17 years		
	1993–1994[1]	1999–2000	2008–2009	1993–1994[1]	1999–2000	2008–2009	1993–1994[1]	1999–2000	2008–2009
	Percent of children without a usual source of health care[2]								
All children[3]	7.7	6.9	5.6	5.2	4.6	4.3	9.0	8.0	6.2
Sex									
Male	8.1	6.7	5.8	5.3	4.5	4.9	9.6	7.8	6.2
Female	7.3	7.1	5.4	5.0	4.7	3.8	8.5	8.2	6.2
Race[4]									
White only	7.0	6.3	5.5	4.7	4.4	4.2	8.3	7.2	6.1
Black or African American only	10.3	7.7	5.9	7.6	4.4	4.2	11.9	9.1	6.8
American Indian or Alaska Native only	*9.3	*9.4	*	*	*	*	*8.7	*9.4	*
Asian only	9.7	10.0	5.1	*3.4	*5.8	*2.8	13.5	12.2	6.3
Native Hawaiian or Other Pacific Islander only	- - -	*	*	- - -	*	*	- - -	*	*
2 or more races	- - -	*4.9	*4.5	- - -	*	*	- - -	*7.2	*5.5
Hispanic origin and race[4]									
Hispanic or Latino	14.3	14.2	9.4	9.3	9.0	6.6	17.7	17.2	11.1
Not Hispanic or Latino	6.7	5.5	4.5	4.4	3.6	3.6	7.8	6.3	5.0
White only	5.7	4.7	4.1	3.7	3.3	3.3	6.7	5.4	4.5
Black or African American only	10.2	7.6	5.7	7.7	4.5	4.2	11.6	9.0	6.5
Percent of poverty level[5]									
Below 100%	13.9	13.1	8.6	9.4	7.6	7.5	16.8	16.2	9.4
100%–199%	9.8	10.6	8.3	6.7	7.5	5.1	11.6	12.2	10.1
200%–399%	3.7	4.8	4.6	1.9	3.2	3.6	4.5	5.6	5.1
400% or more	3.7	2.6	2.1	*1.6	1.5	*1.6	5.0	3.0	2.3
Hispanic origin and race and percent of poverty level[4,5]									
Hispanic or Latino:									
Below 100%	19.6	19.4	11.8	12.7	11.6	9.5	24.8	24.5	13.5
100%–199%	15.3	17.1	11.5	9.9	11.3	7.3	18.9	20.4	14.0
200%–399%	5.2	8.3	6.0	*	*5.0	*2.8	6.7	10.1	7.7
400% or more	*	*3.8	*2.5	*	*	*	*	*5.0	*
Not Hispanic or Latino:									
White only:									
Below 100%	10.2	10.7	*6.1	6.5	*6.3	*5.7	12.7	13.1	*6.4
100%–199%	8.7	7.8	7.6	6.3	5.7	*4.4	10.1	8.8	9.3
200%–399%	3.3	4.0	3.8	1.6	2.7	*3.3	4.0	4.6	4.1
400% or more	4.0	2.3	1.9	*1.7	*1.5	*	5.4	2.6	2.0
Black or African American only:									
Below 100%	13.7	9.4	6.2	10.9	*4.7	*5.0	15.5	11.8	6.9
100%–199%	9.1	9.7	5.6	*6.0	*6.4	*	10.8	11.2	7.5
200%–399%	5.0	5.0	6.7	*	*	*6.5	6.2	5.7	6.8
400% or more	*	*3.5	*	*	*	*	*	*4.0	*
Health insurance status at the time of interview[6]									
Insured	5.0	3.9	3.3	3.3	2.6	2.9	5.9	4.5	3.5
Private	3.8	3.4	2.6	1.9	2.2	*1.7	4.6	3.9	2.9
Medicaid	8.9	5.3	4.4	6.4	3.5	3.9	11.3	6.7	4.7
Uninsured	23.5	29.3	29.5	18.0	20.8	22.3	26.0	32.9	32.3
Health insurance status prior to interview[6]									
Insured continuously all 12 months	4.6	3.6	3.0	3.1	2.3	2.9	5.5	4.2	3.1
Uninsured for any period up to 12 months	15.3	15.0	12.9	10.9	12.5	11.1	18.1	16.4	13.9
Uninsured more than 12 months	27.6	35.8	35.2	21.4	26.8	25.8	30.0	39.1	38.3

See footnotes at end of table.

Table 74 (page 2 of 2). No usual source of health care among children under 18 years of age, by selected characteristics: United States, average annual, selected years 1993–1994 through 2008–2009

[Data are based on household interviews of a sample of the civilian noninstitutionalized population]

Characteristic	Under 18 years			Under 6 years			6–17 years		
	1993–1994[1]	1999–2000	2008–2009	1993–1994[1]	1999–2000	2008–2009	1993–1994[1]	1999–2000	2008–2009
Percent of poverty level and health insurance status prior to interview[5,6]	Percent of children without a usual source of health care[2]								
Below 100%:									
Insured continuously all 12 months	8.6	5.7	4.4	5.8	*2.7	4.5	10.7	7.5	4.4
Uninsured for any period up to 12 months . .	21.7	19.8	15.8	18.0	*16.0	*18.8	23.7	21.9	*
Uninsured more than 12 months	31.2	42.7	40.1	25.5	31.0	33.1	33.4	47.1	42.6
100%–199%:									
Insured continuously all 12 months	5.6	5.2	3.8	3.7	3.7	*3.0	6.7	6.0	4.2
Uninsured for any period up to 12 months . .	14.5	15.4	14.5	*9.7	*14.4	*8.6	18.0	15.9	17.2
Uninsured more than 12 months	27.6	34.4	38.0	21.4	26.4	*29.3	30.2	37.4	40.4
200%–399%:									
Insured continuously all 12 months	2.8	3.2	2.9	1.5	2.1	*2.8	3.4	3.7	2.9
Uninsured for any period up to 12 months . .	9.1	11.1	9.7	*	*8.4	*	11.6	12.7	*10.6
Uninsured more than 12 months	18.2	27.1	29.3	*9.7	*20.3	*	21.0	29.4	34.7
400% or more:									
Insured continuously all 12 months	3.1	2.0	1.8	*	*1.2	*	4.3	2.4	1.9
Uninsured for any period up to 12 months . .	*	*10.3	*	*	*	*	*	*	*
Uninsured more than 12 months	*	*30.0	*	*	*	*	*	*33.3	*
Geographic region									
Northeast.	4.1	2.8	2.7	2.9	2.3	*2.7	4.8	3.0	2.6
Midwest.	5.2	5.3	4.8	4.1	3.7	4.2	5.9	6.0	5.1
South	10.9	8.5	6.6	7.3	5.8	4.8	12.7	9.8	7.5
West	8.6	9.7	6.9	5.3	5.7	4.8	10.6	11.7	8.1
Location of residence[7]									
Within MSA	7.7	6.8	5.6	5.0	4.7	4.3	9.2	7.8	6.2
Outside MSA	7.8	7.4	5.7	6.0	4.2	4.3	8.7	8.7	6.4

* Estimates are considered unreliable. Data preceded by an asterisk have a relative standard error (RSE) of 20%–30%. Data not shown have an RSE greater than 30%.

- - - Data not available.

[1]Data prior to 1997 are not strictly comparable with data for later years due to the 1997 questionnaire redesign. See Appendix I, National Health Interview Survey.

[2]Persons who report the emergency department as the place of their usual source of care are defined as having no usual source of care. See Appendix II, Usual source of care.

[3]Includes all other races not shown separately and unknown health insurance status.

[4]The race groups white, black, American Indian or Alaska Native, Asian, Native Hawaiian or Other Pacific Islander, and 2 or more races include persons of Hispanic and non-Hispanic origin. Persons of Hispanic origin may be of any race. Starting with 1999 data, race-specific estimates are tabulated according to the 1997 Revisions to the Standards for the Classification of Federal Data on Race and Ethnicity and are not strictly comparable with estimates for earlier years. The five single-race categories plus multiple-race categories shown in the table conform to the 1997 Standards. Starting with 1999 data, race-specific estimates are for persons who reported only one racial group; the category 2 or more races includes persons who reported more than one racial group. Prior to 1999, data were tabulated according to the 1977 Standards with four racial groups and the Asian only category included Native Hawaiian or Other Pacific Islander. Estimates for single-race categories prior to 1999 included persons who reported one race or, if they reported more than one race, identified one race as best representing their race. Starting with 2003 data, race responses of other race and unspecified multiple race were treated as missing, and then race was imputed if these were the only race responses. Almost all persons with a race response of other race were of Hispanic origin. See Appendix II, Hispanic origin; Race.

[5]Percent of poverty level is based on family income and family size and composition using U.S. Census Bureau poverty thresholds. Missing family income data were imputed starting in 1993. See Appendix II, Family income; Poverty; Table VII.

[6]Health insurance categories are mutually exclusive. Persons who reported both Medicaid and private coverage are classified as having private coverage. Medicaid includes other public assistance through 1996. Starting with 1997 data, state-sponsored health plan coverage is included as Medicaid coverage. Starting with 1999 data, coverage by the Children's Health Insurance Program (CHIP) is included with Medicaid coverage. In addition to private and Medicaid, the insured category also includes military, other government, and Medicare coverage. Persons not covered by private insurance, Medicaid, CHIP, public assistance (through 1996), state-sponsored or other government-sponsored health plans (starting in 1997), Medicare, or military plans are considered to have no health insurance coverage. Persons with only Indian Health Service coverage are considered to have no health insurance coverage. Health insurance status was unknown for 8%–9% of children in 1993–1996 and about 1% in 1997–2009. See Appendix II, Health insurance coverage.

[7]MSA is metropolitan statistical area. Starting with 2005–2006 data, MSA status is determined using 2000 census data and the 2000 standards for defining MSAs. For data prior to 2005, see Appendix II, Metropolitan statistical area (MSA) for the applicable standards.

NOTES: Standard errors are available in the spreadsheet version of this table. Available from: http://www.cdc.gov/nchs/hus.htm. Data for additional years are available. See Appendix III.

SOURCE: CDC/NCHS, National Health Interview Survey, access to care and health insurance supplements (1993–1996). Starting in 1997, data are from the family core and sample child questionnaires.

Table 75 (page 1 of 2). No usual source of health care among adults 18–64 years of age, by selected characteristics: United States, average annual, selected years 1993–1994 through 2008–2009

[Data are based on household interviews of a sample of the civilian noninstitutionalized population]

Characteristic	1993–1994[1]	1995–1996[1]	1997–1998	1999–2000	2001–2002	2006–2007	2008–2009
	Percent of adults without a usual source of health care[2]						
18–64 years[3]	18.9	16.9	17.7	17.8	16.4	18.5	19.5
Age							
18–44 years	21.7	19.6	21.1	21.6	20.6	23.5	25.0
18–24 years	26.6	22.6	27.0	27.2	27.2	28.7	29.6
25–44 years	20.3	18.8	19.3	19.9	18.5	21.8	23.4
45–64 years	12.8	11.3	11.2	10.9	9.2	11.2	11.6
45–54 years	14.1	12.2	12.6	12.0	10.3	13.3	13.6
55–64 years	11.1	9.8	9.0	9.2	7.6	8.3	9.0
Sex							
Male	23.9	21.4	23.6	24.1	21.6	23.9	25.3
Female	14.1	12.6	12.0	11.8	11.4	13.3	13.8
Race[4]							
White only	18.4	16.5	17.0	16.7	15.4	18.3	18.9
Black or African American only	20.0	18.3	19.4	19.2	16.9	19.8	21.5
American Indian or Alaska Native only	19.7	16.5	21.3	19.2	16.3	24.4	24.8
Asian only	24.8	21.5	21.7	22.1	20.1	17.3	19.4
Native Hawaiian or Other Pacific Islander only	- - -	- - -	- - -	*	*	*	*
2 or more races	- - -	- - -	- - -	21.0	20.1	20.4	26.1
American Indian or Alaska Native; White	- - -	- - -	- - -	25.8	18.1	19.3	25.9
Hispanic origin and race[4]							
Hispanic or Latino	30.3	27.4	30.4	32.6	32.5	34.3	32.8
Mexican	32.4	29.8	35.9	36.5	36.5	39.0	36.1
Not Hispanic or Latino	17.7	15.7	16.2	15.8	14.0	15.9	17.1
White only	17.1	15.0	15.4	14.9	13.1	15.2	16.0
Black or African American only	19.7	18.1	19.3	19.2	16.8	18.9	21.4
Percent of poverty level[5]							
Below 100%	29.5	26.1	29.1	29.6	29.3	30.6	32.7
100%–199%	25.4	22.9	25.6	27.1	25.6	28.6	30.3
200%–399%	15.6	13.4	16.6	17.2	16.0	18.5	19.7
400% or more	13.4	13.8	11.6	11.6	9.6	10.4	10.6
Hispanic origin and race and percent of poverty level[4,5]							
Hispanic or Latino:							
Below 100%	40.0	34.3	42.8	44.4	46.3	46.7	44.1
100%–199%	36.9	32.9	35.4	40.6	40.0	42.1	40.7
200%–399%	20.7	19.5	23.6	26.9	27.9	29.5	27.9
400% or more	13.8	16.3	14.4	16.1	13.7	15.9	16.6
Not Hispanic or Latino:							
White only:							
Below 100%	28.2	23.6	25.0	24.2	23.4	25.0	27.8
100%–199%	23.3	20.7	22.4	23.0	20.7	24.5	26.0
200%–399%	14.8	12.5	15.4	15.3	13.6	16.2	17.7
400% or more	13.4	13.7	11.3	11.2	9.1	10.0	9.9
Black or African American only:							
Below 100%	24.7	21.9	23.9	23.7	22.8	26.5	29.4
100%–199%	22.3	22.1	25.3	24.4	20.4	23.4	27.6
200%–399%	16.5	14.5	17.6	18.2	16.2	18.0	19.9
400% or more	11.7	12.6	11.2	12.0	9.6	9.1	11.2
Health insurance status at the time of interview[6]							
Insured	13.3	11.4	11.4	10.9	9.1	9.9	10.4
Private	13.1	11.3	11.5	11.1	9.0	9.8	10.3
Medicaid	16.3	13.0	10.3	9.9	11.1	11.5	12.1
Uninsured	43.1	41.8	46.7	49.2	49.1	52.8	54.1
Health insurance status prior to interview[6]							
Insured continuously all 12 months	12.7	10.8	10.6	10.3	8.3	9.0	9.5
Uninsured for any period up to 12 months	30.9	29.6	30.7	31.2	33.3	33.6	36.7
Uninsured more than 12 months	46.9	44.8	51.4	54.8	54.6	57.9	57.2

See footnotes at end of table.

Table 75 (page 2 of 2). No usual source of health care among adults 18–64 years of age, by selected characteristics: United States, average annual, selected years 1993–1994 through 2008–2009

[Data are based on household interviews of a sample of the civilian noninstitutionalized population]

Characteristic	1993–1994[1]	1995–1996[1]	1997–1998	1999–2000	2001–2002	2006–2007	2008–2009
Percent of poverty level and health insurance status prior to interview[5,6]	Percent of adults without a usual source of health care[2]						
Below 100%:							
Insured continuously all 12 months	16.7	13.3	13.1	11.6	11.5	11.6	13.5
Uninsured for any period up to 12 months . .	33.6	28.5	33.0	31.9	36.5	34.5	38.9
Uninsured more than 12 months	50.1	46.1	54.3	57.1	58.8	62.6	63.4
100%–199%:							
Insured continuously all 12 months	14.7	12.2	13.0	12.3	11.0	10.5	13.0
Uninsured for any period up to 12 months . .	30.9	31.1	31.1	34.6	35.1	36.6	37.1
Uninsured more than 12 months	47.6	43.8	51.1	54.9	54.5	58.4	58.3
200%–399%:							
Insured continuously all 12 months	11.7	9.4	10.6	10.6	8.3	9.5	9.9
Uninsured for any period up to 12 months . .	29.2	28.3	30.1	29.0	32.0	33.4	37.0
Uninsured more than 12 months	44.5	44.7	50.9	53.6	53.4	55.3	54.1
400% or more:							
Insured continuously all 12 months	11.8	11.8	9.5	9.3	7.2	7.8	7.6
Uninsured for any period up to 12 months . .	31.5	32.3	28.6	30.2	30.7	29.1	33.8
Uninsured more than 12 months	36.5	45.5	44.6	51.8	47.0	51.5	48.1
Disability measure[7]							
Any basic actions difficulty or complex activity limitation	- - -	- - -	15.5	14.1	13.2	15.7	17.1
Any basic actions difficulty	- - -	- - -	15.7	14.1	13.1	15.8	17.1
Any complex activity limitation.	- - -	- - -	13.1	11.6	10.4	12.6	13.8
No disability	- - -	- - -	18.2	18.8	17.5	19.5	20.3
Geographic region							
Northeast.	14.7	13.4	13.3	12.8	11.9	13.1	12.9
Midwest.	16.2	14.7	15.1	17.0	14.1	16.2	17.3
South	21.8	18.7	20.7	19.7	18.3	21.4	22.5
West	21.1	19.9	20.2	20.1	19.9	20.5	21.8
Location of residence							
Within MSA[8]	19.3	17.3	17.9	18.1	16.6	18.9	19.5
Outside MSA[8]	17.5	15.4	17.0	16.8	15.4	16.5	19.4

* Estimates are considered unreliable. Data not shown have a relative standard error of greater than 30%.

- - - Data not available.

[1]Data prior to 1997 are not strictly comparable with data for later years due to the 1997 questionnaire redesign. See Appendix I, National Health Interview Survey.

[2]Persons who report the emergency department as the place of their usual source of care are defined as having no usual source of care. See Appendix II, Usual source of care.

[3]Includes all other races not shown separately, unknown health insurance status, and unknown disability status.

[4]The race groups, white, black, American Indian or Alaska Native, Asian, Native Hawaiian or Other Pacific Islander, and 2 or more races, include persons of Hispanic and non-Hispanic origin. Persons of Hispanic origin may be of any race. Starting with 1999 data, race-specific estimates are tabulated according to the 1997 Revisions to the Standards for the Classification of Federal Data on Race and Ethnicity and are not strictly comparable with estimates for earlier years. The five single-race categories plus multiple-race categories shown in the table conform to the 1997 Standards. Starting with 1999 data, race-specific estimates are for persons who reported only one racial group; the category 2 or more races includes persons who reported more than one racial group. Prior to 1999, data were tabulated according to the 1977 Standards with four racial groups and the Asian only category included Native Hawaiian or Other Pacific Islander. Estimates for single-race categories prior to 1999 included persons who reported one race or, if they reported more than one race, identified one race as best representing their race. Starting with 2003 data, race responses of other race and unspecified multiple race were treated as missing, and then race was imputed if these were the only race responses. Almost all persons with a race response of other race were of Hispanic origin. See Appendix II, Hispanic origin; Race.

[5]Percent of poverty level is based on family income and family size and composition using U.S. Census Bureau poverty thresholds. Missing family income data were imputed starting in 1993. See Appendix II, Family income; Poverty; Table VII.

[6]Health insurance categories are mutually exclusive. Persons who reported both Medicaid and private coverage are classified as having private coverage. Medicaid includes other public assistance through 1996. Starting with 1997 data, state-sponsored health plan coverage is included as Medicaid coverage. Starting with 1999 data, coverage by the Children's Health Insurance Program (CHIP) is included with Medicaid coverage. In addition to private and Medicaid, the insured category also includes military, other government, and Medicare coverage. Persons not covered by private insurance, Medicaid, CHIP, public assistance (through 1996), state-sponsored or other government-sponsored health plans (starting in 1997), Medicare, or military plans are considered to have no health insurance coverage. Persons with only Indian Health Service coverage are considered to have no health insurance coverage. In 1993–1996, health insurance status was unknown for 8%–9% of adults in the sample. In 1997–2009, health insurance status was unknown for about 1% of adults. See Appendix II, Health insurance coverage.

[7]Any basic actions difficulty or complex activity limitation is defined as having one or more of the following limitations or difficulties: movement difficulty, emotional difficulty, sensory (seeing or hearing) difficulty, cognitive difficulty, self-care (ADL or IADL) limitation, social limitation, or work limitation. For more information, see Appendix II, Basic actions difficulty; Complex activity limitation. Starting with 2007 data, the hearing question, a component of the basic actions difficulty measure, was revised. Consequently, data prior to 2007 are not comparable with data for 2007 and beyond. For more information on the impact of the revised hearing question, see Appendix II, Hearing trouble.

[8]MSA is metropolitan statistical area. Starting with 2005–2006 data, MSA status is determined using 2000 census data and the 2000 standards for defining MSAs. For data prior to 2005, see Appendix II, Metropolitan statistical area (MSA) for the applicable standards.

NOTES: Standard errors are available in the spreadsheet version of this table. Available from: http://www.cdc.gov/nchs/hus.htm. Data for additional years are available. See Appendix III.

SOURCE: CDC/NCHS, National Health Interview Survey, access to care and health insurance supplements (1993–1996). Starting in 1997, data are from the family core and sample adult questionnaires.

Table 76 (page 1 of 3). Reduced access to medical care, dental care, and prescription drugs during the past 12 months due to cost, by selected characteristics: United States, selected years 1997–2009

[Data are based on household interviews of a sample of the civilian noninstitutionalized population]

Characteristic	Did not get or delayed medical care due to cost[1]			Did not get prescription drugs due to cost[2]			Did not get dental care due to cost[3]		
	1997	2008	2009	1997	2008	2009	1997	2008	2009
	Percent								
Total[4]	8.3	10.4	11.4	4.8	8.0	8.4	8.6	12.6	13.3
Age									
Under 19 years	4.5	5.4	5.4	2.1	3.1	3.2	6.0	6.9	7.0
Under 18 years	4.4	5.4	5.2	2.2	3.1	3.2	6.0	7.0	7.1
Under 6 years	3.3	4.2	4.4	1.6	2.7	2.1	3.9	4.0	4.9
6–17 years	4.9	6.0	5.7	2.4	3.3	3.7	6.8	8.1	7.9
18–64 years	10.7	13.6	15.1	6.3	10.7	11.2	10.6	15.9	16.8
18–44 years	11.0	13.6	15.1	6.9	10.9	11.7	11.7	16.6	18.2
18–24 years	10.2	12.5	13.8	6.7	9.4	9.8	11.6	13.4	16.3
25–34 years	11.4	15.0	16.1	6.9	11.9	12.8	12.3	20.1	19.9
35–44 years	11.0	13.0	15.2	7.1	10.9	11.9	11.2	15.5	17.7
45–64 years	10.1	13.5	15.1	5.1	10.5	10.6	8.4	14.9	14.9
45–54 years	10.6	13.9	16.0	5.6	11.3	11.4	9.4	16.6	16.4
55–64 years	9.3	13.1	14.0	4.2	9.5	9.6	7.0	12.8	13.0
65 years and over	4.6	4.5	5.1	2.8	3.9	4.2	3.5	5.6	6.2
65–74 years	5.0	5.1	6.0	3.4	4.8	5.0	4.2	7.4	8.0
75 years and over	4.1	3.8	4.0	2.0	2.8	3.1	2.6	3.6	4.1
18–64 years									
Sex									
Male	9.3	12.2	14.1	5.1	8.8	9.4	8.8	13.9	14.6
Female	12.0	14.9	16.1	7.4	12.6	13.0	12.4	17.9	18.9
Race[5]									
White only	10.8	13.8	15.2	5.9	10.3	10.9	10.6	15.8	16.7
Black or African American only	10.8	14.6	16.7	9.5	15.0	14.5	10.8	18.6	19.0
American Indian or Alaska Native only	14.5	17.1	17.3	*10.1	*16.5	*14.3	18.8	25.5	22.5
Asian only	6.3	6.2	7.5	*2.8	4.9	4.7	7.8	8.0	9.3
Native Hawaiian or Other Pacific Islander only	*	*	*	*	*	*	*	*	*
2 or more races	- - -	18.1	25.0	- - -	*12.0	19.2	- - -	23.5	28.5
Hispanic origin and race[5]									
Hispanic or Latino	10.5	13.9	16.4	6.7	13.4	14.3	11.5	20.8	22.2
Mexican	9.7	14.2	15.9	6.5	13.0	14.0	11.3	21.4	22.2
Not Hispanic or Latino	10.7	13.5	14.9	6.3	10.3	10.7	10.5	15.1	15.8
White only	10.9	13.8	14.9	5.9	9.8	10.2	10.5	14.9	15.5
Black or African American only	10.8	14.7	16.7	9.5	14.8	14.7	10.8	18.2	19.0
Education[6]									
No high school diploma or GED	16.2	19.9	21.2	11.5	18.2	19.3	14.5	23.7	26.6
High school diploma or GED	11.1	14.7	17.0	7.0	13.2	14.0	11.4	19.3	19.7
Some college or more	9.2	12.3	13.7	4.3	8.5	8.8	8.8	13.7	13.7
Percent of poverty level[7]									
Below 100%	19.6	21.9	24.8	14.8	19.6	20.5	19.4	27.2	30.0
100%–199%	17.9	22.5	24.0	11.6	20.4	18.8	18.3	27.9	27.8
200%–399%	10.5	15.0	16.8	5.5	10.7	12.2	10.2	16.9	17.9
400% or more	4.6	6.7	7.2	1.7	4.3	4.1	4.5	7.1	6.8
Hispanic origin and race and percent of poverty level[5,7]									
Hispanic or Latino:									
Below 100%	14.6	17.0	23.2	10.6	19.1	21.0	16.1	25.5	28.8
100%–199%	12.2	17.0	18.1	8.1	17.0	15.1	13.5	27.8	26.3
200%–399%	8.0	13.1	14.7	4.4	11.0	14.6	9.2	18.3	22.1
400% or more	5.1	7.4	8.3	*	*6.9	*4.0	4.5	11.2	7.4
Not Hispanic or Latino:									
White only:									
Below 100%	24.3	26.3	27.2	17.3	20.9	20.9	23.4	28.9	32.0
100%–199%	20.9	26.8	27.8	12.4	22.4	21.0	20.6	29.7	30.2
200%–399%	11.4	16.3	18.1	5.4	10.3	11.9	10.6	17.2	17.8
400% or more	4.6	6.9	7.1	1.7	4.0	3.8	4.5	6.9	6.6
Black or African American only:									
Below 100%	16.1	21.0	23.2	14.9	20.5	20.9	14.8	29.2	28.5
100%–199%	14.3	20.8	22.5	13.9	21.4	19.4	16.4	25.8	25.2
200%–399%	8.8	12.7	14.1	7.0	13.9	12.7	8.6	14.7	15.5
400% or more	4.6	7.1	9.0	*2.9	*6.0	6.9	4.3	7.5	8.6

See footnotes at end of table.

Table 76 (page 2 of 3). Reduced access to medical care, dental care, and prescription drugs during the past 12 months due to cost, by selected characteristics: United States, selected years 1997–2009

[Data are based on household interviews of a sample of the civilian noninstitutionalized population]

Characteristic	Did not get or delayed medical care due to cost[1]			Did not get prescription drugs due to cost[2]			Did not get dental care due to cost[3]		
	1997	2008	2009	1997	2008	2009	1997	2008	2009
Health insurance status at the time of interview[8]				Percent					
Insured	6.8	8.8	9.5	3.7	6.8	7.0	7.2	11.0	10.8
Private	6.0	7.8	8.6	2.9	5.5	5.7	6.2	8.9	8.6
Medicaid	11.9	14.1	13.6	11.1	14.3	13.5	14.8	22.6	22.1
Uninsured	27.6	33.1	36.5	18.0	27.0	26.7	26.1	36.3	39.0
Health insurance status prior to interview[8]									
Insured continuously all 12 months	5.5	7.3	7.9	2.8	5.6	6.0	6.0	9.5	9.5
Uninsured for any period up to 12 months	28.7	34.9	37.1	17.7	27.1	24.9	25.2	33.4	34.0
Uninsured more than 12 months	30.6	34.6	37.7	18.9	27.4	27.9	28.0	37.9	41.2
Percent of poverty level and health insurance status prior to interview[7,8]									
Below 100%:									
Insured continuously all 12 months	9.4	10.7	11.4	8.1	9.9	11.9	10.7	17.5	20.2
Uninsured for any period up to 12 months	31.9	37.7	37.9	25.5	36.6	30.1	31.6	43.9	38.4
Uninsured more than 12 months	32.4	36.3	41.1	21.6	31.8	31.7	29.4	39.5	43.7
100%–199%:									
Insured continuously all 12 months	9.5	12.3	12.6	6.0	11.3	9.6	11.0	18.4	15.8
Uninsured for any period up to 12 months	33.6	39.9	38.5	20.5	33.6	27.4	28.2	36.9	40.0
Uninsured more than 12 months	30.0	34.2	38.7	19.5	30.5	32.5	29.3	40.5	44.8
200%–399%:									
Insured continuously all 12 months	6.1	9.1	10.0	2.9	6.8	8.1	6.8	11.0	11.3
Uninsured for any period up to 12 months	27.1	34.5	39.6	14.0	21.1	22.9	21.6	31.1	30.9
Uninsured more than 12 months	31.3	33.7	34.1	17.3	23.4	23.5	26.5	36.6	39.2
400% or more:									
Insured continuously all 12 months	3.1	4.5	4.9	0.8	2.7	2.6	3.1	5.1	4.6
Uninsured for any period up to 12 months	20.8	27.4	30.2	10.7	20.2	19.9	19.3	23.8	26.7
Uninsured more than 12 months	25.5	34.6	35.0	13.5	19.3	15.8	23.6	30.8	29.4
Disability measure[9]									
Any basic actions difficulty or complex activity limitation	23.3	28.8	30.2	14.8	21.4	21.8	19.8	27.3	27.8
Any basic actions difficulty	24.2	29.7	31.1	15.3	21.7	22.0	20.1	27.6	27.9
Any complex activity limitation	25.7	31.0	31.8	19.4	25.8	26.5	23.2	30.8	31.9
No disability	9.0	11.7	13.8	3.4	6.9	7.5	7.5	11.8	12.9
Geographic region									
Northeast	8.8	9.7	10.7	4.9	7.9	8.7	8.9	11.9	12.4
Midwest	10.5	13.8	16.4	5.9	10.5	11.4	9.7	14.9	15.5
South	11.8	15.4	16.2	7.3	13.0	13.0	10.9	17.9	18.6
West	10.8	13.4	15.6	6.3	9.6	10.2	13.1	17.0	18.8
Location of residence									
Within MSA[10]	10.2	13.1	14.8	5.9	10.3	10.8	10.0	15.6	16.4
Outside MSA[10]	12.5	16.4	17.1	7.9	13.1	13.6	12.9	17.8	19.2

See footnotes at end of table.

[Data are based on household interviews of a sample of the civilian noninstitutionalized population]

---

* Estimates are considered unreliable. Data preceded by an asterisk have a relative standard error (RSE) of 20%–30%. Data not shown have an RSE of greater than 30%.

- - - Data not available.

[1]Based on persons responding yes to the question, "During the past 12 months was there any time when person needed medical care but did not get it because person couldn't afford it?" or "During the past 12 months has medical care been delayed because of worry about the cost?"

[2]Based on persons responding yes to the question, "During the past 12 months was there any time when you needed prescription medicine but didn't get it because you couldn't afford it?"

[3]Based on person responding yes to the question, "During the past 12 months was there any time when you needed dental care (including checkups) but didn't get it because you couldn't afford it?"

[4]Includes all other races not shown separately, unknown health insurance status, unknown education level, and unknown disability status.

[5]The race groups, white, black, American Indian or Alaska Native, Asian, Native Hawaiian or Other Pacific Islander, and 2 or more races, include persons of Hispanic and non-Hispanic origin. Persons of Hispanic origin may be of any race. Starting with 1999 data, race-specific estimates are tabulated according to the 1997 Revisions to the Standards for the Classification of Federal Data on Race and Ethnicity and are not strictly comparable with estimates for earlier years. The five single-race categories plus multiple-race categories shown in the table conform to the 1997 Standards. Starting with 1999 data, race-specific estimates are for persons who reported only one racial group; the category 2 or more races includes persons who reported more than one racial group. Prior to 1999, data were tabulated according to the 1977 Standards with four racial groups and the Asian only category included Native Hawaiian or Other Pacific Islander. Estimates for single-race categories prior to 1999 included persons who reported one race or, if they reported more than one race, identified one race as best representing their race. Starting with 2003 data, race responses of other race and unspecified multiple race were treated as missing, and then race was imputed if these were the only race responses. Almost all persons with a race response of other race were of Hispanic origin. See Appendix II, Hispanic origin; Race.

[6]Estimates are for persons 25–64 years of age. GED is General Educational Development high school equivalency diploma. See Appendix II, Education.

[7]Percent of poverty level is based on family income and family size and composition using U.S. Census Bureau poverty thresholds. Missing family income data were imputed for 1997 and beyond. See Appendix II, Family income; Poverty; Table VII.

[8]For information on the health insurance categories see Appendix II, Health Insurance Coverage.

[9]Any basic actions difficulty or complex activity limitation is defined as having one or more of the following limitations or difficulties: movement difficulty, emotional difficulty, sensory (seeing or hearing) difficulty, cognitive difficulty, self-care (ADL or IADL) limitation, social limitation, or work limitation. For more information, see Appendix II, Basic actions difficulty; Complex activity limitation. Starting with 2007 data, the hearing question, a component of the basic actions difficulty measure, was revised. Consequently, data prior to 2007 are not comparable with data for 2007 and beyond. For more information on the impact of the revised hearing question, see Appendix II, Hearing trouble.

[10]MSA is metropolitan statistical area. Starting with 2006 data, MSA status is determined using 2000 census data and the 2000 standards for defining MSAs. For data prior to 2006, see Appendix II, Metropolitan statistical area (MSA) for the applicable standards.

NOTES: Standard errors and additional data years are available in the spreadsheet version of this table. Available from: http://www.cdc.gov/nchs/hus.htm. Data for additional years are available. See Appendix III.

SOURCE: CDC/NCHS, National Health Interview Survey, family core, sample child, and sample adult questionnaires.

Table 77. Reduced access to medical care during the past 12 months due to cost, by state: 25 largest states and United States, average annual, selected years 1997–1998 through 2008–2009

[Data are based on household interviews of a sample of the civilian noninstitutionalized population]

State	Did not get or delayed medical care due to cost[1]			Did not get prescription drugs due to cost[2]			Did not get dental care due to cost[3]		
	1997–1998	2001–2002	2008–2009	1997–1998	2001–2002	2008–2009	1997–1998	2001–2002	2008–2009
	Percent								
Total, United States	7.9	7.6	10.9	4.5	5.8	8.2	8.1	8.6	12.9
Alabama.	7.6	8.1	10.8	6.8	9.0	9.9	8.7	10.5	12.7
Arizona.	8.0	7.1	13.8	4.1	5.4	9.3	9.4	9.1	18.1
California	6.8	6.4	9.4	3.9	5.0	6.8	8.3	8.0	12.8
Colorado.	6.4	8.1	14.6	3.1	4.8	7.3	8.9	11.4	14.1
Florida	9.8	9.3	13.7	4.8	6.4	10.5	7.2	8.3	17.3
Georgia	8.0	7.6	11.6	4.2	3.8	8.8	5.8	5.0	12.6
Illinois.	6.1	6.4	9.1	3.0	4.4	6.7	5.7	7.0	10.2
Indiana.	9.0	8.5	14.3	5.1	7.2	10.3	7.2	7.3	13.7
Kentucky	11.5	10.2	13.0	6.3	9.6	11.4	7.9	10.8	16.1
Maryland	8.0	7.5	8.6	5.8	6.6	7.0	9.8	8.3	8.9
Massachusetts	5.1	5.4	6.2	1.7	4.8	4.7	5.0	6.2	6.8
Michigan.	7.2	7.0	13.2	3.8	5.8	9.7	7.5	7.8	14.4
Minnesota.	8.1	6.6	11.1	3.6	3.7	6.4	8.7	8.0	12.0
Missouri	7.1	6.1	12.9	4.3	5.4	10.4	7.3	7.5	14.2
New Jersey.	7.2	5.4	7.8	3.8	4.5	6.6	7.3	6.8	10.2
New York	6.4	6.1	6.7	2.8	4.0	5.5	5.6	7.1	7.4
North Carolina.	7.8	7.8	11.3	4.0	6.0	8.2	8.2	7.4	9.6
Ohio.	9.2	8.2	11.0	5.0	6.3	6.7	8.8	10.2	11.4
Pennsylvania.	5.9	6.1	9.6	4.3	3.8	7.9	7.4	6.6	12.0
South Carolina	7.6	7.8	10.8	5.2	6.5	9.0	*5.7	7.9	*11.8
Tennessee	10.0	8.0	11.5	8.0	6.1	11.0	10.5	7.9	*14.3
Texas.	7.9	8.9	14.5	4.7	8.5	12.0	8.8	11.3	18.6
Virginia.	6.2	6.7	10.2	4.1	4.8	6.7	8.3	6.3	9.8
Washington.	8.6	9.0	12.1	4.8	6.2	8.0	11.6	11.7	17.0
Wisconsin.	6.5	5.8	10.6	*3.0	3.9	6.2	5.5	7.5	10.9

* Estimates are considered unreliable. Data preceded by an asterisk have a relative standard error (RSE) of 20%–30%.
[1]Based on persons responding yes to the question, "During the past 12 months was there any time when person needed medical care but did not get it because person couldn't afford it?" or "During the past 12 months has medical care been delayed because of worry about the cost?"
[2]Based on persons responding yes to the question, "During the past 12 months was there any time when you needed prescription medicine but didn't get it because you couldn't afford it?"
[3]Based on person responding yes to the question, "During the past 12 months was there any time when you needed dental care (including check ups) but didn't get it because you couldn't afford it?"

NOTES: Data are for the 25 states with the largest populations in 2008–2009. Standard errors are available in the spreadsheet version of this table. Available from: http://www.cdc.gov/nchs/hus.htm. See related Table 76. Data for additional years are available. See Appendix III.

SOURCE: CDC/NCHS, National Health Interview Survey, family core, sample child, and sample adult questionnaires.

Table 78 (page 1 of 2). No health care visits to an office or clinic within the past 12 months among children under 18 years of age, by selected characteristics: United States, average annual, selected years 1997–1998 through 2008–2009

[Data are based on household interviews of a sample of the civilian noninstitutionalized population]

Characteristic	Under 18 years			Under 6 years			6–17 years		
	1997–1998	2001–2002	2008–2009	1997–1998	2001–2002	2008–2009	1997–1998	2001–2002	2008–2009
	Percent of children without a health care visit [1]								
All children [2]	12.8	12.1	10.5	5.7	6.3	5.3	16.3	14.9	13.2
Sex									
Male	12.9	12.3	10.7	4.9	6.4	5.5	16.8	15.1	13.5
Female	12.7	11.9	10.3	6.5	6.1	5.1	15.8	14.6	12.9
Race [3]									
White only	12.2	11.5	10.3	5.5	6.4	5.2	15.5	13.9	12.9
Black or African American only	14.3	13.3	11.1	6.5	5.9	6.3	18.1	18.1	13.6
American Indian or Alaska Native only	13.8	*18.6	*11.5	*	*	*	*17.6	*23.0	*12.4
Asian only	16.3	15.6	13.1	*5.6	*6.8	*4.0	22.1	20.5	17.7
Native Hawaiian or Other Pacific Islander only	- - -	*	*	- - -	*	*	- - -	*	*
2 or more races	- - -	8.3	8.6	- - -	*3.3	*4.2	- - -	12.4	11.6
Hispanic origin and race [3]									
Hispanic or Latino	19.3	18.8	14.9	9.7	9.6	7.7	25.3	24.0	19.3
Not Hispanic or Latino	11.6	10.6	9.3	4.8	5.4	4.6	14.9	13.0	11.6
White only	10.7	9.7	8.5	4.3	5.3	4.1	13.7	11.7	10.6
Black or African American only	14.5	13.4	11.4	6.5	6.0	6.4	18.3	16.8	13.9
Percent of poverty level [4]									
Below 100%	17.6	17.3	13.7	8.1	9.1	8.3	23.6	21.8	17.3
100%–199%	16.2	14.8	14.4	7.2	7.4	6.3	20.8	18.7	18.7
200%–399%	11.7	11.2	9.8	4.9	5.4	4.5	14.8	13.8	12.3
400% or more	7.4	7.7	5.6	3.0	4.1	*2.5	9.5	9.3	7.0
Hispanic origin and race and percent of poverty level [3,4]									
Hispanic or Latino:									
Below 100%	23.2	22.1	15.4	11.7	10.4	8.6	31.1	29.4	20.3
100%–199%	20.9	21.3	17.7	9.7	12.3	10.0	28.1	26.2	22.2
200%–399%	15.7	15.5	12.4	8.0	*7.3	*4.3	19.7	20.0	16.9
400% or more	7.8	9.7	9.7	*	*	*	9.3	12.5	12.9
Not Hispanic or Latino:									
White only:									
Below 100%	14.0	13.2	13.4	*5.6	*8.6	*	19.7	15.6	16.9
100%–199%	14.1	11.8	12.8	6.0	*6.0	*	18.0	14.8	17.2
200%–399%	10.9	10.2	8.7	4.3	4.8	*4.5	13.9	12.5	10.7
400% or more	7.2	7.4	4.8	*2.8	4.2	*	9.1	8.6	6.0
Black or African American only:									
Below 100%	15.8	16.1	11.8	7.6	*7.8	*8.0	20.5	20.3	14.2
100%–199%	16.4	13.3	13.4	*7.7	*4.4	*	20.4	17.5	17.2
200%–399%	13.3	12.2	10.5	*4.9	*6.5	*	16.7	14.6	12.5
400% or more	8.3	8.9	*7.7	*	*	*	10.7	11.5	*9.2
Health insurance status at the time of interview [5]									
Insured	10.4	9.8	8.2	4.5	4.7	4.1	13.4	12.3	10.4
Private	10.4	9.5	7.7	4.3	4.3	3.7	13.1	11.8	9.5
Medicaid	10.1	10.3	9.1	5.0	5.5	4.7	14.4	13.3	12.1
Uninsured	28.8	31.9	34.4	14.6	21.0	20.8	34.9	36.3	39.8
Health insurance status prior to interview [5]									
Insured continuously all 12 months	10.3	9.5	7.8	4.4	4.6	4.1	13.2	12.0	9.8
Uninsured for any period up to 12 months	15.9	17.7	17.2	7.7	10.3	7.4	20.9	21.9	22.1
Uninsured more than 12 months	34.9	41.4	42.9	19.9	30.2	29.7	40.2	45.3	47.1

See footnotes at end of table.

Table 78 (page 2 of 2). No health care visits to an office or clinic within the past 12 months among children under 18 years of age, by selected characteristics: United States, average annual, selected years 1997–1998 through 2008–2009

[Data are based on household interviews of a sample of the civilian noninstitutionalized population]

Characteristic	Under 18 years			Under 6 years			6–17 years		
	1997–1998	2001–2002	2008–2009	1997–1998	2001–2002	2008–2009	1997–1998	2001–2002	2008–2009
Percent of poverty level and health insurance status prior to interview[4,5]	Percent of children without a health care visit[1]								
Below 100%:									
Insured continuously all 12 months	12.6	11.7	9.3	5.7	6.1	5.9	17.6	14.9	11.7
Uninsured for any period up to 12 months . .	19.9	21.8	17.0	*9.9	*14.4	*7.9	26.1	26.6	22.7
Uninsured more than 12 months	39.9	48.2	52.9	24.9	*28.0	*44.9	45.2	55.7	55.7
100%–199%:									
Insured continuously all 12 months	12.6	10.9	9.8	4.8	4.2	4.3	16.7	14.5	13.0
Uninsured for any period up to 12 months . .	15.6	18.9	20.6	*8.7	*10.7	*8.4	20.2	23.2	26.2
Uninsured more than 12 months	33.7	41.3	43.4	21.3	35.4	*31.0	37.9	43.6	46.8
200%–399%:									
Insured continuously all 12 months	10.5	10.0	8.2	4.5	4.6	4.0	13.2	12.4	10.3
Uninsured for any period up to 12 months . .	12.8	14.5	13.9	*	*7.1	*	17.2	18.7	17.5
Uninsured more than 12 months	29.9	30.8	33.8	*11.8	*24.2	*	36.5	32.9	40.7
400% or more:									
Insured continuously all 12 months	7.0	7.2	5.1	2.9	3.9	*2.4	8.8	8.7	6.3
Uninsured for any period up to 12 months . .	*10.8	*11.4	*14.3	*	*	*	*15.1	*14.1	*18.6
Uninsured more than 12 months	*28.8	*38.4	*27.0	*	*	*	*37.7	*40.3	*33.4
Geographic region									
Northeast	7.0	6.0	5.3	3.1	3.9	*3.2	8.9	6.9	6.3
Midwest	12.2	10.3	9.9	5.9	5.1	*4.9	15.3	12.8	12.5
South	14.3	14.0	11.1	5.6	7.0	5.1	18.5	17.4	14.3
West	16.3	16.0	13.8	7.9	8.1	7.3	20.7	20.0	17.3
Location of residence									
Within MSA[6]	12.3	11.7	10.2	5.4	6.1	4.9	15.9	14.5	12.9
Outside MSA[6]	14.6	13.5	12.0	6.9	6.9	*7.2	17.9	16.3	14.4

* Estimates are considered unreliable. Data preceded by an asterisk have a relative standard error (RSE) of 20%–30%. Data not shown have an RSE of greater than 30%.

- - - Data not available.

[1]Respondents were asked how many times a doctor or other health care professional was seen in the past 12 months at a doctor's office, clinic, or some other place. Excluded are visits to emergency rooms, hospitalizations, home visits, and telephone calls. Starting with 2000 data, dental visits were also excluded. See Appendix II, Health care contact.

[2]Includes all other races not shown separately and unknown health insurance status.

[3]The race groups, white, black, American Indian or Alaska Native, Asian, Native Hawaiian or Other Pacific Islander, and 2 or more races, include persons of Hispanic and non-Hispanic origin. Persons of Hispanic origin may be of any race. Starting with 1999 data, race-specific estimates are tabulated according to the 1997 Revisions to the Standards for the Classification of Federal Data on Race and Ethnicity and are not strictly comparable with estimates for earlier years. The five single-race categories plus multiple-race categories shown in the table conform to the 1997 Standards. Starting with 1999 data, race-specific estimates are for persons who reported only one racial group; the category 2 or more races includes persons who reported more than one racial group. Prior to 1999, data were tabulated according to the 1977 Standards with four racial groups and the Asian only category included Native Hawaiian or Other Pacific Islander. Estimates for single-race categories prior to 1999 included persons who reported one race or, if they reported more than one race, identified one race as best representing their race. Starting with 2003 data, race responses of other race and unspecified multiple race were treated as missing, and then race was imputed if these were the only race responses. Almost all persons with a race response of other race were of Hispanic origin. See Appendix II, Hispanic origin; Race.

[4]Percent of poverty level is based on family income and family size and composition using U.S. Census Bureau poverty thresholds. Missing family income data were imputed starting in 1997. See Appendix II, Family income; Poverty; Table VII.

[5]Health insurance categories are mutually exclusive. Persons who reported both Medicaid and private coverage are classified as having private coverage. Starting with 1997 data, state-sponsored health plan coverage is included as Medicaid coverage. Starting with 1999 data, coverage by the Children's Health Insurance Program (CHIP) is included with Medicaid coverage. In addition to private and Medicaid, the insured category also includes military, other government, and Medicare coverage. Persons not covered by private insurance, Medicaid, CHIP, state-sponsored or other government-sponsored health plans (starting in 1997), Medicare, or military plans are considered to have no health insurance coverage. Persons with only Indian Health Service coverage are considered to have no health insurance coverage. See Appendix II, Health insurance coverage.

[6]MSA is metropolitan statistical area. Starting with 2005–2006 data, MSA status is determined using 2000 census data and the 2000 standards for defining MSAs. For data prior to 2005, see Appendix II, Metropolitan statistical area (MSA) for the applicable standards.

NOTES: In 1997 the National Health Interview Survey questionnaire was redesigned. See Appendix I, National Health Interview Survey. Standard errors for selected years are available in the spreadsheet version of this table. Available from: http://www.cdc.gov/nchs/hus.htm. Data for additional years are available. See Appendix III.

SOURCE: CDC/NCHS, National Health Interview Survey, family core and sample child questionnaires.

Table 79 (page 1 of 3). Health care visits to doctor offices, emergency departments, and home visits within the past 12 months, by selected characteristics: United States, selected years 1997–2009

[Data are based on household interviews of a sample of the civilian noninstitutionalized population]

Characteristic	Number of health care visits[1]											
	None			1–3 visits			4–9 visits			10 or more visits		
	1997	2008	2009	1997	2008	2009	1997	2008	2009	1997	2008	2009
	Percent distribution											
Total, age-adjusted[2,3]	16.5	15.5	15.4	46.2	46.8	46.7	23.6	24.8	24.7	13.7	12.9	13.2
Total, crude[2]	16.5	15.3	15.2	46.5	46.7	46.6	23.5	24.9	24.9	13.5	13.1	13.4
Age												
Under 18 years	11.8	10.1	9.1	54.1	56.6	56.9	25.2	26.1	27.4	8.9	7.3	6.5
Under 6 years	5.0	4.6	4.4	44.9	49.2	50.5	37.0	36.7	37.3	13.0	9.5	7.8
6–17 years	15.3	12.9	11.6	58.7	60.3	60.3	19.3	20.6	22.3	6.8	6.2	5.9
18–44 years	21.7	22.7	22.7	46.7	46.3	45.7	19.0	19.4	19.3	12.6	11.7	12.3
18–24 years	22.0	24.3	24.0	46.8	46.8	47.4	20.0	19.7	19.4	11.2	9.2	9.1
25–44 years	21.6	22.1	22.2	46.7	46.1	45.1	18.7	19.2	19.3	13.0	12.5	13.4
45–64 years	16.9	14.4	15.4	42.9	44.5	43.6	24.7	25.7	24.9	15.5	15.5	16.1
45–54 years	17.9	17.7	18.0	43.9	45.0	44.5	23.4	23.5	23.0	14.8	13.8	14.5
55–64 years	15.3	9.9	12.0	41.3	43.8	42.6	26.7	28.6	27.3	16.7	17.7	18.1
65 years and over	8.9	5.6	4.7	34.7	32.8	34.7	32.5	37.6	36.1	23.8	24.0	24.5
65–74 years	9.8	7.0	5.6	36.9	35.7	37.6	31.6	36.4	34.6	21.6	20.9	22.2
75 years and over	7.7	3.9	3.7	31.8	29.4	31.1	33.8	39.1	38.0	26.6	27.6	27.2
Sex[3]												
Male	21.3	20.3	20.3	47.1	47.5	47.1	20.6	22.2	22.0	11.0	10.0	10.6
Female	11.8	10.8	10.5	45.4	46.2	46.4	26.5	27.3	27.4	16.3	15.8	15.7
Race[3,4]												
White only	16.0	15.4	15.1	46.1	46.2	46.5	23.9	25.1	25.0	14.0	13.3	13.5
Black or African American only	16.8	15.4	14.6	46.1	48.3	46.8	23.2	24.2	24.8	13.9	12.2	13.8
American Indian or Alaska Native only	17.1	15.4	21.7	38.0	42.8	50.1	24.2	29.1	18.4	20.7	12.7	9.9
Asian only	22.8	18.2	20.8	49.1	53.7	50.6	19.7	20.9	20.7	8.3	7.2	8.0
Native Hawaiian or Other Pacific Islander only	- - -	*	*	- - -	*	*	- - -	*	*	- - -	*	*
2 or more races	- - -	11.9	16.2	- - -	44.9	41.4	- - -	25.2	28.9	- - -	18.0	13.4
Hispanic origin and race[3,4]												
Hispanic or Latino	24.9	24.3	23.8	42.3	44.0	44.3	20.3	20.6	21.2	12.5	11.1	10.8
Mexican	28.9	26.6	25.9	40.8	43.4	44.5	18.5	19.1	20.1	11.8	11.0	9.5
Not Hispanic or Latino	15.4	13.7	13.7	46.7	47.3	47.2	24.0	25.6	25.5	13.9	13.4	13.7
White only	14.7	13.1	12.9	46.6	46.7	47.0	24.4	26.2	25.9	14.3	14.0	14.2
Black or African American only	16.9	15.2	14.4	46.1	48.7	46.6	23.1	23.9	25.2	13.8	12.1	13.8
Percent of poverty level[3,5]												
Below 100%	20.6	19.1	19.4	37.8	39.3	39.2	22.7	23.9	23.5	18.9	17.6	17.9
100%–199%	20.1	22.2	19.6	43.3	41.4	43.4	21.7	22.0	23.0	14.9	14.4	14.0
200%–399%	16.4	16.0	16.3	47.2	47.3	47.0	23.6	24.6	24.1	12.8	12.1	12.5
400% or more	12.8	10.3	10.9	49.8	51.4	50.3	24.9	26.5	26.7	12.5	11.8	12.1

See footnotes at end of table.

Table 79 (page 2 of 3).

Table 79 (page 2 of 3). Health care visits to doctor offices, emergency departments, and home visits within the past 12 months, by selected characteristics: United States, selected years 1997–2009

[Data are based on household interviews of a sample of the civilian noninstitutionalized population]

Characteristic	Number of health care visits[1]											
	None			1–3 visits			4–9 visits			10 or more visits		
	1997	2008	2009	1997	2008	2009	1997	2008	2009	1997	2008	2009
Hispanic origin and race and percent of poverty level[3,4,5]	Percent distribution											
Hispanic or Latino:												
Below 100%	30.2	26.8	26.7	34.8	39.8	38.6	19.9	19.2	20.3	15.0	14.3	14.4
100%–199%	28.7	29.7	28.8	39.7	39.1	42.0	20.4	19.8	18.8	11.2	11.5	10.4
200%–399%	20.7	23.8	21.4	47.4	46.4	47.2	19.8	20.4	22.3	12.1	9.4	9.1
400% or more	15.2	14.8	14.7	50.4	52.2	51.8	22.6	22.9	24.1	11.8	10.2	9.5
Not Hispanic or Latino:												
White only:												
Below 100%	17.0	16.2	15.8	38.3	37.4	40.4	23.9	26.2	24.4	20.9	20.3	19.4
100%–199%	17.3	19.2	15.9	44.1	40.5	42.7	22.2	23.2	25.1	16.3	17.0	16.3
200%–399%	15.4	14.5	14.9	46.9	46.1	46.4	24.3	26.1	24.7	13.4	13.2	14.1
400% or more	12.5	9.5	10.1	49.1	50.9	49.7	25.5	27.2	27.4	13.0	12.5	12.8
Black or African American only:												
Below 100%	17.4	16.6	15.0	38.5	43.0	38.1	23.4	22.6	26.3	20.7	17.8	20.7
100%–199%	18.8	18.9	16.7	43.7	46.3	45.4	22.9	22.7	25.2	14.5	12.2	12.7
200%–399%	16.6	14.4	16.1	49.7	52.0	48.5	22.9	23.1	24.2	10.8	10.5	11.3
400% or more	14.0	11.5	10.1	54.3	52.9	53.6	22.7	25.7	25.7	9.0	9.9	10.6
Health insurance status at the time of interview[6,7]												
Under 65 years:												
Insured	14.3	12.3	12.1	49.0	50.1	50.0	23.6	24.9	25.1	13.1	12.7	12.8
Private	14.7	12.5	12.6	50.6	52.3	52.4	23.1	24.6	24.7	11.6	10.5	10.3
Medicaid	9.8	11.3	9.1	35.5	38.0	38.8	26.5	25.7	27.3	28.2	25.0	24.9
Uninsured	33.7	39.0	38.8	42.8	43.4	42.2	15.3	12.7	12.8	8.2	5.0	6.2
Health insurance status prior to interview[6,7]												
Under 65 years:												
Insured continuously all 12 months	14.1	12.1	12.0	49.2	50.2	50.2	23.6	25.1	25.2	13.0	12.6	12.7
Uninsured for any period up to 12 months	18.9	19.0	20.8	46.0	47.9	46.4	20.8	22.0	20.7	14.4	11.1	12.0
Uninsured more than 12 months	39.0	46.2	43.7	41.4	40.7	40.7	13.2	9.5	10.9	6.4	3.6	4.7
Percent of poverty level and health insurance status prior to interview[5,6,7]												
Under 65 years:												
Below 100%:												
Insured continuously all 12 months	13.8	12.3	10.7	39.7	40.8	41.3	25.2	26.2	26.5	21.4	20.7	21.5
Uninsured for any period up to 12 months	19.7	17.2	18.6	37.6	44.5	44.8	21.9	22.9	19.4	20.9	15.5	17.2
Uninsured more than 12 months	41.2	49.0	47.4	39.9	37.9	37.5	12.2	9.9	10.5	6.6	*3.2	4.5
100%–199%:												
Insured continuously all 12 months	16.0	14.9	12.8	46.4	44.7	47.1	21.9	23.5	25.3	15.8	16.9	14.8
Uninsured for any period up to 12 months	18.8	23.5	21.6	45.1	43.4	42.8	21.0	22.5	21.5	15.0	10.7	14.1
Uninsured more than 12 months	38.7	48.1	44.4	41.0	39.4	40.7	14.0	9.6	9.8	6.3	2.9	5.1
200%–399%:												
Insured continuously all 12 months	15.1	13.4	13.6	49.4	49.7	49.6	23.4	25.1	24.3	12.1	11.7	12.5
Uninsured for any period up to 12 months	17.9	17.7	22.1	49.3	52.5	47.8	20.0	20.5	20.6	12.8	9.3	9.5
Uninsured more than 12 months	37.0	41.6	41.2	43.8	44.1	44.2	12.6	9.4	10.2	6.6	4.8	4.4
400% or more:												
Insured continuously all 12 months	12.4	9.9	10.7	52.2	54.1	53.0	23.9	25.3	25.6	11.5	10.7	10.7
Uninsured for any period up to 12 months	17.2	14.8	20.2	50.0	51.7	50.9	24.2	21.9	21.2	*8.5	11.6	*7.7
Uninsured more than 12 months	35.1	42.6	34.8	44.1	43.6	41.2	15.1	*10.0	19.4	*5.7	*	*
Respondent-assessed health status[3]												
Fair or poor	7.8	9.7	9.6	23.3	30.3	22.4	29.0	25.8	30.4	39.9	34.2	37.6
Good to excellent	17.2	16.1	16.0	48.4	48.8	49.0	23.3	24.5	24.6	11.1	10.5	10.5

See footnotes at end of table.

Table 79 (page 3 of 3). Health care visits to doctor offices, emergency departments, and home visits within the past 12 months, by selected characteristics: United States, selected years 1997–2009

[Data are based on household interviews of a sample of the civilian noninstitutionalized population]

Characteristic	Number of health care visits[1]											
	None			1–3 visits			4–9 visits			10 or more visits		
	1997	2008	2009	1997	2008	2009	1997	2008	2009	1997	2008	2009
Disability measure among adults 18 years of age and over[3,8]				Percent distribution								
Any basic actions difficulty or complex activity limitation	11.1	10.8	10.6	32.0	31.7	29.8	27.9	28.7	29.0	29.1	28.8	30.7
Any basic actions difficulty	11.1	10.6	10.7	31.9	32.2	29.3	27.5	28.5	29.5	29.4	28.7	30.6
Any complex activity limitation	7.1	7.7	7.2	23.7	22.0	21.3	27.5	27.0	28.6	41.7	43.2	42.9
No disability	20.9	19.4	19.8	49.6	49.6	49.8	20.8	22.8	21.9	8.7	8.2	8.5
Geographic region[3]												
Northeast	13.2	11.2	11.7	45.9	48.9	47.3	26.0	26.5	25.9	14.9	13.4	15.1
Midwest	15.9	14.8	14.5	47.7	48.2	47.1	22.8	23.7	24.5	13.6	13.3	13.9
South	17.2	15.6	15.6	46.1	45.8	45.4	23.3	26.0	25.8	13.5	12.7	13.2
West	19.1	19.1	18.5	44.8	45.6	48.1	22.8	22.7	22.5	13.3	12.5	11.0
Location of residence[3,9]												
Within MSA	16.2	15.5	15.2	46.4	46.9	47.1	23.7	24.9	24.6	13.7	12.7	13.0
Outside MSA	17.3	15.7	15.9	45.4	46.5	45.0	23.3	24.0	25.3	13.9	13.8	13.8

* Estimates are considered unreliable. Data preceded by an asterisk have a relative standard error (RSE) of 20%–30%. Data not shown have an RSE greater than 30%.

- - - Data not available.

[1]This table presents a summary measure of health care visits to doctor offices, emergency departments, and home visits during a 12-month period. See Appendix II, Emergency department visit; Health care contact; Home visit.

[2]Includes all other races not shown separately, unknown health insurance status, and unknown disability status.

[3]Estimates are age-adjusted to the year 2000 standard population using six age groups: Under 18 years, 18–44 years, 45–54 years, 55–64 years, 65–74 years, and 75 years and over. The disability measure is age-adjusted using the five adult age groups. See Appendix II, Age adjustment.

[4]The race groups white, black, American Indian or Alaska Native, Asian, Native Hawaiian or Other Pacific Islander, and 2 or more races include persons of Hispanic and non-Hispanic origin. Persons of Hispanic origin may be of any race. Starting with 1999 data, race-specific estimates are tabulated according to the 1997 Revisions to the Standards for the Classification of Federal Data on Race and Ethnicity and are not strictly comparable with estimates for earlier years. The five single-race categories plus multiple-race categories shown in the table conform to the 1997 Standards. Starting with 1999 data, race-specific estimates are for persons who reported only one racial group; the category 2 or more races includes persons who reported more than one racial group. Prior to 1999, data were tabulated according to the 1977 Standards with four racial groups and the Asian only category included Native Hawaiian or Other Pacific Islander. Estimates for single-race categories prior to 1999 included persons who reported one race or, if they reported more than one race, identified one race as best representing their race. Starting with 2003 data, race responses of other race and unspecified multiple race were treated as missing, and then race was imputed if these were the only race responses. Almost all persons with a race response of other race were of Hispanic origin. See Appendix II, Hispanic origin; Race.

[5]Percent of poverty level is based on family income and family size and composition using U.S. Census Bureau poverty thresholds. Missing family income data were imputed for 1997 and beyond. See Appendix II, Family income; Poverty; Table VII.

[6]Estimates for persons under 65 years of age are age-adjusted to the year 2000 standard population using four age groups: Under 18 years, 18–44 years, 45–54 years, and 55–64 years. See Appendix II, Age adjustment.

[7]Health insurance categories are mutually exclusive. Persons who reported both Medicaid and private coverage are classified as having private coverage. Starting with 1997 data, state-sponsored health plan coverage is included as Medicaid coverage. Starting with 1999 data, coverage by the Children's Health Insurance Program (CHIP) is included with Medicaid coverage. In addition to private and Medicaid, the insured category also includes military plans, other government-sponsored health plans, and Medicare, not shown separately. Persons not covered by private insurance, Medicaid, CHIP, state-sponsored or other government-sponsored health plans (starting in 1997), Medicare, or military plans are considered to have no health insurance coverage. Persons with only Indian Health Service coverage are considered to have no health insurance coverage. See Appendix II, Health insurance coverage.

[8]Any basic actions difficulty or complex activity limitation is defined as having one or more of the following limitations or difficulties: movement difficulty, emotional difficulty, sensory (seeing or hearing) difficulty, cognitive difficulty, self-care (ADL or IADL) limitation, social limitation, or work limitation. For more information, see Appendix II, Basic actions difficulty; Complex activity limitation. Starting with 2007 data, the hearing question, a component of the basic actions difficulty measure, was revised. Consequently, data prior to 2007 are not comparable with data for 2007 and beyond. For more information on the impact of the revised hearing question, see Appendix II, Hearing trouble.

[9]MSA is metropolitan statistical area. Starting with 2006 data, MSA status is determined using 2000 census data and the 2000 standards for defining MSAs. For data prior to 2006, see Appendix II, Metropolitan statistical area (MSA) for the applicable standards.

NOTES: In 1997, the National Health Interview Survey questionnaire was redesigned. See Appendix I, National Health Interview Survey. Standard errors are available in the spreadsheet version of this table. See http://www.cdc.gov/nchs/hus.htm. Data for additional years are available. See Appendix III.

SOURCE: CDC/NCHS, National Health Interview Survey, family core and sample adult questionnaires.

Table 80. Influenza vaccination among adults 65 years of age and over: Selected Organisation for Economic Co-operation and Development (OECD) countries, 1998–2007

[Data are based on reporting by OECD countries]

Country	1998	1999	2000	2001	2002	2003	2004	2005	2006	2007
	Percent receiving influenza vaccination during past 12 months									
Australia	- - -	69.0	74.0	78.0	76.9	76.9	79.1	- - -	77.5	- - -
Austria	- - -	23.7	- - -	- - -	- - -	- - -	- - -	- - -	36.1	- - -
Belgium	- - -	- - -	- - -	58.0	- - -	- - -	65.0	- - -	- - -	- - -
Canada	- - -	- - -	63.0	67.0	- - -	67.0	- - -	71.0	- - -	- - -
Czech Republic	- - -	- - -	- - -	- - -	16.5	- - -	- - -	- - -	- - -	- - -
Denmark	- - -	- - -	- - -	- - -	29.8	44.9	50.8	55.3	53.7	- - -
Finland	- - -	- - -	- - -	25.0	43.0	45.0	46.0	52.0	46.0	48.4
France	61.0	58.0	65.0	65.0	67.0	65.0	68.0	68.0	68.0	69.0
Germany [1]	- - -	44.6	- - -	55.8	- - -	48.0	- - -	63.0	60.0	56.0
Hungary	- - -	- - -	- - -	- - -	36.8	38.9	37.9	37.1	34.0	34.2
Ireland	- - -	- - -	- - -	- - -	- - -	62.2	61.4	63.0	60.6	61.7
Italy	- - -	40.7	50.7	55.2	60.3	63.4	66.6	68.3	66.6	64.9
Japan	- - -	- - -	- - -	28.0	35.0	43.0	48.0	49.0	48.0	- - -
Luxembourg	- - -	- - -	- - -	42.8	46.0	49.1	51.0	55.4	52.0	54.1
Netherlands	72.0	72.0	76.0	76.0	78.0	77.0	73.0	77.0	75.0	77.0
Portugal	31.3	39.0	- - -	41.9	36.9	46.9	39.0	41.6	50.4	- - -
Republic of Korea	- - -	- - -	- - -	- - -	- - -	- - -	75.7	77.2	- - -	- - -
Slovak Republic	- - -	- - -	20.7	31.5	- - -	37.9	22.9	29.3	25.7	33.4
Spain	63.5	59.8	61.5	61.9	67.2	68.0	68.6	70.1	67.6	62.3
Switzerland	41.0	46.0	51.0	54.0	55.0	58.0	57.0	59.0	61.0	56.0
United Kingdom	- - -	- - -	65.0	68.0	69.0	71.0	71.0	75.0	75.1	73.5
United States	63.3	65.7	64.4	63.1	65.7	65.5	64.6	59.7	64.3	66.7

- - - Data not available.

[1] 1998 data for Germany are for adults 69 years of age and over. Starting with 1999 data, data are for adults 60 years of age and over.

NOTES: Data are for adults 65 years of age and over. Countries estimate influenza vaccination coverage using different methods. Therefore, estimates may not be directly comparable across countries and comparisons among them should be made with caution. See the OECD Health Statistics portal, available from: http://www.ecosante.fr/index2.php?base=OCDE&langs=ENG&langh=ENG&valeur=&source=1, for more information on the sources and methods for collecting influenza immunization data.

SOURCE: Organisation for Economic Co-operation and Development (OECD): OECD Health Data 2009, http://www.oecd.org/els/health/.

Table 81 (page 1 of 3). Vaccination coverage among children 19–35 months of age for selected diseases, by race, Hispanic origin, poverty level, and location of residence in metropolitan statistical area (MSA): United States, selected years 1995–2009

[Data are based on telephone interviews of a sample of the civilian noninstitutionalized population, supplemented by a survey of immunization providers for interview participants]

| | | Race and Hispanic origin[1] | | | | | | | Poverty level | | Location of residence | | |
| | | Not Hispanic or Latino | | | | | | | | | Inside MSA[2] | | |
Vaccination and year	All	White	Black or African American	American Indian or Alaska Native	Asian[3]	Native Hawaiian or Other Pacific Islander[3]	2 or more races	Hispanic or Latino	Below poverty level	At or above poverty level	Central city	Remaining area	Outside MSA[2]
					Percent of children 19–35 months of age								
Combined series (4:3:1:4:3:1:4):[4]													
2009	44	45	40	- - -	39	- - -	41	46	41	46	45	45	42
Combined series (4:3:1:3:3:1:4):[5]													
2007	67	67	62	75	69	*	66	67	65	67	67	68	63
2008	68	68	66	63	74	*	76	69	63	71	70	69	65
2009	64	64	58	- - -	55	- - -	57	67	61	65	- - -	- - -	- - -
Combined series (4:3:1:3:3:1):[6]													
2002	66	66	62	- - -	74	- - -	61	66	62	66	64	68	61
2006	77	78	74	75	76	- - -	75	77	73	78	77	78	75
2007	77	78	75	83	79	*	76	78	75	78	77	78	76
2008	76	75	73	77	82	*	79	78	72	78	77	76	74
2009	70	69	67	73	70	- - -	67	73	68	70	- - -	- - -	- - -
DTP/DT/DTaP (4 doses or more):[7]													
1995	78	80	74	71	84	- - -	- - -	75	71	81	77	79	78
2000	82	84	76	75	85	- - -	- - -	79	76	84	80	83	83
2005	86	87	84	*	89	*	86	84	82	87	85	87	85
2006	85	87	81	83	86	*	84	85	81	87	84	86	85
2007	85	85	82	86	88	*	84	84	81	86	85	85	83
2008	85	85	80	82	92	*	88	85	80	87	85	85	82
2009	84	86	79	82	87	93	82	83	80	86	84	84	84
Polio (3 doses or more):													
1995	88	89	84	86	90	- - -	- - -	87	85	89	87	88	89
2000	90	91	87	90	93	- - -	- - -	88	87	90	88	90	91
2005	92	91	91	*	93	*	94	92	90	92	91	93	92
2006	93	93	90	91	92	96	92	93	92	93	93	93	93
2007	93	93	91	95	95	87	92	93	92	93	92	93	94
2008	94	94	92	91	97	*	94	94	92	94	94	94	93
2009	93	93	91	92	94	97	93	93	92	93	94	92	92
Measles, Mumps, Rubella:													
1995	90	91	87	88	95	- - -	- - -	88	86	91	90	90	89
2000	91	92	88	87	90	- - -	- - -	90	89	91	90	91	91
2005	92	91	92	90	92	90	94	91	89	92	92	92	90
2006	92	93	91	89	95	94	91	92	91	93	93	93	92
2007	92	92	92	96	94	88	95	93	91	93	92	93	92
2008	92	91	92	96	95	97	94	93	92	92	93	92	90
2009	90	91	88	95	91	97	89	89	89	91	91	89	89
Hib (3 doses or more):[8]													
1995	91	93	88	93	90	- - -	- - -	89	88	93	91	92	92
2000	93	95	93	90	92	- - -	- - -	91	90	95	92	94	95
2005	94	94	93	88	89	91	95	94	92	95	93	94	94
2006	93	94	91	94	90	96	91	94	91	94	93	94	92
2007	93	93	91	95	91	*	90	94	91	93	92	94	92
2008	91	91	89	89	93	96	90	92	88	92	91	92	89
Hib (primary series plus booster dose):[8]													
2009	55	55	51	- - -	55	- - -	54	55	51	57	56	55	53
Hepatitis B (3 doses or more):													
1995	68	68	66	52	80	- - -	- - -	70	65	69	69	71	59
2000	90	91	89	91	91	- - -	- - -	88	87	91	89	90	92
2005	93	93	93	90	93	*	94	93	91	94	92	94	93
2006	93	94	92	95	92	97	92	94	93	94	93	94	93
2007	93	93	91	97	94	*	92	94	92	93	92	93	94
2008	94	93	92	92	98	*	95	94	91	94	93	94	93
2009	92	92	92	93	93	96	93	93	92	93	93	92	92

See footnotes at end of table.

Table 81 (page 2 of 3). Vaccination coverage among children 19–35 months of age for selected diseases, by race, Hispanic origin, poverty level, and location of residence in metropolitan statistical area (MSA): United States, selected years 1995–2009

[Data are based on telephone interviews of a sample of the civilian noninstitutionalized population, supplemented by a survey of immunization providers for interview participants]

| | | Race and Hispanic origin[1] | | | | | | | Poverty level | | Location of residence | | |
| | | | Not Hispanic or Latino | | | | | | | | Inside MSA[2] | | |
Vaccination and year	All	White	Black or African American	American Indian or Alaska Native	Asian[3]	Native Hawaiian or Other Pacific Islander[3]	2 or more races	Hispanic or Latino	Below poverty level	At or above poverty level	Central city	Remaining area	Outside MSA[2]
						Percent of children 19–35 months of age							
Varicella:[9]													
1998	43	42	42	28	53	- - -	- - -	47	41	44	45	45	34
2000	68	66	67	62	77	- - -	- - -	70	64	69	69	70	60
2005	88	86	91	82	92	*	90	89	87	88	88	88	86
2006	89	89	89	85	93	90	91	90	88	90	90	90	86
2007	90	89	90	95	94	89	92	91	89	90	90	90	89
2008	91	90	90	94	94	92	91	92	90	91	92	90	88
2009	90	89	88	89	90	98	91	91	89	90	91	89	89
PCV (4 doses or more):[10]													
2005	54	57	46	*	56	*	54	51	45	57	52	58	48
2006	68	71	61	63	65	*	71	67	62	71	69	71	62
2007	75	77	70	80	75	*	74	75	73	76	75	77	71
2008	80	81	76	71	82	*	85	79	74	83	81	81	75
2009	80	83	73	76	73	- - -	73	81	75	83	80	82	82

| | Not Hispanic or Latino | | | | Hispanic or Latino | |
| | White | | Black or African American | | | |
Vaccination and year	Below poverty level	At or above poverty level	Below poverty level	At or above poverty level	Below poverty level	At or above poverty level
			Percent of children 19–35 months of age			
Combined series (4:3:1:4:3:1:4):[4]						
2009	43	46	38	44	44	49
Combined series (4:3:1:3:3:1:4):[5]						
2007	60	68	60	64	69	66
2008	59	70	63	69	64	73
2009	62	65	55	63	66	68
Combined series (4:3:1:3:3:1):[6]						
2005	70	77	74	80	76	75
2006	69	79	72	77	76	78
2007	70	79	74	77	78	79
2008	68	77	70	75	75	81
2009	68	69	64	71	71	74

See footnotes at end of table.

Table 81 (page 3 of 3). Vaccination coverage among children 19–35 months of age for selected diseases, by race, Hispanic origin, poverty level, and location of residence in metropolitan statistical area (MSA): United States, selected years 1995–2009

[Data are based on telephone interviews of a sample of the civilian noninstitutionalized population, supplemented by a survey of immunization providers for interview participants]

- - - Data not available.

* Estimates are considered unreliable. For data prior to 2007, percents not shown if the unweighted sample size for the numerator was less than 30, or the confidence interval half-width divided by the estimate was greater than 50%, or the confidence interval half-width was greater than 10. Starting with 2007 data, percents not shown if the unweighted sample size for the denominator was less than 30, or the confidence interval half-width divided by the estimate was greater than 60%, or the confidence interval half-width was greater than 10.

[1]Persons of Hispanic origin may be of any race. Starting with 2002 data, estimates were tabulated using the 1997 Revisions to the Standards for the Classification of Federal Data on Race and Ethnicity. Estimates for earlier years were tabulated using the 1977 Standards on Race and Ethnicity. See Appendix II, Hispanic origin; Race.

[2]MSA is metropolitan statistical area. See Appendix II, Metropolitan statistical area.

[3]Prior to data year 2002, the category Asian included Native Hawaiian and Other Pacific Islander.

[4]The 4:3:1:4:3:1:4 combined series consists of 4 or more doses of diphtheria and tetanus toxoids and pertussis vaccine (DTP), diphtheria and tetanus toxoids (DT), or diphtheria and tetanus toxoids and acellular pertussis vaccine (DTaP); 3 or more doses of any poliovirus vaccine; 1 or more doses of a measles-containing vaccine (MCV); 3 or more doses or 4 or more doses of *Haemophilus influenzae* type b vaccine (Hib) depending on Hib vaccine product type (primary series plus booster dose); 3 or more doses of hepatitis B vaccine; 1 or more doses of varicella vaccine; and 4 or more doses of pneumococcal conjugate vaccine (PCV). The vaccine shortage that ended in September 2004 might have reduced coverage with the fourth dose of PCV among children in the 2007 National Immunization Survey (NIS) cohort. Also see footnote 8 for additional information on (Hib) vaccination.

[5]The 4:3:1:3:3:1:4 combined series consists of 4 or more doses of diphtheria and tetanus toxoids and pertussis vaccine (DTP), diphtheria and tetanus toxoids (DT), or diphtheria and tetanus toxoids and acellular pertussis vaccine (DTaP); 3 or more doses of any poliovirus vaccine; 1 or more doses of a measles-containing vaccine (MCV); 3 or more doses of *Haemophilus influenzae* type b vaccine (Hib); 3 or more doses of hepatitis B vaccine; 1 or more doses of varicella vaccine; and 4 or more doses of pneumococcal conjugate vaccine (PCV). The vaccine shortage that ended in September 2004 might have reduced coverage with the fourth dose of PCV among children in the 2007 NIS cohort.

[6]The 4:3:1:3:3:1 combined series consists of 4 or more doses of diphtheria and tetanus toxoids and pertussis vaccine (DTP), diphtheria and tetanus toxoids (DT), or diphtheria and tetanus toxoids and acellular pertussis vaccine (DTaP); 3 or more doses of any poliovirus vaccine; 1 or more doses of a measles-containing vaccine (MCV); 3 or more doses of *Haemophilus influenzae* type b vaccine (Hib); 3 or more doses of hepatitis B vaccine; and 1 or more doses of varicella vaccine.

[7]Diphtheria and tetanus toxoids and pertussis vaccine (DTP), diphtheria and tetanus toxoids (DT), and diphtheria and tetanus toxoids and acellular pertussis vaccine (DTaP).

[8]*Haemophilus influenzae* type b vaccine (Hib). Before January 2009, NIS did not distinguish between Hib vaccine product types; therefore, children who received 3 doses of a vaccine product that requires 4 doses were misclassified as fully vaccinated. In addition, there was a Hib vaccine shortage during December 2007–September 2009. For more information, see Changes in measurement of *Haemophilus influenzae* serotype b (Hib) vaccination coverage—National Immunization Survey, United States, 2009. MMWR 59(33); 1069–72. Available from: http://www.cdc.gov/mmwr/preview/mmwrhtml/mm5933a3.htm?s_cid=mm5933a3_e%0d%0a.

[9]Recommended in 1996. Data collection for varicella began in July 1996.

[10]PCV is pneumococcal conjugate vaccine. Recommended in 2000. Data collection for PCV began in July 2001. Data for 4 doses of PCV are not available prior to 2005.

NOTES: Final estimates from the National Immunization Survey include an adjustment for children with missing immunization provider data. Poverty level is based on family income and family size using U.S. Census Bureau poverty thresholds. In 2009, 5% of 17,313 children with provider-reported vaccination history data, 7% of Hispanic, 4% of non-Hispanic white, and 6% of non-Hispanic black children were missing information about poverty level and were omitted from the estimates of vaccination coverage by poverty level. See Appendix II, Poverty. See Appendix I, National Immunization Survey. Additional information on childhood immunizations is available from: http://www.cdc.gov/vaccines/recs/schedules/child-schedule.htm#printable. Data for additional years are available. See Appendix III.

SOURCE: CDC/NCHS and National Center for Immunization and Respiratory Diseases, National Immunization Survey. Available from: http://www.cdc.gov/vaccines/stats-surv/imz-coverage.htm#nis and http://www.cdc.gov/nchs/nis.htm.

Table 82 (page 1 of 2). Vaccination coverage among children 19–35 months of age, by state and selected urban area: United States, selected years 2002–2009

[Data are based on telephone interviews of a sample of the civilian noninstitutionalized population, supplemented by a survey of immunization providers for interview participants]

State and selected urban area	2002	2004	2005	2006	2007	2008	2009
	Percent of children 19–35 months of age with 4:3:1:3:3:1 series [1]						
United States	66	76	76	77	77	76	70
Alabama	73	80	82	79	78	75	73
Jefferson County (Birmingham)	74	81	85	- - -	- - -	- - -	- - -
Alaska	56	66	68	67	70	69	64
Arizona	59	73	75	71	75	76	70
Maricopa County (Phoenix)	62	72	76	68	- - -	- - -	- - -
Arkansas	68	81	64	73	72	76	63
California	67	79	74	79	77	79	75
Alameda County	- - -	- - -	71	- - -	76	- - -	- - -
Fresno County	- - -	- - -	- - -	73	- - -	- - -	- - -
Los Angeles County (Los Angeles)	72	77	78	79	78	76	78
Northern CA	- - -	- - -	- - -	71	- - -	69	- - -
Santa Clara County (Santa Clara)	75	80	- - -	78	- - -	81	- - -
San Bernadino County	- - -	- - -	63	- - -	70	- - -	- - -
San Diego County (San Diego)	71	74	- - -	80	- - -	- - -	- - -
Colorado	56	73	79	76	78	79	65
Denver	- - -	- - -	79	- - -	- - -	- - -	- - -
Connecticut	73	85	82	82	87	70	47
Delaware	70	80	82	80	80	72	65
District of Columbia	68	80	72	79	82	78	75
Florida	66	85	78	79	80	80	75
Dade County (Miami)	60	73	- - -	80	76	78	- - -
Duval County (Jacksonville)	70	69	77	76	- - -	- - -	- - -
Orange County	- - -	- - -	- - -	- - -	- - -	79	- - -
Georgia	77	82	82	81	80	72	69
Fulton/DeKalb Counties (Atlanta)	75	81	72	75	- - -	- - -	- - -
Hawaii	69	80	78	79	88	77	67
Idaho	53	70	68	68	66	60	52
Illinois	58	74	77	74	74	75	73
Chicago	58	71	70	77	71	78	72
Madison/St. Clair County	- - -	- - -	- - -	- - -	- - -	75	- - -
Indiana	59	68	70	76	74	76	66
Lake County	- - -	- - -	- - -	- - -	- - -	- - -	65
Marion County (Indianapolis)	62	74	- - -	77	71	- - -	72
Iowa	58	76	76	79	76	75	66
Kansas	55	66	72	70	76	77	77
Eastern KS	- - -	- - -	- - -	74	- - -	- - -	- - -
Kentucky	64	77	71	80	78	74	66
Louisiana	62	70	74	70	77	82	77
Orleans Parish (New Orleans)	53	68	- - -	- - -	- - -	- - -	- - -
Maine	62	74	76	76	73	74	53
Maryland	71	76	79	78	91	80	80
Baltimore City	69	80	77	72	- - -	75	63
Massachusetts	78	84	91	84	78	82	81
Boston	71	79	- - -	82	- - -	- - -	- - -
Michigan	72	79	81	78	79	75	71
Detroit	60	66	71	65	- - -	- - -	- - -
Minnesota	62	78	78	78	81	75	58
Twin Cities	- - -	- - -	- - -	- - -	- - -	75	- - -
Mississippi	64	80	79	73	77	76	73
Missouri	60	75	73	81	76	73	61
St. Louis County	- - -	- - -	74	- - -	- - -	- - -	- - -
Montana	49	65	65	66	65	59	55
Nebraska	64	73	84	75	83	72	60
Nevada	65	65	63	60	63	68	59
Clark County	- - -	- - -	59	- - -	- - -	- - -	- - -
New Hampshire	66	78	77	76	91	81	79
New Jersey	66	74	72	76	81	69	67
Newark	50	64	67	68	- - -	- - -	- - -
New Mexico	59	79	75	72	76	77	68
New York	67	78	74	77	78	73	69
New York City	71	77	71	72	76	75	72
North Carolina	70	78	82	82	77	71	56

See footnotes at end of table.

Table 82 (page 2 of 2). Vaccination coverage among children 19–35 months of age, by state and selected urban area: United States, selected years 2002–2009

[Data are based on telephone interviews of a sample of the civilian noninstitutionalized population, supplemented by a survey of immunization providers for interview participants]

State and selected urban area	2002	2004	2005	2006	2007	2008	2009
	Percent of children 19–35 months of age with 4:3:1:3:3:1 series [1]						
North Dakota	56	71	79	80	77	70	56
Ohio	64	71	78	75	78	82	74
Cuyahoga County (Cleveland)	65	78	77	77	- - -	- - -	- - -
Franklin County (Columbus)	69	79	81	- - -	- - -	- - -	- - -
Oklahoma	60	71	72	78	79	72	70
Oregon	60	74	65	74	71	71	65
Pennsylvania	68	82	77	79	79	78	69
Allegheny County	- - -	- - -	- - -	74	- - -	- - -	- - -
Philadelphia	68	75	77	80	82	80	74
Rhode Island	81	82	80	81	76	78	51
South Carolina	74	77	76	81	80	78	67
South Dakota	62	73	80	74	77	77	75
Tennessee	67	79	80	77	79	81	74
Davidson County (Nashville)	67	88	81	- - -	- - -	- - -	- - -
Shelby County (Memphis)	61	71	74	73	- - -	- - -	- - -
Texas	65	69	77	75	77	78	74
Bexar County (San Antonio)	72	73	71	75	80	76	71
Dallas County (Dallas)	68	67	73	73	72	74	74
El Paso County (El Paso)	61	64	69	69	77	75	71
Houston	56	62	77	70	73	72	70
Utah	61	68	68	78	74	77	70
Vermont	58	67	63	75	67	65	65
Virginia	65	74	82	77	76	73	70
Washington	52	67	66	71	69	74	70
Eastern WA	- - -	- - -	- - -	72	- - -	- - -	- - -
Eastern/Western WA	- - -	- - -	- - -	- - -	- - -	76	67
King County (Seattle)	56	74	69	71	- - -	- - -	- - -
Western WA	- - -	- - -	- - -	- - -	71	- - -	- - -
West Virginia	66	76	68	68	76	77	65
Wisconsin	68	78	77	81	77	80	59
Milwaukee County (Milwaukee)	60	73	74	78	- - -	- - -	- - -
Wyoming	54	64	67	63	70	65	62

- - - Data not available.

[1]The 4:3:1:3:3:1 combined series consists of 4 or more doses of diphtheria and tetanus toxoids and pertussis vaccine (DTP), diphtheria and tetanus toxoids (DT), or diphtheria and tetanus toxoids and acellular pertussis vaccine (DTaP); 3 or more doses of any poliovirus vaccine; 1 or more doses of a measles-containing vaccine (MCV); 3 or more doses of *Haemophilus influenzae* type b vaccine (Hib) regardless of vaccine brand type; 3 or more doses of hepatitis B vaccine; and 1 or more doses of varicella vaccine. The 4:3:1:3:3:1 combined series is the most complete series for which long-term state trend data are currently available. See Table 81 for additional data on childhood vaccinations.

NOTES: Urban areas were originally selected because they were at risk for undervaccination. Final estimates from the National Immunization Survey include an adjustment for children with missing immunization provider data. Additional information on childhood immunizations is available from: http://www.cdc.gov/vaccines/recs/schedules/child-schedule.htm#printable. Data for additional years are available. See Appendix III.

SOURCE: CDC/NCHS and National Center for Immunization and Respiratory Diseases, National Immunization Survey. Available from: http://www.cdc.gov/vaccines/stats-surv/imz-coverage.htm#nis and http://www.cdc.gov/nchs/nis.htm.

Table 83. Vaccination coverage among adolescents 13–17 years of age for selected diseases, by selected characteristics: United States, 2006–2009

[Data are based on telephone interviews of a sample of the civilian noninstitutionalized population, supplemented by a survey of immunization providers for interview participants]

Vaccination coverage	2006[1]	2007[1]	2008	2009
	Percent of adolescents 13–17 years			
Measles, mumps, rubella (2 doses or more) . .	86.9	88.9	89.3	89.1
Hepatitis B (3 doses or more)	81.3	87.6	87.9	89.9
History of varicella or received varicella vaccine (2 doses or more)[2]	- - -	- - -	73.5	75.7
Td or Tdap (1 dose or more)[3]	60.1	72.3	72.2	76.2
Tdap (1 dose or more)[3]	10.8	30.4	40.8	55.6
Meningococcal conjugate vaccine (MCV4) (1 dose or more)[4]	11.7	32.4	41.8	53.6
Quadrivalent human papillomavirus (HPV4) (1 dose or more)[5]	- - -	25.1	37.2	44.3
Quadrivalent human papillomavirus (HPV4) (3 doses or more)[5]	- - -	- - -	17.9	26.7

Vaccination coverage, 2009	Race and Hispanic origin[6]					Poverty level[7]		Location of residence		
	Not Hispanic or Latino							Inside MSA[8]		
	White	Black or African American	American Indian or Alaska Native	Asian	Hispanic or Latino	Below poverty level	At or above poverty level	Central city	Remaining area	Outside MSA[8]
	Percent of adolescents 13–17 years									
Measles, mumps, rubella (2 doses or more) . .	90.2	86.3	90.4	92.9	87.6	87.8	89.3	88.5	90.2	87.5
Hepatitis B (3 doses or more)	90.2	88.9	89.7	89.5	90.0	88.3	90.3	89.2	91.6	86.9
History of varicella or received varicella vaccine (2 doses or more)[2]	77.0	71.3	71.9	72.6	74.9	74.4	75.9	- - -	- - -	- - -
Td or Tdap (1 dose or more)[3]	76.5	72.5	78.0	84.5	76.7	71.8	77.0	79.7	77.3	64.4
Tdap (1 dose or more)[3]	55.8	52.7	59.3	64.3	55.6	52.8	56.1	60.1	55.0	46.3
Meningococcal conjugate vaccine (MCV4) (1 dose or more)[4]	53.1	53.0	46.9	58.8	55.9	52.5	53.8	58.3	55.9	36.0
Quadrivalent human papillomavirus (HPV4) (1 dose or more)[5]	43.9	44.6	52.3	41.5	45.5	51.9	42.5	49.4	42.5	37.5
Quadrivalent human papillomavirus (HPV4) (3 doses or more)[5]	29.1	23.1	29.6	22.1	23.4	25.5	26.8	- - -	- - -	- - -

- - - Data not available.

[1]For 2006 and 2007, data were only collected in the 4th quarter of the year. Starting with 2008, data were collected for the entire year.

[2]Varicella is chickenpox.

[3]Td or Tdap refers to tetanus toxoid-diphtheria vaccine (Td) or tetanus toxoid, reduced diphtheria toxoid, and acellular pertussis vaccine (Tdap) received since the age of 10 years.

[4]Includes persons receiving MCV4 or meningococcal-unknown type vaccine.

[5]Percents reported among females.

[6]Persons of Hispanic origin may be of any race. Estimates were tabulated using the 1997 Revisions to the Standards for the Classification of Federal Data on Race and Ethnicity. Data for Native Hawaiian and Other Pacific Islander persons and persons of multiple races were not included because of small sample sizes. See Appendix II, Hispanic origin; Race.

[7]Poverty level is based on family income and family size using U.S. Census Bureau poverty thresholds. In 2009, less than 1% (unweighted) of adolescents with provider-reported vaccination data were missing information about poverty level and were not included in the estimates of vaccination coverage by poverty level. See Appendix II, Poverty.

[8]MSA is metropolitan statistical area. See Appendix II, Metropolitan statistical area.

NOTES: Vaccination coverage estimates are based on provider-verified responses from parents who live in households with telephones. Complex statistical methods are used to adjust vaccination estimates to account for adolescents whose parents refuse to participate in the survey, for adolescents who live in households without telephones, or for adolescents whose vaccination histories cannot be verified through their providers. Detailed vaccination data among adolescents, by race and Hispanic origin, percent of poverty level, and MSA were not available prior to 2008. Interpretation of vaccination data needs to take into account when specific vaccines were licensed and recommended for use among adolescents. HPV4 vaccine was licensed by the U.S. Food and Drug Administration in June 2006. For the initial recommendations on HPV4 vaccination, see: CDC. Quadrivalent human papillomavirus vaccine: Recommendations of the Advisory Committee on Immunization Practices. MMWR 2007;56(RR–02):1–24. Available from: http://www.cdc.gov/mmwr/preview/mmwrhtml/rr5602a1.htm?s_cid=rr5602a1_e. MCV4 vaccine was licensed for use by the U.S. Food and Drug Administration in January 2005. For the initial recommendations on MCV4 vaccination, see: CDC. Prevention and control of meningococcal disease: Recommendations of the Advisory Committee on Immunization Practices. MMWR 2005;54(RR–07):1–21. Available from: http://www.cdc.gov/mmwr/preview/mmwrhtml/rr5407a1.htm. Tdap vaccines were licensed by the U.S. Food and Drug Administration in May and June of 2005. For the initial recommendations on Tdap vaccination, see: CDC. Preventing tetanus, diphtheria, and pertussis among adolescents: Use of tetanus toxoid, reduced diphtheria toxoid and acellular pertussis vaccines. Recommendations of the Advisory Committee on Immunization Practices. MMWR 2006;55(RR–03):1–34. Available from: http://www.cdc.gov/mmwr/preview/mmwrhtml/rr5503a1.htm. See Appendix I, National Immunization Survey. Additional information on the recommended schedule for adolescent vaccination is available from: http://www.cdc.gov/vaccines/recs/schedules/child-schedule.htm#printable.

SOURCE: CDC/NCHS and National Center for Immunization and Respiratory Diseases, National Immunization Survey. Available from: http://www.cdc.gov/vaccines/stats-surv/imz-coverage.htm#nisteen.

Table 84 (page 1 of 2). Influenza vaccination among adults 18 years of age and over, by selected characteristics: United States, selected years 1989–2009

[Data are based on household interviews of a sample of the civilian noninstitutionalized population]

Characteristic	1989	1995	2000	2005	2006	2007	2008	2009
	Percent receiving influenza vaccination during past 12 months[1]							
18 years and over, age-adjusted[2,3]	9.6	23.7	28.7	21.6	27.4	29.9	32.1	34.1
18 years and over, crude[3]	9.1	23.0	28.4	21.4	27.6	30.1	32.6	34.7
Age								
18–49 years	3.4	13.1	17.1	10.7	15.6	17.8	20.1	23.0
50 years and over	19.9	41.9	47.9	38.1	45.9	48.5	50.7	51.1
50–64 years.	10.6	27.0	34.6	23.0	33.2	36.2	39.6	40.7
65 years and over	30.4	58.2	64.4	59.7	64.3	66.7	67.2	66.8
65–74 years.	28.0	54.9	61.1	53.7	60.1	61.6	60.9	61.5
75 years and over	34.2	63.0	68.4	66.3	69.2	72.6	74.3	73.2
50 years and over								
Sex								
Male.	19.2	40.2	45.9	34.7	43.2	45.6	47.6	49.2
Female.	20.6	43.4	49.5	40.9	48.3	51.0	53.5	52.8
Race[4]								
White only.	20.9	43.6	49.8	39.7	47.2	49.9	52.1	52.4
Black or African American only	12.5	28.2	33.2	26.9	34.9	38.2	41.1	41.7
American Indian or Alaska Native only.	26.2	*	43.6	*22.9	56.3	45.8	49.3	42.8
Asian only.	*9.2	35.6	43.3	30.6	44.8	45.3	47.1	50.4
Native Hawaiian or Other Pacific Islander only	- - -	- - -	*	*	*	*	*	*
2 or more races.	- - -	- - -	50.7	30.4	40.2	44.8	46.3	47.7
Hispanic origin and race[4]								
Hispanic or Latino	13.2	33.8	34.4	24.7	31.7	35.5	38.0	40.3
Mexican.	13.0	35.4	33.0	26.1	33.5	36.1	36.5	40.4
Not Hispanic or Latino	20.3	42.4	48.8	39.1	47.1	49.6	51.9	52.1
White only.	21.3	44.3	50.6	41.0	48.6	51.3	53.6	53.7
Black or African American only.	12.4	28.5	33.2	26.9	35.1	38.1	41.0	41.7
Percent of poverty level[5]								
Below 100%.	19.6	39.7	44.1	35.8	42.1	44.8	44.4	45.2
100%–199%.	24.0	43.2	50.7	41.2	47.5	47.9	52.0	49.4
200%–399%.	20.5	43.7	51.5	42.1	48.0	50.7	51.8	52.6
400% or more	17.5	39.3	44.3	33.9	44.4	48.0	50.8	52.0
Hispanic origin and race and percent of poverty level[4,5]								
Hispanic or Latino:								
Below 100%	12.7	29.7	35.8	22.3	30.9	41.1	37.0	42.2
100%–199%	20.4	34.7	35.6	27.5	32.0	42.7	41.3	32.4
200%–399%	12.7	34.2	33.7	22.3	33.8	31.3	34.5	41.1
400% or more	*9.8	39.1	32.2	26.6	29.5	28.9	39.9	48.7
Not Hispanic or Latino:								
White only:								
Below 100%.	22.5	44.4	48.6	42.2	47.8	47.4	49.3	49.8
100%–199%.	26.1	46.7	54.8	46.1	51.7	50.8	57.0	54.3
200%–399%.	21.6	45.4	54.6	46.4	50.8	54.3	54.6	55.0
400% or more.	18.1	40.8	46.0	35.1	45.9	50.2	52.3	53.3
Black or African American only:								
Below 100%.	14.6	31.8	35.5	28.9	34.8	38.9	36.7	37.8
100%–199%.	12.0	28.3	37.9	27.4	35.0	35.6	38.4	41.8
200%–399%.	14.1	29.0	31.0	25.7	36.2	41.2	44.1	45.1
400% or more.	*8.8	*20.0	28.7	26.2	34.6	36.2	42.9	41.0

See footnotes at end of table.

Table 84 (page 2 of 2). Influenza vaccination among adults 18 years of age and over, by selected characteristics: United States, selected years 1989–2009

[Data are based on household interviews of a sample of the civilian noninstitutionalized population]

Characteristic	1989	1995	2000	2005	2006	2007	2008	2009
Disability measure[6]	Percent receiving influenza vaccination during past 12 months[1]							
Any basic actions difficulty or complex activity limitation	- - -	- - -	55.2	46.5	53.4	55.8	57.2	56.9
Any basic actions difficulty	- - -	- - -	55.3	46.7	53.7	56.0	57.6	57.1
Any complex activity limitation	- - -	- - -	57.1	50.3	56.0	56.8	58.9	58.8
No disability	- - -	- - -	41.3	29.7	38.4	41.6	44.8	46.0
Geographic region								
Northeast	17.9	39.7	45.9	38.4	44.1	49.0	52.7	52.0
Midwest	20.0	43.2	49.3	39.9	49.4	51.4	53.7	52.9
South	20.2	41.4	46.8	37.3	43.9	47.2	49.4	50.9
West	21.8	43.8	50.1	36.8	47.3	46.9	48.1	48.8
Location of residence[7]								
Within MSA	18.9	41.6	47.1	37.2	44.9	47.1	50.2	51.0
Outside MSA	23.3	42.9	50.2	41.0	49.7	53.7	53.0	51.6

* Estimates are considered unreliable. Data preceded by an asterisk have a relative standard error (RSE) of 20%–30%. Data not shown have an RSE greater than 30%.

- - - Data not available.

[1]Respondents were asked, "During the past 12 months, have you had a flu shot? A flu shot is usually given in the fall and protects against influenza for the flu season." Beginning in September 2003, respondents were asked about influenza vaccination by nasal spray (sometimes called by the brand name FluMist™) during the past 12 months, in addition to the question regarding the flu shot. Starting with 2005 data, receipt of nasal spray or flu shot was included in the calculation of influenza vaccination estimates.

[2]Estimates are age-adjusted to the year 2000 standard population using four age groups: 18–49 years, 50–64 years, 65–74 years, and 75 years and over. See Appendix II, Age adjustment.

[3]Includes all other races not shown separately, unknown disability status, and unknown poverty level in 1989.

[4]The race groups white, black, American Indian or Alaska Native, Asian, Native Hawaiian or Other Pacific Islander, and 2 or more races include persons of Hispanic and non-Hispanic origin. Persons of Hispanic origin may be of any race. Starting with 1999 data, race-specific estimates are tabulated according to the 1997 Revisions to the Standards for Federal Data on Race and Ethnicity and are not strictly comparable with estimates for earlier years. The five single-race categories plus multiple-race categories shown in the table conform to the 1997 Standards. Starting with 1999 data, race-specific estimates are for persons who reported only one racial group; the category 2 or more races includes persons who reported more than one racial group. Prior to 1999, data were tabulated according to the 1977 Standards with four racial groups and the Asian only category included Native Hawaiian or Other Pacific Islander. Estimates for single-race categories prior to 1999 included persons who reported one race or, if they reported more than one race, identified one race as best representing their race. Starting with 2003 data, race responses of other race and unspecified multiple race were treated as missing, and then race was imputed if these were the only race responses. Almost all persons with a race response of other race were of Hispanic origin. See Appendix II, Hispanic origin; Race.

[5]Percent of poverty level is based on family income and family size and composition using U.S. Census Bureau poverty thresholds. Poverty level was unknown for 11% of persons 18 years and over in 1989. Missing family income data were imputed for 1997 and beyond. See Appendix II, Family Income; Poverty; Table VII.

[6]Any basic actions difficulty or complex activity limitation is defined as having one or more of the following limitations or difficulties: movement difficulty, emotional difficulty, sensory (seeing or hearing) difficulty, cognitive difficulty, self-care (ADL or IADL) limitation, social limitation, or work limitation. For more information, see Appendix II, Basic actions difficulty; Complex activity limitation. Starting with 2007 data, the hearing question, a component of the basic actions difficulty measure, was revised. Consequently, data prior to 2007 are not comparable with data for 2007 and beyond. For more information on the impact of the revised hearing question, see Appendix II, Hearing trouble.

[7]MSA is metropolitan statistical area. Starting with 2006 data, MSA status is determined using 2000 census data and the 2000 standards for defining MSAs. For data prior to 2006, see Appendix II, Metropolitan statistical area (MSA) for the applicable standards.

NOTES: In 2000, the Advisory Committee on Immunization Practices (ACIP) of the Centers for Disease Control and Prevention (CDC) recommended universal influenza vaccination for persons 50 years and over. Medicare reimbursement for the costs of the vaccine and its administration began in 1993. Currently, ACIP recommends vaccination of all children age 6 months to 18 years, adults age 50 and over, and persons at high risk. See http://www.cdc.gov/flu/professionals/acip/index.htm for more information. Standard errors for selected years are available in the spreadsheet version of this table. Available from: http://www.cdc.gov/nchs/hus.htm. Data for additional years are available. See Appendix III.

SOURCE: CDC/NCHS, National Health Interview Survey. Data are from the Immunization Supplement (1981), the Health Promotion and Disease Prevention Supplement (1991), and the Year 2000 Supplement (1993–1995). Starting in 1997, data are from the sample adult questionnaire.

Table 85 (page 1 of 2). Pneumococcal vaccination among adults 18 years of age and over, by selected characteristics: United States, selected years 1989–2009

[Data are based on household interviews of a sample of the civilian noninstitutionalized population]

Characteristic	1989	1995	2000	2005	2006	2007	2008	2009
	Percent ever receiving pneumococcal vaccination [1]							
18 years and over, age-adjusted [2,3]	4.6	12.0	15.4	16.7	17.0	16.7	18.3	19.0
18 years and over, crude [3]	4.4	11.7	15.1	16.5	17.0	16.7	18.5	19.3
Age								
18–49 years	2.1	6.5	5.4	5.8	5.7	5.3	6.8	7.5
50–64 years	4.4	10.0	14.7	17.1	18.2	17.3	18.5	19.2
65 years and over	14.1	34.0	53.1	56.2	57.1	57.7	60.0	60.6
65–74 years.	13.1	31.4	48.2	49.4	52.0	51.8	52.5	54.6
75 years and over	15.7	37.8	59.1	63.9	63.0	64.4	68.7	68.0
High-risk group [4]								
Total, 18–64 years.	- - -	- - -	18.3	22.6	23.1	24.4	24.9	17.4
18–49 years.	- - -	- - -	12.2	15.0	13.5	16.0	16.0	11.2
50–64 years.	- - -	- - -	26.0	30.6	32.5	32.2	33.9	28.2
65 years and over								
Sex								
Male.	13.9	34.6	52.1	53.4	54.3	55.1	56.4	59.2
Female.	14.3	33.6	53.9	58.4	59.2	59.6	62.8	61.7
Race [5]								
White only.	14.8	35.3	55.6	58.4	60.0	60.1	62.5	63.1
Black or African American only	6.4	21.9	30.6	40.2	35.5	43.7	44.1	44.2
American Indian or Alaska Native only.	31.2	*	70.1	*	*57.5	*	66.9	*
Asian only.	*	*23.4	40.9	35.0	35.6	33.4	45.7	44.8
Native Hawaiian or Other Pacific Islander only	- - -	- - -	*	*	*	*	*	*
2 or more races.	- - -	- - -	55.6	64.8	63.6	55.8	*35.9	67.9
Hispanic origin and race [5]								
Hispanic or Latino	9.8	23.2	30.4	27.5	33.3	31.8	36.4	40.1
Mexican.	12.9	*18.8	32.0	31.3	29.3	34.3	39.5	42.8
Not Hispanic or Latino	14.3	34.5	54.4	58.1	58.7	59.6	61.8	62.2
White only	15.0	35.9	56.8	60.6	62.0	62.2	64.5	64.8
Black or African American only.	6.2	21.8	30.6	40.4	35.6	44.0	44.5	44.7
Percent of poverty level [6]								
Below 100%	11.2	28.7	40.6	46.7	45.4	48.7	46.5	48.5
100%–199%	15.1	30.7	51.4	54.5	55.8	55.6	59.5	60.6
200%–399%	15.1	36.1	55.8	60.8	59.9	59.8	61.4	62.9
400% or more	15.5	39.5	56.9	55.3	59.3	59.8	62.8	61.5
Hispanic origin and race and percent of poverty level [5,6]								
Hispanic or Latino:								
Below 100%	*	*14.1	23.8	20.9	24.5	*22.4	*25.7	32.6
100%–199%	*11.0	*15.6	32.3	26.9	30.9	37.9	32.9	41.8
200%–399%	*11.1	*34.4	37.6	35.2	42.3	29.6	44.8	40.0
400% or more	*	*55.1	*26.4	*25.2	*38.2	*33.7	42.4	49.1
Not Hispanic or Latino:								
White only:								
Below 100%.	13.3	32.5	47.9	55.6	56.0	59.7	60.4	61.0
100%–199%	16.0	33.5	56.1	60.5	61.6	60.8	66.3	66.3
200%–399%	15.7	37.1	57.6	64.1	62.6	63.4	64.5	66.3
400% or more.	15.9	39.3	59.5	57.4	63.0	62.4	64.1	62.9
Black or African American only:								
Below 100%.	*5.0	*22.6	28.8	42.3	38.4	40.7	37.6	33.8
100%–199%	7.8	*20.9	28.1	36.6	36.2	41.9	43.5	46.9
200%–399%	*5.9	*21.7	35.5	41.6	40.0	48.7	44.5	49.3
400% or more.	*	*	*32.6	44.6	*24.7	43.6	56.5	45.8

See footnotes at end of table.

Table 85 (page 2 of 2). Pneumococcal vaccination among adults 18 years of age and over, by selected characteristics: United States, selected years 1989–2009

[Data are based on household interviews of a sample of the civilian noninstitutionalized population]

Characteristic	1989	1995	2000	2005	2006	2007	2008	2009
Any basic actions difficulty or complex activity limitation[7]			Percent ever receiving pneumococcal vaccination[1]					
Any basic actions difficulty or complex activity limitation	- - -	- - -	56.6	61.6	61.4	64.2	64.9	65.9
Any basic actions difficulty	- - -	- - -	56.8	61.6	61.6	64.4	65.1	66.0
Any complex activity limitation	- - -	- - -	58.0	63.3	61.6	63.9	67.0	67.8
No disability	- - -	- - -	48.0	47.8	50.0	47.0	53.4	53.1
Geographic region								
Northeast	10.4	28.2	51.2	55.8	53.7	54.6	60.9	58.5
Midwest	13.7	31.0	52.6	58.5	61.5	60.6	63.8	58.4
South	14.9	35.9	51.3	57.4	55.7	58.5	59.8	61.9
West	17.9	41.1	59.7	51.4	57.2	55.6	55.4	63.0
Location of residence[8]								
Within MSA	13.1	33.8	52.4	55.1	56.6	56.5	59.1	60.0
Outside MSA	17.1	34.8	55.4	59.8	58.9	61.7	63.2	62.9

- - - Data not available.

* Estimates are considered unreliable. Data preceded by an asterisk have a relative standard error (RSE) of 20%–30%. Data not shown have an RSE of greater than 30%.

[1]Respondents were asked, "Have you ever had a pneumonia shot? This shot is usually given only once or twice in a person's lifetime and is different from the flu shot. It is also called the pneumococcal vaccine."

[2]Estimates are age-adjusted to the year 2000 standard population using four age groups: 18–49 years, 50–64 years, 65–74 years, and 75 years and over. See Appendix II, Age adjustment.

[3]Includes all other races not shown separately, unknown poverty level in 1989, and unknown disability status.

[4]High-risk group membership is based on recommendations of the Advisory Committee on Immunization Practices (ACIP). The high-risk group includes persons who reported diabetes, cancer, heart, lung, liver, or kidney disease. Starting in 2009, this group also includes persons who reported asthma or cigarette smoking to be consistent with the revised ACIP recommendation. For more information on high-risk groups see the adult vaccination schedule available from: http://www.cdc.gov/mmwr/preview/mmwrhtml/mm5901a5.htm.

[5]The race groups white, black, American Indian or Alaska Native, Asian, Native Hawaiian or Other Pacific Islander, and 2 or more races include persons of Hispanic and non-Hispanic origin. Persons of Hispanic origin may be of any race. Starting with 1999 data, race-specific estimates are tabulated according to the 1997 Revisions to the Standards for Federal Data on Race and Ethnicity and are not strictly comparable with estimates for earlier years. The five single-race categories plus multiple-race categories shown in the table conform to the 1997 Standards. Starting with 1999 data, race-specific estimates are for persons who reported only one racial group; the category 2 or more races includes persons who reported more than one racial group. Prior to 1999, data were tabulated according to the 1977 Standards with four racial groups and the Asian only category included Native Hawaiian or Other Pacific Islander. Estimates for single-race categories prior to 1999 included persons who reported one race or, if they reported more than one race, identified one race as best representing their race. Starting with 2003 data, race responses of other race and unspecified multiple race were treated as missing, and then race was imputed if these were the only race responses. Almost all persons with a race response of other race were of Hispanic origin. See Appendix II, Hispanic origin; Race.

[6]Percent of poverty level is based on family income and family size and composition using U.S. Census Bureau poverty thresholds. Poverty level was unknown for 11% of persons 18 years of age and over in 1989. Missing family income data were imputed for 1997 and beyond. See Appendix II, Family Income; Poverty; Table VII.

[7]Any basic actions difficulty or complex activity limitation is defined as having one or more of the following limitations or difficulties: movement difficulty, emotional difficulty, sensory (seeing or hearing) difficulty, cognitive difficulty, self-care (ADL or IADL) limitation, social limitation, or work limitation. For more information, see Appendix II, Basic actions difficulty; Complex activity limitation. Starting with 2007 data, the hearing question, a component of the basic actions difficulty measure, was revised. Consequently, data prior to 2007 are not comparable with 2007 data. For more information on the impact of the revised hearing question, see Appendix II, Hearing trouble.

[8]MSA is metropolitan statistical area. Starting with 2006 data, MSA status is determined using 2000 census data and the 2000 standards for defining MSAs. For data prior to 2006, see Appendix II, Metropolitan statistical area (MSA) for the applicable standards.

NOTES: In 1997, the Advisory Committee on Immunization Practices (ACIP) of the Centers for Disease Control and Prevention (CDC) recommended universal pneumonia vaccination for persons 65 years of age and over. A pneumococcal polysaccharide vaccine was first licensed in 1977. Medicare reimbursement for the costs of the vaccine and its administration began in 1981. CDC. Prevention of pneumococcal disease: Recommendations of the advisory committee on immunization practices (ACIP). MMWR 1997;46(RR–08);1–24. Available from: http://www.cdc.gov/mmwr/preview/mmwrhtml/00047135.htm. Pneumococcal vaccination among adults 19–64 years is recommended for those with other risk factors (medical, occupational, lifestyle, or other indications). Recommended adult immunization schedule United States, October 2007-September 2008. Available from: http://www.cdc.gov/mmwr/pdf/wk/mm5641-Immunization.pdf. Standard errors for selected years are available in the spreadsheet version of this table. Available from: http://www.cdc.gov/nchs/hus.htm. Data for additional years are available. See Appendix III.

SOURCE: CDC/NCHS, National Health Interview Survey. Data are from the Immunization Supplement (1981), the Health Promotion and Disease Prevention Supplement (1991), and the Year 2000 Supplement (1993–1995). Starting in 1997, data are from the sample adult questionnaire.

Table 86 (page 1 of 3). Use of mammography among women 40 years of age and over, by selected characteristics: United States, selected years 1987–2008

[Data are based on household interviews of a sample of the civilian noninstitutionalized population]

Characteristic	1987	1990	1993	1994	1999	2000	2003	2005	2008
	Percent of women having a mammogram within the past 2 years [1]								
40 years and over, age-adjusted [2,3]	29.0	51.7	59.7	61.0	70.3	70.4	69.5	66.6	67.1
40 years and over, crude [2]	28.7	51.4	59.7	60.9	70.3	70.4	69.7	66.8	67.6
50 years and over, age-adjusted [2,3]	27.3	49.8	59.7	60.9	72.1	73.7	72.4	68.2	70.3
50 years and over, crude [2]	27.4	49.7	59.7	60.6	71.9	73.6	72.4	68.4	70.5
Age									
40–49 years	31.9	55.1	59.9	61.3	67.2	64.3	64.4	63.5	61.5
50–64 years	31.7	56.0	65.1	66.5	76.5	78.7	76.2	71.8	74.2
65 years and over	22.8	43.4	54.2	55.0	66.8	67.9	67.7	63.8	65.5
65–74 years	26.6	48.7	64.2	63.0	73.9	74.0	74.6	72.5	72.6
75 years and over	17.3	35.8	41.0	44.6	58.9	61.3	60.6	54.7	57.9
Race [4]									
40 years and over, crude:									
White only	29.6	52.2	60.0	60.6	70.6	71.4	70.1	67.4	67.9
Black or African American only	24.0	46.4	59.1	64.3	71.0	67.8	70.4	64.9	68.0
American Indian or Alaska Native only	*	43.2	49.8	65.8	63.0	47.4	63.1	72.8	62.7
Asian only	*	46.0	55.1	55.8	58.3	53.5	57.6	54.6	66.1
Native Hawaiian or Other Pacific Islander only	- - -	- - -	- - -	- - -	*	*	*	*	*
2 or more races	- - -	- - -	- - -	- - -	70.2	69.2	65.3	63.7	55.2
Hispanic origin and race [4]									
40 years and over, crude:									
Hispanic or Latina	18.3	45.2	50.9	51.9	65.7	61.2	65.0	58.8	61.2
Not Hispanic or Latina	29.4	51.8	60.3	61.5	70.7	71.1	70.1	67.5	68.3
White only	30.3	52.7	60.6	61.3	71.1	72.2	70.5	68.3	68.7
Black or African American only	23.8	46.0	59.2	64.4	71.0	67.9	70.5	65.2	68.3
Age, Hispanic origin, and race [4]									
40–49 years:									
Hispanic or Latina	*15.3	45.1	52.6	47.5	61.6	54.1	59.4	54.2	54.1
Not Hispanic or Latina:									
White only	34.3	57.0	61.6	62.0	68.3	67.2	65.2	65.5	64.1
Black or African American only	27.8	48.4	55.6	67.2	69.2	60.9	68.2	62.1	59.5
50–64 years:									
Hispanic or Latina	23.0	47.5	59.2	60.1	69.7	66.5	69.4	61.5	71.3
Not Hispanic or Latina:									
White only	33.6	58.1	66.2	67.5	77.9	80.6	77.2	73.5	74.1
Black or African American only	26.4	48.4	65.5	63.6	75.0	77.7	76.2	71.6	76.7
65 years and over:									
Hispanic or Latina	*	41.1	*35.7	48.0	67.2	68.3	69.5	63.8	59.0
Not Hispanic or Latina:									
White only	24.0	43.8	54.7	54.9	66.8	68.3	68.1	64.7	66.1
Black or African American only	14.1	39.7	56.3	61.0	68.1	65.5	65.4	60.5	66.4
Age and percent of poverty level [5]									
40 years and over, crude:									
Below 100%	14.6	30.8	41.1	44.2	57.4	54.8	55.4	48.5	51.4
100%–199%	20.9	39.1	47.5	48.6	59.5	58.1	60.8	55.3	55.8
200%–399%	29.7	53.3	63.2	65.0	69.1	68.8	69.9	67.2	64.4
400% or more	42.9	68.7	74.1	74.1	79.8	81.5	77.7	76.6	79.0
40–49 years:									
Below 100%	18.6	32.2	36.1	43.0	51.3	47.4	50.6	42.5	46.6
100%–199%	18.4	39.0	47.8	47.6	52.8	43.6	54.0	49.8	46.5
200%–399%	31.2	55.2	63.0	64.5	63.0	60.2	63.0	61.8	56.8
400% or more	44.1	68.9	69.6	69.9	77.4	75.8	71.6	73.6	72.5
50–64 years:									
Below 100%	14.6	29.9	47.3	46.2	63.3	61.7	58.3	50.4	57.5
100%–199%	24.2	39.8	47.0	49.0	64.9	68.3	64.0	58.8	58.9
200%–399%	29.7	56.2	66.1	69.6	74.8	75.1	74.1	70.7	69.8
400% or more	44.7	71.6	78.7	78.0	83.4	86.9	84.9	80.6	84.3
65 years and over:									
Below 100%	13.1	30.8	40.4	43.9	57.6	54.8	57.0	52.3	49.1
100%–199%	19.9	38.6	47.6	48.8	60.2	60.3	62.8	56.1	59.4
200%–399%	27.7	47.4	60.3	61.0	70.0	71.1	72.3	68.6	65.0
400% or more	34.7	61.2	71.3	73.0	76.7	81.9	73.0	72.6	78.3

See footnotes at end of table.

Table 86 (page 2 of 3). Use of mammography among women 40 years of age and over, by selected characteristics: United States, selected years 1987–2008

[Data are based on household interviews of a sample of the civilian noninstitutionalized population]

Characteristic	1987	1990	1993	1994	1999	2000	2003	2005	2008
Health insurance status at the time of interview[6]			Percent of women having a mammogram within the past 2 years[1]						
40–64 years:									
Insured	- - -	- - -	66.2	68.3	75.5	76.0	75.1	72.5	73.4
Private	- - -	- - -	67.1	69.4	76.3	77.1	76.3	74.5	74.2
Medicaid.	- - -	- - -	51.9	54.5	62.5	61.7	63.5	55.6	64.2
Uninsured	- - -	- - -	36.0	34.0	44.8	40.7	41.5	38.1	39.7
Health insurance status prior to interview[6]									
40–64 years:									
Insured continuously all 12 months.	- - -	- - -	66.6	68.6	76.1	76.8	75.6	73.1	74.1
Uninsured for any period up to 12 months.	- - -	- - -	49.4	49.9	57.1	53.0	56.0	51.3	55.3
Uninsured more than 12 months	- - -	- - -	28.4	26.6	38.9	34.0	37.0	32.9	34.6
Age and education[7]									
40 years and over, crude:									
No high school diploma or GED	17.8	36.4	46.4	48.2	56.7	57.7	58.1	52.8	53.8
High school diploma or GED.	31.3	52.7	59.0	61.0	69.2	69.7	67.8	64.9	65.2
Some college or more	37.7	62.8	69.5	69.7	77.3	76.2	75.1	72.7	73.4
40–49 years:									
No high school diploma or GED. . . .	15.1	38.5	43.6	50.4	48.8	46.8	53.3	51.2	46.9
High school diploma or GED	32.6	53.1	56.6	55.8	60.8	59.0	60.8	58.8	57.2
Some college or more.	39.2	62.3	66.1	68.7	74.4	70.6	68.1	68.3	66.3
50–64 years:									
No high school diploma or GED. . . .	21.2	41.0	51.4	51.6	62.3	66.5	63.4	56.9	64.9
High school diploma or GED	33.8	56.5	62.4	67.8	77.2	76.6	71.8	70.1	70.4
Some college or more.	40.5	68.0	78.5	74.7	81.2	84.2	82.7	77.0	78.5
65 years and over:									
No high school diploma or GED. . . .	16.5	33.0	44.2	45.6	56.6	57.4	56.9	50.7	49.2
High school diploma or GED	25.9	47.5	57.4	59.1	68.4	71.8	69.7	64.3	65.7
Some college or more.	32.3	56.7	64.8	64.3	77.1	74.1	75.1	73.0	75.6
Disability measure[8]									
40 years and over, crude:									
Any basic actions difficulty or complex activity limitation	- - -	- - -	- - -	- - -	67.6	67.8	67.2	63.5	63.9
Any basic actions difficulty	- - -	- - -	- - -	- - -	67.1	67.9	67.3	63.5	63.9
Any complex activity limitation.	- - -	- - -	- - -	- - -	64.8	64.1	62.3	59.9	60.2
No disability	- - -	- - -	- - -	- - -	72.3	72.6	71.8	69.8	71.1

See footnotes at end of table.

[Data are based on household interviews of a sample of the civilian noninstitutionalized population]

* Estimates are considered unreliable. Data preceded by an asterisk have a relative standard error (RSE) of 20%–30%. Data not shown have an RSE greater than 30%.

- - - Data not available.

[1]Questions concerning use of mammography differed slightly on the National Health Interview Survey across the years for which data are shown. See Appendix II, Mammography.

[2]Includes all other races not shown separately, unknown poverty level in 1987, unknown health insurance status, unknown education level, and unknown disability status.

[3]Estimates for women 40 years of age and over are age-adjusted to the year 2000 standard population using four age groups: 40–49 years, 50–64 years, 65–74 years, and 75 years and over. Estimates for women 50 years of age and over are age-adjusted using three age groups. See Appendix II, Age adjustment.

[4]The race groups, white, black, American Indian or Alaska Native, Asian, Native Hawaiian or Other Pacific Islander, and 2 or more races, include persons of Hispanic and non-Hispanic origin. Persons of Hispanic origin may be of any race. Starting with 1999 data, race-specific estimates are tabulated according to the 1997 Revisions to the Standards for the Classification of Federal Data on Race and Ethnicity and are not strictly comparable with estimates for earlier years. The five single-race categories plus multiple-race categories shown in the table conform to the 1997 Standards. Starting with 1999 data, race-specific estimates are for persons who reported only one racial group; the category 2 or more races includes persons who reported more than one racial group. Prior to 1999, data were tabulated according to the 1977 Standards with four racial groups and the Asian only category included Native Hawaiian or Other Pacific Islander. Estimates for single-race categories prior to 1999 included persons who reported one race or, if they reported more than one race, identified one race as best representing their race. Starting with 2003 data, race responses of other race and unspecified multiple race were treated as missing, and then race was imputed if these were the only race responses. Almost all persons with a race response of other race were of Hispanic origin. See Appendix II, Hispanic origin; Race.

[5]Percent of poverty level is based on family income and family size and composition using U.S. Census Bureau poverty thresholds. Poverty level was unknown for 11% of women 40 years of age and over in 1987. Missing family income data were imputed for 1997 and beyond. See Appendix II, Family income; Poverty; Table VII.

[6]Health insurance categories are mutually exclusive. Persons who reported both Medicaid and private coverage are classified as having private coverage. Starting with 1997 data, state-sponsored health plan coverage is included as Medicaid coverage. Starting with 1999 data, coverage by the Children's Health Insurance Program (CHIP) is included with Medicaid coverage. In addition to private and Medicaid, the insured category also includes military plans, other government-sponsored health plans, and Medicare, not shown separately. Persons not covered by private insurance, Medicaid, CHIP, public assistance (through 1996), state-sponsored or other government-sponsored health plans (starting in 1997), Medicare, or military plans are considered to have no health insurance coverage. Persons with only Indian Health Service coverage are considered to have no health insurance coverage. See Appendix II, Health insurance coverage.

[7]Education categories shown are for 1998 and subsequent years. GED is General Educational Development high school equivalency diploma. In years prior to 1998, the following categories based on number of years of school completed were used: less than 12 years, 12 years, 13 years or more. See Appendix II, Education.

[8]Any basic actions difficulty or complex activity limitation is defined as having one or more of the following limitations or difficulties: movement difficulty, emotional difficulty, sensory (seeing or hearing) difficulty, cognitive difficulty, self-care (ADL or IADL) limitation, social limitation, or work limitation. For more information, see Appendix II, Basic actions difficulty; Complex activity limitation. Starting with 2007 data, the hearing question, a component of the basic actions difficulty measure, was revised. Consequently, data prior to 2007 are not comparable with 2007 data and beyond. For more information on the impact of the revised hearing question, see Appendix II, Hearing trouble.

NOTES: Standard errors are available in the spreadsheet version of this table. Available from: http://www.cdc.gov/nchs/hus.htm. Data starting in 1997 are not strictly comparable with data for earlier years due to the 1997 questionnaire redesign. See Appendix I, National Health Interview Survey. Data for additional years are available. See Appendix III. Data have been revised and differ from previous editions of *Health, United States*.

SOURCE: CDC/NCHS, National Health Interview Survey. Data are from the following supplements: cancer control (1987), health promotion and disease prevention (1990–1991), and year 2000 objectives (1993–1994). Starting in 1998, data are from the family core and sample adult questionnaires.

Table 87 (page 1 of 5). Use of Pap smears among women 18 years of age and over, by selected characteristics: United States, selected years 1987–2008

[Data are based on household interviews of a sample of the civilian noninstitutionalized population]

Characteristic	1987	1993	1994	1999	2000	2003	2005	2008
	Percent of women having a Pap smear within the past 3 years[1]							
18 years and over, age-adjusted[2,3]	74.1	77.7	76.8	80.8	81.3	79.2	77.9	75.6
18 years and over, crude[2]	74.4	77.7	76.8	80.8	81.2	79.0	77.7	75.1
Age								
18–44 years	83.3	84.6	82.8	86.8	84.9	83.9	83.6	81.8
18–24 years	74.8	78.8	76.6	76.8	73.5	75.1	74.5	70.5
25–44 years	86.3	86.3	84.6	89.9	88.5	86.8	86.8	85.7
45–64 years	70.5	77.2	77.4	81.7	84.6	81.3	80.6	78.8
45–54 years	75.7	82.1	81.9	83.8	86.3	83.6	83.4	81.0
55–64 years	65.2	70.6	71.0	78.4	82.0	77.8	76.8	76.0
65 years and over	50.8	57.6	57.3	61.0	64.5	60.8	54.9	50.0
65–74 years	57.9	64.7	64.9	70.0	71.6	70.1	66.3	61.6
75 years and over	40.4	48.0	47.3	50.8	56.7	51.1	42.7	37.5
Race[4]								
18 years and over, crude:								
White only	74.1	77.3	76.2	80.6	81.3	78.7	77.7	74.9
Black or African American only	80.7	82.7	83.5	85.7	85.1	84.0	81.1	80.1
American Indian or Alaska Native only	85.4	78.1	73.5	92.2	76.8	84.8	75.2	69.4
Asian only	51.9	68.8	66.4	64.4	66.4	68.3	64.1	65.1
Native Hawaiian or Other Pacific Islander only	- - -	- - -	- - -	*	*	*	*	*
2 or more races	- - -	- - -	- - -	86.9	80.0	81.6	86.2	77.1
Hispanic origin and race[4]								
18 years and over, crude:								
Hispanic or Latina	67.6	77.2	74.4	76.3	77.0	75.4	75.5	75.4
Not Hispanic or Latina	74.9	77.8	77.0	81.3	81.7	79.5	78.0	75.1
White only	74.7	77.3	76.5	81.0	81.8	79.3	78.1	74.9
Black or African American only	80.9	82.7	83.8	86.0	85.1	83.8	81.2	80.0
Age, Hispanic origin, and race[4]								
18–44 years:								
Hispanic or Latina	73.9	80.9	80.6	77.0	78.1	75.9	76.5	77.9
Not Hispanic or Latina:								
White only	84.5	85.3	82.9	88.7	86.6	85.8	85.8	83.8
Black or African American only	89.1	88.0	89.1	90.8	88.5	88.6	86.4	83.5
45–64 years:								
Hispanic or Latina	57.7	75.8	70.1	79.5	77.8	77.9	78.4	78.2
Not Hispanic or Latina:								
White only	71.2	77.2	77.5	81.9	85.9	81.4	81.4	79.0
Black or African American only	76.2	80.3	82.2	84.6	85.7	84.7	80.5	82.1
65 years and over:								
Hispanic or Latina	41.7	57.1	43.8	63.7	66.8	64.6	60.0	52.6
Not Hispanic or Latina:								
White only	51.8	57.1	58.2	60.5	64.2	60.7	54.1	49.0
Black or African American only	44.8	61.2	59.5	64.5	67.2	59.6	60.1	58.7
Age and percent of poverty level[5]								
18 years and over, crude:								
Below 100%	64.3	70.3	68.8	73.6	72.0	70.5	68.7	68.9
100%–199%	68.2	71.2	68.8	72.5	73.4	71.4	69.0	65.0
200%–399%	77.6	80.6	80.1	80.6	80.2	78.6	77.9	72.5
400% or more	83.6	85.1	85.4	87.6	89.1	86.6	85.7	84.4
18–44 years:								
Below 100%	77.1	77.0	78.9	79.7	77.1	77.1	76.2	76.5
100%–199%	80.4	81.9	78.2	84.0	79.4	79.5	78.1	75.5
200%–399%	84.8	86.6	84.5	86.7	86.1	84.0	85.5	82.6
400% or more	88.9	91.3	88.7	91.1	89.8	89.5	88.7	87.0
45–64 years:								
Below 100%	53.6	66.5	62.0	73.1	73.6	66.0	65.9	66.2
100%–199%	60.4	64.8	66.2	70.4	76.1	71.4	69.6	65.6
200%–399%	71.0	79.5	80.3	79.9	80.0	80.8	79.3	75.3
400% or more	79.1	83.9	84.0	87.4	91.5	87.5	87.4	87.1
65 years and over:								
Below 100%	33.2	47.4	44.0	51.9	53.7	52.6	44.4	41.6
100%–199%	50.4	55.7	51.5	54.7	61.0	55.4	49.5	43.5
200%–399%	58.0	59.7	63.7	64.0	65.1	62.4	56.8	45.8
400% or more	65.2	67.5	76.2	70.4	75.4	70.2	64.6	65.7

See footnotes at end of table.

Table 87 (page 2 of 5). Use of Pap smears among women 18 years of age and over, by selected characteristics: United States, selected years 1987–2008

[Data are based on household interviews of a sample of the civilian noninstitutionalized population]

Characteristic	1987	1993	1994	1999	2000	2003	2005	2008
Health insurance status at the time of interview[6]			Percent of women having a Pap smear within the past 3 years[1]					
18–64 years, crude:								
Insured	- - -	84.7	83.8	87.2	87.8	86.4	85.6	83.4
Private	- - -	84.8	83.6	87.5	88.0	87.0	86.5	84.2
Medicaid	- - -	82.7	86.2	84.2	85.8	82.8	80.9	80.3
Uninsured	- - -	69.4	68.6	73.3	70.4	66.6	67.7	67.1
Health insurance status prior to interview[6]								
18–64 years, crude:								
Insured continuously all 12 months	- - -	84.8	83.7	87.3	88.0	86.6	85.8	83.7
Uninsured for any period up to 12 months	- - -	81.8	83.4	83.5	83.7	81.8	81.3	78.9
Uninsured more than 12 months	- - -	65.1	63.6	68.8	65.1	60.2	62.0	62.1
Age and education[7]								
25 years and over, crude:								
No high school diploma or GED	57.1	61.9	60.9	66.1	69.9	64.9	64.1	60.6
High school diploma or GED	76.4	78.2	76.0	79.3	79.8	75.9	73.8	69.5
Some college or more	84.0	84.4	85.2	87.8	88.0	86.2	84.6	82.6
25–44 years:								
No high school diploma or GED	75.1	73.6	73.6	79.0	79.6	71.7	75.5	76.2
High school diploma or GED	85.6	85.4	82.4	87.6	86.2	84.3	83.1	80.0
Some college or more	90.1	89.8	89.1	93.0	91.4	90.8	90.5	89.3
45–64 years:								
No high school diploma or GED	58.0	65.6	66.1	71.6	75.7	71.4	69.7	70.4
High school diploma or GED	72.3	77.6	75.9	79.8	81.8	77.6	79.0	73.9
Some college or more	80.1	83.0	84.7	85.7	89.1	86.2	84.1	83.0
65 years and over:								
No high school diploma or GED	44.0	50.7	47.7	51.8	56.6	52.5	46.0	36.7
High school diploma or GED	55.4	61.6	61.2	63.7	66.9	61.2	52.5	49.3
Some college or more	59.4	62.3	66.5	68.8	69.8	67.8	63.8	59.0
Disability measure[8]								
18 years and over, crude:								
Any basic actions difficulty or complex activity limitation	- - -	- - -	- - -	74.4	75.4	72.7	69.1	66.1
Any basic actions difficulty	- - -	- - -	- - -	74.3	75.1	72.6	69.1	66.2
Any complex activity limitation	- - -	- - -	- - -	69.3	71.0	67.6	62.2	60.1
No disability	- - -	- - -	- - -	83.8	84.1	82.5	82.6	80.4

See footnotes at end of table.

Table 87 (page 3 of 5). **Use of Pap smears among women 18 years of age and over, by selected characteristics: United States, selected years 1987–2008**

[Data are based on household interviews of a sample of the civilian noninstitutionalized population]

Characteristic	1987	1993	1994	1999	2000	2003	2005	2008
	Percent of women having a Pap smear within the past 3 years, among those who have not had a hysterectomy[9]							
18 years and over, age-adjusted[2,3]	77.3	78.7	78.0	81.6	82.7	- - -	79.6	78.2
18 years and over, crude[2]	77.8	80.0	79.1	82.6	83.3	- - -	80.8	79.4
Age								
18–44 years	85.1	84.7	83.2	86.3	84.9	- - -	83.8	81.9
18–24 years	76.4	79.0	76.8	75.5	73.6	- - -	74.6	70.7
25–44 years	88.1	86.5	85.2	89.7	88.7	- - -	87.3	86.0
45–64 years	75.8	79.2	79.8	83.8	86.9	- - -	83.4	84.0
45–54 years	80.9	82.9	83.5	85.5	87.6	- - -	85.7	83.9
55–64 years	70.5	73.6	73.7	80.6	85.5	- - -	79.6	84.1
65 years and over	55.4	59.7	59.3	63.7	68.6	- - -	59.3	56.3
65–74 years	62.8	67.9	67.4	71.9	75.9	- - -	72.4	69.9
75 years and over	44.4	49.9	49.4	54.7	60.9	- - -	46.3	42.2
Race[4]								
18 years and over, crude:								
White only	77.8	79.9	78.8	82.8	83.7	- - -	81.2	79.7
Black or African American only	82.3	83.3	85.0	87.2	86.8	- - -	82.2	82.7
American Indian or Alaska Native only	85.9	78.2	79.6	94.1	77.7	- - -	75.6	74.8
Asian only	52.5	69.6	67.9	63.4	66.9	- - -	64.8	65.7
Native Hawaiian or Other Pacific Islander only	- - -	- - -	- - -	*	*77.1	- - -	*	*
2 or more races	- - -	- - -	- - -	87.5	82.2	- - -	88.8	81.6
Hispanic origin and race[4]								
18 years and over, crude:								
Hispanic or Latina	69.8	77.3	78.0	75.1	78.0	- - -	76.0	77.5
Not Hispanic or Latina	78.5	80.2	79.3	83.5	84.0	- - -	81.5	79.7
White only	78.6	80.2	78.9	83.6	84.4	- - -	82.2	80.3
Black or African American only	82.4	83.4	84.9	87.5	86.8	- - -	82.4	82.6
Age, Hispanic origin, and race[4]								
18–44 years:								
Hispanic or Latina	75.1	80.2	81.0	76.0	77.9	- - -	76.6	78.4
Not Hispanic or Latina:								
White only	86.5	85.7	83.3	88.3	86.6	- - -	86.2	83.9
Black or African American only	90.3	87.6	89.1	90.6	88.7	- - -	86.3	83.5
45–64 years:								
Hispanic or Latina	62.4	75.3	78.1	77.8	81.0	- - -	78.6	81.2
Not Hispanic or Latina:								
White only	77.0	79.3	79.7	84.7	88.5	- - -	85.1	85.0
Black or African American only	78.0	81.1	82.1	86.6	87.4	- - -	80.7	86.0
65 years and over:								
Hispanic or Latina	43.8	58.9	52.0	60.9	71.2	- - -	60.5	53.9
Not Hispanic or Latina:								
White only	56.8	60.0	60.4	63.8	68.0	- - -	59.5	56.5
Black or African American only	46.3	55.8	57.1	65.1	72.1	- - -	59.3	64.1
Age and percent of poverty level[5]								
18 years and over, crude:								
Below 100%	67.5	71.7	72.4	74.8	73.8	- - -	70.5	72.5
100%–199%	71.6	73.7	71.9	75.2	75.7	- - -	72.8	69.9
200%–399%	81.0	83.0	82.2	82.5	83.0	- - -	81.5	77.5
400% or more	87.0	87.8	87.1	88.9	90.5	- - -	88.3	87.9
18–44 years:								
Below 100%	79.3	77.2	79.7	79.0	76.8	- - -	76.2	76.7
100%–199%	81.8	82.1	78.7	83.7	79.2	- - -	78.2	75.5
200%–399%	86.6	86.5	84.8	86.2	86.0	- - -	86.1	82.5
400% or more	90.2	91.9	88.8	90.6	90.0	- - -	88.8	87.3
45–64 years:								
Below 100%	58.0	65.8	65.8	74.7	75.6	- - -	64.9	71.0
100%–199%	66.1	64.2	68.4	72.2	78.2	- - -	71.9	70.5
200%–399%	76.9	82.2	82.8	81.2	81.7	- - -	81.7	79.8
400% or more	84.4	86.6	86.2	89.7	93.7	- - -	90.9	92.5
65 years and over:								
Below 100%	36.4	47.5	45.9	53.5	55.9	- - -	43.9	44.8
100%–199%	54.6	56.6	53.4	56.3	63.3	- - -	54.5	49.1
200%–399%	62.8	63.5	66.7	68.3	71.8	- - -	61.5	53.5
400% or more	73.0	71.7	78.8	72.9	78.6	- - -	70.6	71.0

See footnotes at end of table.

Table 87 (page 4 of 5). Use of Pap smears among women 18 years of age and over, by selected characteristics: United States, selected years 1987–2008

[Data are based on household interviews of a sample of the civilian noninstitutionalized population]

Characteristic	1987	1993	1994	1999	2000	2003	2005	2008
Health insurance status at the time of interview[6]	Percent of women having a Pap smear within the past 3 years, among those who have not had a hysterectomy[9]							
18–64 years, crude:								
Insured	- - -	85.9	85.2	87.8	88.7	- - -	87.1	85.9
Private	- - -	86.0	85.0	88.1	88.8	- - -	87.9	86.7
Medicaid	- - -	83.9	87.0	84.2	86.9	- - -	82.7	82.7
Uninsured	- - -	70.2	70.2	74.3	70.8	- - -	68.2	68.1
Health insurance status prior to interview[6]								
18–64 years, crude:								
Insured continuously all 12 months	- - -	86.1	85.1	88.0	88.9	- - -	87.2	86.3
Uninsured for any period up to 12 months	- - -	81.7	83.8	84.4	84.4	- - -	82.8	81.0
Uninsured more than 12 months	- - -	66.5	65.7	69.9	65.5	- - -	62.9	62.7
Age and education[7]								
25 years and over, crude:								
No high school diploma or GED	61.7	63.2	64.4	68.3	72.5	- - -	67.0	67.6
High school diploma or GED	80.0	80.2	78.1	81.2	82.7	- - -	77.2	73.9
Some college or more	86.7	86.7	87.0	89.9	90.1	- - -	88.3	86.9
25–44 years:								
No high school diploma or GED	77.3	73.1	76.3	78.4	78.6	- - -	74.9	76.5
High school diploma or GED	87.6	85.6	82.5	87.4	86.2	- - -	83.5	79.5
Some college or more	91.5	90.0	89.4	92.9	91.7	- - -	91.2	89.8
45–64 years:								
No high school diploma or GED	63.9	65.5	68.1	73.2	77.5	- - -	70.5	75.0
High school diploma or GED	77.0	78.8	78.5	81.6	84.1	- - -	80.2	78.5
Some college or more	85.5	86.2	86.4	87.7	91.0	- - -	88.0	87.9
65 years and over:								
No high school diploma or GED	48.4	51.3	48.8	52.7	59.7	- - -	49.3	43.2
High school diploma or GED	60.4	63.8	62.5	65.0	71.3	- - -	56.9	53.9
Some college or more	63.6	65.7	70.2	75.6	74.9	- - -	70.0	66.2
Disability measure[8]								
18 years and over, crude:								
Any basic actions difficulty or complex activity limitation	- - -	- - -	- - -	77.8	78.6	- - -	73.8	73.7
Any basic actions difficulty	- - -	- - -	- - -	77.8	78.5	- - -	74.0	74.1
Any complex activity limitation	- - -	- - -	- - -	73.9	73.9	- - -	67.7	68.4
No disability	- - -	- - -	- - -	84.5	85.1	- - -	84.0	82.1

See footnotes at end of table.

Table 87 (page 5 of 5). Use of Pap smears among women 18 years of age and over, by selected characteristics: United States, selected years 1987–2008

[Data are based on household interviews of a sample of the civilian noninstitutionalized population]

- - - Data not available.

* Estimates are considered unreliable. Data preceded by an asterisk have a relative standard error (RSE) of 20%–30%. Data not shown have an RSE of greater than 30%.

[1]Questions concerning use of Pap smears differed slightly on the National Health Interview Survey across the years for which data are shown. See Appendix II, Pap smear.

[2]Includes all other races not shown separately, unknown poverty level in 1987, unknown health insurance status, unknown education level, and unknown disability status.

[3]Estimates are age-adjusted to the year 2000 standard population using five age groups: 18–44 years, 45–54 years, 55–64 years, 65–74 years, and 75 years and over. Age-adjusted estimates in this table may differ from other age-adjusted estimates based on the same data and presented elsewhere if different age groups are used in the adjustment procedure. See Appendix II, Age adjustment.

[4]The race groups, white, black, American Indian or Alaska Native, Asian, Native Hawaiian or Other Pacific Islander, and 2 or more races, include persons of Hispanic and non-Hispanic origin. Persons of Hispanic origin may be of any race. Starting with 1999 data, race-specific estimates are tabulated according to the 1997 Revisions to the Standards for the Classification of Federal Data on Race and Ethnicity and are not strictly comparable with estimates for earlier years. The five single-race categories plus multiple-race categories shown in the table conform to the 1997 Standards. Starting with 1999 data, race-specific estimates are for persons who reported only one racial group; the category 2 or more races includes persons who reported more than one racial group. Prior to 1999, data were tabulated according to the 1977 Standards with four racial groups and the Asian only category included Native Hawaiian or Other Pacific Islander. Estimates for single-race categories prior to 1999 included persons who reported one race or, if they reported more than one race, identified one race as best representing their race. Starting with 2003 data, race responses of other race and unspecified multiple race were treated as missing, and then race was imputed if these were the only race responses. Almost all persons with a race response of other race were of Hispanic origin. See Appendix II, Hispanic origin; Race.

[5]Percent of poverty level is based on family income and family size and composition using U.S. Census Bureau poverty thresholds. Missing family income data were imputed for 1993 and beyond. See Appendix II, Family income; Poverty; Table VII.

[6]Health insurance categories are mutually exclusive. Persons who reported both Medicaid and private coverage are classified as having private coverage. Starting with 1997 data, state-sponsored health plan coverage is included as Medicaid coverage. Starting with 1999 data, coverage by the Children's Health Insurance Program (CHIP) is included with Medicaid coverage. In addition to private and Medicaid, the insured category also includes military plans, other government-sponsored health plans, and Medicare, not shown separately. Persons not covered by private insurance, Medicaid, CHIP, public assistance (through 1996), state-sponsored or other government-sponsored health plans (starting in 1997), Medicare, or military plans are considered to have no health insurance coverage. Persons with only Indian Health Service coverage are considered to have no health insurance coverage. See Appendix II, Health insurance coverage.

[7]Education categories shown are for 1998 and subsequent years. GED is General Educational Development high school equivalency diploma. In years prior to 1998, the following categories based on number of years of school completed were used: less than 12 years, 12 years, 13 years or more. See Appendix II, Education.

[8]Any basic actions difficulty or complex activity limitation is defined as having one or more of the following limitations or difficulties: movement difficulty, emotional difficulty, sensory (seeing or hearing) difficulty, cognitive difficulty, self-care (ADL or IADL) limitation, social limitation, or work limitation. For more information, see Appendix II, Basic actions difficulty; Complex activity limitation. Starting with 2007 data, the hearing question, a component of the basic actions difficulty measure, was revised. Consequently, data prior to 2007 are not comparable with data for 2007 and beyond. For more information on the impact of the revised hearing question, see Appendix II, Hearing trouble.

[9]The U.S. Preventive Services Task Force recommends against routine Pap smear screening in women who have had a total hysterectomy for benign disease. Therefore, Pap smear screening estimates are presented among women who have not had a hysterectomy, in addition to the estimates among all women. Questions concerning hysterectomy differed slightly on the National Health Interview Survey across the years for which data are shown. See Appendix II, Pap smear.

NOTES: Standard errors are available in the spreadsheet version of this table. Available from: http://www.cdc.gov/nchs/hus.htm. Data starting in 1997 are not strictly comparable with data for earlier years due to the 1997 questionnaire redesign. See Appendix I, National Health Interview Survey. Data for additional years are available. See Appendix III.

SOURCE: CDC/NCHS, National Health Interview Survey. Data are from the following supplements: cancer control (1987), year 2000 objectives (1993–1994). Starting in 1998, data are from the family core and sample adult questionnaires.

Table 88 (page 1 of 3). Emergency department visits within the past 12 months among children under 18 years of age, by selected characteristics: United States, selected years 1997–2009

[Data are based on household interviews of a sample of the civilian noninstitutionalized population]

Characteristic	Under 18 years			Under 6 years			6–17 years		
	1997	2008	2009	1997	2008	2009	1997	2008	2009
	Percent of children with one or more emergency department visits [1]								
All children [2]	19.9	20.9	20.8	24.3	27.4	25.9	17.7	17.5	18.2
Sex									
Male	21.5	21.9	22.2	25.2	28.5	25.6	19.6	18.5	20.3
Female	18.3	19.7	19.4	23.3	26.2	26.2	15.7	16.4	15.9
Race [3]									
White only	19.4	20.2	19.8	22.6	25.9	24.6	17.8	17.3	17.3
Black or African American only	24.0	24.2	26.9	33.1	33.0	34.2	19.4	19.8	23.2
American Indian or Alaska Native only	*24.1	35.6	*23.1	*24.3	*	*	*24.0	32.7	*20.7
Asian only	12.6	12.0	11.4	20.8	21.7	14.0	8.6	*7.4	10.0
Native Hawaiian or Other Pacific Islander only	- - -	*	*	- - -	*	*	- - -	*	*
2 or more races	- - -	23.7	25.2	- - -	33.7	28.6	- - -	16.5	22.9
Hispanic origin and race [3]									
Hispanic or Latino	21.1	21.6	20.2	25.7	30.1	27.5	18.1	16.4	15.7
Not Hispanic or Latino	19.7	20.7	21.0	24.0	26.5	25.3	17.6	17.8	18.8
White only	19.2	20.0	19.8	22.2	24.5	23.7	17.7	17.7	18.0
Black or African American only	23.6	24.3	26.5	32.7	33.4	33.1	19.2	19.9	23.2
Percent of poverty level [4]									
Below 100%	25.1	27.7	26.6	29.5	35.1	33.9	22.2	22.8	21.9
100%–199%	22.0	22.2	23.3	28.0	28.9	28.9	19.0	18.5	20.4
200%–399%	18.0	20.1	18.9	21.4	27.1	23.3	16.4	16.7	16.8
400% or more	16.3	16.1	16.0	19.1	19.7	17.9	15.1	14.5	15.1
Hispanic origin and race and percent of poverty level [3,4]									
Hispanic or Latino:									
Percent of poverty level:									
Below 100%	21.9	25.4	24.6	25.0	33.3	29.9	19.6	19.4	20.9
100%–199%	20.8	21.8	18.7	28.8	29.9	27.3	15.6	17.0	13.6
200%–399%	21.4	16.7	16.9	24.6	27.1	26.1	19.6	10.6	12.2
400% or more	17.7	21.7	16.5	*20.2	26.3	*22.7	16.4	19.5	*12.2
Not Hispanic or Latino:									
White only:									
Percent of poverty level:									
Below 100%	25.5	27.7	27.8	27.2	32.6	36.1	24.4	24.2	22.6
100%–199%	22.3	22.5	24.7	25.8	27.6	29.0	20.7	20.0	22.5
200%–399%	17.8	21.3	18.3	20.9	27.4	21.8	16.3	18.3	16.6
400% or more	16.5	15.5	16.2	19.0	17.2	17.4	15.4	14.8	15.7
Black or African American only:									
Percent of poverty level:									
Below 100%	29.3	30.4	28.4	39.5	40.4	39.4	23.0	24.9	21.1
100%–199%	22.5	22.9	26.8	31.7	26.6	27.6	18.5	20.8	26.4
200%–399%	18.5	21.9	27.9	23.9	32.4	32.1	16.3	17.8	26.1
400% or more	16.1	16.7	16.9	*18.8	*32.0	*19.6	15.2	*11.0	15.7
Health insurance status at the time of interview [5]									
Insured	19.8	21.2	21.1	24.4	27.8	25.7	17.5	17.7	18.7
Private	17.5	16.8	16.6	20.9	21.5	18.7	15.9	14.6	15.6
Medicaid	28.2	29.1	27.8	33.0	36.5	32.7	24.1	24.3	24.4
Uninsured	20.2	18.4	16.8	23.0	24.1	27.4	18.9	15.8	13.0
Health insurance status prior to interview [5]									
Insured continuously all 12 months	19.6	20.9	20.8	24.1	27.3	25.4	17.3	17.5	18.3
Uninsured for any period up to 12 months	24.0	26.7	25.8	27.1	37.5	32.4	21.9	21.2	22.5
Uninsured more than 12 months	18.4	14.5	14.2	19.3	*15.8	*24.1	18.1	14.1	11.4

See footnotes at end of table.

Table 88 (page 2 of 3). **Emergency department visits within the past 12 months among children under 18 years of age, by selected characteristics: United States, selected years 1997–2009**

[Data are based on household interviews of a sample of the civilian noninstitutionalized population]

Characteristic	Under 18 years			Under 6 years			6–17 years		
	1997	2008	2009	1997	2008	2009	1997	2008	2009
Percent of poverty level and health insurance status prior to interview[4,5]	Percent of children with one or more emergency department visits[1]								
Below 100%:									
Insured continuously all 12 months	26.3	28.9	27.1	30.9	36.2	33.8	22.8	23.8	22.4
Uninsured for any period up to 12 months . .	26.5	33.8	28.3	29.7	48.4	36.3	24.4	*24.9	*23.1
Uninsured more than 12 months	17.5	*	*19.6	*16.0	*	*	18.0	*	*17.6
100%–199%:									
Insured continuously all 12 months	21.8	22.8	23.8	28.0	29.5	28.1	18.6	18.7	21.4
Uninsured for any period up to 12 months . .	24.5	24.9	28.4	29.7	33.6	34.8	21.0	21.0	25.4
Uninsured more than 12 months	19.5	*17.2	*10.3	*22.5	*	*	18.6	*17.1	*
200%–399%:									
Insured continuously all 12 months	17.7	20.0	19.0	21.2	26.9	23.0	16.1	16.6	16.9
Uninsured for any period up to 12 months . .	21.1	25.8	22.9	*19.5	*33.0	*28.1	22.1	22.7	*20.6
Uninsured more than 12 months	19.2	*14.9	*11.8	*22.7	*	*	17.6	*11.3	*
400% or more:									
Insured continuously all 12 months	16.2	16.0	16.0	18.9	19.0	18.0	15.1	14.7	15.1
Uninsured for any period up to 12 months . .	*19.2	*18.4	*	*	*	*	*	*	*
Uninsured more than 12 months	*	*	*	*	*	*	*	*	*
Geographic region									
Northeast.	18.5	21.3	21.9	20.7	26.8	25.9	17.4	18.9	19.9
Midwest.	19.5	22.0	22.0	26.0	26.8	27.1	16.4	19.5	19.3
South	21.8	21.5	22.3	25.6	29.4	28.6	19.9	17.3	19.0
West	18.5	18.6	16.6	23.5	25.5	20.9	15.9	14.7	14.4
Location of residence[6]									
Within MSA	19.7	19.9	20.2	23.9	26.2	25.2	17.4	16.7	17.5
Outside MSA	20.8	25.7	24.2	26.2	33.5	29.7	18.6	21.6	21.6
	Percent of children with two or more emergency department visits[1]								
All children[2]	7.1	7.1	6.7	9.6	9.4	8.9	5.8	5.9	5.6
Sex									
Male	7.3	7.3	7.0	9.9	9.3	9.7	6.0	6.2	5.5
Female	6.9	6.9	6.5	9.4	9.6	8.0	5.7	5.6	5.7
Race[3]									
White only	6.6	6.8	5.9	8.4	8.9	7.9	5.7	5.7	4.9
Black or African American only.	9.6	8.2	10.6	14.9	9.7	14.1	6.9	7.4	8.8
American Indian and Alaska Native only	*	*15.3	*	*	*	*	*	*	*
Asian only	*5.7	*4.0	*3.4	*12.9	*	*	*	*	*
Native Hawaiian and Other Pacific Islander only	- - -	*	*	- - -	*	*	- - -	*	*
2 or more races	- - -	*9.3	11.0	- - -	*15.0	*13.3	- - -	*	*9.5
Hispanic origin and race[3]									
Hispanic or Latino.	8.9	8.1	6.7	11.8	11.3	9.7	7.0	6.1	4.8
Not Hispanic or Latino.	6.8	6.8	6.7	9.2	8.8	8.6	5.7	5.9	5.8
White only.	6.2	6.4	5.7	7.8	8.0	7.5	5.5	5.5	4.9
Black or African American only	9.3	8.2	10.5	14.6	9.9	13.4	6.8	7.3	9.0
Percent of poverty level[4]									
Below 100%.	11.1	10.7	11.4	14.5	12.6	15.3	8.9	9.4	8.8
100%–199%.	8.3	9.1	7.4	12.2	12.5	9.6	6.3	7.3	6.3
200%–399%.	6.2	6.5	5.2	7.4	8.6	6.1	5.6	5.4	4.8
400% or more	4.0	3.8	4.0	5.0	4.8	4.9	3.6	3.3	3.6

See footnotes at end of table.

Table 88 (page 3 of 3). Emergency department visits within the past 12 months among children under 18 years of age, by selected characteristics: United States, selected years 1997–2009

[Data are based on household interviews of a sample of the civilian noninstitutionalized population]

Characteristic	Under 18 years			Under 6 years			6–17 years		
	1997	2008	2009	1997	2008	2009	1997	2008	2009
Hispanic origin and race and percent of poverty level[3,4]	Percent of children with two or more emergency department visits[1]								
Hispanic or Latino:									
Percent of poverty level:									
Below 100%	10.4	11.2	8.6	13.9	13.6	12.2	8.0	*9.4	6.1
100%–199%	8.2	9.0	6.3	12.0	14.0	9.3	5.7	*6.1	*4.5
200%–399%	8.5	4.6	5.2	10.0	*7.5	*	*7.6	*3.0	*4.2
400% or more	*5.0	*4.3	*4.5	*	*	*	*	*	*
Not Hispanic or Latino:									
White only:									
Percent of poverty level:									
Below 100%	10.7	10.6	13.3	12.2	*13.6	18.8	9.8	*8.4	*9.8
100%–199%	8.0	8.8	7.0	11.2	*10.4	*7.6	6.4	*8.0	6.7
200%–399%	6.0	7.0	4.6	6.7	8.9	5.8	5.6	6.1	4.1
400% or more	3.7	3.5	3.8	4.6	*3.9	*4.4	3.3	3.3	3.5
Black or African American only:									
Percent of poverty level:									
Below 100%	12.7	10.0	12.7	19.1	*10.6	17.1	8.8	*9.7	9.7
100%–199%	9.2	9.0	11.5	*13.5	*9.6	*16.1	*7.2	*8.6	*9.5
200%–399%	5.8	*6.4	*7.8	*8.9	*9.2	*	*4.5	*5.3	*8.4
400% or more	*	*5.4	*6.9	*	*	*	*	*	*
Health insurance status at the time of interview[5]									
Insured	7.0	7.2	6.8	9.6	9.7	8.9	5.7	5.9	5.6
Private	5.2	4.9	4.2	6.8	6.2	4.7	4.5	4.2	4.0
Medicaid	13.1	11.5	10.6	16.2	14.5	13.7	10.4	9.6	8.5
Uninsured	7.7	6.3	5.7	9.8	*6.4	*7.4	6.8	*6.2	5.0
Health insurance status prior to interview[5]									
Insured continuously all 12 months	6.9	7.1	6.6	9.4	9.6	8.8	5.7	5.8	5.5
Uninsured for any period up to 12 months	8.5	8.6	9.2	11.5	*11.8	11.7	6.6	*6.9	*7.9
Uninsured more than 12 months	6.8	*6.2	*3.7	*8.6	*	*	6.2	*	*3.8
Geographic region									
Northeast	6.2	7.6	6.4	7.6	10.5	*7.1	5.4	*6.4	6.0
Midwest	6.6	7.5	7.2	10.4	8.8	8.1	4.8	6.8	6.7
South	8.0	7.0	7.7	10.1	9.2	11.7	6.9	5.9	5.6
West	7.1	6.5	5.0	10.0	9.8	6.7	5.6	4.6	4.1
Location of residence[6]									
Within MSA	7.2	6.7	6.4	9.6	8.8	9.0	5.9	5.6	5.1
Outside MSA	6.8	9.2	8.2	9.7	12.7	8.4	5.6	7.4	8.0

* Estimates are considered unreliable. Data preceded by an asterisk have a relative standard error (RSE) of 20%–30%. Data not shown have an RSE greater than 30%.

- - - Data not available.

[1] See Appendix II, Emergency department visit.

[2] Includes all other races not shown separately and unknown health insurance status.

[3] The race groups white, black, American Indian or Alaska Native, Asian, Native Hawaiian or Other Pacific Islander, and 2 or more races include persons of Hispanic and non-Hispanic origin. Persons of Hispanic origin may be of any race. Starting with 1999 data, race-specific estimates are tabulated according to the 1997 Revisions to the Standards for the Classification of Federal Data on Race and Ethnicity and are not strictly comparable with estimates for earlier years. The five single-race categories plus multiple-race categories shown in the table conform to the 1997 Standards. Starting with 1999 data, race-specific estimates are for persons who reported only one racial group; the category 2 or more races includes persons who reported more than one racial group. Prior to 1999, data were tabulated according to the 1977 Standards with four racial groups and the Asian only category included Native Hawaiian or Other Pacific Islander. Estimates for single-race categories prior to 1999 included persons who reported one race or, if they reported more than one race, identified one race as best representing their race. Starting with 2003 data, race responses of other race and unspecified multiple race were treated as missing, and then race was imputed if these were the only race responses. Almost all persons with a race response of other race were of Hispanic origin. See Appendix II, Hispanic origin; Race.

[4] Percent of poverty level is based on family income and family size and composition using U.S. Census Bureau poverty thresholds. Missing family income data were imputed for 1997 and beyond. See Appendix II, Family income; Poverty; Table VII.

[5] Health insurance categories are mutually exclusive. Persons who reported both Medicaid and private coverage are classified as having private coverage. Starting with 1997 data, state-sponsored health plan coverage is included as Medicaid coverage. Starting with 1999 data, coverage by the Children's Health Insurance Program (CHIP) is included with Medicaid coverage. In addition to private and Medicaid, the insured category also includes military, other government, and Medicare coverage. Persons not covered by private insurance, Medicaid, CHIP, state-sponsored or other government-sponsored health plans (starting in 1997), Medicare, or military plans are considered to have no health insurance coverage. Persons with only Indian Health Service coverage are considered to have no health insurance coverage. See Appendix II, Health insurance coverage.

[6] MSA is metropolitan statistical area. Starting with 2006 data, MSA status is determined using 2000 census data and the 2000 standards for defining MSAs. For data prior to 2006, see Appendix II, Metropolitan statistical area (MSA) for the applicable standards.

NOTES: Standard errors are available in the spreadsheet version of this table. Available from: http://www.cdc.gov/nchs/hus.htm. Some data have been revised and differ from previous editions of Health, United States. Data for additional years are available. See Appendix III.

SOURCE: CDC/NCHS, National Health Interview Survey, family core and sample child questionnaires.

[Data are based on household interviews of a sample of the civilian noninstitutionalized population]

Characteristic	One or more emergency department visits				Two or more emergency department visits			
	1997	2000	2008	2009	1997	2000	2008	2009
	Percent of adults with emergency department visits [1]							
18 years and over, age-adjusted [2,3]	19.6	20.2	20.7	21.4	6.7	6.9	7.4	8.1
18 years and over, crude [2]	19.6	20.1	20.5	21.2	6.7	6.8	7.3	8.0
Age								
18–44 years	20.7	20.5	21.5	22.0	6.8	7.0	7.8	8.8
18–24 years	26.3	25.7	24.1	24.6	9.1	8.8	9.1	9.1
25–44 years	19.0	18.8	20.6	21.1	6.2	6.4	7.4	8.7
45–64 years	16.2	17.6	17.6	18.4	5.6	5.6	5.7	6.8
45–54 years	15.7	17.9	17.1	18.0	5.5	5.8	5.7	7.0
55–64 years	16.9	17.0	18.2	18.9	5.7	5.3	5.8	6.5
65 years and over	22.0	23.7	23.4	24.9	8.1	8.6	9.1	8.4
65–74 years	20.3	21.6	20.7	21.6	7.1	7.4	7.9	6.7
75 years and over	24.3	26.2	26.4	28.8	9.3	10.0	10.5	10.4
Sex [3]								
Male	19.1	18.7	19.3	19.9	5.9	5.7	6.3	7.1
Female	20.2	21.6	22.1	22.9	7.5	7.9	8.6	9.1
Race [3,4]								
White only	19.0	19.4	20.4	20.4	6.2	6.4	7.3	7.6
Black or African American only	25.9	26.5	25.1	31.1	11.1	10.8	10.3	13.2
American Indian or Alaska Native only	24.8	30.3	30.2	23.5	13.1	*12.6	*10.1	*10.2
Asian only	11.6	13.6	11.5	13.2	*2.9	*3.8	2.2	3.2
Native Hawaiian or Other Pacific Islander only	- - -	*	*	*	- - -	*	*	*
2 or more races	- - -	32.5	24.7	23.6	- - -	11.3	*8.2	10.7
American Indian or Alaska Native; White	- - -	33.9	32.7	28.0	- - -	*9.4	*	*13.9
Hispanic origin and race [3,4]								
Hispanic or Latino	19.2	18.3	19.3	19.5	7.4	7.0	7.1	7.2
Mexican	17.8	17.4	18.9	16.9	6.4	7.1	6.2	6.1
Not Hispanic or Latino	19.7	20.6	21.2	21.9	6.7	6.9	7.6	8.4
White only	19.1	19.8	21.0	20.8	6.2	6.4	7.5	7.9
Black or African American only	25.9	26.5	25.6	31.3	11.0	10.8	10.5	13.3
Percent of poverty level [3,5]								
Below 100%	28.1	29.0	30.0	31.5	12.8	13.3	14.1	15.7
100%–199%	23.8	23.9	24.3	26.6	9.3	9.6	10.4	11.0
200%–399%	18.3	19.8	19.8	20.8	5.9	6.3	6.7	7.8
400% or more	15.9	16.8	16.9	16.3	3.9	4.5	4.6	4.7
Hispanic origin and race and percent of poverty level [3,4,5]								
Hispanic or Latino:								
Below 100%	22.1	22.4	21.3	23.9	9.8	9.7	9.0	10.8
100%–199%	19.2	18.1	18.4	20.0	8.1	6.7	7.9	7.6
200%–399%	18.5	17.3	20.2	19.0	6.0	7.4	5.9	6.2
400% or more	14.6	16.4	17.7	13.5	*3.8	*4.3	*6.1	*4.0
Not Hispanic or Latino:								
White only:								
Below 100%	29.5	30.1	34.6	32.4	13.0	13.9	16.3	15.3
100%–199%	24.3	25.5	26.1	28.3	9.1	10.4	12.0	12.2
200%–399%	18.1	20.1	20.0	20.6	5.8	6.3	7.0	8.3
400% or more	15.8	16.3	17.2	16.1	3.8	4.1	4.4	4.8
Black or African American only:								
Below 100%	34.6	35.4	35.2	41.8	17.5	17.4	18.6	24.1
100%–199%	29.2	28.5	29.9	34.1	12.8	12.2	11.6	14.5
200%–399%	20.8	23.2	21.3	28.7	8.1	8.0	7.9	9.4
400% or more	18.2	22.6	19.6	22.7	5.9	8.8	6.6	7.3

See footnotes at end of table.

Table 89 (page 2 of 3). Emergency department visits within the past 12 months among adults 18 years of age and over, by selected characteristics: United States, selected years 1997–2009

[Data are based on household interviews of a sample of the civilian noninstitutionalized population]

Characteristic	One or more emergency department visits				Two or more emergency department visits			
	1997	2000	2008	2009	1997	2000	2008	2009
Health insurance status at the time of interview[6,7]	Percent of adults with emergency department visits[1]							
18–64 years:								
Insured	18.8	19.5	20.3	20.5	6.1	6.4	7.0	7.8
Private	16.9	17.6	17.0	16.7	4.7	5.1	4.9	5.1
Medicaid	37.6	42.2	39.7	41.5	19.7	21.0	20.2	22.9
Uninsured	20.0	19.3	19.1	21.2	7.5	6.9	7.4	9.0
Health insurance status prior to interview[6,7]								
18–64 years:								
Insured continuously all 12 months	18.3	19.0	19.7	19.8	5.8	6.1	6.7	7.4
Uninsured for any period up to 12 months	25.5	28.2	27.4	27.3	9.4	10.3	11.4	11.7
Uninsured more than 12 months	18.9	17.3	16.7	20.2	7.1	6.4	6.3	8.8
Percent of poverty level and health insurance status prior to interview[5,6,7]								
18–64 years:								
Below 100%:								
Insured continuously all 12 months	30.2	31.6	33.3	35.0	14.7	15.4	17.0	20.3
Uninsured for any period up to 12 months	34.1	43.7	38.6	36.8	16.1	18.1	18.9	18.1
Uninsured more than 12 months	20.8	20.5	19.7	24.1	8.1	9.1	8.2	9.9
100%–199%:								
Insured continuously all 12 months	24.5	25.5	26.0	27.6	8.9	10.2	10.9	11.3
Uninsured for any period up to 12 months	28.7	27.7	27.9	31.7	12.3	11.7	14.6	14.9
Uninsured more than 12 months	19.0	17.4	16.8	20.7	8.3	6.4	5.9	7.9
200%–399%:								
Insured continuously all 12 months	17.5	19.5	19.3	20.3	5.3	6.3	6.4	7.1
Uninsured for any period up to 12 months	21.6	24.6	23.0	21.2	6.6	7.3	7.7	9.4
Uninsured more than 12 months	16.8	15.6	16.7	18.1	5.9	4.5	5.2	9.6
400% or more:								
Insured continuously all 12 months	14.9	15.5	15.9	14.4	3.7	3.7	3.9	3.9
Uninsured for any period up to 12 months	18.0	20.1	24.6	22.2	*3.1	6.4	*6.9	*
Uninsured more than 12 months	19.1	15.8	*11.0	15.0	*	*5.2	*6.5	*5.6
Disability measure[3,8]								
Any basic actions difficulty or complex activity limitation	30.8	32.0	33.1	35.9	13.5	14.6	15.0	17.9
Any basic actions difficulty	30.5	32.4	33.1	36.0	13.5	14.9	14.9	18.2
Any complex activity limitation	39.7	41.5	41.8	44.8	19.9	21.2	22.7	25.0
No disability	14.5	15.3	15.3	15.3	3.7	3.9	4.3	4.4
Geographic region[3]								
Northeast	19.5	20.0	21.3	21.0	6.9	6.2	7.0	8.2
Midwest	19.3	20.1	21.2	22.2	6.2	6.9	7.7	8.6
South	20.9	21.2	21.4	22.6	7.3	7.6	8.2	9.1
West	17.7	18.6	18.4	19.1	6.0	6.3	6.3	6.2
Location of residence[3]								
Within MSA[9]	19.1	19.6	20.1	20.9	6.4	6.6	7.2	7.8
Outside MSA[9]	21.5	22.5	23.9	24.0	7.8	7.8	8.8	9.6

See footnotes at end of table.

Table 89 (page 3 of 3). Emergency department visits within the past 12 months among adults 18 years of age and over, by selected characteristics: United States, selected years 1997–2009

[Data are based on household interviews of a sample of the civilian noninstitutionalized population]

* Estimates are considered unreliable. Data preceded by an asterisk have a relative standard error (RSE) of 20%–30%. Data not shown have an RSE of greater than 30%.

- - - Data not available.

[1]See Appendix II, Emergency department visit.

[2]Includes all other races not shown separately, unknown health insurance status, and unknown disability status.

[3]Estimates are for persons 18 years of age and over and are age-adjusted to the year 2000 standard population using five age groups: 18–44 years, 45–54 years, 55–64 years, 65–74 years, and 75 years and over. See Appendix II, Age adjustment.

[4]The race groups, white, black, American Indian or Alaska Native, Asian, Native Hawaiian or Other Pacific Islander, and 2 or more races, include persons of Hispanic and non-Hispanic origin. Persons of Hispanic origin may be of any race. Starting with 1999 data, race-specific estimates are tabulated according to the 1997 Revisions to the Standards for the Classification of Federal Data on Race and Ethnicity and are not strictly comparable with estimates for earlier years. The five single-race categories plus multiple-race categories shown in the table conform to the 1997 Standards. Starting with 1999 data, race-specific estimates are for persons who reported only one racial group; the category 2 or more races includes persons who reported more than one racial group. Prior to 1999, data were tabulated according to the 1977 Standards with four racial groups, and the Asian only category included Native Hawaiian or Other Pacific Islander. Estimates for single-race categories prior to 1999 included persons who reported one race or, if they reported more than one race, identified one race as best representing their race. Starting with 2003 data, race responses of other race and unspecified multiple race were treated as missing, and then race was imputed if these were the only race responses. Almost all persons with a race response of other race were of Hispanic origin. See Appendix II, Hispanic origin; Race.

[5]Percent of poverty level is based on family income and family size and composition using U.S. Census Bureau poverty thresholds. Missing family income data were imputed for 1997 and beyond. See Appendix II, Family income; Poverty; Table VII.

[6]Estimates for persons 18–64 years of age are age-adjusted to the year 2000 standard population using three age groups: 18–44 years, 45–54 years, and 55–64 years. See Appendix II, Age adjustment.

[7]Health insurance categories are mutually exclusive. Persons who reported both Medicaid and private coverage are classified as having private coverage. Starting with 1997 data, state-sponsored health plan coverage is included as Medicaid coverage. Starting with 1999 data, coverage by the Children's Health Insurance Program (CHIP) is included with Medicaid coverage. In addition to private and Medicaid, the insured category also includes military plans, other government-sponsored health plans, and Medicare, not shown separately. Persons not covered by private insurance, Medicaid, CHIP, state-sponsored or other government-sponsored health plans (starting in 1997), Medicare, or military plans are considered to have no health insurance coverage. Persons with only Indian Health Service coverage are considered to have no health insurance coverage. See Appendix II, Health insurance coverage.

[8]Any basic actions difficulty or complex activity limitation is defined as having one or more of the following limitations or difficulties: movement difficulty, emotional difficulty, sensory (seeing or hearing) difficulty, cognitive difficulty, self-care (ADL or IADL) limitation, social limitation, or work limitation. For more information, see Appendix II, Basic actions difficulty; Complex activity limitation. Starting with 2007 data, the hearing question, a component of the basic actions difficulty measure, was revised. Consequently, data prior to 2007 are not comparable with data for 2007 and beyond. For more information on the impact of the revised hearing question, see Appendix II, Hearing trouble.

[9]MSA is metropolitan statistical area. Starting with 2006 data, MSA status is determined using 2000 census data and the 2000 standards for defining MSAs. For data prior to 2006, see Appendix II, Metropolitan statistical area (MSA) for the applicable standards.

NOTES: Standard errors are available in the spreadsheet version of this table. Available from: http://www.cdc.gov/nchs/hus.htm. Data for additional years are available. See Appendix III.

SOURCE: CDC/NCHS, National Health Interview Survey, family core and sample adult questionnaires.

Table 90 (page 1 of 2). Injury-related visits to hospital emergency departments, by sex, age, and intent and mechanism of injury: United States, average annual, selected years 1995–1996 through 2007–2008

[Data are based on reporting by a sample of hospital emergency departments]

Sex, age, and intent and mechanism of injury[1]	1995–1996	1999–2000	2007–2008[2]	1995–1996	1999–2000	2007–2008[2]
Both sexes	Injury-related visits in thousands			Injury-related visits per 10,000 persons		
All ages[3,4]	33,191	35,316	28,699	1,231.9	1,266.6	960.9
Male						
All ages[3,4]	18,788	19,596	15,332	1,406.5	1,423.4	1,039.7
Under 18 years[3]	5,985	6,020	4,602	1,644.9	1,624.4	1,216.8
Unintentional injuries[5]	5,432	5,421	3,995	1,492.9	1,462.8	1,056.3
Falls	1,402	1,303	1,305	385.2	351.6	345.0
Struck by or against objects or persons	1,011	1,377	850	277.9	371.5	224.6
Motor vehicle traffic	450	432	265	123.7	116.6	70.0
Cut or pierce	493	455	264	135.6	122.8	69.8
Intentional injuries	290	242	198	79.7	65.4	52.2
18–24 years[3]	2,882	2,927	2,305	2,259.7	2,177.6	1,547.4
Unintentional injuries[5]	2,419	2,404	1,788	1,896.7	1,788.5	1,200.6
Falls	299	307	309	234.8	228.1	207.7
Struck by or against objects or persons	387	401	280	303.2	298.2	188.0
Motor vehicle traffic	347	469	366	272.4	348.6	245.8
Cut or pierce	304	394	190	238.7	293.0	127.8
Intentional injuries	335	322	308	262.4	239.8	206.9
25–44 years[3]	6,794	6,688	4,471	1,622.3	1,604.1	1,072.7
Unintentional injuries[5]	5,720	5,503	3,531	1,365.7	1,320.0	847.0
Falls	817	850	677	195.2	204.0	162.5
Struck by or against objects or persons	619	781	384	147.8	187.3	92.1
Motor vehicle traffic	909	848	638	217.0	203.3	153.0
Cut or pierce	860	762	426	205.3	182.8	102.2
Intentional injuries	697	511	350	166.4	122.5	83.9
45–64 years[3]	2,034	2,634	2,707	795.1	893.1	718.3
Unintentional injuries[5]	1,821	2,315	2,223	711.9	785.1	590.0
Falls	445	582	651	174.1	197.4	172.8
Struck by or against objects or persons	186	232	205	72.6	78.8	54.3
Motor vehicle traffic	244	316	331	95.5	107.1	87.9
Cut or pierce	203	294	309	79.2	99.6	81.9
Intentional injuries	86	99	145	33.5	33.5	38.4
65 years and over[3]	1,093	1,327	1,247	797.1	925.2	768.6
Unintentional injuries[5]	1,004	1,203	1,073	732.1	838.2	661.7
Falls	505	579	638	368.3	403.2	393.2
Struck by or against objects or persons	*39	*112	*52	*28.4	*77.8	*32.3
Motor vehicle traffic	99	*114	93	72.2	*79.6	57.4
Cut or pierce	*81	102	81	*59.1	71.3	50.0
Intentional injuries	*	*	*	*	*	*

See footnotes at end of table.

Table 90 (page 2 of 2). Injury-related visits to hospital emergency departments, by sex, age, and intent and mechanism of injury: United States, average annual, selected years 1995–1996 through 2007–2008

[Data are based on reporting by a sample of hospital emergency departments]

Sex, age, and intent and mechanism of injury[1]	1995–1996	1999–2000	2007–2008[2]	1995–1996	1999–2000	2007–2008[2]
Female	Injury-related visits in thousands			Injury-related visits per 10,000 persons		
All ages[3,4]	14,403	15,720	13,367	1,050.5	1,104.7	874.2
Under 18 years[3]	4,097	4,095	3,062	1,183.2	1,161.0	848.2
Unintentional injuries[5]	3,741	3,713	2,690	1,080.3	1,052.7	745.3
Falls	1,040	1,025	1,014	300.3	290.7	280.9
Struck by or against objects or persons	477	728	391	137.7	206.5	108.3
Motor vehicle traffic	447	430	282	129.1	122.0	78.2
Cut or pierce	253	232	145	72.9	65.7	40.1
Intentional injuries	220	149	163	63.5	42.3	45.1
18–24 years[3]	1,721	1,957	1,698	1,376.8	1,487.5	1,186.5
Unintentional injuries[5]	1,405	1,564	1,318	1,123.4	1,189.1	921.0
Falls	268	234	301	214.0	177.9	210.5
Struck by or against objects or persons	134	170	106	107.1	129.5	74.0
Motor vehicle traffic	373	469	378	298.0	356.8	264.5
Cut or pierce	131	156	89	105.0	118.2	61.9
Intentional injuries	239	219	209	191.2	166.7	145.8
25–44 years[3]	4,515	4,900	3,733	1,064.5	1,159.6	905.4
Unintentional injuries[5]	3,845	3,951	2,865	906.6	935.0	694.7
Falls	817	947	900	192.7	224.1	218.2
Struck by or against objects or persons	380	382	216	89.5	90.5	52.4
Motor vehicle traffic	871	788	572	205.3	186.4	138.8
Cut or pierce	338	434	214	79.6	102.6	51.8
Intentional injuries	418	425	345	98.6	100.7	83.6
45–64 years[3]	2,025	2,569	2,681	744.2	822.2	677.5
Unintentional injuries[5]	1,810	2,168	2,209	665.2	693.9	558.3
Falls	600	749	886	220.7	239.9	223.9
Struck by or against objects or persons	159	192	171	58.4	61.4	43.2
Motor vehicle traffic	343	324	345	126.0	103.7	87.3
Cut or pierce	127	175	163	46.7	55.9	41.1
Intentional injuries	*64	125	130	*23.4	40.0	32.9
65 years and over[3]	2,045	2,199	2,193	1,039.0	1,082.7	989.9
Unintentional injuries[5]	1,900	2,005	1,978	965.5	986.9	892.5
Falls	1,220	1,219	1,463	619.7	600.2	660.1
Struck by or against objects or persons	82	103	91	41.9	50.5	41.2
Motor vehicle traffic	169	132	116	85.7	65.1	52.5
Cut or pierce	*42	72	*64	*21.2	*35.3	*28.8
Intentional injuries	*	*	*	*	*	*

* Estimates are considered unreliable. Data preceded by an asterisk have a relative standard error (RSE) of 20%–30%. Data not shown have an RSE of greater than 30%.

[1]Intent and mechanism of injury are based on the first-listed external cause of injury code (E code). Intentional injuries include suicide attempts and assaults. See Appendix II, External cause of injury; Injury-related visit; and Table X for a listing of E codes.

[2]Estimates for 2005–2006 (available in the spreadsheet version) and 2007–2008 were limited to those visits that were initial visits for the condition. This was determined using an imputed variable indicating that the visit was or was not the initial visit in 2005 and 2006, and in 2007 and 2008 this was determined by using the initial visit data collected on the questionnaire. Limiting the estimates to initial visits decreases the total number of injury-related visits by 12% in 2006–2007. No similar variable indicating initial visits was available for 1995–1996 or 1999–2000 data. Therefore, estimates for 2005 and beyond are not directly comparable with 1995–1996 and 1999–2000 estimates.

[3]Includes all injury-related visits not shown separately in table, including those with undetermined intent (1.2% in 2007–2008) and insufficient or no information to code cause of injury (9.8% in 2007–2008).

[4]Rates are age-adjusted to the year 2000 standard population using six age groups: under 18 years, 18–24 years, 25–44 years, 45–64 years, 65–74 years, and 75 years and over. See Appendix II, Age adjustment.

[5]Includes unintentional injury-related visits with mechanism of injury not shown in table.

NOTES: An emergency department visit was considered injury related if the physician's diagnosis was injury related (ICD–9–CM 800–909.2, 909.4, 909.9–994.9, 995.50–995.59, and 995.80–995.85) or an external cause (E code) of injury code was present (ICD–9–CM E800-E869, E880-E929, and E950-E999). For visits with both an ICD and E code present on the record, both variables had to be injury-related for the visit to be considered injury-related. Visits with a first-listed diagnosis or E code describing a complication or adverse effect of medical care are excluded. For more information on injury-related visits, see Bergen G, Chen LH, Warner M, Fingerhut LA. Injury in the United States: 2007 Chartbook. Hyattsville, MD: NCHS. 2008. Available from: http://www.cdc.gov/nchs/data/misc/injury2007.pdf. Rates were calculated using estimates of the civilian population of the United States including institutionalized persons. The population estimates used are the same used for rates calculated for the National Hospital Discharge Survey. Population data are from unpublished tabulations provided by the U.S. Census Bureau. Rates prior to 2001 were calculated using population estimates based on the 1990 census. Rates for 2005 and beyond were calculated using postcensal population estimates based on the 2000 census. Data for additional years are available. See Appendix III.

SOURCE: CDC/NCHS, National Hospital Ambulatory Medical Care Survey.

Table 91 (page 1 of 3). Visits to physician offices, hospital outpatient departments, and hospital emergency departments, by selected characteristics: United States, selected years 1995–2008

[Data are based on reporting by a sample of office-based physicians, hospital outpatient departments, and hospital emergency departments]

Age, sex, and race	All places[1]				Physician offices			
	1995	2000	2007	2008	1995	2000	2007	2008
	Number of visits in thousands							
Total.	860,859	1,014,848	1,200,017	1,189,619	697,082	823,542	994,321	955,969
Under 18 years	194,644	212,165	240,813	225,531	150,351	163,459	194,959	171,744
18–44 years	285,184	315,774	335,440	328,438	219,065	243,011	257,257	243,979
45–64 years	188,320	255,894	334,088	341,595	159,531	216,783	283,890	284,110
45–54 years.	104,891	142,233	170,514	169,674	88,266	119,474	141,478	137,776
55–64 years.	83,429	113,661	163,574	171,921	71,264	97,309	142,412	146,335
65 years and over	192,712	231,014	289,675	294,054	168,135	200,289	258,214	256,135
65–74 years.	102,605	116,505	142,528	144,878	90,544	102,447	127,805	127,125
75 years and over.	90,106	114,510	147,147	149,177	77,591	97,842	130,409	129,010
	Number of visits per 100 persons							
Total, age-adjusted[2].	334	374	402	393	271	304	332	315
Total, crude.	329	370	405	398	266	300	336	320
Under 18 years	275	293	327	306	213	226	264	233
18–44 years	264	291	304	298	203	224	233	221
45–64 years	364	422	439	441	309	358	373	367
45–54 years.	339	385	392	386	286	323	325	313
55–64 years.	401	481	503	513	343	412	438	437
65 years and over	612	706	799	790	534	612	712	688
65–74 years.	560	656	746	729	494	577	669	639
75 years and over.	683	766	859	860	588	654	761	743
Sex and age								
Male, age-adjusted[2].	290	325	351	334	232	261	290	265
Male, crude.	277	314	345	330	220	251	285	262
Under 18 years.	273	302	331	307	209	231	268	233
18–44 years	190	203	205	188	139	148	151	131
45–54 years.	275	316	321	319	229	260	262	255
55–64 years.	351	428	452	441	300	367	396	373
65–74 years.	508	614	732	687	445	539	661	604
75 years and over.	711	771	888	886	616	670	801	768
Female, age-adjusted[2].	377	420	452	451	309	345	374	363
Female, crude.	378	424	462	464	310	348	384	376
Under 18 years.	277	285	321	304	217	221	261	232
18–44 years	336	377	402	407	265	298	315	311
45–54 years.	400	451	460	450	339	384	386	369
55–64 years.	446	529	550	580	382	453	477	496
65–74 years.	603	692	758	765	534	609	676	669
75 years and over.	666	763	840	843	571	645	735	728
Race and age[3]								
White, age-adjusted[2]	339	380	398	395	282	315	335	324
White, crude	338	381	407	406	281	316	345	336
Under 18 years.	295	306	330	312	237	243	273	246
18–44 years	267	301	298	299	211	239	235	230
45–54 years.	334	386	381	387	286	330	324	325
55–64 years.	397	480	498	512	345	416	442	446
65–74 years.	557	641	735	729	496	568	666	648
75 years and over.	689	764	856	855	598	658	765	743
Black or African American, age-adjusted. . .	309	353	475	443	204	239	339	296
Black or African American, crude.	281	324	450	421	178	214	317	276
Under 18 years.	193	264	351	335	100	167	247	208
18–44 years	260	257	380	343	158	149	241	201
45–54 years.	387	383	490	445	281	269	341	289
55–64 years.	414	495	592	589	294	373	444	422
65–74 years.	553	656	900	809	429	512	748	636
75 years and over.	534	745	966	942	395	568	769	762

See footnotes at end of table.

Table 91 (page 2 of 3). **Visits to physician offices, hospital outpatient departments, and hospital emergency departments, by selected characteristics: United States, selected years 1995–2008**

[Data are based on reporting by a sample of office-based physicians, hospital outpatient departments, and hospital emergency departments]

Age, sex, and race	Hospital outpatient departments				Hospital emergency departments			
	1995	2000	2007	2008	1995	2000	2007	2008
	Number of visits in thousands							
Total	67,232	83,289	88,894	109,889	96,545	108,017	116,802	123,761
Under 18 years	17,636	21,076	18,962	25,907	26,657	27,630	26,893	27,880
18–44 years	24,299	26,947	30,300	34,174	41,820	45,816	47,883	50,285
45–64 years	14,811	20,772	25,707	31,150	13,978	18,339	24,491	26,335
45–54 years	8,029	11,558	14,138	16,257	8,595	11,201	14,898	15,641
55–64 years	6,782	9,214	11,569	14,893	5,383	7,138	9,593	10,694
65 years and over	10,486	14,494	13,926	18,658	14,090	16,232	17,535	19,261
65–74 years	6,004	7,515	7,815	10,273	6,057	6,543	6,908	7,479
75 years and over	4,482	6,979	6,111	8,385	8,033	9,690	10,627	11,781
	Number of visits per 100 persons							
Total, age-adjusted[2]	26	31	30	36	37	40	40	42
Total, crude	26	30	30	37	37	39	39	41
Under 18 years	25	29	26	35	38	38	36	38
18–44 years	22	25	27	31	39	42	43	46
45–64 years	29	34	34	40	27	30	32	34
45–54 years	26	31	32	37	28	30	34	36
55–64 years	33	39	36	44	26	30	29	32
65 years and over	33	44	38	50	45	50	48	52
65–74 years	33	42	41	52	33	37	36	38
75 years and over	34	47	36	48	61	65	62	68
Sex and age								
Male, age-adjusted[2]	21	26	23	29	37	38	37	39
Male, crude	21	25	23	29	36	38	37	39
Under 18 years	25	29	25	34	40	41	38	39
18–44 years	14	17	16	18	37	38	37	39
45–54 years	20	26	26	28	26	30	34	35
55–64 years	26	32	27	37	25	30	29	31
65–74 years	29	38	35	44	34	36	36	38
75 years and over	34	42	30	50	61	59	56	68
Female, age-adjusted[2]	31	35	36	44	37	41	42	44
Female, crude	31	35	37	44	37	41	42	44
Under 18 years	25	29	26	36	35	35	35	36
18–44 years	31	33	38	44	40	46	49	53
45–54 years	32	36	39	45	29	31	35	36
55–64 years	38	45	43	51	26	31	30	33
65–74 years	36	46	46	58	32	37	36	37
75 years and over	34	49	39	47	61	69	66	68
Race and age[3]								
White, age-adjusted[2]	23	28	26	33	34	37	36	38
White, crude	23	28	26	33	34	37	36	37
Under 18 years	23	27	23	32	35	36	34	34
18–44 years	20	23	24	28	36	39	39	41
45–54 years	23	28	28	32	25	28	30	31
55–64 years	28	36	30	38	24	28	27	28
65–74 years	29	38	36	47	32	35	33	35
75 years and over	31	44	31	46	60	63	60	67
Black or African American, age-adjusted . . .	48	51	60	69	58	62	76	78
Black or African American, crude	45	48	58	68	58	62	75	77
Under 18 years	39	40	44	61	53	57	60	65
18–44 years	38	40	52	55	64	68	87	87
45–54 years	55	61	*73	80	51	53	76	76
55–64 years	73	70	*87	99	47	52	61	68
65–74 years	*77	85	*83	101	47	59	69	73
75 years and over	66	85	*97	*87	73	92	100	93

See footnotes at end of table.

Table 91 (page 3 of 3). Visits to physician offices, hospital outpatient departments, and hospital emergency departments, by selected characteristics: United States, selected years 1995–2008

[Data are based on reporting by a sample of office-based physicians, hospital outpatient departments, and hospital emergency departments]

* Estimates are considered unreliable. Data preceded by an asterisk have a relative standard error of 20%–30%.

[1] All places includes visits to physician offices and hospital outpatient and emergency departments.

[2] Estimates are age-adjusted to the year 2000 standard population using six age groups: under 18 years, 18–44 years, 45–54 years, 55–64 years, 65–74 years, and 75 years and over. See Appendix II, Age adjustment.

[3] Estimates by racial group should be used with caution because information on race was collected from medical records. In 2008, race data were missing and imputed for 30% of ambulatory care visits, including 33% of visits to physician offices, 21% of visits to hospital outpatient departments, and 16% of visits to hospital emergency departments. Information on the race imputation process used in each data year is available in the public use file documentaiton. Available from: http://www.cdc.gov/nchs/ahcd.htm. Starting with 1999 data, the instruction for the race item on the Patient Record Form was changed so that more than one race could be recorded. In previous years only one race could be checked. Estimates for race in this table are for visits where only one race was recorded. Because of the small number of responses with more than one racial group checked, estimates for visits with multiple races checked are unreliable and are not presented.

NOTES: Rates for 1995–2000 were computed using 1990-based postcensal estimates of the civilian noninstitutionalized population as of July 1, adjusted for net underenumeration using the 1990 National Population Adjustment Matrix from the U.S. Census Bureau. Starting with 2001 data, rates were computed using 2000-based postcensal estimates of the civilian noninstitutionalized population as of July 1. The difference between rates for 2000 computed using 1990-based postcensal estimates and 2000 census counts is minimal. More information is available from: http://www.cdc.gov/nchs/ahcd.htm. Rates will be overestimated to the extent that visits by institutionalized persons are counted in the numerator (for example, hospital emergency department visits by nursing home residents) and institutionalized persons are omitted from the denominator (the civilian noninstitutionalized population). Starting with *Health, United States, 2005*, data for physician offices for 2001 and beyond use a revised weighting scheme. See Appendix I, National Ambulatory Medical Care Survey (NAMCS) and National Hospital Ambulatory Medical Care Survey (NHAMCS). Data for additional years are available. See Appendix III.

SOURCE: CDC/NCHS, National Ambulatory Medical Care Survey and National Hospital Ambulatory Medical Care Survey.

Table 92 (page 1 of 2). Visits to primary care generalist and specialist physicians, by selected characteristics and type of physician: United States, selected years 1980–2008

[Data are based on reporting by a sample of office-based physicians]

| Age, sex, and race | \| Type of primary care generalist physician[1] |||||||||||| |
| | All primary care generalists |||| General and family practice |||| Internal medicine |||| |
	1980	1990	2000	2008	1980	1990	2000	2008	1980	1990	2000	2008
	Percent of all physician office visits												
Total	66.2	63.6	58.9	59.6	33.5	29.9	24.1	23.2	12.1	13.8	15.3	16.0
Under 18 years.	77.8	79.5	79.7	84.9	26.1	26.5	19.9	16.9	2.0	2.9	*	*
18–44 years.	65.3	65.2	62.1	67.9	34.3	31.9	28.2	29.4	8.6	11.8	12.7	13.4
45–64 years.	60.2	55.5	51.2	51.5	36.3	32.1	26.4	26.0	19.5	18.6	20.1	20.5
45–54 years	60.2	55.6	52.3	53.5	37.4	32.0	27.8	28.4	17.1	17.1	18.7	19.0
55–64 years	60.2	55.5	49.9	49.7	35.4	32.1	24.7	23.9	21.8	20.0	21.7	21.9
65 years and over.	61.6	52.6	46.5	43.9	37.5	28.1	20.2	18.5	22.7	23.3	24.5	23.6
65–74 years	61.2	52.7	46.6	44.1	37.4	28.1	19.7	20.3	22.1	23.0	24.5	21.9
75 years and over	62.3	52.4	46.4	43.6	37.6	28.0	20.8	16.8	23.5	23.7	24.5	25.3
Sex and age												
Male:												
Under 18 years	77.3	78.1	77.7	84.2	25.6	24.1	18.3	16.4	2.0	3.0	*	*
18–44 years	50.8	51.8	51.5	57.9	38.0	35.9	34.2	37.1	11.5	15.0	14.4	19.3
45–64 years	55.6	50.6	49.4	46.6	34.4	31.0	28.7	27.4	20.5	19.2	19.8	19.2
65 years and over	58.2	51.2	43.1	39.5	35.6	27.7	19.3	18.2	22.3	23.3	23.8	21.3
Female:												
Under 18 years	78.5	81.1	82.0	85.5	26.6	29.1	21.7	17.4	2.0	2.8	*	*
18–44 years	72.1	71.3	67.2	72.1	32.5	30.0	25.3	26.1	7.3	10.3	11.9	10.9
45–64 years	63.4	58.8	52.5	54.9	37.7	32.8	24.9	25.1	18.9	18.2	20.2	21.3
65 years and over	63.9	53.5	48.9	47.0	38.7	28.3	20.9	18.7	22.9	23.3	25.0	25.3
Race and age[2]												
White:												
Under 18 years	77.6	79.2	78.5	84.0	26.4	27.1	21.2	17.9	2.0	2.3	*	*
18–44 years	64.8	64.4	61.4	66.6	34.5	31.9	29.2	30.7	8.6	10.6	11.0	12.8
45–64 years	59.6	54.2	49.3	51.9	36.0	31.5	27.3	26.8	19.2	17.6	17.1	20.1
65 years and over	61.4	51.9	45.1	43.5	36.6	27.5	20.3	18.9	23.3	23.1	23.0	23.0
Black or African American:												
Under 18 years	79.9	85.5	87.3	90.0	23.7	20.2	*	*14.3	*2.2	9.8	*	*
18–44 years	68.5	68.3	65.0	74.9	31.7	31.9	22.0	25.9	9.0	18.1	20.9	*15.9
45–64 years	66.1	61.6	61.7	51.0	38.6	31.2	23.3	20.3	22.6	26.9	35.9	25.9
65 years and over	64.6	58.6	52.8	52.9	49.0	28.9	*18.5	18.1	14.2	28.7	33.4	31.7

See footnotes at end of table.

Table 92 (page 2 of 2). Visits to primary care generalist and specialist physicians, by selected characteristics and type of physician: United States, selected years 1980–2008

[Data are based on reporting by a sample of office-based physicians]

Age, sex, and race	Type of primary care generalist physician[1]								Specialty care physicians			
	Obstetrics and gynecology				Pediatrics							
	1980	1990	2000	2008	1980	1990	2000	2008	1980	1990	2000	2008
	Percent of all physician office visits											
Total	9.6	8.7	7.8	8.3	10.9	11.2	11.7	12.1	33.8	36.4	41.1	40.4
Under 18 years	1.3	1.2	*1.1	1.2	48.5	48.9	57.3	65.8	22.2	20.5	20.3	15.1
18–44 years	21.7	20.8	20.4	24.1	0.7	0.7	*0.9	1.1	34.7	34.8	37.9	32.1
45–64 years	4.2	4.6	4.5	5.0	*	*	*	*	39.8	44.5	48.8	48.5
45–54 years	5.6	6.3	5.6	6.1	*	*	*	*	39.8	44.4	47.7	46.5
55–64 years	2.9	3.1	3.3	3.9	*	*	*	*	39.8	44.5	50.1	50.3
65 years and over	1.4	1.1	1.5	*1.7	*	*	*	*	38.4	47.4	53.5	56.1
65–74 years	1.7	1.6	2.0	*1.9	*	*	*	*	38.8	47.3	53.4	55.9
75 years and over	1.0	*0.6	*1.0	*	*	*	*	*	37.7	47.6	53.6	56.4
Sex and age												
Male:												
Under 18 years	...	...	...	- - -	49.4	50.7	58.0	66.8	22.7	21.9	22.3	15.8
18–44 years	...	...	...	- - -	1.0	0.7	*1.7	*	49.2	48.2	48.5	42.1
45–64 years	...	...	...	- - -	*	*	*	*	44.4	49.4	50.6	53.4
65 years and over	...	...	...	- - -	*	*	*	*	41.8	48.8	56.9	60.5
Female:												
Under 18 years	2.5	2.3	2.1	2.4	47.4	46.9	56.5	64.7	21.5	18.9	18.0	14.5
18–44 years	31.7	30.4	29.6	34.1	0.6	0.7	*	1.0	27.9	28.7	32.8	27.9
45–64 years	6.7	7.7	7.3	8.3	*	*	*	*	36.6	41.2	47.5	45.1
65 years and over	2.1	1.8	2.6	*3.0	*	*	*	*	36.1	46.5	51.1	53.0
Race and age[2]												
White:												
Under 18 years	1.1	1.0	*1.2	1.1	48.2	48.8	54.7	63.8	22.4	20.8	21.5	16.0
18–44 years	21.0	21.1	20.4	22.0	0.7	0.7	*0.8	*1.1	35.2	35.6	38.6	33.4
45–64 years	4.1	4.8	4.7	4.9	*	*	*	*	40.4	45.8	50.7	48.1
65 years and over	1.4	1.2	1.5	*1.6	*	*	*	*	38.6	48.1	54.9	56.5
Black or African American:												
Under 18 years	2.8	*3.4	*	*	51.2	52.1	75.0	73.4	20.1	14.5	*12.7	*10.0
18–44 years	27.1	17.9	20.7	31.6	*	*	*	*	31.5	31.7	35.0	25.1
45–64 years	4.8	3.5	*2.4	*4.8	*	*	*	*	33.9	38.4	38.3	49.0
65 years and over	*	*	*	*	*	*	*	*	35.4	41.4	47.2	47.1

* Estimates are considered unreliable. Data preceded by an asterisk have a relative standard error (RSE) of 20%–30%. Data not shown have a RSE of greater than 30%.

... Category not applicable.

- - - Data not available.

[1]Type of physician is based on physician's self-designated primary area of practice. Primary care generalist physicians are defined as practitioners in the fields of general and family practice, general internal medicine, general obstetrics and gynecology, and general pediatrics and exclude primary care specialists. Primary care generalists in general and family practice exclude primary care specialities, such as sports medicine and geriatrics. Primary care internal medicine physicians exclude internal medicine specialists, such as allergists, cardiologists, and endocrinologists. Primary care obstetrics and gynecology physicians exclude obstetrics and gynecology specialities, such as gynecological oncology, maternal and fetal medicine, obstetrics and gynecology critical care medicine, and reproductive endocrinology. Primary care pediatricians exclude pediatric specialists, such as adolescent medicine specialists, neonatologists, pediatric allergists, and pediatric cardiologists. See Appendix II, Physician specialty.

[2]Estimates by racial group should be used with caution because information on race was collected from medical records. In 2008, race data were missing and imputed for 33% of visits to physician offices. Information on the race imputation process used in each data year is available in the public use file documentaiton. Available from: http://www.cdc.gov/nchs/ahcd.htm. Starting with 1999 data, the instruction for the race item on the Patient Record Form was changed so that more than one race could be recorded. In previous years only one racial category could be checked. Estimates for racial groups presented in this table are for visits where only one race was recorded. Because of the small number of responses with more than one racial group checked, estimates for visits with multiple races checked are unreliable and are not presented.

NOTES: This table presents data on visits to physician offices and excludes visits to other sites, such as hospital outpatient and emergency departments. See Appendix II, Office visits. In 1980, the survey excluded Alaska and Hawaii. Data for all other years include all 50 states and the District of Columbia. Visits with specialty of physician unknown are excluded. Starting with *Health, United States, 2005*, data for 2001 and later years for physician offices use a revised weighting scheme. See Appendix I, National Ambulatory Medical Care Survey (NAMCS). Data for additional years are available. See Appendix III.

SOURCE: CDC/NCHS, National Ambulatory Medical Care Survey.

Table 93 (page 1 of 2). Dental visits in the past year, by selected characteristics: United States, selected years 1997–2009

[Data are based on household interviews of a sample of the civilian noninstitutionalized population]

Characteristic	2 years and over			2–17 years			18–64 years			65 years and over[1]		
	1997	2008	2009	1997	2008	2009	1997	2008	2009	1997	2008	2009
	Percent of persons with a dental visit in the past year[2]											
Total[3]	65.1	63.9	65.4	72.7	77.3	78.4	64.1	60.4	62.0	54.8	57.6	59.6
Sex												
Male	62.9	61.3	62.6	72.3	76.8	77.6	60.4	56.4	57.9	55.4	56.4	58.4
Female	67.1	66.5	68.0	73.0	77.9	79.3	67.7	64.4	65.9	54.4	58.6	60.5
Race[4]												
White only	66.4	64.9	66.3	74.0	77.6	79.1	65.7	61.8	63.1	56.8	59.4	61.8
Black or African American only	58.9	58.7	59.9	68.8	78.5	76.7	57.0	52.7	55.9	35.4	39.5	38.1
American Indian or Alaska Native only	55.1	55.2	53.1	66.8	70.7	68.5	49.9	48.5	47.3	*	*39.9	*44.2
Asian only	62.5	64.7	67.6	69.9	74.8	76.2	60.3	61.6	65.8	53.9	65.7	62.1
Native Hawaiian or Other Pacific Islander only	- - -	*	*	- - -	*	*	- - -	*	*	- - -	*	*
2 or more races	- - -	62.1	63.5	- - -	72.9	80.0	- - -	55.1	50.0	- - -	*35.0	58.5
Black or African American; White	- - -	63.3	67.1	- - -	65.6	78.7	- - -	58.9	45.3	- - -	*	*
American Indian or Alaska Native; White	- - -	52.1	56.0	- - -	77.7	76.5	- - -	45.0	47.9	- - -	*	58.3
Hispanic origin and race[4]												
Hispanic or Latino	54.0	53.3	56.0	61.0	69.9	73.0	50.8	45.6	48.1	47.8	46.2	47.9
Not Hispanic or Latino	66.4	65.9	67.1	74.7	79.3	80.0	65.7	63.0	64.5	55.2	58.5	60.5
White only	68.0	67.4	68.6	76.4	80.2	81.4	67.5	65.2	66.3	57.2	60.3	62.8
Black or African American only	58.8	58.8	59.8	68.8	78.6	76.7	56.9	52.9	55.9	35.3	39.3	38.4
Percent of poverty level[5]												
Below 100%	50.5	49.5	51.7	62.0	70.1	71.7	46.9	41.3	42.7	31.5	31.1	39.0
100%–199%	50.8	49.1	52.8	62.5	70.1	75.2	48.3	40.9	45.3	40.8	41.2	42.3
200%–399%	66.2	61.8	63.3	76.1	78.1	77.1	63.4	56.7	59.1	60.7	58.5	60.9
400% or more	78.9	78.5	79.5	85.7	86.9	87.8	77.7	76.6	77.9	74.7	77.9	77.5
Hispanic origin and race and percent of poverty level[4,5]												
Hispanic or Latino:												
Below 100%	45.7	48.8	51.7	55.9	68.1	71.7	39.2	36.1	37.6	33.6	32.4	42.7
100%–199%	47.2	46.0	51.7	53.8	66.2	72.4	43.5	33.7	41.4	47.9	44.9	37.5
200%–399%	61.2	55.1	57.1	70.5	72.0	73.8	57.5	48.6	51.3	57.0	49.6	54.4
400% or more	73.0	68.2	69.2	82.4	81.1	76.9	70.8	65.3	67.1	64.9	62.2	63.5
Not Hispanic or Latino:												
White only:												
Below 100%	51.7	48.6	51.3	64.4	67.5	69.6	50.6	45.3	46.3	32.0	31.4	42.2
100%–199%	52.4	49.2	52.7	66.1	71.3	76.2	50.4	43.5	46.4	42.2	41.1	44.4
200%–399%	67.5	63.5	64.7	77.1	79.4	79.1	65.0	59.1	60.7	61.9	60.5	62.4
400% or more	79.7	80.2	81.1	86.8	88.1	89.9	78.5	78.4	79.4	75.5	79.4	79.4
Black or African American only:												
Below 100%	52.8	51.4	52.6	66.1	76.4	74.0	46.2	38.3	42.1	27.7	23.1	28.8
100%–199%	48.7	52.1	53.0	61.2	74.6	79.2	46.3	43.2	45.1	26.9	37.2	26.9
200%–399%	63.3	59.8	61.6	75.0	82.1	74.4	60.7	53.6	59.5	41.5	42.5	46.7
400% or more	74.6	72.9	74.3	81.8	85.2	85.0	73.4	71.3	74.1	66.1	60.3	55.3

See footnotes at end of table.

[Data are based on household interviews of a sample of the civilian noninstitutionalized population]

Characteristic	2 years and over			2–17 years			18–64 years			65 years and over[1]		
	1997	2008	2009	1997	2008	2009	1997	2008	2009	1997	2008	2009
Disability measure[6]	Percent of persons with a dental visit in the past year[2]											
Any basic actions difficulty or complex activity limitation.	...	...	...	...	...	...	55.1	52.3	55.8	49.0	50.1	53.3
Any basic actions difficulty.	...	...	...	...	...	...	54.7	52.8	56.1	48.7	49.8	53.6
Any complex activity limitation	...	...	...	...	...	...	51.0	44.9	50.4	44.6	42.0	47.6
No disability.	...	...	...	...	...	...	67.4	63.4	64.4	64.2	70.7	70.2
Geographic region												
Northeast	69.6	70.9	71.1	77.5	82.4	82.6	69.6	68.4	69.3	55.5	63.8	60.9
Midwest	68.4	66.2	67.6	76.4	79.0	80.5	67.4	63.3	64.2	57.6	57.3	62.0
South	60.2	59.2	60.8	68.0	75.3	76.8	59.4	55.2	56.7	49.0	51.0	54.0
West	65.0	63.9	65.9	71.5	75.0	75.8	62.9	59.8	62.4	61.9	63.8	65.2
Location of residence[7]												
Within MSA	66.7	65.1	66.5	73.6	77.7	79.0	65.7	61.5	63.1	57.6	60.3	61.8
Outside MSA	59.1	57.9	59.5	69.3	75.1	75.5	58.0	54.5	55.9	46.1	48.3	51.3

* Estimates are considered unreliable. Data preceded by an asterisk have a relative standard error (RSE) of 20%–30%. Data not shown have an RSE greater than 30%.

- - - Data not available.

. . . Category not applicable.

[1]Based on the 1997–2009 National Health Interview Surveys, about 24%–30% of persons 65 years and over were edentulous (having lost all their natural teeth). In 1997–2009, about 69%–73% of older dentate persons compared with 17%–21% of older edentate persons had a dental visit in the past year.

[2]Respondents were asked "About how long has it been since you last saw or talked to a dentist?" See Appendix II, Dental visit.

[3]Includes all other races not shown separately and unknown disability status.

[4]The race groups white, black, American Indian or Alaska Native, Asian, Native Hawaiian or Other Pacific Islander, and 2 or more races include persons of Hispanic and non-Hispanic origin. Persons of Hispanic origin may be of any race. Starting with 1999 data, race-specific estimates are tabulated according to the 1997 Revisions to the Standards for the Classification of Federal Data on Race and Ethnicity and are not strictly comparable with estimates for earlier years. The five single-race categories plus multiple-race categories shown in the table conform to the 1997 Standards. Starting with 1999 data, race-specific estimates are for persons who reported only one racial group; the category 2 or more races includes persons who reported more than one racial group. Prior to 1999, data were tabulated according to the 1977 Standards with four racial groups, and the Asian only category included Native Hawaiian or Other Pacific Islander. Estimates for single-race categories prior to 1999 included persons who reported one race or, if they reported more than one race, identified one race as best representing their race. Starting with 2003 data, race responses of other race and unspecified multiple race were treated as missing, and then race was imputed if these were the only race responses. Almost all persons with a race response of other race were of Hispanic origin. See Appendix II, Hispanic origin; Race.

[5]Percent of poverty level is based on family income and family size and composition using U.S. Census Bureau poverty thresholds. Missing family income data were imputed for 1997 and beyond. See Appendix II, Family income; Poverty; Table VII.

[6]Any basic actions difficulty or complex activity limitation is defined as having one or more of the following limitations or difficulties: movement difficulty, emotional difficulty, sensory (seeing or hearing) difficulty, cognitive difficulty, self-care (ADL or IADL) limitation, social limitation, or work limitation. For more information, see Appendix II, Basic actions difficulty; Complex activity limitation. Starting with 2007 data, the hearing question, a component of the basic actions difficulty measure, was revised. Consequently, data prior to 2007 are not comparable with data for 2007 and beyond. For more information on the impact of the revised hearing question, see Appendix II, Hearing trouble.

[7]MSA is metropolitan statistical area. Starting with 2006 data, MSA status is determined using 2000 census data and the 2000 standards for defining MSAs. For data prior to 2006, see Appendix II, Metropolitan statistical area (MSA) for the applicable standards.

NOTES: In 1997 the National Health Interview Survey questionnaire was redesigned. See Appendix I, National Health Interview Survey. Standard errors for selected years are available in the spreadsheet version of this table. Available from: http://www.cdc.gov/nchs/hus.htm. Data for additional years are available. See Appendix III.

SOURCE: CDC/NCHS, National Health Interview Survey, sample child and sample adult questionnaires.

Table 94. Prescription drug use in the past month, by sex, age, race and Hispanic origin: United States, selected years 1988–1994 through 2005–2008

[Data are based on a sample of the civilian noninstitutionalized population]

| | All persons[1] | | Not Hispanic or Latino | | | | Mexican[2,3] | |
| | | | White only[2] | | Black or African American only[2] | | | |
Sex and age	1988–1994	2005–2008	1988–1994	2005–2008	1988–1994	2005–2008	1988–1994	2005–2008
	Percent of population with at least one prescription drug in past month							
Both sexes, age-adjusted[4]	39.1	47.2	41.1	52.0	36.9	42.1	31.7	32.2
Male	32.7	41.8	34.2	46.1	31.1	37.2	27.5	28.8
Female	45.0	52.4	47.6	57.9	41.4	46.0	36.0	35.6
Both sexes, crude	37.8	47.9	41.4	55.0	31.2	39.5	24.0	24.5
Male	30.6	41.7	33.5	48.4	25.5	33.9	20.1	21.4
Female	44.6	53.9	48.9	61.5	36.2	44.4	28.1	27.9
Under 18 years	20.5	25.3	22.9	29.9	14.8	20.8	16.1	17.0
18–44 years	31.3	37.8	34.3	45.1	27.8	29.4	21.1	17.7
45–64 years	54.8	64.8	55.5	67.7	57.5	62.6	48.1	50.1
65 years and over	73.6	90.1	74.0	91.1	74.5	89.1	67.7	76.7
Male:								
Under 18 years	20.4	25.3	22.3	29.2	15.5	23.4	16.3	17.3
18–44 years	21.5	27.5	23.5	33.3	21.1	20.9	14.9	14.2
45–64 years	47.2	59.3	48.1	62.3	48.2	54.7	43.8	46.0
65 years and over	67.2	89.7	67.4	91.6	64.4	85.1	61.3	67.8
Female:								
Under 18 years	20.6	25.2	23.6	30.7	14.2	18.1	16.0	16.7
18–44 years	40.7	47.9	44.7	56.6	33.4	36.6	28.1	22.0
45–64 years	62.0	70.2	62.6	73.0	64.4	69.1	52.2	54.1
65 years and over	78.3	90.5	78.8	90.7	81.3	91.7	73.0	83.9
	Percent of population with three or more prescription drugs in past month							
Both sexes, age-adjusted[4]	11.8	20.8	12.4	22.3	12.6	20.0	9.0	13.8
Male	9.4	18.3	9.9	19.5	10.2	17.5	7.0	11.6
Female	13.9	23.2	14.6	25.1	14.3	21.8	11.0	15.9
Both sexes, crude	11.0	21.4	12.5	25.3	9.2	17.5	4.8	7.8
Male	8.3	17.8	9.5	21.3	7.0	14.4	3.4	6.1
Female	13.6	24.8	15.4	29.1	11.1	20.2	6.4	9.7
Under 18 years	2.4	4.4	3.2	5.3	1.5	3.6	*1.2	2.7
18–44 years	5.7	9.8	6.3	12.1	5.4	7.3	3.0	2.7
45–64 years	20.0	34.1	20.9	35.6	21.9	34.5	16.0	24.5
65 years and over	35.3	65.0	35.0	65.7	41.2	67.0	31.3	52.5
Male:								
Under 18 years	2.6	5.0	3.3	5.7	1.7	5.3	*	3.5
18–44 years	3.6	6.2	4.1	8.0	4.2	*4.9	*1.8	*1.5
45–64 years	15.1	28.6	15.8	29.4	18.7	29.0	11.6	19.7
65 years and over	31.3	64.6	30.9	66.3	31.7	61.5	27.6	45.0
Female:								
Under 18 years	2.3	3.8	3.0	4.8	*1.2	*1.9	*1.5	1.8
18–44 years	7.6	13.3	8.5	16.1	6.4	9.4	4.3	4.1
45–64 years	24.7	39.4	25.8	41.8	24.3	39.1	20.3	29.0
65 years and over	38.2	65.3	38.0	65.3	47.7	70.6	34.5	58.6

* Estimates are considered unreliable. Data preceded by an asterisk have a relative standard error (RSE) of 20%–30%. Data not shown have an RSE greater than 30%.

[1]Includes persons of all races and Hispanic origins, not just those shown separately.

[2]Starting with 1999 data, race-specific estimates are tabulated according to the 1997 Revisions to the Standards for the Classification of Federal Data on Race and Ethnicity and are not strictly comparable with estimates for earlier years. The two non-Hispanic race categories shown in the table conform to the 1997 Standards. Starting with 1999 data, race-specific estimates are for persons who reported only one racial group. Prior to data year 1999, estimates were tabulated according to the 1977 Standards. Estimates for single-race categories prior to 1999 included persons who reported one race or, if they reported more than one race, identified one race as best representing their race. See Appendix II, Hispanic origin; Race.

[3]Persons of Mexican origin may be of any race.

[4]Age-adjusted to the 2000 standard population using four age groups: Under 18 years, 18–44 years, 45–64 years, and 65 years and over. Age-adjusted estimates in this table may differ from other age-adjusted estimates based on the same data and presented elsewhere if different age groups are used in the adjustment procedure. See Appendix II, Age adjustment.

NOTES: See Appendix II, Drug. Standard errors are available in the spreadsheet version of this table. Available from: http://www.cdc.gov/nchs/hus.htm. Data for additional years are available. See Appendix III.

SOURCE: CDC/NCHS, National Health and Nutrition Examination Survey.

Table 95 (page 1 of 3). Selected prescription drug classes used in the past month, by sex and age: United States, selected years 1988–1994 through 2005–2008

[Data are based on a sample of the civilian noninstitutionalized population]

Age group and Multum Lexicon Plus® therapeutic class[1] (primary indications for use)	Total 1988–1994	Total 1999–2002	Total 2005–2008	Male 1988–1994	Male 1999–2002	Male 2005–2008	Female 1988–1994	Female 1999–2002	Female 2005–2008
All ages	Percent of population with at least one prescription drug in drug class in past month								
Antihyperlipidemic agents (high cholesterol)	1.7	6.5	11.4	1.5	7.1	12.0	1.8	5.8	10.8
Analgesics (pain relief)	7.2	9.4	9.0	5.4	7.3	7.7	9.0	11.3	10.2
Antidepressants (depression and related disorders)	1.8	6.4	8.9	1.2	4.4	5.0	2.3	8.3	12.7
Beta-adrenergic blocking agents (high blood pressure, heart disease)	3.1	4.4	7.3	2.7	4.1	6.8	3.5	4.6	7.6
Proton pump inhibitors (gastrointestinal reflux, ulcers)	*	3.8	6.3	*	3.4	5.6	*	4.2	6.9
ACE inhibitors (high blood pressure, heart disease)	2.4	4.6	5.9	2.4	4.7	6.3	2.4	4.5	5.6
Sex hormones (contraceptives, menopause, hot flashes)	...	...	...	...	...	...	9.9	15.3	9.7
Diuretics (high blood pressure, heart disease, kidney disease)	3.4	4.1	5.3	2.3	3.1	4.5	4.4	5.1	6.1
Thyroid drugs (hyper- and hypothyroidism)	2.3	4.0	5.2	0.8	1.5	1.7	3.7	6.3	8.5
Antidiabetic agents (diabetes)	2.6	3.7	5.2	2.5	3.7	4.8	2.6	3.8	5.5
Bronchodilators (asthma, breathing)	2.6	3.5	4.9	2.5	3.1	4.5	2.7	3.8	5.2
Anxiolytics, sedatives, and hypnotics (generalized anxiety and related disorders)	2.8	3.3	4.5	1.9	2.6	3.2	3.6	4.0	5.7
Antihypertensive combinations (high blood pressure)	2.4	2.9	4.1	1.4	1.9	3.0	3.3	3.8	5.1
Calcium channel blocking agents (high blood pressure, heart disease)	3.6	4.2	4.0	3.4	3.5	3.6	3.8	4.8	4.4
Antihistamines (allergies)	2.7	4.5	3.8	2.2	4.0	2.9	3.2	4.9	4.6
Under 18 years									
Bronchodilators (asthma, breathing)	3.0	4.0	5.4	3.3	4.4	6.0	2.7	3.6	4.7
Penicillins (bacterial infections)	6.1	5.1	3.8	5.9	5.2	3.4	6.4	5.0	4.2
CNS stimulants (attention deficit disorder, hyperactivity)	*0.8	2.9	3.7	*1.2	4.4	4.8	*	1.4	2.6
Antihistamines (allergies)	2.0	4.4	2.9	2.1	4.9	3.0	1.9	3.9	2.7
Leukotriene modifiers (asthma, allergies)	...	0.7	2.9	...	*0.9	3.3	...	*	*2.4
Upper respiratory combinations (cough and cold, congestion)	2.3	2.3	1.8	2.6	*2.4	1.6	2.0	*2.2	1.9
Respiratory inhalant products (asthma, chronic obstructive pulmonary disease, and related disorders)	*0.7	1.7	1.8	*	1.8	2.4	*	1.5	1.3
Adrenal cortical steroids (anti-inflammatory)	*0.5	0.8	1.6	*	*0.7	2.1	*0.5	0.9	1.1
Antidepressants (depression and related disorders)	*	1.8	1.5	*	2.2	*1.5	*	*1.5	*1.6
Analgesics (pain relief)	1.2	1.4	1.4	*1.2	1.3	1.0	1.4	1.6	2.0
Cephalosporins (bacterial infections)	1.8	1.2	1.1	1.8	*1.3	1.1	1.8	1.1	*1.2
Macrolide derivatives (bacterial infections)	1.0	1.2	*0.9	*0.7	*1.3	*1.1	*1.3	*1.1	*
18–44 years									
Antidepressants (depression and related disorders)	1.6	6.0	7.8	*1.0	3.6	3.6	2.3	8.5	11.9
Analgesics (pain relief)	7.2	8.0	7.7	5.1	6.0	6.5	9.1	9.9	8.9
Sex hormones (contraceptives, menopause, hot flashes)	...	...	...	...	...	...	11.7	13.7	15.7
Proton pump inhibitors (gastrointestinal reflux, ulcers)	*	2.3	3.5	*	2.4	2.8	*	2.2	4.2
Bronchodilators (asthma, breathing)	1.4	2.2	3.3	*1.1	1.6	2.3	*1.8	2.8	4.2
Antihistamines (allergies)	2.5	3.9	3.2	1.8	3.6	*1.7	3.2	4.2	4.6
Anxiolytics, sedatives, and hypnotics (generalized anxiety and related disorders)	1.4	2.1	3.2	*1.0	*1.7	2.1	1.9	2.5	4.3
Anticonvulsants (epilepsy, seizure, and related disorders)	0.8	1.6	2.9	*0.6	1.6	*2.0	1.0	*1.5	3.8
Thyroid drugs (hyper- and hypothyroidism)	1.4	1.8	2.8	*	*	*	2.1	3.0	4.9
Antihyperlipidemic agents (high cholesterol)	*0.4	1.3	2.5	*	2.0	3.1	*	*	*2.0
Antidiabetic agents (diabetes)	*1.0	1.5	2.1	*	*1.5	1.7	*1.0	*1.6	2.4
ACE inhibitors (high blood pressure, heart disease)	0.7	1.4	1.9	*0.9	1.5	1.7	*0.6	*1.2	2.0
Penicillins (bacterial infections)	3.1	2.2	1.8	2.3	1.8	*1.1	3.8	2.7	2.5
Muscle relaxants (muscle spasm and related disorders)	1.0	1.3	1.6	*1.3	*1.1	*1.1	*0.7	*1.4	2.0
Beta-adrenergic blocking agents (high blood pressure, heart disease)	1.1	*1.2	1.4	*0.9	*1.3	*1.2	1.3	*	1.5

See footnotes at end of table.

Table 95 (page 2 of 3). Selected prescription drug classes used in the past month, by sex and age: United States, selected years 1988–1994 through 2005–2008

[Data are based on a sample of the civilian noninstitutionalized population]

Age group and Multum Lexicon Plus® therapeutic class[1] (primary indications for use)	Total 1988–1994	Total 1999–2002	Total 2005–2008	Male 1988–1994	Male 1999–2002	Male 2005–2008	Female 1988–1994	Female 1999–2002	Female 2005–2008
	Percent of population with at least one prescription drug in drug class in past month								
45–64 years									
Antihyperlipidemic agents (high cholesterol)	4.3	13.8	19.6	4.4	17.2	21.2	4.2	10.7	18.0
Antidepressants (depression and related disorders)	3.5	10.5	15.3	*2.3	7.0	8.5	4.6	13.8	21.9
Analgesics (pain relief)	11.9	16.0	14.0	9.2	13.5	12.3	14.3	18.3	15.7
Beta-adrenergic blocking agents (high blood pressure, heart disease)	6.6	8.7	11.0	7.0	7.8	10.5	6.2	9.5	11.6
Proton pump inhibitors (gastrointestinal reflux, ulcers)	*	7.7	10.9	*	6.7	10.6	*	8.6	11.2
ACE inhibitors (high blood pressure, heart disease)	5.2	8.8	10.3	5.7	9.8	11.4	4.6	7.9	9.3
Antidiabetic agents (diabetes)	5.5	7.0	9.4	5.9	7.8	9.5	5.1	6.3	9.3
Thyroid drugs (hyper- and hypothyroidism)	4.7	6.6	8.5	*1.2	*2.7	*2.9	8.1	10.2	13.9
Sex hormones (contraceptives, menopause, hot flashes)	. . .	. . .	. . .	. . .	. . .	. . .	19.9	30.3	11.2
Antihypertensive combinations (high blood pressure)	5.3	5.6	8.1	3.3	*3.7	6.3	7.1	7.3	9.7
Anxiolytics, sedatives, and hypnotics (generalized anxiety and related disorders)	6.0	6.2	7.8	4.3	4.9	6.2	7.5	7.4	9.3
Diuretics (high blood pressure, heart disease, kidney disease)	6.1	6.6	6.7	4.8	4.8	6.0	7.3	8.3	7.5
Calcium channel blocking agents (high blood pressure, heart disease)	7.0	6.7	6.1	8.2	5.9	5.3	5.9	7.5	6.9
Anticonvulsants (epilepsy, seizure, and related disorders)	2.7	4.3	6.0	*2.5	3.5	5.0	2.9	5.1	7.0
65 years and over									
Antihyperlipidemic agents (high cholesterol)	5.9	23.4	44.5	5.3	24.3	50.6	6.4	22.7	40.0
Beta-adrenergic blocking agents (high blood pressure, heart disease)	11.8	15.9	32.0	10.4	17.5	34.8	12.8	14.8	29.9
Diuretics (high blood pressure, heart disease, kidney disease)	16.2	19.2	24.5	12.2	17.1	24.6	19.1	20.7	24.4
ACE inhibitors (high blood pressure, heart disease)	9.5	16.9	21.0	9.8	18.0	25.1	9.3	16.1	18.1
Analgesics (pain relief)	13.8	18.4	18.1	11.4	15.0	17.8	15.6	20.9	18.3
Calcium channel blocking agents (high blood pressure, heart disease)	16.1	19.1	17.1	14.5	17.4	17.3	17.3	20.4	17.0
Proton pump inhibitors (gastrointestinal reflux, ulcers)	*	9.7	17.0	*	9.2	16.9	*	10.1	17.1
Antidiabetic agents (diabetes)	9.0	12.4	16.0	9.0	12.9	15.9	9.0	12.0	16.1
Thyroid drugs (hyper- and hypothyroidism)	7.1	14.3	15.5	3.5	6.7	6.2	9.8	19.9	22.4
Antidepressants (depression and related disorders)	3.0	9.3	14.2	*2.3	7.2	10.0	3.5	10.8	17.3
Antihypertensive combinations (high blood pressure)	9.6	9.8	13.2	6.0	7.4	9.6	12.2	11.6	15.8
Angiotensin II inhibitors (high blood pressure, heart disease)	. . .	4.8	10.7	. . .	4.1	9.7	. . .	5.3	11.5
Anxiolytics, sedatives, and hypnotics (generalized anxiety and related disorders)	7.8	7.8	9.8	6.1	5.4	7.1	9.1	9.5	11.8
Bisphosphonates (osteoporosis and related disorders)	*	4.0	8.4	*	*	*	*	6.5	13.8
Antiadrenergic agents, peripherally acting (prostate conditions)[2]	. . .	. . .	. . .	2.8	12.5	15.9	. . .	. . .	. . .
65–74 years									
Antihyperlipidemic agents (high cholesterol)	7.3	26.2	44.3	6.2	26.6	52.1	8.1	25.9	38.2
Beta-adrenergic blocking agents (high blood pressure, heart disease)	11.3	14.8	29.0	10.6	16.0	32.2	11.9	13.9	26.4
Diuretics (high blood pressure, heart disease, kidney disease)	14.2	15.9	21.0	10.8	14.6	19.6	17.0	16.9	22.1
ACE inhibitors (high blood pressure, heart disease)	9.6	17.2	19.5	10.6	18.1	24.2	8.9	16.4	15.8
Analgesics (pain relief)	13.0	18.5	18.6	10.5	14.9	16.5	15.0	21.4	20.3
Antidiabetic agents (diabetes)	8.8	12.9	17.8	8.0	13.8	18.2	9.4	12.0	17.5
Proton pump inhibitors (gastrointestinal reflux, ulcers)	*	9.6	16.9	*	8.4	17.0	*	10.5	16.8
Antidepressants (depression and related disorders)	2.8	9.3	15.0	*2.3	5.8	9.6	3.1	12.1	19.3
Calcium channel blocking agents (high blood pressure, heart disease)	15.0	16.1	14.0	14.0	15.3	15.5	15.8	16.8	12.9
Antihypertensive combinations (high blood pressure)	8.1	8.0	13.7	4.8	*6.7	11.0	10.8	9.0	15.8
Thyroid drugs (hyper- and hypothyroidism)	6.6	13.1	13.1	*3.8	*5.0	4.3	8.9	19.9	19.9
Angiotensin II inhibitors (high blood pressure, heart disease)	. . .	4.2	9.7	. . .	*3.5	9.2	. . .	4.9	10.1
Anxiolytics, sedatives, and hypnotics (generalized anxiety and related disorders)	6.9	7.7	9.4	6.0	*4.2	6.8	7.6	10.5	11.4
Antiadrenergic agents, peripherally acting (prostate conditions)[2]	. . .	. . .	. . .	*2.6	13.1	13.1	. . .	. . .	. . .
Bisphosphonates (osteoporosis and related disorders)	*	*3.1	7.2	*	*	*	*	*5.3	12.5
Anticonvulsants (epilepsy, seizure, and related disorders)	3.0	4.2	7.1	*2.7	*3.6	5.7	3.2	*4.7	8.2

See footnotes at end of table.

Table 95 (page 3 of 3). Selected prescription drug classes used in the past month, by sex and age: United States, selected years 1988–1994 through 2005–2008

[Data are based on a sample of the civilian noninstitutionalized population]

Age group and Multum Lexicon Plus® therapeutic class[1] (primary indications for use)	Total			Male			Female		
	1988–1994	1999–2002	2005–2008	1988–1994	1999–2002	2005–2008	1988–1994	1999–2002	2005–2008
75 years and over	Percent of population with at least one prescription drug in drug class in past month								
Antihyperlipidemic agents (high cholesterol)	3.8	19.9	44.8	*3.5	21.1	48.7	4.0	19.2	42.0
Beta-adrenergic blocking agents (high blood pressure, heart disease)	12.5	17.3	35.6	9.8	19.6	38.1	14.1	15.8	33.8
Diuretics (high blood pressure, heart disease, kidney disease)	19.2	23.2	28.7	14.7	20.5	31.1	21.9	24.9	27.0
ACE inhibitors (high blood pressure, heart disease)	9.3	16.4	22.9	8.5	17.7	26.2	9.8	15.6	20.6
Calcium channel blocking agents (high blood pressure, heart disease)	17.8	22.8	20.8	15.3	20.5	19.6	19.2	24.2	21.6
Thyroid drugs (hyper- and hypothyroidism)	8.0	15.8	18.5	3.0	9.2	8.7	10.9	20.0	25.2
Analgesics (pain relief)	15.1	18.4	17.5	13.0	15.1	19.5	16.3	20.4	16.1
Proton pump inhibitors (gastrointestinal reflux, ulcers)	*	9.9	17.3	*	10.2	16.8	*	9.8	17.6
Antidiabetic agents (diabetes)	9.3	11.8	13.9	10.7	11.5	12.9	8.5	12.0	14.5
Antidepressants (depression and related disorders)	3.4	9.3	13.3	*2.3	9.2	10.6	4.0	9.4	15.1
Antihypertensive combinations (high blood pressure)	11.9	12.0	12.6	8.3	*8.2	7.8	14.0	14.4	15.9
Antiplatelet agents (blood thinning, reduce or prevent blood clots)	4.4	5.0	11.7	*4.2	6.7	14.6	4.6	3.9	9.7
Angiotensin II inhibitors (high blood pressure, heart disease)	. . .	5.4	11.9	. . .	*4.9	10.2	. . .	5.8	13.0
Anticoagulants (blood thinning, reduce or prevent blood clots)	2.9	7.2	10.4	3.7	7.6	14.3	*2.4	6.9	7.7
Anxiolytics, sedatives, and hypnotics (generalized anxiety and related disorders)	9.2	7.9	10.3	6.3	7.1	7.5	10.9	8.4	12.3
Bisphosphonates (osteoporosis and related disorders)	*	5.1	10.0	*	*	*	*	7.9	15.4
Minerals and electrolytes mineral deficiencies)	7.5	8.1	8.4	5.6	6.6	6.8	8.7	9.0	9.6
Antiadrenergic agents, peripherally acting (prostate conditions)[2]	. . .	. . .	. . .	*3.1	11.7	19.5	. . .	. . .	. . .

* Estimates are considered unreliable. Data preceded by an asterisk have a relative standard error (RSE) of 20%–30%. Data not shown have an RSE greater than 30%.

. . . Category not applicable.

[1]The drug therapeutic class is based on Lexicon Plus®, a proprietary database of Cerner Multum, Inc. Lexicon Plus is a comprehensive database of all prescription and some nonprescription drug products available in the U.S. drug market. Data on prescription drug use are collected by the National Health and Nutrition Examination Survey. Respondents were asked if they had taken a prescription drug in the past month. Those who answered "yes" were asked to show the interviewer the medication containers for all prescriptions. If no container was available, the respondent was asked to verbally report the name of the medication. Each drug's complete name was recorded and classified. Data presented here are based on the second level classification of prescription drugs. Up to four classes are assigned to each drug. Drugs classified into more than one class were counted in each class. For more information, see http://www.cdc.gov/nchs/nhanes/nhanes2007-2008/RXQ_DRUG.htm. See Appendix II, Multum Lexicon Plus® therapeutic class.

[2]Although some antiadrenergic agents are used to treat high blood pressure, they are generally used currently to treat prostate hyperplasia and related conditions.

NOTES: Some drug classes were not available in 1988–1994 and are coded as not applicable. See Appendix II, Drug. Standard errors are available in the spreadsheet version of this table. Available from: http://www.cdc.gov/nchs/hus.htm. Data for additional years are available. See Appendix III.

SOURCE: CDC/NCHS, National Health and Nutrition Examination Survey.

Table 96 (page 1 of 2). Dietary supplement use among persons 20 years of age and over, by selected characteristics: United States, selected years 1988–1994 through 2005–2008

[Data are based on interviews of a sample of the civilian noninstitutionalized population]

Sex, age, race and Hispanic origin[1], and percent of poverty level	Any supplement use in past month[2]			Any vitamin D supplement use in past month[3]			Any folate (folic acid) supplement use in past month[4]		
	1988–1994	1999–2002	2005–2008	1988–1994	1999–2002	2005–2008	1988–1994	1999–2002	2005–2008
20 years and over, age-adjusted[5]				Percent of population					
Both sexes[6]	42.1	52.3	50.9	28.4	37.3	38.0	30.3	38.1	37.5
Male	35.7	46.8	44.4	24.3	31.8	32.2	26.2	33.6	32.9
Female	47.8	57.4	56.9	32.2	42.3	43.4	34.2	42.2	42.0
Not Hispanic or Latino:									
White only, male	37.5	52.1	48.7	26.1	35.7	35.8	28.2	37.7	36.6
White only, female	50.9	63.4	61.3	35.4	48.3	47.7	37.7	48.2	46.1
Black or African American only, male	29.5	30.4	31.0	18.5	19.8	22.6	18.2	20.7	23.0
Black or African American only, female	38.2	39.7	43.0	22.7	26.6	30.5	23.7	27.5	30.3
Mexican male	28.9	31.2	30.0	17.1	19.3	19.6	18.6	21.1	19.2
Mexican female	36.8	44.0	41.5	21.9	29.2	28.1	23.3	27.9	26.5
Percent of poverty level:[7]									
Below 100%	30.0	37.8	33.5	16.8	24.5	23.2	18.3	24.1	21.7
100%–199%	36.0	42.7	43.9	23.3	27.7	30.3	24.1	27.7	30.4
200%–399%	44.0	53.6	52.5	30.2	38.7	39.4	32.5	39.6	38.8
400% or more	51.0	63.9	60.8	35.8	48.0	47.7	38.5	49.2	47.3
20 years and over, crude									
Both sexes[6]	41.8	52.1	51.3	28.4	37.3	38.3	30.3	38.0	37.8
Male	35.3	46.2	44.2	24.2	31.6	32.1	26.0	33.4	32.8
Female	47.7	57.6	57.8	32.2	42.5	44.1	34.3	42.3	42.5
Not Hispanic or Latino:									
White only, male	37.4	52.4	49.7	26.0	36.0	36.4	28.1	38.0	37.3
White only, female	51.1	64.1	63.3	35.4	48.9	49.1	37.7	48.5	47.2
Black or African American only, male	28.9	29.7	30.3	18.8	19.6	22.6	18.5	20.5	22.7
Black or African American only, female	37.0	39.5	42.4	22.9	26.5	30.4	23.9	27.6	30.1
Mexican male	25.6	27.0	24.1	15.5	17.0	16.0	17.1	18.3	15.7
Mexican female	34.9	40.1	37.6	21.9	26.5	26.5	23.1	26.1	25.8
Percent of poverty level:[7]									
Below 100%	29.4	36.3	31.9	17.1	23.7	22.4	18.4	23.6	21.2
100%–199%	36.8	43.5	45.2	24.0	28.1	31.3	24.9	28.0	31.1
200%–399%	43.6	53.2	53.1	30.4	38.3	39.9	32.7	39.3	39.1
400% or more	50.8	63.7	61.0	36.0	47.9	47.6	38.7	49.4	47.3
Male									
20–34 years	31.0	34.4	31.2	21.9	24.3	22.9	23.5	24.7	23.0
35–44 years	36.8	45.0	38.4	26.3	30.8	29.2	28.5	34.0	29.6
45–54 years	32.8	48.8	47.0	23.6	35.1	32.4	25.3	37.1	33.9
55–64 years	42.9	57.0	56.6	28.1	39.1	42.1	30.2	40.9	43.0
65–74 years	39.4	59.9	60.0	24.4	36.8	43.7	26.3	39.4	44.3
75 years and over	40.9	59.2	64.0	23.0	36.0	44.7	24.1	37.7	45.1
Female									
20–34 years	43.6	47.7	44.4	33.1	35.3	35.6	35.5	37.0	35.6
35–44 years	46.5	54.3	49.7	32.2	39.0	37.9	34.8	40.7	38.2
45–54 years	47.8	60.4	60.3	32.3	45.6	44.9	33.7	46.1	43.2
55–64 years	52.3	66.7	70.2	33.4	50.6	53.8	35.8	48.2	52.0
65–74 years	52.9	66.4	75.5	30.0	48.7	57.7	31.2	43.6	52.1
75 years and over	54.0	68.2	71.1	29.8	48.9	50.6	30.7	44.8	44.8

See footnotes at end of table.

Table 96 (page 2 of 2). Dietary supplement use among persons 20 years of age and over, by selected characteristics: United States, selected years 1988–1994 through 2005–2008

[Data are based on interviews of a sample of the civilian noninstitutionalized population]

[1]Persons of Mexican origin may be of any race. Starting with 1999 data, race-specific estimates are tabulated according to the 1997 Revisions to the Standards for the Classification of Federal Data on Race and Ethnicity and are not strictly comparable with estimates for earlier years. The two non-Hispanic race categories shown in the table conform to the 1997 Standards. Starting with 1999 data, race-specific estimates are for persons who reported only one racial group. Prior to data year 1999, estimates were tabulated according to the 1977 Standards. Estimates for single-race categories prior to 1999 included persons who reported one race or, if they reported more than one race, identified one race as best representing their race. See Appendix II, Hispanic origin; Race.

[2]Respondents were asked "Have you used or taken any vitamins, minerals, or other dietary supplements in the past month?" To facilitate their response, respondents were shown a card with some examples of different types of dietary supplements. The question wording differs slightly on the earlier, 1988–1994, survey. See Appendix II, Dietary supplement.

[3]Includes supplements with vitamin D, cholecalciferol, calciferol, ergocalciferol, or calcitriol as an ingredient.

[4]Includes supplements with folate or folic acid as an ingredient.

[5]Age-adjusted to the 2000 standard population using five age groups: 20–34 years, 35–44 years, 45–54 years, 55–64 years, and 65 years and over. Age-adjusted estimates may differ from other age-adjusted estimates based on the same data and presented elsewhere if different age groups are used in the adjustment procedure. See Appendix II, Age adjustment.

[6]Includes persons of all races and Hispanic origins, not just those shown separately.

[7]Percent of poverty level is based on family income and family size. Persons with unknown percent of poverty level are excluded (5% in 2005–2008). See Appendix II, Family income; Poverty.

NOTES: For more information see Appendix II, Dietary supplement. Standard errors are available in the spreadsheet version of this table. Available from: http://www.cdc.gov/nchs/hus.htm. Data for additional years are available. See Appendix III. Data have been revised and differ from previous editions of *Health, United States*.

SOURCE: CDC/NCHS, National Health and Nutrition Examination Survey.

Table 97. Admissions to mental health organizations, by type of service and organization: United States, selected years 1986–2004

[Data are based on inventories of mental health organizations]

Service and organization	1986	1990	2002	2004	1986	1990	2002	2004
24-hour hospital and residential treatment	Admissions in thousands[1]				Admissions per 100,000 civilian population[2]			
All organizations	1,819	2,110	2,158	2,713	759.9	833.0	738.9	910.5
State and county mental hospitals.	333	283	234	266	139.1	111.6	80.1	89.1
Private psychiatric hospitals	235	411	477	599	98.0	162.4	163.3	200.9
Nonfederal general hospital psychiatric services[3]	849	962	1,087	1,533	354.8	379.9	372.2	514.6
Department of Veterans Affairs medical centers[4]	180	203	158	- - -	75.1	80.3	54.1	- - -
Residential treatment centers for emotionally disturbed children	25	50	63	61	10.2	19.8	21.6	20.3
All other organizations[5]	198	200	139	255	82.7	79.0	47.6	85.5
Less than 24-hour care[6]								
All organizations	2,955	3,377	4,099	4,667	1,233.4	1,333.3	1,403.2	1,566.6
State and county mental hospitals.	68	50	62	130	28.4	19.7	21.2	43.6
Private psychiatric hospitals	132	163	598	447	55.2	64.5	204.7	150.1
Nonfederal general hospital psychiatric services	533	661	681	900	222.4	260.8	233.0	302.2
Department of Veterans Affairs medical centers[4]	133	235	99	- - -	55.3	92.8	33.9	- - -
Residential treatment centers for emotionally disturbed children	67	100	222	194	28.1	39.3	75.8	65.2
All other organizations[5]	2,022	2,168	2,438	2,995	844.0	856.2	834.3	1,005.4

- - - Data not available.

[1]Admissions sometimes are referred to as additions. See Appendix II, Admission.

[2]Civilian population estimates for 2000 and beyond are based on the 2000 census as of July 1; population estimates for 1992–1998 are 1990 postcensal estimates.

[3]These data exclude mental health care provided in nonpsychiatric units of hospitals such as general medical units.

[4]Department of Veterans Affairs medical centers (VA general hospital psychiatric services and VA psychiatric outpatient clinics) were dropped from the survey as of 2004.

[5]Includes freestanding psychiatric outpatient clinics, partial care organizations, and multiservice mental health organizations. See Appendix I, Survey of Mental Health Organizations.

[6]Formerly reported as partial care and outpatient treatment, the survey format was changed in 1994 and the reporting of these services was combined due to similarities in the care provided. These data exclude private office-based mental health care.

NOTES: Data for additional years are available. See Appendix III.

SOURCE: Substance Abuse and Mental Health Services Administration, Center for Mental Health Services (CMHS). Revised 1990, 1992, 1994, 1998, 2000, and 2002 estimates from the Survey of Mental Health Organizations; 2004 Survey of Mental Health Organizations, unpublished data.

Table 98 (page 1 of 3). Persons with hospital stays in the past year, by selected characteristics: United States, selected years 1997–2009

[Data are based on household interviews of a sample of the civilian noninstitutionalized population]

Characteristic	One or more hospital stays[1]				Two or more hospital stays[1]			
	1997	2000	2008	2009	1997	2000	2008	2009
	Percent							
1 year and over, age-adjusted[2,3]	7.8	7.6	7.2	7.3	1.8	1.8	1.8	1.8
1 year and over, crude[2]	7.7	7.5	7.3	7.4	1.7	1.8	1.8	1.9
Age								
1–17 years	2.8	2.5	2.6	2.2	0.5	0.4	0.5	0.4
1–5 years	3.9	3.8	3.9	3.3	0.7	0.7	0.8	0.7
6–17 years	2.3	1.9	2.0	1.8	0.4	0.3	0.3	0.3
18–44 years	7.4	7.0	6.4	6.7	1.2	1.1	1.1	1.2
18–24 years	7.9	7.0	5.4	6.3	1.3	1.1	0.8	1.1
25–44 years	7.3	7.0	6.8	6.8	1.2	1.2	1.2	1.3
45–64 years	8.2	8.4	7.9	8.5	2.2	2.2	2.4	2.4
45–54 years	6.9	7.3	6.9	7.4	1.7	1.8	2.1	2.1
55–64 years	10.2	10.0	9.2	9.9	2.9	2.8	2.8	2.8
65 years and over	18.0	18.2	17.5	17.1	5.4	5.8	5.7	5.2
65–74 years	16.1	16.1	14.2	14.3	4.8	4.9	4.5	4.2
75 years and over	20.4	20.7	21.3	20.4	6.2	6.8	7.1	6.4
75–84 years	19.8	20.1	19.2	19.0	6.1	6.2	6.3	5.8
85 years and over	22.8	23.4	27.4	24.8	6.2	9.0	9.4	7.9
1–64 years								
Total, 1–64 years[2,4]	6.3	6.1	5.7	5.9	1.3	1.2	1.2	1.3
Sex								
Male, crude	4.4	4.2	4.2	4.4	0.9	1.0	1.1	1.1
1–17 years	2.9	2.4	2.8	2.3	0.6	0.4	0.5	0.5
18–44 years	3.6	3.1	3.2	3.4	0.6	0.6	0.6	0.8
45–54 years	6.0	7.0	5.8	6.2	1.4	1.8	2.0	2.0
55–64 years	11.1	10.2	8.5	9.7	3.0	3.0	2.6	2.6
Female, crude	8.0	7.9	7.5	7.7	1.6	1.5	1.5	1.6
1–17 years	2.6	2.5	2.3	2.1	0.5	0.4	0.4	*0.3
18–44 years	11.2	10.8	9.7	9.9	1.8	1.7	1.5	1.7
45–54 years	7.6	7.6	7.9	8.5	2.0	1.9	2.2	2.2
55–64 years	9.4	9.8	9.9	10.1	2.9	2.7	2.9	3.0
Race[4,5]								
White only	6.2	5.9	5.5	5.8	1.2	1.1	1.1	1.2
Black or African American only	7.6	7.4	7.1	6.9	1.9	1.9	2.0	1.8
American Indian or Alaska Native only	7.6	7.0	8.4	8.8	*	*	*	*
Asian only	3.9	3.9	4.0	3.6	*0.5	*0.6	*0.6	*0.6
Native Hawaiian or Other Pacific Islander only	- - -	*	*	*	- - -	*	*	*
2 or more races	- - -	8.8	8.4	7.2	- - -	*1.6	*	*2.2
Hispanic origin and race[4,5]								
Hispanic or Latino	6.8	5.5	5.1	5.7	1.3	0.9	1.0	1.4
Not Hispanic or Latino	6.2	6.1	5.8	5.9	1.3	1.3	1.3	1.3
White only	6.1	6.0	5.6	5.8	1.2	1.2	1.2	1.2
Black or African American only	7.5	7.4	7.2	6.9	1.9	1.9	2.0	1.8
Percent of poverty level[4,6]								
Below 100%	10.3	9.1	8.9	9.5	2.8	2.6	2.8	2.9
100%–199%	7.3	7.3	6.9	7.1	1.7	1.9	1.9	2.0
200%–399%	6.0	6.0	5.6	5.6	1.2	1.1	1.0	1.1
400% or more	4.7	5.0	4.5	4.4	0.7	0.8	0.7	0.7
Hispanic origin and race and percent of poverty level[4,5,6]								
Hispanic or Latino:								
Below 100%	9.1	7.4	7.2	8.0	2.0	1.6	1.8	1.9
100%–199%	5.9	5.4	5.5	5.9	1.0	0.8	1.1	2.0
200%–399%	5.9	4.6	3.7	4.9	1.1	0.7	*0.6	1.0
400% or more	5.5	4.7	4.5	3.8	*1.1	*0.6	*0.8	*0.9
Not Hispanic or Latino:								
White only:								
Below 100%	10.7	9.6	9.6	10.2	3.2	2.7	3.3	3.4
100%–199%	7.7	7.8	7.1	7.7	1.8	2.2	2.1	2.2
200%–399%	6.1	6.1	5.9	5.8	1.2	1.1	1.1	1.0
400% or more	4.7	5.0	4.5	4.6	0.7	0.8	0.7	0.8
Black or African American only:								
Below 100%	11.4	10.8	10.0	10.3	3.3	3.4	3.7	3.2
100%–199%	8.0	8.5	8.2	7.4	2.1	2.3	2.5	2.0
200%–399%	6.2	6.1	6.1	5.8	1.5	1.3	1.3	1.6
400% or more	4.7	5.8	5.2	4.6	*0.9	*1.3	*1.4	*0.8

See footnotes at end of table.

Table 98 (page 2 of 3). Persons with hospital stays in the past year, by selected characteristics: United States, selected years 1997–2009

[Data are based on household interviews of a sample of the civilian noninstitutionalized population]

Characteristic	One or more hospital stays[1]				Two or more hospital stays[1]			
	1997	2000	2008	2009	1997	2000	2008	2009
Health insurance status at the time of interview[4,7]	Percent							
Insured	6.6	6.4	6.0	6.3	1.3	1.3	1.3	1.3
Private	5.6	5.5	4.9	4.9	1.0	1.0	0.8	0.8
Medicaid	16.1	15.9	13.0	14.5	4.9	4.7	4.5	4.6
Uninsured	4.8	4.5	4.3	4.2	1.0	0.9	0.9	1.0
Health insurance status prior to interview[4,7]								
Insured continuously all 12 months	6.5	6.3	5.9	6.2	1.3	1.2	1.2	1.3
Uninsured for any period up to 12 months	8.5	8.4	8.6	7.3	1.8	1.9	2.0	2.0
Uninsured more than 12 months	3.8	3.5	3.2	3.5	0.8	0.8	0.7	0.9
Percent of poverty level and health insurance status prior to interview[4,6,7]								
Below 100%:								
Insured continuously all 12 months	12.4	10.7	10.5	11.9	3.7	3.1	3.6	3.7
Uninsured for any period up to 12 months	13.7	13.4	13.8	11.9	3.4	*3.4	5.0	*3.1
Uninsured more than 12 months	4.9	5.0	3.9	4.6	1.0	*1.6	*0.8	1.3
100%–199%:								
Insured continuously all 12 months	8.5	8.6	8.0	8.7	2.0	2.3	2.5	2.5
Uninsured for any period up to 12 months	9.3	9.1	8.7	8.0	*1.9	*2.2	*1.4	2.6
Uninsured more than 12 months	3.8	3.2	3.7	3.2	*0.7	*0.7	*0.8	*0.8
200%–399%:								
Insured continuously all 12 months	6.3	6.4	5.9	6.1	1.3	1.2	1.1	1.1
Uninsured for any period up to 12 months	7.0	6.6	7.9	5.9	*1.5	*1.3	*1.3	*1.4
Uninsured more than 12 months	3.3	2.8	2.6	3.2	*0.7	*0.4	*	*
400% or more:								
Insured continuously all 12 months	4.9	5.1	4.6	4.5	0.7	0.8	0.7	0.7
Uninsured for any period up to 12 months	3.9	6.0	5.8	3.8	*	*	*1.6	*
Uninsured more than 12 months	*	*2.1	*1.5	*2.4	*	*	*	*
Disability measure among adults 18–64 years[4,8]								
Any basic actions difficulty or complex activity limitation	14.1	15.1	13.8	15.4	4.1	4.4	4.0	5.1
Any basic actions difficulty	13.9	15.1	13.5	15.0	4.1	4.4	3.8	5.0
Any complex activity limitation	21.5	22.6	20.6	23.0	7.7	8.8	7.9	8.7
No disability	5.8	5.6	4.7	5.2	0.6	0.7	0.7	0.6
Geographic region[4]								
Northeast	6.0	5.5	5.4	5.4	1.2	1.0	1.1	1.0
Midwest	6.5	6.3	5.9	6.6	1.5	1.3	1.2	1.6
South	6.8	6.6	6.3	6.2	1.4	1.5	1.5	1.4
West	5.4	5.2	4.8	4.9	0.8	0.9	0.9	1.0
Location of residence[4]								
Within MSA[9]	6.1	5.8	5.6	5.7	1.2	1.1	1.2	1.2
Outside MSA[9]	7.0	6.9	6.3	6.9	1.6	1.5	1.5	1.8
65 years and over								
Total 65 years and over[2,10]	18.1	18.3	17.6	17.2	5.4	5.8	5.7	5.2
65–74 years	16.1	16.1	14.2	14.3	4.8	4.9	4.5	4.2
75 years and over	20.4	20.7	21.3	20.4	6.2	6.8	7.1	6.4
Sex[10]								
Male	19.0	19.5	18.6	18.1	5.8	5.8	6.1	5.5
Female	17.5	17.4	16.8	16.6	5.1	5.7	5.4	5.0

See footnotes at end of table.

Table 98 (page 3 of 3). Persons with hospital stays in the past year, by selected characteristics: United States, selected years 1997–2009

[Data are based on household interviews of a sample of the civilian noninstitutionalized population]

Characteristic	One or more hospital stays[1]				Two or more hospital stays[1]			
	1997	2000	2008	2009	1997	2000	2008	2009
Hispanic origin and race[5,10]	Percent							
Hispanic or Latino	17.3	16.6	16.9	14.3	6.2	6.4	5.3	4.4
Not Hispanic or Latino	18.2	18.4	17.6	17.4	5.4	5.8	5.8	5.3
White only	18.3	18.4	17.9	17.4	5.4	5.7	5.8	5.2
Black or African American only	18.9	19.8	18.5	19.4	5.5	7.5	7.4	6.7
Percent of poverty level[6,10]								
Below 100%	20.9	20.9	21.4	19.5	6.4	7.5	9.1	6.3
100%–199%	19.6	19.2	18.8	18.7	6.5	6.6	6.6	6.4
200%–399%	17.3	18.1	17.3	16.4	4.9	5.8	5.8	4.7
400% or more	16.6	16.0	15.8	16.7	4.7	4.2	4.0	4.8
Disability measure[8,10]								
Any basic actions difficulty or complex activity limitation	22.6	24.7	23.8	24.3	7.2	8.6	9.0	8.4
Any basic actions difficulty	22.7	24.7	23.8	24.5	7.2	8.7	8.8	8.6
Any complex activity limitation	29.0	31.5	31.0	31.4	10.8	12.2	13.5	11.6
No disability	7.8	9.7	8.1	7.7	1.1	1.9	*1.7	*1.3
Geographic region[10]								
Northeast	17.2	16.6	17.0	17.5	5.1	4.5	5.0	5.1
Midwest	18.2	19.5	18.9	18.2	5.6	7.2	6.0	5.5
South	19.4	19.5	19.1	17.7	6.1	6.3	6.6	5.9
West	16.5	16.4	13.9	14.9	4.4	4.4	4.5	4.0
Location of residence[10]								
Within MSA[9]	17.8	17.8	17.4	16.8	5.2	5.4	5.7	5.0
Outside MSA[9]	19.1	19.6	18.1	18.8	6.3	6.9	6.0	6.1

* Estimates are considered unreliable. Data preceded by an asterisk have a relative standard error (RSE) of 20%–30%. Data not shown have an RSE of greater than 30%.

- - - Data not available.

[1]These estimates exclude hospitalizations for institutionalized persons and those who died while hospitalized. See Appendix II, Hospital utilization.

[2]Includes all other races not shown separately, unknown health insurance status, and unknown disability status.

[3]Estimates are for persons 1 year of age and over and are age-adjusted to the year 2000 standard population using six age groups: 1–17 years, 18–44 years, 45–54 years, 55–64 years, 65–74 years, and 75 years and over. See Appendix II, Age adjustment.

[4]Estimates are for persons 1–64 years of age and are age-adjusted to the year 2000 standard population using four age groups: 1–17 years, 18–44 years, 45–54 years, and 55–64 years. The disability measure is age-adjusted using the three adult age groups. See Appendix II, Age adjustment.

[5]The race groups, white, black, American Indian or Alaska Native, Asian, Native Hawaiian or Other Pacific Islander, and 2 or more races, include persons of Hispanic and non-Hispanic origin. Persons of Hispanic origin may be of any race. Starting with 1999 data, race-specific estimates are tabulated according to the 1997 Revisions to the Standards for Federal Data on Race and Ethnicity and are not strictly comparable with estimates for earlier years. The five single-race categories plus multiple-race categories shown in the table conform to the 1997 Standards. Starting with 1999 data, race-specific estimates are for persons who reported only one racial group; the category 2 or more races includes persons who reported more than one racial group. Prior to 1999, data were tabulated according to the 1977 Standards with four racial groups, and the Asian only category included Native Hawaiian or Other Pacific Islander. Estimates for single-race categories prior to 1999 included persons who reported one race or, if they reported more than one race, identified one race as best representing their race. Starting with 2003 data, race responses of other race and unspecified multiple race were treated as missing, and then race was imputed if these were the only race responses. Almost all persons with a race response of other race were of Hispanic origin. See Appendix II, Hispanic origin; Race.

[6]Percent of poverty level is based on family income and family size and composition using U.S. Census Bureau poverty thresholds. Missing family income data were imputed for 1997 and beyond. See Appendix II, Family income; Poverty; Table VII.

[7]Health insurance categories are mutually exclusive. Persons who reported both Medicaid and private coverage are classified as having private coverage. Starting with 1997 data, state-sponsored health plan coverage is included as Medicaid coverage. Starting with 1999 data, coverage by the Children's Health Insurance Program (CHIP) is included with Medicaid coverage. In addition to private and Medicaid, the insured category also includes military, other government, and Medicare coverage. Persons not covered by private insurance, Medicaid, CHIP, state-sponsored or other government-sponsored health plans (starting in 1997), Medicare, or military plans are considered to have no health insurance coverage. Persons with only Indian Health Service coverage are considered to have no health insurance coverage. See Appendix II, Health insurance coverage.

[8]Any basic actions difficulty or complex activity limitation is defined as having one or more of the following limitations or difficulties: movement difficulty, emotional difficulty, sensory (seeing or hearing) difficulty, cognitive difficulty, self-care (ADL or IADL) limitation, social limitation, or work limitation. For more information, see Appendix II, Basic actions difficulty; Complex activity limitation. Starting with 2007 data, the hearing question, a component of the basic actions difficulty measure, was revised. Consequently, data prior to 2007 are not comparable with data for 2007 and beyond. For more information on the impact of the revised hearing question, see Appendix II, Hearing trouble.

[9]MSA is metropolitan statistical area. Starting with 2006 data, MSA status is determined using 2000 census data and the 2000 standards for defining MSAs. For data prior to 2006, see Appendix II, Metropolitan statistical area (MSA) for the applicable standards.

[10]Estimates are for persons 65 years of age and over and are age-adjusted to the year 2000 standard population using two age groups: 65–74 years and 75 years and over. See Appendix II, Age adjustment.

NOTES: Standard errors are available in the spreadsheet version of this table. Available from: http://www.cdc.gov/nchs/hus.htm. Data for additional years are available. See Appendix III.

SOURCE: CDC/NCHS, National Health Interview Survey, family core and sample adult questionnaires.

Table 99 (page 1 of 3). Discharges, days of care, and average length of stay in nonfederal short-stay hospitals, by selected characteristics: United States, selected years 1980–2007

[Data are based on a sample of hospital records]

Characteristic	1980[1]	1985[1]	1990	1995	2000	2005	2006	2007
	Discharges per 10,000 population							
Total, age-adjusted[2]	1,744.5	1,522.3	1,252.4	1,180.2	1,132.8	1,162.4	1,153.1	1,124.0
Total, crude.	1,676.8	1,484.1	1,222.7	1,157.4	1,128.3	1,174.4	1,168.7	1,143.9
Age								
Under 18 years	756.5	614.0	463.5	423.7	402.6	411.0	393.9	376.7
Under 1 year	2,317.6	2,137.9	1,915.3	1,977.6	2,027.6	1,949.3	1,818.4	1,639.3
1–4 years	864.6	650.2	466.9	457.1	458.0	429.7	418.8	389.9
5–17 years	609.3	477.4	334.1	290.2	268.6	286.5	276.0	271.5
18–44 years	1,578.8	1,301.2	1,026.6	914.3	849.4	898.0	906.7	888.8
18–24 years	1,570.3	1,297.8	1,065.3	928.9	854.1	862.4	870.4	846.1
25–44 years	1,582.8	1,302.5	1,013.8	909.9	847.9	910.3	919.3	903.8
25–34 years	1,682.9	1,416.9	1,140.3	1,015.0	942.5	1,007.8	1,011.2	1,003.5
35–44 years	1,438.3	1,153.1	868.8	808.0	764.8	821.5	834.6	810.4
45–64 years	1,947.6	1,707.8	1,354.5	1,185.4	1,114.2	1,147.0	1,161.2	1,143.9
45–54 years	1,750.2	1,470.7	1,123.9	984.7	920.8	964.3	970.5	959.3
55–64 years	2,153.6	1,948.0	1,632.6	1,483.4	1,415.0	1,402.4	1,422.1	1,391.2
65 years and over	3,836.9	3,698.0	3,341.2	3,477.4	3,533.6	3,595.6	3,507.9	3,395.1
65–74 years	3,158.4	2,972.6	2,616.3	2,600.0	2,546.0	2,628.9	2,533.6	2,439.9
75 years and over	4,893.0	4,756.1	4,340.3	4,590.7	4,619.6	4,588.4	4,512.6	4,392.4
75–84 years	4,638.6	4,464.2	3,957.0	4,155.7	4,124.4	4,131.7	4,025.9	3,983.3
85 years and over	5,764.6	5,728.9	5,606.3	5,925.1	6,050.9	5,758.1	5,711.4	5,358.9
Sex[2]								
Male	1,543.9	1,382.5	1,130.0	1,048.5	990.8	1,013.0	1,000.5	973.8
Female.	1,951.9	1,675.6	1,389.5	1,317.3	1,277.3	1,319.6	1,312.3	1,280.6
Sex and age								
Male, all ages	1,390.4	1,240.2	1,002.2	941.7	910.6	959.0	954.9	936.7
Under 18 years	762.6	626.4	463.1	431.3	408.6	412.2	401.5	385.6
18–44 years	950.9	776.9	579.2	507.2	450.0	471.1	476.8	460.8
45–64 years	1,953.1	1,775.6	1,402.7	1,212.0	1,127.4	1,148.8	1,175.7	1,156.6
65–74 years	3,474.1	3,255.2	2,877.6	2,762.2	2,649.1	2,742.6	2,584.3	2,559.3
75–84 years	5,093.5	5,031.8	4,417.3	4,361.1	4,294.1	4,388.1	4,220.3	4,162.6
85 years and over	6,372.3	6,406.9	6,420.9	6,387.9	6,166.6	5,984.1	5,983.5	5,440.6
Female, all ages	1,944.0	1,712.2	1,431.7	1,362.9	1,336.6	1,382.2	1,375.3	1,344.0
Under 18 years	750.2	601.0	464.1	415.7	396.2	409.8	385.9	367.3
18–44 years	2,180.2	1,808.3	1,468.0	1,318.0	1,248.1	1,330.9	1,343.5	1,324.5
45–64 years	1,942.5	1,645.9	1,309.7	1,160.5	1,101.7	1,145.3	1,147.3	1,131.7
65–74 years	2,916.6	2,754.8	2,411.2	2,469.4	2,461.0	2,533.1	2,490.7	2,338.4
75–84 years	4,370.4	4,130.4	3,678.9	4,024.1	4,013.5	3,957.7	3,893.0	3,859.8
85 years and over	5,500.3	5,458.0	5,289.6	5,743.7	6,003.3	5,654.4	5,584.1	5,320.0
Geographic region[2]								
Northeast	1,622.9	1,428.7	1,332.2	1,335.3	1,274.8	1,245.9	1,261.4	1,274.6
Midwest	1,925.2	1,584.7	1,287.5	1,132.8	1,109.2	1,174.9	1,168.0	1,125.5
South.	1,814.1	1,569.4	1,325.0	1,252.4	1,209.2	1,202.5	1,198.8	1,139.9
West	1,519.7	1,469.6	1,006.6	967.4	894.0	1,005.9	964.1	966.0

See footnotes at end of table.

Table 99 (page 2 of 3). Discharges, days of care, and average length of stay in nonfederal short-stay hospitals, by selected characteristics: United States, selected years 1980–2007

[Data are based on a sample of hospital records]

Characteristic	1980[1]	1985[1]	1990	1995	2000	2005	2006	2007
	Days of care per 10,000 population							
Total, age-adjusted[2]	13,027.0	10,017.9	8,189.3	6,386.2	5,576.8	5,541.7	5,474.7	5,404.1
Total, crude.	12,166.8	9,576.6	7,840.5	6,201.7	5,546.5	5,620.9	5,577.8	5,539.4
Age								
Under 18 years.	3,415.1	2,812.3	2,263.1	1,846.7	1,789.7	1,918.3	1,857.6	1,785.0
Under 1 year.	13,213.9	14,141.2	11,484.7	10,834.5	11,524.0	12,131.6	11,624.2	8,466.7
1–4 years	3,333.5	2,280.4	1,700.1	1,525.6	1,482.2	1,355.3	1,405.4	1,280.3
5–17 years	2,698.5	2,049.8	1,633.2	1,240.3	1,172.1	1,300.9	1,239.1	1,406.4
18–44 years	8,323.6	6,294.7	4,676.7	3,517.2	3,093.8	3,305.0	3,360.6	3,258.0
18–24 years	7,174.6	5,287.2	4,015.9	2,987.4	2,679.5	2,819.9	2,889.4	2,738.7
25–44 years	8,861.4	6,685.2	4,895.5	3,676.4	3,225.5	3,472.8	3,524.5	3,439.7
25–34 years.	8,497.5	6,688.9	4,939.7	3,536.1	3,161.7	3,434.3	3,462.2	3,423.1
35–44 years.	9,386.6	6,680.4	4,844.8	3,812.3	3,281.5	3,507.9	3,581.9	3,455.2
45–64 years.	15,969.5	12,015.9	9,139.3	6,574.5	5,515.4	5,717.3	5,793.0	5,868.2
45–54 years	13,167.2	9,692.8	6,996.6	5,162.0	4,374.2	4,711.2	4,667.4	4,745.9
55–64 years	18,895.4	14,369.5	11,722.6	8,671.6	7,290.8	7,124.0	7,333.6	7,371.8
65 years and over.	40,983.5	32,279.7	28,956.1	23,736.5	21,118.9	19,882.8	19,197.5	18,951.7
65–74 years	31,470.3	24,373.3	20,878.2	16,847.0	14,389.7	13,985.3	13,170.2	13,274.8
75 years and over.	55,788.2	43,812.7	40,090.8	32,478.1	28,518.6	25,939.4	25,413.1	24,878.5
75–84 years	51,836.2	40,521.6	35,995.1	28,947.5	25,397.8	23,155.3	22,671.7	22,658.1
85 years and over.	69,332.0	54,782.4	53,616.9	43,305.9	37,537.8	33,071.5	32,165.5	30,124.5
Sex[2]								
Male	12,475.8	9,792.1	8,057.8	6,239.0	5,358.8	5,301.3	5,208.8	5,157.4
Female.	13,662.9	10,340.4	8,404.5	6,548.8	5,809.7	5,828.7	5,764.2	5,685.1
Sex and age								
Male, all ages.	10,674.1	8,518.8	6,943.0	5,507.5	4,860.8	4,979.7	4,947.3	4,937.6
Under 18 years	3,473.1	2,942.7	2,335.7	1,998.0	1,955.7	2,006.2	1,968.0	1,858.1
18–44 years	6,102.4	4,746.6	3,517.4	2,729.7	2,175.0	2,282.7	2,375.6	2,241.8
45–64 years	15,894.9	12,290.1	9,434.2	6,822.7	5,704.4	5,773.5	6,004.3	6,103.5
65–74 years	33,697.6	26,220.5	22,515.5	17,697.4	14,897.4	14,502.6	13,262.1	13,666.7
75–84 years	54,723.3	44,087.4	38,257.8	29,642.6	26,616.7	25,106.9	23,972.7	23,894.6
85 years and over	77,013.1	58,609.5	60,347.3	45,263.6	37,765.3	35,179.0	32,604.0	31,480.6
Female, all ages.	13,560.1	10,566.3	8,691.1	6,863.4	6,202.7	6,239.5	6,186.8	6,121.1
Under 18 years	3,354.5	2,675.5	2,186.8	1,687.9	1,615.1	1,826.1	1,741.8	1,708.3
18–44 years	10,450.7	7,792.0	5,820.3	4,297.9	4,010.8	4,341.8	4,361.5	4,292.3
45–64 years	16,037.1	11,765.5	8,865.1	6,341.7	5,336.4	5,663.9	5,592.2	5,644.3
65–74 years	29,764.7	22,949.2	19,592.7	16,162.0	13,971.3	13,549.0	13,092.4	12,942.1
75–84 years	50,133.3	38,424.7	34,628.3	28,502.5	24,601.0	21,830.1	21,782.1	21,806.2
85 years and over	65,990.5	53,253.6	51,000.5	42,538.6	37,444.4	32,103.5	31,960.3	29,479.5
Geographic region[2]								
Northeast.	14,024.4	11,143.1	10,266.8	8,389.7	7,185.9	6,636.5	6,608.5	7,284.4
Midwest	14,871.9	10,803.6	8,306.5	5,908.8	5,005.3	4,954.3	4,893.5	4,775.3
South.	12,713.5	9,642.6	8,204.1	6,659.9	5,925.1	5,830.4	5,844.8	5,555.7
West	9,635.2	8,300.7	5,755.1	4,510.6	4,082.0	4,690.3	4,451.6	4,184.5

See footnotes at end of table.

Table 99 (page 3 of 3). Discharges, days of care, and average length of stay in nonfederal short-stay hospitals, by selected characteristics: United States, selected years 1980–2007

[Data are based on a sample of hospital records]

Characteristic	1980[1]	1985[1]	1990	1995	2000	2005	2006	2007
	Average length of stay in days							
Total, age-adjusted[2]	7.5	6.6	6.5	5.4	4.9	4.8	4.7	4.8
Total, crude	7.3	6.5	6.4	5.4	4.9	4.8	4.8	4.8
Age								
Under 18 years	4.5	4.6	4.9	4.4	4.4	4.7	4.7	4.7
Under 1 year	5.7	6.6	6.0	5.5	5.7	6.2	6.4	5.2
1–4 years	3.9	3.5	3.6	3.3	3.2	3.2	3.4	3.3
5–17 years	4.4	4.3	4.9	4.3	4.4	4.5	4.5	5.2
18–44 years	5.3	4.8	4.6	3.8	3.6	3.7	3.7	3.7
18–24 years	4.6	4.1	3.8	3.2	3.1	3.3	3.3	3.2
25–44 years	5.6	5.1	4.8	4.0	3.8	3.8	3.8	3.8
25–34 years	5.0	4.7	4.3	3.5	3.4	3.4	3.4	3.4
35–44 years	6.5	5.8	5.6	4.7	4.3	4.3	4.3	4.3
45–64 years	8.2	7.0	6.7	5.5	5.0	5.0	5.0	5.1
45–54 years	7.5	6.6	6.2	5.2	4.8	4.9	4.8	4.9
55–64 years	8.8	7.4	7.2	5.8	5.2	5.1	5.2	5.3
65 years and over	10.7	8.7	8.7	6.8	6.0	5.5	5.5	5.6
65–74 years	10.0	8.2	8.0	6.5	5.7	5.3	5.2	5.4
75 years and over	11.4	9.2	9.2	7.1	6.2	5.7	5.6	5.7
75–84 years	11.2	9.1	9.1	7.0	6.2	5.6	5.6	5.7
85 years and over	12.0	9.6	9.6	7.3	6.2	5.7	5.6	5.6
Sex[2]								
Male	8.1	7.1	7.1	6.0	5.4	5.2	5.2	5.3
Female	7.0	6.2	6.0	5.0	4.5	4.4	4.4	4.4
Sex and age								
Male, all ages	7.7	6.9	6.9	5.8	5.3	5.2	5.2	5.3
Under 18 years	4.6	4.7	5.0	4.6	4.8	4.9	4.9	4.8
18–44 years	6.4	6.1	6.1	5.4	4.8	4.8	5.0	4.9
45–64 years	8.1	6.9	6.7	5.6	5.1	5.0	5.1	5.3
65–74 years	9.7	8.1	7.8	6.4	5.6	5.3	5.1	5.3
75–84 years	10.7	8.8	8.7	6.8	6.2	5.7	5.7	5.7
85 years and over	12.1	9.1	9.4	7.1	6.1	5.9	5.4	5.8
Female, all ages	7.0	6.2	6.1	5.0	4.6	4.5	4.5	4.6
Under 18 years	4.5	4.5	4.7	4.1	4.1	4.5	4.5	4.7
18–44 years	4.8	4.3	4.0	3.3	3.2	3.3	3.2	3.2
45–64 years	8.3	7.1	6.8	5.5	4.8	4.9	4.9	5.0
65–74 years	10.2	8.3	8.1	6.5	5.7	5.3	5.3	5.5
75–84 years	11.5	9.3	9.4	7.1	6.1	5.5	5.6	5.6
85 years and over	12.0	9.8	9.6	7.4	6.2	5.7	5.7	5.5
Geographic region[2]								
Northeast	8.6	7.8	7.7	6.3	5.6	5.3	5.2	5.7
Midwest	7.7	6.8	6.5	5.2	4.5	4.2	4.2	4.2
South	7.0	6.1	6.2	5.3	4.9	4.8	4.9	4.9
West	6.3	5.6	5.7	4.7	4.6	4.7	4.6	4.3

[1]Comparisons of data from 1980–1985 with data from subsequent years should be made with caution because estimates of change may reflect improvements in the survey design rather than true changes in hospital use. See Appendix I, National Hospital Discharge Survey.

[2]Estimates are age-adjusted to the year 2000 standard population using six age groups: under 18 years, 18–44 years, 45–54 years, 55–64 years, 65–74 years, and 75 years and over. See Appendix II, Age adjustment.

NOTES: Excludes newborn infants. Rates are based on the civilian population as of July 1. Starting with *Health, United States, 2003*, rates for 2000 and beyond are based on the 2000 census. Rates for 1990–1999 use population estimates based on the 1990 census adjusted for net underenumeration using the 1990 National Population Adjustment Matrix from the U.S. Census Bureau. Rates for 1990–1999 are not strictly comparable with rates for 2000 and beyond because population estimates for 1990–1999 have not been revised to reflect the 2000 census. See Appendix I, National Hospital Discharge Survey; Population Census and Population Estimates. Data for additional years are available. See Appendix III.

SOURCE: CDC/NCHS, National Hospital Discharge Survey.

Table 100 (page 1 of 3). **Discharges in nonfederal short-stay hospitals, by sex, age, and selected first-listed diagnosis: United States, selected years 1990–2007**

(Data are based on a sample of hospital records)

Age and first-listed diagnosis	Both sexes			Male			Female		
	1990	2000	2007	1990	2000	2007	1990	2000	2007
	Number in thousands								
All ages[1]	30,788	31,706	34,369	12,280	12,514	13,834	18,508	19,192	20,535
Under 18 years[1]	3,072	2,912	2,784	1,572	1,515	1,458	1,500	1,397	1,325
Dehydration	63	114	108	32	64	*56	31	50	52
Acute bronchitis and bronchiolitis	114	201	138	67	116	80	47	85	58
Pneumonia	221	182	150	126	95	83	95	87	67
Asthma	182	214	*157	111	129	*94	71	85	*64
Appendicitis	83	86	98	50	48	63	34	38	34
Injury	329	243	225	210	156	145	119	87	80
Fracture	117	100	87	76	68	57	42	32	30
Complications of care and adverse effects	41	*52	*42	22	*29	*23	19	*23	*19
18–44 years[1]	11,138	9,439	9,969	3,120	2,498	2,607	8,018	6,941	7,362
HIV/AIDS	*20	47	41	*15	32	27	*	15	14
Cancer, all	181	117	111	64	41	39	116	76	72
Childbirth	. . .	. . .	. . .	. . .	. . .	. . .	3,815	3,588	3,986
Uterine fibroids	. . .	. . .	. . .	. . .	. . .	. . .	110	121	85
Diabetes	105	127	147	61	72	82	44	55	66
Alcohol and drug	284	330	280	199	217	183	84	*112	97
Schizophrenia, mood disorders, delusional disorders, nonorganic psychoses	384	*596	650	184	*296	325	200	*300	325
Schizophrenia	145	*160	161	88	*104	103	57	*56	58
Mood disorders	211	*399	445	83	*172	196	128	*227	*249
Heart disease	236	242	245	163	148	144	73	95	101
Ischemic heart disease	129	109	79	95	79	55	34	31	25
Pneumonia	136	121	82	69	55	43	67	66	39
Asthma	106	100	80	27	30	26	79	70	54
Intervertebral disc disorders	222	138	97	138	81	53	84	58	44
Injury	935	509	532	641	346	370	294	164	162
Fracture	302	198	222	217	141	164	85	57	57
Poisoning and toxic effects	124	95	110	54	37	51	70	57	59
Complications of care and adverse effects	135	135	185	63	62	78	72	73	108
45–64 years[1]	6,244	6,958	8,753	3,115	3,424	4,316	3,129	3,534	4,437
HIV/AIDS	*3	*20	33	*3	*15	26	*	*	*7
Cancer, all	545	393	484	236	189	231	309	204	253
Colorectal cancer	59	49	46	33	27	23	26	22	23
Lung/bronchus/tracheal cancer	101	43	64	60	26	31	41	17	33
Breast cancer[2]	. . .	. . .	. . .	. . .	. . .	. . .	69	45	40
Prostate cancer	. . .	. . .	. . .	19	29	52	. . .	. . .	. . .
Uterine fibroids	. . .	. . .	. . .	. . .	. . .	. . .	70	114	87
Diabetes	134	207	220	65	114	112	70	93	108
Alcohol and drug	100	146	227	77	102	167	23	44	60
Schizophrenia, mood disorders, delusional disorders, nonorganic psychoses	152	267	409	56	*120	178	95	146	230
Schizophrenia	47	80	131	19	*44	64	28	36	67
Mood disorders	91	*168	255	32	*66	103	58	*103	151
Heart disease	1,100	1,271	1,205	704	802	753	397	470	452
Ischemic heart disease	739	789	607	502	539	414	237	251	192
Heart attack	233	242	198	165	178	139	68	64	59
Arrhythmias	131	157	207	79	97	125	53	60	82
Heart failure	122	196	227	68	102	125	54	94	102
Hypertension	75	119	148	38	53	71	37	65	77
Stroke	162	229	223	91	116	120	72	113	103
Pneumonia	154	220	219	76	104	106	79	117	113
Chronic obstructive pulmonary disease	73	192	200	39	94	94	34	99	105
Asthma	86	84	123	26	19	36	59	65	87
Osteoarthritis	87	150	317	36	63	138	51	87	179
Intervertebral disc disorders	145	132	145	82	68	71	63	64	74
Injury	334	299	420	178	155	239	157	144	181
Fracture	149	164	205	74	77	110	75	87	95
Poisoning and toxic effects	29	39	76	10	17	37	19	23	39
Internal organ injury	36	28	49	23	18	32	14	10	17
Complications of care and adverse effects	148	215	345	79	110	168	69	105	176

See footnotes at end of table.

Table 100 (page 2 of 3). **Discharges in nonfederal short-stay hospitals, by sex, age, and selected first-listed diagnosis: United States, selected years 1990–2007**

(Data are based on a sample of hospital records)

	Discharges								
	Both sexes			Male			Female		
Age and first-listed diagnosis	1990	2000	2007	1990	2000	2007	1990	2000	2007
	Number in thousands								
65–74 years[1]	4,689	4,678	4,722	2,268	2,199	2,274	2,421	2,479	2,447
Septicemia	49	65	119	27	33	50	21	32	68
Cancer, all	436	292	294	222	146	150	214	146	144
Colorectal cancer	48	42	36	24	25	19	24	17	17
Lung/bronchus/tracheal cancer	77	48	54	50	23	30	26	25	24
Breast cancer[2]	. . .	. . .	. . .	. . .	. . .	. . .	42	31	17
Prostate cancer	. . .	. . .	. . .	40	31	29	. . .	. . .	. . .
Diabetes	93	85	96	34	39	53	59	47	43
Schizophrenia, mood disorders, delusional disorders, nonorganic psychoses	59	68	59	20	*28	22	39	40	37
Dementia and Alzheimer's disease	10	*21	20	4	*13	*8	*6	*7	12
Heart disease	1,000	1,111	881	547	586	513	453	525	367
Ischemic heart disease	576	564	389	331	329	246	245	235	143
Heart attack	185	184	126	110	104	79	75	81	48
Arrhythmias	124	188	179	67	90	105	57	99	74
Heart failure	188	242	201	93	113	108	95	128	93
Hypertension	39	39	66	13	14	22	26	26	44
Stroke	222	233	192	108	109	100	114	124	92
Pneumonia	176	223	169	90	106	82	86	117	87
Chronic obstructive pulmonary disease	81	188	179	41	85	85	40	103	95
Gallstones	79	61	37	30	25	15	49	36	23
Kidney disease	18	35	100	9	17	50	9	18	50
Urinary tract infection	54	47	79	17	16	29	37	31	50
Hyperplasia of the prostate	. . .	. . .	. . .	113	45	19	. . .	. . .	. . .
Osteoarthritis	122	186	251	44	86	102	78	101	149
Injury	193	187	180	71	70	79	122	117	101
Fracture	120	116	115	36	39	43	85	77	72
Hip fracture	48	49	45	12	*17	19	36	32	26
Complications of care and adverse effects	125	147	186	68	79	95	57	68	91
75–84 years[1]	3,949	5,119	5,188	1,660	2,107	2,211	2,289	3,013	2,976
Septicemia	54	85	156	24	38	69	30	46	87
Cancer, all	300	241	218	158	104	102	142	137	116
Colorectal cancer	50	41	37	20	18	18	29	23	19
Lung/bronchus/tracheal cancer	36	33	40	22	16	19	*15	18	21
Breast cancer[2]	. . .	. . .	. . .	. . .	. . .	. . .	24	23	11
Prostate cancer	. . .	. . .	. . .	37	13	*8	. . .	. . .	. . .
Diabetes	44	79	97	17	33	49	27	45	48
Schizophrenia, mood disorders, delusional disorders, nonorganic psychoses	39	51	34	*10	*15	*12	28	36	22
Dementia and Alzheimer's disease	20	45	47	9	18	*21	11	27	26
Heart disease	865	1,185	1,052	377	521	502	488	664	550
Ischemic heart disease	382	517	350	177	259	192	205	258	158
Heart attack	156	207	135	83	104	70	73	103	65
Arrhythmias	133	219	260	58	86	110	76	134	150
Heart failure	261	327	305	108	133	139	153	194	165
Hypertension	23	49	53	*	*14	16	19	35	38
Stroke	258	317	227	104	137	95	154	181	132
Pneumonia	224	327	248	112	153	123	112	175	125
Chronic obstructive pulmonary disease	55	181	172	34	88	78	22	93	94
Gallstones	48	49	50	20	20	21	28	29	30
Kidney disease	24	47	127	10	24	61	*14	23	66
Urinary tract infection	86	106	152	25	36	41	61	71	111
Hyperplasia of the prostate	. . .	. . .	. . .	69	33	20	. . .	. . .	. . .
Osteoarthritis	69	125	183	25	38	68	44	87	115
Injury	259	284	282	58	84	87	201	200	195
Fracture	195	211	197	35	57	52	161	154	144
Hip fracture	115	123	91	20	34	27	95	89	65
Complications of care and adverse effects	81	126	131	38	67	68	43	59	63

See footnotes at end of table.

Table 100 (page 3 of 3). **Discharges in nonfederal short-stay hospitals, by sex, age, and selected first-listed diagnosis: United States, selected years 1990–2007**

(Data are based on a sample of hospital records)

	Discharges								
	Both sexes			Male			Female		
Age and first-listed diagnosis	1990	2000	2007	1990	2000	2007	1990	2000	2007
	Number in thousands								
85 years and over[1]	1,694	2,599	2,954	543	771	967	1,151	1,828	1,987
Septicemia	41	66	118	12	26	45	29	40	73
Cancer, all	77	84	84	31	31	37	45	52	47
Colorectal cancer	14	21	18	*5	*7	4	9	14	13
Lung/bronchus/tracheal cancer	*6	5	*13	*	*3	*5	*	*3	*
Breast cancer[2]	. . .	. . .	. . .	. . .	. . .	. . .	*9	*6	*3
Prostate cancer	. . .	. . .	. . .	*7	*6	*	. . .	. . .	. . .
Diabetes	16	28	35	*5	*7	*11	11	21	24
Schizophrenia, mood disorders, delusional disorders, nonorganic psychoses	*8	*16	*13	*	*	*4	*7	*13	*
Dementia and Alzheimer's disease	15	46	43	*2	12	16	13	34	27
Heart disease	335	558	561	112	176	194	223	382	367
Ischemic heart disease	128	183	146	49	67	57	79	117	89
Heart attack	60	108	85	23	37	30	37	71	55
Arrhythmias	51	100	123	16	31	46	35	69	77
Heart failure	126	206	214	39	57	68	87	149	146
Hypertension	*5	18	28	*	*2	*7	*4	15	21
Stroke	129	161	138	35	50	39	95	111	100
Pneumonia	151	221	199	64	76	70	88	145	129
Chronic obstructive pulmonary disease	13	56	61	*6	19	25	*7	37	36
Gallstones	18	17	22	*6	*4	*7	13	*13	15
Kidney disease	14	21	84	8	*9	32	*6	*13	51
Urinary tract infection	65	82	138	20	19	30	45	63	108
Hyperplasia of the prostate	. . .	. . .	. . .	13	*9	*6	. . .	. . .	. . .
Osteoarthritis	13	24	32	*	*	*8	8	17	24
Injury	164	234	273	37	44	64	127	190	209
Fracture	133	194	220	28	32	45	104	162	174
Hip fracture	82	118	128	19	18	26	63	100	102
Complications of care and adverse effects	29	34	48	11	11	21	18	23	27

* Estimates are considered unreliable. Data preceded by an asterisk have a relative standard error (RSE) of 20%–30%. Data not shown have an RSE greater than 30%.

. . . Category not applicable.

[1] Includes discharges with first-listed diagnoses not shown in table.

[2] Shown for women only.

NOTES: Excludes newborn infants. Diagnostic categories are based on the *International Classification of Diseases, 9th Revision, Clinical Modification* (ICD–9–CM). See Appendix II, Diagnosis; Human immunodeficiency virus (HIV) disease; *International Classification of Diseases, 9th Revision, Clinical Modification*; Table XI for ICD–9–CM codes. Additional data and diagnosis categories are available from: http://www.cdc.gov/nchs/hdi.htm. Data for additional years are available. See Appendix III.

SOURCE: CDC/NCHS, National Hospital Discharge Survey.

Table 101 (page 1 of 3). Discharge rate in nonfederal short-stay hospitals, by sex, age, and selected first-listed diagnosis: United States, selected years 1990–2007

[Data are based on a sample of hospital records]

Age and first-listed diagnosis	Discharges								
	Both sexes			Male			Female		
	1990	2000	2007	1990	2000	2007	1990	2000	2007
	Number per 10,000 population								
All ages, age-adjusted[1,2]	1,252.4	1,132.8	1,124.0	1,130.0	990.8	973.8	1,389.5	1,277.3	1,280.6
All ages, crude[2]	1,222.7	1,128.3	1,143.9	1,002.2	910.6	936.7	1,431.7	1,336.6	1,344.0
Under 18 years[2]	463.5	402.6	376.7	463.1	408.6	385.6	464.1	396.2	367.3
Dehydration	9.5	15.7	14.6	9.4	17.2	*14.7	9.7	14.2	14.5
Acute bronchitis and bronchiolitis	17.2	27.8	18.7	19.6	31.4	21.2	14.6	24.1	16.0
Pneumonia	33.3	25.2	20.3	37.0	25.7	22.0	29.5	24.6	18.5
Asthma	27.5	29.6	*21.3	32.7	34.8	*24.7	22.0	24.0	*17.6
Appendicitis	12.6	11.9	13.2	14.6	13.0	16.8	10.5	10.8	9.5
Injury	49.7	33.6	30.4	62.0	42.0	38.4	36.8	24.8	22.1
Fracture	17.7	13.8	11.8	22.3	18.3	14.9	12.9	9.0	8.4
Complications of care and adverse effects	6.2	*7.3	*5.7	6.5	*7.9	*6.1	5.9	*6.6	*5.2
18–44 years[2]	1,026.6	849.4	888.8	579.2	450.0	460.8	1,468.0	1,248.1	1,324.5
HIV/AIDS	*1.8	4.3	3.7	*2.8	5.8	4.8	*	2.8	2.5
Cancer, all	16.6	10.5	9.9	11.9	7.3	6.8	21.3	13.7	13.0
Childbirth	. . .	. . .	. . .	. . .	. . .	. . .	698.6	645.2	717.1
Uterine fibroids	. . .	. . .	. . .	. . .	. . .	. . .	20.2	21.7	15.3
Diabetes	9.7	11.5	13.1	11.3	13.0	14.4	8.1	9.9	11.8
Alcohol and drug	26.2	29.7	25.0	37.0	39.1	32.4	15.5	*20.2	17.5
Schizophrenia, mood disorders, delusional disorders, nonorganic psychoses	35.4	*53.6	58.0	34.1	*53.2	57.5	36.7	*53.9	58.5
Schizophrenia	13.4	*14.4	14.3	16.4	*18.6	18.2	10.5	*10.1	10.4
Mood disorders	19.4	*35.9	39.7	15.4	*31.0	34.6	23.4	*40.9	*44.8
Heart disease	21.7	21.8	21.8	30.2	26.6	25.4	13.4	17.0	18.2
Ischemic heart disease	11.9	9.9	7.1	17.7	14.2	9.7	6.3	5.6	4.4
Pneumonia	12.5	10.9	7.3	12.8	10.0	7.6	12.2	11.9	7.1
Asthma	9.8	9.0	7.1	5.1	5.4	4.6	14.4	12.6	9.8
Intervertebral disc disorders	20.5	12.5	8.6	25.6	14.5	9.4	15.4	10.4	7.9
Injury	86.2	45.8	47.4	119.0	62.3	65.3	53.8	29.4	29.2
Fracture	27.8	17.8	19.8	40.2	25.4	29.1	15.5	10.2	10.3
Poisoning and toxic effects	11.4	8.5	9.8	10.0	6.7	8.9	12.7	10.3	10.7
Complications of care and adverse effects	12.5	12.2	16.5	11.7	11.2	13.7	13.3	13.1	19.4
45–64 years[2]	1,354.5	1,114.2	1,143.9	1,402.7	1,127.4	1,156.6	1,309.7	1,101.7	1,131.7
HIV/AIDS	*0.6	*3.2	4.3	*1.2	*4.9	7.0	*	*	*1.7
Cancer, all	118.3	62.9	63.2	106.3	62.1	61.9	129.5	63.6	64.4
Colorectal cancer	12.7	7.9	6.0	14.8	8.9	6.3	10.8	6.9	5.8
Lung/bronchus/tracheal cancer	21.8	6.9	8.4	26.8	8.6	8.3	17.2	5.2	8.5
Breast cancer[3]	. . .	. . .	. . .	. . .	. . .	. . .	29.0	14.2	10.3
Prostate cancer	. . .	. . .	. . .	8.5	9.6	13.9	. . .	. . .	. . .
Uterine fibroids	. . .	. . .	. . .	. . .	. . .	. . .	29.3	35.6	22.1
Diabetes	29.1	33.1	28.8	29.1	37.4	30.0	29.2	29.0	27.5
Alcohol and drug	21.7	23.3	29.7	34.6	33.5	44.6	9.6	13.7	15.4
Schizophrenia, mood disorders, delusional disorders, nonorganic psychoses	32.9	42.7	53.4	25.4	*39.6	47.8	39.8	45.6	58.8
Schizophrenia	10.1	12.8	17.1	8.4	*14.4	17.0	11.7	11.3	17.1
Mood disorders	19.6	*26.9	33.3	14.5	*21.6	27.6	24.4	*32.0	38.6
Heart disease	238.7	203.6	157.4	316.8	264.0	201.7	166.1	146.4	115.2
Ischemic heart disease	160.3	126.4	79.3	226.1	177.3	111.0	99.2	78.2	49.1
Heart attack	50.6	38.8	25.8	74.4	58.7	37.1	28.4	19.9	15.0
Arrhythmias	28.5	25.1	27.0	35.5	31.8	33.4	22.1	18.7	20.9
Heart failure	26.4	31.4	29.7	30.7	33.5	33.5	22.4	29.3	26.0
Hypertension	16.3	19.0	19.3	16.9	17.6	18.9	15.6	20.3	19.6
Stroke	35.2	36.7	29.1	40.8	38.3	32.0	30.1	35.2	26.3
Pneumonia	33.5	35.3	28.6	34.0	34.2	28.4	33.0	36.4	28.7
Chronic obstructive pulmonary disease	15.8	30.8	26.1	17.4	30.8	25.3	14.3	30.8	26.9
Asthma	18.6	13.4	16.0	11.8	6.2	9.6	24.9	20.2	22.1
Osteoarthritis	18.9	24.0	41.4	16.3	20.8	36.9	21.2	27.0	45.8
Intervertebral disc disorders	31.5	21.2	18.9	36.8	22.5	19.1	26.5	20.0	18.8
Injury	72.5	47.9	54.9	79.9	51.2	64.1	65.6	44.7	46.2
Fracture	32.4	26.2	26.8	33.4	25.3	29.4	31.5	27.0	24.2
Poisoning and toxic effects	6.3	6.3	10.0	4.5	5.5	10.0	8.0	7.1	10.0
Internal organ injury	7.9	4.5	6.4	10.2	5.9	8.7	5.7	3.2	4.3
Complications of care and adverse effects	32.0	34.5	45.0	35.6	36.3	45.1	28.7	32.7	45.0

See footnotes at end of table.

[Data are based on a sample of hospital records]

	Discharges								
	Both sexes			Male			Female		
Age and first-listed diagnosis	1990	2000	2007	1990	2000	2007	1990	2000	2007
	Number per 10,000 population								
65–74 years[2]	2,616.3	2,546.0	2,439.9	2,877.6	2,649.1	2,559.3	2,411.2	2,461.0	2,338.4
Septicemia	27.2	35.6	61.3	34.9	40.1	56.6	21.2	32.0	65.2
Cancer, all	243.1	159.0	151.8	281.4	176.4	168.4	213.0	144.7	137.8
Colorectal cancer	27.0	22.8	18.6	30.6	29.9	21.1	24.1	16.9	16.5
Lung/bronchus/tracheal cancer	42.9	26.1	27.7	63.9	28.2	33.5	26.4	24.5	22.8
Breast cancer[3]	...	...	...	...	...	...	42.3	31.2	16.4
Prostate cancer	...	...	...	50.6	37.1	32.9	...	...	...
Diabetes	51.8	46.4	49.7	43.6	46.8	60.1	58.3	46.2	40.8
Schizophrenia, mood disorders, delusional disorders, nonorganic psychoses	32.7	37.1	30.5	25.3	*34.2	25.0	38.6	39.6	35.1
Dementia and Alzheimer's disease	5.6	*11.2	10.4	4.9	*16.2	*9.3	*6.1	*7.0	11.3
Heart disease	558.1	604.8	455.0	694.2	706.4	577.7	451.3	521.0	350.9
Ischemic heart disease	321.3	307.0	200.9	419.9	396.5	276.9	243.9	233.2	136.4
Heart attack	103.3	100.3	65.2	139.8	124.7	88.5	74.6	80.2	45.5
Arrhythmias	69.1	102.6	92.6	84.7	108.3	117.9	56.9	97.9	71.1
Heart failure	105.2	131.6	104.0	118.0	136.4	121.9	95.1	127.6	88.9
Hypertension	21.8	21.5	34.3	16.2	16.5	25.1	26.2	25.5	42.1
Stroke	123.9	127.1	99.3	137.5	131.8	112.3	113.1	123.2	88.3
Pneumonia	98.1	121.3	87.1	113.6	127.7	92.0	85.9	116.1	82.9
Chronic obstructive pulmonary disease	45.3	102.3	92.6	52.6	102.6	95.2	39.6	102.0	90.4
Gallstones	44.2	33.4	19.4	38.2	30.2	16.7	48.9	36.0	21.6
Kidney disease	9.9	19.1	51.4	11.0	21.0	55.9	9.0	17.5	47.6
Urinary tract infection	30.2	25.5	41.1	21.7	19.7	32.7	36.9	30.3	48.2
Hyperplasia of the prostate	...	...	...	143.5	53.6	21.0	...	...	...
Osteoarthritis	68.0	101.4	129.8	55.2	103.1	114.6	78.0	100.1	142.8
Injury	107.7	101.5	93.0	90.7	83.8	89.2	121.1	116.2	96.2
Fracture	67.2	63.3	59.4	45.2	46.8	48.8	84.4	76.9	68.3
Hip fracture	26.7	26.4	23.1	15.3	*20.0	20.9	35.7	31.7	25.0
Complications of care and adverse effects	69.7	80.0	96.0	85.7	95.7	107.0	57.2	67.1	86.6
75–84 years[2]	3,957.0	4,124.4	3,983.3	4,417.3	4,294.1	4,162.6	3,678.9	4,013.5	3,859.8
Septicemia	53.9	68.3	120.0	63.8	78.1	130.2	47.9	61.9	113.0
Cancer, all	300.3	194.0	167.4	420.8	211.0	191.9	227.6	182.9	150.6
Colorectal cancer	49.8	33.0	28.4	54.0	37.5	34.5	47.3	30.1	24.3
Lung/bronchus/tracheal cancer	36.5	27.0	30.8	57.2	32.2	35.5	*24.0	23.6	27.6
Breast cancer[3]	...	...	...	...	...	...	38.7	30.8	14.8
Prostate cancer	...	...	...	99.2	27.4	*15.2	...	...	...
Diabetes	44.3	63.4	74.4	44.8	68.1	92.5	44.0	60.3	61.9
Schizophrenia, mood disorders, delusional disorders, nonorganic psychoses	38.8	41.4	26.0	*27.3	*30.6	*22.6	45.7	48.5	28.3
Dementia and Alzheimer's disease	20.0	36.5	36.1	22.8	36.8	*39.1	18.3	36.3	34.1
Heart disease	866.6	954.8	807.7	1,003.8	1,062.5	945.2	783.7	884.3	712.9
Ischemic heart disease	382.4	416.7	268.8	470.5	528.5	360.9	329.1	343.6	205.4
Heart attack	155.9	166.9	103.8	220.9	212.8	131.2	116.7	136.9	84.1
Arrhythmias	133.4	176.8	199.5	153.3	174.4	207.5	121.4	178.3	194.0
Heart failure	261.4	263.1	233.9	286.2	271.1	262.4	246.4	257.9	214.3
Hypertension	22.6	39.7	40.8	*	*28.4	29.5	30.7	47.1	48.7
Stroke	259.0	255.5	174.3	277.7	278.4	178.2	247.7	240.6	171.7
Pneumonia	224.6	263.5	190.4	297.8	310.8	231.0	180.4	232.6	162.4
Chronic obstructive pulmonary disease	55.4	146.2	131.9	89.4	179.6	146.8	34.8	124.3	121.6
Gallstones	47.6	39.6	38.4	51.9	41.4	38.6	45.0	38.5	38.3
Kidney disease	24.5	37.6	97.3	27.6	48.7	114.2	*22.6	30.4	85.6
Urinary tract infection	86.0	85.6	116.9	66.6	72.5	77.2	97.8	94.2	144.3
Hyperplasia of the prostate	...	...	...	183.3	67.2	37.1	...	...	...
Osteoarthritis	68.6	100.6	140.6	65.2	76.5	127.7	70.7	116.4	149.5
Injury	259.1	229.1	216.3	153.4	171.7	162.9	323.0	266.6	253.1
Fracture	195.8	170.2	151.0	92.6	116.4	98.3	258.1	205.4	187.3
Hip fracture	115.2	99.0	70.1	53.7	68.6	50.4	152.4	118.8	83.7
Complications of care and adverse effects	81.5	101.4	100.6	101.4	136.0	127.9	69.4	78.8	81.7

See footnotes at end of table.

Table 101 (page 3 of 3). Discharge rate in nonfederal short-stay hospitals, by sex, age, and selected first-listed diagnosis: United States, selected years 1990–2007

[Data are based on a sample of hospital records]

	Discharges								
	Both sexes			Male			Female		
Age and first-listed diagnosis	1990	2000	2007	1990	2000	2007	1990	2000	2007
	Number per 10,000 population								
85 years and over[2]	5,606.3	6,050.9	5,358.9	6,420.9	6,166.6	5,440.6	5,289.6	6,003.3	5,320.0
Septicemia	135.6	153.9	213.3	139.0	207.3	250.5	134.3	131.9	195.6
Cancer, all	254.0	194.5	151.7	370.6	250.5	206.1	208.7	171.5	125.8
Colorectal cancer	47.6	49.7	32.0	*59.1	*58.8	23.5	43.2	45.9	36.1
Lung/bronchus/tracheal cancer	*19.1	12.1	*23.9	*	*20.9	*29.7	*	*8.5	*
Breast cancer[3]	. . .	. . .	. . .				*41.7	*20.5	*7.3
Prostate cancer	. . .	. . .	. . .	*87.8	*49.3	*	. . .	. . .	. . .
Diabetes	53.0	65.6	63.4	*53.5	*54.2	*60.1	52.8	70.3	65.0
Schizophrenia, mood disorders, delusional disorders, nonorganic psychoses	*27.9	*37.3	*23.5	*	*	*20.6	*30.7	*43.0	*
Dementia and Alzheimer's disease	49.7	107.0	77.7	*28.9	94.3	89.6	57.7	112.2	72.1
Heart disease	1,107.0	1,298.2	1,017.5	1,320.3	1,407.4	1,092.9	1,024.1	1,253.4	981.7
Ischemic heart disease	423.0	427.2	265.1	581.6	534.4	321.0	361.3	383.2	238.5
Heart attack	199.8	251.1	154.7	274.2	296.0	168.1	170.9	232.7	148.4
Arrhythmias	167.2	232.4	222.7	189.6	247.1	259.6	158.5	226.4	205.2
Heart failure	416.7	480.4	387.3	460.5	455.7	382.4	399.7	490.5	389.7
Hypertension	*17.9	41.1	51.4	*	*18.3	*39.5	*19.3	50.4	57.0
Stroke	427.2	373.8	250.9	408.2	396.7	218.2	434.6	364.3	266.5
Pneumonia	501.0	514.9	360.5	753.7	607.8	394.0	402.8	476.8	344.5
Chronic obstructive pulmonary disease	44.1	130.9	111.2	*72.9	150.4	143.1	*32.9	123.0	96.1
Gallstones	60.7	39.2	39.6	*68.2	*29.7	*40.5	57.8	*43.1	39.2
Kidney disease	47.1	49.5	151.7	92.4	*68.1	182.3	*29.4	*41.9	137.1
Urinary tract infection	216.5	191.5	250.5	239.3	153.1	167.9	207.6	207.2	289.7
Hyperplasia of the prostate	. . .	. . .	. . .	158.6	*69.9	*32.6	. . .	. . .	. . .
Osteoarthritis	44.5	56.0	57.5	*	*	*44.2	35.8	57.3	63.9
Injury	542.0	545.5	495.8	435.4	355.6	360.7	583.4	623.5	560.0
Fracture	439.0	450.9	398.7	335.7	252.4	256.0	479.2	532.4	466.5
Hip fracture	272.3	275.1	231.4	224.4	146.5	146.5	291.0	327.9	271.8
Complications of care and adverse effects	96.6	79.1	86.3	132.3	90.5	115.7	82.7	74.4	72.4

* Estimates are considered unreliable. Data preceded by an asterisk have a relative standard error (RSE) of 20%–30%. Data not shown have an RSE greater than 30%.

. . . Category not applicable.

[1]Estimates are age-adjusted to the year 2000 standard population using six age groups: under 18 years, 18–44 years, 45–54 years, 55–64 years, 65–74 years, and 75 years and over. See Appendix II, Age adjustment.

[2]Includes discharges with first-listed diagnoses not shown in table.

[3]Shown for women only.

NOTES: Excludes newborn infants. Diagnostic categories are based on the *International Classification of Diseases, 9th Revision, Clinical Modification* (ICD–9–CM). See Appendix II, Diagnosis; Human immunodeficiency virus (HIV) disease; *International Classification of Diseases, 9th Revision, Clinical Modification*; Table XI for ICD–9–CM codes. Rates are based on the civilian population as of July 1. Starting with *Health, United States, 2003*, rates for 2000 and beyond are based on the 2000 census. Rates for 1990–1999 use population estimates based on the 1990 census adjusted for net underenumeration using the 1990 National Population Adjustment Matrix from the U.S. Census Bureau. Rates for 1990–1999 are not strictly comparable with rates for 2000 and beyond because population estimates for 1990–1999 have not been revised to reflect the 2000 census. See Appendix I, National Hospital Discharge Survey; Population Census and Population Estimates. Additional data and diagnosis categories are available from: http://www.cdc.gov/nchs/hdi.htm. Data for additional years are available. See Appendix III.

SOURCE: CDC/NCHS, National Hospital Discharge Survey.

Table 102 (page 1 of 3). Average length of stay in nonfederal short-stay hospitals, by sex, age, and selected first-listed diagnosis: United States, selected years 1990–2007

[Data are based on a sample of hospital records]

Age and first-listed diagnosis	Average length of stay[1]								
	Both sexes			Male			Female		
	1990	2000	2007	1990	2000	2007	1990	2000	2007
	Number of days								
All ages, crude[2]	6.4	4.9	4.8	6.9	5.3	5.3	6.1	4.6	4.6
Under 18 years[2]	4.9	4.4	4.7	5.0	4.8	4.8	4.7	4.1	4.7
Dehydration	3.0	2.2	2.1	2.9	2.2	*2.2	3.0	2.1	2.0
Acute bronchitis and bronchiolitis	3.7	3.1	2.9	3.6	3.0	3.0	3.8	*3.3	2.8
Pneumonia	4.6	3.6	3.2	4.6	3.4	2.9	4.7	3.9	3.6
Asthma	2.9	2.2	*2.4	2.8	2.1	*2.4	3.1	2.3	*2.4
Appendicitis	4.0	3.2	*3.2	3.9	2.9	*3.3	4.0	3.5	*3.0
Injury	4.1	3.8	3.4	4.2	4.1	3.2	3.8	*3.2	*3.9
Fracture	4.5	3.5	2.8	4.2	3.9	2.7	5.0	2.5	*2.8
Complications of care and adverse effects	*5.3	*5.7	*7.0	*6.0	*5.5	*	*4.5	*5.9	*
18–44 years[2]	4.6	3.6	3.7	6.1	4.8	4.9	4.0	3.2	3.2
HIV/AIDS	*10.7	*8.8	8.3	*10.6	*9.4	8.3	*	*7.5	*8.3
Cancer, all	7.8	6.3	5.9	8.4	7.9	*7.8	7.5	5.4	4.8
Childbirth	. . .	. . .	. . .	. . .	. . .	. . .	2.8	2.5	2.6
Uterine fibroids	. . .	. . .	. . .	. . .	. . .	. . .	4.2	2.5	2.4
Diabetes	5.8	3.9	3.8	6.2	3.7	3.6	5.2	4.3	4.0
Alcohol and drug	9.0	*5.0	4.5	8.9	4.8	4.4	9.1	*5.3	*4.6
Schizophrenia, mood disorders, delusional disorders, nonorganic psychoses	14.3	*7.9	6.8	13.8	*8.2	7.2	14.8	*7.6	6.4
Schizophrenia	15.4	*11.0	9.5	15.3	*10.6	9.5	15.6	*11.9	9.4
Mood disorders	14.3	*6.6	5.7	*13.2	*6.6	5.9	15.0	*6.5	*5.6
Heart disease	5.4	3.6	3.9	5.4	3.5	3.5	5.4	3.7	4.4
Ischemic heart disease	4.6	3.0	2.9	4.8	2.8	2.7	4.1	3.6	3.5
Pneumonia	6.9	5.1	4.7	7.8	5.0	5.2	6.0	5.2	4.0
Asthma	4.4	2.9	3.2	3.8	2.5	2.9	4.6	3.1	3.3
Intervertebral disc disorders	4.4	2.3	2.6	4.2	2.2	2.4	4.7	2.3	2.9
Injury	5.1	4.3	4.2	5.0	4.5	4.4	5.3	4.1	3.7
Fracture	6.0	4.9	4.4	5.6	5.0	4.4	6.9	4.4	4.3
Poisoning and toxic effects	2.7	2.5	2.6	2.7	2.8	2.6	2.7	2.4	2.6
Complications of care and adverse effects	5.6	4.7	5.4	5.3	4.9	5.4	*5.9	4.6	5.4
45–64 years[2]	6.7	5.0	5.1	6.7	5.1	5.3	6.8	4.8	5.0
HIV/AIDS	*	*	8.5	*	*	8.5	*	*	*
Cancer, all	8.8	6.2	6.2	9.3	6.8	6.6	8.4	5.6	5.8
Colorectal cancer	13.3	7.4	8.6	*13.0	7.4	*9.1	*13.6	7.4	*8.0
Lung/bronchus/tracheal cancer	7.7	6.2	6.0	7.1	6.0	6.4	8.6	6.4	5.6
Breast cancer[3]	. . .	. . .	. . .	. . .	. . .	. . .	4.3	2.0	2.4
Prostate cancer	. . .	. . .	. . .	7.3	3.2	2.6	. . .	. . .	. . .
Uterine fibroids	. . .	. . .	. . .	. . .	. . .	. . .	4.5	2.8	2.5
Diabetes	8.1	5.6	5.3	7.3	6.0	5.3	8.9	5.2	5.2
Alcohol and drug	8.5	4.8	4.7	8.6	4.6	4.8	8.3	*5.0	4.3
Schizophrenia, mood disorders, delusional disorders, nonorganic psychoses	14.6	9.1	9.2	13.7	*8.8	9.3	15.2	9.4	9.1
Schizophrenia	15.6	*11.9	12.6	14.2	*11.4	11.7	16.5	*12.5	*13.4
Mood disorders	14.7	*7.9	7.5	13.4	*7.3	8.1	15.4	*8.3	7.1
Heart disease	5.9	3.9	3.9	5.8	3.8	3.8	6.1	4.1	4.0
Ischemic heart disease	5.7	3.7	3.4	5.7	3.6	3.3	5.8	3.8	3.4
Heart attack	7.5	4.8	4.2	7.5	4.7	4.1	7.6	5.0	4.5
Arrhythmias	4.6	2.9	3.2	4.6	2.8	3.3	4.6	2.9	3.2
Heart failure	7.0	4.9	4.9	6.9	5.2	5.0	7.3	4.7	4.8
Hypertension	3.9	2.2	2.5	*4.3	2.0	2.5	3.6	2.4	2.4
Stroke	10.3	5.3	5.4	10.0	5.2	5.5	10.7	5.5	5.3
Pneumonia	8.0	5.8	5.1	8.0	6.0	4.6	7.9	5.7	5.5
Chronic obstructive pulmonary disease	6.5	4.7	4.2	6.8	5.0	4.0	6.2	4.4	4.4
Asthma	5.2	3.9	4.0	5.3	*3.2	3.9	5.2	4.0	4.0
Osteoarthritis	7.4	3.9	3.4	7.1	3.6	3.2	7.5	4.1	3.5
Intervertebral disc disorders	5.2	2.8	2.9	5.0	2.6	2.7	5.4	3.1	3.0
Injury	6.5	5.1	5.3	6.6	5.5	5.4	6.4	4.6	5.2
Fracture	7.6	5.6	5.7	7.2	6.4	6.1	7.9	4.9	5.3
Poisoning and toxic effects	4.9	3.0	3.0	*	*2.9	3.1	4.3	3.1	2.9
Internal organ injury	*8.3	7.6	7.5	*	8.3	6.9	*8.1	*	*
Complications of care and adverse effects	7.9	6.1	6.0	8.4	5.9	6.3	7.4	6.4	5.8

See footnotes at end of table.

Table 102 (page 2 of 3). Average length of stay in nonfederal short-stay hospitals, by sex, age, and selected first-listed diagnosis: United States, selected years 1990–2007

[Data are based on a sample of hospital records]

| | Average length of stay[1] | | | | | | | | |
| | Both sexes | | | Male | | | Female | | |
Age and first-listed diagnosis	1990	2000	2007	1990	2000	2007	1990	2000	2007
	Number of days								
65–74 years[2]	8.0	5.7	5.4	7.8	5.6	5.3	8.1	5.7	5.5
Septicemia	*15.9	8.6	10.2	*	8.5	10.4	14.4	8.8	10.1
Cancer, all	9.4	7.0	6.8	9.9	6.9	7.2	9.0	7.1	6.3
Colorectal cancer	12.9	9.1	8.0	11.3	9.2	8.1	14.5	9.0	7.9
Lung/bronchus/tracheal cancer	9.2	7.0	7.8	8.7	6.8	8.3	10.2	*7.1	*7.2
Breast cancer[3]	...	...	...	...	...	...	4.4	*	2.8
Prostate cancer	...	...	...	6.5	3.8	2.4	...	...	...
Diabetes	8.4	5.9	5.3	9.1	6.2	5.1	8.0	5.6	*5.5
Schizophrenia, mood disorders, delusional disorders, nonorganic psychoses	16.6	11.7	10.7	17.4	*11.7	9.4	16.3	11.7	11.5
Dementia and Alzheimer's disease	*12.6	*9.3	9.0	*10.4	*9.6	*11.4	*14.0	*8.9	7.4
Heart disease	7.0	4.8	4.6	7.0	4.7	4.4	7.0	4.9	4.8
Ischemic heart disease	6.6	4.6	4.3	6.8	4.3	4.3	6.3	4.9	4.2
Heart attack	8.4	5.9	5.8	8.8	5.3	5.8	7.8	6.6	5.8
Arrhythmias	5.7	3.8	3.5	5.6	3.8	3.4	5.8	3.7	3.6
Heart failure	8.4	5.5	5.1	7.9	5.7	5.0	8.8	5.4	5.3
Hypertension	4.3	2.6	2.9	*4.6	*2.7	*3.0	4.1	2.4	2.8
Stroke	8.4	4.7	5.1	8.3	4.5	5.2	8.5	4.8	5.0
Pneumonia	9.5	6.4	5.2	9.5	6.4	5.0	9.5	6.3	5.3
Chronic obstructive pulmonary disease	8.2	4.8	4.6	8.6	4.5	4.6	7.7	5.0	4.6
Gallstones	6.6	4.4	4.2	6.9	*5.2	5.0	6.5	3.9	3.7
Kidney disease	10.4	7.6	6.0	8.4	6.9	5.8	*12.4	8.2	6.3
Urinary tract infection	8.0	4.8	5.1	7.2	5.1	5.0	8.4	4.7	5.2
Hyperplasia of the prostate	...	...	...	4.5	2.8	*2.5	...	...	...
Osteoarthritis	9.3	4.7	3.6	8.8	4.7	3.6	9.5	4.7	3.7
Injury	9.2	5.6	5.4	8.4	5.7	5.9	9.7	5.6	5.1
Fracture	11.1	5.9	5.7	10.2	6.4	6.2	11.5	5.7	5.4
Hip fracture	*15.5	7.1	6.3	*11.8	*7.9	*7.3	*16.7	6.7	5.7
Complications of care and adverse effects	7.8	6.4	6.5	7.3	6.1	6.1	8.5	6.8	6.8
75–84 years[2]	9.1	6.2	5.7	8.7	6.2	5.7	9.4	6.1	5.6
Septicemia	12.1	7.9	8.5	12.9	7.4	8.6	11.5	8.4	8.4
Cancer, all	10.4	7.2	7.1	9.3	7.2	7.1	11.7	7.2	7.1
Colorectal cancer	12.9	9.0	8.2	12.5	*9.3	8.0	13.2	8.8	8.4
Lung/bronchus/tracheal cancer	9.5	6.5	7.2	9.6	6.2	7.7	*9.4	6.9	6.8
Breast cancer[3]	...	...	...	...	...	...	5.7	*3.2	2.1
Prostate cancer	...	...	...	6.6	*5.1	*4.9	...	...	...
Diabetes	12.5	6.0	*7.0	11.7	6.4	*7.1	13.1	5.6	*6.9
Schizophrenia, mood disorders, delusional disorders, nonorganic psychoses	15.8	10.8	10.0	*15.7	*11.6	*9.1	15.8	10.4	10.4
Dementia and Alzheimer's disease	*15.3	8.2	8.1	*12.8	7.6	*7.7	*	8.6	8.5
Heart disease	8.0	5.3	4.7	8.1	5.4	4.7	7.8	5.3	4.7
Ischemic heart disease	7.9	5.1	4.4	8.5	5.2	4.5	7.4	5.1	4.4
Heart attack	9.7	6.2	5.8	10.1	5.8	6.1	9.3	6.6	5.5
Arrhythmias	6.6	4.2	4.0	6.5	4.3	4.1	6.7	4.1	3.9
Heart failure	8.0	5.9	5.2	7.7	6.1	5.1	8.2	5.8	5.3
Hypertension	6.0	2.6	3.1	*	*2.1	*	*5.6	2.8	2.8
Stroke	10.4	5.9	4.8	10.0	5.7	4.8	10.6	6.0	4.8
Pneumonia	10.4	6.3	5.4	9.8	6.4	5.3	11.0	6.3	5.4
Chronic obstructive pulmonary disease	8.0	4.9	4.4	6.6	4.8	4.5	*10.1	4.9	4.4
Gallstones	8.5	5.3	5.9	8.0	5.6	5.9	8.8	5.1	5.9
Kidney disease	10.5	7.4	6.6	11.0	8.2	6.3	*10.1	6.6	6.8
Urinary tract infection	11.0	5.2	4.8	8.1	5.5	4.9	12.3	5.1	4.7
Hyperplasia of the prostate	...	...	...	6.0	3.1	2.4	...	...	...
Osteoarthritis	10.1	4.6	4.4	9.9	4.4	5.1	10.2	4.7	4.1
Injury	10.1	6.8	5.6	8.9	*8.2	5.7	10.4	6.3	5.6
Fracture	11.0	7.4	5.7	10.0	*	6.2	11.2	6.7	5.5
Hip fracture	12.1	7.7	6.2	10.4	7.8	6.5	12.5	7.6	6.1
Complications of care and adverse effects	12.5	7.1	6.5	14.0	8.1	6.0	11.2	6.0	7.1

See footnotes at end of table.

Table 102 (page 3 of 3). Average length of stay in nonfederal short-stay hospitals, by sex, age, and selected first-listed diagnosis: United States, selected years 1990–2007

[Data are based on a sample of hospital records]

Age and first-listed diagnosis	Average length of stay[1]								
	Both sexes			Male			Female		
	1990	2000	2007	1990	2000	2007	1990	2000	2007
	Number of days								
85 years and over[2]	9.6	6.2	5.6	9.4	6.1	5.8	9.6	6.2	5.5
Septicemia	12.6	6.9	7.2	*11.8	6.7	6.8	12.9	6.9	7.4
Cancer, all	12.1	7.5	6.5	13.4	8.6	6.2	11.3	6.8	6.8
Colorectal cancer	22.4	*10.1	10.2	*	*	*11.4	*21.1	8.2	9.8
Lung/bronchus/tracheal cancer	*	*8.0	*5.9	*	*5.9	*	*	*	*
Breast cancer[3]	. . .	. . .	. . .	. . .	. . .	. . .	*5.3	*	*
Prostate cancer	. . .	. . .	. . .	*7.5	*	*	. . .	. . .	. . .
Diabetes	9.1	5.5	*6.3	*	*	*	9.2	4.9	6.0
Schizophrenia, mood disorders, delusional disorders, nonorganic psychoses	*	*10.5	*	*	*	*	*	*10.8	*
Dementia and Alzheimer's disease	11.4	7.9	7.1	*	*8.8	*7.9	*11.0	*7.6	6.6
Heart disease	8.1	5.2	4.8	7.8	5.1	5.0	8.2	5.3	4.7
Ischemic heart disease	7.5	5.4	4.6	6.8	5.4	4.6	7.9	5.4	4.6
Heart attack	9.8	6.7	5.8	8.9	6.4	6.0	10.3	6.9	5.7
Arrhythmias	8.3	4.4	4.2	*9.6	4.3	4.4	7.7	4.4	4.1
Heart failure	8.6	5.3	4.9	8.0	4.9	5.1	8.8	5.5	4.8
Hypertension	*	*4.2	2.8	*	*	*2.9	*	*	*2.8
Stroke	9.6	5.3	5.3	9.6	5.6	4.9	9.5	5.1	5.4
Pneumonia	10.9	7.0	5.8	11.1	6.1	5.6	10.7	7.5	5.9
Chronic obstructive pulmonary disease	*9.0	5.7	4.6	*7.8	5.5	4.1	*	5.7	4.9
Gallstones	10.3	5.8	6.9	*9.3	*5.6	*7.3	10.7	*5.9	*6.7
Kidney disease	*12.6	8.5	6.6	*	*9.0	7.0	*13.8	*8.2	6.4
Urinary tract infection	10.2	5.6	4.8	9.3	5.7	4.0	10.7	5.5	5.1
Hyperplasia of the prostate	. . .	. . .	. . .	6.6	*3.7	*3.9	. . .	. . .	. . .
Osteoarthritis	10.5	4.7	4.5	*	*	*3.9	*9.6	4.4	4.7
Injury	10.5	5.9	5.5	11.0	6.4	6.1	10.3	5.8	5.3
Fracture	11.1	6.1	5.5	11.2	6.4	6.3	11.1	6.0	5.3
Hip fracture	12.7	6.5	5.9	12.6	6.8	6.7	12.7	6.5	5.6
Complications of care and adverse effects	*11.7	*8.2	6.0	*10.7	*6.4	*6.5	*12.3	*9.1	5.5

* Estimates are considered unreliable. Data preceded by an asterisk have a relative standard error (RSE) of 20%–30%. Data not shown have an RSE greater than 30%.

. . . Category not applicable.

[1]Average length of stay is calculated by dividing days of care by number of discharges. See Appendix II, Average length of stay; Days of care.
[2]Includes discharges with first-listed diagnoses not shown in table.
[3]Shown for women only.

NOTES: Excludes newborn infants. Diagnostic categories are based on the *International Classification of Diseases, 9th Revision, Clinical Modification* (ICD–9–CM). See Appendix II, Diagnosis; Human immunodeficiency virus (HIV) disease; *International Classification of Diseases, 9th Revision, Clinical Modification*; Table XI for ICD–9–CM codes. Rates are based on the civilian population as of July 1. Starting with *Health, United States, 2003*, rates for 2000 and beyond are based on the 2000 census. Rates for 1990–1999 use population estimates based on the 1990 census adjusted for net underenumeration using the 1990 National Population Adjustment Matrix from the U.S. Census Bureau. Rates for 1990–1999 are not strictly comparable with rates for 2000 and beyond because population estimates for 1990–1999 have not been revised to reflect the 2000 census. See Appendix I, National Hospital Discharge Survey; Population Census and Population Estimates. Additional data and diagnosis categories are available from: http://www.cdc.gov/nchs/hdi.htm. Data for additional years are available. See Appendix III.

SOURCE: CDC/NCHS, National Hospital Discharge Survey.

Table 103 (page 1 of 4). Discharges with at least one procedure in nonfederal short-stay hospitals, by sex, age, and selected procedures: United States, selected years 1990–2007

[Data are based on a sample of hospital records]

Age and procedure (any listed)	Both sexes			Male			Female		
	1990	2000	2007	1990	2000	2007	1990	2000	2007
18 years and over					Percent				
Hospital discharges with at least one procedure, crude[1]	67.4	62.1	63.1	65.2	59.2	59.5	68.7	63.9	65.4
					Number per 10,000 population				
Hospital discharges with at least one procedure, age-adjusted[1,2]	1,020.1	859.9	875.6	882.2	701.4	694.6	1,176.4	1,026.2	1,066.1
Hospital discharges with at least one procedure, crude[1]	1,006.4	856.8	879.1	788.1	648.4	670.1	1,205.9	1,049.8	1,075.7
Operations on vessels of heart	28.3	41.2	37.4	41.9	56.9	52.2	15.8	26.7	23.4
Coronary angioplasty or arthrectomy	14.0	26.2	26.7	20.5	34.9	36.5	8.0	18.1	17.4
Coronary artery stent insertion	…	21.7	24.0	…	28.7	33.2	…	15.3	15.3
Drug-eluting stent insertion	…	…	16.6	…	…	22.7	…	…	10.9
Coronary artery bypass graft (CABG)	14.1	15.0	10.2	21.2	21.8	14.9	7.7	8.7	5.8
Cardiac catheterization	52.1	57.8	46.2	68.3	72.1	57.4	37.4	44.6	35.6
Pacemaker	8.6	8.5	8.8	10.1	8.5	9.2	7.1	8.5	8.5
Carotid (neck arteries) endarterectomy	3.6	5.9	4.0	4.1	6.6	4.8	3.1	5.3	3.2
Endoscopy of small intestine	40.8	42.5	42.8	38.6	39.1	38.0	42.8	45.6	47.2
Endoscopy of large intestine	27.9	25.0	21.5	22.5	20.2	18.2	32.8	29.4	24.6
Gall bladder removal	27.9	19.6	17.4	16.5	13.3	12.7	38.2	25.5	21.9
Laparoscopic gall bladder removal	…	14.8	14.2	…	9.2	9.1	…	20.1	18.9
Treatment of intra-abdominal scar tissue	17.0	14.4	15.3	6.5	5.7	8.2	26.6	22.4	22.0
Reduction of fracture	27.6	24.9	24.7	27.3	22.0	22.9	27.8	27.7	26.3
Excision of intervertebral disc and spinal fusion	18.7	18.2	19.5	22.3	20.0	20.2	15.4	16.4	18.8
Total hip replacement	6.4	7.3	9.7	5.4	6.8	9.2	7.3	7.7	10.2
Partial hip replacement	4.8	5.0	10.5	2.0	2.3	8.6	7.3	7.6	12.2
Total knee replacement	6.7	13.8	22.7	4.9	11.0	17.1	8.4	16.4	27.9
CAT scan	68.4	29.2	21.3	68.6	27.4	20.1	68.2	30.9	22.5
Arteriography and angiocardiography with contrast	59.7	63.0	53.6	75.6	76.2	62.2	45.2	50.7	45.6
Diagnostic ultrasound	72.3	36.9	34.4	62.1	33.1	31.5	81.7	40.4	37.1
Magnetic resonance imaging	9.5	9.2	9.7	9.4	8.2	8.5	9.6	10.2	10.9
Mechanical ventilation	17.6	23.0	27.5	18.8	23.9	30.1	16.4	22.1	25.1
18–44 years					Percent				
Hospital discharges with at least one procedure[1]	73.0	71.7	72.6	62.6	55.9	55.4	77.0	77.4	78.7
					Number per 10,000 population				
Hospital discharges with at least one procedure[1]	749.3	609.1	645.1	362.8	251.6	255.2	1,130.6	965.9	1,042.0
Operations on vessels of heart	3.0	3.9	3.5	4.9	5.5	4.9	*1.2	2.3	2.2
Coronary angioplasty or arthrectomy	1.9	3.0	3.0	3.0	4.3	4.2	*0.8	1.6	*1.8
Coronary artery stent insertion	…	2.5	2.6	…	3.6	3.7	…	1.4	*1.6
Drug-eluting stent insertion	…	…	1.6	…	…	2.1	…	…	*1.0
Coronary artery bypass graft (CABG)	1.0	0.9	0.5	*1.8	1.1	*0.6	*	*0.7	*
Cardiac catheterization	9.0	8.5	7.1	12.5	11.0	8.2	5.5	5.9	6.1
Endoscopy of small intestine	13.1	10.3	12.9	13.2	10.4	10.9	13.0	10.2	14.9
Endoscopy of large intestine	6.9	5.5	6.1	5.6	4.7	5.3	8.1	6.3	7.0
Gall bladder removal	18.7	11.9	11.9	6.2	4.3	5.9	31.0	19.4	18.0
Laparoscopic gall bladder removal	…	9.9	10.8	…	3.0	4.9	…	16.8	16.9
Treatment of intra-abdominal scar tissue	14.1	10.8	10.5	2.0	1.5	2.1	26.0	20.1	19.1
Hysterectomy	…	…	…	…	…	…	63.3	55.7	44.8
Abdominal hysterectomy	…	…	…	…	…	…	47.1	34.6	22.7
Vaginal hysterectomy	…	…	…	…	…	…	15.8	19.1	16.1
Forceps, vacuum, and breech delivery	…	…	…	…	…	…	77.5	59.9	54.0
Episiotomy	…	…	…	…	…	…	293.3	160.8	74.6
Other procedures inducing or assisting delivery	…	…	…	…	…	…	387.9	384.2	415.8
Medical induction of labor	…	…	…	…	…	…	41.1	77.7	116.2
Cesarean section	…	…	…	…	…	…	167.1	149.5	235.3
Reduction of fracture	19.1	13.7	14.5	27.9	19.0	21.5	10.4	8.4	7.4
Excision of intervertebral disc and spinal fusion	17.0	14.1	10.6	21.5	16.2	11.1	12.6	12.1	10.0
CAT scan	27.5	10.6	8.5	32.3	11.0	8.8	22.7	10.3	8.3
Arteriography and angiocardiography with contrast	12.5	10.3	10.2	17.4	12.9	10.8	7.6	7.7	9.6
Diagnostic ultrasound	34.2	11.6	9.3	19.3	8.3	6.9	48.9	14.9	11.8
Magnetic resonance imaging	4.9	3.8	3.3	4.9	3.6	2.2	4.9	*4.0	*4.4
Mechanical ventilation	4.6	7.0	9.2	5.4	8.2	11.0	3.8	5.8	7.4

See footnotes at end of table.

Table 103 (page 2 of 4). **Discharges with at least one procedure in nonfederal short-stay hospitals, by sex, age, and selected procedures: United States, selected years 1990–2007**

[Data are based on a sample of hospital records]

Age and procedure (any listed)	Both sexes			Male			Female		
	1990	2000	2007	1990	2000	2007	1990	2000	2007
45–64 years					Percent				
Hospital discharges with at least one procedure [1]	68.2	62.3	62.7	68.9	63.4	63.5	67.6	61.3	61.9
				Number per 10,000 population					
Hospital discharges with at least one procedure [1]	924.2	694.6	716.7	965.9	714.4	734.1	885.4	675.9	700.1
Operations on vessels of heart	53.0	57.7	45.8	83.2	88.5	69.1	24.8	28.4	23.6
Coronary angioplasty or arthrectomy	29.4	37.5	33.5	45.3	55.9	50.1	14.5	20.0	17.8
Coronary artery stent insertion	...	31.1	30.3	...	46.5	45.7	...	16.5	15.6
Drug-eluting stent insertion	...	...	20.3	...	...	30.3	...	...	10.8
Coronary artery bypass graft (CABG)	23.4	20.3	11.7	37.5	32.5	18.1	10.3	8.6	5.5
Cardiac catheterization	98.2	83.0	59.1	136.8	113.9	79.7	62.3	53.7	39.5
Pacemaker	7.8	4.0	4.3	10.9	5.2	5.5	*4.9	2.8	3.3
Carotid (neck arteries) endarterectomy	4.0	5.2	3.1	5.2	5.2	3.9	3.0	*5.2	*2.3
Endoscopy of small intestine	45.0	36.4	37.8	46.3	40.7	38.0	43.8	32.3	37.7
Endoscopy of large intestine	28.5	19.3	18.4	25.4	18.1	16.7	31.4	20.4	20.1
Gall bladder removal	36.4	20.6	16.7	22.3	16.3	13.8	49.5	24.6	19.5
Laparoscopic gall bladder removal	...	15.3	13.1	...	12.1	9.4	...	18.5	16.7
Treatment of intra-abdominal scar tissue	17.1	15.0	16.6	9.5	7.0	10.4	24.2	22.6	22.6
Removal of prostate	...	...	...	35.8	15.6	19.9	...	...	...
Transurethral prostatectomy	...	...	...	30.4	7.0	*4.8	...	...	...
Hysterectomy	...	...	...	...	...	...	76.4	78.2	54.2
Abdominal hysterectomy	...	...	...	...	...	...	58.4	53.2	32.7
Vaginal hysterectomy	...	...	...	...	...	...	17.6	21.6	14.9
Reduction of fracture	20.3	18.5	19.0	19.5	17.6	19.3	21.0	19.3	18.7
Excision of intervertebral disc and spinal fusion	26.1	25.7	27.5	29.4	27.1	28.4	23.1	24.4	26.7
Total hip replacement	6.2	8.1	11.1	5.7	9.1	11.6	6.5	7.2	10.5
Partial hip replacement	*	*1.3	9.3	*	*0.8	8.6	*	*1.7	9.9
Total knee replacement	6.7	12.7	26.0	5.8	8.7	20.5	*7.4	16.4	31.3
Mastectomy	...	...	...	...	...	...	21.2	10.6	8.3
CAT scan	65.4	25.2	19.7	69.9	25.9	19.5	61.2	24.5	20.0
Arteriography and angiocardiography with contrast	105.4	85.3	64.0	138.5	111.4	81.4	74.6	60.7	47.5
Diagnostic ultrasound	69.5	34.3	33.2	73.8	38.0	35.0	65.5	30.9	31.5
Magnetic resonance imaging	10.9	8.9	9.9	10.7	9.4	9.3	11.0	8.4	10.5
Mechanical ventilation	17.6	21.2	26.5	18.6	22.9	30.7	16.7	19.6	22.4
65–74 years					Percent				
Hospital discharges with at least one procedure [1]	66.5	61.3	63.3	69.3	63.9	65.2	63.8	58.9	61.5
				Number per 10,000 population					
Hospital discharges with at least one procedure [1]	1,739.4	1,559.8	1,544.0	1,994.1	1,692.3	1,668.7	1,539.4	1,450.6	1,438.1
Operations on vessels of heart	97.0	139.8	127.4	148.9	195.3	187.0	56.3	94.1	76.9
Coronary angioplasty or arthrectomy	44.1	86.3	86.7	64.9	116.0	122.6	27.8	61.9	56.3
Coronary artery stent insertion	...	71.7	77.9	...	94.9	110.5	...	52.5	50.1
Drug-eluting stent insertion	...	...	58.3	...	...	82.5	...	...	37.7
Coronary artery bypass graft (CABG)	52.1	53.9	39.2	83.1	79.7	62.1	27.7	32.6	19.8
Cardiac catheterization	164.0	174.2	137.9	213.8	222.7	179.5	124.9	134.2	102.7
Pacemaker	24.6	22.5	22.9	32.1	22.8	29.4	18.7	22.3	17.3
Carotid (neck arteries) endarterectomy	14.6	24.1	17.0	18.0	29.5	23.4	11.9	19.6	11.6
Endoscopy of small intestine	92.8	106.6	91.6	91.5	102.4	93.1	93.7	110.0	90.3
Endoscopy of large intestine	70.3	64.8	46.3	62.5	59.7	43.4	76.5	69.0	48.8
Gall bladder removal	45.0	42.1	27.9	42.0	37.9	24.5	47.4	45.5	30.8
Laparoscopic gall bladder removal	...	29.5	20.5	...	24.4	15.9	...	33.7	24.5
Treatment of intra-abdominal scar tissue	23.1	21.4	27.0	17.1	14.5	23.5	27.7	27.1	29.9
Removal of prostate	...	...	...	201.1	83.7	54.8	...	...	...
Transurethral prostatectomy	...	...	...	180.9	59.4	24.4	...	...	...
Hysterectomy	...	...	...	...	...	...	37.4	35.9	26.5
Abdominal hysterectomy	...	...	...	...	...	...	20.8	20.5	15.2
Vaginal hysterectomy	...	...	...	...	...	...	16.5	14.7	10.2
Reduction of fracture	36.2	36.4	32.6	24.3	26.2	21.1	45.5	44.8	42.3
Excision of intervertebral disc and spinal fusion	16.3	21.1	37.7	14.2	22.5	43.2	18.0	20.0	33.0
Total hip replacement	24.0	25.4	33.5	23.0	26.4	33.7	24.9	24.5	33.2
Partial hip replacement	8.9	7.6	21.6	*4.0	*	19.9	*12.7	10.5	23.0
Total knee replacement	33.2	65.4	91.1	26.4	64.5	71.8	38.6	66.0	107.5
Mastectomy	...	...	...	...	...	...	30.7	22.7	12.5
CAT scan	153.7	64.3	*43.0	163.4	65.7	*46.7	146.1	63.1	*39.9
Arteriography and angiocardiography with contrast	184.5	186.2	154.6	239.0	231.9	193.3	141.7	148.5	121.8
Diagnostic ultrasound	155.2	92.7	81.5	165.2	94.1	95.8	147.4	91.6	69.4
Magnetic resonance imaging	20.6	17.2	20.9	19.2	*14.6	*22.2	21.7	*19.3	19.9
Mechanical ventilation	48.6	60.0	71.1	58.7	70.3	76.9	40.6	51.6	66.2

See footnotes at end of table.

Table 103 (page 3 of 4).

Table 103 (page 3 of 4). Discharges with at least one procedure in nonfederal short-stay hospitals, by sex, age, and selected procedures: United States, selected years 1990–2007

[Data are based on a sample of hospital records]

Age and procedure (any listed)	Both sexes			Male			Female		
	1990	2000	2007	1990	2000	2007	1990	2000	2007
75–84 years					Percent				
Hospital discharges with at least one procedure[1]	59.0	53.6	55.3	61.7	56.3	56.6	57.0	51.8	54.2
					Number per 10,000 population				
Hospital discharges with at least one procedure[1]	2,332.9	2,212.3	2,201.0	2,723.9	2,416.5	2,357.4	2,096.7	2,078.8	2,093.2
Operations on vessels of heart	69.1	143.2	140.9	107.6	202.5	200.8	45.8	104.5	99.6
Coronary angioplasty or arthrectomy	22.4	84.7	95.7	33.7	109.3	133.6	15.7	68.7	69.7
Coronary artery stent insertion	. . .	69.8	86.9	. . .	86.5	123.1	. . .	58.8	62.1
Drug-eluting stent insertion	. . .	. . .	61.8	. . .	. . .	85.9	. . .	. . .	45.1
Coronary artery bypass graft (CABG)	47.0	57.7	42.0	74.7	90.5	60.9	30.3	36.2	28.9
Cardiac catheterization	116.6	190.2	163.7	166.0	236.9	211.3	86.8	159.6	131.0
Pacemaker	50.8	58.1	54.0	70.6	72.2	58.8	38.8	48.9	50.7
Carotid (neck arteries) endarterectomy	19.8	32.8	21.4	24.2	45.5	25.5	*17.1	24.5	18.6
Endoscopy of small intestine	171.4	189.7	178.0	188.9	193.8	172.3	160.8	187.0	182.0
Endoscopy of large intestine	131.1	123.7	94.3	126.1	113.8	88.7	134.1	130.1	98.2
Gall bladder removal	51.8	43.4	44.5	64.4	46.7	47.6	44.2	41.3	42.5
Laparoscopic gall bladder removal	. . .	28.9	31.5	. . .	29.6	32.1	. . .	28.5	31.0
Treatment of intra-abdominal scar tissue	34.0	28.6	29.9	28.2	26.3	28.7	37.5	30.2	30.7
Removal of prostate	. . .	. . .	. . .	273.5	98.0	45.9	. . .	. . .	. . .
Transurethral prostatectomy	. . .	. . .	. . .	257.5	89.0	41.6	. . .	. . .	. . .
Hysterectomy	. . .	. . .	. . .	. . .	. . .	. . .	28.5	25.5	23.5
Abdominal hysterectomy	. . .	. . .	. . .	. . .	. . .	. . .	18.8	16.2	11.4
Vaginal hysterectomy	. . .	. . .	. . .	. . .	. . .	. . .	*9.4	8.1	*
Reduction of fracture	86.2	80.1	69.0	43.4	57.2	44.1	112.1	95.0	86.1
Excision of intervertebral disc and spinal fusion	12.0	17.4	25.2	*13.2	*20.4	26.2	11.3	15.3	24.4
Total hip replacement	30.7	26.3	37.6	*26.9	*21.3	35.9	33.1	29.6	38.9
Partial hip replacement	43.6	36.6	35.6	*14.3	20.0	31.1	61.2	47.5	38.7
Total knee replacement	28.4	59.3	86.9	*19.5	48.7	72.8	33.9	66.3	96.5
Mastectomy	. . .	. . .	. . .	. . .	. . .	. . .	29.2	22.0	12.9
CAT scan	279.7	119.2	*73.4	307.2	127.9	*78.1	263.0	113.5	*70.1
Arteriography and angiocardiography with contrast	141.0	219.2	195.0	192.3	287.9	237.9	109.9	174.3	165.5
Diagnostic ultrasound	273.5	134.1	131.3	315.7	142.8	129.0	248.0	128.4	132.8
Magnetic resonance imaging	30.5	*37.3	36.5	43.0	*33.6	*32.5	*23.0	*39.8	*39.3
Mechanical ventilation	79.8	91.1	95.1	110.3	106.5	114.3	61.3	80.9	81.9
85 years and over					Percent				
Hospital discharges with at least one procedure[1]	49.3	44.6	45.5	52.4	45.4	46.0	47.8	44.3	45.2
					Number per 10,000 population				
Hospital discharges with at least one procedure[1]	2,762.1	2,700.5	2,435.8	3,367.3	2,797.9	2,500.7	2,526.8	2,660.6	2,404.9
Operations on vessels of heart	*14.0	51.1	50.0	*	83.0	87.7	*	38.0	32.1
Coronary angioplasty or arthrectomy	*	36.3	38.6	*	*52.9	60.6	*	29.5	28.2
Coronary artery stent insertion	. . .	31.6	31.9	. . .	*48.9	52.5	. . .	*24.4	22.2
Drug-eluting stent insertion	. . .	. . .	18.0	. . .	. . .	*28.0	. . .	. . .	*13.2
Coronary artery bypass graft (CABG)	*	*15.1	11.4	*	*30.1	27.1	*	*9.0	*
Cardiac catheterization	*23.7	87.7	61.9	*	122.8	85.7	*19.0	73.2	50.6
Pacemaker	79.5	82.9	82.9	120.4	104.3	118.5	63.5	74.2	65.9
Carotid (neck arteries) endarterectomy	*	*12.0	*9.6	*	*	*	*	*4.8	*6.1
Endoscopy of small intestine	228.8	262.4	229.0	288.7	245.1	226.4	205.5	269.5	230.3
Endoscopy of large intestine	180.8	158.1	116.9	188.0	133.3	122.8	178.0	168.3	114.1
Gall bladder removal	46.4	40.9	40.1	*68.4	*42.9	*45.1	37.8	*40.1	*37.7
Laparoscopic gall bladder removal	. . .	*30.4	33.2	. . .	*	*36.4	. . .	*30.5	*31.6
Treatment of intra-abdominal scar tissue	29.6	24.3	19.7	*	*16.4	18.3	33.7	*27.5	*20.4
Removal of prostate	. . .	. . .	. . .	257.2	*113.0	39.5	. . .	. . .	. . .
Transurethral prostatectomy	. . .	. . .	. . .	247.1	*110.0	37.0	. . .	. . .	. . .
Hysterectomy	. . .	. . .	. . .	. . .	. . .	. . .	*	*	*
Abdominal hysterectomy	. . .	. . .	. . .	. . .	. . .	. . .	*	*	*
Vaginal hysterectomy	. . .	. . .	. . .	. . .	. . .	. . .	*	*	*
Reduction of fracture	196.2	200.5	178.6	150.6	93.8	89.8	213.9	244.3	220.9
Excision of intervertebral disc and spinal fusion	*	*2.3	*11.1	*	*	*	*	*	*
Total hip replacement	*27.8	*20.7	19.7	*	*	*	*23.2	*26.3	*23.1
Partial hip replacement	67.4	82.2	75.6	*52.9	*44.1	65.2	73.1	97.9	80.6
Total knee replacement	*12.4	*22.9	25.5	*	*	*27.9	*	*16.2	24.3
Mastectomy	. . .	. . .	. . .	. . .	. . .	. . .	*28.9	*15.7	*
CAT scan	378.4	158.7	*105.3	401.2	141.4	*87.3	369.5	165.9	*113.9
Arteriography and angiocardiography with contrast	50.6	120.8	106.1	*87.6	164.4	118.9	36.2	102.8	100.0
Diagnostic ultrasound	327.7	208.5	166.6	394.5	181.4	128.1	301.7	219.6	*184.8
Magnetic resonance imaging	*18.5	*40.4	35.8	*	*	*54.1	*16.2	*	27.2
Mechanical ventilation	91.5	106.0	101.7	97.9	116.5	136.8	89.1	101.7	85.1

See footnotes at end of table.

[Data are based on a sample of hospital records]

. . . Category not applicable.

*Estimates are considered unreliable. Data preceded by an asterisk have a relative standard error (RSE) of 20%–30%. Data not shown have an RSE of greater than 30%.

[1]Includes discharges for procedures not shown separately.

[2]Estimates are age-adjusted to the year 2000 standard population using five age groups: 18–44 years, 45–54 years, 55–64 years, 65–74 years, and 75 years and over. See Appendix II, Age adjustment.

NOTES: Excludes newborn infants. Up to four procedures were coded for each hospital discharge. If more than one procedure with the same code (e.g., a coronary artery bypass graft) was performed during the hospital stay, it was counted only once (any listed). Procedure categories are based on the *International Classification of Diseases, 9th Revision, Clinical Modification* (ICD–9–CM). See Appendix II, *International Classification of Diseases, 9th Revision, Clinical Modification*; Procedure; Table XII for ICD–9–CM codes. Rates are based on the civilian population as of July 1. Starting with *Health, United States, 2003*, rates for 2000 and beyond are based on the 2000 census. Rates for 1990–1999 use population estimates based on the 1990 census adjusted for net underenumeration using the 1990 National Population Adjustment Matrix from the U.S. Census Bureau. Rates for 1990–1999 are not strictly comparable with rates for 2000 and beyond because population estimates for 1990–1999 have not been revised to reflect the 2000 census. See Appendix I, National Hospital Discharge Survey; Population Census and Population Estimates. Data for additional years are available. See Appendix III.

SOURCE: CDC/NCHS, National Hospital Discharge Survey.

Table 104. Hospital admissions, average length of stay, outpatient visits, and outpatient surgery by type of ownership and size of hospital: United States, selected years 1975–2008

[Data are based on reporting by a census of hospitals]

Type of ownership and size of hospital	1975	1980	1990	1995	2000	2006	2007	2008
Admissions				Number in thousands				
All hospitals	36,157	38,892	33,774	33,282	34,891	37,189	37,120	37,529
Federal	1,913	2,044	1,759	1,559	1,034	1,008	981	956
Nonfederal[1]	34,243	36,848	32,015	31,723	33,946	36,180	36,139	36,573
Community[2]	33,435	36,143	31,181	30,945	33,089	35,378	35,346	35,761
Nonprofit	23,722	25,566	22,878	22,557	24,453	25,798	25,752	25,899
For profit	2,646	3,165	3,066	3,428	4,141	4,732	4,626	4,839
State-local government	7,067	7,413	5,236	4,961	4,496	4,848	4,967	5,023
6–24 beds	174	159	95	124	141	192	200	205
25–49 beds	1,431	1,254	870	944	995	1,188	1,170	1,218
50–99 beds	3,675	3,700	2,474	2,299	2,355	2,301	2,295	2,319
100–199 beds	7,017	7,162	5,833	6,288	6,735	6,662	6,341	6,304
200–299 beds	6,174	6,596	6,333	6,495	6,702	7,008	7,009	6,867
300–399 beds	4,739	5,358	5,091	4,693	5,135	5,721	5,637	5,894
400–499 beds	3,689	4,401	3,644	3,413	3,617	3,872	4,044	3,895
500 beds or more	6,537	7,513	6,840	6,690	7,410	8,435	8,650	9,059
Average length of stay[3]				Number of days				
All hospitals	11.4	10.0	9.1	7.8	6.8	6.4	6.3	6.3
Federal	20.3	16.8	14.9	13.1	12.8	11.2	11.5	11.9
Nonfederal[1]	10.8	9.6	8.8	7.5	6.6	6.3	6.2	6.2
Community[2]	7.7	7.6	7.2	6.5	5.8	5.6	5.5	5.5
Nonprofit	7.8	7.7	7.3	6.4	5.7	5.4	5.4	5.4
For profit	6.6	6.5	6.4	5.8	5.4	5.2	5.2	5.3
State-local government	7.6	7.3	7.7	7.4	6.7	6.5	6.4	6.3
6–24 beds	5.6	5.3	5.4	5.5	4.3	4.0	4.0	4.1
25–49 beds	6.0	5.8	6.1	5.7	5.1	4.9	4.9	5.2
50–99 beds	6.8	6.7	7.2	7.0	6.5	6.3	6.3	6.4
100–199 beds	7.1	7.0	7.1	6.4	5.7	5.5	5.5	5.5
200–299 beds	7.5	7.4	6.9	6.2	5.7	5.2	5.2	5.1
300–399 beds	7.8	7.6	7.0	6.1	5.5	5.4	5.3	5.3
400–499 beds	8.1	7.9	7.3	6.3	5.6	5.4	5.3	5.3
500 beds or more	9.1	8.7	8.1	7.1	6.3	5.9	5.9	5.8
Outpatient visits[4]				Number in thousands				
All hospitals	254,844	262,951	368,184	483,195	592,673	690,425	693,510	709,960
Federal	51,957	50,566	58,527	59,934	63,402	83,974	82,187	78,640
Nonfederal[1]	202,887	212,385	309,657	423,261	531,972	606,452	611,323	631,320
Community[2]	190,672	202,310	301,329	414,345	521,405	599,553	603,300	624,098
Nonprofit	131,435	142,156	221,073	303,851	393,168	453,501	455,825	469,804
For profit	7,713	9,696	20,110	31,940	43,378	44,207	43,943	44,897
State-local government	51,525	50,459	60,146	78,554	84,858	101,845	103,532	109,398
6–24 beds	915	1,155	1,471	3,644	4,555	7,803	7,698	8,383
25–49 beds	5,855	6,227	10,812	19,465	27,007	37,054	39,176	40,729
50–99 beds	16,303	17,976	27,582	38,597	49,385	52,975	54,312	56,743
100–199 beds	35,156	36,453	58,940	91,312	114,183	124,426	119,455	119,780
200–299 beds	32,772	36,073	60,561	84,080	99,248	103,431	106,535	107,977
300–399 beds	29,169	30,495	43,699	54,277	73,444	82,916	81,671	90,620
400–499 beds	22,127	25,501	33,394	44,284	52,205	60,440	60,604	57,643
500 beds or more	48,375	48,430	64,870	78,685	101,378	130,508	133,849	142,223
Outpatient surgery				Percent of total surgeries[5]				
Community hospitals[2]	- - -	16.3	50.5	58.1	62.7	63.1	62.7	63.2

- - - Data not available.

[1]The category of nonfederal hospitals comprises psychiatric, tuberculosis and other respiratory diseases hospitals, and long-term and short-term general and other special hospitals. See Appendix II, Hospital.

[2]Community hospitals are nonfederal short-term general and special hospitals whose facilities and services are available to the public. See Appendix II, Hospital.

[3]Average length of stay is calculated as the number of inpatient days divided by the number of admissions. See Appendix II, Average length of stay.

[4]Outpatient visits include visits to the emergency department, outpatient department, referred visits (pharmacy, EKG, radiology), and outpatient surgery. See Appendix II, Outpatient visit.

[5]Total surgeries is a measure of patients with at least one surgical procedure. Persons with multiple surgical procedures during the same outpatient visit or inpatient stay are counted only once. See Appendix II, Outpatient surgery.

NOTE: Data have been revised and differ from previous editions of *Health, United States*.

SOURCE: American Hospital Association (AHA) Annual Survey of Hospitals. Hospital Statistics, 1976, 1981, 1991–2010 editions. Chicago, IL. (Copyrights 1976, 1981, 1991–2010: Used with the permission of Health Forum LLC, an affiliate of the AHA.)

Table 105. Persons employed in health service sites, by site and sex: United States, selected years 2000–2009

[Data are based on household interviews of a sample of the civilian noninstitutionalized population]

Site	2000	2003	2004	2005	2006	2007	2008	2009
Both sexes				Number of persons in thousands				
All employed civilians [1]	136,891	137,736	139,252	141,730	144,427	146,047	145,362	139,877
All health service sites [2]	12,211	13,615	13,817	14,052	14,352	14,687	15,108	15,478
Offices and clinics of physicians	1,387	1,673	1,727	1,801	1,785	1,720	1,562	1,555
Offices and clinics of dentists	672	771	780	792	852	843	774	801
Offices and clinics of chiropractors	120	142	156	163	163	144	139	136
Offices and clinics of optometrists	95	92	93	98	98	114	110	117
Offices and clinics of other health practitioners [3]	143	250	274	275	292	299	195	220
Outpatient care centers	772	873	885	901	919	881	1,107	1,102
Home health care services	548	741	750	795	928	959	881	967
Other health care services [4]	1,027	943	976	1,045	1,096	1,334	1,647	1,747
Hospitals	5,202	5,652	5,700	5,719	5,712	5,955	6,241	6,265
Nursing care facilities	1,593	1,877	1,858	1,848	1,807	1,689	1,779	1,869
Residential care facilities, without nursing	652	601	618	615	700	749	673	699
Men								
All health service sites [2]	2,756	2,986	3,067	3,097	3,187	3,316	3,352	3,382
Offices and clinics of physicians	354	414	424	418	421	417	375	373
Offices and clinics of dentists	158	163	158	156	173	161	136	142
Offices and clinics of chiropractors	32	53	63	68	61	54	58	52
Offices and clinics of optometrists	26	29	24	27	29	26	24	25
Offices and clinics of other health practitioners [3]	38	63	69	80	80	71	52	46
Outpatient care centers	186	200	203	201	199	216	266	261
Home health care services	45	56	65	81	91	96	96	106
Other health care services [4]	304	297	314	311	344	399	470	505
Hospitals	1,241	1,263	1,333	1,347	1,337	1,464	1,451	1,438
Nursing care facilities	195	267	251	246	263	217	231	252
Residential care facilities, without nursing	177	181	164	162	189	195	193	182
Women								
All health service sites [2]	9,457	10,631	10,750	10,958	11,167	11,370	11,755	12,096
Offices and clinics of physicians	1,034	1,259	1,302	1,383	1,364	1,303	1,187	1,182
Offices and clinics of dentists	514	607	623	637	679	681	638	659
Offices and clinics of chiropractors	88	90	93	95	102	90	81	85
Offices and clinics of optometrists	69	64	69	71	69	88	86	92
Offices and clinics of other health practitioners [3]	106	186	204	195	213	228	143	174
Outpatient care centers	586	673	683	700	720	665	841	841
Home health care services	503	685	685	713	837	863	785	861
Other health care services [4]	723	646	662	734	752	935	1,176	1,241
Hospitals	3,961	4,390	4,366	4,372	4,376	4,491	4,790	4,827
Nursing care facilities	1,398	1,611	1,607	1,602	1,544	1,472	1,548	1,617
Residential care facilities, without nursing	475	420	454	453	511	554	480	517
Both sexes				Percent of employed civilians				
All health service sites	8.9	9.9	9.9	9.9	9.9	10.1	10.4	11.1
				Percent distribution				
All health service sites	100.0	100.0	100.0	100.0	100.0	100.0	100.0	100.0
Offices and clinics of physicians	11.4	12.3	12.5	12.8	12.4	11.7	10.3	10.0
Offices and clinics of dentists	5.5	5.7	5.6	5.6	5.9	5.7	5.1	5.2
Offices and clinics of chiropractors	1.0	1.0	1.1	1.2	1.1	1.0	0.9	0.9
Offices and clinics of optometrists	0.8	0.7	0.7	0.7	0.7	0.8	0.7	0.8
Offices and clinics of other health practitioners [3]	1.2	1.8	2.0	2.0	2.0	2.0	1.3	1.4
Outpatient care centers	6.3	6.4	6.4	6.4	6.4	6.0	7.3	7.1
Home health care services	4.5	5.4	5.4	5.7	6.5	6.5	5.8	6.2
Other health care services [4]	8.4	6.9	7.1	7.4	7.6	9.1	10.9	11.3
Hospitals	42.6	41.5	41.3	40.7	39.8	40.5	41.3	40.5
Nursing care facilities	13.0	13.8	13.4	13.2	12.6	11.5	11.8	12.1
Residential care facilities, without nursing	5.3	4.4	4.5	4.4	4.9	5.1	4.5	4.5

[1]Excludes workers under 16 years of age.
[2]Data for health service sites for men and women may not sum to total for all health service sites for both sexes due to rounding.
[3]Includes health service sites such as psychologists' offices, nutritionists' offices, speech defect clinics, midwives offices or clinics, and other offices and clinics. Complete list of clinics under this category is available from: http://www.census.gov/hhes/www/ioindex/ioindex02/cens02_7970_8470.html, Census Industry Code 808.
[4]Includes health service sites such as clinical laboratories, blood banks, CT-SCAN (computer tomography) centers, radiology laboratories, and other offices and clinics. Complete list of clinics under this category is available from: http://www.census.gov/hhes/www/ioindex/ioindex02/cens02_7970_8470.html, Census Industry Code 818.

NOTES: Annual data are based on data collected each month and averaged over the year. Health service sites are based on the North American Industry Classification System. See Appendix II, Industry of employment, Table IX for codes for industries. Data for additional years are available. See Appendix III.

SOURCE: U.S. Department of Labor, Bureau of Labor Statistics, Current Population Survey: Employment and Earnings, January 2010, available from: http://www.bls.gov/cps/cpsa2009.pdf.

Table 106. Active physicians and physicians in patient care, by state: United States, selected years 1975–2008

[Data are based on reporting by physicians]

State	Active physicians[1,2]						Physicians in patient care[1,2,3]					
	1975	1985	1995	2000[4]	2007	2008	1975	1985	1995	2000	2007	2008
	Number per 10,000 civilian population											
United States	15.3	20.7	24.2	25.8	27.4	27.7	13.5	18.0	21.3	22.7	25.3	25.7
Alabama	9.2	14.2	18.4	19.8	21.6	21.6	8.6	13.1	17.0	18.2	20.5	20.6
Alaska	8.4	13.0	15.7	18.5	24.2	24.2	7.8	12.1	14.2	16.3	20.6	20.6
Arizona	16.7	20.2	21.4	20.9	22.3	22.3	14.1	17.1	18.2	17.6	20.6	20.6
Arkansas	9.1	13.8	17.3	18.8	20.4	20.4	8.5	12.8	16.0	17.3	19.3	19.4
California	18.8	23.7	23.7	23.8	26.1	26.2	17.3	21.5	21.7	21.6	24.2	24.4
Colorado	17.3	20.7	23.7	24.0	26.6	26.6	15.0	17.7	20.6	20.9	24.7	24.7
Connecticut	19.8	27.6	32.8	33.7	36.1	36.6	17.7	24.3	29.5	30.3	33.0	33.5
Delaware	14.3	19.7	23.4	24.7	26.2	26.4	12.7	17.1	19.7	21.0	24.4	24.7
District of Columbia	39.6	55.3	63.6	62.5	73.2	74.9	34.6	45.6	53.6	54.5	63.8	65.9
Florida	15.2	20.2	22.9	24.1	25.5	25.8	13.4	17.8	20.3	21.2	23.9	24.2
Georgia	11.5	16.2	19.7	20.4	21.4	21.4	10.6	14.7	18.0	18.6	20.0	20.1
Hawaii	16.2	21.5	24.8	26.4	31.7	31.8	14.7	19.8	22.8	24.0	29.4	29.6
Idaho	9.5	12.1	13.9	15.8	17.9	17.9	8.9	11.4	13.1	14.4	17.0	17.0
Illinois	14.5	20.5	24.8	26.1	27.7	27.8	13.1	18.2	22.1	23.1	25.7	25.8
Indiana	10.6	14.7	18.4	20.0	22.1	22.2	9.6	13.2	16.6	18.0	20.8	21.0
Iowa	11.4	15.6	19.2	19.8	21.4	21.5	9.4	12.4	15.1	15.5	19.2	19.5
Kansas	12.8	17.3	20.8	21.8	23.6	23.8	11.2	15.1	18.0	18.8	22.0	22.0
Kentucky	10.9	15.1	19.2	20.6	23.0	23.1	10.1	13.9	18.0	19.1	21.6	21.7
Louisiana	11.4	17.3	21.7	23.8	25.5	25.3	10.5	16.1	20.3	22.4	24.4	24.2
Maine	12.8	18.7	22.3	26.8	31.5	31.1	10.7	15.6	18.2	21.7	28.5	28.2
Maryland	18.6	30.4	34.1	35.4	40.0	40.2	16.5	24.9	29.9	31.1	35.1	35.3
Massachusetts	20.8	30.2	37.5	38.6	43.2	43.6	18.3	25.4	33.2	34.4	39.1	39.7
Michigan	15.4	20.8	24.8	26.3	28.1	28.5	12.0	16.0	19.0	20.2	25.1	25.5
Minnesota	14.9	20.5	23.4	24.9	28.4	28.8	13.7	18.5	21.5	23.0	26.6	27.0
Mississippi	8.4	11.8	13.9	16.6	18.1	18.2	8.0	11.1	13.0	15.2	17.1	17.3
Missouri	15.0	20.5	23.9	24.7	26.2	26.2	11.6	16.3	19.7	20.2	24.0	24.1
Montana	10.6	14.0	18.4	20.4	22.9	23.0	10.1	13.2	17.1	18.8	21.9	21.9
Nebraska	12.1	15.7	19.8	21.7	24.1	24.7	10.9	14.4	18.3	20.1	22.5	23.1
Nevada	11.9	16.0	16.7	18.0	19.6	19.7	10.9	14.5	14.6	15.9	18.5	18.5
New Hampshire	14.3	18.1	21.5	23.8	27.7	28.6	13.1	16.7	19.8	21.7	26.0	26.9
New Jersey	16.2	23.4	29.3	31.1	33.0	32.9	14.0	19.8	24.9	26.2	30.1	30.0
New Mexico	12.2	17.0	20.2	20.9	23.8	23.9	10.1	14.7	18.0	18.5	22.2	22.3
New York	22.7	29.0	35.3	36.2	38.2	37.8	20.2	25.2	31.6	32.3	35.1	34.8
North Carolina	11.7	16.9	21.1	22.3	24.7	25.0	10.6	15.0	19.4	20.5	23.1	23.4
North Dakota	9.7	15.8	20.5	19.2	24.5	24.7	9.2	14.9	18.9	19.8	23.4	23.6
Ohio	14.1	19.9	23.8	25.4	28.0	28.2	12.2	16.8	20.0	21.3	25.6	25.9
Oklahoma	11.6	16.1	18.8	19.4	20.7	20.9	9.4	12.9	14.7	14.8	18.7	18.9
Oregon	15.6	19.7	21.6	22.9	27.3	27.8	13.8	17.6	19.5	20.5	25.6	26.1
Pennsylvania	16.6	23.6	30.1	31.6	32.9	33.1	13.9	19.2	24.6	25.4	29.3	29.6
Rhode Island	17.8	23.3	30.4	32.5	36.8	37.0	16.1	20.2	26.7	28.8	34.0	34.5
South Carolina	10.0	14.7	18.9	21.0	22.9	22.8	9.3	13.6	17.6	19.4	21.7	21.7
South Dakota	8.2	13.4	16.7	19.2	22.4	22.8	7.7	12.3	15.7	17.7	21.3	21.8
Tennessee	12.4	17.7	22.5	23.6	25.9	26.0	11.3	16.2	20.8	21.8	24.4	24.6
Texas	12.5	16.8	19.4	20.3	21.4	21.5	11.0	14.7	17.3	17.9	20.0	20.2
Utah	14.1	17.2	19.2	19.6	20.9	20.8	13.0	15.5	17.6	17.8	19.5	19.3
Vermont	18.2	23.8	26.9	32.0	36.0	36.0	15.5	20.3	24.2	28.8	33.2	33.3
Virginia	12.9	19.5	22.5	23.9	26.9	27.2	11.9	17.8	20.8	22.0	25.1	25.5
Washington	15.3	20.2	22.5	23.7	26.8	27.0	13.6	17.9	20.2	21.2	24.8	25.1
West Virginia	11.0	16.3	21.0	23.5	25.5	25.7	10.0	14.6	17.9	19.5	23.1	23.3
Wisconsin	12.5	17.7	21.5	23.1	26.1	26.2	11.4	15.9	19.6	20.9	24.5	24.6
Wyoming	9.5	12.9	15.3	17.3	19.5	19.9	8.9	12.0	13.9	15.7	18.4	18.7

[1]Includes active doctors of medicine (MDs) and active doctors of osteopathy (DOs). See Appendix II, Physician.
[2]Starting with 2003 data, federal and nonfederal physicians are included. Data prior to 2003 included nonfederal physicians only.
[3]Prior to 2006, excludes DOs. Excludes physicians in medical teaching, administration, research, and other nonpatient care activities. Includes residents.
[4]Data for doctors of osteopathy are as of January 2001.

NOTES: Data for MDs are as of December 31. Data for DOs are as of May 31.

SOURCE: American Medical Association (AMA): Physician distribution and medical licensure in the U.S., 1975; Physician characteristics and distribution in the U.S., 1986 edition; 1996–1997 edition; 2008–2010 edition; Department of Physician Practice and Communication Information, Division of Survey and Data Resources, AMA. (Copyrights 1976, 1986, 1997, 2004, 2008, 2009, 2010: Used with the permission of the AMA); American Osteopathic Association: 1975–1976 Yearbook and Directory of Osteopathic Physicians, 1985–1986 Yearbook and Directory of Osteopathic Physicians; American Association of Colleges of Osteopathic Medicine: Annual Statistical Report, 1996; American Osteopathic Association: Factsheet 2006, 2006; Osteopathic Medical Profession Report 2007 and 2008; and unpublished data.

Table 107. Doctors of medicine, by place of medical education and activity: United States and outlying U.S. areas, selected years 1975–2008

[Data are based on reporting by physicians]

Place of medical education and activity	1975	1985	1995	2000	2005	2006	2007	2008
	Number of doctors of medicine							
Total doctors of medicine	393,742	552,716	720,325	813,770	902,053	921,904	941,304	954,224
Active doctors of medicine[1]	340,280	497,140	625,443	692,368	762,438	766,836	776,554	784,199
Place of medical education:								
U.S. medical graduates	- - -	392,007	481,137	527,931	571,798	574,315	580,336	586,421
International medical graduates[2]	- - -	105,133	144,306	164,437	190,640	192,521	196,218	197,778
Activity:								
Patient care[3,4]	287,837	431,527	564,074	631,431	718,473	723,118	732,234	740,867
Office-based practice	213,334	329,041	427,275	490,398	563,225	560,411	562,897	556,818
General and family practice	46,347	53,862	59,932	67,534	74,999	74,900	75,952	75,443
Cardiovascular diseases	5,046	9,054	13,739	16,300	17,519	17,480	17,504	17,352
Dermatology	3,442	5,325	6,959	7,969	8,795	8,920	9,036	9,066
Gastroenterology	1,696	4,135	7,300	8,515	9,742	9,881	10,042	10,119
Internal medicine	28,188	52,712	72,612	88,699	107,028	107,284	108,552	107,943
Pediatrics	12,687	22,392	33,890	42,215	51,854	51,815	52,095	51,719
Pulmonary diseases	1,166	3,035	4,964	6,095	7,321	7,377	7,490	7,535
General surgery	19,710	24,708	24,086	24,475	26,079	25,592	25,434	24,640
Obstetrics and gynecology	15,613	23,525	29,111	31,726	34,659	34,225	34,405	33,968
Ophthalmology	8,795	12,212	14,596	15,598	16,580	15,765	15,852	15,656
Orthopedic surgery	8,148	13,033	17,136	17,367	19,115	19,220	19,299	19,110
Otolaryngology	4,297	5,751	7,139	7,581	8,206	8,199	8,177	8,034
Plastic surgery	1,706	3,299	4,612	5,308	6,011	6,016	6,100	6,093
Urological surgery	5,025	7,081	7,991	8,460	8,955	8,850	8,796	8,656
Anesthesiology	8,970	15,285	23,770	27,624	31,887	31,746	31,617	31,389
Diagnostic radiology	1,978	7,735	12,751	14,622	17,618	17,577	17,327	17,197
Emergency medicine	- - -	- - -	11,700	14,541	20,173	20,055	20,036	19,965
Neurology	1,862	4,691	7,623	8,559	10,400	10,423	10,476	10,386
Pathology, anatomical/clinical	4,195	6,877	9,031	10,267	11,747	11,465	11,191	10,738
Psychiatry	12,173	18,521	23,334	24,955	27,638	27,387	27,492	26,521
Radiology	6,970	7,355	5,994	6,674	7,049	6,954	6,913	6,809
Other specialty	15,320	28,453	29,005	35,314	39,850	39,280	39,111	38,479
Hospital-based practice	74,503	102,486	136,799	141,033	155,248	162,707	169,337	184,049
Residents and interns[5]	53,527	72,159	93,650	95,125	95,391	97,102	98,688	108,073
Full-time hospital staff	20,976	30,327	43,149	45,908	59,857	65,605	70,649	75,976
Other professional activity[6]	24,252	44,046	40,290	41,556	43,965	43,718	44,320	43,332
Inactive	21,449	38,646	72,326	75,168	99,823	108,344	111,551	119,239
Not classified	26,145	13,950	20,579	45,136	39,304	46,252	52,740	50,347
Unknown address	5,868	2,980	1,977	1,098	488	472	459	439

- - - Data not available.

[1]Doctors of medicine who are inactive, have unknown address, or primary specialty not classified are excluded. See Appendix II, Physician.
[2]International medical graduates received their medical education in schools outside the United States and Canada.
[3]Specialty information is based on the physician's self-designated primary area of practice. Categories include generalists and specialists. See Appendix II, Physician specialty.
[4]Starting with 2003 data, estimates include federal and nonfederal doctors of medicine. Prior to 2003, estimates were for nonfederal doctors of medicine only. See Health, United States, 2004, Table 103 for data on federal doctors of medicine.
[5]Starting with 1990 data, clinical fellows are included in this category. In prior years, clinical fellows were included in the other professional activity category.
[6]Includes medical teaching, administration, research, and other. Prior to 1990, this category also included clinical fellows.

NOTES: Data for doctors of medicine are as of December 31, except for 1990–1994 data, which are as of January 1. Outlying areas include Puerto Rico, the U.S. Virgin Islands, and the Pacific islands of Canton, Caroline, Guam, Mariana, Marshall, American Samoa, and Wake.

SOURCE: American Medical Association (AMA). Distribution of physicians in the United States, 1970; Physician distribution and medical licensure in the U.S., 1975; Physician characteristics and distribution in the U.S., 1981, 1986, 1989, 1990, 1992, 1993, 1994, 1995–1996, 1996–1997, 1997–1998, 1999, 2000–2001, 2001–2002, 2002–2003, 2003–2004, 2004–2010 editions, Department of Physician Practice and Communications Information, Division of Survey and Data Resources, AMA. (Copyrights 1971, 1976, 1982, 1986, 1989, 1990, 1992, 1993, 1994, 1996, 1997, 1997, 1982, 1986, 1989, 1990, 1992, 1993, 1994, 1996–2010: Used with the permission of the AMA.)

Table 108. Doctors of medicine in primary care, by specialty: United States and outlying U.S. areas, selected years 1949–2008

[Data are based on reporting by physicians]

Specialty	1949[1]	1960[1]	1970	1980	1990	1995	2000	2004	2008
					Number				
Total doctors of medicine[2]	201,277	260,484	334,028	467,679	615,421	720,325	813,770	884,974	954,224
Active doctors of medicine[3]	191,577	247,257	310,845	414,916	547,310	625,443	692,368	744,143	784,199
General primary care specialists	113,222	125,359	134,354	170,705	213,514	241,329	274,653	296,495	305,264
General practice/family medicine	95,980	88,023	57,948	60,049	70,480	75,976	86,312	91,164	93,761
Internal medicine	12,453	26,209	39,924	58,462	76,295	88,240	101,353	111,800	115,314
Obstetrics/Gynecology	- - -	- - -	18,532	24,612	30,220	33,519	35,922	37,779	38,272
Pediatrics	4,789	11,127	17,950	27,582	36,519	43,594	51,066	55,752	57,917
Primary care subspecialists	- - -	- - -	3,161	16,642	30,911	39,659	52,294	62,322	71,794
Family medicine	- - -	- - -	- - -	- - -	- - -	236	483	768	1,193
Internal medicine	- - -	- - -	1,948	13,069	22,054	26,928	34,831	41,471	47,779
Obstetrics/Gynecology	- - -	- - -	344	1,693	3,477	4,133	4,319	4,280	4,363
Pediatrics	- - -	- - -	869	1,880	5,380	8,362	12,661	15,803	18,459
					Percent of active doctors of medicine				
General primary care specialist	59.1	50.7	43.2	41.1	39.0	38.6	39.7	39.8	38.9
General practice/family medicine	50.1	35.6	18.6	14.5	12.9	12.1	12.5	12.3	12.0
Internal medicine	6.5	10.6	12.8	14.1	13.9	14.1	14.6	15.0	14.7
Obstetrics/Gynecology	- - -	- - -	6.0	5.9	5.5	5.4	5.2	5.1	4.9
Pediatrics	2.5	4.5	5.8	6.6	6.7	7.0	7.4	7.5	9.2
Primary care subspecialists	- - -	- - -	1.0	4.0	5.6	6.3	7.6	8.4	9.2
Family medicine	- - -	- - -	0.0	0.0	0.0	0.0	0.1	0.1	0.2
Internal medicine	- - -	- - -	0.6	3.1	4.0	4.3	5.0	5.6	6.1
Obstetrics/Gynecology	- - -	- - -	0.1	0.4	0.6	0.7	0.6	0.6	0.6
Pediatrics	- - -	- - -	0.3	0.5	1.0	1.3	1.8	2.1	2.4

- - - Data not available.

0.0 Percent greater than zero but less than 0.05.

[1]Estimated by the Bureau of Health Professions, Health Resources Administration. Active doctors of medicine (MDs) include those with address unknown and primary specialty not classified.

[2]Includes MDs engaged in federal and nonfederal patient care (office-based or hospital-based) and other professional activities.

[3]Starting with 1970 data, MDs who are inactive, have unknown address, or primary specialty not classified are excluded. Also see Table 108. See Appendix II, Physician.

NOTES: See Appendix II, Physician specialty. Data are as of December 31 except for 1990–1994 data, which are as of January 1, and 1949 data, which are as of midyear. Outlying areas include Puerto Rico, the U.S. Virgin Islands, and the Pacific islands of Canton, Caroline, Guam, Mariana, Marshall, American Samoa, and Wake. Data have been revised and differ from previous editions of *Health, United States*.

SOURCE: Health Manpower Source Book: Medical Specialists, USDHEW, 1962; American Medical Association (AMA). Distribution of physicians in the United States, 1970; Physician characteristics and distribution in the U.S., 1981, 1992, 1996–1997, 1997–1998, 1999, 2000–2001, 2001–2002, 2002–2003, 2003–2004, 2004, 2005, 2006, 2007, 2008, 2009 editions, Department of Physician Practice and Communications Information, Division of Survey and Data Resources, AMA. (Copyrights 1971, 1982, 1992, 1996, 1997, 1999, 2000, 2001, 2002, 2003, 2004, 2005, 2006, 2007, 2008, 2009: Used with the permission of the AMA.)

Table 109. Active dentists, by state: United States, selected years 1993–2007

[Data are based on reporting by dentists]

State	1993	1996	2000	2003	2006	2007	1993	1996	2000	2003	2006	2007
	Number of dentists						Number of dentists per 10,000 civilian population					
United States	155,087	160,388	166,383	173,574	179,594	181,725	6.1	6.1	6.1	6.0	6.0	6.0
Alabama	1,779	1,861	1,912	1,972	2,032	2,032	4.3	4.4	4.3	4.4	4.4	4.4
Alaska	421	454	467	476	513	519	7.5	7.7	7.5	7.3	7.7	7.6
Arizona	2,032	2,140	2,322	2,643	3,107	3,225	5.3	4.9	4.5	4.7	5.0	5.1
Arkansas	1,001	1,030	1,080	1,119	1,146	1,162	4.2	4.1	4.0	4.1	4.1	4.1
California	20,909	21,661	22,963	25,496	26,887	27,654	6.8	6.8	6.8	7.2	7.4	7.6
Colorado	2,503	2,634	2,818	2,953	3,139	3,181	7.3	6.9	6.6	6.5	6.6	6.5
Connecticut	2,587	2,644	2,636	2,668	2,694	2,710	7.9	8.1	7.7	7.7	7.7	7.7
Delaware	331	356	357	372	395	403	4.8	4.9	4.6	4.6	4.6	4.7
District of Columbia	810	745	728	660	609	614	13.9	13.8	12.7	11.7	10.5	10.4
Florida	7,110	7,582	8,170	8,747	9,450	9,640	5.3	5.3	5.1	5.1	5.2	5.3
Georgia	3,251	3,389	3,611	3,811	4,167	4,295	4.9	4.7	4.4	4.4	4.5	4.5
Hawaii	976	1,012	992	1,026	1,046	1,043	8.8	8.9	8.2	8.2	8.1	8.1
Idaho	573	621	678	756	834	863	5.4	5.2	5.2	5.5	5.7	5.8
Illinois	7,978	8,169	8,205	8,211	8,249	8,268	6.9	6.9	6.6	6.5	6.4	6.4
Indiana	2,716	2,788	2,867	2,967	3,013	3,035	4.8	4.8	4.7	4.8	4.8	4.8
Iowa	1,545	1,526	1,564	1,579	1,583	1,610	5.5	5.4	5.3	5.4	5.3	5.4
Kansas	1,316	1,325	1,329	1,397	1,417	1,437	5.3	5.2	4.9	5.1	5.1	5.2
Kentucky	2,129	2,177	2,258	2,307	2,340	2,356	5.7	5.6	5.6	5.6	5.6	5.6
Louisiana	2,029	2,070	2,086	2,141	2,102	2,118	4.8	4.8	4.7	4.8	4.9	4.9
Maine	592	596	601	617	650	662	4.8	4.8	4.7	4.7	4.9	5.0
Maryland	3,753	3,900	3,986	4,147	4,132	4,212	7.7	7.8	7.5	7.5	7.4	7.5
Massachusetts	4,652	4,912	5,137	5,248	5,299	5,314	7.8	8.1	8.1	8.2	8.2	8.2
Michigan	5,884	5,911	5,913	6,154	6,141	6,126	6.2	6.2	5.9	6.1	6.1	6.1
Minnesota	2,913	2,912	2,960	3,014	3,137	3,196	6.5	6.3	6.0	6.0	6.1	6.1
Mississippi	1,040	1,075	1,115	1,158	1,173	1,190	4.0	4.0	3.9	4.0	4.0	4.1
Missouri	2,773	2,757	2,680	2,771	2,803	2,813	5.4	5.2	4.8	4.9	4.8	4.8
Montana	476	482	485	499	525	549	5.8	5.5	5.4	5.4	5.6	5.7
Nebraska	1,054	1,090	1,087	1,107	1,116	1,111	6.6	6.6	6.4	6.4	6.3	6.3
Nevada	570	605	763	921	1,185	1,285	4.3	3.8	3.8	4.1	4.7	5.0
New Hampshire	642	669	707	761	821	830	5.8	5.8	5.7	5.9	6.2	6.3
New Jersey	6,144	6,436	6,607	6,854	7,113	7,042	7.9	8.1	7.9	7.9	8.2	8.1
New Mexico	719	770	809	844	871	907	4.6	4.5	4.4	4.5	4.5	4.6
New York	14,395	14,968	15,159	15,231	15,110	15,184	8.0	8.2	8.0	7.9	7.8	7.9
North Carolina	2,968	3,178	3,394	3,692	4,031	4,108	4.4	4.4	4.2	4.4	4.6	4.5
North Dakota	315	332	300	314	323	326	5.0	5.2	4.7	5.0	5.1	5.1
Ohio	5,981	6,079	6,108	6,053	6,081	6,063	5.4	5.4	5.4	5.3	5.3	5.3
Oklahoma	1,584	1,641	1,683	1,722	1,774	1,804	5.0	5.0	4.9	4.9	5.0	5.0
Oregon	2,034	2,149	2,273	2,360	2,506	2,551	6.8	6.7	6.6	6.6	6.8	6.8
Pennsylvania	7,915	7,988	8,031	7,993	7,907	7,747	6.6	6.6	6.5	6.5	6.4	6.2
Rhode Island	581	591	589	586	596	569	5.8	6.0	5.6	5.4	5.6	5.4
South Carolina	1,601	1,656	1,803	1,912	2,006	2,026	4.5	4.5	4.5	4.6	4.6	4.6
South Dakota	347	353	359	363	387	397	4.9	4.8	4.8	4.8	4.9	5.0
Tennessee	2,748	2,814	2,993	3,031	3,031	3,076	5.5	5.3	5.3	5.2	5.0	5.0
Texas	8,860	9,274	9,873	10,309	10,758	10,981	5.1	4.9	4.7	4.7	4.6	4.6
Utah	1,162	1,233	1,398	1,531	1,671	1,713	6.4	6.2	6.3	6.5	6.6	6.5
Vermont	323	345	353	361	360	361	5.7	5.9	5.8	5.8	5.8	5.8
Virginia	3,686	3,805	4,036	4,209	4,489	4,563	5.9	5.8	5.7	5.7	5.9	5.9
Washington	3,271	3,495	3,860	4,209	4,510	4,528	6.4	6.4	6.5	6.9	7.1	7.0
West Virginia	816	836	828	824	854	847	4.5	4.6	4.6	4.6	4.7	4.7
Wisconsin	3,054	3,077	3,119	3,178	3,199	3,186	6.1	6.0	5.8	5.8	5.8	5.7
Wyoming	235	252	267	265	281	269	5.1	5.3	5.4	5.3	5.5	5.1

NOTES: The data include professionally active dentists only. Professionally active dentist occupation categories include active practitioners; dental school faculty or staff; armed forces dentists; government-employed dentists at the federal, state, or local levels; interns and residents; and other health or dental organization staff members. U.S. totals include dentists with unknown state of practice not shown separately. Rates were calculated using the number of dentists from ADA and civilian population data from AMA, to be consistent with Table 106.

SOURCE: American Dental Association (ADA), Survey Center, Distribution of Dentists in the United States: Historical Report, 1993–2001, Table 1; p. 6 (number of dentists); Distribution of Dentists in the United States by Region and State, 2003, Table 1; p. 6–7 (number of dentists); Distribution of Dentists in the United States by Region and State, 2006, Table 1; p. 6–7 (number of dentists); Distribution of Dentists in the United States by Region and State, 2007, Table 1; p. 6–7 (number of dentists) (© 2003, 2005, 2008, 2009 American Dental Association. All rights reserved. Reprinted by permission). American Medical Association (AMA). Physician characteristics and distribution in the U.S., 2009 and previous editions (number of civilian population) (© 1994, 1997, 2002, 2005, 2008, 2009: Used with the permission of the AMA).

Table 110. Health care employees and wages, by selected occupations: United States, selected years 2001–2009

[Data are based on a semiannual mail survey of nonfarm establishments]

Occupation title	Number of employees[1]				AAPC[2]	Mean hourly wage[3]				AAPC[2]
	2001	2003	2006	2009	2001–2009	2001	2003	2006	2009	2001–2009
Health care practitioner and technical occupations										
Audiologists	11,040	10,030	10,910	12,590	1.7	$23.89	$25.23	$29.38	$32.14	3.8
Cardiovascular technologists and technicians	40,990	43,300	43,870	48,070	2.0	17.55	18.44	21.15	23.91	3.9
Dental hygienists	149,880	146,360	166,380	173,900	1.9	27.30	28.13	30.01	32.63	2.3
Diagnostic medical sonographers. . . .	32,990	37,240	44,340	51,630	5.8	23.08	24.39	27.94	30.60	3.6
Dietetic technicians.	28,940	26,870	24,450	24,510	–2.1	11.23	11.64	12.55	13.72	2.5
Dietitians and nutritionists	43,200	46,190	51,230	53,220	2.6	19.74	20.68	23.02	25.59	3.3
Emergency medical technicians and paramedics	170,690	181,750	196,190	217,920	3.1	12.24	12.95	14.13	15.88	3.3
Licensed practical and licensed vocational nurses	683,790	682,590	720,380	728,670	0.8	15.14	15.97	18.05	19.66	3.3
Nuclear medicine technologists	17,360	17,550	19,270	21,670	2.8	24.65	26.57	30.29	32.91	3.7
Occupational therapists.	77,080	81,380	88,570	97,840	3.0	25.10	25.87	30.05	33.98	3.9
Opticians, dispensing	63,120	63,780	65,190	60,840	–0.5	13.49	13.74	15.49	16.73	2.7
Pharmacists.	223,630	215,030	239,920	267,860	2.3	35.02	37.80	44.95	51.27	4.9
Pharmacy technicians.	207,140	211,270	282,450	331,890	6.1	10.82	11.47	12.75	13.92	3.2
Physical therapists	126,450	134,970	156,100	174,490	4.1	28.43	29.02	32.72	36.64	3.2
Physician assistants	56,200	60,030	62,960	76,900	4.0	30.00	31.15	35.71	40.78	3.9
Psychiatric technicians	59,750	56,000	58,940	70,730	2.1	12.94	13.60	14.64	14.77	1.7
Radiation therapists	13,460	13,990	14,290	15,570	1.8	25.71	30.83	32.49	37.18	4.7
Radiologic technologists and technicians.	168,240	173,030	190,180	213,560	3.0	18.68	20.03	23.71	26.05	4.2
Recreational therapists	26,830	22,860	24,130	21,960	–2.5	14.92	15.82	17.55	19.84	3.6
Registered nurses	2,217,990	2,246,430	2,417,150	2,583,770	1.9	23.19	24.63	28.71	31.99	4.1
Respiratory therapists	82,930	87,180	99,330	107,270	3.3	19.17	20.07	23.37	26.06	3.9
Respiratory therapy technicians	28,700	25,470	18,710	15,100	–7.7	16.93	17.11	19.17	21.96	3.3
Speech-language pathologists	83,110	86,640	98,690	111,640	3.8	24.20	25.10	29.25	32.86	3.9
Health care support occupations										
Dental assistants	267,840	272,030	277,040	294,020	1.2	13.29	13.57	14.83	16.35	2.6
Home health aides	560,190	583,880	751,480	955,220	6.9	8.90	9.22	9.66	10.39	2.0
Massage therapists.	26,440	29,940	41,920	55,920	9.8	15.93	16.49	18.93	19.13	2.3
Medical assistants	345,930	362,670	409,570	495,970	4.6	11.71	11.99	13.07	14.16	2.4
Medical equipment preparers.	33,540	37,140	42,740	47,070	4.3	11.29	11.66	12.97	14.32	3.0
Medical transcriptionists	94,090	97,810	86,790	82,810	–1.6	12.99	13.59	14.74	16.03	2.7
Nursing aides, orderlies, and attendants	1,307,600	1,341,650	1,376,660	1,438,010	1.2	9.54	10.12	11.04	12.01	2.9
Occupational therapist aides	7,560	6,060	7,780	8,040	0.8	11.70	12.21	13.35	13.89	2.2
Occupational therapist assistants . . .	17,520	18,940	23,700	26,680	5.4	17.39	18.04	20.25	24.44	4.3
Pharmacy aides	58,130	61,170	47,810	52,230	–1.3	9.22	9.42	10.07	10.74	1.9
Physical therapist aides	35,250	36,870	45,520	44,160	2.9	10.45	10.71	11.20	12.01	1.8
Physical therapist assistants	47,810	52,440	59,350	63,750	3.7	17.18	17.67	19.91	23.36	3.9
Psychiatric aides	59,640	57,770	57,000	62,610	0.6	11.42	11.48	12.01	13.19	1.8

[1]Estimates do not include self-employed, owners and partners in unincorporated firms, household workers, or unpaid family workers and were rounded to the nearest 10.

[2]AAPC is average annual percent change. See Appendix II, Average annual rate of change (percentage change).

[3]The mean hourly wage rate for an occupation is the total wages that all workers in the occupation earn in an hour divided by the total employment of the occupation. More information is available from: http://www.bls.gov/oes/current/oes_tec.htm.

NOTES: This table includes both full-time and part-time wage and salary workers. This table excludes occupations such as dentists, physicians, and chiropractors, which have a large percentage of workers who are self-employed. Challenges in using Occupational Employment Statistics (OES) data as a time series include changes in the occupational, industrial, and geographical classification systems, changes in theway data are collected, changes in the survey reference period, and changes in mean wage estimation methodology, as well as permanent features of the methodology. See Appendix I, Occupational Employment Statistics. Data for additional years are available. See Appendix III.

SOURCE: U.S. Department of Labor, Bureau of Labor Statistics. Occupational Employment Statistics. Available from: http://www.bls.gov/oes/current/oes_nat.htm#29-0000.

Table 111. First-year enrollment and graduates of health professions schools, and number of schools, by selected profession: United States, selected academic years 1980–1981 through 2007–2008

[Data are based on reporting by health professions associations]

Profession	1980–1981	1990–1991	2000–2001	2006–2007	2007–2008
First-year enrollment			Number		
Dentistry	6,030	4,001	4,327	4,733	4,770
Medicine (Allopathic)[1,2]	17,186	16,876	16,699	17,826	18,287
Medicine (Osteopathic)[3]	1,496	1,950	2,927	4,055	4,528
Optometry[1]	1,174	1,245	1,384	1,434	1,443
Pharmacy[1,4]	7,377	8,267	8,382	10,992	11,557
Podiatry[5]	695	561	475	647	666
Public Health[1,6]	- - -	4,392	5,840	7,382	7,481
Graduates					
Dentistry	5,550	3,995	4,367	4,714	4,796
Medicine (Allopathic)[1]	15,632	15,427	15,796	16,143	16,167
Medicine (Osteopathic)	1,151	1,534	2,510	3,000	3,364
Optometry[1]	1,092	1,224	1,310	1,291	1,317
Pharmacy[1]	7,323	7,122	7,000	9,812	10,500
Podiatry	597	591	531	331	444
Public Health[1]	3,168	3,995	5,747	7,315	7,482
Schools					
Dentistry	60	56	55	56	56
Medicine (Allopathic)[1]	126	126	125	126	126
Medicine (Osteopathic)	14	15	19	20	25
Optometry[1]	13	17	17	17	17
Pharmacy[1]	72	74	82	100	102
Podiatry	5	7	7	7	8
Public Health[1]	21	25	28	38	40

- - - Data not available.

[1] Includes data from schools in Puerto Rico.

[2] Includes new entrants and those repeating the initial year.

[3] May also include persons enrolled in first-year classes for data years 1980–1981 and 2006–2007.

[4] Starting with 2005–2006 data, first-year enrollment for pharmacy schools include Pharm.D.1 enrollments only. Prior to 2005, first-year enrollment data include both Pharm.D.1, B.S. Pharmacy, and B.Pharm. enrollments. Includes second from last year for baccalaureate and third from last year for Pharm.D.1 and does not include first-year enrollees in accelerated programs. In 2006, one pharmacy school did not report enrollment data.

[5] First-year enrollment data for podiatry in 1980–1981 are reported as of the beginning of the academic year.

[6] Starting with 2005–2006 data, first-year enrollment data for public health schools include Spring, Summer, and Fall enrollment. Prior to 2005–2006, the data are for Fall enrollment only and are not directly comparable to 2005–2006 data.

NOTES: Data on the number of schools and first-year enrollments are reported as of the beginning of the academic year, while data on the number of graduates are reported as of the end of the academic year. Some numbers in this table have been revised and differ from previous editions of Health, United States.

SOURCE: American Dental Association (ADA): 2008–2009 Survey of Dental Education: Academic Programs, Enrollments, and Graduates - vol 1, Chicago, IL. 2010. Table 10; p. 23 (number of first-year students) and Table 22; p. 46 (number of dental school graduates and number of dental schools). Available from: http://www.ada.org/goto/edreports (© 2010 American Dental Association. All rights reserved. Reprinted by permission); Association of American Medical Colleges: FACTS - Applicants, Matriculants, Graduates, and Residency Applicants, Applicants and Matriculants data. Available from: http://www.aamc.org. Association of American Medical Colleges: AAMC Data Book, Medical Schools and Teaching Hospitals by the Numbers, Washington, DC. 2005, 2006, and 2009 (© 2005, 2006, and 2009: Used with the permission of the AAMC); American Association of Colleges of Osteopathic Medicine: A Report on a Survey of Osteopathic Medical School Growth, 2007–2008, Chevy Chase, MD. Fast Facts about Osteopathic Medical Education. Available from: http://www.aacom.org/data. Reprinted with permission from AACOM, All rights reserved; Association of Schools and Colleges of Optometry: Annual Student Data Report Academic Years 2000–2001, 2001–2002, 2005–2006, 2006–2007, and 2007–2008 and unpublished data. Available from: http://www.opted.org; American Association of Colleges of Pharmacy: Fall 2005 - Fall 2008 editions of the Profile of Pharmacy Students. Available from: http://www.aacp.org; American Association of Colleges of Podiatric Medicine: Applicant, Matriculant, and Graduate Statistics, 2006, 2007, and 2008. Available from: http://www.aacpm.org. Association of Schools of Public Health: Annual Data Reports, 2007. Washington, DC. Available from: http://www.asph.org/document.cfm?page=749. Bureau of Health Professions: United States Health Personnel FACTBOOK. Health Resources and Services Administration. Rockville, MD. 2003.

Table 112 (page 1 of 2). Total enrollment in schools for selected health occupations, by race and Hispanic origin: United States, selected academic years 1980–1981 through 2007–2008

[Data are based on reporting by health professions associations]

Occupation, race, and Hispanic origin	1980–1981	1990–1991	2000–2001	2007–2008	1980–1981	1990–1991	2000–2001	2007–2008
Dentistry	Number of students				Percent distribution of students			
All races[1]	22,842	15,951	17,349	19,342	100.0	100.0	100.0	100.0
Not Hispanic or Latino:								
White	19,947	11,185	10,997	11,723	87.3	70.1	63.4	60.6
Black or African American	1,022	940	832	1,147	4.5	5.9	4.8	5.9
Hispanic or Latino[2]	780	1,254	925	1,214	3.4	7.9	5.3	6.3
American Indian or Alaska Native	53	53	112	118	0.2	0.3	0.6	0.6
Asian or Pacific Islander	1,040	2,519	4,295	4,387	4.6	15.8	24.8	22.7
Medicine (Allopathic)[3]								
All races[1]	65,189	65,163	69,414	74,518	100.0	100.0	100.0	100.0
Not Hispanic or Latino:								
White	55,434	47,893	42,154	46,496	85.0	73.5	60.7	62.4
Black or African American	3,708	4,241	4,881	5,386	5.7	6.5	7.0	7.2
Mexican	951	1,109	1,655	1,936	1.5	1.7	2.4	2.6
Puerto Rican	1,127	1,253	1,228	1,561	1.7	1.9	1.8	2.1
Other Hispanic or Latino[4]	683	1,176	1,307	2,320	1.0	1.8	1.9	3.1
American Indian or Alaska Native[5]	221	277	530	657	0.3	0.4	0.8	0.9
Asian or Pacific Islander	1,924	8,436	13,264	16,045	3.0	12.9	19.1	21.5
Medicine (Osteopathic)[6]								
All races[1]	4,940	6,792	10,817	15,634	100.0	100.0	100.0	100.0
White, Non-Hispanic	4,688	5,680	7,940	11,028	94.9	83.6	73.4	70.5
Black or African American	94	217	400	600	1.9	3.2	3.7	3.8
Hispanic or Latino	52	277	381	569	1.1	4.1	3.5	3.6
American Indian or Alaska Native	19	36	72	102	0.4	0.5	0.7	0.7
Asian or Pacific Islander	87	582	1,734	2,713	1.8	8.6	16.0	17.4
Optometry								
All races[1]	4,540	4,762	5,428	5,556	100.0	100.0	100.0	100.0
Not Hispanic or Latino:								
White	4,108	3,575	3,338	3,349	90.5	75.1	61.5	60.3
Black or African American	57	135	126	172	1.3	2.8	2.3	3.1
Hispanic or Latino	80	295	268	255	1.8	6.2	4.9	4.6
American Indian or Alaska Native	12	21	27	19	0.3	0.4	0.5	0.3
Asian or Pacific Islander	243	603	1,373	1,397	5.4	12.7	25.3	25.1
Pharmacy[7]								
All races[1]	21,628	29,797	34,481	50,691	100.0	100.0	100.0	100.0
Not Hispanic or Latino:								
White	19,153	21,717	20,409	30,165	88.6	72.9	59.2	59.5
Black or African American	945	2,103	3,132	3,229	4.4	7.1	9.1	6.4
Hispanic or Latino	459	1,118	1,255	2,044	2.1	3.8	3.6	4.0
American Indian or Alaska Native	36	85	137	248	0.2	0.3	0.4	0.5
Asian or Pacific Islander	1,035	3,346	7,392	10,974	4.8	11.2	21.4	21.6

See footnotes at end of table.

Table 112 (page 2 of 2). Total enrollment in schools for selected health occupations, by race and Hispanic origin: United States, selected academic years 1980–1981 through 2007–2008

[Data are based on reporting by health professions associations]

Occupation, race, and Hispanic origin	1980–1981	1990–1991	2000–2001	2007–2008	1980–1981	1990–1991	2000–2001	2007–2008
Podiatry	Number of students				Percent distribution of students			
All races [1]	2,577	2,221	1,968	2,095	100.0	100.0	100.0	100.0
Not Hispanic or Latino:								
White	2,353	1,671	1,305	1,304	91.3	75.2	66.3	62.2
Black or African American	110	235	177	225	4.3	10.6	9.0	10.7
Hispanic or Latino	39	149	103	113	1.5	6.7	5.2	5.4
American Indian or Alaska Native	6	7	12	10	0.2	0.3	0.6	0.5
Asian or Pacific Islander	69	159	272	247	2.7	7.2	14.0	11.8
Public health								
All races [1]	- - -	- - -	16,777	22,604	- - -	- - -	100.0	100.0
Not Hispanic or Latino:								
White	- - -	- - -	8,569	11,064	- - -	- - -	65.0	59.3
Black or African American	- - -	- - -	1,280	2,177	- - -	- - -	9.7	11.7
Hispanic or Latino	- - -	- - -	1,037	1,637	- - -	- - -	7.9	8.8
American Indian or Alaska Native	- - -	- - -	97	134	- - -	- - -	0.7	0.7
Asian or Pacific Islander	- - -	- - -	1,660	2,326	- - -	- - -	12.6	12.5

- - - Data not available.

[1]Includes other and unknown races; may also include foreign students.

[2]Includes students from the University of Puerto Rico.

[3]Starting with 2002–2003 data, allopathic medical students had the option of reporting both their race and ethnicity alone or in combination with some other race or ethnicity, allowing multiple responses. Therefore, the data prior to 2002 are not directly comparable to later data. Total enrollments include unduplicated number of enrollments only. Therefore, the data for 2006–2007 and subsequent years are not directly comparable to earlier years.

[4]Includes Cuban students.

[5]Starting with 2000–2001, data include American Indian, Alaska Native, and Native Hawaiian; for previous years included American Indian and Alaska Native only.

[6]Starting with 2006, students could be reported in multiple race/ethnicity categories. All racial/ethnic groups will not add to the total enrollment. Percentages do not total to 100%. Other/unknown are not listed and students designating multiple race/ethnicity may be counted in more than one category.

[7]Prior to 2000–2001, total enrollment data were only for students in the final three years of pharmacy education. Starting with 2000–2001, pharmacy data are for all students. Starting in 2005, enrollments include PharmD.1. only. In 2006–2007, one pharmacy school did not report enrollment data.

NOTES: Total enrollment data are collected at the beginning of the academic year. The race categories' summed totals may not add up to the total number of students for all races. Some numbers have been revised and differ from previous editions of Health, United States.

SOURCE: American Dental Association (ADA): 2007–2008 Survey of Dental Education: Academic Programs, Enrollments, and Graduates - vol 1, Chicago, IL. 2008. Table 19; p. 43 (number of first-year students) and available from: http://www.ada.org/goto/edreports (Copyright© 2009 American Dental Association. All rights reserved. Reprinted by permission); Association of American Medical Colleges: FACTS - Applicants, Matriculants, Graduates, and Residency Applicants, Applicants and Matriculants data. Available from: http://www.aamc.org. Association of American Medical Colleges: AAMC Data Book, Medical Schools and Teaching Hospitals by the Numbers, Washington, DC. 2005, 2006, and 2009 (Copyright 2005, 2006, and 2009: Used with the permission of the AAMC); American Association of Colleges of Osteopathic Medicine (AACOM). A Report on a Survey of Osteopathic Medical School Growth, 2007–2008, Chevy Chase, MD. Fast Facts about Osteopathic Medical Education. Available from: http://www.aacom.org/data. Reprinted with permission from AACOM. All rights reserved; Association of Schools and Colleges of Optometry: Annual Student Data Report Academic Years 1980–1981, 1990–1991, 2000–2001, and 2007–2008. Available from: http://www.opted.org; American Association of Colleges of Pharmacy: Fall 2005 - Fall 2008 editions of the Profile of Pharmacy Students, Available from: http://www.aacp.org; American Association of Colleges of Podiatric Medicine: Applicant, Matriculant, and Graduate Statistics, 2006, 2007, and 2008. Available from: http://www.aacpm.org; Association of Schools of Public Health: Annual Data Reports, 2008. Washington, DC. Available from: http://www.asph.org/document.cfm?page=749; Bureau of Health Professions: United States Health Personnel FACTBOOK. Health Resources and Services Administration. Rockville, MD. 2003.

Table 113. Hospitals, beds, and occupancy rates, by type of ownership and size of hospital: United States, selected years 1975–2008

[Data are based on reporting by a census of hospitals]

Type of ownership and size of hospital	1975	1980	1990	1995	2000	2007	2008
Hospitals				Number			
All hospitals	7,156	6,965	6,649	6,291	5,810	5,708	5,815
Federal	382	359	337	299	245	213	213
Nonfederal[1]	6,774	6,606	6,312	5,992	5,565	5,495	5,602
Community[2]	5,875	5,830	5,384	5,194	4,915	4,897	5,010
Nonprofit	3,339	3,322	3,191	3,092	3,003	2,913	2,923
For profit	775	730	749	752	749	873	982
State-local government	1,761	1,778	1,444	1,350	1,163	1,111	1,105
6–24 beds	299	259	226	278	288	360	389
25–49 beds	1,155	1,029	935	922	910	1,076	1,151
50–99 beds	1,481	1,462	1,263	1,139	1,055	971	995
100–199 beds	1,363	1,370	1,306	1,324	1,236	1,083	1,070
200–299 beds	678	715	739	718	656	613	596
300–399 beds	378	412	408	354	341	343	355
400–499 beds	230	266	222	195	182	191	184
500 beds or more	291	317	285	264	247	260	270
Beds							
All hospitals	1,465,828	1,364,516	1,213,327	1,080,601	983,628	945,199	951,045
Federal	131,946	117,328	98,255	77,079	53,067	45,744	45,992
Nonfederal[1]	1,333,882	1,247,188	1,115,072	1,003,522	930,561	899,455	905,053
Community[2]	941,844	988,387	927,360	872,736	823,560	800,892	808,069
Nonprofit	658,195	692,459	656,755	609,729	582,988	553,748	556,651
For profit	73,495	87,033	101,377	105,737	109,883	115,742	120,887
State-local government	210,154	208,895	169,228	157,270	130,689	131,402	130,531
6–24 beds	5,615	4,932	4,427	5,085	5,156	6,238	6,726
25–49 beds	41,783	37,478	35,420	34,352	33,333	34,350	37,142
50–99 beds	106,776	105,278	90,394	82,024	75,865	69,974	71,477
100–199 beds	192,438	192,892	183,867	187,381	175,778	155,291	153,488
200–299 beds	164,405	172,390	179,670	175,240	159,807	149,546	144,895
300–399 beds	127,728	139,434	138,938	121,136	117,220	118,160	122,363
400–499 beds	101,278	117,724	98,833	86,459	80,763	84,136	80,815
500 beds or more	201,821	218,259	195,811	181,059	175,638	183,197	191,163
Occupancy rate[3]				Percent			
All hospitals	76.7	77.7	69.5	65.7	66.1	68.3	68.2
Federal	80.7	80.1	72.9	72.6	68.2	67.7	67.9
Nonfederal[1]	76.3	77.4	69.2	65.1	65.9	68.3	68.2
Community[2]	75.0	75.6	66.8	62.8	63.9	66.6	66.4
Nonprofit	77.5	78.2	69.3	64.5	65.5	68.6	68.4
For profit	65.9	65.2	52.8	51.8	55.9	57.2	57.8
State-local government	70.4	71.1	65.3	63.7	63.2	66.5	66.1
6–24 beds	48.0	46.8	32.3	36.9	31.7	34.7	33.8
25–49 beds	56.7	52.8	41.3	42.6	41.3	46.2	46.7
50–99 beds	64.7	64.2	53.8	54.1	54.8	56.2	56.6
100–199 beds	71.2	71.4	61.5	58.8	60.0	61.8	61.9
200–299 beds	77.1	77.4	67.1	63.1	65.0	66.6	66.4
300–399 beds	79.7	79.7	70.0	64.8	65.7	69.6	69.4
400–499 beds	81.1	81.2	73.5	68.1	69.1	70.2	74.2
500 beds or more	80.9	82.1	77.3	71.4	72.2	75.8	74.9

[1]The category of nonfederal hospitals comprises psychiatric hospitals, tuberculosis and other respiratory diseases hospitals, and long-term and short-term general and other special hospitals. See Appendix II, Hospital.
[2]Community hospitals are nonfederal short-term general and special hospitals whose facilities and services are available to the public. See Appendix II, Hospital.
[3]Estimated percentage of staffed beds that are occupied. Occupancy rate is calculated as the average daily census (from the American Hospital Association) divided by the number of hospital beds. See Appendix II, Occupancy rate.

SOURCE: American Hospital Association (AHA) Annual Survey of Hospitals. Hospital Statistics, 1976, 1981, 1991–2010 editions. Chicago, IL. (Copyrights 1976, 1981, 1991–2010: Used with the permission of Health Forum LLC, an affiliate of the AHA.)

Table 114. Mental health organizations and beds for 24-hour hospital and residential treatment, by type of organization: United States, selected years 1986–2004

[Data are based on inventories of mental health organizations]

Type of organization	1986	1990	1994	1998	2000	2002	2004
	Number of mental health organizations						
All organizations............................	3,512	3,942	3,853	3,741	3,211	3,044	2,891
State and county mental hospitals..............	285	278	270	237	229	227	237
Private psychiatric hospitals...................	314	464	432	347	271	255	264
Nonfederal general hospital psychiatric services	1,351	1,577	1,539	1,595	1,325	1,231	1,230
Department of Veterans Affairs medical centers[1]............................	139	131	136	124	134	132	- - -
Residential treatment centers for emotionally disturbed children............................	437	501	472	462	476	510	458
All other organizations[2]......................	986	991	1,004	976	776	689	702
	Number of beds						
All organizations............................	267,613	325,529	293,139	269,148	214,186	211,040	212,231
State and county mental hospitals..............	119,033	102,307	84,063	71,266	61,833	57,314	57,034
Private psychiatric hospitals...................	30,201	45,952	42,742	31,731	26,402	24,996	28,422
Nonfederal general hospital psychiatric services	45,808	53,576	53,455	54,775	40,410	40,520	41,403
Department of Veterans Affairs medical centers[1]............................	26,874	24,779	21,346	17,173	8,989	9,581	- - -
Residential treatment centers for emotionally disturbed children............................	24,547	35,170	32,691	32,040	33,508	39,407	33,835
All other organizations[2]......................	21,150	63,745	58,842	62,163	43,044	39,222	51,536
	Beds per 100,000 civilian population[3]						
All organizations............................	111.7	128.5	110.9	94.0	74.8	72.2	71.2
State and county mental hospitals..............	49.7	40.4	31.8	24.9	21.6	19.6	19.1
Private psychiatric hospitals...................	12.6	18.1	16.2	11.1	9.2	8.6	9.5
Nonfederal general hospital psychiatric services	19.1	21.2	20.2	19.1	14.1	13.9	13.9
Department of Veterans Affairs medical centers[1]............................	11.2	9.9	8.1	6.0	3.1	3.3	- - -
Residential treatment centers for emotionally disturbed children............................	10.3	13.9	12.4	11.2	11.7	13.5	11.4
All other organizations[2]......................	8.8	25.2	22.2	21.7	15.0	13.4	17.3

- - - Data not available.

[1]Department of Veterans Affairs medical centers (VA general hospital psychiatric services and VA psychiatric outpatient clinics) were dropped from the survey as of 2004.

[2]Includes freestanding psychiatric outpatient clinics, partial care organizations, and multiservice mental health organizations. See Appendix I, Survey of Mental Health Organizations.

[3]Civilian population estimates for 2000 and beyond are based on the 2000 census as of July 1; population estimates for 1992–1998 are 1990 postcensal estimates.

NOTES: Data for additional years are available. See Appendix III.

SOURCE: Substance Abuse and Mental Health Services Administration, Center for Mental Health Services (CMHS), Survey of Mental Health Organizations.

Table 115. Community hospital beds and average annual percent change, by state: United States, selected years 1960–2008

[Data are based on reporting by a census of hospitals]

State	1960	1970	1980	1990	2000	2008	1960–1970	1970–1980	1980–1990	1990–2000	2000–2008
	Beds per 1,000 resident population [1]						Average annual percent change [2]				
United States	3.6	4.3	4.5	3.7	2.9	2.7	1.8	0.5	−1.9	−2.4	−0.9
Alabama	2.8	4.3	5.1	4.6	3.7	3.3	4.4	1.7	−1.0	−2.2	−1.4
Alaska	2.4	2.3	2.7	2.3	2.3	2.3	−0.4	1.6	−1.6	–	–
Arizona	3.0	4.1	3.6	2.7	2.1	2.0	3.2	−1.3	−2.8	−2.5	−0.6
Arkansas	2.9	4.2	5.0	4.6	3.7	3.4	3.8	1.8	−0.8	−2.2	−1.1
California	3.0	3.8	3.6	2.7	2.1	1.9	2.4	−0.5	−2.8	−2.5	−1.2
Colorado	3.8	4.6	4.2	3.2	2.2	2.0	1.9	−0.9	−2.7	−3.7	−1.2
Connecticut	3.4	3.4	3.5	2.9	2.3	2.3	–	0.3	−1.9	−2.3	–
Delaware	3.7	3.7	3.6	3.0	2.3	2.4	–	−0.3	−1.8	−2.6	0.5
District of Columbia	5.9	7.4	7.3	7.6	5.8	5.7	2.3	−0.1	0.4	−2.7	−0.2
Florida	3.1	4.4	5.1	3.9	3.2	2.9	3.6	1.5	−2.6	−2.0	−1.2
Georgia	2.8	3.8	4.6	4.0	2.9	2.6	3.1	1.9	−1.4	−3.2	−1.4
Hawaii	3.7	3.4	3.1	2.7	2.5	2.4	−0.8	−0.9	−1.4	−0.8	−0.5
Idaho	3.2	4.0	3.7	3.2	2.7	2.2	2.3	−0.8	−1.4	−1.7	−2.5
Illinois	4.0	4.7	5.1	4.0	3.0	2.7	1.6	0.8	−2.4	−2.8	−1.3
Indiana	3.1	4.0	4.5	3.9	3.2	2.8	2.6	1.2	−1.4	−2.0	−1.7
Iowa	3.9	5.6	5.7	5.1	4.0	3.5	3.7	0.2	−1.1	−2.4	−1.7
Kansas	4.2	5.4	5.8	4.8	4.0	3.7	2.5	0.7	−1.9	−1.8	−1.0
Kentucky	3.0	4.0	4.5	4.3	3.7	3.3	2.9	1.2	−0.5	−1.5	−1.4
Louisiana	3.9	4.2	4.8	4.6	3.9	3.6	0.7	1.3	−0.4	−1.6	−1.0
Maine	3.4	4.7	4.7	3.7	2.9	2.7	3.3	–	−2.4	−2.4	−0.9
Maryland	3.3	3.1	3.6	2.8	2.1	2.1	−0.6	1.5	−2.5	−2.8	–
Massachusetts	4.2	4.4	4.4	3.6	2.6	2.4	0.5	–	−2.0	−3.2	−1.0
Michigan	3.3	4.3	4.4	3.7	2.6	2.5	2.7	0.2	−1.7	−3.5	−0.5
Minnesota	4.8	6.1	5.7	4.4	3.4	3.0	2.4	−0.7	−2.6	−2.5	−1.6
Mississippi	2.9	4.4	5.3	5.0	4.8	4.5	4.3	1.9	−0.6	−0.4	−0.8
Missouri	3.9	5.1	5.7	4.8	3.6	3.2	2.7	1.1	−1.7	−2.8	−1.5
Montana	5.1	5.8	5.9	5.8	4.7	3.9	1.3	0.2	−0.2	−2.1	−2.3
Nebraska	4.4	6.2	6.0	5.5	4.8	4.1	3.5	−0.3	−0.9	−1.4	−2.0
Nevada	3.9	4.2	4.2	2.8	1.9	2.0	0.7	–	−4.0	−3.8	0.6
New Hampshire	4.4	4.0	3.9	3.1	2.3	2.2	−0.9	−0.3	−2.3	−2.9	−0.6
New Jersey	3.1	3.6	4.2	3.7	3.0	2.4	1.5	1.6	−1.3	−2.1	−2.8
New Mexico	2.9	3.5	3.1	2.8	1.9	2.0	1.9	−1.2	−1.0	−3.8	0.6
New York	4.3	4.6	4.5	4.1	3.5	3.1	0.7	−0.2	−0.9	−1.6	−1.5
North Carolina	3.4	3.8	4.2	3.3	2.9	2.5	1.1	1.0	−2.4	−1.3	−1.8
North Dakota	5.2	6.8	7.4	7.0	6.0	5.4	2.7	0.8	−0.6	−1.5	−1.3
Ohio	3.4	4.2	4.7	4.0	3.0	2.9	2.1	1.1	−1.6	−2.8	−0.4
Oklahoma	3.2	4.5	4.6	4.0	3.2	3.0	3.5	0.2	−1.4	−2.2	−0.8
Oregon	3.5	4.0	3.5	2.8	1.9	1.8	1.3	−1.3	−2.2	−3.8	−0.7
Pennsylvania	4.1	4.7	4.8	4.4	3.4	3.2	1.4	0.2	−0.9	−2.5	−0.8
Rhode Island	3.7	4.0	3.8	3.2	2.3	2.3	0.8	−0.5	−1.7	−3.2	–
South Carolina	2.9	3.7	3.9	3.3	2.9	2.8	2.5	0.5	−1.7	−1.3	−0.4
South Dakota	4.5	5.6	5.5	6.1	5.7	5.1	2.2	−0.2	1.0	−0.7	−1.4
Tennessee	3.4	4.7	5.5	4.8	3.6	3.4	3.3	1.6	−1.4	−2.8	−0.7
Texas	3.3	4.3	4.7	3.5	2.7	2.5	2.7	0.9	−2.9	−2.6	−1.0
Utah	2.8	3.6	3.1	2.6	1.9	1.8	2.5	−1.5	−1.7	−3.1	−0.7
Vermont	4.5	4.5	4.4	3.0	2.7	2.1	–	−0.2	−3.8	−1.0	−3.1
Virginia	3.0	3.7	4.1	3.3	2.4	2.3	2.1	1.0	−2.1	−3.1	−0.5
Washington	3.3	3.5	3.1	2.5	1.9	1.7	0.6	−1.2	−2.1	−2.7	−1.4
West Virginia	4.1	5.4	5.5	4.7	4.4	4.1	2.8	0.2	−1.6	−0.7	−0.9
Wisconsin	4.3	5.2	4.9	3.8	2.9	2.4	1.9	−0.6	−2.5	−2.7	−2.3
Wyoming	4.6	5.5	3.6	4.8	3.9	3.9	1.8	−4.1	2.9	−2.1	–

– Quantity zero.
[1] Civilian population for 1997 and earlier years.
[2] See Appendix II, Average annual rate of change (percentage change).

NOTE: The types of facilities included in the category of community hospitals have changed over time. See Appendix II, Hospital.

SOURCE: American Hospital Association (AHA): Hospitals. JAHA 35(15):383–430, 1961 (Copyright 1961: Used with permission of AHA); AHA Annual Survey of Hospitals for 1970 and 1980 unpublished; Hospital Statistics 1991–1992, 2001–2010 editions. Chicago, IL. (Copyrights 1971, 1981, 1991, 2001–2010: Used with permission of Health Forum LLC, an affiliate of the AHA.)

Table 116. Occupancy rates in community hospitals and average annual percent change, by state: United States, selected years 1960–2008

[Data are based on reporting by a census of hospitals]

State	1960	1970	1980	1990	2000	2008	1960–1970	1970–1980	1980–1990	1990–2000	2000–2008
	Occupancy rate[1]						Average annual percent change[2]				
United States	75	77	75	67	64	66	0.3	−0.3	−1.1	−0.5	0.4
Alabama	71	80	73	63	60	63	1.2	−0.9	−1.5	−0.5	0.6
Alaska.	54	59	58	50	57	61	0.9	−0.2	−1.5	1.3	0.9
Arizona	74	73	74	62	63	67	−0.1	0.1	−1.8	0.2	0.8
Arkansas.	70	74	70	62	59	56	0.6	−0.6	−1.2	−0.5	−0.7
California.	74	71	69	64	66	71	−0.4	−0.3	−0.7	0.3	0.9
Colorado	81	74	72	64	58	60	−0.9	−0.3	−1.2	−1.0	0.4
Connecticut	78	83	80	77	75	80	0.6	−0.4	−0.4	−0.3	0.8
Delaware.	70	79	82	77	75	81	1.2	0.4	−0.6	−0.3	1.0
District of Columbia	81	78	83	75	74	78	−0.4	0.6	−1.0	−0.1	0.7
Florida.	74	76	72	62	61	63	0.3	−0.5	−1.5	−0.2	0.4
Georgia.	72	77	70	66	63	66	0.7	−0.9	−0.6	−0.5	0.6
Hawaii.	62	76	75	85	76	75	2.1	−0.1	1.3	−1.1	−0.2
Idaho	56	66	65	56	53	53	1.7	−0.2	−1.5	−0.5	0.0
Illinois.	76	79	75	66	60	64	0.4	−0.5	−1.3	−0.9	0.8
Indiana.	80	80	78	61	56	60	–	−0.3	−2.4	−0.9	0.9
Iowa.	73	72	69	62	58	59	−0.1	−0.4	−1.1	−0.7	0.2
Kansas	69	71	69	56	53	55	0.3	−0.3	−2.1	−0.5	0.5
Kentucky	73	80	77	62	62	62	0.9	−0.4	−2.1	–	0.0
Louisiana.	68	74	70	57	56	58	0.8	−0.6	−2.0	−0.2	0.4
Maine	73	73	75	72	64	66	–	0.3	−0.4	−1.2	0.4
Maryland.	74	79	84	79	73	75	0.7	0.6	−0.6	−0.8	0.3
Massachusetts.	76	80	82	74	71	73	0.5	0.2	−1.0	−0.4	0.3
Michigan	81	81	78	66	65	69	–	−0.4	−1.7	−0.2	0.7
Minnesota	72	74	74	67	67	68	0.3	–	−1.0	–	0.2
Mississippi.	63	74	71	59	59	59	1.6	−0.4	−1.8	–	0.0
Missouri.	76	79	75	62	58	64	0.4	−0.5	−1.9	−0.7	1.2
Montana	60	66	66	61	67	66	1.0	–	−0.8	0.9	−0.2
Nebraska.	66	70	67	58	59	59	0.6	−0.4	−1.4	0.2	0.0
Nevada	71	73	69	60	71	69	0.3	−0.6	−1.4	1.7	−0.4
New Hampshire	67	73	73	67	59	64	0.9	–	−0.9	−1.3	1.0
New Jersey	78	83	83	80	69	73	0.6	–	−0.4	−1.5	0.7
New Mexico.	65	70	66	58	58	56	0.7	−0.6	−1.3	–	−0.4
New York.	79	83	86	86	79	80	0.5	0.4	–	−0.8	0.2
North Carolina	74	79	78	73	70	71	0.7	−0.1	−0.7	−0.4	0.2
North Dakota	71	67	69	64	60	59	−0.6	0.3	−0.7	−0.6	−0.2
Ohio	81	82	79	65	61	63	0.1	−0.4	−1.9	−0.6	0.4
Oklahoma	71	73	68	58	56	61	0.3	−0.7	−1.6	−0.4	1.1
Oregon	66	69	69	57	59	62	0.4	–	−1.9	0.3	0.6
Pennsylvania.	76	82	80	73	68	70	0.8	−0.2	−0.9	−0.7	0.4
Rhode Island	76	83	86	79	72	74	0.9	0.4	−0.8	−0.9	0.3
South Carolina.	77	76	77	71	69	65	−0.1	0.1	−0.8	−0.3	−0.7
South Dakota.	66	66	61	62	65	67	–	−0.8	0.2	0.5	0.4
Tennessee.	76	78	76	64	56	64	0.3	−0.3	−1.7	−1.3	1.7
Texas	68	73	70	57	59	60	0.7	−0.4	−2.0	0.3	0.2
Utah	70	74	70	59	56	57	0.6	−0.6	−1.7	−0.5	0.2
Vermont	69	76	74	67	67	69	1.0	−0.3	−1.0	–	0.4
Virginia	78	81	78	67	68	69	0.4	−0.4	−1.5	0.1	0.2
Washington	63	70	72	63	60	64	1.1	0.3	−1.3	−0.5	0.8
West Virginia	75	79	76	63	61	61	0.5	−0.4	−1.9	−0.3	0.0
Wisconsin	74	73	74	65	60	63	−0.1	0.1	−1.3	−0.8	0.6
Wyoming.	61	63	57	54	56	55	0.3	−1.0	−0.5	0.4	−0.2

– Quantity zero.

0.0 Rate greater than zero but less than 0.05.

[1]Estimated percent of staffed beds that are occupied. Occupancy rate is calculated as the average daily census (inpatient days divided by 365) divided by the number of hospital beds. See Appendix II, Occupancy rate.

[2]See Appendix II, Average annual rate of change (percent change).

NOTE: The types of facilities included in the category of community hospitals have changed over time. See Appendix II, Hospital.

SOURCE: American Hospital Association (AHA): Hospitals. JAHA 35(15):383–430, 1961. (Copyright 1961: Used with permission of AHA); AHA Annual Survey of Hospitals, 1970 and 1980 unpublished; Hospital Statistics 1991–1992, 2001–2010 editions. Chicago, IL. (Copyright 1971, 1981, 1991, 2001–2010: Used with permission of Health Forum LLC, an affiliate of the AHA.)

Table 117 (page 1 of 2). Nursing homes, beds, residents, and occupancy rates, by state: United States, selected years 1995–2009

[Data are based on a census of certified nursing facilities]

State	Nursing homes				Beds			
	1995	2000	2008	2009	1995	2000	2008	2009
United States	16,389	16,886	15,730	15,700	1,751,302	1,795,388	1,703,846	1,705,808
Alabama	221	225	232	231	23,353	25,248	26,824	26,854
Alaska.	15	15	15	15	814	821	725	716
Arizona	152	150	133	135	16,162	17,458	16,033	16,073
Arkansas.	256	255	232	230	29,952	25,715	24,477	24,413
California.	1,382	1,369	1,255	1,252	140,203	131,762	122,554	121,699
Colorado	219	225	212	210	19,912	20,240	19,956	19,867
Connecticut	267	259	241	240	32,827	32,433	29,678	29,306
Delaware.	42	43	45	46	4,739	4,906	4,870	4,953
District of Columbia	19	20	18	19	3,206	3,078	2,645	2,765
Florida.	627	732	676	676	72,656	83,365	82,067	81,887
Georgia.	352	363	359	360	38,097	39,817	39,762	39,993
Hawaii.	34	45	48	47	2,513	4,006	4,256	4,241
Idaho	76	84	78	79	5,747	6,181	6,034	6,176
Illinois.	827	869	791	794	103,230	110,766	101,790	102,123
Indiana	556	564	510	504	59,538	56,762	57,107	57,450
Iowa	419	467	451	447	39,959	37,034	33,658	33,301
Kansas	429	392	346	341	30,016	27,067	26,011	25,732
Kentucky.	288	307	287	287	23,221	25,341	25,769	25,996
Louisiana.	337	337	285	282	37,769	39,430	36,096	35,602
Maine	132	126	112	109	9,243	8,248	7,243	7,113
Maryland	218	255	230	231	28,394	31,495	29,231	29,100
Massachusetts.	550	526	433	429	54,532	56,030	49,323	49,126
Michigan	432	439	425	428	49,473	50,696	47,323	47,271
Minnesota	432	433	390	385	43,865	42,149	34,117	32,956
Mississippi.	183	190	203	202	16,059	17,068	18,346	18,458
Missouri.	546	551	516	513	52,679	54,829	55,028	55,361
Montana	100	104	91	90	7,210	7,667	7,081	7,053
Nebraska.	231	236	224	225	18,169	17,877	16,198	16,214
Nevada	42	51	48	49	3,998	5,547	5,675	5,719
New Hampshire	74	83	80	80	7,412	7,837	7,718	7,742
New Jersey	300	361	361	360	43,967	52,195	51,132	51,159
New Mexico.	83	80	70	70	6,969	7,289	6,780	6,760
New York.	624	665	652	640	107,750	120,514	120,336	121,769
North Carolina	391	410	422	423	38,322	41,376	43,770	44,106
North Dakota	87	88	83	84	7,125	6,954	6,395	6,339
Ohio	943	1,009	955	961	106,884	105,038	93,039	93,359
Oklahoma	405	392	323	316	33,918	33,903	29,786	29,269
Oregon	161	150	138	137	13,885	13,500	12,473	12,313
Pennsylvania	726	770	711	711	92,625	95,063	87,878	88,861
Rhode Island	94	99	86	86	9,612	10,271	8,868	
South Carolina.	166	178	175	177	16,682	18,102	18,798	19,085
South Dakota.	114	114	110	109	8,296	7,844	6,591	6,900
Tennessee.	322	349	319	318	37,074	38,593	36,943	37,185
Texas	1,266	1,215	1,145	1,165	123,056	125,052	126,732	128,984
Utah	91	93	93	96	7,101	7,651	7,967	8,027
Vermont	23	44	40	40	1,862	3,743	3,268	3,293
Virginia	271	278	281	281	30,070	30,595	31,908	31,972
Washington	285	277	238	233	28,464	25,905	22,314	22,050
West Virginia	129	139	130	128	10,903	11,413	10,895	10,843
Wisconsin	413	420	393	391	48,754	46,395	37,385	36,482
Wyoming.	37	40	39	38	3,035	3,119	2,993	2,974

See footnotes at end of table.

Table 117 (page 2 of 2). Nursing homes, beds, residents, and occupancy rates, by state: United States, selected years 1995–2009

[Data are based on a census of certified nursing facilities]

State	Residents				Occupancy rate[1]			
	1995	2000	2008	2009	1995	2000	2008	2009
United States	1,479,550	1,480,076	1,412,540	1,401,718	84.5	82.4	82.9	82.2
Alabama	21,691	23,089	23,205	23,186	92.9	91.4	86.5	86.3
Alaska	634	595	616	633	77.9	72.5	85.0	88.4
Arizona	12,382	13,253	12,201	11,908	76.6	75.9	76.1	74.1
Arkansas	20,823	19,317	17,753	17,801	69.5	75.1	72.5	72.9
California	109,805	106,460	103,487	102,747	78.3	80.8	84.4	84.4
Colorado	17,055	17,045	16,464	16,288	85.7	84.2	82.5	82.0
Connecticut	29,948	29,657	26,819	26,253	91.2	91.4	90.4	89.6
Delaware	3,819	3,900	3,999	4,256	80.6	79.5	82.1	85.9
District of Columbia	2,576	2,858	2,437	2,531	80.3	92.9	92.1	91.5
Florida	61,845	69,050	71,833	71,657	85.1	82.8	87.5	87.5
Georgia	35,933	36,559	35,276	34,899	94.3	91.8	88.7	87.3
Hawaii	2,413	3,558	3,840	3,841	96.0	88.8	90.2	90.6
Idaho	4,697	4,640	4,522	4,419	81.7	75.1	74.9	71.6
Illinois	83,696	83,604	76,282	75,673	81.1	75.5	74.9	74.1
Indiana	44,328	42,328	39,536	39,190	74.5	74.6	69.2	68.2
Iowa	27,506	29,204	26,292	25,814	68.8	78.9	78.1	77.5
Kansas	25,140	22,230	19,301	19,029	83.8	82.1	74.2	74.0
Kentucky	20,696	22,730	23,233	23,318	89.1	89.7	90.2	89.7
Louisiana	32,493	30,735	25,875	25,077	86.0	77.9	71.7	70.4
Maine	8,587	7,298	6,591	6,485	92.9	88.5	91.0	91.2
Maryland	24,716	25,629	25,243	25,025	87.0	81.4	86.4	86.0
Massachusetts	49,765	49,805	43,684	43,227	91.3	88.9	88.6	88.0
Michigan	43,271	42,615	40,224	40,306	87.5	84.1	85.0	85.3
Minnesota	41,163	38,813	31,056	30,073	93.8	92.1	91.0	91.3
Mississippi	15,247	15,815	16,246	16,294	94.9	92.7	88.6	88.3
Missouri	39,891	38,586	37,510	37,588	75.7	70.4	68.2	67.9
Montana	6,415	5,973	5,137	5,077	89.0	77.9	72.5	72.0
Nebraska	16,166	14,989	12,899	12,627	89.0	83.8	79.6	77.9
Nevada	3,645	3,657	4,724	4,699	91.2	65.9	83.2	82.2
New Hampshire	6,877	7,158	6,953	6,941	92.8	91.3	90.1	89.7
New Jersey	40,397	45,837	45,946	45,788	91.9	87.8	89.9	89.5
New Mexico	6,051	6,503	5,695	5,569	86.8	89.2	84.0	82.4
New York	103,409	112,957	110,940	109,867	96.0	93.7	92.2	90.2
North Carolina	35,511	36,658	38,025	37,587	92.7	88.6	86.9	85.2
North Dakota	6,868	6,343	5,847	5,777	96.4	91.2	91.4	91.1
Ohio	79,026	81,946	81,395	80,185	73.9	78.0	87.5	85.9
Oklahoma	26,377	23,833	19,518	19,209	77.8	70.3	65.5	65.6
Oregon	11,673	9,990	8,113	7,708	84.1	74.0	65.0	62.6
Pennsylvania	84,843	83,880	79,710	80,562	91.6	88.2	90.7	90.7
Rhode Island	8,823	9,041	7,955	8,040	91.8	88.0	89.7	91.2
South Carolina	14,568	15,739	17,004	17,148	87.3	86.9	90.5	89.9
South Dakota	7,926	7,059	6,528	6,476	95.5	90.0	99.0	93.9
Tennessee	33,929	34,714	32,288	31,876	91.5	89.9	87.4	85.7
Texas	89,354	85,275	90,385	90,534	72.6	68.2	71.3	70.2
Utah	5,832	5,703	5,456	5,358	82.1	74.5	68.5	66.8
Vermont	1,792	3,349	2,992	2,980	96.2	89.5	91.6	90.5
Virginia	28,119	27,091	28,279	28,392	93.5	88.5	88.6	88.8
Washington	24,954	21,158	18,760	18,188	87.7	81.7	84.1	82.5
West Virginia	10,216	10,334	9,710	9,613	93.7	90.5	89.1	88.7
Wisconsin	43,998	38,911	32,325	31,619	90.2	83.9	86.5	86.7
Wyoming	2,661	2,605	2,431	2,380	87.7	83.5	81.2	80.0

[1]Percentage of beds occupied (number of nursing home residents per 100 nursing home beds).

NOTES: See Appendix I, Online Survey Certification and Reporting Database (OSCAR). Annual numbers of nursing homes, beds, and residents are based on a 15-month OSCAR reporting cycle. Data for additional years are available. See Appendix III.

SOURCE: Cowles CM ed., 2009 Nursing Home Statistical Yearbook. McMinnville, OR: Cowles Research Group, 2010 and previous editions; and Cowles Research Group, unpublished data. Based on data from the Centers for Medicare & Medicaid Services' Online Survey Certification and Reporting (OSCAR) database.

Table 118 (page 1 of 2). Certified intermediate care facilities and specialty hospitals, number of facilities and beds, by state: United States, selected years 1995–2009

[Data are based on a census of certified facilities]

	Facilities											
	ICF/MR[1]		Hospitals									
			Long-term		Psychiatric		Rehabilitation		Children's		CAH[2]	
State	1995	2009	1995	2009	1995	2009	1995	2009	1995	2009	1995	2009
						Number						
United States	7,106	6,437	175	427	689	502	190	225	70	77	. . .	1,311
Alabama	8	5	2	7	10	11	5	7	1	2	. . .	3
Alaska	6	0	0	1	3	2	0	0	0	0	. . .	13
Arizona	12	12	3	8	11	7	4	7	1	2	. . .	15
Arkansas	40	41	0	8	9	8	6	8	1	1	. . .	29
California	687	1,171	8	19	64	33	12	5	7	10	. . .	29
Colorado	7	3	5	8	9	9	5	3	2	1	. . .	29
Connecticut	145	114	5	3	10	6	1	1	1	1	. . .	0
Delaware	6	2	0	1	3	4	1	0	1	1	. . .	0
District of Columbia	122	85	0	2	2	3	1	1	1	1	. . .	0
Florida	110	102	10	19	43	24	13	13	2	2	. . .	11
Georgia	12	9	5	15	28	15	2	3	1	2	. . .	34
Hawaii	15	18	1	1	1	1	1	1	1	1	. . .	9
Idaho	48	66	0	3	6	5	1	1	0	0	. . .	26
Illinois	315	310	4	6	19	14	3	4	2	2	. . .	51
Indiana	578	547	5	14	30	22	6	6	0	0	. . .	35
Iowa	116	139	0	1	4	4	0	0	0	0	. . .	82
Kansas	47	32	2	5	10	4	4	4	0	1	. . .	83
Kentucky	9	12	0	7	13	11	4	5	0	0	. . .	30
Louisiana	454	548	13	39	40	37	9	21	1	1	. . .	27
Maine	42	17	0	0	4	4	1	1	0	0	. . .	15
Maryland	5	4	4	4	14	9	3	2	2	2	. . .	0
Massachusetts	8	6	21	17	18	15	5	8	2	2	. . .	3
Michigan	503	1	2	19	15	10	4	4	1	1	. . .	36
Minnesota	348	218	1	2	6	7	0	1	3	3	. . .	79
Mississippi	12	14	1	10	4	5	1	0	0	0	. . .	27
Missouri	26	18	3	9	17	14	2	4	3	3	. . .	36
Montana	3	1	0	1	2	2	0	0	0	0	. . .	47
Nebraska	4	3	1	2	5	3	1	1	2	2	. . .	65
Nevada	14	9	2	6	5	6	2	3	0	0	. . .	10
New Hampshire	7	1	0	0	3	2	2	2	0	0	. . .	13
New Jersey	10	8	3	6	14	17	8	8	1	2	. . .	0
New Mexico	32	42	2	3	6	2	5	5	1	0	. . .	6
New York	892	568	7	4	35	28	4	0	2	1	. . .	13
North Carolina	320	332	2	7	15	10	1	2	0	0	. . .	22
North Dakota	65	66	1	2	1	3	1	0	0	0	. . .	36
Ohio	416	426	5	23	19	15	0	3	8	6	. . .	34
Oklahoma	37	84	4	13	18	10	3	2	2	2	. . .	34
Oregon	2	1	0	1	4	3	0	0	0	0	. . .	25
Pennsylvania	252	200	5	23	31	24	17	17	5	5	. . .	13
Rhode Island	55	5	2	1	3	2	1	1	0	0	. . .	0
South Carolina	174	89	1	6	9	8	3	6	0	0	. . .	5
South Dakota	10	1	0	1	2	1	0	0	0	1	. . .	38
Tennessee	74	86	2	9	16	11	5	6	3	2	. . .	17
Texas	879	867	35	74	52	36	28	42	7	8	. . .	76
Utah	14	15	1	3	7	3	1	1	1	1	. . .	10
Vermont	6	1	0	0	2	1	0	0	0	0	. . .	8
Virginia	20	39	3	5	19	9	4	7	2	3	. . .	7
Washington	28	14	2	2	4	5	1	1	2	2	. . .	38
West Virginia	63	67	0	2	5	4	6	5	0	0	. . .	18
Wisconsin	44	16	1	5	17	11	2	2	1	3	. . .	59
Wyoming	4	2	1	0	2	2	1	1	0	0	. . .	15

See footnotes at end of table.

Table 118 (page 2 of 2). Certified intermediate care facilities and specialty hospitals, number of facilities and beds, by state: United States, selected years 1995–2009

[Data are based on a census of certified facilities]

	Beds											
	ICF/MR[1]		Hospitals									
			Long-term		Psychiatric		Rehabilitation		Children's		CAH[2]	
State	1995	2009	1995	2009	1995	2009	1995	2009	1995	2009	1995	2009
	Number											
United States	159,557	110,719	21,373	29,366	105,165	69,161	13,731	14,533	12,719	12,929	...	32,604
Alabama	981	281	341	429	1,760	1,050	289	392	225	434	...	75
Alaska	121	0	0	60	244	205	0	0	0	0	...	217
Arizona	690	242	203	557	955	941	211	371	15	250	...	314
Arkansas	1,802	1,691	0	283	730	787	446	463	280	280	...	763
California	14,334	11,142	1,477	1,881	7,737	4,938	838	367	1,346	1,797	...	1,019
Colorado	382	99	1,264	420	1,375	943	271	226	378	253	...	606
Connecticut	1,350	1,126	796	687	1,990	1,012	60	60	98	129	...	0
Delaware	405	285	0	35	514	478	60	0	97	180	...	0
District of Columbia	797	515	0	171	583	800	160	160	279	279	...	0
Florida	3,495	3,060	745	1,119	5,385	2,865	833	1,022	376	424	...	265
Georgia	2,240	1,647	372	713	4,103	2,735	108	168	235	483	...	857
Hawaii	207	91	13	9	88	88	100	100	232	207	...	88
Idaho	541	534	0	140	221	263	54	56	0	0	...	507
Illinois	13,001	10,569	1,385	916	3,172	2,223	371	448	351	339	...	1,224
Indiana	7,387	4,189	265	649	2,213	1,466	388	316	0	0	...	956
Iowa	3,679	3,127	0	50	522	287	0	0	0	0	...	2,401
Kansas	2,233	993	54	167	1,717	718	217	257	0	34	...	1,928
Kentucky	1,203	915	0	557	2,086	1,697	225	288	0	0	...	735
Louisiana	6,847	6,517	797	1,979	3,868	2,048	435	588	188	201	...	677
Maine	555	191	0	0	551	392	80	100	0	0	...	373
Maryland	1,042	463	465	465	3,846	1,788	352	131	165	150	...	0
Massachusetts	2,707	1,954	4,218	3,857	2,137	1,596	636	1,064	458	421	...	69
Michigan	3,556	272	249	1,000	3,280	1,253	340	240	260	228	...	874
Minnesota	5,162	1,899	264	356	1,432	442	0	16	329	339	...	2,150
Mississippi	2,131	2,739	25	393	316	1,709	110	0	0	0	...	774
Missouri	1,659	1,147	317	556	1,969	1,892	120	237	592	432	...	867
Montana	188	107	0	40	54	194	0	0	0	0	...	957
Nebraska	761	261	192	148	767	488	60	72	142	200	...	1,418
Nevada	229	121	79	413	407	589	122	189	0	0	...	211
New Hampshire	78	25	0	0	423	341	152	152	0	0	...	346
New Jersey	4,637	3,622	476	412	3,486	3,249	848	774	60	120	...	0
New Mexico	604	272	86	106	397	124	194	212	37	0	...	149
New York	15,379	8,925	1,351	1,010	14,199	6,378	428	0	404	92	...	290
North Carolina	5,294	5,174	182	419	2,941	3,705	80	213	0	0	...	750
North Dakota	721	637	68	72	328	303	88	0	0	0	...	805
Ohio	8,936	7,366	683	1,573	3,079	1,776	0	199	2,535	1,356	...	830
Oklahoma	3,132	2,062	194	636	1,726	638	219	107	168	160	...	764
Oregon	546	76	0	28	670	701	0	0	0	0	...	830
Pennsylvania	7,412	4,544	369	1,355	7,334	3,454	1,574	1,365	721	1,042	...	345
Rhode Island	297	51	1,062	495	371	177	82	82	0	0	...	0
South Carolina	3,550	1,864	166	308	1,089	1,093	213	344	0	0	...	125
South Dakota	558	240	0	24	145	320	0	0	0	114	...	775
Tennessee	2,590	1,189	125	329	1,721	1,253	350	370	395	200	...	391
Texas	15,868	12,949	1,803	3,869	6,561	4,305	1,838	2,478	1,447	1,631	...	1,677
Utah	965	855	34	111	741	486	50	84	194	232	...	221
Vermont	36	6	0	0	164	149	0	0	0	0	...	194
Virginia	2,758	2,001	892	236	1,677	1,345	231	288	250	296	...	175
Washington	1,482	940	97	69	1,541	1,417	102	102	276	276	...	1,138
West Virginia	782	517	0	60	564	485	246	270	0	0	...	722
Wisconsin	4,083	1,009	34	204	1,720	1,491	135	121	186	350	...	1,438
Wyoming	164	218	230	0	266	84	15	41	0	0	...	314

. . . Category not applicable.
[1]ICF/MR is intermediate care facilities for persons with mental retardation.
[2]CAH is critical access hospital. CAHs were created as part of the Balanced Budget Act of 1997.

NOTES: See Appendix I, Online Survey Certification and Reporting Database (OSCAR). Facilities are surveyed periodically, usually at least every 12 months. Data for additional years are available. See Appendix III.

SOURCE: Centers for Medicare & Medicaid Services' Online Survey Certification and Reporting (OSCAR) database.

Table 119. Medicare-certified providers and suppliers: United States, selected years 1975–2008

[Data are compiled from various Centers for Medicare & Medicaid Services data systems]

Providers or suppliers	1975	1980	1985	1990	1996	1999	2003	2005	2007	2008
					Number of providers or suppliers					
Skilled nursing facilities	- - -	5,052	6,451	8,937	- - -	14,913	14,838	15,006	15,054	15,032
Home health agencies	2,242	2,924	5,679	5,730	8,437	7,857	6,928	8,090	9,024	9,407
Clinical Lab Improvement Act Facilities	- - -	- - -	- - -	- - -	159,907	171,018	176,947	196,296	206,065	210,872
End-stage renal disease facilities . . .	- - -	999	1,393	1,937	2,876	3,787	4,309	4,755	5,095	5,317
Outpatient physical therapy	117	419	854	1,195	2,302	2,867	2,961	2,962	2,915	2,781
Portable X-ray	132	216	308	443	555	666	641	553	550	547
Rural health clinics	- - -	391	428	551	2,775	3,453	3,306	3,661	3,781	3,757
Comprehensive outpatient rehabilitation facilities	- - -	- - -	72	186	307	522	587	634	539	476
Ambulatory surgical centers.	- - -	- - -	336	1,197	2,112	2,894	3,597	4,445	4,964	5,174
Hospices	- - -	- - -	164	825	1,927	2,326	2,323	2,872	3,255	3,346

- - - Data not available.

NOTES: Data for 1975–1990 are as of July 1. Data for 1996–1999 and 2004–2008 are as of December 31. Data for 2001, 2002, and 2003 are as of December 2000, December 2001, and December 2002, respectively. Data for additional years are available. See Appendix III.

SOURCE: Centers for Medicare & Medicaid Services (CMS). 2009 CMS Statistics. Baltimore, MD: CMS; 2009 and previous editions. Available from: http://www.cms.hhs.gov/DataCompendium/.

Table 120 (page 1 of 2). Number of magnetic resonance imaging (MRI) units and computed tomography (CT) scanners: Selected countries, selected years 1990–2007

[Data are based on reporting by the Organisation for Economic Co-operation and Development (OECD) countries]

Country	1990	1995	2000	2005	2006	2007	1990	1995	2000	2005	2006	2007
	Number of MRI units per million population						Number of CT scanners per million population					
Australia[1]	0.6	2.9	3.5	4.2	4.8	5.1	13.8	20.5	26.1	51.0	56.0	- - -
Austria	- - -	- - -	10.9	16.2	16.8	17.7	- - -	- - -	25.8	29.6	29.8	29.8
Belgium	2.0	3.3	6.0	7.0	7.1	7.5	16.1	- - -	21.8	38.7	39.8	41.6
Canada[2]	0.7	1.4	2.5	5.7	6.2	6.7	7.1	8.0	- - -	11.5	12.0	12.7
Czech Republic[3]	- - -	1.0	1.7	3.1	3.8	4.4	- - -	6.7	9.6	12.3	13.1	12.9
Denmark	2.5	- - -	5.4	- - -	- - -	- - -	4.3	7.3	11.4	13.8	15.8	17.4
Finland	1.8	4.3	9.9	14.7	15.2	15.3	9.8	11.7	13.5	14.7	14.8	16.4
France	0.8	2.1	2.6	4.7	5.3	5.7	6.7	9.2	9.5	9.8	10.0	10.3
Germany[4]	- - -	- - -	- - -	- - -	- - -	- - -	- - -	- - -	- - -	- - -	- - -	- - -
Greece	0.4	- - -	- - -	13.2	- - -	- - -	6.5	- - -	- - -	25.8	- - -	- - -
Hungary[5]	0.1	1.0	1.8	2.6	2.6	2.8	1.9	4.6	5.7	7.1	7.2	7.3
Iceland	3.9	7.5	10.7	20.3	19.7	19.3	11.8	18.7	21.3	23.7	26.3	32.1
Ireland	- - -	- - -	- - -	- - -	8.0	8.5	4.3	- - -	- - -	10.6	12.8	14.3
Italy[6]	1.3	- - -	7.7	15.0	16.9	18.6	6.0	- - -	21.0	27.7	29.1	30.3
Japan[7]	6.1	- - -	- - -	40.1	- - -	- - -	55.2	- - -	- - -	- - -	- - -	- - -
Luxembourg	2.6	2.4	2.3	10.8	10.7	10.5	5.2	26.6	25.2	28.2	27.7	27.3
Mexico	- - -	- - -	- - -	1.3	1.4	1.5	- - -	- - -	- - -	3.3	3.4	4.0
Netherlands[8]	0.9	3.9	- - -	6.6	- - -	- - -	7.3	- - -	- - -	8.2	8.4	- - -
New Zealand	- - -	- - -	- - -	- - -	- - -	8.8	3.6	- - -	8.8	- - -	- - -	12.3
Poland	- - -	- - -	- - -	2.0	1.9	2.7	- - -	- - -	4.4	7.9	9.2	9.7
Portugal[9]	0.8	- - -	- - -	- - -	5.8	8.9	4.6	- - -	- - -	26.2	25.8	26.0
Republic of Korea	- - -	3.9	5.4	12.1	13.6	16.0	- - -	15.5	28.4	32.3	33.7	37.1
Slovak Republic[10]	- - -	- - -	- - -	4.3	4.5	5.7	- - -	- - -	- - -	11.3	12.1	13.7
Spain[11]	- - -	2.7	4.8	8.1	8.8	9.3	- - -	8.3	12.0	13.5	13.9	14.6
Sweden	1.5	6.8	- - -	- - -	- - -	- - -	10.5	- - -	- - -	- - -	- - -	- - -
Switzerland	- - -	- - -	12.9	14.4	14.0	14.4	- - -	- - -	18.5	18.2	18.7	18.7
Turkey	- - -	- - -	- - -	- - -	3.5	5.6	1.6	- - -	- - -	- - -	7.8	8.1
United Kingdom[12]	- - -	- - -	4.7	5.4	5.6	8.2	- - -	- - -	4.5	7.5	7.6	- - -
United States[13]	- - -	12.3	- - -	- - -	26.5	25.9	- - -	- - -	- - -	- - -	34.0	34.3
	Number of MRI units						Number of CT scanners					
Australia[1]	11	52	67	86	100	108	235	370	500	1,040	1,160	- - -
Austria	- - -	- - -	88	133	139	147	- - -	- - -	209	244	247	248
Belgium	20	33	61	73	75	80	160	- - -	223	406	420	442
Canada[2]	19	40	76	185	201	222	198	234	- - -	373	392	419
Czech Republic[3]	- - -	10	17	32	39	45	- - -	69	99	126	134	133
Denmark	13	- - -	29	- - -	- - -	- - -	22	38	61	75	86	95
Finland	9	22	51	77	80	81	49	60	70	77	78	87
France	45	123	156	288	325	350	379	534	563	595	615	635
Germany[4]	- - -	184	405	585	635	673	- - -	702	999	1,271	1,304	1,340
Greece	4	- - -	- - -	147	- - -	- - -	66	- - -	- - -	286	- - -	- - -
Hungary[5]	1	10	18	26	26	28	20	47	58	72	73	73
Iceland	1	2	3	6	6	6	3	5	6	7	8	10
Ireland	- - -	- - -	- - -	- - -	34	37	15	- - -	- - -	44	54	62
Italy[6]	72	- - -	442	870	986	1,097	340	- - -	1,203	1,613	1,703	1,785
Japan[7]	756	- - -	- - -	5,128	- - -	- - -	6,821	- - -	- - -	- - -	- - -	- - -
Luxembourg	1	1	1	5	5	5	2	11	11	13	13	13
Mexico	- - -	- - -	- - -	139	147	161	- - -	- - -	- - -	347	356	422
Netherlands[8]	13	60	- - -	107	- - -	- - -	109	- - -	- - -	134	137	- - -
New Zealand	- - -	- - -	- - -	- - -	- - -	37	12	- - -	34	- - -	- - -	52
Poland	- - -	- - -	- - -	77	74	103	- - -	- - -	169	303	352	368
Portugal[9]	8	- - -	- - -	- - -	61	94	45	- - -	- - -	277	273	276
Republic of Korea	- - -	174	254	584	657	777	- - -	699	1,334	1,557	1,629	1,799
Slovak Republic[10]	- - -	- - -	- - -	23	24	31	- - -	- - -	- - -	61	65	74
Spain[11]	- - -	107	194	350	386	417	- - -	327	483	587	611	654
Sweden	13	60	- - -	- - -	- - -	- - -	90	- - -	- - -	- - -	- - -	- - -
Switzerland	- - -	- - -	93	107	105	109	- - -	- - -	133	135	140	141
Turkey	- - -	- - -	- - -	- - -	254	395	89	- - -	- - -	- - -	566	569
United Kingdom[12]	- - -	- - -	277	326	342	500	- - -	- - -	264	450	458	- - -
United States[13]	- - -	3,265	- - -	- - -	7,930	7,810	- - -	- - -	- - -	- - -	10,150	10,335

See footnotes at end of table.

Table 120 (page 2 of 2). Number of magnetic resonance imaging (MRI) units and computed tomography (CT) scanners: Selected countries, selected years 1990–2007

[Data are based on reporting by the Organisation for Economic Co-operation and Development (OECD) countries]

- - - Data not available.

[1]Starting with 2000 data, the number of MRI units include only those that are approved for billing to Medicare (Australia's national health program). In 1999, approved units represented approximately 60% of total units.

[2]The number of units in freestanding imaging facilities was imputed for years prior to 2003 based on data collected in the 2003 National Survey of Selected Medical Imaging Equipment, conducted by the Canadian Institute for Health Information. MRI units in Quebec are not included in 2000.

[3]Prior to 2000, the data include only equipment of Health Sector establishments.

[4]Data include equipment installed in all types of hospitals.

[5]Equipment used in military hospitals and the health institutes of Hungarian State Railways are not included.

[6]1990 data include only equipment in public and private hospitals.

[7]Prior to 2000, the data include only equipment in hospitals.

[8]2005 data are the number of hospitals reporting to have an MRI unit.

[9]Data do not include equipment in all the private sectors.

[10]Data include devices in hospitals and do not include equipment in other health care facilities.

[11]Data include equipment available in hospitals and do not include equipment in other health care facilities.

[12]Data include devices in public sector establishments only.

[13]Data are from the MRI Census and are comparable to the OECD definition. The devices in U.S. territories are not included.

NOTES: Data for additional years are available. Countries use different methods for collecting data. Therefore, estimates may not be directly comparable across countries and comparisons among them should be made with caution. See Appendix III.

SOURCE: Organisation for Economic Co-operation and Development (OECD); 2007 Computed Tomography (CT) and Magnetic Resonance Imaging (MRI) Census. Benchmark Report: IMV, Limited, Medical Information Division.

Table 121. Total health expenditures as a percent of gross domestic product, and per capita health expenditures in dollars, by selected countries: Selected years 1960–2007

[Data compiled by the Organisation for Economic Co-operation and Development (OECD)]

Country	1960	1970	1980	1990	1995	2000	2003	2004	2005	2006	2007[1]
						Health expenditures as a percent of gross domestic product					
Australia	3.8	- - -	6.3	6.9	7.4	8.3	8.5	8.8	8.7	8.8	8.9
Austria	4.3	5.2	7.4	8.3	9.5	9.9	10.3	10.4	10.4	10.2	10.1
Belgium	- - -	3.9	6.3	7.2	8.2	8.6	10.2	10.5	10.3	10.0	10.2
Canada	5.4	6.9	7.0	8.9	9.0	8.8	9.8	9.8	9.9	10.0	10.1
Czech Republic	- - -	- - -	- - -	4.7	7.0	6.5	7.4	7.4	7.2	7.0	6.8
Denmark	- - -	- - -	8.9	8.3	8.1	8.3	9.3	9.5	9.5	9.6	9.8
Finland	3.8	5.5	6.3	7.7	7.9	7.2	8.1	8.2	8.5	8.3	8.2
France	3.8	5.4	7.0	8.4	10.4	10.1	10.9	11.0	11.1	11.0	11.0
Germany	- - -	6.0	8.4	8.3	10.1	10.3	10.8	10.6	10.7	10.5	10.4
Greece	- - -	5.4	5.9	6.6	8.6	7.9	9.0	8.7	9.4	9.5	9.6
Hungary	- - -	- - -	- - -	- - -	7.3	6.9	8.3	8.0	8.3	8.1	7.4
Iceland	3.0	4.7	6.3	7.8	8.2	9.5	10.4	9.9	9.4	9.1	9.3
Ireland	3.7	5.1	8.3	6.1	6.7	6.3	7.3	7.5	7.3	7.1	7.6
Italy	- - -	- - -	- - -	7.7	7.3	8.1	8.3	8.7	8.9	9.0	8.7
Japan	3.0	4.6	6.5	6.0	6.9	7.7	8.1	8.0	8.2	8.1	- - -
Luxembourg	- - -	3.1	5.2	5.4	5.6	5.8	7.5	8.1	7.7	7.3	- - -
Mexico	- - -	- - -	- - -	4.4	5.1	5.1	5.8	5.8	5.8	5.8	5.9
Netherlands	- - -	- - -	7.4	8.0	8.3	8.0	9.8	10.0	9.8	9.7	9.8
New Zealand	- - -	5.2	5.9	6.9	7.2	7.7	8.0	8.4	8.8	9.2	9.0
Norway	2.9	4.4	7.0	7.6	7.9	8.4	10.0	9.7	9.1	8.6	8.9
Poland	- - -	- - -	- - -	4.8	5.5	5.5	6.2	6.2	6.2	6.2	6.4
Portugal	- - -	2.5	5.3	5.9	7.8	8.8	9.7	10.0	10.2	9.9	- - -
Republic of Korea	- - -	- - -	4.1	4.3	4.1	4.7	5.3	5.3	5.7	6.0	6.3
Slovak Republic	- - -	- - -	- - -	- - -	- - -	5.5	5.8	7.2	7.0	7.3	7.7
Spain	1.5	3.5	5.3	6.5	7.4	7.2	8.1	8.2	8.3	8.4	8.5
Sweden	- - -	6.8	8.9	8.2	8.0	8.2	9.4	9.2	9.2	9.1	9.1
Switzerland	4.9	5.4	7.3	8.2	9.6	10.2	11.3	11.3	11.2	10.8	10.8
Turkey	- - -	- - -	2.4	2.7	2.5	4.9	6.0	5.9	5.7	- - -	- - -
United Kingdom	3.9	4.5	5.6	5.9	6.8	7.0	7.8	8.1	8.2	8.5	8.4
United States[2]	5.2	7.1	9.0	12.2	13.6	13.6	15.6	15.6	15.7	15.8	16.0
						Per capita health expenditures[3]					
Australia	$ 90	- - -	$ 644	$1,203	$1,610	$2,263	$2,664	$2,870	$2,979	$3,167	$3,357
Austria	77	$196	783	1,618	2,216	2,824	3,200	3,392	3,472	3,608	3,763
Belgium	- - -	150	643	1,357	1,853	2,377	3,059	3,272	3,301	3,356	3,595
Canada	125	301	780	1,738	2,057	2,516	3,066	3,220	3,464	3,696	3,895
Czech Republic	- - -	- - -	- - -	559	899	980	1,339	1,422	1,477	1,535	1,626
Denmark	- - -	- - -	896	1,544	1,871	2,378	2,832	3,055	3,152	3,357	3,512
Finland	63	185	571	1,366	1,481	1,853	2,254	2,459	2,590	2,709	2,840
France	69	194	668	1,449	2,101	2,542	2,985	3,115	3,303	3,423	3,601
Germany	- - -	269	971	1,768	2,274	2,671	3,088	3,160	3,348	3,464	3,588
Greece	- - -	161	491	853	1,263	1,449	2,029	2,092	2,352	2,547	2,727
Hungary	- - -	- - -	- - -	- - -	660	852	1,284	1,305	1,411	1,457	1,388
Iceland	57	175	755	1,666	1,909	2,736	3,196	3,335	3,304	3,207	3,319
Ireland	43	117	513	791	1,203	1,805	2,521	2,753	2,831	3,001	3,424
Italy	- - -	- - -	- - -	1,359	1,538	2,052	2,271	2,399	2,536	2,673	2,686
Japan	30	152	585	1,125	1,551	1,967	2,224	2,337	2,474	2,581	- - -
Luxembourg	- - -	- - -	- - -	- - -	1,910	2,553	3,580	4,080	4,021	4,162	- - -
Mexico	- - -	- - -	- - -	296	386	508	629	670	724	777	823
Netherlands	- - -	- - -	728	1,416	1,798	2,337	3,099	3,310	3,450	3,611	3,837
New Zealand	- - -	215	509	990	1,245	1,605	1,846	2,043	2,180	2,398	2,454
Norway	49	144	668	1,369	1,862	3,039	3,837	4,079	4,301	4,507	4,763
Poland	- - -	- - -	- - -	289	411	583	748	808	857	920	1,035
Portugal	- - -	48	276	636	1,035	1,509	1,823	1,912	2,098	2,150	- - -
Republic of Korea	- - -	- - -	107	357	525	809	1,068	1,155	1,296	1,491	1,688
Slovak Republic	- - -	- - -	- - -	- - -	- - -	603	792	1,058	1,139	1,322	1,555
Spain	16	95	363	872	1,193	1,536	2,017	2,126	2,267	2,466	2,671
Sweden	- - -	312	946	1,596	1,745	2,283	2,829	2,950	2,958	3,124	3,323
Switzerland	166	346	1,017	2,033	2,568	3,217	3,779	3,938	4,015	4,165	4,417
Turkey	- - -	- - -	70	155	173	432	502	576	618	- - -	- - -
United Kingdom	84	160	470	963	1,349	1,833	2,324	2,557	2,693	2,885	2,992
United States[2]	149	356	1,091	2,810	3,748	4,704	5,851	6,194	6,558	6,933	7,290

- - - Data not available.

[1] For some countries, data are preliminary estimates. See: http://www.ecosante.org/oecd.htm for more information.

[2] The Organisation for Economic Co-operation and Development (OECD) estimates for the United States differ from the National Health Expenditures estimates shown in Table 123 because of differences in methodology.

[3] Per capita health expenditures for each country have been adjusted to U.S. dollars using gross domestic product purchasing power parities for each year. See Appendix II, Gross domestic product; Purchasing power parities.

NOTES: These data include revisions in health expenditures and differ from previous editions of Health, United States. Trends should be interpreted with caution due to data series breaks and changes in methodology. Data for additional years are available. Please see Appendix III.

SOURCE: The Organisation for Economic Co-operation and Development Health Data File 2008, incorporating revisions to the annual update. Available from: http://www.ecosante.org/oecd.htm.

Table 122. Gross domestic product, federal, and state and local government expenditures, national health expenditures, and average annual percent change: United States, selected years 1960–2008

[Data are compiled from various sources by the Centers for Medicare & Medicaid Services]

Gross domestic product, government expenditures, and national health expenditures	1960	1970	1980	1990	2000	2006	2007	2008
	Amount in billions							
Gross domestic product (GDP)	$ 526	$1,038	$2,788	$ 5,801	$ 9,952	$ 13,399	$ 14,078	$ 14,441
Implicit price deflator for GDP[1]	18.6	24.3	47.8	72.2	88.6	103.3	106.2	108.5
All federal government expenditures	$ 86.8	$201.6	$589.5	$1,259.2	$1,871.9	$2,728.3	$2,897.2	$3,118.0
All state and local government expenditures	40.2	113.0	329.4	731.8	1,281.3	1,778.6	1,905.6	2,014.4
National health expenditures	$ 27.5	$ 74.9	$253.4	$ 714.2	$1,352.9	$2,112.5	$2,239.7	$2,338.7
Private	20.7	46.8	147.0	427.4	756.5	1,136.8	1,201.0	1,232.0
Public	6.7	28.1	106.4	286.8	596.4	975.7	1,038.7	1,106.7
Federal government	2.9	17.7	71.6	193.9	417.6	709.6	755.3	816.9
State and local government	3.9	10.4	34.8	92.9	178.8	266.1	283.4	289.8
	Amount per capita							
National health expenditures	$ 148	$ 356	$1,100	$ 2,814	$ 4,789	$ 7,071	$ 7,423	$ 7,681
Private	111	222	638	1,684	2,678	3,805	3,980	4,046
Public	36	134	462	1,130	2,111	3,266	3,443	3,635
Federal government	15	84	311	764	1,478	2,375	2,503	2,683
State and local government	21	49	151	366	633	891	939	952
	Percent							
National health expenditures as percent of GDP	5.2	7.2	9.1	12.3	13.6	15.8	15.9	16.2
Health expenditures as a percent of total government expenditures								
All federal government	3.3	8.8	12.1	15.4	22.3	26.0	26.1	26.2
All state and local government	9.7	9.2	10.6	12.7	14.0	15.0	14.9	14.4
	Percent distribution							
National health expenditures	100.0	100.0	100.0	100.0	100.0	100.0	100.0	100.0
Private	75.5	62.5	58.0	59.8	55.9	53.8	53.6	52.7
Public	24.5	37.5	42.0	40.2	44.1	46.2	46.4	47.3
Federal government	10.4	23.7	28.2	27.2	30.9	33.6	33.7	34.9
State and local government	14.1	13.8	13.7	13.0	13.2	12.6	12.7	12.4
	Average annual percent change from previous year shown[2]							
GDP	...	7.0	10.4	7.6	5.5	5.1	5.1	2.6
Federal government expenditures	...	8.8	11.3	7.9	4.0	6.5	6.2	7.6
State and local government expenditures	...	10.9	11.3	8.3	5.8	5.6	7.1	5.7
National health expenditures	...	10.5	13.0	10.9	6.6	7.7	6.0	4.4
Private	...	8.5	12.1	11.3	5.9	7.0	5.6	2.6
Public	...	15.3	14.2	10.4	7.6	8.6	6.5	6.5
Federal government	...	20.0	15.0	10.5	8.0	9.2	6.4	8.2
State and local government	...	10.3	12.9	10.3	6.8	6.9	6.5	2.2
National health expenditures, per capita	...	9.2	11.9	9.9	5.5	6.7	5.0	3.5
Private	...	7.2	11.1	10.2	4.7	6.0	4.6	1.7
Public	...	13.9	13.2	9.4	6.4	7.5	5.4	5.6
Federal government	...	18.6	13.9	9.4	6.8	8.2	5.4	7.2
State and local government	...	9.0	11.9	9.2	5.6	5.9	5.5	1.3

... Category not applicable.

[1] Year 2005 = 100. Last revised December 23, 2008, by the Bureau of Economic Analysis.

[2] See Appendix II, Average annual rate of change (percent change).

NOTES: Dollar amounts shown are in current dollars. The data reflect U.S. Census Bureau resident population estimates as of July 2008, excluding the Armed Forces overseas. See Appendix II, Gross domestic product (GDP); Health expenditures, national. Percents are calculated using unrounded data. Estimates may not add to totals because of rounding. Data have been revised and differ from previous editions of *Health, United States*. Data for additional years are available. See Appendix III.

SOURCE: Centers for Medicare & Medicaid Services, Office of the Actuary, National Health Statistics Group, National Health Expenditure Accounts, National health expenditures, 2008. Available from: http://www.cms.hhs.gov/NationalHealthExpendData/; U.S. Department of Commerce, Bureau of Economic Analysis, National Economic Accounts, National Income and Product Accounts Tables 1.1.9, 3.2, 3.3 accessed on June 17, 2010. Available from: http://www.bea.gov/national/nipaweb/SelectTable.asp?Selected=N/.

Table 123. Consumer Price Index and average annual percent change for all items, selected items, and medical care components: United States, selected years 1960–2009

[Data are based on reporting by samples of providers and other retail outlets]

Items and medical care components	1960	1970	1980	1990	1995	2000	2005	2008	2009
	Consumer Price Index (CPI)								
All items	29.6	38.8	82.4	130.7	152.4	172.2	195.3	215.3	214.5
All items less medical care	30.2	39.2	82.8	128.8	148.6	167.3	188.7	207.8	206.6
Services	24.1	35.0	77.9	139.2	168.7	195.3	230.1	255.5	259.2
Food	30.0	39.2	86.8	132.4	148.4	167.8	190.7	214.1	218.0
Apparel	45.7	59.2	90.9	124.1	132.0	129.6	119.5	118.9	120.1
Housing	- - -	36.4	81.1	128.5	148.5	169.6	195.7	216.3	217.1
Energy	22.4	25.5	86.0	102.1	105.2	124.6	177.1	236.7	193.1
Medical care	22.3	34.0	74.9	162.8	220.5	260.8	323.2	364.1	375.6
Components of medical care									
Medical care services	19.5	32.3	74.8	162.7	224.2	266.0	336.7	384.9	397.3
Professional services	- - -	37.0	77.9	156.1	201.0	237.7	281.7	311.0	319.4
Physicians' services	21.9	34.5	76.5	160.8	208.8	244.7	287.5	311.3	320.8
Dental services	27.0	39.2	78.9	155.8	206.8	258.5	324.0	376.9	388.1
Eyeglasses and eye care[1]	- - -	- - -	- - -	117.3	137.0	149.7	163.2	174.1	175.5
Services by other medical professionals[1]	- - -	- - -	- - -	120.2	143.9	161.9	186.8	205.5	209.8
Hospital and related services	- - -	- - -	69.2	178.0	257.8	317.3	439.9	534.0	567.9
Hospital services[2]	- - -	- - -	- - -	- - -	- - -	115.9	161.6	197.2	210.7
Inpatient hospital services[2,3]	- - -	- - -	- - -	- - -	- - -	113.8	156.6	190.8	203.6
Outpatient hospital services[1,3]	- - -	- - -	- - -	138.7	204.6	263.8	373.0	456.8	490.6
Hospital rooms	9.3	23.6	68.0	175.4	251.2	- - -	- - -	- - -	- - -
Other inpatient services[1]	- - -	- - -	- - -	142.7	206.8	- - -	- - -	- - -	- - -
Nursing homes and adult day care[2]	- - -	- - -	- - -	- - -	- - -	117.0	145.0	165.3	171.6
Health insurance[4]	- - -	- - -	- - -	- - -	- - -	- - -	- - -	114.2	110.5
Medical care commodities	46.9	46.5	75.4	163.4	204.5	238.1	276.0	296.0	305.1
Prescription drugs[5]	54.0	47.4	72.5	181.7	235.0	285.4	349.0	378.3	391.1
Nonprescription drugs and medical supplies[1]	- - -	- - -	- - -	120.6	140.5	149.5	151.7	158.3	161.4
Internal and respiratory over-the-counter drugs	- - -	42.3	74.9	145.9	167.0	176.9	179.7	188.7	193.0
Nonprescription medical equipment and supplies	- - -	- - -	79.2	138.0	166.3	178.1	180.6	185.6	188.2
	Average annual percent change from previous year shown								
All items	. . .	2.7	7.8	9.7	3.1	2.5	6.5	3.8	−0.4
All items excluding medical care	. . .	2.6	7.8	9.2	2.9	2.4	6.2	3.8	−0.6
All services	. . .	3.8	8.3	12.3	3.9	3.0	8.5	3.5	1.4
Food	. . .	2.7	8.3	8.8	2.3	2.5	6.6	5.5	1.8
Apparel	. . .	2.6	4.4	6.4	1.2	−0.4	−4	−0.1	1.0
Housing	. . .	- - -	8.3	9.6	2.9	2.7	7.4	3.2	0.4
Energy	. . .	1.3	12.9	3.5	0.6	3.4	19.2	13.9	−18.4
Medical care	. . .	4.3	8.2	16.8	6.3	3.4	11.3	3.7	3.2
Components of medical care									
Medical care services	. . .	5.2	8.8	16.8	6.6	3.5	12.5	4.2	3.2
Professional services	. . .	- - -	7.7	14.9	5.2	3.4	8.9	3.4	2.7
Physicians' services	. . .	4.6	8.3	16.0	5.4	3.2	8.4	2.7	3.0
Dental services	. . .	3.8	7.2	14.6	5.8	4.6	12	5.1	3.0
Eyeglasses and eye care[1]	. . .	- - -	- - -	- - -	3.2	1.8	4.4	1.4	0.8
Services by other medical professionals[1]	. . .	- - -	- - -	- - -	3.7	2.4	7.4	4.1	2.1
Hospital and related services	. . .	- - -	- - -	20.8	7.7	4.2	17.7	7.0	6.4
Hospital services[2]	. . .	- - -	- - -	- - -	- - -	- - -	18.1	7.4	6.9
Inpatient hospital services[2,3]	. . .	- - -	- - -	- - -	- - -	- - -	17.3	7.1	6.7
Outpatient hospital services[1,3]	. . .	- - -	- - -	- - -	8.1	5.2	18.9	7.7	7.4
Hospital rooms	. . .	9.8	11.2	20.9	7.4	- - -	- - -	- - -	- - -
Other inpatient services[1]	. . .	- - -	- - -	- - -	7.7	- - -	- - -	- - -	- - -
Nursing homes and adult day care[2]	. . .	- - -	- - -	- - -	- - -	- - -	11.3	3.6	3.8
Health insurance[4]	. . .	- - -	- - -	- - -	- - -	- - -	- - -	0.6	−3.2
Medical care commodities	. . .	−0.1	5.0	16.7	4.6	3.1	7.7	2.1	3.1
Prescription drugs[5]	. . .	−1.3	4.3	20.2	5.3	4.0	10.6	2.5	3.4
Nonprescription drugs and medical supplies[1]	. . .	- - -	- - -	- - -	3.1	1.2	0.7	0.9	2.0
Internal and respiratory over-the-counter drugs	. . .	- - -	5.9	14.3	2.7	1.2	0.8	1.2	2.3
Nonprescription medical equipment and supplies	. . .	- - -	- - -	11.7	3.8	1.4	0.7	0.3	1.3

- - - Data not available.   . . . Category not applicable.

[1]December 1986 = 100.
[2]December 1996 = 100.
[3]Special index based on a substantially smaller sample.
[4]December 2005 = 100.   [5]Prior to 2006, this category included medical supplies.

NOTES: CPI for all urban consumers (CPI-U) U.S. city average, detailed expenditure categories. 1982–1984 = 100, except where noted. Data are not seasonally adjusted. See Appendix I, Consumer Price Index. See Appendix II, Consumer Price Index.

SOURCE: U.S. Department of Labor, Bureau of Labor Statistics, Consumer Price Index. Various releases. 2009 data available from: http://www.bls.gov/cpi/cpid09av.pdf.

Table 124. Growth in personal health care expenditures and percent distribution of factors affecting growth: United States, 1960–2008

[Data are compiled from various sources by the Centers for Medicare & Medicaid Services]

Period	Average annual percent increase	All factors	Factors affecting growth			
			Inflation[1]		Population	Intensity[2]
			Economy-wide	Medical		
			Percent distribution[3]			
1960–2008	9.7	100	40	16	11	33
1960–1965	8.3	100	17	10	18	55
1965–1970	12.7	100	33	12	8	46
1970–1975	12.3	100	55	1	8	36
1975–1980	13.8	100	55	12	7	26
1980–1985	11.6	100	46	32	9	13
1985–1990	10.3	100	32	26	10	32
1990–1995	7.3	100	35	29	16	21
1995–2000	5.7	100	30	17	18	35
1995–1996	5.4	100	36	19	19	26
1996–1997	5.4	100	33	7	20	41
1997–1998	5.3	100	22	21	20	38
1998–1999	5.7	100	26	22	18	34
1999–2000	6.7	100	33	16	15	36
2000–2005	7.8	100	32	18	12	38
2000–2001	8.7	100	27	18	12	43
2001–2002	8.2	100	20	27	12	41
2002–2003	8.0	100	28	20	11	41
2003–2004	7.1	100	41	18	14	28
2004–2005	6.8	100	50	3	14	33
2005–2006	6.5	100	51	3	16	31
2006–2007	5.9	100	49	9	17	25
2007–2008	4.6	100	47	20	20	13

[1]Total inflation is economy-wide, and medical inflation is the medical inflation above economy-wide inflation.
[2]Intensity is the residual percent of growth that cannot be attributed to inflation or population growth. It represents changes in the use or kinds of services and supplies.
[3]Percents may not sum to 100 due to rounding.

NOTES: These data include revisions in health expenditures for 1975 and subsequent years and revisions in population for 2000 and subsequent years. The implicit price deflator for Gross domestic product (GDP) is used to measure economy-wide inflation for all years 1960–2008. See Appendix II, Health expenditures, national; Gross domestic product (GDP). All indexes used to calculate the factors affecting growth were rebased in 2003 with base year 2000. Data have been revised and differ from previous editions of *Health, United States*.

SOURCE: Centers for Medicare & Medicaid Services, Office of the Actuary, National Health Statistics Group, National Health Expenditure Accounts, National health expenditures, 2008. Available from: http://www.cms.hhs.gov/NationalHealthExpendData/; unpublished data.

[Data are compiled from various sources by the Centers for Medicare & Medicaid Services]

Type of national health expenditure	1960	1970	1980	1990	2000	2005	2006	2007	2008
					Amount in billions				
National health expenditures	$27.5	$74.9	$253.4	$714.2	$1,352.9	$1,982.5	$2,112.5	$2,239.7	$2,338.7
Health services and supplies	24.9	67.1	233.5	666.8	1,264.1	1,851.9	1,975.4	2,089.7	2,181.3
Personal health care	23.3	62.9	214.8	607.6	1,139.2	1,655.2	1,762.9	1,866.4	1,952.3
Hospital care	9.2	27.6	101.0	251.6	416.9	607.5	649.4	687.6	718.4
Professional services	8.3	20.6	67.3	216.8	426.8	621.5	658.4	697.5	731.2
Physician and clinical services	5.4	14.0	47.1	157.5	288.6	422.4	446.5	472.6	496.2
Other professional services	0.4	0.7	3.6	18.2	39.1	55.9	58.4	62.2	65.7
Dental services	2.0	4.7	13.3	31.5	62.0	86.3	90.7	96.4	101.2
Other personal health care	0.6	1.2	3.3	9.6	37.1	56.9	62.7	66.3	68.1
Nursing home and home health	0.9	4.3	20.9	65.2	125.8	168.8	178.1	191.7	203.1
Home health care[1]	0.1	0.2	2.4	12.6	30.5	48.1	53.0	59.3	64.7
Nursing home care[1]	0.8	4.0	18.5	52.6	95.3	120.7	125.1	132.4	138.4
Retail outlet sales of medical products	4.9	10.5	25.7	74.0	169.8	257.4	277.0	289.7	299.6
Prescription drugs	2.7	5.5	12.0	40.3	120.6	199.7	217.0	226.8	234.1
Other medical products	2.3	5.0	13.6	33.7	49.2	57.7	60.0	62.9	65.5
Government administration and net cost of private health insurance	1.2	2.8	12.2	39.3	81.8	140.3	152.0	158.4	159.6
Government public health activities[2]	0.4	1.4	6.4	20.0	43.0	56.4	60.6	64.8	69.4
Investment	2.6	7.8	19.9	47.3	88.8	130.6	137.1	150.0	157.5
Research[3]	0.7	2.0	5.4	12.7	25.6	40.7	41.8	42.5	43.6
Structures and equipment	1.9	5.8	14.5	34.7	63.2	90.0	95.3	107.5	113.9
					Average annual percent change from previous year shown				
National health expenditures	...	10.5	13.0	10.9	6.6	7.9	6.6	6.0	4.4
Health services and supplies	...	10.4	13.3	11.1	6.6	7.9	6.7	5.8	4.4
Personal health care	...	10.4	13.1	11.0	6.5	7.8	6.5	5.9	4.6
Hospital care	...	11.6	13.9	9.6	5.2	7.8	6.9	5.9	4.5
Professional services	...	9.5	12.5	12.4	7.0	7.8	5.9	5.9	4.8
Physician and clinical services	...	10.1	12.9	12.8	6.2	7.9	5.7	5.8	5.0
Other professional services	...	6.6	17.1	17.5	8.0	7.4	4.4	6.5	5.6
Dental services	...	9.1	11.1	9.0	7.0	6.9	5.1	6.2	5.1
Other personal health care	...	7.3	10.1	11.4	14.5	8.9	10.3	5.8	2.6
Nursing home and home health	...	17.2	17.2	12.1	6.8	6.1	5.6	7.6	6.0
Home health care[1]	...	14.5	26.9	18.1	9.3	9.5	10.3	11.8	9.0
Nursing home care[1]	...	17.4	16.4	11.0	6.1	4.8	3.7	5.8	4.6
Retail outlet sales of medical products	...	7.8	9.4	11.2	8.7	8.7	7.6	4.6	3.4
Prescription drugs	...	7.5	8.2	12.8	11.6	10.6	8.7	4.5	3.2
Other medical products	...	8.1	10.6	9.5	3.8	3.3	4.0	4.8	4.1
Government administration and net cost of private health insurance	...	8.6	16.0	12.4	7.6	11.4	8.3	4.3	0.7
Government public health activities[2]	...	13.8	16.9	12.0	8.0	5.5	7.4	7.1	7.1
Investment	...	11.7	9.9	9.0	6.5	8.0	5.0	9.4	5.0
Research[3]	...	10.9	10.8	8.9	7.3	9.7	2.9	1.6	2.6
Structures and equipment	...	11.9	9.5	9.1	6.2	7.3	5.9	12.9	5.9

See footnotes at end of table.

Table 125 (page 2 of 2). National health expenditures, average annual percent change, and percent distribution, by type of expenditure: United States, selected years 1960–2008

[Data are compiled from various sources by the Centers for Medicare & Medicaid Services]

Type of national health expenditure	1960	1970	1980	1990	2000	2005	2006	2007	2008
					Percent distribution				
National health expenditures	100.0	100.0	100.0	100.0	100.0	100.0	100.0	100.0	100.0
Health services and supplies	90.6	89.6	92.1	93.4	93.4	93.4	93.5	93.3	93.3
Personal health care	84.8	84.1	84.8	85.1	84.2	83.5	83.4	83.3	83.5
Hospital care	33.4	36.9	39.9	35.2	30.8	30.6	30.7	30.7	30.7
Professional services	30.3	27.6	26.5	30.4	31.5	31.4	31.2	31.1	31.3
Physician and clinical services	19.5	18.7	18.6	22.1	21.3	21.3	21.1	21.1	21.2
Other professional services	1.4	1.0	1.4	2.5	2.9	2.8	2.8	2.8	2.8
Dental services	7.1	6.2	5.3	4.4	4.6	4.4	4.3	4.3	4.3
Other personal health care	2.2	1.7	1.3	1.3	2.7	2.9	3.0	3.0	2.9
Nursing home and home health	3.2	5.7	8.2	9.1	9.3	8.5	8.4	8.6	8.7
Home health care[1]	0.2	0.3	0.9	1.8	2.3	2.4	2.5	2.6	2.8
Nursing home care[1]	3.0	5.4	7.3	7.4	7.0	6.1	5.9	5.9	5.9
Retail outlet sales of medical products	18.0	14.0	10.1	10.4	12.6	13.0	13.1	12.9	12.8
Prescription drugs	9.7	7.3	4.8	5.6	8.9	10.1	10.3	10.1	10.0
Other medical products	8.3	6.6	5.4	4.7	3.6	2.9	2.8	2.8	2.8
Government administration and net cost of private health insurance	4.4	3.7	4.8	5.5	6.0	7.1	7.2	7.1	6.8
Government public health activities[2]	1.3	1.8	2.5	2.8	3.2	2.8	2.9	2.9	3.0
Investment	9.4	10.4	7.9	6.6	6.6	6.6	6.5	6.7	6.7
Research[3]	2.5	2.6	2.1	1.8	1.9	2.1	2.0	1.9	1.9
Structures and equipment	6.9	7.8	5.7	4.9	4.7	4.5	4.5	4.8	4.9

. . . Category not applicable.

[1]Freestanding facilities only. Additional services of this type are provided in hospital-based facilities and counted as hospital care.

[2]Includes personal care services delivered by government public health agencies.

[3]Research and development expenditures of drug companies and other manufacturers and providers of medical equipment and supplies are excluded. They are included in the expenditure class in which the product falls because such expenditures are covered by the payment received for that product. See Appendix II, Health expenditures, national.

NOTES: Percents are calculated using unrounded data. Data have been revised and differ from previous editions of *Health, United States*.

SOURCE: Centers for Medicare & Medicaid Services, Office of the Actuary, National Health Statistics Group, National Health Expenditure Accounts, National health expenditures, 2008. Available from: http://www.cms.hhs.gov/NationalHealthExpendData/.

Table 126 (page 1 of 2). Personal health care expenditures, by source of funds and type of expenditure: United States, selected years 1960–2008

[Data are compiled from various sources by the Centers for Medicare & Medicaid Services]

Type of personal health care expenditures and source of funds	1960	1970	1980	1990	2000	2006	2007	2008
				Amount				
Per capita.	$ 125	$ 299	$ 932	$2,394	$ 4,032	$ 5,901	$ 6,186	$ 6,411
				Amount in billions				
All personal health care expenditures[1]. .	$ 23.3	$ 62.9	$214.8	$607.6	$1,139.2	$1,762.9	$1,866.4	$1,952.3
Personal health care implicit price deflator[2]	- - -	13.3	28.7	58.6	83.0	103.4	106.9	110.2
				Percent distribution				
All sources of funds.	100.0	100.0	100.0	100.0	100.0	100.0	100.0	100.0
Out-of-pocket payments	55.2	39.6	27.1	22.4	16.9	14.5	14.5	14.2
Private health insurance	21.4	22.3	28.5	33.7	35.4	36.0	35.6	35.4
Other private funds	2.0	2.8	4.3	5.0	5.0	4.2	4.3	3.9
Government[3].	21.4	35.3	40.1	38.9	42.7	45.3	·45.5	46.5
Medicare	. . .	11.6	16.8	17.5	18.9	21.7	21.9	22.8
Medicaid	. . .	8.0	11.5	11.5	16.4	16.2	16.3	16.2
CHIP[4]	. . .	. . .	. . .	. . .	0.2	0.4	0.4	0.5
				Amount in billions				
Hospital care expenditures[5]	$ 9.2	$ 27.6	$101.0	$251.6	$ 416.9	$ 649.4	$ 687.6	$ 718.4
				Percent distribution				
All sources of funds.	100.0	100.0	100.0	100.0	100.0	100.0	100.0	100.0
Out-of-pocket payments	20.7	9.0	5.4	4.5	3.3	3.2	3.2	3.2
Private health insurance	35.8	32.5	36.6	38.9	34.6	36.1	35.8	36.1
Other private funds	1.2	3.2	5.0	4.1	5.3	4.7	4.9	3.8
Government[3].	42.2	55.2	53.0	52.5	56.9	55.9	56.0	56.9
Medicare	. . .	19.4	26.1	27.0	29.8	28.9	28.5	29.4
Medicaid	. . .	9.6	9.1	10.6	17.0	17.1	17.4	17.1
CHIP[4]	. . .	. . .	. . .	. . .	0.2	0.4	0.4	0.4
				Amount in billions				
Physician and clinical services expenditures.	$ 5.4	$ 14.0	$ 47.1	$157.5	$ 288.6	$ 446.5	$ 472.6	$ 496.2
				Percent distribution				
All sources of funds.	100.0	100.0	100.0	100.0	100.0	100.0	100.0	100.0
Out-of-pocket payments	61.7	46.2	30.4	19.2	11.1	10.4	10.4	10.1
Private health insurance	29.8	30.1	35.5	42.7	47.3	49.3	49.2	48.7
Other private funds	1.4	1.6	3.9	7.2	7.7	6.5	6.5	6.4
Government[3].	7.2	22.1	30.2	31.0	33.8	33.9	33.8	34.7
Medicare	. . .	11.8	17.0	18.6	20.2	20.4	20.2	20.7
Medicaid	. . .	4.6	5.2	4.5	6.6	7.0	7.0	7.3
CHIP[4]	. . .	. . .	. . .	. . .	0.3	0.4	0.5	0.5
				Amount in billions				
Nursing home expenditures[6]	$ 0.8	$ 4.0	$ 18.5	$ 52.6	$ 95.3	$ 125.1	$ 132.4	$ 138.4
				Percent distribution				
All sources of funds.	100.0	100.0	100.0	100.0	100.0	100.0	100.0	100.0
Out-of-pocket payments	77.3	52.0	35.7	36.1	30.1	26.0	26.8	26.7
Private health insurance	0.0	0.2	1.1	5.6	8.3	7.4	7.4	7.4
Other private funds	6.3	4.8	4.0	7.2	4.8	3.6	3.9	3.7
Government[3].	16.4	43.0	59.2	51.1	56.8	63.0	61.9	62.2
Medicare	. . .	3.5	1.7	3.2	10.6	16.8	17.6	18.6
Medicaid	. . .	23.3	55.4	45.8	44.1	43.6	41.4	40.6
CHIP[4]	. . .	. . .	. . .	. . .	0.0	0.0	0.0	0.0

See footnotes at end of table.

[Data are compiled from various sources by the Centers for Medicare & Medicaid Services]

Type of personal health care expenditures and source of funds	1960	1970	1980	1990	2000	2006	2007	2008
				Amount in billions				
Home health expenditures	$ 0.1	$ 0.2	$ 2.4	$ 12.6	$ 30.5	$ 53.0	$ 59.3	$ 64.7
				Percent distribution				
All sources of funds.	100.0	100.0	100.0	100.0	100.0	100.0	100.0	100.0
Out-of-pocket payments	12.5	9.4	15.2	17.9	17.9	10.9	10.2	10.1
Private health insurance	2.5	3.0	14.7	22.9	22.7	10.6	9.6	9.0
Other private funds	66.7	38.7	15.6	7.7	4.0	2.1	1.9	1.8
Government[3]	17.4	48.8	54.5	51.6	55.4	76.4	78.3	79.1
Medicare	. . .	26.7	26.8	26.0	28.0	39.7	40.8	41.2
Medicaid	. . .	6.7	11.7	17.1	22.1	33.5	34.3	34.7
CHIP[4]	. . .	. . .	. . .	. . .	0.0	0.0	0.0	0.0
				Amount in billions				
Prescription drug expenditures	$ 2.7	$ 5.5	$ 12.0	$ 40.3	$120.6	$217.0	$226.8	$234.1
				Percent distribution				
All sources of funds.	100.0	100.0	100.0	100.0	100.0	100.0	100.0	100.0
Out-of-pocket payments	96.0	82.4	70.3	55.5	27.7	21.6	21.6	20.7
Private health insurance	1.3	8.8	14.8	26.4	49.3	44.3	43.1	42.1
Other private funds	0.0	0.0	0.0	0.0	0.0	0.0	0.0	0.0
Government[3]	2.7	8.8	14.9	18.1	23.0	34.1	35.3	37.2
Medicare	. . .	0.0	0.0	0.5	1.7	18.2	20.3	22.2
Medicaid	. . .	7.6	11.7	12.6	16.7	8.8	8.3	8.3
CHIP[4]	. . .	. . .	. . .	. . .	0.3	0.7	0.7	0.7
				Amount in billions				
Dental services expenditures	$ 2.0	$ 4.7	$ 13.3	$ 31.5	$ 62.0	$ 90.7	$ 96.4	$101.2
				Percent distribution				
All sources of funds.	100.0	100.0	100.0	100.0	100.0	100.0	100.0	100.0
Out-of-pocket payments	97.2	91.0	66.4	48.5	44.6	44.3	44.3	44.1
Private health insurance	1.9	4.5	28.6	48.5	50.5	49.6	49.3	48.6
Other private funds	0.0	0.0	0.2	0.2	0.3	0.1	0.1	0.1
Government[3]	0.9	4.5	4.8	2.8	4.6	6.0	6.3	7.2
Medicare	. . .	0.0	0.0	0.0	0.1	0.1	0.2	0.2
Medicaid	. . .	3.5	3.8	2.4	3.7	4.8	5.2	5.9
CHIP[4]	. . .	. . .	. . .	. . .	0.4	0.7	0.6	0.7
				Amount in billions				
All other personal health care expenditures[7]	$ 3.3	$ 6.9	$ 20.5	$ 61.5	$125.4	$181.1	$191.5	$199.3
				Percent distribution				
All sources of funds.	100.0	100.0	100.0	100.0	100.0	100.0	100.0	100.0
Out-of-pocket payments	78.1	73.0	69.2	58.1	41.2	34.3	34.3	34.1
Private health insurance	1.3	2.4	6.7	12.7	13.1	13.2	13.2	13.3
Other private funds	5.6	5.0	5.6	6.4	5.5	5.1	5.1	5.1
Government[3]	15.0	19.6	18.5	22.7	40.2	47.4	47.3	47.5
Medicare	. . .	1.0	3.5	6.9	9.9	11.9	12.0	12.8
Medicaid	. . .	3.0	3.0	6.4	20.4	26.7	27.0	27.0
CHIP[4]	. . .	. . .	. . .	. . .	0.2	0.4	0.4	0.5

. . . Category not applicable.

0.0 Quantity more than zero but less than 0.05.

[1]Includes all expenditures for specified health services and supplies other than expenses for program administration, net cost of private health insurance, and government public health activities.

[2]Constructed from the Producer Price Index for hospital care, Nursing Home Input Price Index for nursing home care, and Consumer Price Indices specific to each of the remaining personal health care components.

[3]Includes other government expenditures for these health care services, for example, care funded by the Department of Veterans Affairs, and state and locally financed subsidies to hospitals.

[4]Children's Health Insurance Program (CHIP). Medicaid CHIP expansions are included.

[5]Includes expenditures for hospital-based nursing home and home health agency care.

[6]Includes expenditures for care in freestanding nursing homes. Expenditures for care in hospital-based nursing homes are included with hospital care.

[7]Includes expenditures for other professional services, other nondurable medical products, durable medical equipment, and other personal health care, not shown separately. See Appendix II, Health expenditures, national.

NOTES: Percents may not add to totals because of rounding. The Medicare and Medicaid programs began coverage in 1965. The Children's Health Insurance Program began coverage in 1997. Data have been revised and differ from previous editions of *Health, United States*.

SOURCE: Centers for Medicare & Medicaid Services, Office of the Actuary, National Health Statistics Group, National Health Expenditure Accounts, National health expenditures, 2008. Available from: http://www.cms.hhs.gov/NationalHealthExpendData/.

Table 127 (page 1 of 2). Personal health care expenditures, by age: United States, selected years 1987–2004

[Data are compiled from various sources by the Centers for Medicare & Medicaid Services]

Type of personal health care expenditures and age	1987	1996	1999	2002	2004	1987	1996	1999	2002	2004
All personal health care expenditures[1]	Amount in billions					Amount per capita				
Total	$442.8	$910.3	$1,068.3	$1,341.2	$1,551.3	$ 1,796	$ 3,354	$ 3,818	$ 4,652	$ 5,276
Under 19 years	59.0	121.0	143.0	184.2	206.0	868	1,623	1,872	2,385	2,650
19–44 years	126.0	239.1	276.1	337.6	368.7	1,223	2,216	2,550	3,094	3,370
45–54 years	42.0	106.3	136.1	179.7	217.2	1,781	3,197	3,703	4,487	5,210
55–64 years	58.2	106.4	133.6	174.7	227.8	2,636	4,878	5,581	6,533	7,787
65–74 years	69.7	133.7	146.6	173.0	197.1	3,998	7,174	8,042	9,562	10,778
75–84 years	56.3	127.5	144.9	182.6	208.9	5,984	11,199	12,054	14,578	16,389
85 years and over	31.6	76.3	88.0	109.4	125.4	10,562	19,577	20,992	23,985	25,691
Hospital care expenditures[2]										
Total	190.5	352.2	395.0	488.6	566.9	773	1,298	1,412	1,695	1,928
Under 19 years	22.7	43.1	49.2	67.3	77.8	335	578	645	872	1,000
19–44 years	55.5	93.8	103.6	129.0	143.4	538	869	957	1,182	1,311
45–54 years	17.6	36.7	44.2	56.8	71.1	744	1,103	1,204	1,417	1,706
55–64 years	27.7	44.3	51.8	62.1	80.5	1,254	2,028	2,165	2,322	2,752
65–74 years	32.7	59.1	60.1	68.2	76.6	1,879	3,171	3,297	3,772	4,191
75–84 years	24.2	52.6	58.5	70.4	78.8	2,575	4,619	4,867	5,619	6,178
85 years and over	10.1	22.7	27.5	34.9	38.7	3,368	5,838	6,548	7,645	7,916
Physician and clinical services expenditures										
Total	111.7	229.4	269.6	337.9	393.7	453	845	964	1,172	1,339
Under 19 years	18.6	39.3	44.6	55.6	58.5	274	527	585	719	753
19–44 years	36.3	71.5	79.6	97.7	105.0	352	663	735	896	960
45–54 years	10.8	30.1	38.2	47.5	61.0	456	906	1,039	1,186	1,463
55–64 years	14.0	28.6	35.0	44.8	60.6	634	1,312	1,461	1,676	2,070
65–74 years	18.3	31.4	36.4	43.2	49.7	1,053	1,686	1,996	2,386	2,716
75–84 years	10.8	21.7	27.1	37.2	44.1	1,148	1,907	2,257	2,969	3,463
85 years and over	2.9	6.8	8.7	11.9	14.8	970	1,740	2,082	2,616	3,037
Nursing home expenditures[3]										
Total	36.3	79.6	90.5	105.7	115.0	147	293	323	367	391
Under 19 years	0.4	1.0	1.2	1.3	1.4	6	14	16	16	18
19–44 years	3.7	7.2	7.0	7.7	7.9	36	67	64	70	72
45–54 years	1.4	3.2	4.3	5.9	7.0	59	96	116	147	168
55–64 years	1.5	3.5	4.8	6.6	8.0	69	160	201	248	272
65–74 years	3.9	10.3	11.4	13.5	14.8	226	550	624	743	809
75–84 years	10.8	23.7	26.7	30.9	33.4	1,145	2,079	2,224	2,469	2,623
85 years and over	14.6	30.7	35.2	39.9	42.5	4,882	7,888	8,392	8,746	8,706

See footnotes at end of table.

[Data are compiled from various sources by the Centers for Medicare & Medicaid Services]

Type of personal health care expenditures and age	1987	1996	1999	2002	2004	1987	1996	1999	2002	2004
Home health expenditures	Amount in billions					Amount per capita				
Total	$ 6.7	$ 33.6	$ 31.5	$ 34.2	$ 42.7	$ 27	$ 124	$ 113	$ 119	$ 145
Under 19 years	0.6	3.3	3.2	4.0	4.9	9	44	42	51	63
19–44 years	1.7	4.4	4.9	5.6	6.4	16	41	46	51	58
45–54 years	0.3	3.3	3.9	3.8	4.5	11	98	105	94	108
55–64 years	0.7	2.2	2.5	2.5	3.2	30	99	103	94	110
65–74 years	1.2	5.2	3.8	4.3	5.2	68	279	208	235	285
75–84 years	1.5	8.7	6.8	7.3	9.4	164	764	567	585	734
85 years and over	0.7	6.6	6.5	6.8	9.1	249	1,693	1,546	1,497	1,869
Prescription drug expenditures										
Total	26.9	68.5	104.7	157.9	189.7	109	253	374	548	645
Under 19 years	2.8	6.5	9.5	13.8	16.3	41	87	124	178	210
19–44 years	6.4	18.3	27.8	36.5	40.3	62	169	256	334	368
45–54 years	3.6	10.7	18.8	31.9	36.1	153	322	513	796	866
55–64 years	5.0	11.5	18.5	30.4	41.3	225	528	772	1,138	1,412
65–74 years	5.0	11.8	15.9	21.3	25.2	287	635	870	1,178	1,379
75–84 years	3.3	7.3	10.7	17.2	20.8	351	637	886	1,372	1,630
85 years and over	0.9	2.5	3.6	6.9	9.7	300	631	856	1,506	1,980
Dental services expenditures										
Total	25.3	46.8	57.1	73.3	81.5	102	172	204	254	277
Under 19 years	6.6	13.9	17.1	21.6	24.8	97	186	224	280	319
19–44 years	10.1	16.3	18.8	23.3	25.1	98	151	174	214	229
45–54 years	3.3	7.6	9.2	12.1	12.8	140	229	251	302	308
55–64 years	2.7	4.3	5.8	8.7	10.4	123	198	242	325	355
65–74 years	1.8	3.1	4.0	4.5	4.9	105	165	218	249	267
75–84 years	0.6	1.4	1.8	2.7	2.9	60	121	152	213	227
85 years and over	0.1	0.2	0.4	0.4	0.6	47	53	86	94	117
All other personal health care expenditures[4]										
Total	45.5	100.1	119.8	143.5	161.8	184	369	429	498	550
Under 19 years	7.3	14.0	18.1	20.7	22.3	108	187	237	269	288
19–44 years	12.4	27.5	34.4	37.9	40.7	121	256	317	347	372
45–54 years	5.1	14.7	17.5	21.8	24.6	218	443	475	544	591
55–64 years	6.6	12.1	15.2	19.5	23.8	300	553	636	731	815
65–74 years	6.6	12.8	15.1	18.1	20.7	380	686	831	998	1,131
75–84 years	5.1	12.2	13.2	16.9	19.5	540	1,073	1,101	1,351	1,533
85 years and over	2.2	6.8	6.2	8.6	10.1	747	1,733	1,483	1,881	2,065

[1]Includes all expenditures for specified health services and supplies other than expenses for government administration, net cost of private health insurance, and government public health activities.
[2]Includes expenditures for hospital-based nursing home and home health agency care.
[3]Includes expenditures for care in freestanding nursing homes. Expenditures for care in hospital-based nursing homes are included in hospital care expenditures.
[4]Includes expenditures for other professional services, other non-durable medical products, durable medical equipment, and other personal health care, not shown separately. See Appendix II, Health expenditures, national.

NOTES: Estimates of personal health care expenditures presented in this table are based on National Health Expenditures 2005 vintage estimates, and therefore may not match National Health Expenditures 2008 vintage estimates for total personal health care and other services that are published elsewhere in *Health, United States*.

SOURCE: Centers for Medicare & Medicaid Services, Office of the Actuary, National Health Statistics Group, National Health Expenditure Accounts, National health expenditures, 2004. Available from: http://www.cms.hhs.gov/NationalHealthExpendData/.

Table 128. National health expenditures for mental health services, average annual percent change and percent distribution, by type of expenditure: United States, selected years 1986–2003

[Data are compiled from various sources by the Substance Abuse and Mental Health Services Administration]

Type of expenditure	1986	1990	1995	2000	2002	2003
	Amount in millions					
Total expenditures	$33,125	$46,456	$61,763	$79,203	$93,135	$100,321
Total, all service providers	29,355	40,636	52,163	57,740	65,790	69,918
General non-specialty hospitals	5,469	7,613	11,125	12,069	14,729	15,927
General hospital specialty units	3,038	5,729	7,953	6,445	6,455	6,568
General hospital non-specialty units.	2,432	1,885	3,171	5,624	8,274	9,359
Specialty hospitals.	8,251	11,069	11,473	11,005	11,328	11,673
All physicians	3,753	5,827	8,261	10,445	12,541	13,748
Psychiatrists	2,681	4,276	5,924	7,569	8,678	9,802
Non-psychiatric physicians	1,072	1,551	2,337	2,876	3,863	3,946
Other professionals	3,099	4,261	5,191	6,251	7,567	8,370
Freestanding nursing homes	4,754	5,496	5,261	5,310	5,964	6,234
Freestanding home health	113	221	592	612	749	823
Multi-service mental health organizations. . . .	3,916	6,148	10,260	12,048	12,913	13,143
Retail prescription drug	2,191	3,340	5,754	16,417	20,949	23,259
Insurance administration	1,579	2,480	3,847	5,046	6,395	7,145
	Amount in inflation-adjusted millions					
Total expenditures, inflation-adjusted dollars	$46,491	$56,938	$67,057	$79,203	$89,392	$ 94,284
	Deflator (2000 = 1.00)					
GDP implicit price deflator [1]	0.71	0.82	0.92	1.00	1.04	1.06
	Average annual percent change from previous year shown					
Total expenditures	. . .	8.8	5.9	5.1	8.4	7.7
Total, all service providers	. . .	8.5	5.1	2.1	6.7	6.3
General non-specialty hospitals	. . .	8.6	7.9	1.6	10.5	8.1
General hospital specialty units	. . .	17.2	6.8	−4.1	0.1	1.8
General hospital non-specialty units.	. . .	−6.2	11.0	12.1	21.3	13.1
Specialty hospitals.	. . .	7.6	0.7	−0.8	1.5	3.0
All physicians	. . .	11.6	7.2	4.8	9.6	9.6
Psychiatrists	. . .	12.4	6.7	5.0	7.1	13.0
Non-psychiatric physicians	. . .	9.7	8.6	4.2	15.9	2.1
Other professionals	. . .	8.3	4.0	3.8	10.0	10.6
Freestanding nursing homes	. . .	3.7	−0.9	0.2	6.0	4.5
Freestanding home health	. . .	18.4	21.7	0.7	10.7	9.9
Multi-service mental health organizations. . . .	. . .	11.9	10.8	3.3	3.5	1.8
Retail prescription drug	. . .	11.1	11.5	23.3	13.0	11.0
Insurance administration	. . .	11.9	9.2	5.6	12.6	11.7
	Percent distribution					
Total expenditures	100.0	100.0	100.0	100.0	100.0	100.0
Total, all service providers	88.6	87.5	84.5	72.9	70.6	69.7
General non-specialty hospitals	16.5	16.4	18.0	15.2	15.8	15.9
General hospital specialty units	9.2	12.3	12.9	8.1	6.9	6.5
General hospital non-specialty units.	7.3	4.1	5.1	7.1	8.9	9.3
Specialty hospitals.	24.9	23.8	18.6	13.9	12.2	11.6
All physicians	11.3	12.5	13.4	13.2	13.5	13.7
Psychiatrists	8.1	9.2	9.6	9.6	9.3	9.8
Non-psychiatric physicians	3.2	3.3	3.8	3.6	4.1	3.9
Other professionals	9.4	9.2	8.4	7.9	8.1	8.3
Freestanding nursing homes	14.4	11.8	8.5	6.7	6.4	6.2
Freestanding home health	0.3	0.5	1.0	0.8	0.8	0.8
Multi-service mental health organizations. . . .	11.8	13.2	16.6	15.2	13.9	13.1
Retail prescription drug	6.6	7.2	9.3	20.7	22.5	23.2
Insurance administration	4.8	5.3	6.2	6.4	6.9	7.1

. . . Category not applicable.

[1]Gross domestic product (GDP) implicit price deflator developed by the U.S. Department of Commerce, Bureau of Economic Analysis. Table 1.1.9 Implicit price deflator for gross domestic product is available from: http://www.bea.gov/national/nipaweb/TableView.asp?SelectedTable=13&Freq=Qtr&FirstYear=2008&LastYear=2010, accessed September 13, 2006.

NOTES: Additional data on specialty and non-specialty providers are available in the Internet version of this table. Available from: http://www.cdc.gov/nchs/hus.htm. Specialty providers include general hospital specialty units, specialty hospitals, psychiatrists, other professionals, multi-service mental health organizations, and specialty substance abuse centers. Non-specialty providers include general hospital non-specialty units, non-psychiatric physicians, freestanding nursing homes, and freestanding home health providers. Data for additional years are available. See Appendix III.

SOURCE: Mark TL, Levit KR, Coffey RM, McKusick DR, Harwood HJ, King EC, et al. National Expenditures for Mental Health Services and Substance Abuse Treatment, 1993–2003. SAMHSA pub no SMA 07–4227. Rockville, MD: Substance Abuse and Mental Health Services Administration, 2007 and unpublished data.

Table 129. National health expenditures for substance abuse treatment, average annual percent change and percent distribution, by type of expenditure: United States, selected years 1986–2003

[Data are compiled from various sources by the Substance Abuse and Mental Health Services Administration]

Type of expenditure	1986	1990	1995	2000	2002	2003
	Amount in millions					
Total expenditures	$ 9,302	$12,075	$15,561	$17,545	$19,867	$20,740
Total, all service providers	8,777	11,378	14,590	16,473	18,558	19,335
General non-specialty hospitals	2,995	3,167	3,764	3,649	4,132	4,359
General hospital specialty units	2,240	2,089	3,320	2,739	2,859	2,890
General hospital non-specialty units	755	1,078	444	911	1,272	1,470
Specialty hospitals	1,453	1,346	1,315	736	738	676
All physicians	685	904	1,048	1,413	1,554	1,672
Psychiatrists	237	328	410	510	428	540
Non-psychiatric physicians	448	577	638	902	1,127	1,131
Other professionals	1,451	1,685	1,652	2,076	2,372	2,636
Freestanding nursing homes	106	126	179	254	292	301
Freestanding home health	2	3	16	10	3	4
Multi-service mental health organizations	325	657	1,012	1,492	1,312	1,246
Specialty substance abuse centers	1,761	3,490	5,605	6,845	8,156	8,441
Retail prescription drug	14	19	33	67	89	98
Insurance administration	512	679	937	1,005	1,220	1,307
	Amount in inflation-adjusted millions					
Total expenditures, inflation-adjusted dollars	$13,056	$14,800	$16,895	$17,545	$19,068	$19,492
	Deflator (2000 = 1.00)					
GDP implicit price deflator [1]	0.71	0.82	0.92	1.00	1.04	1.06
	Average annual percent change from previous year shown					
Total expenditures	. . .	6.7	5.2	2.4	6.4	4.4
Total, all service providers	. . .	6.7	5.1	2.5	6.1	4.2
General non-specialty hospitals	. . .	1.4	3.5	−0.6	6.4	5.5
General hospital specialty units	. . .	−1.7	9.7	−3.8	2.2	1.1
General hospital non-specialty units	. . .	9.3	−16.3	15.4	18.2	15.5
Specialty hospitals	. . .	−1.9	−0.5	−11.0	0.1	−8.4
All physicians	. . .	7.2	3.0	6.2	4.9	7.5
Psychiatrists	. . .	8.4	4.6	4.5	−8.4	26.2
Non-psychiatric physicians	. . .	6.5	2.0	7.2	11.7	0.4
Other professionals	. . .	3.8	−17.6	26.6	6.9	11.2
Freestanding nursing homes	. . .	4.3	7.3	7.3	7.3	3.2
Freestanding home health	. . .	15.9	36.6	−9.2	−43.1	11.9
Multi-service mental health organizations	. . .	19.3	9.0	8.1	−6.2	−5.0
Specialty substance abuse centers	. . .	18.7	9.9	4.1	9.2	3.5
Retail prescription drug	. . .	9.0	11.6	15.0	15.0	11.3
Insurance administration	. . .	7.3	6.7	1.4	10.1	7.2
	Percent distribution					
Total expenditures	100.0	100.0	100.0	100.0	100.0	100.0
Total, all service providers	94.4	94.2	93.8	93.9	93.4	93.2
General non-specialty hospitals	32.2	26.2	24.2	20.8	20.8	21.0
General hospital specialty units	24.1	17.3	21.3	15.6	14.4	13.9
General hospital non-specialty units	8.1	8.9	2.9	5.2	6.4	7.1
Specialty hospitals	15.6	11.1	8.5	4.2	3.7	3.3
All physicians	7.4	7.5	6.7	8.1	7.8	8.1
Psychiatrists	2.6	2.7	2.6	2.9	2.2	2.6
Non-psychiatric physicians	4.8	4.8	4.1	5.1	5.7	5.5
Other professionals	15.6	14.0	4.1	11.8	11.9	12.7
Freestanding nursing homes	1.1	1.0	1.1	1.4	1.5	1.5
Freestanding home health	0.0	0.0	0.1	0.1	0.0	0.0
Multi-service mental health organizations	3.5	5.4	6.5	8.5	6.6	6.0
Specialty substance abuse centers	18.9	28.9	36.0	39.0	41.1	40.7
Retail prescription drug	0.1	0.2	0.2	0.4	0.4	0.5
Insurance administration	5.5	5.6	6.0	5.7	6.1	6.3

. . . Category not applicable.

0.0 Quantity is greater than zero but less than 0.05.

[1]Gross domestic product (GDP) implicit price deflator developed by the U.S. Department of Commerce, Bureau of Economic Analysis. Table 1.1.9 Implicit price deflator for gross domestic product is available from: http://www.bea.gov/national/nipaweb/TableView.asp?SelectedTable=13&Freq=Qtr&FirstYear=2008&LastYear=2010, accessed September 13, 2006.

NOTES: Additional data on specialty and non-specialty providers are available in the internet version of this table. Available from: http://www.cdc.gov/nchs/hus.htm. Specialty providers include general hospital specialty units, specialty hospitals, psychiatrists, other professionals, multi-service mental health organizations, and specialty substance abuse centers. Non-specialty providers include general hospital non-specialty units, non-psychiatric physicians, freestanding nursing homes, and freestanding home health providers. Data for additional years are available. See Appendix III.

SOURCE: Mark TL, Levit KR, Coffey RM, McKusick DR, Harwood HJ, King EC, et al. National Expenditures for Mental Health Services and Substance Abuse Treatment, 1993–2003. SAMHSA pub no SMA 07–4227. Rockville, MD: Substance Abuse and Mental Health Services Administration, 2007 and unpublished data.

Table 130 (page 1 of 3). Expenses for health care and prescribed medicine, by selected population characteristics: United States, selected years 1987–2007

[Data are based on household interviews of a sample of the noninstitutionalized population and a sample of medical providers]

| | Population in millions[2] | | | Total expenses[1] | | | | | | | |
| | | | | Percent of persons with expense | | | | Mean annual expense per person with expense[3] | | | |
Characteristic	1997	2000	2007	1987	1997	2000	2007	1987	1997	2000	2007
All ages	271.3	278.4	301.3	84.5	84.1	83.5	84.9	$2,850	$3,131	$3,250	$4,404
Under 65 years:											
Total	237.1	243.6	262.6	83.2	82.5	81.8	83.1	2,219	2,374	2,561	3,499
Under 6 years.	23.8	24.1	24.3	88.9	88.0	86.7	88.7	1,885	1,108	1,353	1,860
6–17 years	48.1	48.4	49.6	80.2	81.7	80.0	84.0	1,243	1,244	1,345	1,496
18–44 years	108.9	109.0	111.0	81.5	78.3	77.7	77.3	1,951	2,152	2,293	2,754
45–64 years	56.3	62.1	77.7	87.0	89.2	88.5	89.2	3,777	4,167	4,288	6,138
Sex											
Male	118.0	120.9	131.2	78.8	77.6	76.6	78.8	2,093	2,145	2,451	3,252
Female	119.1	122.7	131.4	87.5	87.4	87.0	87.5	2,327	2,575	2,656	3,721
Hispanic origin and race[4]											
Hispanic or Latino	29.4	32.0	43.7	71.0	69.5	69.0	70.2	1,770	1,976	1,744	2,252
Not Hispanic or Latino:											
White.	166.2	169.2	166.7	86.9	87.2	86.6	88.0	2,226	2,547	2,679	3,747
Black or African American . .	31.3	32.1	33.4	72.2	72.1	71.3	77.4	2,684	1,904	2,719	3,630
Asian[5]	. . .	. . .	11.8	. . .	. . .	. . .	79.2	. . .	. . .	. . .	3,278
Other[5]	10.2	10.2	6.9	72.8	75.8	76.0	83.0	1,473	1,578	2,183	3,619
Insurance status[6]											
Any private insurance	174.0	181.6	178.5	86.5	86.5	85.9	88.7	2,128	2,419	2,439	3,646
Public insurance only	29.8	29.7	44.3	82.4	83.3	83.6	83.9	3,569	2,885	3,887	3,760
Uninsured all year	33.3	32.3	39.9	61.8	61.1	57.3	57.2	1,387	1,418	1,806	2,057
65 years and over:											
Total	34.2	34.8	38.7	93.7	95.2	95.5	96.5	7,040	7,681	7,392	9,696
Sex											
Male	14.6	15.0	16.5	92.0	94.5	93.4	95.3	7,204	8,632	7,926	9,819
Female	19.6	19.8	22.2	94.9	95.7	97.1	97.4	6,925	6,981	7,003	9,608
Hispanic origin and race[4]											
Hispanic or Latino	1.7	1.9	2.7	82.5	94.2	92.5	92.4	6,704	8,038	6,633	10,770
Not Hispanic or Latino:											
White.	28.8	28.9	30.9	94.9	95.9	95.9	97.3	6,931	7,720	7,503	9,663
Black or African American . .	2.8	2.9	3.3	88.5	92.2	94.0	95.4	8,485	7,565	7,109	9,810
Asian[5]	. . .	. . .	1.3	. . .	. . .	. . .	89.5	. . .	. . .	. . .	7,644
Other[5]	*	*	*	*	*	*	*	*	*	*	*
Insurance status[7]											
Medicare only	8.8	12.0	14.0	85.9	92.1	94.8	94.6	5,546	7,077	6,347	9,153
Medicare and private insurance.	21.7	19.2	19.0	95.4	97.0	96.0	98.4	6,965	7,491	7,579	9,386
Medicare and other public coverage	3.2	3.2	5.1	94.4	93.2	96.3	97.0	10,818	10,826	10,142	12,646

See footnotes at end of table.

Table 130 (page 2 of 3). Expenses for health care and prescribed medicine, by selected population characteristics: United States, selected years 1987–2007

[Data are based on household interviews of a sample of the noninstitutionalized population and a sample of medical providers]

| | Prescribed medicine expenses[8] | | | | | | | |
| | Percent of persons with expense | | | | Mean annual out-of-pocket expense per person with out-of-pocket expense[3] | | | |
Characteristic	1987	1997	2000	2007	1987	1997	2000	2007
All ages	57.3	62.1	62.3	61.7	$168	$261	$330	$347
Under 65 years:								
Total	54.0	58.7	58.5	57.5	124	185	240	273
Under 6 years.	61.8	61.3	56.9	50.4	44	45	45	43
6–17 years.	44.3	48.2	46.2	44.9	82	70	84	110
18–44 years	51.3	55.9	56.0	53.0	97	158	182	217
45–64 years	65.3	71.8	73.3	74.4	235	344	451	440
Sex								
Male	46.5	51.5	51.3	51.7	115	164	211	253
Female	61.4	65.8	65.6	63.3	131	200	262	288
Hispanic origin and race[4]								
Hispanic or Latino	41.6	47.7	45.0	43.9	89	123	176	192
Not Hispanic or Latino:								
White.	57.7	63.1	63.8	63.4	130	200	258	298
Black or African American . .	44.1	50.0	47.6	51.6	109	149	197	240
Asian[5]	. . .	. . .	. . .	42.6	. . .	. . .	. . .	192
Other[5]	41.1	44.8	47.8	57.1	91	160	169	242
Insurance status[6]								
Any private insurance	56.5	61.6	61.6	62.6	128	176	206	271
Public insurance only	56.5	62.0	62.4	56.3	86	182	343	194
Uninsured all year	35.1	40.2	37.6	36.4	137	266	397	422
65 years and over:								
Total	81.6	86.0	88.3	90.0	387	624	750	668
Sex								
Male	78.0	82.8	83.9	87.2	359	562	562	614
Female	84.0	88.3	91.5	92.1	403	666	880	706
Hispanic origin and race[4]								
Hispanic or Latino	74.7	87.5	83.9	83.7	*511	509	632	491
Not Hispanic or Latino:								
White.	82.3	86.7	89.0	91.1	394	645	778	707
Black or African American . .	79.5	85.3	85.3	89.6	303	518	640	481
Asian[5]	. . .	. . .	. . .	82.2	. . .	. . .	. . .	547
Other[5]	*	*	*	*	*	*	*	*
Insurance status[7]								
Medicare only	70.6	82.1	87.7	87.0	427	721	896	711
Medicare and private insurance.	83.4	88.1	89.0	93.0	401	633	693	726
Medicare and other public coverage	88.2	85.0	88.5	91.4	146	349	593	337

See footnotes at end of table.

Table 130 (page 3 of 3). Expenses for health care and prescribed medicine, by selected population characteristics: United States, selected years 1987–2007

[Data are based on household interviews of a sample of the noninstitutionalized population and a sample of medical providers]

. . . Category not applicable.

* Estimates are considered unreliable. Data preceded by an asterisk have a relative standard error equal to or greater than 30%. Data not shown if based on fewer than 100 sample cases.

[1]Includes expenses for inpatient hospital and physician services, ambulatory physician and nonphysician services, prescribed medicines, home health services, dental services, and other medical equipment, supplies, and services that were purchased or rented during the year. Excludes expenses for over-the-counter medications, phone contacts with health providers, and premiums for health insurance.

[2]Includes persons in the civilian noninstitutionalized population for all or part of the year. Expenditures for persons in this population for only part of the year are restricted to those incurred during periods of eligibility (e.g., expenses incurred during periods of institutionalization and military service are not included in estimates).

[3]Estimates of expenses were converted to 2007 dollars using the Consumer Price Index (all items) and differ from previous editions of Health, United States. See Appendix II, Consumer Price Index (CPI).

[4]Persons of Hispanic origin may be of any race. Starting with 2002 data, MEPS respondents were allowed to report multiple races and these persons are included in the Other category. As a result, there is a slight increase in percentage of persons classified in the Other category in 2002 compared with prior years.

[5]Prior to 2002 Asians were categorized with Pacific Islanders and tabulated in the Other category. Starting in 2002, MEPS allowed respondents to classify themselves as non-Hispanic Asian-only.

[6]Any private insurance includes individuals with insurance that provided coverage for hospital and physician care at any time during the year, other than Medicare, Medicaid, or other public coverage for hospital or physician services. Public insurance only includes individuals who were not covered by private insurance at any time during the year but were covered by Medicare, Medicaid, other public coverage for hospital or physician services, and/or CHAMPUS/CHAMPVA (TRICARE) at any point during the year. Uninsured includes persons not covered by either private or public insurance throughout the entire year or period of eligibility for the survey. Individuals with Indian Health Service coverage only are considered uninsured.

[7]Populations do not add to total because uninsured persons and persons with unknown insurance status were excluded.

[8]Includes expenses for all prescribed medications that were purchased or refilled during the survey year.

NOTES: 1987 estimates are based on the National Medical Expenditure Survey (NMES); estimates for other years are based on the Medical Expenditure Panel Survey (MEPS). Because expenditures in NMES were based primarily on charges and those for MEPS were based on payments, NMES data were adjusted to be more comparable to MEPS using estimated charge to payment ratios for 1987. Overall, this resulted in an approximate 11% reduction from the unadjusted 1987 NMES expenditure estimates. For a detailed explanation of this adjustment, see Zuvekas S, Cohen J. A guide to comparing health care expenditures in the 1996 MEPS to the 1987 NMES. Inquiry 2002;39(1):76–86. See Appendix I, Medical Expenditure Panel Survey (MEPS). Data for additional years are available. See Appendix III.

SOURCE: Agency for Healthcare Research and Quality, Center for Financing, Access, and Cost Trends. 1987 National Medical Expenditure Survey and 1996–2007 Medical Expenditure Panel Surveys.

Table 131 (page 1 of 3). Sources of payment for health care, by selected population characteristics: United States, selected years 1987–2007

[Data are based on household interviews of a sample of the noninstitutionalized population and a sample of medical providers]

| | | Source of payment for health care | | | | | | | |
| | | Out of pocket | | | | Private insurance[1] | | | |
Characteristic	All sources	1987	1997	2000	2007	1987	1997	2000	2007
		Percent distribution							
All ages	100.0	24.8	19.4	19.4	16.2	36.6	40.3	40.3	41.6
Under 65 years:									
Total	100.0	26.2	21.1	20.3	17.5	46.6	53.1	52.5	56.2
Under 6 years	100.0	18.5	14.2	10.3	9.9	39.5	49.3	51.2	39.4
6–17 years	100.0	35.7	29.0	27.7	23.5	47.3	53.2	48.8	46.6
18–44 years	100.0	27.4	21.1	19.9	19.2	46.8	52.9	51.2	54.6
45–64 years	100.0	24.0	20.1	20.2	16.4	47.8	53.6	54.5	60.0
Sex									
Male	100.0	24.5	21.3	18.1	16.3	44.6	50.3	52.2	56.9
Female	100.0	27.5	21.0	22.1	18.4	48.1	55.1	52.7	55.6
Hispanic origin and race[2]									
Hispanic or Latino	100.0	22.0	18.8	20.5	18.7	36.1	42.3	45.8	41.6
Not Hispanic or Latino:									
White	100.0	28.2	21.8	21.7	18.9	50.1	55.8	55.1	59.7
Black or African American	100.0	15.5	17.1	11.8	10.7	30.0	42.3	40.5	39.9
Asian[3]	100.0	. . .	. . .	. . .	13.8	. . .	. . .	. . .	78.5
Other[3]	100.0	27.2	21.2	17.0	12.4	46.7	45.2	51.2	51.1
Insurance status									
Any private insurance[4]	100.0	29.0	21.6	21.2	18.3	60.0	67.6	70.2	74.1
Public insurance only[5]	100.0	8.9	10.6	9.8	7.1	. . .	. . .	. . .	. . .
Uninsured all year[6]	100.0	40.6	41.3	40.4	37.8	. . .	. . .	. . .	. . .
65 years and over	100.0	22.0	16.3	17.5	13.6	15.8	16.5	14.9	10.8
Sex									
Male	100.0	21.7	14.2	14.2	13.3	17.6	20.1	16.8	11.2
Female	100.0	22.2	18.1	20.2	13.8	14.4	13.2	13.3	10.4
Hispanic origin and race[2]									
Hispanic or Latino	100.0	*13.5	13.6	13.9	7.3	*4.7	5.9	8.4	4.9
Not Hispanic or Latino:									
White	100.0	23.7	17.0	18.3	14.7	16.7	17.9	15.2	11.1
Black or African American	100.0	11.2	11.4	13.6	7.9	*11.9	8.8	9.3	10.4
Asian[3]	100.0	. . .	. . .	. . .	17.0	. . .	. . .	. . .	12.4
Other[3]	100.0	*	*	*	*	*	*	*	*
Insurance status									
Medicare only	100.0	29.8	19.8	22.2	14.9	. . .	. . .	. . .	. . .
Medicare and private insurance	100.0	23.4	17.3	17.0	15.8	18.9	25.7	25.3	21.0
Medicare and other public coverage	100.0	*6.2	5.2	9.1	4.7	. . .	. . .	. . .	. . .

See footnotes at end of table.

Table 131 (page 2 of 3). Sources of payment for health care, by selected population characteristics: United States, selected years 1987–2007

[Data are based on household interviews of a sample of the noninstitutionalized population and a sample of medical providers]

	Source of payment for health care							
	Public sources[7]				Other[8]			
Characteristic	1987	1997	2000	2007	1987	1997	2000	2007
	Percent distribution							
All ages	34.1	34.4	35.4	37.4	4.5	5.9	5.0	4.8
Under 65 years:								
Total	21.3	18.1	21.3	20.8	6.0	7.7	6.0	5.6
Under 6 years	35.8	25.4	33.6	40.9	6.2	11.2	4.9	*9.7
6–17 years	11.8	14.1	20.1	24.9	5.2	3.7	3.4	5.0
18–44 years	19.4	15.7	21.1	19.9	6.4	10.3	7.8	6.4
45–64 years	22.4	20.3	20.2	18.8	5.8	6.0	5.2	4.9
Sex								
Male	23.9	19.5	23.5	21.1	7.1	8.9	6.3	5.7
Female	19.2	17.0	19.5	20.5	5.2	6.8	5.7	5.5
Hispanic origin and race[2]								
Hispanic or Latino	35.8	28.9	27.5	31.2	6.0	10.0	6.2	8.5
Not Hispanic or Latino:								
White	15.9	15.3	18.0	16.3	5.8	7.1	5.2	5.1
Black or African American . .	47.2	30.7	38.8	43.0	7.3	9.9	8.8	6.4
Asian[3]	. . .	. . .	. . .	*4.8	. . .	. . .	. . .	*2.9
Other[3]	21.0	23.7	19.0	28.1	5.1	9.9	*12.8	*8.5
Insurance status								
Any private insurance[4]	6.2	6.6	5.3	5.5	4.8	4.2	3.3	2.0
Public insurance only[5]	87.2	80.7	84.4	87.5	3.9	8.7	5.8	5.3
Uninsured all year[6]	28.6	7.5	*21.2	9.8	30.9	51.1	38.4	52.4
65 years and over	60.8	64.8	64.7	72.5	1.5	2.5	2.9	3.2
Sex								
Male	58.8	63.4	66.9	72.6	*1.9	2.3	2.2	2.9
Female	62.3	65.9	63.0	72.3	1.1	2.7	3.5	3.4
Hispanic origin and race[2]								
Hispanic or Latino	80.2	77.8	75.6	86.1	*1.6	*2.7	*2.2	1.7
Not Hispanic or Latino:								
White	58.0	62.6	64.1	70.7	1.6	2.5	2.4	3.5
Black or African American . .	76.3	77.6	68.3	79.8	0.6	2.2	*8.9	1.9
Asian[3]	. . .	. . .	. . .	67.2	. . .	. . .	. . .	*3.4
Other[3]	*	*	*	*	*	*	*	*
Insurance status								
Medicare only	68.8	72.4	72.2	77.1	1.4	7.7	5.7	8.0
Medicare and private insurance	56.1	56.3	57.1	62.6	1.6	0.6	*0.6	0.5
Medicare and other public coverage	92.9	92.7	87.3	94.1	1.0	*2.1	*3.6	*0.9

See footnotes at end of table.

Table 131 (page 3 of 3). Sources of payment for health care, by selected population characteristics: United States, selected years 1987–2007

[Data are based on household interviews of a sample of the noninstitutionalized population and a sample of medical providers]

. . . Category not applicable.

* Estimates are considered unreliable. Data preceded by an asterisk have a relative standard error equal to or greater than 30%. Data not shown if based on fewer than 100 sample cases.

[1]Private insurance includes any type of private insurance payments reported for people with private health insurance coverage during the year.

[2]Persons of Hispanic origin may be of any race. Starting with 2002 data, MEPS respondents were allowed to report multiple races and these persons are included in the Other category. As a result, there is a slight increase in the percent of persons classified in the Other category in 2002 compared with prior years.

[3]Prior to 2002 Asians were categorized with Pacific Islanders and tabulated in the Other category. Starting in 2002, MEPS allowed respondents to classify themselves as non-Hispanic Asian-only.

[4]Includes individuals with insurance that provided coverage for hospital and physician care at any time during the year, other than Medicare, Medicaid, or other public coverage for hospital or physician services.

[5]Includes individuals who were not covered by private insurance at any time during the year but were covered by Medicare, Medicaid, other public coverage for hospital or physician services, and/or CHAMPUS/CHAMPVA (TRICARE) at any point during the year.

[6]Includes individuals not covered by either private or public insurance throughout the entire year or period of eligibility for the survey. However, some expenses for the uninsured were paid by sources that were not defined as health insurance coverage, such as the Department of Veterans Affairs, community and neighborhood clinics, the Indian Health Service, state and local health departments, state programs other than Medicaid, Workers' Compensation, and other unclassified sources (e.g., automobile, homeowners', or liability insurance). Individuals with Indian Health Service coverage only are considered uninsured.

[7]Public sources include payments made by Medicare, Medicaid, the Department of Veterans Affairs, other federal sources (e.g., Indian Health Service, military treatment facilities, and other care provided by the federal government), CHAMPUS/CHAMPVA (TRICARE), and various state and local sources (e.g., community and neighborhood clinics, state and local health departments, and state programs other than Medicaid).

[8]Other sources includes Workers' Compensation, unclassified sources (automobile, home, or liability insurance, and other miscellaneous or unknown sources), Medicaid payments reported for people who were not enrolled in the program at any time during the year, and any type of private insurance payments reported for people without private health insurance coverage during the year.

NOTES: 1987 estimates are based on the National Medical Expenditure Survey (NMES); estimates for other years are based on the Medical Expenditure Panel Survey (MEPS). Because expenditures in NMES were based primarily on charges and those for MEPS were based on payments, NMES data were adjusted to be more comparable to MEPS using estimated charge to payment ratios for 1987. Overall, this resulted in an approximate 11% reduction from the unadjusted 1987 NMES expenditure estimates. For a detailed explanation of this adjustment, see Zuvekas S, Cohen J. A guide to comparing health care expenditures in the 1996 MEPS to the 1987 NMES. Inquiry 2002;39(1):76–86. Percents sum to 100 across sources within years. See Appendix I, Medical Expenditure Panel Survey (MEPS). Data for additional years are available. See Appendix III.

SOURCE: Agency for Healthcare Research and Quality, Center for Financing, Access, and Cost Trends. 1987 National Medical Expenditure Survey and 1996–2007 Medical Expenditure Panel Surveys.

Table 132. Out-of-pocket health care expenses among persons with medical expenses, by age: United States, selected years 1987–2007

[Data are based on household interviews for a sample of the noninstitutionalized population and a sample of medical providers]

Age and year	Percent of persons with expenses	Total	Amount paid out of pocket among persons with expenses[1]					
			$0	$1–99	$100–499	$500–999	$1,000–1,999	$2,000+
All ages			Percent distribution					
1987	84.5	100.0	10.4	20.5	37.1	15.0	9.7	7.4
2000	83.5	100.0	6.9	27.3	34.5	14.4	9.5	7.4
2004	84.7	100.0	8.8	22.9	31.3	14.9	11.8	10.5
2005	84.7	100.0	8.7	21.8	31.8	15.7	11.8	10.2
2006	84.6	100.0	8.7	22.0	31.8	15.6	12.0	9.7
2007	84.9	100.0	9.8	23.0	32.0	15.3	11.2	8.7
Under 6 years								
1987	88.9	100.0	19.2	28.7	39.7	8.0	2.7	1.7
2000	86.7	100.0	16.7	52.2	25.6	3.8	1.3	0.5
2004	90.0	100.0	26.0	41.4	25.6	4.3	2.1	0.6
2005	88.9	100.0	27.2	37.2	27.2	5.9	1.7	0.7
2006	89.2	100.0	27.1	40.1	25.9	4.4	1.5	1.0
2007	88.7	100.0	30.2	37.0	24.5	4.8	2.1	1.3
6–17 years								
1987	80.2	100.0	15.5	27.9	37.4	9.1	5.3	4.9
2000	80.0	100.0	14.7	38.0	32.6	6.5	3.9	4.3
2004	83.9	100.0	18.7	34.9	29.6	8.3	4.4	4.2
2005	83.0	100.0	18.6	33.4	31.0	8.7	4.5	3.9
2006	83.6	100.0	19.2	33.6	29.8	8.2	3.9	5.3
2007	84.0	100.0	21.6	33.5	29.7	7.3	3.9	3.9
18–44 years								
1987	81.5	100.0	10.1	22.7	39.7	14.5	8.0	5.1
2000	77.7	100.0	5.8	30.0	39.8	13.6	6.5	4.2
2004	77.0	100.0	7.2	25.8	37.8	14.4	9.0	5.8
2005	77.1	100.0	7.0	25.5	38.2	14.7	8.7	5.9
2006	76.9	100.0	6.8	24.9	38.5	14.9	8.7	6.1
2007	77.3	100.0	7.7	27.2	37.3	14.0	8.4	5.3
45–64 years								
1987	87.0	100.0	5.7	13.0	36.6	20.4	14.3	10.1
2000	88.5	100.0	2.6	16.3	35.6	20.3	14.8	10.4
2004	88.9	100.0	2.7	13.7	31.1	21.2	17.0	14.2
2005	89.7	100.0	2.4	13.3	30.1	21.8	18.4	14.0
2006	89.2	100.0	2.7	13.4	31.0	21.1	17.5	14.3
2007	89.2	100.0	2.9	14.6	31.3	21.4	16.6	13.2
65–74 years								
1987	92.8	100.0	5.3	10.3	28.0	22.3	18.6	15.4
2000	94.7	100.0	1.5	10.2	28.0	22.4	20.9	17.0
2004	96.6	100.0	1.5	8.6	23.5	19.3	21.1	26.0
2005	95.9	100.0	1.7	6.7	25.1	21.8	21.3	23.4
2006	95.7	100.0	1.7	7.7	24.1	22.5	25.4	18.7
2007	95.8	100.0	2.7	9.0	29.5	23.8	20.0	15.1
75 years and over								
1987	95.1	100.0	5.6	7.7	25.6	19.7	20.1	21.2
2000	96.5	100.0	2.6	10.3	25.4	22.4	19.3	19.9
2004	97.7	100.0	1.8	6.2	19.6	17.4	25.2	29.7
2005	97.4	100.0	1.6	6.7	21.6	19.9	20.9	29.3
2006	97.6	100.0	1.7	6.9	23.3	22.3	24.5	21.3
2007	97.3	100.0	1.9	9.0	26.3	20.3	21.9	20.6

[1]Estimates of expenses were converted to 2007 dollars using the Consumer Price Index (all items) and differ from previous editions of *Health, United States*. See Appendix II, Consumer Price Index (CPI).

NOTES: Includes persons in the civilian noninstitutionalized population for all or part of the year. Expenses for persons in this population for only part of the year are restricted to those incurred during periods of eligibility (e.g., expenses incurred during periods of institutionalization and military service are not included in estimates). Out-of-pocket expenses include expenditures for inpatient hospital and physician services, ambulatory physician and nonphysician services, prescribed medicines, home health services, dental services, and various other medical equipment, supplies, and services that were purchased or rented during the year. Out-of-pocket expenses for over-the-counter medications, phone contacts with health providers, and premiums for health insurance policies are not included in these estimates. 1987 estimates are based on the National Medical Expenditure Survey (NMES); estimates for other years are based on the Medical Expenditure Panel Survey (MEPS). Because expenditures in NMES were based primarily on charges and those for MEPS were based on payments, NMES data were adjusted to be more comparable to MEPS using estimated charge to payment ratios for 1987. Overall, this resulted in an approximate 11% reduction from the unadjusted 1987 NMES expenditure estimates. For a detailed explanation of this adjustment, see Zuvekas S, Cohen J. A guide to comparing health care expenditures in the 1996 MEPS to the 1987 NMES. Inquiry 2002;39(1):76–86. See Appendix I, Medical Expenditure Panel Survey (MEPS). Data for additional years are available. See Appendix III.

SOURCE: Agency for Healthcare Research and Quality, Center for Financing, Access, and Cost Trends. 1987 National Medical Expenditure Survey and 1997–2007 Medical Expenditure Panel Surveys.

Table 133 (page 1 of 2). Expenditures for health services and supplies and percent distribution, by type of payer: United States, selected years 1987–2008

[Data are compiled from various sources by the Centers for Medicare & Medicaid Services]

Type of payer	1987	1990	1995	2000	2004	2005	2006	2007	2008
					Amount in billions				
Total[1]	$477.8	$666.8	$952.5	$1,264.1	$1,733.6	$1,851.9	$1,975.4	$2,089.7	$2,181.3
Private	333.4	457.1	602.4	821.1	1,051.7	1,115.3	1,174.9	1,236.4	1,265.0
Private business	122.1	177.3	243.4	342.2	444.2	472.4	484.3	503.2	509.4
Employer contribution to private health insurance premiums	84.2	128.7	175.8	251.0	338.6	362.7	369.6	383.3	387.8
Private employer contribution to Medicare hospital insurance trust fund[2]	24.6	29.4	43.1	62.3	68.6	72.5	77.3	81.3	82.7
Workers compensation and temporary disability insurance and industrial inplant health services	13.3	19.2	24.4	29.0	37.0	37.2	37.5	38.6	38.9
Household	188.9	251.0	317.5	425.1	546.2	578.5	620.3	656.9	685.0
Employee contribution to private health insurance premiums and individual policy premiums	43.9	69.0	99.0	133.6	195.3	205.5	221.6	233.5	246.1
Employee and self-employment contributions and voluntary premiums paid to Medicare hospital insurance trust fund[2]	29.5	35.6	56.0	82.6	91.4	96.5	107.1	112.7	117.3
Premiums paid by individuals to Medicare supplementary medical insurance trust fund	6.2	10.2	16.4	16.3	24.6	29.0	36.7	40.4	43.9
Out-of-pocket health spending	109.2	136.1	146.1	192.6	234.8	247.5	254.9	270.3	277.8
Other private revenues	22.4	28.8	41.5	53.8	61.3	64.4	70.2	76.2	70.6
Public	144.4	209.7	350.2	443.0	681.8	736.6	800.6	853.3	916.2
Federal government	73.9	110.6	197.3	235.7	387.1	413.5	455.9	485.9	536.3
Employer contributions to private health insurance premiums	4.9	9.9	11.4	14.3	21.6	23.1	24.3	24.6	25.1
Medicaid[3]	28.1	43.2	88.1	119.7	175.1	182.8	180.6	191.8	208.2
Other[4]	22.3	28.5	37.9	50.1	79.6	83.7	89.8	95.9	103.4
State and local government	70.5	99.1	152.8	207.4	294.7	323.0	344.6	367.4	380.0
Employer contributions to private health insurance premiums	16.0	26.2	38.8	55.9	90.6	99.7	108.3	114.4	120.4
Medicaid[3]	22.8	31.6	60.1	85.1	122.1	137.2	138.9	147.5	147.4
Other[5]	28.6	37.2	48.3	58.9	72.9	76.7	87.5	94.8	100.9
					Percent distribution				
Total	100.0	100.0	100.0	100.0	100.0	100.0	100.0	100.0	100.0
Private	69.8	68.6	63.2	65.0	60.7	60.2	59.5	59.2	58.0
Private business	25.6	26.6	25.5	27.1	25.6	25.5	24.5	24.1	23.4
Employer contribution to private health insurance premiums	17.6	19.3	18.5	19.9	19.5	19.6	18.7	18.3	17.8
Private employer contribution to Medicare hospital insurance trust fund[2]	5.2	4.4	4.5	4.9	4.0	3.9	3.9	3.9	3.8
Workers compensation and temporary disability insurance and industrial inplant health services	2.8	2.9	2.6	2.3	2.1	2.0	1.9	1.8	1.8
Household	39.5	37.6	33.3	33.6	31.5	31.2	31.4	31.4	31.4
Employee contribution to private health insurance premiums and individual policy premiums	9.2	10.4	10.4	10.6	11.3	11.1	11.2	11.2	11.3
Employee and self-employment contributions and voluntary premiums paid to Medicare hospital insurance trust fund[2]	6.2	5.3	5.9	6.5	5.3	5.2	5.4	5.4	5.4
Premiums paid by individuals to Medicare supplementary medical insurance trust fund	1.3	1.5	1.7	1.3	1.4	1.6	1.9	1.9	2.0
Out-of-pocket health spending	22.9	20.4	15.3	15.2	13.5	13.4	12.9	12.9	12.7
Other private revenues	4.7	4.3	4.4	4.3	3.5	3.5	3.6	3.6	3.2

See footnotes at end of table.

Table 133 (page 2 of 2). Expenditures for health services and supplies and percent distribution, by type of payer: United States, selected years 1987–2008

[Data are compiled from various sources by the Centers for Medicare & Medicaid Services]

Type of payer	1987	1990	1995	2000	2004	2005	2006	2007	2008
	Percent distribution								
Public	30.2	31.4	36.8	35.0	39.3	39.8	40.5	40.8	42.0
Federal government..................	15.5	16.6	20.7	18.6	22.3	22.3	23.1	23.3	24.6
Employer contributions to private health insurance premiums	1.0	1.5	1.2	1.1	1.2	1.2	1.2	1.2	1.2
Medicaid[3]	5.9	6.5	9.2	9.5	10.1	9.9	9.1	9.2	9.5
Other[4]	4.7	4.3	4.0	4.0	4.6	4.5	4.5	4.6	4.7
State and local government	14.7	14.9	16.0	16.4	17.0	17.4	17.4	17.6	17.4
Employer contributions to private health insurance premiums	3.3	3.9	4.1	4.4	5.2	5.4	5.5	5.5	5.5
Medicaid[3]	4.8	4.7	6.3	6.7	7.0	7.4	7.0	7.1	6.8
Other[5]	6.0	5.6	5.1	4.7	4.2	4.1	4.4	4.5	4.6

[1]Excludes research and construction.
[2]Includes one-half of self-employment contribution to Medicare hospital insurance trust fund and taxation of Social Security benefits.
[3]Includes Medicaid buy-in premiums for Medicare.
[4]Includes expenditures for Medicare (with adjustments for contributions by employers and individuals and premiums paid to the Medicare insurance trust fund), maternal and child health, vocational rehabilitation, Substance Abuse and Mental Health Services Administration, Indian Health Service, federal workers' miscellaneous general hospital and medical programs, public health activities, Department of Defense, Department of Veterans Affairs, and Children's Health Insurance Program (CHIP).
[5]Includes other public and general assistance, maternal and child health, vocational rehabilitation, public health activities, hospital subsidies, and state phase-down payments. See Appendix II, Health expenditure, national.

NOTES: This table disaggregates health expenditures according to four classes of payers: businesses, households (individuals), federal government, and state and local governments, with a small amount of revenue coming from nonpatient revenue sources such as philanthropy. Where businesses or households pay dedicated funds into government health programs (for example, Medicare) or employers and employees share in the cost of health premiums, these costs are assigned to businesses or households accordingly. This results in a lower share of expenditures being assigned to the federal government than for tabulations of expenditures by source of funds. Estimates of national health expenditure by source of funds aim to track government-sponsored health programs over time and do not delineate the role of business employers in paying for health care. Estimates may not sum to totals because of rounding. Data have been revised and differ from previous editions of *Health, United States*. Data for additional years are available. See Appendix III.

SOURCE: Centers for Medicare & Medicaid Services, Office of the Actuary, National Health Statistics Group. Businesses, Households, and Governments, 1987–2008. Available from: http://www.cms.hhs.gov/NationalHealthExpendData/.

Table 134 (page 1 of 2). Employers' costs per employee-hour worked for total compensation, wages and salaries, and health insurance, by selected characteristics: United States, selected years 1991–2010

[Data are based on surveys of a sample of employers]

Characteristic	1991	1994	1996	2000	2006	2007	2008	2009	2010
	Total compensation per employee-hour worked								
State and local government	$22.31	$25.27	$25.73	$29.05	$36.96	$38.66	$37.84	$39.51	$39.81
Total private industry	15.40	17.08	17.49	19.85	25.09	25.91	26.76	27.46	27.73
Industry:									
Goods producing	18.48	20.85	21.27	23.55	29.36	30.12	31.38	32.29	32.42
Service providing	14.31	15.82	16.28	18.72	24.05	24.84	25.63	26.37	26.77
Occupational group:[1]									
White collar	18.15	20.26	21.10	24.19	- - -	- - -	- - -	- - -	- - -
Blue collar	15.15	16.92	17.04	18.73	- - -	- - -	- - -	- - -	- - -
Service	7.82	8.38	8.61	9.72	- - -	- - -	- - -	- - -	- - -
Management, professional, and related	- - -	- - -	- - -	- - -	44.32	46.05	47.55	48.82	48.80
Sales and office	- - -	- - -	- - -	- - -	19.93	20.55	21.15	21.40	21.77
Service	- - -	- - -	- - -	- - -	12.3	12.87	13.27	13.53	13.71
Natural resources, construction, and maintenance	- - -	- - -	- - -	- - -	28.07	28.96	30.13	30.97	31.10
Production, transportation, and material moving	- - -	- - -	- - -	- - -	21.19	22.22	23.07	23.28	23.72
Census region:									
Northeast	17.56	20.03	20.57	22.67	28.75	29.56	30.56	31.73	32.13
Midwest	15.05	16.26	16.30	19.22	24.65	25.16	25.98	26.44	26.75
South	13.68	15.05	15.62	17.81	22.35	23.17	23.90	24.45	24.72
West	15.97	18.08	18.78	20.88	26.56	27.77	28.70	29.53	29.52
Union status:									
Union	19.76	23.26	23.31	25.88	34.07	35.27	36.28	36.59	37.16
Nonunion	14.54	16.04	16.61	19.07	24.03	24.82	25.64	26.39	26.67
Establishment employment size:									
1–99 employees	13.38	14.58	14.85	17.16	20.43	21.29	22.23	22.56	22.84
100 or more	17.34	19.45	20.09	22.81	30.34	30.86	31.68	32.83	33.33
100–499	14.31	15.88	16.61	19.30	25.91	26.31	26.80	28.19	28.55
500 or more	20.60	23.35	24.03	26.93	35.94	36.48	37.60	38.71	39.76
	Wages and salaries as a percent of total compensation								
State and local government	69.6	69.5	69.8	70.8	67.6	67.0	65.9	65.7	65.9
Total private industry	72.3	71.1	71.9	73.0	70.7	70.8	70.6	70.8	70.6
Industry:									
Goods producing	68.7	66.5	67.6	69.0	66.2	66.8	66.7	66.9	66.7
Service providing	73.9	73.1	73.8	74.5	72.0	72.0	71.8	71.9	71.6
Occupational group:[1]									
White collar	73.8	72.7	73.2	74.0	- - -	- - -	- - -	- - -	- - -
Blue collar	68.4	66.8	68.1	69.4	- - -	- - -	- - -	- - -	- - -
Service	76.2	75.5	75.8	77.9	- - -	- - -	- - -	- - -	- - -
Management, professional, and related	- - -	- - -	- - -	- - -	70.9	71.1	71.0	71.1	70.7
Sales and office	- - -	- - -	- - -	- - -	72.2	72.1	72.0	71.8	71.6
Service	- - -	- - -	- - -	- - -	75.3	75.0	74.8	75.3	75.4
Natural resources, construction, and maintenance	- - -	- - -	- - -	- - -	68.0	68.3	68.3	68.2	68.0
Production, transportation, and material moving	- - -	- - -	- - -	- - -	66.7	66.8	66.6	67.0	66.8
Census region:									
Northeast	72.0	70.5	70.9	72.2	70.0	69.7	69.8	69.6	69.0
Midwest	71.1	69.7	71.1	72.4	69.4	69.9	69.8	70.3	70.0
South	73.3	72.1	72.7	73.5	72.1	72.0	71.8	71.9	71.8
West	72.8	72.0	73.1	74.0	71.0	71.0	70.8	71.1	71.1
Union status:									
Union	65.9	63.5	64.0	65.2	62.3	62.2	61.9	62.2	61.6
Nonunion	74.1	72.9	73.6	74.4	72.1	72.2	72.1	72.2	72.0
Establishment employment size:									
1–99 employees	74.7	73.5	74.7	75.5	73.7	73.8	73.8	74.0	73.6
100 or more	70.5	69.3	69.9	71.0	68.4	68.5	68.2	68.4	68.2
100–499	72.1	71.6	71.6	72.8	70.0	70.1	69.8	70.0	70.0
500 or more	69.3	67.6	68.6	69.4	66.9	67.1	66.9	67.0	66.5

See footnotes at end of table.

Table 134 (page 2 of 2). **Employers' costs per employee-hour worked for total compensation, wages and salaries, and health insurance, by selected characteristics: United States, selected years 1991–2010**

[Data are based on surveys of a sample of employers]

Characteristic	1991	1994	1996	2000	2006	2007	2008	2009	2010
				Health insurance as a percent of total compensation					
State and local government	6.9	8.2	7.7	7.8	10.6	10.9	11.0	10.9	11.4
Total private industry	6.0	6.7	5.9	5.5	6.9	7.1	7.2	7.3	7.5
Industry:									
Goods producing	6.9	8.1	7.2	6.9	8.4	8.4	8.5	8.7	8.9
Service providing	5.5	6.0	5.4	4.9	6.4	6.7	6.8	6.9	7.2
Occupational group: [1]									
White collar	5.6	6.2	5.5	5.0	- - -	- - -	- - -	- - -	- - -
Blue collar	7.0	8.0	7.2	6.8	- - -	- - -	- - -	- - -	- - -
Service	4.6	5.4	4.8	4.3	- - -	- - -	- - -	- - -	- - -
Management, professional, and related	- - -	- - -	- - -	- - -	5.6	5.8	5.8	6.0	6.2
Sales and office	- - -	- - -	- - -	- - -	7.5	7.8	7.9	8.3	8.6
Service	- - -	- - -	- - -	- - -	6.2	6.7	6.8	6.7	6.7
Natural resources, construction, and maintenance	- - -	- - -	- - -	- - -	7.7	7.6	7.6	7.9	8.0
Production, transportation, and material moving	- - -	- - -	- - -	- - -	9.0	9.3	9.6	9.7	9.9
Census region:									
Northeast	6.2	6.9	6.2	5.6	6.7	6.9	6.9	7.2	7.5
Midwest	6.3	7.3	6.3	5.8	7.6	7.8	7.9	8.1	8.3
South	5.5	6.3	5.9	5.4	6.7	6.9	6.9	7.0	7.2
West	5.8	6.1	5.2	5.0	6.4	6.7	6.9	6.9	7.1
Union status:									
Union	8.2	9.8	8.8	8.4	10.3	10.8	10.9	11.4	11.8
Nonunion	5.4	5.9	5.3	5.0	6.3	6.4	6.5	6.6	6.8
Establishment employment size:									
1–99 employees	5.1	5.7	5.0	4.8	6.0	6.1	6.1	6.3	6.4
100 or more	6.6	7.3	6.6	6.0	7.5	7.8	8.0	8.1	8.4
100–499	6.3	6.5	6.3	5.6	7.4	7.7	7.9	7.9	8.3
500 or more	6.8	7.9	6.9	6.4	7.6	7.9	8.0	8.2	8.5

- - - Data not available.

[1]Starting with 2004 data, sample establishments were classified by industry categories based on the North American Industry Classification (NAICS) system, as defined by the U.S. Office of Management and Budget. Within a sample establishment, specific job categories were selected and classified into about 840 occupational classifications according to the 2000 Standard Occupational Classification (SOC) system. Individual occupations were combined to represent one of five higher-level aggregations, such as management, professional, and related occupations. NAICS and SOC have replaced the 1987 Standard Industrial Classification System (SIC) and the Occupational Classification System (OCS). For more detailed information on NAICS and SOC, including background and definitions, see Appendix I, National Compensation Survey and http://www.bls.gov/soc/home.htm.

NOTES: Costs are calculated annually from March survey data. Total compensation includes wages and salaries and benefits. See Appendix II, Employer costs for employee compensation; Industry of Employment. Data for additional years are available. See Appendix III.

SOURCE: U.S. Department of Labor, Bureau of Labor Statistics, National Compensation Survey, Employer Costs for Employee Compensation—March 2009 and previous editions; Pub no 10–0774, June 9, 2010. Washington, DC. Available from: http://www.bls.gov/ncs/ect/home.htm.

Table 135 (page 1 of 3). Private health insurance coverage among persons under 65 years of age, by selected characteristics: United States, selected years 1984–2009

[Data are based on household interviews of a sample of the civilian noninstitutionalized population]

Characteristic	Private health insurance[1]									
	1984[2]	1989[2]	1995[2]	1997	2000[3]	2005	2006	2007	2008	2009
	Number in millions									
Total[4]	157.5	162.7	164.2	165.8	174.0	174.7	171.2	174.1	171.9	166.7
	Percent of population									
Total[4]	76.8	75.9	71.3	70.7	71.5	68.2	66.3	66.8	65.6	63.3
Age										
Under 19 years	72.6	71.9	65.4	66.1	66.7	62.3	59.5	59.9	58.6	56.1
Under 6 years	68.1	67.9	59.5	61.3	62.7	56.6	54.7	54.1	53.2	50.1
6–18 years	74.8	73.9	68.3	68.4	68.5	64.9	61.7	62.6	61.1	59.0
Under 18 years	72.6	71.8	65.2	66.1	66.6	62.1	59.4	59.8	58.4	55.8
6–17 years	74.9	74.0	68.3	68.5	68.5	64.7	61.7	62.6	61.1	58.8
18–44 years	76.5	75.5	70.9	69.4	70.5	66.6	65.0	65.5	64.4	61.7
18–24 years	67.4	64.5	60.8	59.3	60.3	58.0	57.0	59.0	56.2	54.4
25–34 years	77.4	75.9	70.1	68.1	70.1	65.1	63.0	63.5	62.7	60.0
35–44 years	83.9	82.7	77.7	76.4	77.0	73.7	72.0	71.7	71.7	68.4
45–64 years	83.3	82.5	80.1	79.0	78.7	76.9	75.2	75.5	74.3	72.6
45–54 years	83.3	83.4	80.9	80.4	80.0	77.4	75.1	75.4	74.8	72.6
55–64 years	83.3	81.6	79.0	76.9	76.7	76.2	75.4	75.5	73.6	72.6
Sex										
Male	77.3	76.1	71.6	70.9	71.6	68.0	65.9	66.4	65.3	62.9
Female	76.2	75.7	70.9	70.5	71.3	68.4	66.7	67.1	65.9	63.7
Sex and marital status[5]										
Male:										
Married	85.0	84.2	80.2	81.6	81.5	79.6	78.1	78.1	77.7	75.8
Divorced, separated, widowed	65.5	64.6	62.4	59.9	62.2	56.7	55.4	55.8	56.0	52.9
Never married	71.3	68.3	65.4	63.3	63.8	60.2	57.8	59.8	57.9	54.9
Female:										
Married	83.8	83.5	79.3	81.0	81.0	79.3	78.6	78.4	77.7	76.7
Divorced, separated, widowed	63.1	63.6	61.7	59.1	63.2	59.9	56.3	57.0	56.3	54.2
Never married	72.2	70.0	66.2	63.8	64.2	61.5	59.0	60.8	58.8	56.4
Race[6]										
White only	79.9	79.1	74.5	74.2	75.7	70.9	69.1	69.7	68.5	66.3
Black or African American only	58.1	57.7	53.0	54.7	55.9	52.9	51.3	51.8	50.0	47.4
American Indian or Alaska Native only	49.1	45.5	45.3	39.4	43.7	43.0	36.3	36.4	30.7	35.9
Asian only	69.9	71.9	68.4	68.0	72.1	72.2	72.1	73.2	74.3	71.3
Native Hawaiian or Other Pacific Islander only	- - -	- - -	- - -	- - -	*	*	*	*	*	*
2 or more races	- - -	- - -	- - -	- - -	61.4	57.6	54.0	52.7	58.0	47.8
Hispanic origin and race[6]										
Hispanic or Latino	55.7	51.5	46.4	46.4	47.8	42.4	40.0	41.7	39.9	37.3
Mexican	53.3	46.8	42.6	42.3	45.4	39.7	36.5	37.9	36.8	34.7
Puerto Rican	48.4	45.6	47.6	47.0	51.1	48.5	46.1	54.2	48.2	46.2
Cuban	72.5	70.3	63.6	71.0	63.9	58.1	63.4	64.8	57.9	54.3
Other Hispanic or Latino	61.6	61.0	51.4	49.9	50.7	45.6	44.3	44.3	43.5	39.7
Not Hispanic or Latino	78.7	78.5	74.4	74.0	75.2	73.0	71.3	71.7	70.8	68.6
White only	82.4	82.5	78.6	78.1	79.5	77.3	75.6	76.2	75.3	73.3
Black or African American only	58.2	57.7	53.4	54.9	56.0	53.1	52.2	52.3	50.6	48.0
Age and percent of poverty level[7]										
Under 65 years:										
Below 100%	32.2	27.0	22.6	23.3	25.2	21.4	21.4	21.4	19.2	15.3
100%–199%	70.3	64.3	55.3	53.5	50.1	44.7	42.8	40.0	38.1	37.4
100%–133%	59.4	52.8	41.7	40.2	39.3	36.0	33.7	29.7	27.3	26.5
134%–199%	75.2	69.5	62.7	60.2	55.4	49.5	48.0	45.6	43.8	43.4
200%–399%	89.3	89.2	86.4	80.8	78.1	74.8	74.9	73.2	72.3	70.6
400% or more	95.4	94.6	93.2	91.8	91.9	90.6	89.8	91.0	90.1	90.2

See footnotes at end of table.

Table 135 (page 2 of 3). Private health insurance coverage among persons under 65 years of age, by selected characteristics: United States, selected years 1984–2009

[Data are based on household interviews of a sample of the civilian noninstitutionalized population]

Characteristic	Private health insurance[1]									
	1984[2]	1989[2]	1995[2]	1997	2000[3]	2005	2006	2007	2008	2009
	Percent of population									
Under 19 years:										
Below 100%.	29.6	24.1	19.0	19.3	20.3	15.0	15.0	14.1	12.4	9.7
100%–199%.	73.6	68.5	55.8	54.7	49.5	41.6	38.5	35.7	34.1	34.0
100%–133%.	63.8	56.9	42.5	40.1	37.1	32.6	29.1	25.5	23.3	21.3
134%–199%.	78.4	74.0	64.4	62.5	56.2	47.0	44.8	41.8	40.1	41.4
200%–399%.	91.1	92.1	89.1	83.5	80.8	76.6	77.1	75.8	73.7	73.2
400% or more	96.2	96.2	93.3	93.3	93.0	92.5	91.4	93.2	92.0	91.8
Under 18 years:										
Below 100%.	28.5	22.3	16.9	18.3	19.5	14.2	14.0	12.7	11.3	9.3
100%–199%.	73.9	68.9	56.1	54.7	49.4	41.4	38.3	35.6	34.1	34.0
100%–133%.	63.9	57.3	42.3	39.4	36.8	32.1	29.1	25.6	23.3	21.1
134%–199%.	78.6	74.5	64.9	62.9	56.3	47.0	44.6	41.6	40.0	41.3
200%–399%.	91.3	92.3	89.2	83.7	81.1	76.6	77.3	76.0	73.8	73.0
400% or more	96.1	96.5	93.1	93.5	93.1	92.5	91.6	93.4	92.2	91.8
18–64 years:										
Below 100%.	35.0	30.8	27.0	26.8	29.1	25.9	26.1	26.8	24.0	19.2
100%–199%.	68.3	61.5	54.8	52.8	50.5	46.5	45.1	42.5	40.2	39.1
100%–133%.	56.6	50.0	41.4	40.6	40.9	38.4	36.5	32.2	29.6	29.4
134%–199%.	73.3	66.6	61.5	58.7	54.9	50.7	49.5	47.7	45.8	44.5
200%–399%.	88.3	87.6	85.0	79.4	76.7	74.0	73.9	72.0	71.7	69.6
400% or more	95.2	94.4	93.2	91.3	91.6	90.1	89.3	90.4	89.6	89.8
Disability measure among adults 18–64 years[8]										
Any basic actions difficulty or complex activity limitation.	- - -	- - -	- - -	61.6	63.1	58.1	56.4	56.4	53.2	51.6
Any basic actions difficulty.	- - -	- - -	- - -	62.3	63.9	58.8	57.1	56.9	54.3	52.3
Any complex activity limitation	- - -	- - -	- - -	47.9	48.4	44.0	41.7	40.3	37.0	36.0
No disability.	- - -	- - -	- - -	77.4	77.2	73.7	72.5	72.9	73.3	70.4
Geographic region										
Northeast	80.5	82.0	75.4	74.2	76.3	74.0	70.8	72.2	71.3	69.7
Midwest	80.6	81.5	77.3	77.1	78.8	74.6	71.7	72.0	69.9	67.5
South	74.3	71.4	66.9	67.3	66.8	62.5	61.8	62.6	62.1	59.3
West	71.9	71.2	67.5	65.4	66.5	65.6	64.6	64.0	62.8	60.6
Location of residence[9]										
Within MSA.	77.5	76.5	72.1	71.2	72.3	69.0	67.5	67.8	66.5	64.6
Outside MSA.	75.2	73.8	67.9	68.4	67.8	64.6	60.3	61.0	61.1	56.2

See footnotes at end of table.

Table 135 (page 3 of 3). Private health insurance coverage among persons under 65 years of age, by selected characteristics: United States, selected years 1984–2009

[Data are based on household interviews of a sample of the civilian noninstitutionalized population]

- - - Data not available.

*Estimates are considered unreliable. Data not shown have a relative standard error of greater than 30%.

[1]Any private health insurance coverage (both individual and insurance obtained through the workplace) at the time of interview; includes those who also had another type of coverage.

[2]Data prior to 1997 are not strictly comparable with data for later years due to the 1997 questionnaire redesign. See Appendix I, National Health Interview Survey and Appendix II, Health insurance coverage.

[3]Estimates for 2000–2002 were calculated using 2000-based sample weights and may differ from estimates in other reports that used 1990-based sample weights for 2000–2002 estimates.

[4]Includes all other races not shown separately, those with unknown marital status, unknown disability status, and, in 1984 and 1989, persons with unknown poverty level.

[5]Includes persons 14–64 years of age.

[6]The race groups, white, black, American Indian or Alaska Native, Asian, Native Hawaiian or Other Pacific Islander, and 2 or more races, include persons of Hispanic and non-Hispanic origin. Persons of Hispanic origin may be of any race. Starting with 1999 data, race-specific estimates are tabulated according to the 1997 Revisions to the Standards for the Classification of Federal Data on Race and Ethnicity and are not strictly comparable with estimates for earlier years. The five single-race categories plus multiple-race categories shown in the table conform to the 1997 Standards. Starting with 1999 data, race-specific estimates are for persons who reported only one racial group; the category 2 or more races includes persons who reported more than one racial group. Prior to 1999, data were tabulated according to the 1977 Standards with four racial groups and the Asian only category including Native Hawaiian or Other Pacific Islander. Estimates for single-race categories prior to 1999 included persons who reported one race or, if they reported more than one race, identified one race as best representing their race. Starting with 2003 data, race responses of other race and unspecified multiple race were treated as missing, and then race was imputed if these were the only race responses. Almost all persons with a race response of other race were of Hispanic origin. See Appendix II, Hispanic origin; Race.

[7]Percent of poverty level is based on family income and family size and composition using U.S. Census Bureau poverty thresholds. Poverty level was unknown for 10%–11% of persons under 65 years of age in 1984 and 1989. Missing family income data were imputed for 1995 and beyond. See Appendix II, Family income; Poverty; Table VII.

[8]Any basic actions difficulty or complex activity limitation is defined as having one or more of the following limitations or difficulties: movement difficulty, emotional difficulty, sensory (seeing or hearing) difficulty, cognitive difficulty, self-care (ADL or IADL) limitation, social limitation, or work limitation. For more information, see Appendix II, Basic actions difficulty; Complex activity limitation. Starting with 2007 data, the hearing question, a component of the basic actions difficulty measure, was revised. Consequently, data prior to 2007 are not comparable with data for 2007 and beyond. For more information on the impact of the revised hearing question, see Appendix II, Hearing trouble.

[9]MSA is metropolitan statistical area. Starting with 2006 data, MSA status is determined using 2000 census data and the 2000 standards for defining MSAs. For data prior to 2006, see Appendix II, Metropolitan statistical area (MSA) for the applicable standards.

NOTES: Private health insurance coverage is at the time of interview. The number of persons with private coverage was calculated by multiplying the percentage with private coverage by the number of persons under age 65 in the civilian non-institutionalized U.S. population. Percentages were calculated with unknown values excluded from denominators. See Appendix II, Health insurance coverage. Standard errors are available in the spreadsheet version of this table. Available from: http://www.cdc.gov/nchs/hus.htm. Data for additional years are available. See Appendix III.

SOURCE: CDC/NCHS, National Health Interview Survey, health insurance supplements (1984, 1989, 1994–1996). Starting with 1997, data are from the family core and the sample adult questionnaires.

Table 136 (page 1 of 3). Private health insurance coverage obtained through the workplace among persons under 65 years of age, by selected characteristics: United States, selected years 1984–2009

[Data are based on household interviews of a sample of the civilian noninstitutionalized population]

Characteristic	Private insurance obtained through workplace[1]									
	1984[2]	1989[2]	1995[2]	1997	1998	2000[3]	2005	2007	2008	2009
	Number in millions									
Total[4]	141.8	146.3	150.7	153.6	157.4	160.8	160.1	157.9	155.6	150.2
	Percent of population									
Total[4]	69.1	68.3	65.4	66.4	67.5	67.1	63.6	61.6	60.5	58.0
Age										
Under 19 years	66.4	65.6	60.5	62.8	64.1	63.1	58.7	55.8	54.5	52.0
Under 6 years	62.1	62.3	55.1	58.3	61.1	58.9	53.4	50.8	49.6	46.3
6–18 years	68.4	67.3	63.1	64.9	65.5	64.9	61.1	58.1	56.9	54.8
Under 18 years	66.5	65.8	60.4	62.8	64.3	63.0	58.6	55.8	54.4	51.8
6–17 years	68.7	67.7	63.3	65.1	65.9	65.0	61.1	58.3	56.9	54.7
18–44 years	69.6	68.4	65.3	65.7	66.8	66.5	62.2	60.3	59.4	56.6
18–24 years	58.7	55.3	53.5	54.9	56.1	55.5	52.1	52.3	49.5	47.4
25–34 years	71.2	69.5	65.0	64.6	67.0	66.4	61.1	59.0	58.4	55.5
35–44 years	77.4	76.2	72.7	72.7	72.6	73.2	69.9	67.0	67.0	64.3
45–64 years	71.8	71.6	72.2	72.8	72.9	72.9	70.9	69.2	68.0	65.7
45–54 years	74.6	74.4	74.7	75.6	75.2	75.6	72.6	70.4	69.5	67.1
55–64 years	69.0	68.3	68.4	68.4	69.3	68.6	68.6	67.7	66.2	64.0
Sex										
Male	69.8	68.7	65.9	66.7	67.6	67.3	63.6	61.3	60.3	57.6
Female	68.4	67.9	64.9	66.2	67.3	66.9	63.6	61.9	60.8	58.4
Sex and marital status[5]										
Male:										
Married	77.9	76.9	74.9	77.4	77.8	77.5	75.3	73.3	72.7	70.6
Divorced, separated, widowed	58.0	57.3	56.4	55.2	56.4	57.4	51.9	50.8	51.0	48.0
Never married	61.5	58.8	58.2	58.4	59.1	58.8	54.9	53.5	51.9	48.8
Female:										
Married	76.1	75.5	73.2	76.4	76.9	76.3	74.2	72.7	72.2	70.7
Divorced, separated, widowed	51.9	54.9	54.6	53.8	55.4	57.8	54.3	51.3	51.4	48.6
Never married	63.5	60.9	59.2	59.6	59.2	60.1	56.3	55.1	53.0	50.6
Race[6]										
White only	72.0	71.2	68.4	69.7	70.9	71.0	66.1	64.2	63.0	60.6
Black or African American only	52.4	52.8	49.3	52.6	52.1	53.4	50.6	49.1	47.7	45.3
American Indian or Alaska Native only	45.8	40.9	40.2	37.2	41.3	41.7	39.9	35.1	29.4	33.6
Asian only	59.0	61.1	59.6	61.7	64.4	65.8	64.4	64.6	66.2	62.5
Native Hawaiian or Other Pacific Islander only	- - -	- - -	- - -	- - -	- - -	*	*	*	*	*
2 or more races	- - -	- - -	- - -	- - -	- - -	59.8	54.8	49.7	54.3	45.0
Hispanic origin and race[6]										
Hispanic or Latino	52.0	47.3	43.4	43.9	45.9	45.3	40.0	38.8	37.6	34.9
Mexican	50.5	44.2	40.9	40.8	42.4	43.6	37.6	35.7	35.2	32.6
Puerto Rican	45.9	42.3	44.5	45.1	49.6	49.4	46.2	51.2	45.9	42.9
Cuban	57.4	56.5	54.0	58.4	60.3	53.6	53.5	54.7	49.2	46.4
Other Hispanic or Latino	57.4	54.7	46.7	47.0	48.6	47.3	42.6	40.8	39.8	36.9
Not Hispanic or Latino	70.7	70.5	68.2	69.5	70.5	70.6	68.0	66.1	65.2	62.8
White only	74.0	74.1	72.1	73.3	74.4	74.5	71.9	70.2	69.0	66.8
Black or African American only	52.5	52.8	49.8	52.9	52.3	53.6	50.9	49.5	48.2	45.9
Age and percent of poverty level[7]										
Under 65 years:										
Below 100%	24.1	19.8	17.5	20.0	20.2	21.0	17.8	17.4	15.5	11.9
100%–199%	61.7	56.1	49.3	48.9	48.7	45.4	40.1	35.5	33.8	33.3
100%–133%	50.0	44.3	36.0	35.9	37.6	35.0	31.4	25.4	23.9	22.7
134%–199%	66.9	61.5	56.6	55.4	54.6	50.6	44.9	40.8	39.1	39.3
200%–399%	82.8	82.2	80.5	76.5	76.4	73.4	69.8	67.7	66.8	64.7
400% or more	88.8	87.8	86.7	87.4	87.3	87.9	86.1	85.5	84.6	84.1

See footnotes at end of table.

[Data are based on household interviews of a sample of the civilian noninstitutionalized population]

Characteristic	Private insurance obtained through workplace[1]									
	1984[2]	1989[2]	1995[2]	1997	1998	2000[3]	2005	2007	2008	2009
	Percent of population									
Under 19 years:										
Below 100%.	23.6	18.6	15.1	17.0	17.2	17.1	13.3	12.1	11.3	7.9
100%–199%.	67.0	62.1	50.5	51.2	51.8	45.8	38.3	32.7	31.4	31.9
100%–133%.	56.1	49.9	37.4	36.7	39.2	33.7	29.2	22.6	21.1	19.8
134%–199%.	72.3	67.9	58.8	59.0	58.8	52.3	43.7	38.7	37.2	38.9
200%–399%.	85.7	86.0	83.9	80.0	80.0	76.9	72.4	71.2	68.3	67.7
400% or more	90.8	90.3	87.5	89.7	88.7	89.5	88.3	87.5	86.9	86.0
Under 18 years:										
Below 100%.	23.0	17.5	13.6	16.2	16.8	16.6	12.5	11.2	10.3	7.5
100%–199%.	67.5	62.5	50.9	51.2	52.1	45.8	38.2	32.7	31.4	32.0
100%–133%.	56.3	50.3	37.2	36.0	39.6	33.5	28.7	22.7	21.1	19.8
134%–199%.	72.8	68.4	59.6	59.4	58.9	52.5	43.9	38.6	37.1	38.9
200%–399%.	85.9	86.4	84.1	80.2	80.3	77.1	72.4	71.5	68.4	67.6
400% or more	90.7	90.5	87.1	89.8	89.0	89.7	88.5	87.7	87.1	86.0
18–64 years:										
Below 100%.	24.8	21.8	20.5	22.7	22.5	24.0	21.2	21.2	18.7	14.8
100%–199%.	58.3	52.3	48.4	47.6	46.8	45.2	41.1	37.0	35.1	34.0
100%–133%.	46.0	40.4	35.3	35.8	36.4	36.0	33.0	27.1	25.5	24.3
134%–199%.	63.6	57.5	55.0	53.2	52.1	49.5	45.4	42.0	40.2	39.4
200%–399%.	81.4	80.2	78.8	74.7	74.5	71.7	68.7	66.2	66.1	63.6
400% or more	88.5	87.5	86.7	86.8	86.9	87.5	85.4	84.9	83.9	83.6
Disability measure among adults 18–64 years[8]										
Any basic actions difficulty or complex activity limitation.	- - -	- - -	- - -	57.3	57.4	58.5	53.3	51.5	49.1	46.7
Any basic actions difficulty.	- - -	- - -	- - -	58.0	57.9	59.1	54.0	52.1	49.9	47.4
Any complex activity limitation	- - -	- - -	- - -	43.3	44.0	43.5	38.9	35.4	33.5	31.1
No disability.	- - -	- - -	- - -	72.5	73.9	72.5	68.5	67.1	67.5	64.8
Geographic region										
Northeast	74.0	75.0	69.8	71.0	73.2	72.5	70.6	68.2	68.0	65.3
Midwest	72.0	73.3	71.2	72.6	73.7	74.9	70.1	68.0	64.7	62.0
South.	66.2	63.6	61.8	62.9	63.4	62.5	58.0	57.2	56.7	54.1
West.	64.7	63.9	60.4	60.7	61.5	61.1	59.7	57.3	56.8	54.5
Location of residence[9]										
Within MSA	70.9	69.6	66.6	67.3	68.6	68.2	64.5	62.7	61.5	59.3
Outside MSA	65.3	63.5	60.7	62.8	63.2	62.6	59.6	55.7	55.1	50.8

See footnotes at end of table.

Table 136 (page 3 of 3). Private health insurance coverage obtained through the workplace among persons under 65 years of age, by selected characteristics: United States, selected years 1984–2009

[Data are based on household interviews of a sample of the civilian noninstitutionalized population]

- - - Data not available.

*Estimates are considered unreliable. Data not shown have a relative standard error of greater than 30%.

[1] Any private insurance at the time of interview that was originally obtained through a present or former employer or union, or, starting with 1997 data, through the workplace, self-employment, or a professional association; includes those who also had another type of coverage.

[2] Data prior to 1997 are not strictly comparable with data for later years due to the 1997 questionnaire redesign. See Appendix I, National Health Interview Survey and Appendix II, Health insurance coverage.

[3] Estimates for 2000–2002 were calculated using 2000-based sample weights and may differ from estimates in other reports that used 1990-based sample weights for 2000–2002 estimates.

[4] Includes all other races not shown separately, those with unknown marital status, unknown disability status, and, in 1984 and 1989, persons with unknown poverty level.

[5] Includes persons 14–64 years of age.

[6] The race groups, white, black, American Indian or Alaska Native, Asian, Native Hawaiian or Other Pacific Islander, and 2 or more races, include persons of Hispanic and non-Hispanic origin. Persons of Hispanic origin may be of any race. Starting with 1999 data, race-specific estimates are tabulated according to the 1997 Revisions to the Standards for the Classification of Federal Data on Race and Ethnicity and are not strictly comparable with estimates for earlier years. The five single-race categories plus multiple-race categories shown in the table conform to the 1997 Standards. Starting with 1999 data, race-specific estimates are for persons who reported only one racial group; the category 2 or more races includes persons who reported more than one racial group. Prior to 1999, data were tabulated according to the 1977 Standards with four racial groups and the Asian only category included Native Hawaiian or Other Pacific Islander. Estimates for single-race categories prior to 1999 included persons who reported one race or, if they reported more than one race, identified one race as best representing their race. Starting with 2003 data, race responses of other race and unspecified multiple race were treated as missing, and then race was imputed if these were the only race responses. Almost all persons with a race response of other race were of Hispanic origin. See Appendix II, Hispanic origin; Race.

[7] Percent of poverty level is based on family income and family size and composition using U.S. Census Bureau poverty thresholds. Poverty level was unknown for 10%–11% of persons under 65 years of age in 1984 and 1989. Missing family income data were imputed for 1995 and beyond. See Appendix II, Family income; Poverty; Table VII.

[8] Any basic actions difficulty or complex activity limitation is defined as having one or more of the following limitations or difficulties: movement difficulty, emotional difficulty, sensory (seeing or hearing) difficulty, cognitive difficulty, self-care (ADL or IADL) limitation, social limitation, or work limitation. For more information, see Appendix II, Basic actions difficulty; Complex activity limitation. Starting with 2007 data, the hearing question, a component of the basic actions difficulty measure, was revised. Consequently, data prior to 2007 are not comparable with data for 2007 and beyond. For more information on the impact of the revised hearing question, see Appendix II, Hearing trouble.

[9] MSA is metropolitan statistical area. Starting with 2006 data, MSA status is determined using 2000 census data and the 2000 standards for defining MSAs. For data prior to 2006, see Appendix II, Metropolitan statistical area (MSA) for the applicable standards.

NOTES: Private coverage through the workplace is at the time of interview. The number of persons with private coverage through the workplace was calculated by multiplying the percentage with private coverage through the workplace by the number of persons under age 65 in the civilian non-institutionalized U.S. population. Percentages were calculated with unknown values excluded from denominators. See Appendix II, Health insurance coverage. Standard errors are available in the spreadsheet version of this table. Available from: http://www.cdc.gov/nchs/hus.htm. Data for additional years are available. See Appendix III.

SOURCE: CDC/NCHS, National Health Interview Survey, health insurance supplements (1984, 1989, 1994–1996). Starting with 1997, data are from the family core and the sample adult questionnaires.

Table 137 (page 1 of 3). Medicaid coverage among persons under 65 years of age, by selected characteristics: United States, selected years 1984–2009

[Data are based on household interviews of a sample of the civilian noninstitutionalized population]

Characteristic	1984[1]	1989[1]	1995[1]	1997	2000[2]	2004(1)[3]	2004(2)[3]	2007[3]	2008[3]	2009[3]
					Number in millions					
Total[4]	14.0	15.4	26.6	22.9	23.2	31.1	31.6	36.2	38.4	42.4
					Percent of population					
Total[4]	6.8	7.2	11.5	9.7	9.5	12.3	12.5	13.9	14.7	16.1
Age										
Under 19 years	11.7	12.2	21.1	18.0	19.2	25.4	25.8	29.3	30.6	33.9
Under 6 years	15.5	15.7	29.3	24.7	24.7	31.8	32.4	36.6	38.1	41.4
6–18 years	9.8	10.5	17.0	14.9	16.8	22.5	22.9	25.9	27.1	30.3
Under 18 years	11.9	12.6	21.5	18.4	19.6	25.9	26.4	29.8	31.3	34.5
6–17 years	10.1	10.9	17.4	15.2	17.2	23.1	23.4	26.4	27.9	30.9
18–44 years	5.1	5.2	7.8	6.6	5.6	7.5	7.7	8.7	9.2	10.3
18–24 years	6.4	6.8	10.4	8.8	8.1	10.3	10.4	11.4	12.2	14.0
25–34 years	5.3	5.2	8.2	6.8	5.5	7.6	7.8	8.5	9.3	10.1
35–44 years	3.5	4.0	5.9	5.2	4.3	5.7	5.8	7.0	7.1	7.7
45–64 years	3.4	4.3	5.6	4.6	4.5	5.4	5.5	5.9	6.4	6.9
45–54 years	3.2	3.8	5.1	4.0	4.2	5.4	5.5	6.0	6.2	7.0
55–64 years	3.6	4.9	6.4	5.6	4.9	5.4	5.5	5.7	6.8	6.8
Sex										
Male	5.4	5.7	9.6	8.4	8.2	10.8	11.0	12.5	13.4	14.4
Female	8.1	8.6	13.4	11.1	10.8	13.7	13.9	15.2	15.9	17.8
Sex and marital status[5]										
Male:										
Married	1.9	1.8	2.9	2.5	2.2	2.9	3.0	3.5	3.6	4.1
Divorced, separated, widowed	4.9	5.4	7.7	5.7	6.1	6.7	6.8	7.8	8.1	8.3
Never married	4.8	5.6	8.1	7.0	7.2	10.2	10.4	11.3	12.1	13.1
Female:										
Married	2.6	3.0	5.2	3.5	3.1	4.2	4.3	4.7	5.2	5.3
Divorced, separated, widowed	16.0	16.1	19.0	14.7	12.7	14.9	15.2	16.3	17.2	18.7
Never married	10.7	11.9	16.5	14.2	13.2	16.9	17.1	18.1	18.7	20.9
Race[6]										
White only	4.6	5.1	8.9	7.4	7.1	10.2	10.4	11.4	12.1	13.7
Black or African American only	20.5	19.0	28.5	22.4	21.2	24.5	24.9	27.7	28.3	29.5
American Indian or Alaska Native only	*28.2	29.7	19.0	19.6	15.1	18.0	18.4	21.2	37.0	29.7
Asian only	*8.7	*8.8	10.5	9.6	7.5	9.6	9.8	8.7	9.2	9.9
Native Hawaiian or Other Pacific Islander only	- - -	- - -	- - -	- - -	*	*	*	*	*	*
2 or more races	- - -	- - -	- - -	- - -	19.1	19.0	19.3	27.9	24.7	30.1
Hispanic origin and race[6]										
Hispanic or Latino	13.3	13.5	21.9	17.6	15.5	21.9	22.5	24.7	24.9	27.6
Mexican	12.2	12.4	21.6	17.2	14.0	21.9	22.4	25.9	25.4	28.4
Puerto Rican	31.5	27.3	33.4	31.0	29.4	28.5	29.1	28.0	31.0	32.1
Cuban	*4.8	*7.7	13.4	7.3	9.2	17.9	17.9	13.3	13.0	16.7
Other Hispanic or Latino	7.9	11.1	18.2	15.3	14.5	19.9	20.8	21.4	22.3	24.6
Not Hispanic or Latino	6.2	6.5	10.2	8.7	8.5	10.5	10.7	11.7	12.6	13.7
White only	3.7	4.1	7.1	6.1	6.1	7.8	7.9	8.5	9.2	10.4
Black or African American only	20.7	19.0	28.1	22.1	21.0	24.1	24.6	27.3	27.9	29.1
Age and percent of poverty level[7]										
Under 65 years:										
Below 100%	33.0	37.6	48.4	40.5	38.4	44.2	45.0	47.6	49.1	51.2
100%–199%	5.3	7.5	14.4	13.0	16.2	21.6	22.0	26.1	27.4	29.0
100%–133%	8.7	11.9	23.1	19.9	22.3	28.8	29.3	34.2	36.1	38.3
134%–199%	3.7	5.6	9.7	9.5	13.1	18.0	18.3	21.8	22.8	23.8
200%–399%	0.8	1.3	2.3	2.7	4.0	6.1	6.1	6.8	7.8	8.0
400% or more	0.2	0.5	0.4	0.8	0.9	1.5	1.5	1.5	1.6	1.7

See footnotes at end of table.

[Data are based on household interviews of a sample of the civilian noninstitutionalized population]

Characteristic	1984[1]	1989[1]	1995[1]	1997	2000[2]	2004(1)[3]	2004(2)[3]	2007[3]	2008[3]	2009[3]
					Percent of population					
Under 19 years:										
Below 100%.	42.0	45.8	63.5	56.4	56.9	67.5	68.9	72.7	73.4	77.5
100%–199%.	6.5	8.6	21.3	20.3	27.8	38.7	39.5	47.2	48.5	52.7
100%–133%.	10.3	13.4	32.4	30.5	36.2	48.9	49.8	56.9	60.0	65.4
134%–199%.	4.7	6.3	14.3	14.8	23.3	33.3	33.9	41.5	42.2	45.4
200%–399%.	1.0	1.7	3.5	4.4	7.6	12.1	12.2	13.3	16.4	16.4
400% or more	*	*1.2	*	1.3	2.1	3.2	3.2	3.0	3.5	3.6
Under 18 years:										
Below 100%.	43.3	47.8	66.0	58.0	58.5	69.2	70.7	75.0	75.3	78.3
100%–199%.	6.6	8.7	21.6	20.8	28.4	39.5	40.2	48.1	49.5	53.5
100%–133%.	10.4	13.5	32.9	31.4	36.7	49.5	50.5	57.7	61.1	66.8
134%–199%.	4.8	6.4	14.4	15.1	23.8	34.1	34.7	42.4	43.1	46.0
200%–399%.	1.0	1.7	3.5	4.5	7.6	12.2	12.3	13.3	16.8	16.8
400% or more	*	*1.1	*	1.3	2.2	3.3	3.3	3.0	3.6	3.7
18–64 years:										
Below 100%.	25.3	29.1	34.8	28.0	24.9	28.6	28.9	30.6	33.0	33.6
100%–199%.	4.5	6.8	10.2	8.6	9.1	11.9	12.2	14.0	15.3	16.2
100%–133%.	7.6	10.8	16.3	13.0	13.1	16.9	17.3	19.8	21.9	23.1
134%–199%.	3.1	5.1	7.2	6.5	7.2	9.5	9.7	11.0	11.8	12.5
200%–399%.	0.7	1.1	1.7	1.9	2.4	3.4	3.4	4.0	4.1	4.6
400% or more	0.2	0.4	0.4	0.7	0.6	1.0	1.0	1.1	1.1	1.2
Disability measure among adults 18–64 years[8]										
Any basic actions difficulty or complex activity limitation.	- - -	- - -	- - -	13.2	12.8	14.7	14.9	16.5	18.6	18.2
Any basic actions difficulty.	- - -	- - -	- - -	12.7	12.2	14.0	14.2	15.9	17.7	17.8
Any complex activity limitation	- - -	- - -	- - -	22.9	23.2	23.9	24.1	28.7	31.0	30.2
No disability.	- - -	- - -	- - -	3.5	3.0	4.5	4.7	5.2	4.9	6.4
Geographic region										
Northeast	8.6	6.6	11.7	11.3	10.6	12.8	13.0	15.4	16.1	17.3
Midwest	7.4	7.6	10.5	8.4	8.0	10.2	10.4	13.7	14.5	16.4
South.	5.1	6.5	11.3	8.7	9.4	12.2	12.4	12.9	13.5	14.8
West.	7.0	8.5	12.9	11.7	10.4	14.2	14.4	14.5	15.7	16.8
Location of residence[9]										
Within MSA.	7.1	7.0	11.3	9.7	8.9	11.7	11.9	13.3	14.2	15.2
Outside MSA.	6.1	7.9	12.3	10.1	11.9	14.8	15.0	17.1	17.2	20.8

See footnotes at end of table.

Table 137 (page 3 of 3). Medicaid coverage among persons under 65 years of age, by selected characteristics: United States, selected years 1984–2009

[Data are based on household interviews of a sample of the civilian noninstitutionalized population]

- - - Data not available.

*Estimates are considered unreliable. Data not shown have a relative standard error of greater than 30%.

[1]Data prior to 1997 are not strictly comparable with data for later years due to the 1997 questionnaire redesign. See Appendix I, National Health Interview Survey and Appendix II, Health insurance coverage.

[2]Estimates for 2000–2002 were calculated using 2000-based sample weights and may differ from estimates in other reports that used 1990-based sample weights for 2000–2002 estimates.

[3]Beginning in quarter 3 of the 2004 NHIS, persons under 65 years with no reported coverage were asked explicitly about Medicaid coverage. Estimates were calculated without and with the additional information from this question in the columns labeled 2004(1) and 2004(2), respectively, and estimates were calculated with the additional information starting with 2005 data.

[4]Includes all other races not shown separately, those with unknown marital status, unknown disability status, and, in 1984 and 1989, persons with unknown poverty level.

[5]Includes persons 14–64 years of age.

[6]The race groups, white, black, American Indian or Alaska Native, Asian, Native Hawaiian or Other Pacific Islander, and 2 or more races, include persons of Hispanic and non-Hispanic origin. Persons of Hispanic origin may be of any race. Starting with 1999 data, race-specific estimates are tabulated according to the 1997 Revisions to the Standards for the Classification of Federal Data on Race and Ethnicity and are not strictly comparable with estimates for earlier years. The five single-race categories plus multiple-race categories shown in the table conform to the 1997 Standards. Starting with 1999 data, race-specific estimates are for persons who reported only one racial group; the category 2 or more races includes persons who reported more than one racial group. Prior to 1999, data were tabulated according to the 1977 Standards with four racial groups and the Asian only category included Native Hawaiian or Other Pacific Islander. Estimates for single-race categories prior to 1999 included persons who reported one race or, if they reported more than one race, identified one race as best representing their race. Starting with 2003 data, race responses of other race and unspecified multiple race were treated as missing, and then race was imputed if these were the only race responses. Almost all persons with a race response of other race were of Hispanic origin. See Appendix II, Hispanic origin; Race.

[7]Percent of poverty level is based on family income and family size and composition using U.S. Census Bureau poverty thresholds. Poverty level was unknown for 10%–11% of persons under 65 years of age in 1984 and 1989. Missing family income data were imputed for 1995 and beyond. See Appendix II, Family income; Poverty; Table VII.

[8]Any basic actions difficulty or complex activity limitation is defined as having one or more of the following limitations or difficulties: movement difficulty, emotional difficulty, sensory (seeing or hearing) difficulty, cognitive difficulty, self-care (ADL or IADL) limitation, social limitation, or work limitation. For more information, see Appendix II, Basic actions difficulty; Complex activity limitation. Starting with 2007 data, the hearing question, a component of the basic actions difficulty measure, was revised. Consequently, data prior to 2007 are not comparable with data for 2007 and beyond. For more information on the impact of the revised hearing question, see Appendix II, Hearing trouble.

[9]MSA is metropolitan statistical area. Starting with 2006 data, MSA status is determined using 2000 census data and the 2000 standards for defining MSAs. For data prior to 2006, see Appendix II, Metropolitan statistical area (MSA) for the applicable standards.

NOTES: The category Medicaid coverage includes persons who had any of the following at the time of interview: Medicaid, other public assistance through 1996, state-sponsored health plan starting in 1997, or Children's Health Insurance Program (CHIP) starting in 1999; it includes those who also had another type of coverage in addition to one of these. In 2007, 11.2% of persons under 65 years of age reported being covered by Medicaid, 1.2% by state-sponsored health plans, and 1.5% by CHIP. The number of persons with Medicaid coverage was calculated by multiplying the percentage with Medicaid coverage by the number of persons under age 65 in the civilian non-institutionalized U.S. population. Percentages were calculated with unknown values excluded from denominators. See Appendix II, Health insurance coverage. Standard errors are available in the spreadsheet version of this table. Available from: http://www.cdc.gov/nchs/hus.htm. Data for additional years are available. See Appendix III.

SOURCE: CDC/NCHS, National Health Interview Survey, health insurance supplements (1984, 1989, 1994–1996). Starting with 1997, data are from the family core and the sample adult questionnaires.

Table 138 (page 1 of 3). No health insurance coverage among persons under 65 years of age, by selected characteristics: United States, selected years 1984–2009

[Data are based on household interviews of a sample of the civilian noninstitutionalized population]

Characteristic	1984[1]	1989[1]	1995[1]	1997	2000[2]	2004(1)[3]	2004(2)[3]	2007[3]	2008[3]	2009[3]
					Number in millions					
Total[4]	29.8	33.4	37.1	41.0	41.4	42.1	41.6	43.3	44.1	46.2
					Percent of population					
Total[4]	14.5	15.6	16.1	17.5	17.0	16.6	16.4	16.6	16.8	17.5
Age										
Under 19 years	14.1	15.0	13.7	14.4	12.9	10.1	9.6	9.4	9.5	8.5
Under 6 years	14.9	15.1	11.8	12.5	11.8	8.9	8.2	7.3	7.6	6.6
6–18 years	13.8	15.0	14.6	15.2	13.4	10.6	10.3	10.4	10.5	9.4
Under 18 years	13.9	14.7	13.4	14.0	12.6	9.7	9.2	9.0	9.0	8.2
6–17 years	13.4	14.5	14.3	14.7	13.0	10.0	9.7	9.9	9.8	9.0
18–44 years	17.1	18.4	20.4	22.4	22.4	23.6	23.5	23.9	24.4	25.9
18–24 years	25.0	27.1	28.0	30.1	30.4	30.1	30.0	27.9	29.0	29.6
25–34 years	16.2	18.3	21.1	23.8	23.3	25.7	25.5	26.1	26.6	27.8
35–44 years	11.2	12.3	15.1	16.7	16.9	17.6	17.5	19.1	19.1	21.4
45–64 years	9.6	10.5	10.9	12.4	12.6	12.9	12.8	13.5	13.6	14.6
45–54 years	10.5	11.0	11.6	12.8	12.8	13.7	13.6	14.9	14.9	16.5
55–64 years	8.7	10.0	9.9	11.8	12.4	11.7	11.6	11.6	11.8	12.2
Sex										
Male	15.3	16.8	17.4	18.7	18.1	18.1	17.9	18.2	18.3	19.4
Female	13.8	14.4	14.8	16.3	15.9	15.2	14.9	15.1	15.4	15.7
Sex and marital status[5]										
Male:										
Married	11.1	12.5	15.0	13.9	14.1	14.5	14.4	15.3	15.4	16.3
Divorced, separated, widowed	24.9	25.0	24.0	28.8	25.8	27.1	27.0	28.1	27.0	29.8
Never married	22.4	25.0	25.6	27.9	27.2	27.6	27.5	27.0	27.6	29.4
Female:										
Married	11.2	11.8	13.6	13.0	13.3	13.2	13.1	13.5	13.5	14.2
Divorced, separated, widowed	19.2	19.1	18.1	23.2	21.3	23.3	23.0	22.6	22.1	22.8
Never married	16.3	18.0	17.5	20.5	21.1	19.6	19.3	19.5	20.7	21.0
Race[6]										
White only	13.6	14.5	15.5	16.4	15.4	16.3	16.1	16.3	16.7	17.1
Black or African American only	19.9	21.6	18.0	20.1	19.5	18.1	17.6	17.0	18.0	18.9
American Indian or Alaska Native only	22.5	28.4	34.3	38.1	38.4	35.0	34.6	38.8	28.4	32.5
Asian only	18.5	16.9	18.6	19.5	17.6	16.7	16.5	15.4	13.9	16.2
Native Hawaiian or Other Pacific Islander only	- - -	- - -	- - -	- - -	*	*	*	*	*	*
2 or more races	- - -	- - -	- - -	- - -	16.8	12.6	12.3	15.0	15.8	18.2
Hispanic origin and race[6]										
Hispanic or Latino	29.5	33.7	31.4	34.5	35.6	35.1	34.4	31.8	33.3	32.9
Mexican	33.8	39.9	35.6	39.4	39.9	38.1	37.6	34.7	36.1	35.0
Puerto Rican	18.3	24.7	17.6	19.0	16.4	21.0	20.4	12.8	16.8	17.8
Cuban	21.6	20.6	22.3	21.1	25.4	22.8	22.8	20.7	28.1	27.8
Other Hispanic or Latino	27.4	25.8	30.2	33.0	33.4	33.3	32.3	32.7	32.5	33.4
Not Hispanic or Latino	13.2	13.7	14.2	15.2	14.0	13.3	13.2	13.7	13.5	14.4
White only	11.9	12.1	13.0	13.8	12.5	12.1	12.0	12.6	12.5	13.2
Black or African American only	19.7	21.5	17.9	20.0	19.5	17.8	17.3	16.8	17.9	18.8
Age and percent of poverty level[7]										
Under 65 years:										
Below 100%	33.9	35.2	29.6	33.7	34.2	31.8	31.0	28.4	29.0	30.4
100%–199%	21.8	25.6	28.3	30.6	31.0	29.4	29.0	30.0	30.6	29.8
100%–133%	28.8	32.3	34.1	36.4	35.8	32.1	31.5	32.3	32.7	30.5
134%–199%	18.7	22.6	25.1	27.7	28.6	28.0	27.7	28.8	29.5	29.4
200%–399%	7.6	8.3	10.0	14.2	15.4	15.7	15.6	16.9	16.6	17.8
400% or more	3.2	4.2	5.4	6.1	5.9	5.9	5.9	5.6	6.2	5.8

See footnotes at end of table.

Table 138 (page 2 of 3). No health insurance coverage among persons under 65 years of age, by selected characteristics: United States, selected years 1984–2009

[Data are based on household interviews of a sample of the civilian noninstitutionalized population]

Characteristic	1984[1]	1989[1]	1995[1]	1997	2000[2]	2004(1)[3]	2004(2)[3]	2007[3]	2008[3]	2009[3]
					Percent of population					
Under 19 years:										
Below 100%.	29.0	31.7	20.4	23.8	22.6	17.2	15.7	12.7	14.0	12.2
100%–199%.	18.0	20.7	22.6	23.7	22.1	16.5	15.8	16.4	16.3	13.0
100%–133%.	24.4	27.6	26.4	28.1	26.7	18.1	17.2	17.9	17.2	13.0
134%–199%.	14.9	17.4	20.1	21.3	19.6	15.7	15.1	15.6	15.8	13.0
200%–399%.	5.1	4.9	6.7	9.7	9.6	8.1	8.0	8.5	8.0	8.0
400% or more	1.8	2.1	4.4	4.0	3.5	2.8	2.8	2.3	2.8	2.4
Under 18 years:										
Below 100%.	28.9	31.6	20.0	23.2	22.0	16.5	15.0	11.9	13.3	11.8
100%–199%.	17.5	20.2	22.0	23.2	21.7	15.8	15.1	15.7	15.5	12.3
100%–133%.	24.0	27.1	26.1	28.0	26.5	17.6	16.7	17.0	16.3	11.9
134%–199%.	14.4	16.9	19.5	20.6	19.0	14.9	14.2	15.0	15.0	12.5
200%–399%.	4.9	4.7	6.6	9.4	9.3	7.7	7.6	8.2	7.5	7.8
400% or more	1.8	1.9	4.6	3.9	3.3	2.6	2.6	2.2	2.7	2.3
18–64 years:										
Below 100%.	37.6	38.2	37.0	41.2	42.4	41.4	41.0	38.6	38.6	42.5
100%–199%.	24.4	28.8	32.0	34.7	36.4	36.7	36.5	37.9	38.9	38.9
100%–133%.	31.9	35.6	39.7	41.4	41.8	40.4	40.1	41.7	42.0	40.4
134%–199%.	21.1	25.9	28.2	31.5	33.9	34.9	34.7	36.1	37.3	38.0
200%–399%.	8.9	10.0	11.7	16.4	18.2	19.1	19.1	20.5	20.2	21.7
400% or more	3.4	4.4	5.5	6.7	6.6	6.8	6.8	6.5	7.1	6.7
Disability measure among adults 18–64 years[8]										
Any basic actions difficulty or complex activity limitation.	- - -	- - -	- - -	20.1	17.6	19.8	19.6	19.6	19.5	21.4
Any basic actions difficulty.	- - -	- - -	- - -	20.1	17.6	20.0	19.8	19.6	19.4	21.2
Any complex activity limitation	- - -	- - -	- - -	20.2	16.1	18.1	17.9	18.3	15.8	19.2
No disability.	- - -	- - -	- - -	17.6	18.5	19.3	19.2	19.9	19.8	21.2
Geographic region										
Northeast	10.2	10.9	13.3	13.5	12.2	11.9	11.8	11.0	11.4	11.4
Midwest	11.3	10.7	12.2	13.2	12.3	12.6	12.4	13.0	13.9	14.6
South	17.7	19.7	19.4	20.9	20.5	20.2	19.9	20.1	20.1	21.2
West.	18.2	18.8	17.9	20.6	20.7	19.1	18.9	18.9	18.8	19.4
Location of residence[9]										
Within MSA.	13.6	15.2	15.5	16.9	16.6	16.4	16.2	16.1	16.4	17.1
Outside MSA.	16.6	17.0	18.6	19.8	18.6	17.4	17.2	19.4	19.1	20.2

See footnotes at end of table.

Table 138 (page 3 of 3). No health insurance coverage among persons under 65 years of age, by selected characteristics: United States, selected years 1984–2009

[Data are based on household interviews of a sample of the civilian noninstitutionalized population]

- - - Data not available.

*Estimates are considered unreliable. Data not shown have a relative standard error of greater than 30%.

[1]Data prior to 1997 are not strictly comparable with data for later years due to the 1997 questionnaire redesign. See Appendix I, National Health Interview Survey and Appendix II, Health insurance coverage.

[2]Estimates for 2000–2002 were calculated using 2000-based sample weights and may differ from estimates in other reports that used 1990-based sample weights for 2000–2002 estimates.

[3]Beginning in quarter 3 of the 2004 NHIS, persons under 65 years with no reported coverage were asked explicitly about Medicaid coverage. Estimates were calculated without and with the additional information from this question in the columns labeled 2004(1) and 2004(2), respectively, and estimates were calculated with the additional information starting with 2005 data.

[4]Includes all other races not shown separately, those with unknown marital status, unknown disability status, and, in 1984 and 1989, persons with unknown poverty level.

[5]Includes persons 14–64 years of age.

[6]The race groups, white, black, American Indian or Alaska Native, Asian, Native Hawaiian or Other Pacific Islander, and 2 or more races, include persons of Hispanic and non-Hispanic origin. Persons of Hispanic origin may be of any race. Starting with 1999 data, race-specific estimates are tabulated according to the 1997 Revisions to the Standards for the Classification of Federal Data on Race and Ethnicity and are not strictly comparable with estimates for earlier years. The five single-race categories plus multiple-race categories shown in the table conform to the 1997 Standards. Starting with 1999 data, race-specific estimates are for persons who reported only one racial group; the category 2 or more races includes persons who reported more than one racial group. Prior to 1999, data were tabulated according to the 1977 Standards with four racial groups and the Asian only category included Native Hawaiian or Other Pacific Islander. Estimates for single-race categories prior to 1999 included persons who reported one race or, if they reported more than one race, identified one race as best representing their race. Starting with 2003 data, race responses of other race and unspecified multiple race were treated as missing, and then race was imputed if these were the only race responses. Almost all persons with a race response of other race were of Hispanic origin. See Appendix II, Hispanic origin; Race.

[7]Percent of poverty level is based on family income and family size and composition using U.S. Census Bureau poverty thresholds. Poverty level was unknown for 10%–11% of persons under 65 years of age in 1984 and 1989. Missing family income data were imputed for 1995 and beyond. See Appendix II, Family income; Poverty; Table VII.

[8]Any basic actions difficulty or complex activity limitation is defined as having one or more of the following limitations or difficulties: movement difficulty, emotional difficulty, sensory (seeing or hearing) difficulty, cognitive difficulty, self-care (ADL or IADL) limitation, social limitation, or work limitation. For more information, see Appendix II, Basic actions difficulty; Complex activity limitation. Starting with 2007 data, the hearing question, a component of the basic actions difficulty measure, was revised. Consequently, data prior to 2007 are not comparable with data for 2007 and beyond. For more information on the impact of the revised hearing question, see Appendix I, Hearing trouble.

[9]MSA is metropolitan statistical area. Starting with 2006 data, MSA status is determined using 2000 census data and the 2000 standards for defining MSAs. For data prior to 2006, see Appendix II, Metropolitan statistical area (MSA) for the applicable standards.

NOTES: Persons not covered by private insurance, Medicaid, Children's Health Insurance Program (CHIP), public assistance (through 1996), state-sponsored or other government-sponsored health plans (starting in 1997), Medicare, or military plans are considered to have no health insurance coverage. Persons with only Indian Health Service coverage are considered to have no health insurance coverage. Health insurance coverage is at the time of interview. The number of persons with no health insurance coverage was calculated by multiplying the percentage with no coverage by the number of persons under age 65 in the civilian non-institutionalized U.S. population. Percentages were calculated with unknown values excluded from denominators. See Appendix II, Health insurance coverage. Standard errors are available in the spreadsheet version of this table. Available from: http://www.cdc.gov/nchs/hus.htm. Data for additional years are available. See Appendix III.

SOURCE: CDC/NCHS, National Health Interview Survey, health insurance supplements (1984, 1989, 1994–1996). Starting with 1997, data are from the family core and the sample adult questionnaires.

Table 139 (page 1 of 2). Health insurance coverage of Medicare beneficiaries 65 years of age and over, by type of coverage and selected characteristics: United States, selected years 1992–2008

[Data are based on household interviews of a sample of noninstitutionalized Medicare beneficiaries]

Characteristic	Medicare Health Maintenance Organization[1]					Medicaid[2]				
	1992	1995	2000	2007	2008	1992	1995	2000	2007	2008
Age	Number in millions									
65 years and over	1.1	2.6	5.9	7.3	8.1	2.7	2.8	2.7	3.3	3.2
	Percent of population									
65 years and over	3.9	8.9	19.3	20.4	22.1	9.4	9.6	9.0	9.2	8.8
65–74 years.	4.2	9.5	20.6	21.0	22.9	7.9	8.8	8.5	8.8	8.2
75–84 years.	3.7	8.3	18.5	20.8	23.0	10.6	9.6	8.9	9.3	9.1
85 years and over	*	7.3	16.3	17.0	16.5	16.6	13.6	11.2	11.4	10.3
Sex										
Male.	4.6	9.2	19.3	21.9	23.6	6.3	6.2	6.3	6.6	5.8
Female.	3.4	8.6	19.3	19.2	20.9	11.6	12.0	10.9	11.4	11.2
Race and Hispanic origin										
White, not Hispanic or Latino . . .	3.6	8.4	18.4	18.5	20.2	5.6	5.4	5.1	5.7	5.4
Black, not Hispanic or Latino . . .	*	7.9	20.7	27.9	28.5	28.5	30.3	23.6	18.8	20.0
Hispanic.	*	15.5	27.5	36.7	37.5	39.0	40.5	28.7	24.4	21.1
Percent of poverty level[3]										
Below 100%	3.6	7.7	18.4	- - -	- - -	22.3	17.2	15.9	- - -	- - -
100%-less than 200%	3.7	9.5	23.4	- - -	- - -	6.7	6.3	8.4	- - -	- - -
200% or more.	4.2	10.1	18.0	- - -	- - -	*	*	*	- - -	- - -
Marital status										
Married.	4.6	9.5	18.7	22.2	24.2	4.0	4.3	4.3	4.1	4.0
Widowed	2.3	7.7	19.4	15.8	17.1	14.9	15.0	13.6	14.3	13.9
Divorced.	*	9.7	24.4	24.5	25.5	23.4	24.5	20.2	18.0	16.8
Never married.	*	*	15.8	21.1	20.7	19.2	19.0	17.0	22.1	18.2

Characteristic	Employer-sponsored plan[4]					Medigap[5]				
	1992	1995	2000	2007	2008	1992	1995	2000	2007	2008
Age	Number in millions									
65 years and over	12.5	11.3	10.7	12.1	12.0	9.9	9.5	7.6	7.9	7.9
	Percent of population									
65 years and over	42.8	38.6	35.2	33.8	32.7	33.9	32.5	25.0	22.0	21.5
65–74 years.	46.9	41.1	36.6	35.1	34.0	31.4	29.9	21.7	20.4	19.6
75–84 years.	38.2	37.1	35.0	33.1	31.2	37.5	35.2	27.8	22.9	22.7
85 years and over	31.6	30.2	29.4	30.2	31.1	38.3	37.6	31.1	26.2	26.3
Sex										
Male.	46.3	42.1	37.7	36.5	35.3	30.6	30.0	23.4	20.2	20.1
Female.	40.4	36.0	33.4	31.6	30.7	36.2	34.4	26.2	23.4	22.7
Race and Hispanic origin										
White, not Hispanic or Latino . . .	45.9	41.3	38.6	36.8	35.4	37.2	36.2	28.3	25.3	24.9
Black, not Hispanic or Latino . . .	25.9	26.7	22.0	25.8	23.2	13.6	10.2	7.5	7.3	6.5
Hispanic.	20.7	16.9	15.8	16.2	19.7	15.8	10.1	11.3	7.7	7.8
Percent of poverty level[3]										
Below 100%	29.0	32.1	28.1	- - -	- - -	30.8	29.8	22.6	- - -	- - -
100%-less than 200%	37.5	32.0	27.0	- - -	- - -	39.3	39.1	28.4	- - -	- - -
200% or more.	58.4	52.8	49.0	- - -	- - -	32.8	32.2	26.2	- - -	- - -
Marital status										
Married.	49.9	44.6	41.0	39.1	38.3	33.0	32.6	25.6	22.1	21.4
Widowed	34.1	30.3	28.7	28.7	27.6	37.5	35.2	26.7	24.3	23.6
Divorced.	27.3	26.6	22.4	22.3	19.3	27.9	24.1	16.9	16.1	18.5
Never married.	38.0	35.1	28.5	28.1	28.9	29.1	26.2	21.9	17.4	14.6

See footnotes at end of table.

Table 139 (page 2 of 2). Health insurance coverage of Medicare beneficiaries 65 years of age and over, by type of coverage and selected characteristics: United States, selected years 1992–2008

[Data are based on household interviews of a sample of noninstitutionalized Medicare beneficiaries]

Characteristic	Medicare fee-for-service only or Other[6]				
	1992	1995	2000	2007	2008
Age	Number in millions				
65 years and over	2.9	3.1	3.5	5.2	5.5
	Percent of population				
65 years and over	9.9	10.5	11.5	14.6	14.9
65–74 years.	9.7	10.7	12.6	14.8	15.2
75–84 years.	10.1	9.9	9.9	14.0	14.0
85 years and over	10.8	11.3	12.1	15.2	15.8
Sex					
Male.	12.2	12.6	13.3	14.8	15.1
Female.	8.3	8.9	10.2	14.4	14.7
Race and Hispanic origin					
White, not Hispanic or Latino . . .	7.7	8.7	9.6	13.7	14.1
Black, not Hispanic or Latino . . .	26.7	25.0	26.1	20.2	21.7
Hispanic.	18.3	17.1	16.7	15.0	13.9
Percent of poverty level[3]					
Below 100%	14.3	13.3	15.1	- - -	- - -
100%-less than 200%	12.9	13.1	12.7	- - -	- - -
200% or more	4.0	4.5	6.3	- - -	- - -
Marital status					
Married.	8.5	9.0	10.5	12.6	12.1
Widowed	11.2	11.9	11.6	16.8	17.7
Divorced.	15.7	15.1	16.1	19.1	20.0
Never married	*	13.1	16.8	11.4	17.7

* Estimates are considered unreliable if the sample cell size is 50 or fewer.
- - - Data not available.
[1]Enrollee has Medicare Health Maintenance Organization (HMO) regardless of other insurance. See Appendix II, Managed care.
[2]Enrolled in Medicaid and not enrolled in a Medicare risk HMO. See Appendix II, Managed care.
[3]Percent of poverty level is based on family income and family size and composition using U.S. Census Bureau poverty thresholds. See Appendix II, Family income; Poverty.
[4]Private insurance plans purchased through employers (own, current, or former employer, family business, union, or former employer or union of spouse) and not enrolled in a Medicare risk HMO or Medicaid.
[5]Supplemental insurance purchased privately or through organizations such as AARP or professional organizations, and not enrolled in a Medicare risk HMO, Medicaid, or employer-sponsored plan.
[6]Medicare fee-for-service only or other public plans (except Medicaid).

NOTES: Data for noninstitutionalized Medicare beneficiaries. Insurance categories are mutually exclusive. Persons with more than one type of coverage are categorized according to the order in which the health insurance categories appear. See Appendix I, Medicare Current Beneficiary Survey (MCBS). Data for additional years are available. See Appendix III.

SOURCE: Centers for Medicare & Medicaid Services, Medicare Current Beneficiary Survey, Access to Care file.

Table 140 (page 1 of 2). Medicare enrollees and expenditures and percent distribution, by Medicare program and type of service: United States and other areas, selected years 1970–2008

[Data are compiled from various sources by the Centers for Medicare & Medicaid Services]

Medicare program and type of service	1970	1980	1990	1995	2000	2003	2004	2005	2006	2007	2008[1]
Enrollees					Number in millions						
Total Medicare[2]	20.4	28.4	34.3	37.6	39.7	41.2	41.9	42.6	43.4	44.3	45.2
Hospital insurance	20.1	28.0	33.7	37.2	39.3	40.7	41.5	42.2	43.1	43.9	44.9
Supplementary medical insurance (SMI)[3]	19.5	27.3	32.6	35.6	37.3	38.6	- - -	- - -	- - -	- - -	- - -
Part B	19.5	27.3	32.6	35.6	37.3	38.6	39.1	39.8	40.4	41.1	41.7
Part D[4]	- - -	- - -	- - -	- - -	- - -	- - -	1.2	1.8	27.0	30.8	32.1
Expenditures					Amount in billions						
Total Medicare	$ 7.5	$ 36.8	$111.0	$184.2	$221.8	$280.8	$308.9	$336.4	$408.3	$431.7	$468.1
Total hospital insurance (HI)	5.3	25.6	67.0	117.6	131.1	154.6	170.6	182.9	191.9	203.1	235.6
HI payments to managed care organizations[5]	- - -	0.0	2.7	6.7	21.4	19.5	20.8	24.9	32.9	39.0	50.6
HI payments for fee-for-service utilization	5.1	25.0	63.4	109.5	105.1	134.5	146.5	156.6	159.6	163.4	172.8
Inpatient hospital	4.8	24.1	56.9	82.3	87.1	109.1	117.0	123.2	124.1	124.2	130.5
Skilled nursing facility	0.2	0.4	2.5	9.1	11.1	14.8	17.2	19.4	20.3	22.5	24.2
Home health agency	0.1	0.5	3.7	16.2	4.0	4.9	5.4	6.0	5.9	6.2	6.6
Hospice	- - -	- - -	0.3	1.9	2.9	5.7	6.8	8.0	9.3	10.5	11.7
Home health agency transfer[6]	- - -	- - -	- - -	- - -	1.7	−2.2	- - -	- - -	- - -	- - -	- - -
Medicare Advantage premiums[7]	- - -	- - -	- - -	- - -	- - -	- - -	- - -	- - -	0.0	0.1	0.9
Accounting error (CY 2005–2008)[8]	- - -	- - -	- - -	- - -	- - -	- - -	- - -	−1.9	−3.9	−2.7	8.5
Administrative expenses[9]	0.2	0.5	0.9	1.4	2.9	2.8	3.3	3.3	3.3	3.2	3.6
Total supplementary medical insurance (SMI)[3]	2.2	11.2	44.0	66.6	90.7	126.1	138.3	153.5	216.4	228.6	232.6
Total Part B	2.2	11.2	44.0	66.6	90.7	126.1	137.9	152.4	169.0	178.9	183.3
Part B payments to managed care organizations[5]	0.0	0.2	2.8	6.6	18.4	17.3	18.7	22.0	31.5	38.9	47.6
Part B payments for fee-for-service utilization[10]	1.9	10.4	39.6	58.4	72.2	104.3	116.2	125.0	130.2	134.6	141.0
Physician/supplies[11]	1.8	8.2	29.6	- - -	- - -	- - -	- - -	- - -	- - -	- - -	- - -
Outpatient hospital[12]	0.1	1.9	8.5	- - -	- - -	- - -	- - -	- - -	- - -	- - -	- - -
Independent laboratory[13]	0.0	0.1	1.5	- - -	- - -	- - -	- - -	- - -	- - -	- - -	- - -
Physician fee schedule	- - -	- - -	- - -	31.7	37.0	48.3	54.1	57.7	58.2	58.9	60.8
Durable medical equipment	- - -	- - -	- - -	3.7	4.7	7.5	7.7	8.0	8.3	8.1	8.9
Laboratory[14]	- - -	- - -	- - -	4.3	4.0	5.5	6.1	6.3	6.7	7.1	7.3
Other[15]	- - -	- - -	- - -	9.9	13.6	22.6	25.0	26.7	28.0	28.9	30.2
Hospital[16]	- - -	- - -	- - -	8.7	8.4	15.3	17.4	19.2	21.3	22.4	23.8
Home health agency	0.0	0.2	0.1	0.2	4.5	5.1	5.9	7.1	7.8	9.2	10.0
Home health agency transfer[6]	- - -	- - -	- - -	- - -	−1.7	2.2	- - -	- - -	- - -	- - -	- - -
Medicare Advantage premiums	- - -	- - -	- - -	- - -	- - -	- - -	- - -	- - -	0.0	0.1	0.1
Accounting error (CY 2005–2008)[8]	- - -	- - -	- - -	- - -	- - -	- - -	- - -	1.9	3.9	2.7	−8.5
Administrative expenses[9]	0.2	0.6	1.5	1.6	1.8	2.4	2.8	2.6	2.9	2.5	3.0
Part D start-up costs[17]	- - -	- - -	- - -	- - -	- - -	- - -	0.2	0.7	0.2	0.0	0.0
Total Part D[4]	- - -	- - -	- - -	- - -	- - -	- - -	0.4	1.1	47.4	49.7	49.3
					Percent distribution of expenditures						
Total hospital insurance (HI)	100.0	100.0	100.0	100.0	100.0	100.0	100.0	100.0	100.0	100.0	100.0
HI payments to managed care organizations[5]	- - -	0.0	4.0	5.7	16.3	12.6	12.2	13.6	17.2	19.2	21.5
HI payments for fee-for-service utilization	97.0	97.9	94.6	93.1	80.2	87.0	85.9	85.6	83.2	80.5	73.4
Inpatient hospital	91.4	94.3	85.0	70.0	66.4	70.6	68.6	67.4	64.6	61.2	55.4
Skilled nursing facility	4.7	1.5	3.7	7.8	8.5	9.6	10.1	10.6	10.6	11.1	10.3
Home health agency	1.0	2.1	5.5	13.8	3.1	3.1	3.2	3.3	3.1	3.1	2.8
Hospice	- - -	- - -	0.5	1.6	2.2	3.7	4.0	4.4	4.9	5.2	5.0
Home health agency transfer[6]	- - -	- - -	- - -	- - -	1.3	−1.4	- - -	- - -	- - -	- - -	- - -
Medicare Advantage premiums[7]	- - -	- - -	- - -	- - -	- - -	- - -	- - -	- - -	0.0	0.0	0.4
Accounting error (CY 2005–2008)[8]	- - -	- - -	- - -	- - -	- - -	- - -	- - -	−1.0	−2.0	−1.3	3.6
Administrative expenses[9]	3.0	2.1	1.4	1.2	2.2	1.8	2.0	1.8	1.7	1.6	1.5

See footnotes at end of table.

Table 140 (page 2 of 2). **Medicare enrollees and expenditures and percent distribution, by Medicare program and type of service: United States and other areas, selected years 1970–2008**

[Data are compiled from various sources by the Centers for Medicare & Medicaid Services]

Medicare program and type of service	1970	1980	1990	1995	2000	2003	2004	2005	2006	2007	2008[1]
					Percent distribution of expenditures						
Total supplementary medical insurance (SMI)[3]	100.0	100.0	100.0	100.0	100.0	100.0	100.0	100.0	100.0	100.0	100.0
Total Part B	100.0	100.0	100.0	100.0	100.0	100.0	99.7	99.3	78.1	78.3	78.8
Part B payments to managed care organizations[5]	1.2	1.8	6.4	9.9	20.2	13.7	13.5	14.3	14.5	17.0	20.5
Part B payments for fee-for-service utilization[10]	88.1	92.8	90.1	87.6	79.6	82.7	84.0	81.5	60.2	58.9	60.6
Physician/supplies[11]	80.9	72.8	67.3	- - -	- - -	- - -	- - -	- - -	- - -	- - -	- - -
Outpatient hospital[12]	5.2	16.9	19.3	- - -	- - -	- - -	- - -	- - -	- - -	- - -	- - -
Independent laboratory[13]	0.5	1.0	3.4	- - -	- - -	- - -	- - -	- - -	- - -	- - -	- - -
Physician fee schedule	- - -	- - -	- - -	47.5	40.8	38.3	39.1	37.6	26.9	25.7	26.1
Durable medical equipment	- - -	- - -	- - -	5.5	5.2	6.0	5.6	5.2	3.8	3.5	3.8
Laboratory[14]	- - -	- - -	- - -	6.4	4.4	4.3	4.4	4.1	3.1	3.1	3.2
Other[15]	- - -	- - -	- - -	14.8	15.0	17.9	18.1	17.4	13.0	12.7	13.0
Hospital[16]	- - -	- - -	- - -	13.0	9.3	12.1	12.6	12.5	9.8	9.8	10.2
Home health agency	1.5	2.1	0.2	0.3	4.9	4.0	4.2	4.6	3.6	4.0	4.3
Home health agency transfer[6]	- - -	- - -	- - -	- - -	−1.9	1.7	- - -	- - -	- - -	- - -	- - -
Medicare Advantage premiums[7]	- - -	- - -	- - -	- - -	- - -	- - -	- - -	- - -	0.0	0.0	0.0
Accounting error (CY 2005–2008)[8]	- - -	- - -	- - -	- - -	- - -	- - -	- - -	1.2	1.8	1.2	−3.6
Administrative expenses[9]	10.7	5.4	3.5	2.4	2.0	1.9	2.0	1.7	1.3	1.1	1.3
Part D start-up costs[17]	- - -	- - -	- - -	- - -	- - -	- - -	0.1	0.4	0.1	0.0	0.0
Total Part D[4]	- - -	- - -	- - -	- - -	- - -	- - -	0.3	0.7	21.9	21.7	21.2

- - - Category not applicable or data not available.
0.0 Quantity greater than 0 but less than 0.05.
[1]Preliminary estimates.
[2]Average number enrolled in the hospital insurance (HI) and/or supplementary medical insurance (SMI) programs for the period. See Appendix II, Medicare.
[3]Starting with 2004 data, the SMI trust fund consists of two separate accounts: Part B (which pays for a portion of the costs of physicians' services, outpatient hospital services, and other related medical and health services for voluntarily enrolled individuals) and Part D (Medicare Prescription Drug Account, which pays private plans to provide prescription drug coverage).
[4]The Medicare Modernization Act, enacted on December 8, 2003, established within SMI two Part D accounts related to prescription drug benefits: the Medicare Prescription Drug Account and the Transitional Assistance Account. The Medicare Prescription Drug Account is used in conjunction with the broad, voluntary prescription drug benefits that began in 2006. The Transitional Assistance Account was used to provide transitional assistance benefits, beginning in 2004 and extending through 2005, for certain low-income beneficiaries prior to the start of the new prescription drug benefit. The amounts shown for Total Part D expenditures—and thus for total SMI expenditures and total Medicare expenditures—for 2006 and later years include estimated amounts for premiums paid directly from Part D beneficiaries to Part D prescription drug plans.
[5]Medicare-approved managed care organizations.
[6]For 1998 to 2003 data, reflects annual home health HI to SMI transfer amounts.
[7]When a beneficiary chooses a Medicare Advantage plan whose monthly premium exceeds the benchmark amount, the additional premiums (that is, amounts beyond those paid by Medicare to the plan) are the responsibility of the beneficiary. Beneficiaries subject to such premiums may choose to either reimburse the plans directly or have the additional premiums deducted from their Social Security checks. The amounts shown here are only those additional premiums deducted from Social Security checks. These amounts are transferred to the HI trust and SMI trust funds and then transferred from the trust funds to the plans.
[8]Represents misallocation of benefit payments between the HI trust fund and the Part B account of the SMI trust fund from May 2005 to September 2007, and the transfer made in June 2008 to correct the misallocation.
[9]Includes expenditures for research, experiments and demonstration projects, peer review activity (performed by Peer Review Organizations from 1983 to 2001 and by Quality Review Organizations from 2002 to present), and to combat and prevent fraud and abuse.
[10]Type-of-service reporting categories for fee-for-service reimbursement differ before and after 1991.
[11]Includes payment for physicians, practitioners, durable medical equipment, and all suppliers other than independent laboratory through 1990. Starting with 1991 data, physician services subject to the physician fee schedule are shown. Payments for laboratory services paid under the laboratory fee schedule and performed in a physician office are included under Laboratory beginning in 1991. Payments for durable medical equipment are shown separately beginning in 1991. The remaining services from the Physician/supplies category are included in Other.
[12]Includes payments for hospital outpatient department services, skilled nursing facility outpatient services, Part B services received as an inpatient in a hospital or skilled nursing facility setting, and other types of outpatient facilities. Starting with 1991 data, payments for hospital outpatient department services, except for laboratory services, are listed under Hospital. Hospital outpatient laboratory services are included in the Laboratory line.
[13]Starting with 1991 data, those independent laboratory services that were paid under the laboratory fee schedule (most of the independent laboratory category) are included in the Laboratory line; the remaining services are included in the Physician fee schedule and Other lines.
[14]Payments for laboratory services paid under the laboratory fee schedule performed in a physician office, independent laboratory, or in a hospital outpatient department.
[15]Includes payments for physician-administered drugs; freestanding ambulatory surgical center facility services; ambulance services; supplies; freestanding end-stage renal disease (ESRD) dialysis facility services; rural health clinics; outpatient rehabilitation facilities; psychiatric hospitals; and federally qualified health centers.
[16]Includes the hospital facility costs for Medicare Part B services that are predominantly in the outpatient department, with the exception of hospital outpatient laboratory services, which are included on the Laboratory line. Physician reimbursement is included on the Physician fee schedule line.
[17]Part D start-up costs were funded through the SMI Part B account in 2004–2008.

NOTES: All data shown are estimates and are subject to revision. Percents may not sum to totals because of rounding. Estimates are for Medicare-covered services furnished to Medicare enrollees residing in the United States, Puerto Rico, Virgin Islands, Guam, other outlying areas, foreign countries, and unknown residence. Estimates in this table have been revised and differ from previous editions of *Health, United States*.

SOURCE: Centers for Medicare & Medicaid Services (CMS), Office of the Actuary, Medicare and Medicaid Cost Estimates Group. Estimates are based on unpublished data from CMS, the Office of the Actuary, and Treasury Department financial statements. Estimates are subject to change as more recent data become available.

Table 141. Medicare enrollees and program payments among fee-for-service Medicare beneficiaries, by sex and age: United States and other areas, selected years 1994–2008

[Data are compiled from administrative data by the Centers for Medicare & Medicaid Services]

Sex and age	1994	1995	1999	2000	2002	2005	2006	2007	2008
	Fee-for-service enrollees in thousands								
Total	34,076	34,062	32,179	32,740	34,977	36,685	35,847	35,490	35,320
Sex									
Male	14,533	14,563	13,872	14,195	15,314	16,251	15,958	15,879	15,890
Female	19,543	19,499	18,307	18,545	19,664	20,433	19,890	19,611	19,430
Age									
Under 65 years	4,031	4,239	4,742	4,907	5,448	6,286	6,225	6,318	6,359
65–74 years	16,713	16,373	14,072	14,230	15,107	15,587	15,179	15,041	15,182
75–84 years	9,845	9,911	9,748	9,919	10,533	10,689	10,298	9,947	9,592
85 years and over	3,486	3,540	3,618	3,684	3,889	4,123	4,146	4,184	4,187
	Fee-for-service program payments in billions								
Total	$ 146.6	$ 159.0	$ 166.7	$ 174.3	$ 215.4	$ 274.1	$ 280.7	$ 288.5	$ 301.1
Sex									
Male	63.9	68.8	73.2	76.2	94.3	121.0	123.6	126.5	131.5
Female	82.6	90.2	93.5	98.0	121.1	153.2	157.0	162.1	169.7
Age									
Under 65 years	18.8	21.0	24.3	25.8	33.2	46.7	48.4	50.9	54.2
65–74 years	55.1	58.1	56.0	57.5	70.0	86.6	87.4	89.1	92.9
75–84 years	50.7	55.3	59.5	62.7	77.1	95.2	96.2	96.4	97.9
85 years and over	21.8	24.6	26.9	28.3	35.1	45.6	48.7	52.1	56.1
	Percent distribution of fee-for-service program payments								
Total	100.0	100.0	100.0	100.0	100.0	100.0	100.0	100.0	100.0
Sex									
Male	43.6	43.2	43.9	43.7	43.8	44.1	44.0	43.8	43.7
Female	56.4	56.8	56.1	56.3	56.2	55.9	56.0	56.2	56.3
Age									
Under 65 years	12.9	13.2	14.6	14.8	15.4	17.0	17.2	17.6	18.0
65–74 years	37.6	36.5	33.6	33.0	32.5	31.6	31.1	30.9	30.9
75–84 years	34.6	34.8	35.7	36.0	35.8	34.7	34.3	33.4	32.5
85 years and over	14.9	15.5	16.1	16.2	16.3	16.6	17.3	18.0	18.6
	Average fee-for-service payment per enrollee [1]								
Total	$ 4,301	$ 4,667	$ 5,180	$ 5,323	$ 6,159	$ 7,473	$ 7,830	$ 8,129	$ 8,526
Sex									
Male	4,397	4,721	5,275	5,370	6,157	7,443	7,747	7,964	8,274
Female	4,229	4,627	5,108	5,286	6,159	7,497	7,896	8,263	8,732
Age									
Under 65 years	4,673	4,960	5,117	5,252	6,102	7,435	7,774	8,058	8,530
65–74 years	3,300	3,548	3,982	4,040	4,635	5,558	5,756	5,924	6,119
75–84 years	5,152	5,576	6,106	6,320	7,317	8,904	9,345	9,696	10,206
85 years and over	6,267	6,950	7,428	7,684	9,019	11,061	11,742	12,440	13,396

[1]Medicare enrollees in managed care are not included in the denominator used to calculate average payments.

NOTES: Table includes data for Medicare enrollees residing in Puerto Rico, U.S. Virgin Islands, Guam, other outlying areas, foreign countries, and unknown residence. Prior to 2004, number of fee-for-service enrollees, fee-for-service program payments, and fee-for-service billing reimbursement were based on a 5% annual Denominator File derived from the Centers for Medicare & Medicaid Services' (CMS) Enrollment Database and the fee-for-service claims for a 5% sample of beneficiaries as recorded in CMS' National Claims History File. Starting with 2004 data, the 100% Denominator File was used. See Appendix I, Medicare Administrative Data; Appendix II, Medicare. Data for additional years are available. See Appendix III.

SOURCE: Centers for Medicare & Medicaid Services, Office of Research, Development, and Information. Health Care Financing Review: Medicare and Medicaid Statistical Supplements for publication years 1996 to 2009. Available from: http://www.cms.hhs.gov/MedicareMedicaidStatSupp/LT/list.asp.

Table 142 (page 1 of 2). Medicare beneficiaries, by race, Hispanic origin, and selected characteristics: United States, selected years 1992–2006

[Data are based on household interviews of a sample of Medicare beneficiaries and Medicare administrative records]

| | All | | | Not Hispanic or Latino | | | | | | Hispanic or Latino | | |
| | | | | White | | | Black or African American | | | | | |
Characteristic	1992	2005	2006	1992	2005	2006	1992	2005	2006	1992	2005	2006
	Number of beneficiaries in millions											
All Medicare beneficiaries	36.8	43.4	43.8	30.9	34.0	34.4	3.3	4.1	4.0	1.9	3.3	3.4
	Percent distribution of beneficiaries											
All Medicare beneficiaries	100.0	100.0	100.0	84.2	78.4	78.4	8.9	9.4	9.1	5.2	7.5	7.8
Medical care use	Percent of beneficiaries with at least one service											
All Medicare beneficiaries:												
Long-term care facility stay	7.7	8.5	8.9	8.0	9.1	9.6	6.2	8.6	8.8	4.2	4.8	5.1
Community-only residents:												
Inpatient hospital.	17.9	17.4	16.7	18.1	17.2	16.2	18.4	19.6	20.0	16.6	17.9	17.1
Outpatient hospital	57.9	74.7	74.7	57.8	75.1	74.9	61.1	73.3	76.8	53.1	72.7	71.4
Physician/supplier[1]	92.4	96.4	97.0	93.0	96.8	97.3	89.1	94.8	96.3	87.9	94.5	95.4
Dental	40.4	45.1	45.6	43.1	49.2	50.0	23.5	22.6	25.2	29.1	33.6	33.1
Prescription medicine	85.2	93.4	94.0	85.5	93.6	94.2	83.1	91.9	92.6	84.6	92.8	94.2
Expenditures	Expenditures per beneficiary											
All Medicare beneficiaries:												
Total health care[2]	$6,716	$14,246	$15,622	$6,816	$14,166	$15,587	$7,043	$16,668	$17,865	$5,784	$13,432	$13,503
Long-term care facility[3]	1,581	2,440	2,566	1,674	2,578	2,729	1,255	2,797	3,035	*758	1,209	986
Community-only residents:												
Total personal health care	5,054	10,597	11,756	4,988	10,499	11,483	5,530	11,373	13,370	4,938	10,938	11,814
Inpatient hospital	2,098	2,566	2,504	2,058	2,534	2,410	2,493	3,136	3,299	1,999	2,103	2,764
Outpatient hospital	504	1,364	1,233	478	1,300	1,172	668	1,578	1,577	511	1,762	1,482
Physician/supplier[1]	1,524	3,125	3,375	1,525	3,128	3,289	1,398	3,155	3,601	1,587	3,430	2,927
Dental	142	327	355	153	354	391	70	203	164	97	214	285
Prescription medicine	468	2,277	3,002	481	2,341	3,014	417	2,118	2,896	389	1,914	2,999
Long-term care facility residents only:												
Long-term care facility[4]	23,054	38,277	39,361	23,177	37,597	38,681	21,272	45,594	43,841	*25,026	*36,913	*49,417
Sex	Percent distribution of beneficiaries											
Both sexes	100.0	100.0	100.0	100.0	100.0	100.0	100.0	100.0	100.0	100.0	100.0	100.0
Male	42.9	44.3	44.4	42.7	44.3	44.5	42.0	41.6	40.2	46.7	46.1	46.9
Female.	57.1	55.7	55.6	57.3	55.7	55.5	58.0	58.4	59.8	53.3	53.9	53.1
Eligibility criteria and age												
All Medicare beneficiaries[5]	100.0	100.0	100.0	100.0	100.0	100.0	100.0	100.0	100.0	100.0	100.0	100.0
Disabled.	10.2	15.6	16.0	8.6	13.1	13.7	19.1	29.3	29.5	16.5	22.6	21.7
Under 45 years	3.5	3.8	3.8	2.9	3.0	3.1	7.6	8.2	7.9	6.9	5.6	4.9
45–64 years	6.5	11.8	12.2	5.8	10.1	10.6	11.5	21.1	21.6	9.6	17.0	16.8
Aged	89.8	84.4	84.1	91.4	86.9	86.2	81.0	70.7	70.5	83.5	77.5	78.4
65–74 years	51.5	43.4	43.2	52.0	43.2	42.6	48.0	40.5	40.2	49.4	46.5	47.7
75–84 years	28.8	29.8	29.4	29.5	31.6	31.2	24.0	22.0	21.3	27.1	23.4	23.0
85 years and over	9.7	11.2	11.5	9.9	12.1	12.4	9.0	8.2	9.0	6.9	7.6	7.7
Living arrangement												
All living arrangements	100.0	100.0	100.0	100.0	100.0	100.0	100.0	100.0	100.0	100.0	100.0	100.0
Alone.	27.0	28.5	28.4	27.5	29.3	29.0	27.7	31.8	32.4	20.2	21.2	22.8
With spouse	51.2	48.9	49.1	53.3	51.6	51.8	33.3	26.3	27.6	50.4	46.0	44.3
With children.	9.1	10.4	10.0	7.7	8.1	7.8	16.8	20.3	19.0	16.6	19.3	17.5
With others.	7.6	7.8	8.0	6.2	6.2	6.6	18.1	17.0	15.5	10.8	11.4	13.1
Long-term care facility	5.1	4.4	4.5	5.3	4.8	4.8	4.0	4.5	5.4	*2.0	*2.1	*2.2

See footnotes at end of table.

[Data are based on household interviews of a sample of Medicare beneficiaries and Medicare administrative records]

| | All | | | Not Hispanic or Latino | | | | | | Hispanic or Latino | | |
| | | | | White | | | Black or African American | | | | | |
Characteristic	1992	2005	2006	1992	2005	2006	1992	2005	2006	1992	2005	2006
Age and limitation of activity[6]						Percent distribution of beneficiaries						
Disabled, under age 65	100.0	100.0	100.0	100.0	100.0	100.0	100.0	100.0	100.0	100.0	100.0	100.0
None	22.7	29.1	30.5	21.8	28.7	30.2	26.2	35.6	37.4	21.2	22.8	25.0
IADL only	39.0	36.3	36.6	38.9	35.9	36.2	35.8	39.6	37.0	46.1	38.8	37.1
1 or 2 ADL	21.2	21.2	19.6	21.5	21.2	20.3	21.2	*15.8	16.3	*20.9	*22.5	*19.2
3–5 ADL	17.2	13.4	13.3	17.9	14.2	13.4	*16.8	*9.0	*9.3	*11.9	*16.0	*18.7
65–74 years	100.0	100.0	100.0	100.0	100.0	100.0	100.0	100.0	100.0	100.0	100.0	100.0
None	67.0	72.2	72.2	68.7	73.6	74.1	55.1	65.8	66.5	59.2	66.0	64.6
IADL only	17.8	14.7	14.9	17.0	14.1	14.6	22.9	15.7	16.0	*20.9	18.7	13.8
1 or 2 ADL	10.4	9.1	8.6	9.6	8.7	8.0	14.4	13.3	*11.3	*15.7	*8.4	*11.4
3–5 ADL	4.8	4.0	4.2	4.6	3.6	3.3	*7.6	*5.2	*6.2	*4.2	*6.8	*10.2
75–84 years	100.0	100.0	100.0	100.0	100.0	100.0	100.0	100.0	100.0	100.0	100.0	100.0
None	46.6	55.6	55.0	47.5	56.7	55.9	42.0	46.2	51.0	44.3	53.6	51.5
IADL only	23.9	21.6	21.8	23.6	21.0	22.0	26.7	25.5	17.0	*27.8	21.6	21.8
1 or 2 ADL	16.5	13.5	13.4	16.8	13.8	13.1	15.3	*10.0	*14.7	*14.9	*12.6	*13.6
3–5 ADL	13.0	9.4	9.8	12.2	8.5	9.0	*15.9	18.3	*17.3	*13.0	*12.2	*13.1
85 years and over	100.0	100.0	100.0	100.0	100.0	100.0	100.0	100.0	100.0	100.0	100.0	100.0
None	19.9	28.1	29.5	20.2	29.1	30.7	*19.6	*23.4	*25.1	*19.7	*26.5	*20.8
IADL only	20.9	25.0	24.4	20.2	25.2	23.8	*22.1	*26.0	*32.2	*24.7	*20.9	*23.7
1 or 2 ADL	23.5	20.2	20.2	23.5	20.2	20.6	*24.3	*15.3	*12.1	*23.7	*22.2	*22.8
3–5 ADL	35.8	26.7	25.8	36.1	25.5	24.9	*34.0	35.3	*30.7	*31.8	*30.4	*32.7

* Estimates are based on 50 persons or fewer or with a relative standard error of 30% or higher and are considered unreliable.

[1]Physician/supplier services include medical and osteopathic doctor and health practitioner visits, diagnostic laboratory and radiology services, medical and surgical services, and durable medical equipment and nondurable medical supplies.

[2]Total health care expenditures by Medicare beneficiaries, including expenses paid by Medicare and all other sources of payment for the following services: inpatient hospital, outpatient hospital, physician/supplier, dental, prescription medicine, home health, and hospice and long-term care facility care. Does not include health insurance premiums.

[3]Expenditures for long-term care in facilities for all beneficiaries include facility room and board expenses for beneficiaries who resided in a facility for the full year, for beneficiaries who resided in a facility for part of the year and in the community for part of the year, and expenditures for short-term facility stays for full-year or part-year community residents. See Appendix II, Long-term care facility.

[4]Expenditures for facility-based long-term care for facility-based beneficiaries include facility room and board expenses for beneficiaries who resided in a facility for the full year and for beneficiaries who resided in a facility for part of the year and in the community for part of the year. It does not include expenditures for short-term facility stays for full-year community residents. See Appendix II, Long-term care facility.

[5]Medicare beneficiaries with end-stage renal disease (ESRD) are included within the subgroups Aged and Disabled. In 2006, less than 1% of Medicare beneficiaries qualified because of ESRD.

[6]Includes data for both community and long-term care facility residents. See Appendix II for definitions of Activities of daily living (ADLs) and Instrumental activities of daily living (IADLs).

NOTES: Percentages and percent distributions are calculated using unrounded numbers. Expenditures include expenses for Medicare beneficiaries paid by Medicare and all other sources of payment. Data for additional years are available. See Appendix III.

SOURCE: Centers for Medicare & Medicaid Services, Medicare Current Beneficiary Survey, Cost and Use file, Health and Health Care of the Medicare Population. Available from: http://www.cms.hhs.gov/mcbs. and unpublished data.

Table 143. Medicaid beneficiaries and payments, by basis of eligibility, and race and Hispanic origin: United States, selected fiscal years 1999–2008

[Data are compiled by the Centers for Medicare & Medicaid Services from the Medicaid Data System]

Basis of eligibility and race and Hispanic origin	1999	2000	2002	2003	2004	2005	2006	2007	2008
Beneficiaries[1]	Number in millions								
All beneficiaries	40.1	42.8	49.3	52.0	55.6	57.3	57.8	56.8	58.2
	Percent of beneficiaries								
Basis of eligibility:									
Aged (65 years and over).	9.4	8.7	7.9	7.8	7.8	7.6	7.6	7.1	7.1
Blind and disabled.	16.7	16.1	15.0	14.8	14.6	14.2	14.4	14.8	14.8
Adults in families with dependent children[2].	18.7	20.5	22.8	22.5	22.5	21.7	21.9	21.8	22.0
Children under age 21[3]	46.9	46.1	47.1	47.8	47.8	47.2	48.0	48.4	47.8
Other Title XIX[4].	8.4	8.6	7.2	7.2	7.3	9.2	8.1	7.8	8.4
Race and Hispanic origin:[5]									
White	- - -	- - -	40.9	41.2	41.1	39.1	39.1	38.6	38.0
Black or African American.	- - -	- - -	22.8	22.4	22.1	21.6	21.8	21.6	21.3
American Indian or Alaska Native	- - -	- - -	1.3	1.4	1.3	1.2	1.2	1.2	1.3
Asian or Pacific Islander.	- - -	- - -	3.4	3.3	3.3	3.5	3.5	3.5	3.3
Hispanic or Latino	- - -	- - -	19.0	19.3	19.4	20.7	21.0	21.6	21.8
Multiple race or unknown	- - -	- - -	12.6	12.5	12.7	13.9	13.3	13.5	14.4
Payments[6]	Amount in billions								
All payments	$ 153.5	$ 168.3	$ 213.5	$ 233.2	$ 257.7	$ 273.2	$ 269.0	$ 276.2	$ 294.2
	Percent distribution								
Total	100.0	100.0	100.0	100.0	100.0	100.0	100.0	100.0	100.0
Basis of eligibility:									
Aged (65 years and over).	27.7	26.4	24.4	23.7	23.1	23.0	21.6	20.7	20.7
Blind and disabled.	42.9	43.2	43.3	43.7	43.3	43.4	43.3	43.3	43.6
Adults in families with dependent children[2].	10.3	10.6	11.0	11.5	12.0	11.8	12.3	12.4	12.7
Children under age 21[3]	15.7	15.9	16.8	17.1	17.2	17.1	18.8	19.4	19.3
Other Title XIX[4].	3.4	3.9	4.5	4.0	4.5	4.6	3.9	4.2	3.9
Race and Hispanic origin:[5]									
White	- - -	- - -	54.1	53.8	53.4	52.7	52.1	50.7	50.2
Black or African American.	- - -	- - -	19.6	19.7	19.8	20.0	20.4	20.8	20.8
American Indian or Alaska Native	- - -	- - -	1.1	1.2	1.2	1.2	1.2	1.2	1.3
Asian or Pacific Islander.	- - -	- - -	2.8	2.4	2.5	2.7	2.8	2.8	2.7
Hispanic or Latino	- - -	- - -	9.7	10.6	10.7	12.2	12.8	13.1	13.7
Multiple race or unknown	- - -	- - -	12.6	12.2	12.3	11.2	10.8	11.4	11.3
Payments per beneficiary[6]	Amount								
All beneficiaries	$ 3,819	$ 3,936	$ 4,328	$ 4,487	$ 4,639	$ 4,764	$ 4,657	$ 4,862	$ 5,051
Basis of eligibility:									
Aged (65 years and over).	11,268	11,929	13,370	13,677	13,687	14,402	13,276	14,141	14,766
Blind and disabled.	9,832	10,559	12,470	13,303	13,714	14,536	13,982	14,194	14,839
Adults in families with dependent children[2].	2,104	2,030	2,093	2,292	2,471	2,585	2,622	2,753	2,912
Children under age 21[3]	1,282	1,358	1,545	1,606	1,664	1,729	1,825	1,951	2,036
Other Title XIX[4].	1,532	1,778	2,718	2,474	2,896	2,383	2,255	2,622	2,335
Race and Hispanic origin:[5]									
White	- - -	- - -	5,721	5,870	6,026	6,429	6,199	6,390	6,674
Black or African American.	- - -	- - -	3,733	3,944	4,158	4,398	4,358	4,669	4,929
American Indian or Alaska Native	- - -	- - -	3,774	4,001	4,320	4,627	4,489	4,826	5,229
Asian or Pacific Islander.	- - -	- - -	3,562	3,327	3,513	3,712	3,696	3,863	4,120
Hispanic or Latino	- - -	- - -	2,215	2,463	2,563	2,822	2,831	2,960	3,177
Multiple race or unknown	- - -	- - -	4,338	4,396	4,493	3,816	3,770	4,106	3,979

- - - Data not available.

[1]Beneficiaries include Medicaid enrollees who received services and those enrolled in managed care plans.

[2]Includes adults who meet the requirements for the Aid to Families with Dependent Children (AFDC) program that were in effect in their state on July 16, 1996, or, at state option, more liberal criteria (with some exceptions). Includes adults in the Temporary Assistance for Needy Families (TANF) program. Starting with 2001 data, includes women in the Breast and Cervical Cancer Prevention and Treatment Program and unemployed adults. For more information on the eligibility requirements, see Appendix II, Medicaid.

[3]Includes children (including those in the foster care system) in the TANF program. For more information on the eligibility requirements, see Appendix II, Medicaid.

[4]Includes some participants in the Supplemental Security Income program and other people deemed medically needy in participating states. Prior to 2001, includes unemployed adults. Excludes foster care children and includes unknown eligibility.

[5]Race and Hispanic origin are as determined on initial Medicaid application. Categories are mutually exclusive. Starting with 2001 data, the Hispanic category included Hispanic persons, regardless of race. Persons indicating more than one race were included in the multiple race category.

[6]Medicaid payments exclude disproportionate share hospital (DSH) payments ($10.7 billion in FY2008) and DSH mental health facility payments ($1.9 billion in FY2008).

NOTES: Data are for fiscal year ending September 30. See Appendix II, Medicaid; Medicaid payments. See Appendix I, Medicaid Statistical Information System (MSIS). For more information, see: http://www.cms.gov/MSIS/Downloads/msisdd2010.pdf. Hawaii and Utah had not reported 2008 data as of the date accessed. Some data have been revised and differ from previous editions of *Health, United States*. Data for additional years are available. See Appendix III.

SOURCE: Centers for Medicare & Medicaid Services, Center for Medicaid and State Operations, Medicaid Statistical Information System (MSIS). MSIS data for 2001–2008 were accessed on July 6, 2010.

Table 144. Medicaid beneficiaries and payments, by type of service: United States, selected fiscal years 1999–2008

[Data are compiled by the Centers for Medicare & Medicaid Services from the Medicaid Data System]

Type of service	1999	2000	2002	2003	2004	2005	2006	2007	2008
Beneficiaries [1]	Number in millions								
All beneficiaries	40.2	42.8	49.3	52.0	55.6	57.3	57.5	56.8	58.2
	Percent of beneficiaries								
Inpatient hospital	11.2	11.5	10.2	10.0	9.8	9.5	10.9	9.0	9.0
Mental health facility	0.2	0.2	0.2	0.2	0.2	0.2	0.2	0.2	0.2
Mentally retarded intermediate care facility	0.3	0.3	0.2	0.2	0.2	0.2	0.2	0.2	0.2
Nursing facility	4.0	4.0	3.6	3.3	3.1	3.0	3.0	2.9	2.8
Physician	45.7	44.7	44.7	44.0	43.1	41.9	40.2	38.8	37.0
Dental	14.0	13.8	16.0	16.4	16.2	16.1	16.4	16.8	16.6
Other practitioner	9.9	11.1	11.3	11.1	10.7	10.2	10.1	9.5	8.8
Outpatient hospital	30.9	30.9	30.1	29.8	28.7	28.2	27.6	26.2	25.2
Clinic	16.8	17.9	19.2	19.6	20.0	20.6	20.5	20.6	20.1
Laboratory and radiological	25.4	26.6	28.5	28.3	28.9	27.7	28.0	27.8	26.6
Home health	2.0	2.3	2.2	2.3	2.1	2.1	2.1	2.1	1.9
Prescribed drugs	49.4	48.0	49.4	50.2	50.3	49.1	47.1	42.1	41.8
Capitated care	51.5	49.7	51.7	53.1	54.2	58.4	61.0	64.5	64.8
Primary care case management	9.7	13.0	14.6	14.5	15.4	14.9	14.8	12.5	15.0
Personal support	10.1	10.6	11.5	11.6	11.3	11.8	11.8	11.6	10.9
Other care [2]	21.6	21.4	22.6	23.1	22.9	21.8	21.6	21.5	21.3
Payments [3]	Amount in billions								
All payments	$ 153.5	$ 168.3	$ 213.5	$ 233.2	$ 257.7	$ 273.2	$ 267.4	$ 276.2	$ 294.2
	Percent distribution								
Total	100.0	100.0	100.0	100.0	100.0	100.0	100.0	100.0	100.0
Inpatient hospital	14.5	14.4	13.6	13.5	13.5	12.8	13.5	13.4	12.5
Mental health facility	1.1	1.1	1.0	0.9	0.9	0.8	0.9	0.9	0.8
Mentally retarded intermediate care facility	6.1	5.6	5.0	4.7	4.3	4.3	4.4	4.3	4.2
Nursing facility	21.7	20.5	18.4	17.3	16.3	16.3	17.0	16.8	16.1
Physician	4.3	4.0	3.9	3.9	4.0	4.1	3.9	3.6	3.5
Dental	0.8	0.8	1.1	1.1	1.1	1.1	1.2	1.2	1.3
Other practitioner	0.3	0.4	0.4	0.4	0.4	0.4	0.4	0.3	0.3
Outpatient hospital	4.0	4.2	4.0	4.0	4.0	3.6	3.8	3.7	3.7
Clinic	3.8	3.7	3.1	3.1	3.2	3.2	3.2	3.1	3.0
Laboratory and radiological	0.8	0.8	1.0	1.0	1.0	1.1	1.1	1.1	1.0
Home health	1.9	1.9	1.8	1.9	1.8	2.0	2.2	2.3	2.2
Prescribed drugs	10.8	11.9	13.3	14.5	15.3	15.6	10.4	8.0	7.9
Capitated care	14.0	14.5	15.8	16.0	16.5	17.0	18.8	21.2	23.0
Primary care case management	0.3	0.1	0.1	0.1	0.2	0.1	0.1	0.1	0.1
Personal support	6.9	6.9	7.2	7.4	7.2	7.5	8.0	8.4	8.3
Other care [2]	8.6	8.8	10.3	10.2	10.3	10.1	11.1	11.6	12.0
Payments per beneficiary [3]	Amount								
Total payment per beneficiary	$ 3,819	$ 3,936	$ 4,328	$ 4,487	$ 4,639	$ 4,764	$ 4,654	$ 4,862	$ 5,051
Inpatient hospital	4,943	4,919	5,771	6,047	6,424	6,401	5,781	7,191	7,070
Mental health facility	18,094	17,800	21,377	20,503	19,928	19,232	17,156	21,407	21,848
Mentally retarded intermediate care facility	76,443	79,330	91,588	95,287	97,497	107,135	110,340	113,735	123,501
Nursing facility	20,568	20,220	22,326	23,882	24,475	26,096	26,531	28,282	29,493
Physician	357	356	378	403	426	467	456	457	485
Dental	214	238	293	305	318	327	329	340	390
Other practitioner	118	139	151	154	160	201	196	170	171
Outpatient hospital	491	533	571	596	639	615	642	695	734
Clinic	860	805	706	720	750	749	731	741	765
Laboratory and radiological	114	113	154	161	168	183	185	185	188
Home health	3,571	3,135	3,689	3,720	3,978	4,493	4,977	5,334	5,684
Prescribed drugs	837	975	1,165	1,293	1,411	1,510	1,030	926	957
Capitated care	1,040	1,148	1,318	1,357	1,415	1,386	1,431	1,598	1,791
Primary care case management	119	30	28	28	58	27	29	33	32
Personal support	2,583	2,543	2,704	2,864	2,946	3,041	3,160	3,534	3,865
Other care [2]	1,508	1,600	1,963	1,975	2,086	2,208	2,388	2,611	2,836

[1]Beneficiaries include Medicaid enrollees who received services and those enrolled in managed care plans.
[2]Unknown services (0.2% of beneficiaries and 0.4% of payments in 2008) are included with Other care.
[3]Medicaid payments exclude disproportionate share hospital (DSH) payments ($10.7 billion in FY2008) and DSH mental health facility payments ($1.9 billion in FY2008).

NOTES: Data are for fiscal year ending September 30. See Appendix II, Medicaid; Medicaid payments. See Appendix I, Medicaid Statistical Information System (MSIS). Beneficiaries receiving more than one type of service are included in each category. For more information on types of services, see: http://www.cms.gov/MSIS/Downloads/msisdd2010.pdf. Hawaii and Utah had not reported 2008 data as of the date accessed. Data for additional years are available. See Appendix III.

SOURCE: Centers for Medicare & Medicaid Services, Center for Medicaid and State Operations, Medicaid Statistical Information System (MSIS). MSIS data for 2007–2008 were accessed on July 2, 2010.

Table 145 (page 1 of 2). Department of Veterans Affairs health care expenditures and use, and persons treated, by selected characteristics: United States, selected fiscal years 1970–2009

[Data are compiled from patient records, enrollment information, and budgetary data by the Department of Veterans Affairs]

Type of expenditure and use	1970	1980	1990	1995	2000	2005[1]	2007[1]	2008[1]	2009[1]
Health care expenditures				Amount in millions					
All expenditures[2]	$1,689	$ 5,981	$11,500	$16,126	$19,327	$30,291	$34,025	$38,282	$42,955
				Percent distribution					
All services	100.0	100.0	100.0	100.0	100.0	100.0	100.0	100.0	100.0
Inpatient hospital	71.3	64.3	57.5	49.0	37.3	24.3	24.0	23.5	22.7
Outpatient care	14.0	19.1	25.3	30.2	45.7	53.4	53.5	53.2	53.5
Nursing home care	5.5	7.1	9.5	10.0	8.2	8.4	8.3	8.1	7.8
All other[3]	9.1	9.6	7.7	10.8	8.8	13.9	14.2	15.2	16.0
Health care use				Number in thousands					
Inpatient hospital discharges[4,5]	787	1,248	1,029	879	579	614	607	622	640
Outpatient visits[6]	7,312	17,971	22,602	27,527	38,370	57,169	62,234	66,484	73,969
Nursing home discharges[5,7]	47	57	75	79	91	61	63	64	65
Inpatients[8]									
Total	- - -	- - -	598	527	417	488	477	492	512
				Percent distribution					
Total	- - -	- - -	100.0	100.0	100.0	100.0	100.0	100.0	100.0
Veterans with service-connected disability	- - -	- - -	38.9	39.3	34.4	37.6	39.9	41.1	42.6
Veterans without service-connected disability	- - -	- - -	60.3	59.9	64.7	61.5	59.1	58.0	56.4
Low income	- - -	- - -	54.8	56.2	41.7	39.9	36.9	35.4	34.8
Veterans receiving aid and attendance or housebound benefits or who are catastrophically disabled[9]	- - -	- - -	- - -	- - -	16.0	12.1	11.3	11.1	10.5
Veterans receiving medical care subject to copayments[10]	- - -	- - -	2.8	2.8	5.2	8.6	9.8	10.0	9.5
Other and unknown[11]	- - -	- - -	2.7	0.9	1.8	1.0	1.0	1.6	1.6
Nonveterans	- - -	- - -	0.8	0.8	0.9	0.9	0.9	0.9	1.0
Outpatients[8]				Number in thousands					
Total	- - -	- - -	2,564	2,790	3,657	5,077	5,221	5,291	5,439
				Percent distribution					
Total	- - -	- - -	100.0	100.0	100.0	100.0	100.0	100.0	100.0
Veterans with service-connected disability	- - -	- - -	38.3	37.5	30.7	31.6	33.8	34.7	37.1
Veterans without service-connected disability	- - -	- - -	49.8	50.5	60.8	62.7	60.8	59.7	57.2
Low income	- - -	- - -	41.1	42.2	37.6	31.8	28.9	27.2	25.9
Veterans receiving aid and attendance or housebound benefits or who are catastrophically disabled[9]	- - -	- - -	- - -	- - -	3.8	3.5	3.5	3.5	3.4
Veterans receiving medical care subject to copayments[10]	- - -	- - -	3.6	4.2	15.4	25.4	25.5	25.2	23.8
Other and unknown[11]	- - -	- - -	5.1	4.1	4.0	2.0	3.0	3.8	4.0
Nonveterans	- - -	- - -	11.8	12.0	8.5	5.7	5.4	5.7	5.7

See footnotes at end of table.

Table 145 (page 2 of 2). Department of Veterans Affairs health care expenditures and use, and persons treated, by selected characteristics: United States, selected fiscal years 1970–2009

[Data are compiled from patient records, enrollment information, and budgetary data by the Department of Veterans Affairs]

- - - Data not available.

[1]Starting with FY2005, the cost report data are taken from a different report than earlier years. The major impact of this change was to assign more cost to outpatient care than inpatient hospital. Also in FY2005, the responsibility for residential rehabilitation programs including domiciliary care was reassigned from extended care to mental health care.

[2]Health care expenditures exclude construction, medical administration, and miscellaneous operating expenses at Department of Veterans Affairs headquarters.

[3]Includes miscellaneous benefits and services, contract hospitals, education and training, subsidies to state veterans hospitals, nursing homes and residential rehabilitation treatment programs (formerly domiciliaries), and the Civilian Health and Medical Program of the Department of Veterans Affairs.

[4]Discharges from medicine, surgery, psychiatry, rehabilitation medicine, spinal cord, and neurology units. Starting with FY2005 data, includes domiciliary care. Does not include long-term stays. One-day dialysis patients were included in 1980. Interfacility transfers were included starting with 1990 data.

[5]Until FY2004, includes Department of Veterans Affairs nursing home and residential rehabilitation treatment programs (formerly domiciliary) stays, and community nursing home care stays.

[6]Hospital outpatient care. Includes the following services: physicians, lab tests, home-based primary care, or outpatient fee-basis care.

[7]Includes state nursing home veteran patients.

[8]Individuals receiving services. Individuals with multiple discharges or visits are only counted once in the inpatient or outpatient category. The inpatient and outpatient totals are not additive because most inpatients are also treated as outpatients.

[9]Includes veterans who are receiving aid and attendance or housebound benefit and veterans who have been determined by the Department of Veterans Affairs to be catastrophically disabled.

[10]Includes veterans who receive medical care subject to copayments according to income level, based on financial means testing.

[11]Includes expenditures for services for veterans who were prisoners of war, exposed to Agent Orange, and other. Prior to FY1994, veterans who reported exposure to Agent Orange were classified as having a service-connected disability. Beginning in FY1994, those veterans reporting Agent Orange exposure but not treated for it were means tested and placed in the low income or other group depending on income.

NOTES: Estimates only relate to health care use paid for by the Veteran's Administration. In 1980 and subsequent years, the FY ended September 30. Starting with FY1995 data, categories for health care expenditures and health care use were revised. In FY1999, a new data reporting system was introduced. At the end of FY2009, the veteran population was estimated at 23.1 million, with 40% age 65 and over, compared with 11% in FY1980. Of all living veterans, 10% had served during World War II, 11% during the Korean conflict, 33% during the Vietnam era, 24% during the Persian Gulf War (service from August 2, 1990 to present), and 26% during peacetime. These percentages sum to more than 100% because some veterans serve during more than one war. These data are from the U.S. Department of Veterans Affairs. See Appendix I, Department of Veterans Affairs, National Patient Care Database, Patient Treatment File, and National Enrollment Database. Data for additional years are available. See Appendix III.

SOURCE: Department of Veterans Affairs (VA), Office of the Assistant Deputy Under Secretary for Health, National Patient Care Database, National Enrollment Database, budgetary data, and unpublished data. Veteran population estimates were provided by the VA's Office of the Actuary.

Table 146 (page 1 of 2). Medicare enrollees, enrollees in managed care, payment per enrollee, and short-stay hospital utilization, by state: United States, selected years 1994–2008

[Data are compiled by the Centers for Medicare & Medicaid Services]

| | | | | | | | Short-stay hospital utilization | | | |
| | Enrollment in thousands[1] | | Percent of enrollees in managed care[2] | | Payment per fee-for-service enrollee | | Discharges per 1,000 enrollees[3] | | Average length of stay in days[3] | |
State	1994	2008	1994	2008	1994	2008	1994	2008	1994	2008
United States[4].	36,190	44,385	7.9	21.9	$4,375	$8,649	345	343	7.5	5.6
Alabama.	633	809	0.8	18.9	4,454	8,306	413	412	7.0	5.4
Alaska.	33	60	0.6	1.0	3,687	7,043	269	229	6.3	5.7
Arizona.	578	870	24.8	36.0	4,442	7,945	292	298	5.9	5.0
Arkansas.	416	509	0.2	12.2	3,719	7,528	366	346	7.0	5.5
California.	3,582	4,492	30.0	34.1	5,219	8,862	366	289	6.1	5.8
Colorado	413	579	17.2	32.1	3,935	7,496	302	284	6.0	4.9
Connecticut	497	549	2.6	14.4	4,426	9,419	287	338	8.1	5.8
Delaware.	99	141	0.2	4.1	4,712	8,959	326	337	8.1	6.2
District of Columbia	80	75	3.9	10.0	5,655	10,215	376	396	10.1	6.9
Florida.	2,584	3,212	13.8	27.0	5,027	10,317	326	355	7.1	5.7
Georgia.	819	1,153	0.4	12.9	4,402	7,857	378	328	6.9	5.6
Hawaii.	146	194	29.8	37.2	3,069	5,531	301	201	9.1	6.9
Idaho	146	214	2.5	24.6	3,045	6,494	274	210	5.2	4.8
Illinois	1,605	1,775	5.5	9.3	4,324	8,893	374	396	7.3	5.4
Indiana	805	964	2.6	12.8	3,945	8,202	345	341	6.9	5.4
Iowa	470	506	3.1	11.8	3,080	6,842	322	285	6.6	5.2
Kansas	378	418	3.3	9.3	3,847	7,864	348	319	6.5	5.3
Kentucky	578	728	2.3	13.7	3,862	8,044	396	380	7.2	5.5
Louisiana.	572	656	0.4	20.4	5,468	9,894	399	385	7.2	5.7
Maine	198	253	0.1	5.7	3,464	6,937	322	266	7.6	5.4
Maryland.	596	745	1.4	7.2	4,997	10,092	362	402	7.5	5.1
Massachusetts.	924	1,019	6.1	18.6	5,147	9,115	350	360	7.6	5.4
Michigan	1,331	1,580	0.7	21.9	4,307	9,448	328	384	7.6	5.6
Minnesota	625	749	19.6	34.2	3,394	7,895	334	345	5.7	4.9
Mississippi.	391	479	0.1	8.5	4,189	9,089	423	398	7.4	5.9
Missouri.	821	966	3.4	18.3	4,191	8,052	349	365	7.3	5.4
Montana	128	160	0.4	15.0	3,114	6,414	306	248	5.9	4.7
Nebraska.	247	271	2.2	11.3	2,926	7,509	281	286	6.3	5.2
Nevada	187	330	19.0	30.2	4,306	8,249	291	292	7.0	5.8
New Hampshire	152	212	0.2	5.2	3,414	7,469	281	255	7.6	5.7
New Jersey	1,158	1,283	2.6	10.5	4,531	9,974	354	373	10.2	6.2
New Mexico.	205	294	13.6	22.8	3,110	6,782	301	261	6.0	5.1
New York.	2,601	2,891	6.2	27.0	4,855	9,545	334	367	11.2	7.1
North Carolina	1,001	1,405	0.5	16.1	3,465	7,853	314	332	8.0	5.5
North Dakota	101	107	0.6	7.7	3,218	7,152	327	267	6.3	5.2
Ohio	1,649	1,841	2.4	25.2	3,982	8,780	350	388	7.1	5.3
Oklahoma	481	578	2.5	13.4	4,098	8,498	355	381	7.0	5.3
Oregon	469	584	27.7	40.3	3,285	6,176	305	225	5.2	4.9
Pennsylvania.	2,053	2,221	3.3	36.7	5,212	8,711	379	388	8.0	5.7
Rhode Island	166	178	7.0	35.7	4,118	8,086	312	335	8.1	5.9
South Carolina	497	724	0.1	13.4	3,777	7,972	319	328	8.3	5.9
South Dakota.	114	132	0.1	9.8	2,952	6,307	356	257	6.1	5.0
Tennessee.	754	1,004	0.3	20.4	4,441	8,103	375	380	7.1	5.4
Texas	2,029	2,802	4.1	17.0	4,703	9,769	333	344	7.2	5.6
Utah	182	264	9.4	27.3	3,443	7,059	238	237	5.4	4.6
Vermont	82	105	0.1	3.2	3,182	7,114	283	207	7.6	5.4
Virginia	803	1,079	1.5	12.2	3,748	7,320	348	325	7.3	5.6
Washington	676	903	12.5	22.0	3,401	6,958	269	248	5.3	4.9
West Virginia	326	373	8.3	22.3	3,798	7,659	420	368	7.1	5.8
Wisconsin	752	874	2.0	24.4	3,246	7,532	310	299	6.8	5.1
Wyoming.	58	76	3.3	5.4	3,537	6,397	315	260	5.6	4.8

See footnotes at end of table.

Table 146 (page 2 of 2). Medicare enrollees, enrollees in managed care, payment per enrollee, and short-stay hospital utilization, by state: United States, selected years 1994–2008

[Data are compiled by the Centers for Medicare & Medicaid Services]

[1]Total persons enrolled in hospital insurance, supplementary medical insurance, or both, as of July 1. Includes fee-for-service and managed care enrollees.
[2]Includes enrollees in Medicare-approved managed care organizations. See Appendix II, Managed care.
[3]Data are for fee-for-service enrollees only.
[4]Includes residents of any of the 50 states and the District of Columbia.

NOTES: Prior to 2004, enrollment and percent of enrollees in managed care were based on a 5% annual Denominator File derived from the Centers for Medicare & Medicaid Services' (CMS') Enrollment Database. Starting with 2004 data, the 100% Denominator File was used. Payments per fee-for-service enrollee are based on fee-for-service billing reimbursement for a 5% sample of Medicare beneficiaries as recorded in CMS' National Claims History File. Short-stay hospital utilization is based on the Medicare Provider Analysis and Review (MEDPAR) stay records for a 20% sample of Medicare beneficiaries. Estimates may not sum to totals because of rounding. State based on residence of the beneficiary. Data for additional years are available. See Appendix III.

SOURCE: Centers for Medicare & Medicaid Services, Office of Research, Development, and Information. Health Care Financing Review: Medicare and Medicaid Statistical Supplements for publication years 1996 to 2009. Available from: http://www.cms.hhs.gov/MedicareMedicaidStatSupp/LT/list.asp.

Table 147. Medicaid beneficiaries, beneficiaries in managed care, payments per beneficiary, and beneficiaries per 100 persons below the poverty level, by state: United States, selected fiscal years 1999–2008

[Data are compiled by the Centers for Medicare & Medicaid Services from the Medicaid Data System]

State	Beneficiaries in thousands[1]		Percent of beneficiaries in managed care[2]		Payments per beneficiary[3]			Beneficiaries per 100 persons below the poverty level	
	2000	2008	2000	2008	2000	2007	2008	1999–2000	2007–2008
United States	42,763	58,239	56	70	$3,936	$4,862	$ 5,051	131	149
Alabama	619	830	60	66	3,860	4,703	4,227	88	124
Alaska................	96	119	–	–	4,876	7,789	8,162	180	226
Arizona	681	1,399	92	91	3,100	3,364	4,707	113	116
Arkansas..............	489	827	57	80	3,086	3,365	3,932	113	214
California..............	7,915	10,515	50	52	2,155	2,898	3,067	162	210
Colorado..............	381	626	90	96	4,747	4,412	4,768	107	122
Connecticut	420	524	72	65	6,762	7,665	7,905	184	178
Delaware..............	115	181	79	64	4,584	5,792	6,290	147	218
District of Columbia	139	168	66	63	5,715	9,080	10,338	179	162
Florida................	2,360	2,871	60	63	3,114	4,529	4,606	136	125
Georgia...............	1,290	1,712	96	92	2,774	3,754	4,009	136	123
Hawaii................	204	- - -	74	79	2,626	4,439	- - -	83	- - -
Idaho	131	233	30	83	4,530	5,204	5,419	75	135
Illinois	1,516	2,317	10	55	5,150	4,765	4,418	115	159
Indiana	705	1,126	67	71	4,224	4,669	4,387	148	129
Iowa	314	498	90	82	4,707	5,447	5,401	149	171
Kansas	263	351	56	84	4,670	6,041	6,541	94	104
Kentucky..............	771	893	81	91	3,780	4,946	5,011	158	128
Louisiana..............	761	1,157	6	69	3,456	3,770	4,316	95	158
Maine	192	306	35	63	6,820	4,493	4,435	155	202
Maryland..............	665	757	81	73	5,396	7,153	7,369	170	155
Massachusetts..........	1,047	1,230	64	60	5,153	7,028	7,310	153	169
Michigan..............	1,352	1,790	100	88	3,611	4,128	5,157	135	157
Minnesota	559	763	63	62	5,857	7,922	8,711	178	152
Mississippi............	605	657	39	72	2,987	4,776	4,751	139	114
Missouri..............	890	1,054	40	97	3,673	4,641	4,957	157	138
Montana	104	113	61	36	4,173	5,537	5,792	73	91
Nebraska..............	229	249	77	84	4,185	5,942	6,165	136	137
Nevada	138	249	39	83	3,733	4,259	4,535	70	95
New Hampshire	97	131	6	78	6,712	8,262	7,137	119	154
New Jersey	822	1,065	59	72	5,724	7,176	7,241	128	136
New Mexico............	376	507	64	62	3,325	5,366	6,028	110	153
New York..............	3,420	4,869	25	65	7,646	8,392	8,840	128	176
North Carolina	1,209	1,785	68	67	3,996	5,383	5,000	122	126
North Dakota	61	74	55	58	5,852	6,894	7,442	87	111
Ohio	1,305	2,062	21	72	5,434	5,879	5,850	103	137
Oklahoma	507	765	69	88	3,163	4,182	4,376	106	157
Oregon	542	487	83	91	3,135	4,636	5,047	132	109
Pennsylvania	1,492	2,134	73	81	4,266	5,543	5,857	141	165
Rhode Island	179	204	69	62	5,982	7,830	8,087	187	178
South Carolina..........	685	871	6	94	3,900	4,772	4,990	157	139
South Dakota...........	102	137	93	99	3,935	4,710	4,923	155	152
Tennessee.............	1,568	1,471	100	100	2,226	4,098	4,324	211	159
Texas	2,603	3,993	34	70	3,487	3,781	4,172	85	101
Utah	224	- - -	90	86	4,277	5,748	- - -	132	- - -
Vermont	139	162	47	91	3,451	5,166	5,445	208	275
Virginia	627	839	59	63	3,960	5,473	5,552	115	113
Washington............	895	1,188	100	89	2,717	4,653	4,912	155	175
West Virginia	335	378	35	45	4,154	6,114	6,360	129	142
Wisconsin	577	1,532	44	52	5,039	4,594	2,996	113	218
Wyoming..............	46	69	–	–	4,609	6,472	7,273	84	126

– Quantity zero.

- - - Data not available.

[1]Beneficiaries include Medicaid enrollees who received services and those enrolled in managed care plans.

[2]Medicaid managed care enrollment data include individuals in state health care reform programs that expand eligibility beyond traditional Medicaid eligibility standards. The managed care enrollment data include enrollees receiving comprehensive and limited benefits. Managed care enrollment as of June 30 of year shown. Starting with 2001 data, U.S. total excludes Puerto Rico and Virgin Islands. Managed care enrollment data may change year to year due to a variety of factors, including changes in waiver programs, outreach efforts, and data reporting practices. For more information, see: http://www.cms.gov/medicaiddatasourcesgeninfo/.

[3]Medicaid payments exclude disproportionate share hospital (DSH) payments ($10.7 billion in FY2008) and DSH mental health facility payments ($1.9 billion in FY2008).

NOTES: See Appendix II, Medicaid; Medicaid payments. See Appendix I, Medicaid Statistical Information System (MSIS). Hawaii and Utah had not reported 2008 data as of the date accessed. Some data have been revised and differ from previous editions of Health, United States. Data for additional years are available. See Appendix III.

SOURCE: Centers for Medicare & Medicaid Services, Center for Medicaid and State Operations, Medicaid Statistical Information System (MSIS). MSIS data for 2007–2008 were accessed on July 2, 2010. Poverty populations are available from: Department of Commerce, U.S. Census Bureau, Housing and Household Economic Statistics Division. Available from: http://www.census.gov/hhes/www/cpstables/032009/pov/new46_100125_01.htm. Managed care enrollment data from Medicaid managed care enrollment report as of June 30, 2008. Available from: http://www.cms.gov/MedicaidDataSourcesGenInfo/04_MdManCrEnrllRep.asp.

Table 148. Persons without health insurance coverage, by state: United States, average annual 1995–1997 through 2006–2008

[Data are based on household interviews of a sample of the civilian noninstitutionalized population]

State	1995–1997	1998–2000	2001–2003	2006–2008
	Percent of population			
United States.	15.7	14.4	15.1	15.5
Alabama	14.0	14.2	13.3	13.0
Alaska.	14.7	18.1	17.8	18.2
Arizona	23.0	19.5	17.3	19.6
Arkansas	21.3	15.3	16.6	17.6
California	20.7	19.2	18.7	18.5
Colorado	15.5	14.1	16.3	16.5
Connecticut	10.6	9.5	10.4	9.6
Delaware	14.1	11.2	10.1	11.4
District of Columbia.	16.1	14.5	13.3	10.4
Florida.	18.9	17.2	17.6	20.5
Georgia	17.8	15.2	16.4	17.7
Hawaii	8.3	9.8	9.9	8.1
Idaho.	16.1	16.5	17.5	15.0
Illinois	11.6	13.3	14.0	13.4
Indiana	11.5	11.3	12.9	11.8
Iowa	11.6	8.2	9.5	9.8
Kansas	11.8	11.0	10.9	12.4
Kentucky	15.0	13.1	13.3	15.0
Louisiana	18.8	19.5	19.4	20.1
Maine	13.5	11.5	10.7	9.5
Maryland	13.4	11.9	13.2	13.2
Massachusetts	12.0	9.2	9.6	7.1
Michigan	10.1	10.6	11.0	11.3
Minnesota	9.1	8.2	8.2	8.7
Mississippi	19.4	15.7	17.0	19.1
Missouri.	13.5	9.0	10.9	12.8
Montana	15.3	18.3	16.1	16.3
Nebraska.	10.4	9.5	10.3	12.5
Nevada	17.3	17.5	18.3	18.5
New Hampshire	10.4	8.6	9.9	10.7
New Jersey	15.8	12.9	13.7	15.1
New Mexico	23.5	22.6	21.3	23.0
New York	16.6	15.3	15.5	13.8
North Carolina	15.3	13.7	16.1	16.6
North Dakota	11.1	12.1	10.5	11.4
Ohio	11.6	10.2	11.7	11.1
Oklahoma	18.0	17.7	18.7	16.9
Oregon	13.7	13.7	14.8	17.0
Pennsylvania	9.8	8.3	10.7	9.8
Rhode Island	11.0	6.9	9.3	10.4
South Carolina	16.2	13.8	13.1	16.1
South Dakota	10.2	12.0	11.0	11.5
Tennessee	14.5	10.8	11.8	14.4
Texas	24.4	22.2	24.6	24.9
Utah	12.4	13.2	13.6	14.5
Vermont.	11.3	10.3	9.9	10.2
Virginia	12.9	12.9	12.5	13.5
Washington	12.4	12.8	14.3	11.8
West Virginia	15.8	15.2	14.8	14.2
Wisconsin	7.9	9.3	9.5	8.9
Wyoming	15.0	15.1	16.5	13.9

[1]The 2004 and 2005 data (available in spreadsheet version) were revised in March 2007. Available from: http://www.census.gov/hhes/www/hlthins/data/usernote/index.html.

NOTES: Questions on health insurance coverage are asked of the previous calendar year. Persons were considered uninsured if they were not covered by any type of health insurance at any time in that year. Ninety-percent confidence intervals for selected years are available in the spreadsheet version of this table. Available from: http://www.cdc.gov/nchs/hus.htm. Starting with 1997 data, people with no coverage other than access to the Indian Health Service are no longer considered covered by health insurance. The effect of this change on the estimate of number uninsured is negligible. Starting with 1999 data, estimates reflect the results of follow-up verification questions which decreased the percent uninsured by 1.2 percentage points. See Appendix I, Current Population Survey. Data for additional years are available. See Appendix III.

SOURCE: U.S. Census Bureau, Current Population Survey, Annual Social and Economic Supplements. DeNavas-Walt C, Proctor BD, Smith JC. Income, poverty, and health insurance coverage in the United States: 2008. Current Population Reports, P–60–236. Washington, DC: U.S. Government Printing Office. 2009. Available from: http://www.census.gov/hhes/www/hlthins/data/usernote/index.html.

Appendix Contents

Appendix II: Tables

Appendix II: Figure

Appendix I. Data Sources

Health, United States consolidates the most current data on the health of the population of the United States, the availability and use of health resources, and health care expenditures. Information was obtained from the data files and published reports of many federal government, private, and global agencies and organizations. In each case, the sponsoring agency or organization collected data using its own methods and procedures. Therefore, data in this report may vary considerably with respect to source, method of collection, definitions, and reference period.

Although a detailed description and comprehensive evaluation of each data source are beyond the scope of this appendix, readers should be aware of the general strengths and weaknesses of the different data collection systems. For example, population-based surveys obtain socioeconomic data, data on family characteristics, and information on the impact of an illness, such as days lost from work or limitation of activity. These data are limited by the amount of information a respondent remembers or is willing to report. For example, a respondent may not know detailed medical information, such as a precise diagnosis or the type of procedure performed, and therefore cannot report that information. In contrast, records-based surveys, which collect data from physician and hospital records, usually contain good diagnostic information but little or no information about the socioeconomic characteristics of individuals or the impact of illnesses on individuals.

Different data collection systems may cover different populations, and understanding these differences is critical to interpreting the resulting data. Data on vital statistics and national expenditures cover the entire population. However, most data on morbidity and the utilization of health resources cover only the civilian noninstitutionalized population and thus may not include data for military personnel, who are usually young; for institutionalized people, including the prison population, who may be of any age; or for nursing home residents, who are usually older.

All data collection systems are subject to error, and records may be incomplete or contain inaccurate information. Respondents may not remember essential information, a question may not mean the same thing to different respondents, and some institutions or individuals may not respond at all. It is not always possible to measure the magnitude of these errors or their effect on the data. Where possible, table notes describe the universe and method of data collection to assist users in evaluating data quality.

Some information is collected in more than one survey, and estimates of the same statistic may vary among surveys because of different survey methodologies, sampling frames, questionnaires, definitions, and tabulation categories. For example, cigarette use is measured by the National Health Interview Survey, the National Survey on Drug Use & Health, the Monitoring the Future Survey, and the Youth Risk Behavior Survey. These surveys use slightly different questions, cover persons of differing ages, and interview in diverse settings (e.g., at school compared with at home), so estimates will differ.

Overall estimates generally have relatively small sampling errors, but estimates for certain population subgroups may be based on a small sample size and have relatively large sampling errors. Numbers of births and deaths from the National Vital Statistics System (NVSS) represent complete counts (except for births in those states where data are based on a 50% sample for certain years). Therefore, these data are not subject to sampling error. However, when the figures are used for analytical purposes, such as the comparison of rates over a period, the number of events that actually occurred may be considered as one of a large series of possible results that could have arisen under the same circumstances. When the number of events is small and the probability of such an event is rare, estimates may be unstable, and considerable caution must be used in interpreting the statistics. Estimates that are unreliable because of large sampling errors or small numbers of events are noted with asterisks in tables, and the criteria used to designate unreliable estimates are indicated in an accompanying footnote.

In this appendix, government data sources are listed alphabetically by data set name, and private and global sources are listed separately. To the extent possible, government data systems are described using a standard format. The Overview is a brief, general statement about the purpose or objectives of the data system. The Selected Content section lists major data elements that are collected or estimated using interpolation or modeling. The Data Years section gives the years that the survey or data system has existed or been fielded. The Coverage section describes the population that the data system represents: for example, residents of the United States, the noninstitutionalized population, persons in specific population groups, or other entities that make up the survey. The Methodology section presents a short description of the methods used to collect data. Sample size and response rates are given for surveys. The Issues Affecting Interpretation section describes major changes in the data collection methodology or other factors that must be considered when analyzing trends: for example, a major survey redesign that may introduce a discontinuity in the trend. For additional information about the methodology, data files, and history of a data source, consult the References and For More Information sections that follow each summary.

Government Sources

Abortion Surveillance System

CDC/National Center for Chronic Disease Prevention and Health Promotion (NCCDPHP)

Overview. The Abortion Surveillance Program documents the number and characteristics of women obtaining legal induced abortions, monitors unintended pregnancy, and assists efforts to identify and reduce preventable causes of morbidity and mortality associated with abortions.

Selected Content. Content includes age, race/ethnicity, marital status, previous live births, period of gestation, and previous induced abortions of women obtaining legal induced abortions.

Data Years. Between 1973 and 1997, the number of abortions is based on reporting from 52 reporting areas: 50 states, the District of Columbia, and New York City. In 1998 and 1999, CDC compiled abortion data from 48 reporting areas. Alaska, California, New Hampshire, and Oklahoma did not report, and data for these areas were not estimated. In 2000–2004, CDC compiled data from 49 reporting areas. Alaska, California, and New Hampshire did not report abortion data to CDC in 2000–2002. In 2003 and 2004, California, New Hampshire, and West Virginia did not report. In 2005 and 2006, California, Louisiana, and New Hampshire did not report.

Coverage. The system includes women of all ages, including adolescents, who obtain legal induced abortions.

Methodology. Starting with 2000 data, the number and characteristics of women who obtain legal induced abortions are provided for 49 reporting areas by central health agencies, such as state health departments and the health departments of New York City and the District of Columbia, and by hospitals and other medical facilities. In general, the procedures are reported by the state in which the procedure is performed (i.e., state of occurrence). Although the total number of legal induced abortions is available for those 49 reporting areas, not all areas collect information on the characteristics of women who obtain abortions. The number of areas reporting each characteristic and the number of areas with complete data for each characteristic vary from year to year. For example, in 2005 the number of areas reporting different women's characteristics ranged from 28 areas reporting adequate data for the Office of Management and Budget (OMB) recommended race categories (accounting for 39% of the total number of reported abortions), 30 areas reporting adequate data on Hispanic ethnicity, and 43 areas reporting marital status, to 48 areas reporting age. Data from reporting areas with more than 15% unknown for a given characteristic are excluded from the analysis of that characteristic.

Issues Affecting Interpretation. The drug mifepristone for medical abortion was approved in September 2000 by the U.S. Food and Drug Administration (FDA) for distribution and use in the United States. The percentage of medical abortions increased from 1% in 2000 to 10% in 2005. Between 1989 and 1997, the total number of abortions reported to CDC was about 10% less than the total estimated independently by the Guttmacher Institute (previously, the Alan Guttmacher Institute, or AGI), a not-for-profit organization for reproductive health research, policy analysis, and public education. Between 1998 and 2005, the total number of abortions reported to CDC was about 34% less than the total estimated by Guttmacher. The three reporting areas (the largest of which was California) that did not report abortions to CDC in 2005 accounted for 18% of all abortions tallied by Guttmacher's 2005 survey. (Also see Appendix I, Guttmacher Institute Abortion Provider Census.)

Reference:

Gamble SB, Strauss LT, Parker WY, Cook DA, Zane SB, Hamdan S. Abortion surveillance—United States, 2005. In: Surveillance Summaries, 28 Nov 2008. MMWR 2008;57(SS–13):1–32. Available from: http://www.cdc.gov/mmwr/preview/mmwrhtml/ss5713a1.htm.

For More Information. See the NCCDPHP surveillance and research website at: http://www.cdc.gov/reproductivehealth/Data_Stats/index.htm.

AIDS Surveillance

CDC/National Center for HIV/AIDS, Viral Hepatitis, STD, and TB Prevention (NCHHSTP)

Overview. Acquired immunodeficiency syndrome (AIDS) surveillance data are used to detect and monitor cases of human immunodeficiency virus (HIV) disease and AIDS in the United States, identify epidemiologic trends, identify unusual cases requiring follow-up, and inform public health efforts to prevent and control the disease.

Selected Content. Data collected on cases diagnosed with AIDS include age, sex, race/ethnicity, mode of exposure, and geographic region.

Data Years. Reports on AIDS cases are available from the beginning of the epidemic that started in 1981.

Coverage. All 50 states, the District of Columbia (D.C.), U.S. dependencies and possessions, and independent nations in free association with the United States report AIDS cases to CDC using a uniform surveillance case definition and case report form. As of April 2008, all states had implemented confidential, name-based HIV infection reporting.

Methodology. AIDS surveillance is conducted by health departments in each state or territory and D.C. Although surveillance activities range from passive to active, most areas employ multifaceted active surveillance programs, which include four major reporting sources of AIDS information: hospitals and hospital-based physicians, physicians in nonhospital practice, public and private clinics, and medical record systems (death certificates, tumor registries, hospital discharge abstracts, and communicable disease reports). Using a standard confidential case report form, the health departments collect information that is then transmitted electronically, without personal identifiers, to CDC.

Adjustments of the estimated data on HIV infection (not AIDS) and AIDS to account for reporting delays are calculated by a maximum likelihood statistical procedure that takes into account the differences in reporting delays among exposure, geographic, racial/ethnic, age, sex, and vital status categories and is based on the assumption that reporting delays in these categories have not changed over time. AIDS surveillance data are provisional and are updated annually.

Issues Affecting Interpretation. Although the completeness of reporting of AIDS cases to state and local health departments differs by geographic region and patient population, studies conducted by state and local health departments indicate that the reporting of AIDS cases in most areas of the United States is more than 85% complete. To assess trends in AIDS cases, deaths, and prevalence, it is preferable to use case data adjusted for reporting delays and presented by year of diagnosis, rather than straight counts of cases presented by year of report.

The definition of AIDS was modified in 1985 and 1987. The case definition for adults and adolescents was modified again in 1993. The revisions incorporated a broader range of AIDS-indicator diseases and conditions and used HIV diagnostic tests to improve the sensitivity and specificity of the definition. Laboratory and diagnostic criteria for the 1987 pediatric case definition were updated in 1994. Effective January 2000, the surveillance case definition for HIV infection was revised to reflect advances in laboratory HIV virologic tests. The definition incorporates the reporting criteria for HIV infection and AIDS into a single case definition for adults and children.

In 2008, changes were made to the case definition for HIV infection. The new case definition combined the two previous case definitions for HIV and AIDS and established a new disease staging classification. This change in the new case definition prompted changes to the title of the report and new terminology diagnoses of HIV infection and AIDS diagnoses throughout the report. The term "HIV/AIDS"— previously used to refer to a new diagnosis of HIV infection regardless of the person's disease stage at the time of diagnosis—was replaced with the term "diagnosis of HIV infection," to reflect implementation of the revised case definition for HIV infection that incorporated the previous case definition for AIDS and established a new disease staging classification.

Decreases in AIDS incidence and in the number of AIDS deaths, first noted in 1996, have been ascribed to the effect of new treatments, which prevent or delay the onset of AIDS and premature death among HIV-infected persons and result in an increase in the number of persons living with HIV and AIDS. A growing number of states require confidential reporting of persons with HIV infection and participate in CDC's integrated HIV/AIDS surveillance system that compiles information on the population of persons newly diagnosed and living with HIV infection.

Reference:

> CDC. HIV/AIDS surveillance report. Atlanta, GA: CDC [published annually]. Available from: http://www.cdc.gov/hiv/topics/surveillance/resources/reports.

For More Information. See the NCHHSTP website at: http://www.cdc.gov/nchhstp.

Census of Fatal Occupational Injuries (CFOI)

Bureau of Labor Statistics (BLS)

Overview. CFOI compiles comprehensive and timely information on fatal work injuries occurring in the 50 states and the District of Columbia (D.C.), to monitor workplace safety and inform private and public health efforts to improve workplace safety.

Selected Content. Information is collected about each workplace fatality, including occupation and other worker characteristics, equipment involved, and circumstances of the event.

Data Years. Data have been collected annually since 1992.

Coverage. The data cover all 50 states and D.C.

Methodology. CFOI is administered by BLS, in conjunction with participating state agencies, to compile counts that are as complete as possible to identify, verify, and profile fatal work injuries. Key information about each workplace fatality (occupation and other worker characteristics, equipment or machinery involved, and circumstances of the event) is obtained by cross-referencing source records. For a fatality to be included in the census, the decedent must have been employed (that is, working for pay, compensation, or profit) at the time of the event, engaged in a legal work activity, or present at the site of the incident as a requirement of his or her job. These criteria are generally broader than those used by federal and state agencies administering specific laws and regulations. Fatalities that occur during a person's commute to or from work are excluded from the census counts. Fatalities to volunteer workers who are exposed to the same work hazards and perform the same duties or functions as paid employees and that meet the CFOI work relationship criteria are included.

Data for CFOI are compiled from various federal, state, and local administrative sources including death certificates, workers' compensation reports and claims, reports to various regulatory agencies, medical examiner reports, police reports, and news reports. Diverse sources are used because studies have shown that no single source captures all job-related fatalities. Source documents are matched so that each fatality is counted only once. To ensure that a fatality occurred while the decedent was at work, information is verified from two or more independent source documents or from a source document and a follow-up questionnaire.

Denominator data for the calculation of fatal injury rates are provided by the Current Population Survey (CPS). CPS and CFOI differ in scope. Where these differences occur, CFOI-adjusted fatal injury counts are used in calculating the rates, to maintain consistency between the rate numerator (number of fatal injuries) and the denominator (annual average employment and/or average hours at work). Workers under 16 years of age are excluded from fatal injury rate data. Starting with 2008 data, volunteers and military personnel also are excluded. Volunteers and military personnel are not included in the CPS data, and CFOI has been unable to obtain reliable hours-worked data for these groups.

Issues Affecting Interpretation. The number of occupational fatalities and fatality rates is revised periodically. States have up to 8 months to update their initial published counts and may identify additional fatal work injuries after data collection has closed for a reference year. Fatalities initially excluded from the published count because of insufficient information to determine work relationship may subsequently be verified as work-related and included in the revised counts and rates. Increases in the published counts over the last 5 years based on additional information have averaged approximately 110 fatalities per year, or less than 2% of the annual total.

Beginning with 2003 data, CFOI began using the North American Industry Classification System (NAICS) to classify industries. Prior to 2003, the program used the Standard Industrial Classification (SIC) system and the U.S. Census Bureau's occupational classification system. Although some titles in SIC and NAICS are similar, there is limited comparability between the two systems because the industry groupings are defined differently. (See Appendix II, Industry of employment.)

Starting with 2008 data, fatal injury rates presented in *Health, United States* are based on hours, rather than employment, and consequently are not directly comparable with earlier injury rate data. Hours-based rates standardize the amount of exposure and are considered more accurate than employment-based rates. Hours-based rates use the average number of employees at work and the average hours each employee works. Employment- and hours-based rates will be similar for groups of workers who usually work full time. Differences in these rates are more likely for groups of workers who have a high percentage of part-time workers, like younger workers. Hours-worked data are provided by CPS. For more information, see: http://www.bls.gov/iif/oshnotice10.htm.

Reference:

Bureau of Labor Statistics. National Census of Fatal Occupational Injuries in 2008 [press release]. USDL–09–0979. Washington, DC: U.S. Department of Labor; 2009 August 20. Available from: http://www.bls.gov/news.release/archives/cfoi_08202009.pdf.

For More Information. See the CFOI website at: http://www.bls.gov/iif/oshcfoi1.htm.

Consumer Price Index (CPI)

Bureau of Labor Statistics (BLS)

Overview. The CPI is designed to produce a monthly measure of the average change in the prices paid by urban consumers for a fixed market basket of goods and services.

Selected Content. Price indexes are available for the United States, the four census regions, size of city, cross-classifications of regions and size-classes, and 26 local areas. For other local areas, data are bimonthly or semiannual. Indexes are available for major groups of consumer expenditures (food and beverages, housing, apparel, transportation, medical care, recreation, education and communications, and other goods and services), for items within each group, and for special categories such as services. Monthly indexes are available for the United States, the four census regions, and some local areas. More detailed item indexes are available for the United States than for regions and local areas. Indexes are available for two population groups: a CPI for All Urban Consumers (CPI–U), which covers approximately 87% of the total population; and a CPI for Urban Wage Earners and Clerical Workers (CPI–W), which covers 32% of the population.

Data Years. Data are available back to 1913. Prior to 1978, the data are based on the CPI–W population.

Coverage. The all-urban index (CPI–U), introduced in 1978, covers residents of metropolitan areas and residents of urban parts of nonmetropolitan areas (about 87% of the U.S. population in 2000).

Methodology. In calculating the index, price changes for the various items in each location are averaged together with weights that represent their importance in the spending of all urban consumers. Local data are aggregated to obtain a U.S. city average.

The index measures price changes from a designated reference date, 1982–1984, which equals 100. An increase of 22%, for example, is shown as 122. Change can also be expressed in dollars; for example, the price of a base period market basket of goods and services bought by all urban consumers has risen from $100 in 1982–1984 to $215 in 2008.

The CPI currently reflects spending patterns based on the Survey of Consumer Expenditures from 2007–2008, the 1990 Census of Population, and the ongoing Point-of-Purchase Survey. Using an improved sample design, prices for the goods and services required to calculate the index are collected in urban areas throughout the country and from retail and service establishments. Data on rents are collected from tenants of rented housing and residents of owner-occupied housing units. Food, fuels, and other goods and services are priced monthly in urban locations. Price information is obtained through visits or calls by trained BLS field representatives using computer-assisted telephone interviews.

Issues Affecting Interpretation. A 1987 revision changed the treatment of health insurance in the cost–weight definitions for medical care items. This change has no effect on the overall index result but provides a clearer picture of the role of health insurance in the CPI. As part of the revision, three new indexes were created by separating previously combined items; for example, eye care is separated from other professional services, and inpatient and outpatient treatment are separated from other hospital and medical care services.

Effective January 1997, the hospital index was restructured by combining the three categories—room, inpatient services, and outpatient services—into one category: hospital services. In addition, new procedures for hospital data collection identify a payor, diagnosis, and the payor's reimbursement arrangement from selected hospital bills.

References:

Bureau of Labor Statistics. BLS handbook of methods. BLS bulletin no 2490. Washington, DC: U.S. Department of Labor; 1997.

Bureau of Labor Statistics. Revising the Consumer Price Index. Mon Labor Rev 1996;119(12).

Ford IK, Ginsburg DH. Medical care in the Consumer Price Index. In: Cutler DM, Berndt ER, eds. Medical care output and productivity. Bureau of Economic Research studies in income and wealth, vol 62. Chicago, IL: University of Chicago Press; 2001. pp 203–19.

For More Information. See the BLS/CPI website at: http://www.bls.gov/cpi.

Current Population Survey (CPS)

Bureau of Labor Statistics (BLS) and U.S. Census Bureau

Overview. CPS provides current estimates and trends in employment, unemployment, and other characteristics of the general labor force, the population as a whole, and various population subgroups.

Selected Content. The CPS interview is divided into three basic parts: (a) household and demographic information, (b) labor force information, and (c) supplement information for months that include supplements. Comprehensive work experience information is gathered on the employment status, occupation, and industry of persons interviewed.

Estimates of poverty and health insurance coverage presented in *Health, United States* from CPS are derived from the Annual Social and Economic Supplement (ASEC), formerly called the Annual Demographic Supplement (ADS) or commonly called the March Supplement. ASEC collects data on family characteristics, household composition, marital status, migration, income from all sources, information on weeks worked, time spent looking for work or on layoff from a job, occupation and industry classification of the job held longest during the year, health insurance coverage, and receipt of noncash benefits such as food stamps, school lunch program, employer-provided group health insurance plan, employer-provided pension plan, personal health insurance, Medicaid, Medicare, CHAMPUS or military health care, and energy assistance.

Data Years. The basic CPS has been conducted since 1945, although some data were collected prior to that time. The U.S. Census Bureau has collected data in the ASEC or ADS since 1947.

Coverage. The 2000-based basic CPS sample was introduced in April 2004, and implementation was completed by July 2005 with coverage in every state and the District of Columbia. The adult universe (i.e., the population of marriageable age) is composed of persons 15 years of age and over in the civilian noninstitutionalized population for CPS labor force data. The sample for the March CPS supplement is expanded to include members of the Armed Forces who are living in a household that includes at least one civilian adult, as well as additional Hispanic households that are not included in the monthly labor force estimates.

Methodology. The basic CPS sample is selected from multiple frames using multiple stages of selection. Each unit is selected with a known probability to represent similar units in the universe. The sample design is state-based, with the sample in each state being independent of the others.

One person generally responds for all eligible members of a household. For those who are employed, employment information is collected on the job held in the reference week. The reference week is defined as the 7-day period, Sunday through Saturday, that includes the 12th of the month. In CPS, a person with two or more jobs is classified according to the job at which he or she worked the greatest number of hours. In general, the BLS publishes labor force data only for persons 16 years of age and over because those under 16 are substantially limited in their labor market activities by compulsory schooling and child labor laws. No upper age limit is used, and full-time students are treated the same as nonstudents.

The additional Hispanic sample is from the previous November's basic CPS sample. If a person is identified as being of Hispanic origin from the November interview and is still residing at the same address in March, that housing unit is eligible for the March survey. This amounts to a near doubling of the Hispanic sample because there is no overlap of housing units between the basic CPS samples in November and March.

For all CPS data files, a single weight is prepared and used to compute the monthly labor force status estimates. An additional weight is prepared for the earnings universe that roughly corresponds to wage and salary workers in the two outgoing rotations. The final weight is the product of the basic weight, the adjustments for special weighting, the noninterview adjustment, the first-stage ratio adjustment factor, and the second-stage ratio adjustment factor. This final weight should be used when producing estimates from the basic CPS data. Differences in the questionnaire, sample, and data uses for the March CPS supplement result in the need for additional adjustment procedures to produce what is called the March Supplement weight.

Sample Size and Response Rate. Beginning with 2001, the Children's Health Insurance Program (CHIP) sample expansion was introduced. This included an increase in the basic CPS sample to 60,000 households per month. Prior to 2001, estimates were based on 50,000 households per month. The expansion also included an additional 12,000 households that were allocated differentially across states, based on prior information of the number of uninsured children in each state, to produce statistically reliable current state data on the number of low-income children who do not have health insurance coverage. In an average month, the nonresponse rate for the basic CPS is about 7%–8%.

Issues Affecting Interpretation. Over the years, the number of income questions has expanded, questions on work experience and other characteristics have been added, and the month of interview was moved to March. In 2002, an ASEC sample increase was implemented, requiring more time for data collection. Thus, additional ASEC interviews are now taking place in February and April. However, even with this sample increase, most of the data collection still occurs in March.

In 1994, major changes were introduced that included a complete redesign of the questionnaire to include new health insurance questions and the introduction of computer-assisted interviewing for the entire survey. In addition, some of the labor force concepts and definitions were revised. Prior to the redesign, CPS data were primarily collected using a paper-and-pencil form. Beginning in 1994, population controls were based on the 1990 census and adjusted for the estimated population undercount. Starting with *Health, United States, 2003*, poverty estimates for data years 2000 and beyond were recalculated based on the expanded CHIP sample, and Census 2000-based population controls were implemented. Starting with 2002 health insurance data, 1997 race standards were implemented that allowed respondents to report more than one race.

Reference:

U.S. Census Bureau. Current Population Survey: Design and methodology, Technical paper 66. Washington, DC: U.S. Census Bureau; 2006. Available from: http://www.census.gov/prod/2006pubs/tp-66.pdf.

For More Information. See the CPS website at: http://www.census.gov/cps.

Department of Veterans Affairs National Patient Care Database, Patient Treatment File, and National Enrollment Database

Department of Veterans Affairs (VA)

Overview. The VA compiles and analyzes multiple data sets on the health and health care of its clients and other veterans to monitor access and quality of care and to conduct program and policy evaluations.

Selected Content. The VA maintains the National Patient Care Database (NPCD), the Patient Treatment File (PTF), and the National Enrollment Database (NED).

The NPCD and PTF are nationwide systems that contain a statistical record for each episode of care provided under VA auspices, in VA and non-VA hospitals, nursing homes, VA residential rehabilitation treatment programs (formerly called domiciliaries), and VA outpatient clinics. Three major extracts are the PTF, the Patient Census File (PCF), and the NPCD.

The PTF collects data at the time of the patient's discharge on each episode of inpatient care provided to patients at VA hospitals, VA nursing homes, VA residential rehabilitation treatment programs, community nursing homes, and other non-VA facilities. The PTF record contains unique patient identifiers, dates of inpatient treatment, date of birth, state and county of residence, type of disposition, place of disposition after discharge, and *International Classification of Diseases, 9th Revision, Clinical Modification* (ICD–9–CM) diagnostic and procedure or operative codes for each episode of care.

The PCF collects data on each patient remaining in a VA medical facility at midnight at the end of each quarter of the fiscal year. The census record includes information similar to that reported in the PTF record.

The NPCD collects data on each instance of medical treatment provided to a veteran in an outpatient setting. The NPCD record includes the age, unique patient identifiers, state and county of residence, VA eligibility code, clinic(s) visited, purpose of visit, and date of visit for each episode of care.

The VA also maintains the NED as the official repository of enrollment information for each veteran enrolled in the VA health care system.

Coverage. U.S. veterans who receive services within the VA medical system are included. Data are available for some nonveterans who receive care at VA facilities.

Methodology. The NPCD and PTF are the source data for the Veterans Health Administration (VHA) Medical SAS Datasets. The NPCD and PTF are also the VHA's centralized relational databases (a data warehouse) that receive encounter data from VHA clinical information systems. The databases are updated daily. Data are collected locally at each VA medical center and transmitted electronically to the VA's Austin Automation Center for use in providing nationwide statistics, reports, and comparisons.

Issues Affecting Interpretation. The databases include users of the VA health care system. VA eligibility is a hierarchy based on service-connected disabilities, income, age, and availability of services. Therefore, different VA programs may serve populations with different sociodemographic characteristics than those served by other health care systems.

For More Information. See the VA Information Resource Center website at: http://www.virec.research.va.gov/Support/Training-NewUsersToolkit/IntroToVAData.htm.

Employee Benefits Survey—See National Compensation Survey

Medicaid Statistical Information System (MSIS)

Centers for Medicare & Medicaid Services (CMS)

Overview. CMS works with its state partners to collect data on each person served by the Medicaid program, to monitor and evaluate access and quality of care, trends in program eligibility, characteristics of enrollees, changes in payment policy, and other program-related issues.

Selected Content. Data collected include claims for services and their associated payments for each Medicaid beneficiary, by type of service. MSIS also collects information on the characteristics of every Medicaid eligible, including eligibility and demographic information.

Data Years. Selected state data are available starting in 1992. MSIS was an optional program until 1999, when the Balanced Budget Act of 1997 mandated that all states use MSIS. Data for the 50 states and the District of Columbia are available starting in 1999.

Coverage. The data include information about all individuals enrolled in the Medicaid program, the services they receive, and the payments made for those services.

Methodology. The primary data sources for Medicaid statistical data are the MSIS and CMS–64 reports.

MSIS is the basic source of state-reported eligibility and claims data on the Medicaid population, its characteristics, utilization, and payments. Beginning in FY 1999, as a result of legislation enacted from the Balanced Budget Act of 1997, states were required to submit individual eligibility and claims data tapes to CMS quarterly, through MSIS. Prior to FY 1999, states were required to submit an annual HCFA–2082 report, designed to collect aggregated statistical data on eligibles, recipients, services, and expenditures during a federal fiscal year (October 1 through September 30), or, at state option, to submit eligibility data and claims through MSIS. The claims data reflect bills adjudicated or processed during the year, rather than services used during the year.

CMS–64, a product of the financial budget and grant system, is a statement of expenditures for the Medicaid program that the states submit to CMS 30 days after each quarter. The report is an accounting statement of actual expenditures made by the states for which they are entitled to receive federal reimbursement under Title XIX for that quarter. The amount claimed on CMS–64 is a summary of expenditures derived from source documents such as invoices, cost reports, and eligibility records.

CMS–64 shows the disposition of Medicaid grant funds for the quarter being reported and for previous years, the recoupments made or refunds received, and income earned on grant funds. The data on CMS–64 are used to reconcile the monetary advance made on the basis of states' funding estimates filed prior to the beginning of the quarter on CMS–37. As such, CMS–64 is the primary source for making adjustments for any identified overpayments and underpayments to the states. Also incorporated into this process are disallowance actions forwarded from other federal financial adjustments. Finally, CMS–64 provides information that forms the basis for a series of Medicaid financial reports and budget analyses. Also included are third-party liability (TPL) collections tables. TPL refers to the legal obligation of certain health care sources to pay the medical claims of Medicaid recipients before Medicaid pays these claims. Medicaid pays only after the TPL sources have met their legal obligation to pay.

Issues Affecting Interpretation. Medicaid tables in *Health, United States* are based on MSIS data. Users of

Medicaid data may note apparent inconsistencies in the data that are primarily due to the difference in information captured in MSIS compared with CMS–64 reports. The most substantive difference is due to payments made to disproportionate share hospitals. Payments to disproportionate share hospitals do not appear in MSIS because states reimburse these hospitals directly and there is no fee-for-service billing. Other, less significant, differences between MSIS and CMS–64 occur because adjudicated claims data are used in MSIS versus actual payments reflected in CMS–64. Differences also may occur because of internal state practices for capturing and reporting these data through two separate systems. Finally, national totals for CMS–64 are different because they include other jurisdictions, such as the Northern Mariana Islands and American Samoa. Starting with 1999 data, MSIS excluded data from Puerto Rico and the U.S. Virgin Islands, which accounted for approximately 1 million eligibles and $250 million in Medicaid payments.

For More Information. See the CMS websites at: http://www.cms.hhs.gov/home/medicaid.asp and http://www.cms.hhs.gov/msis and the Research Data Assistance Center (ResDAC) website at: http://www.resdac.umn.edu/medicaid/data_available.asp. (Also see Appendix II, Medicaid.)

Medical Expenditure Panel Survey (MEPS)

Agency for Healthcare Research and Quality (AHRQ)

Overview. MEPS produces nationally representative estimates of health care use, expenditures, sources of payment, insurance coverage, and quality of care for the U.S. civilian noninstitutionalized population.

Selected Content. MEPS data in *Health, United States* include total health care expenses and prescribed medicine expenses, presented by sociodemographic characteristics, type of health insurance, and sources of payment.

Data Years. The 1977 National Medical Care Expenditure Survey and the 1987 National Medical Expenditure Survey (NMES) are earlier versions of this survey. Since 1996, MEPS has been conducted on an annual basis.

Coverage. The U.S. civilian noninstitutionalized population is the primary population represented. The 1987 and 1996 surveys also had an institutionalized population component.

Methodology. The MEPS–HC is a national probability survey conducted on an annual basis since 1996. The panel design of the survey features five rounds of interviewing covering two full calendar years. MEPS consists of three components: the Household Component (HC), the Medical Provider Component (MPC), and the Insurance Component (IC).

The HC is a nationally representative survey of the civilian noninstitutionalized population drawn from a subsample of households that participated in the prior year's National Health Interview Survey conducted by NCHS. Whenever possible, missing expenditure data are imputed using data collected in the MPC.

The MPC collects data from hospitals, physicians, home health care providers, and pharmacies that were reported in the HC as providing care to MEPS sample persons. Data are collected in the MPC to improve the accuracy of expenditure estimates that would be obtained if derived solely from the HC. The MPC is particularly useful in obtaining expenditure information for persons enrolled in managed care plans and for Medicaid recipients. Sample sizes for the MPC vary from year to year, depending on the HC sample size and the MPC sampling rates for providers.

The IC is a separate component that collects data on the types and costs of workplace health insurance from a sample of about 40,000 business establishments and 3,000 state and local governments each year.

The MEPS predecessor, the 1987 NMES, consisted of two components: the Household Survey (HS) and the Medical Provider Survey (MPS). The NMES–HS component was designed to provide nationally representative estimates of health insurance status, health insurance coverage, and health care use for the U.S. civilian noninstitutionalized population for calendar year 1987. Data from the NMES–MPS component were used in conjunction with HS data to produce estimates of health care expenditures. The NMES–HS consisted of four rounds of household interviews. Income was collected in a special supplement administered early in 1988. Events under the scope of the NMES–MPS included medical services provided by or under the direction of a physician, all hospital events, and home health care.

Sample Size and Response Rate. In recent years, the MEPS annual survey has consisted of approximately 12,500 families and 32,000 individuals. The annual response rate, which reflects nonresponse to the National Health Interview Survey from which the MEPS sample is selected as well as nonresponse and attrition in MEPS, has averaged about 60% in recent years.

Issues Affecting Interpretation. The 1987 estimates are based on NMES, and 1996 and later years estimates are based on MEPS. Because expenditures in NMES were based primarily on charges, whereas those for MEPS were based on payments, data for NMES were adjusted to be more comparable with MEPS by using estimated charge-to-payment ratios for 1987. For a detailed explanation of this adjustment, see Zuvekas and Cohen (2002).

References:

> Hahn B, Lefkowitz D. Annual expenses and sources of payment for health care services. National Medical Expenditure Survey research findings no 14. AHCPR pub no 93–0007. Rockville, MD: Agency for Health Care Policy and Research; 1992.

> Ezzati-Rice TM, Rohde F, Greenblatt J. Sample design of the Medical Expenditure Panel Survey Household Component, 1998–2007. Methodology report no 22. Rockville, MD: Agency for Healthcare Research and Quality; 2008. Available from: http://www.meps.ahrq.gov/mepsweb/data_files/publications/mr22/mr22.shtml.

> Zuvekas SH, Cohen JW. A guide to comparing health care expenditures in the 1996 MEPS to the 1987 NMES. Inquiry 2002;39(1):76–86.

For More Information. See the MEPS website at: http://www.meps.ahrq.gov/mepsweb/.

Medicare Administrative Data

Centers for Medicare & Medicaid Services (CMS)

Overview. CMS collects and synthesizes Medicare enrollment, spending, and claims data to monitor and evaluate access to and quality of care, trends in utilization, changes in payment policy, and other program-related issues.

Selected Content. Data include claims information for services furnished to Medicare beneficiaries and Medicare enrollment data. Claims data include type of service, procedures, diagnoses, dates of service, charge amounts, and payment amounts. Enrollment data include date of birth, sex, race or ethnicity, and reason for entitlement.

Data Years. Some data files are available as far back as 1987, but CMS no longer provides technical support for files with data prior to 1991.

Coverage. Enrollment data are for all persons enrolled in the Medicare program. Claims data include data for Medicare beneficiaries who filed claims.

Methodology. The claims and utilization data files contain extensive utilization information at various levels of summarization for a variety of providers and services. There are many types and levels of these files: the National Claims History files, the Standard Analytic files (SAFs), Medicare Provider and Analysis Review (MEDPAR) files, Medicare enrollment files, and various other files.

The NCH 100% Nearline file contains all institutional and noninstitutional claims and provides records of every Medicare claim submitted, including adjustment claims. SAFs contain final action claims data in which all adjustments have been resolved. These files contain information collected by Medicare to pay for health care services provided to a Medicare beneficiary. SAFs are available for each institutional (inpatient, outpatient, skilled nursing facility, hospice, or home health agency) and noninstitutional (physician and durable medical equipment providers) claim type. The record unit of SAFs is the claim (some episodes of care may have more than one claim). SAFs include the Inpatient SAF, the Skilled Nursing Facility SAF, the Outpatient SAF, the Home Health Agency SAF, the Hospice SAF, the Durable Medical Equipment SAF, and the Physician/Supplier SAF.

MEDPAR files contain inpatient hospital and skilled nursing facility (SNF) final action stay records. Each MEDPAR record represents a stay in an inpatient hospital or SNF. An inpatient stay record summarizes all services rendered to a beneficiary from the time of admission to a facility, through discharge. Each MEDPAR record may represent one claim or multiple claims, depending on the length of a beneficiary's stay and the amount of inpatient services used throughout the stay.

The Denominator file contains demographic and enrollment information about each beneficiary enrolled in Medicare during a calendar year. The information in the Denominator file is frozen in March of the following calendar year. Some of the information contained in this file includes the beneficiary unique identifier, state and county codes, ZIP code, date of birth, date of death, sex, race, age, monthly entitlement indicators (for Medicare Part A, Medicare Part B, or Part A and Part B), reasons for entitlement, state buy-in indicators, and monthly managed care indicators (yes/no). The Denominator file is used to determine beneficiary demographic characteristics, entitlement, and beneficiary participation in Medicare Managed Care Organizations (MCOs).

The Vital Status file contains demographic information about each beneficiary ever entitled to Medicare. Some of the information contained in this file includes the beneficiary unique identifier, state and county codes, ZIP Code, date of birth, date of death, sex, race, and age. Often the Vital Status file is used to obtain recent death information for a cohort of Medicare beneficiaries.

The Group Health Plan (GHP) master file contains data on beneficiaries who are currently enrolled, or have ever been enrolled, in an MCO under contract with CMS. Each record represents one beneficiary, and each beneficiary has one record. Some of the information contained in this file includes the beneficiary unique identifier, date of birth, date of death, state and county, and managed care enrollment information such as dates of membership and MCO contract number. The GHP master file is used to identify the exact MCO in which beneficiaries were enrolled.

Issues Affecting Interpretation. Because Medicare managed care programs may not file claims, files based only on claims data will exclude care for persons enrolled in Medicare managed care programs. In addition, to maintain a manageable file size, some files are based on a sample of enrollees, rather than on all Medicare enrollees. Coding and the interpretation of Medicare coverage rules have also changed over the life of the Medicare program.

For More Information. See the CMS Research Data Assistance Center (ResDAC) website at: http://www.resdac.umn.edu/medicare/index.asp and the CMS website at: http://www.cms.hhs.gov/home/medicare.asp. (Also see Appendix II, Medicare.)

Medicare Current Beneficiary Survey (MCBS)

Centers for Medicare & Medicaid Services (CMS)

Overview. MCBS produces nationally representative estimates of health status, health care use and expenditures, health insurance coverage, and socioeconomic and demographic characteristics of Medicare beneficiaries. It is used to estimate expenditures and sources of payment for all services used by Medicare beneficiaries, including copayments, deductibles, and noncovered services; to ascertain all types of health insurance coverage and relate coverage to sources of payment; and to trace processes over time, such as changes in health status and the effects of program changes.

Selected Content. The survey collects data on the utilization of health services, health and functional status, health care expenditures, and health insurance and beneficiary information (such as income, living arrangement, family assistance, and quality of life).

Data Years. The first round of interviewing was conducted from September through December 1991, and the survey has been in the field continuously since then. The data are designed to support both cross-sectional and longitudinal analyses.

Coverage. MCBS is a continuous survey of a nationally representative sample of aged, institutionalized, and disabled Medicare beneficiaries.

Methodology. The overlapping panel design of the survey allows each sample person to be interviewed three times a year for 4 years, whether he or she resides in the community or a facility or moves between the two settings, using the version of the questionnaire appropriate to the setting. Sample persons are interviewed using computer-assisted personal interviewing (CAPI) survey instruments. Because residents of long-term care facilities often are in poor health, information about institutionalized residents is collected from proxy respondents such as nurses and other primary caregivers affiliated with the facility. The sample is selected from the Medicare enrollment files, with oversampling among disabled persons under 65 years of age and among persons 80 years and over.

MCBS has two components: the Cost and Use file and the Access to Care file. Medicare claims are linked to survey-reported events to produce the Cost and Use file, which provides complete expenditure and source of payment data on all health care services, including those not covered by Medicare. The Access to Care file contains information on beneficiaries' access to health care, satisfaction with care, and usual source of care. The sample for this file represents the always enrolled population—those who participated in the Medicare program for the entire year. In contrast, the Cost and Use file represents the ever enrolled population, including those who entered Medicare and those who died during the year.

Sample Size and Response Rate. Each fall, about one-third of the sample is retired and roughly 6,000 new sample persons are included in the survey; the exact number chosen is based on projections of target samples of 12,000 persons with 3 years of cost and use information distributed appropriately across the sample cells. In the community, response rates for initial interviews range in the mid- to high 80s; once respondents have completed the first interview, their participation in subsequent rounds is 95% or more. In recent rounds, data have been collected from approximately 16,000 beneficiaries. Roughly 90% of the sample is made up of persons who live in the community, with the remaining persons living in long-term care facilities. Response rates for facility interviews approach 100%.

Issues Affecting Interpretation. Because only Medicare enrollees are included in the survey, the survey excludes a small proportion of persons 65 years of age and over who are not enrolled in Medicare. This should be noted when using the MCBS to make estimates of the entire population 65 years and over in the United States.

References:

Adler GS. A profile of the Medicare Current Beneficiary Survey. Health Care Financ Rev 1994;15(4):153–63.

Lo A, Chu A, Apodaca R. Redesign of the Medicare Current Beneficiary Survey sample. Rockville, MD: Westat, Inc.; 2003. Available from: http://www.amstat.org/sections/srms/Proceedings/y2002/Files/JSM2002-000662.pdf.

For More Information. See the MCBS website at: http://www.cms.hhs.gov/MCBS.

Monitoring the Future Study (MTF)

National Institute on Drug Abuse (NIDA)

Overview. MTF is an ongoing study of the behaviors, attitudes, and values of U.S. secondary school students, college students, and young adults.

Selected Content. Data collected include lifetime, annual, and 30-day prevalence of use of specific illegal drugs and substances, inhalants, tobacco, and alcohol. Data are also collected on usage levels, frequency of use, perceived risks associated with use, opinions about whether use is approved or disapproved by others, and opinions about availability of the substances.

Data Years. MTF has been conducted annually since 1975, initially with high school seniors. Ongoing panel studies of representative samples from each graduating class have been conducted by mail since

1976, and annual surveys of 8th and 10th graders were initiated in 1991.

Coverage. MTF surveys a sample of high school seniors, 10th graders, and 8th graders selected to be representative of all seniors, 10th graders, and 8th graders in public and private high schools in the coterminous United States.

Methodology. The survey design is a multistage random sample, with stage 1 being selection of particular geographic areas, stage 2 being selection of one or more schools in each area, and stage 3 being selection of classes within each school. Data are collected using self-administered questionnaires conducted in the classroom by representatives of the Institute for Social Research. Dropouts and students who are absent on the day of the survey are excluded. Recognizing that the dropout population is at higher risk for drug use, this survey was expanded in 1991 to include similar nationally representative samples of 8th and 10th graders, which have lower dropout rates than seniors and include future high-risk 12th grade dropouts. For more information on MTF adjustments for absentees and dropouts, see:

Johnston LD, O'Malley PM, Bachman JG, Schulenberg JE. Monitoring the Future: National survey results on drug use, 1975–2009, vol I: Secondary school students. Appendix A. NIH pub no 10–7584. Bethesda, MD: National Institute on Drug Abuse; 2010. Available from: http://www.monitoringthefuture.org/pubs/monographs/vol1_2009.pdf.

Sample Size and Response Rates. In 2009, a total of 46,097 students in the 8th, 10th, and 12th grades in 389 secondary schools were surveyed. The annual senior samples comprised 14,268 seniors in 125 public and private high schools nationwide. The 10th-grade samples involved 16,320 students in 119 schools, and the 8th-grade samples had 15,509 students in 145 schools. Response rates were 82% for 12th graders, 89% for 10th graders, and 88% for 8th graders and have been relatively constant across time. Absentees constitute virtually all of the nonresponding students.

Issues Affecting Interpretation. Estimates of substance use among youth based on the National Survey on Drug Use & Health (NSDUH) are not directly comparable with estimates based on MTF and the Youth Risk Behavior Surveillance System (YRBSS). In addition to the fact that MTF excludes dropouts and absentees, rates are not directly comparable across these surveys because of differences in populations covered, sample design, questionnaires, and interview setting. NSDUH collects data in residences, whereas MTF and YRBSS collect data in school classrooms. In addition, NSDUH estimates are tabulated by age, whereas MTF and YRBSS estimates are tabulated by grade, representing different ages as well as different populations.

References:

Johnston LD, O'Malley PM, Bachman JG, Schulenberg JE. Monitoring the Future: National results on adolescent drug use. Overview of key findings, 2009. NIH pub no 10–7583. Bethesda, MD: National Institute on Drug Abuse; 2010. Available from: http://www.monitoringthefuture.org/pubs/monographs/overview2009.pdf.

Johnston LD, O'Malley PM, Bachman JG, Schulenberg JE. Monitoring the Future: National survey results on drug use, 1975–2008, vol I: Secondary school students. NIH pub no 09–7402. Bethesda, MD: National Institute on Drug Abuse; 2009. Available from: http://www.monitoringthefuture.org/pubs/monographs/vol1_2008.pdf.

Cowan CD. Coverage, sample design, and weighting in three federal surveys. J Drug Issues 2001;31(3):599–614.

For More Information. See the NIDA website at: http://www.nida.nih.gov/Infofax/HSYouthtrends.html and the MTF website at: http://www.monitoringthefuture.org.

National Ambulatory Medical Care Survey (NAMCS)

CDC/NCHS

Overview. NAMCS is a national survey designed to provide information about the provision and use of medical care services in office-based physician practices in the United States.

Selected Content. Data are collected from medical records on type of providers seen; reason for visit; diagnoses; drugs ordered, provided, or continued; and selected procedures and tests ordered or performed during the visit. Patient data include age, sex, race, and expected source of payment. Data are also collected on selected characteristics of physician practices.

Data Years. NAMCS, which began in 1973, was conducted annually until 1981, once in 1985, and resumed an annual schedule in 1989.

Coverage. The scope of the survey covers patient encounters in the offices of nonfederally employed physicians classified by the American Medical Association (AMA) or American Osteopathic Association (AOA) as office-based patient care physicians. Patient encounters with physicians engaged in prepaid practices—health maintenance organizations (HMOs), independent practice organizations (IPAs), and other prepaid practices—are included in NAMCS. Excluded are visits to hospital-based physicians; visits to specialists in anesthesiology, pathology, and radiology; and visits to physicians who are principally engaged in teaching, research, or administration. Telephone contacts and nonoffice visits are also excluded.

Methodology. A multistage probability design is employed. The first-stage sample consisted of 84 primary sampling units (PSUs) in 1985, and beginning in 1989, 112 PSUs, which were selected from about 1,900 such units into which the United States had been divided. In each sample PSU, a sample of practicing nonfederal office-based physicians is selected from master files maintained by the AMA and the AOA. The final stage involves systematic random samples of office visits during randomly assigned 7-day reporting periods. In 1985, the survey excluded Alaska and Hawaii. Starting in 1989, the survey included all 50 states and the District of Columbia.

The U.S. Census Bureau acts as the data collection agent for NAMCS. Screening interviews are conducted by Census field representatives to obtain information about physicians' office-based practices and to ensure that the practice is within the scope of the survey. Field representatives visit eligible physicians prior to their participation in the survey to provide them with survey materials and instruct them on how to sample patient visits and complete patient record forms. Participants are asked to complete forms for a systematic random sample of approximately 30 office visits occurring during a randomly assigned 1-week period, but increasingly patient record forms are abstracted by field representatives.

Sample data are weighted to produce national estimates. The estimation procedure used in NAMCS has three basic components: inflation by the reciprocal of the probability of selection, adjustment for nonresponse, and ratio adjustment to fixed totals.

Sample Size and Response Rate. In each sample year from 2003 to 2005, 3,000 physicians were sampled, and the response rates were 66%–70%. Data were provided for approximately 25,000 visits per survey year. In sample years 2006 and 2007, 3,500 physicians were sampled, and the response rates were 64%–65%. Data were provided for approximately 29,000 visits in 2006 and almost 33,000 visits in 2007. In 2008, a sample of 3,319 physicians was selected: 2,229 were in scope and 1,334 participated, for a response rate of 59.1%. The response rate has been modified to accommodate the mixture of one- and two-stage samples of providers. Data were provided for 28,741 visits.

Issues Affecting Interpretation. The NAMCS patient record form is modified approximately every 2–4 years to reflect changes in physician practice characteristics, patterns of care, and technological innovations. Examples of recent changes include increasing the number of drugs recorded on the patient record form and adding checkboxes for specific tests or procedures performed. Sample sizes vary by survey year. For some years it is suggested that analysts combine two or more years of data if they wish to examine relatively rare populations or events. Starting with *Health, United States, 2005*, data for survey years 2001–2002 were revised to be consistent with the weighting scheme introduced in the 2003 NAMCS data. For more information on the new weighting scheme, see the "National Ambulatory Medical Care Survey: 2003 Summary" (2005).

Reference:

Hing E, Cherry DK, Woodwell DA. National Ambulatory Medical Care Survey: 2003 summary. Advance data from vital and health statistics; no 365. Hyattsville, MD: NCHS; 2005. Available from: http://www.cdc.gov/nchs/data/ad/ad365.pdf.

For More Information. See the Ambulatory Health Care Data website at: http://www.cdc.gov/nchs/ahcd.htm.

National Compensation Survey (NCS)

Bureau of Labor Statistics (BLS)

Overview. NCS provides comprehensive measures of occupational earnings, compensation cost trends, benefit incidence, and detailed plan provisions.

Selected Content. Detailed occupational earnings are collected for metropolitan and nonmetropolitan areas, for broad geographic regions, and on a national basis. The Employment Cost Index (ECI) and Employer Costs for Employee Compensation (ECEC) are compensation measures derived from NCS. ECI measures changes in labor costs; average hourly employer costs for employee compensation are presented in ECEC. National benefits data are presented for five broad occupational groupings: professional, management, and related; sales and office; service; natural resources, construction, and maintenance; and production, transportation, and material moving. Data are also available by goods- and service-producing industries, union affiliation, and establishment size.

Data Years. NCS replaces three existing BLS surveys: ECI, the Occupational Compensation Survey Program (OCSP), and the Employee Benefits Survey (EBS). ECI and EBS were fully integrated into NCS in 1999. Prior to 1999, EBS was collected for small private establishments (those employing fewer than 100 workers) and from state and local governments regardless of employment size. In odd-numbered years, data were collected for medium and large private establishments (those employing 100 workers or more). ECI was created in the mid-1970s, and EBS was added to an existing data collection effort—the Professional, Administrative, and Technical Pay Survey—in the late 1970s. ECEC was developed in 1987.

Coverage. NCS provides information for the Nation for the nine census divisions and for 152 selected areas (combined statistical areas, metropolitan statistical areas, micropolitan statistical areas, and county clusters). Not all areas have information for all occupations. NCS includes both full- and part-time workers who are paid a wage or salary and includes data for the civilian economy, including both private industry and state and local government. It excludes agriculture, fishing, and forestry industries; private household workers; and the federal government.

Methodology. NCS is conducted quarterly by the BLS's Office of Compensation and Working Conditions. The sample is selected using a three-stage design. The first stage involves the selection of areas for the state and local government sample and the private industry sample. In the second stage, establishments are selected systematically, with the probability of selection proportionate to their relative employment size within the industry. Use of this technique means that the larger an establishment's employment, the greater its chance of selection. The third stage of sampling is a probability sample of occupations within a sampled establishment. This step is performed by the BLS field economist during an interview with the respondent establishment in which selection of an occupation is based on probability of selection proportionate to employment in the establishment and each occupation is classified under its corresponding major occupational group.

Data collection is conducted by BLS field economists. Data are gathered from each establishment on the primary business activity of the establishment; types of occupations; number of employees; wages, salaries, and benefits; hours of work; and duties and responsibilities. Wage data obtained by occupation and work level allows NCS to publish occupational wage statistics for localities, census divisions, and the Nation.

Sample. The sample consists of approximately 152 areas that represent the Nation's almost 370 metropolitan statistical areas and almost 580 micropolitan statistical areas, as defined by the Office of Management and Budget (OMB), and the remaining portions of the 50 states. NCS is in the midst of a 6-year transition from the OMB's December 1993 area definitions to the December 2003 area definitions. During this transition, NCS is surveying additional areas as new areas are being phased into the sample and others are being phased out. For more information, see: http://www.bls.gov/ncs/ncswage2007.htm#AppendixA.

Issues Affecting Interpretation. Because NCS merges separate surveys, trend analyses prior to 2000 should be interpreted with care. The industrial coverage, establishment size coverage, and geographic coverage for EBS have changed since 1990. All surveys conducted from 1979–1989 excluded part-time employees, as well as establishments in Alaska and Hawaii. The surveys conducted from 1979–1986 covered only medium and large private establishments and excluded most of the service industries. Establishments that employed at least 50, 100, or 250 workers (depending on the industry) were included. The survey conducted in 1987 consisted of state and local governments with 50 or more employees. The surveys carried out in 1988 and 1989 included all private-sector establishments that employed 100 or more people.

ECEC switched to new industry and occupation classification systems with the release of the March 2004 data. The North American Industry Classification System (NAICS) is now used to classify industries, and the 2000 Standard Occupational Classification (SOC) system is used to classify occupations. ECEC data based on the 1987 Standard Industrial Classification System and the 1990 Occupational Classification System are no longer produced, and data classified under these coding schemes are not comparable to data classified under NAICS or SOC. The 2007 NAICS is gradually replacing the 2002 NAICS, but this does not affect trends. Beginning with the March 2004 quarter, historical data are available based on NAICS and the 2000

SOC. The historical tables are available from: http://www.bls.gov/ncs/ect/home.htm or upon request from BLS. For more detailed information on NAICS and SOC, including background definitions and implementation schedules, see the BLS websites at: http://www.bls.gov/bls/naics.htm and http://www.bls.gov/soc/home.htm.

The state and local government sample, which is replaced less frequently than the private industry sample, was replaced in its entirety in September 2007. As a result of this replacement, the number of state and local government occupations and establishments increased substantially. The private industry sample is rotated over approximately 5 years, which makes the sample more representative of the economy and reduces respondent burden. Data are collected for the pay period including the 12th day of the survey months of March, June, September, and December. The sample is replaced on a cross-area, cross-industry basis.

References:

Bureau of Labor Statistics. Employer costs for employee compensation—March 2009 [press release]. Washington, DC; U.S. Department of Labor; 2009 June 10. Available from: http://www.bls.gov/news.release/pdf/ecec.pdf.

Wiatrowski WJ. The National Compensation Survey: Compensation statistics for the 21st century. Washington, DC; U.S. Department of Labor, Bureau of Labor Statistics. Compensation and Working Conditions 2000;Winter:5–14. Available from: http://www.bls.gov/opub/cwc/archive/winter2000art1.pdf.

BLS handbook of methods [online], ch 8, National compensation measures. U.S. Bureau of Labor Statistics. 2007. Available from: http://www.bls.gov/opub/hom/pdf/homch8.pdf.

For More Information. See the NCS website at: http://www.bls.gov/ncs.

National Health Expenditure Accounts

Centers for Medicare & Medicaid Services (CMS)

Overview. National Health Expenditure Accounts provide estimates of how much money is spent on different types of health-care-related services and programs in the United States.

Selected Content. National health expenditures measure spending for health care in the United States by type of service delivered (e.g., hospital care, physician services, nursing home care) and source of funding for those services (e.g., private health insurance, Medicare, Medicaid, out-of-pocket spending).

Data Years. Expenditure estimates are available starting from 1960 in data files or published articles.

Methodology. The American Hospital Association data on hospital finances, and the U.S. Census Bureau's Services Annual Survey (SAS), are the primary sources for estimates relating to hospital care. These are supplemented by data on federal hospitals. The salaries of physicians and dentists on the staffs of hospitals, hospital outpatient clinics, hospital-based home health care agencies, and nursing home care provided in the hospital setting are also considered to be components of hospital care. Expenditures for nursing home care and home health care, and for the services of health care professionals (i.e., doctors, chiropractors, private duty nurses, therapists, and podiatrists), are estimated primarily by using a combination of data from SAS and the quinquennial Census of Service Industries.

The estimates of retail spending for prescription drugs are based on industry data on prescription drug transactions from the Census of Retail Trade (U.S. Bureau of the Census) and IMS Health, an organization that collects data from the pharmaceutical industry. Expenditures for other medical nondurables and for vision products and other medical durables purchased in retail outlets are based on input-output (I/O) tables prepared by the U.S. Department of Commerce's Bureau of Economic Analysis, U.S. Bureau of Labor Statistics (BLS), Consumer Expenditure Survey; the 1987 National Medical Expenditure Survey and the Medical Expenditure Panel Surveys conducted by the Agency for Healthcare Research and Quality; and spending by Medicare and Medicaid. Those durable and nondurable products provided to inpatients in hospitals or nursing homes, and those provided by licensed professionals or through home health care agencies, are excluded here but are included with the expenditure estimates for the provider service category.

The construction estimates measured the value put in place in the construction of some medical sector buildings, mainly hospitals and nursing homes; these estimates were derived from the Bureau of the Census C–30 survey of new construction. Medical capital equipment comprises the value of new capital equipment (including software) purchased or put in place by the medical sector during the year.

Expenditures for noncommercial research (the cost of commercial research by drug companies is assumed to be embedded in the price charged for the product; to include this item again would result in double counting) are developed from information gathered by the National Institutes of Health and the National Science Foundation.

Source of funding estimates likewise come from many sources. Data on federal health care programs are taken from administrative records maintained by the servicing agencies. Among the sources used to estimate state and local government spending for health care are the U.S. Census Bureau's Government Finances reports and the National Academy of Social Insurance reports on state-operated workers' compensation programs. Federal, state, and local expenditures for education and training of medical personnel are excluded from these measures where they are separable. For the private financing of health care, data on the financial experience of health insurance organizations come from special CMS analyses of private health insurers and from the BLS survey on the cost of employer-sponsored health insurance and on consumer expenditures.

Information on out-of-pocket spending from the U.S. Bureau of the Census Services Annual Survey; U.S. BLS Consumer Expenditure Survey; the 1987 National Medical Care Expenditure Survey and the Medical Expenditure Panel Surveys conducted by the Agency for Healthcare Research and Quality; and from private surveys conducted by the American Hospital Association, the American Medical Association, the American Dental Association, and IMS Health is used to develop estimates of direct spending by customers.

Reference:

> Hartman M, Martin A, Nuccio O, Catlin A, and the National Health Expenditure Accounts Team. Health spending growth at a historic low in 2008. Health Aff (Millwood) 2010;29(1):147–55.

For More Information. See the CMS National Health Expenditure Accounts website at: http://www.cms.hhs.gov/NationalHealthExpendData.

National Health and Nutrition Examination Survey (NHANES)

CDC/NCHS

Overview. The NHANES program includes a series of cross-sectional, nationally representative health examination surveys conducted in mobile examination units or clinics (MECs). In the first series of surveys, the National Health Examination Survey

(NHES), data were collected on the prevalence of certain chronic diseases, the distributions of various physical and psychological measures, and measures of growth and development. In 1971, a nutrition surveillance component was added, and the survey name was changed to NHANES. See the Data Years section for more information on the survey name and the years it was conducted.

Selected Content. NHANES has collected data on chronic disease prevalence and conditions (including undiagnosed conditions) and risk factors such as obesity and smoking, serum cholesterol levels, hypertension, diet and nutritional status, immunization status, infectious disease prevalence, health insurance, and measures of environmental exposures. Other topics addressed include hearing, vision, mental health, anemia, diabetes, cardiovascular disease, osteoporosis, oral health, pharmaceuticals and dietary supplements used, and physical fitness.

NHES I data were collected on the prevalence of certain chronic diseases, as well as the distribution of various physical and psychological measures, including blood pressure and serum cholesterol levels. NHES II and NHES III focused on factors related to growth and development in children and youth.

For NHANES I, data were collected on indicators of the nutritional and health status of the American people through dietary intake data, biochemical tests, physical measurements, and clinical assessments for evidence of nutritional deficiency. Detailed examinations were conducted by dentists, ophthalmologists, and dermatologists, with an assessment of need for treatment. In addition, data were obtained for a subsample of adults on overall health care needs and behavior, and more detailed examination data were collected on cardiovascular, respiratory, arthritic, and hearing conditions. For NHANES II, the nutrition component was expanded and the medical area focused on diabetes, kidney and liver function, allergy, and speech pathology. The third survey (NHANES III) also included data on antibodies, spirometry, and bone health.

Beginning in 1999 with continuous data collection for NHANES, new topics have included cardiorespiratory fitness, physical functioning, lower extremity disease, full body scan (DXA) for body fat and bone density, and tuberculosis infection.

Data Years. Data have been collected from surveys conducted during 1960–1962 (NHES I), 1963–1965 (NHES II), 1966–1970 (NHES III), 1971–1974 (NHANES I), 1976–1980 (NHANES II), 1982–1984 (Hispanic Health and Nutrition Examination Survey (HHANES)),

and 1988–1994 (NHANES III). Beginning in 1999, the survey has been conducted continuously.

Coverage. With the exception of HHANES (see Methodology, below), NHES and NHANES provide estimates of the health status of the civilian noninstitutionalized population of the United States. NHES II and NHES III examined probability samples of the Nation's noninstitutionalized children 6–11 years of age and 12–17 years, respectively.

The NHANES I target population was the civilian noninstitutionalized population 1–74 years of age residing in the coterminous United States, except for people residing on any of the reservation lands set aside for the use of American Indians.

The NHANES II target population was the civilian noninstitutionalized population 6 months to 74 years of age residing in the United States, including Alaska and Hawaii.

HHANES studied three geographically and ethnically distinct populations: Mexican Americans living in Texas, New Mexico, Arizona, Colorado, and California; Cuban Americans living in Dade County, Florida; and Puerto Ricans living in parts of New York, New Jersey, and Connecticut.

The NHANES III target population was the civilian noninstitutionalized population 2 months of age and over. The sample design provided for oversampling among children 2 months to 5 years of age, persons 60 years and over, black persons, and persons of Mexican origin.

Beginning in 1999, NHANES oversampled low-income persons, adolescents 12–19 years of age, persons 60 years and over, African Americans, and persons of Mexican origin. The sample for data years 1999–2006 is not designed to give a nationally representative sample for the total population of Hispanics residing in the United States. Starting with 2007–2008 data collection, all Hispanics were oversampled, not just Mexican Americans. For more information on the sampling methodology changes, see: http://www.cdc.gov/nchs/nhanes/nhanes2007-2008/sampling_0708.htm.

Methodology. NHANES include clinical examinations, selected medical and laboratory tests, and self-reported data. NHANES and previous surveys interviewed persons in their homes and conducted medical examinations, including laboratory analysis of blood, urine, and other tissue samples. Medical examinations and laboratory tests follow very specific protocols and are as standard as possible to ensure comparability across sites and providers. In 1999–2002, as a substitute for the MEC examinations, a small number of survey participants received an abbreviated health examination in their homes if they were unable to come to the MEC.

For the first program or cycle of NHES I, a highly stratified multistage probability sample was selected to represent the 111 million civilian noninstitutionalized adults 18–79 years of age in the United States at that time. The sample areas consisted of 42 primary sampling units (PSUs) from the 1,900 geographic units. NHES II and NHES III were also multistage stratified probability samples of clusters of households in land-based segments. NHES II and III used the same 40 PSUs.

For NHANES I, the sample areas consisted of 65 PSUs. A subsample of persons 25–74 years of age was selected to receive the more detailed health examination. Groups at high risk of malnutrition were oversampled.

NHANES II used a multistage probability design that involved selection of PSUs, segments (clusters of households) within PSUs, households, eligible persons, and, finally, sample persons. The sample design provided for oversampling among persons 6 months to 5 years of age, 60–74 years, and those living in poverty areas.

HHANES was similar in content and design to NHANES I and II. The major difference between HHANES and the previous national surveys is that HHANES used a probability sample of three special subgroups of the population living in selected areas of the United States, rather than a national probability sample. The three HHANES universes included approximately 84%, 57%, and 59% of the respective 1980 Mexican-, Cuban-, and Puerto Rican-origin populations in the continental United States.

The survey for NHANES III was conducted from 1988 to 1994 and consisted of two phases of equal length and sample size. Phases 1 and 2 comprised random samples of the civilian U.S. population living in households. About 40,000 persons 2 months of age and over were selected and asked to complete an extensive interview and an examination. Participants were selected from households in 81 counties across the United States. Children 2 months to 5 years of age and persons 60 years and over were oversampled to provide precise descriptive information on the health status of selected population groups in the United States.

Beginning in 1999, NHANES became a continuous, annual survey, which allows increased flexibility in survey content. Since April 1999, NHANES has collected data every year from a representative sample of the civilian noninstitutionalized U.S. population, newborns and older, by in-home personal interviews and physical examinations in the MEC. The sample design is a complex, multistage, clustered design using unequal probabilities of selection. The first-stage sample frame for continuous NHANES during 1999–2001 was the list of PSUs selected for the design of the National Health Interview Survey. Typically, an NHANES PSU is a county. For 2002, an independent sample of PSUs (based on current census data) was selected. This independent design was used for the period 2002–2008. For 1999, because of a delay in the start of data collection, 12 distinct PSUs were in the annual sample. For each year in 2000–2008, 15 PSUs were selected. The within-PSU design involves forming secondary sampling units that are nested within census tracts, selecting dwelling units within secondary units, and then selecting sample persons within dwelling units. The final sample person selection involves differential probabilities of selection according to the demographic variables of sex (male or female), race/ethnicity (Hispanic, black, all others), and age. Because of the differential probabilities of selection, dwelling units are screened for potential sample persons. Sample weights are available and should be used in estimating descriptive statistics. The complex design features should be used in estimating standard errors for the descriptive estimates.

The estimation procedure used to produce national statistics for all NHANES involved inflation by the reciprocal of the probability of selection, adjustment for nonresponse, and poststratified ratio adjustment to population totals. Sampling errors also were estimated to measure the reliability of the statistics.

Sample Size and Response Rates. NHES I sampled 7,710 adults. The examination response rate was 87%. NHES II sampled 7,417 children and reported a response rate of 96% for the questionnaire sample and 73% for the examination sample. NHES III sampled 7,514 youth and reported a response rate of 90%.

A sample of 28,043 persons was selected for NHANES I. Household interviews were completed for more than 96% of the persons selected, and about 75% (20,749) were examined. A sample of 27,801 persons was selected for NHANES II; 73% (20,322 persons) were examined.

In HHANES, 9,894 persons in the Southwest were selected (75% or 7,462 were examined); in Dade County, 2,244 persons were selected (60% or 1,357 were examined); and in the Northeast, 3,786 persons were selected (75% or 2,834 were examined). Over the 6-year survey period of NHANES III, 39,695 persons were selected, the household interview response rate was 86%, and the medical examination response rate was 78%.

In the sample selection for NHANES 1999–2000, there were 22,839 dwelling units screened. Of these, 6,005 households had at least one eligible sample person identified for interviewing, for a total of 12,160 eligible sample persons. The overall response rate in NHANES 1999–2000 for those interviewed was 82% (9,965 of 12,160), and the response rate for those examined was 76% (9,282 of 12,160). For NHANES 2001–2002 there were 13,156 persons selected in the sample, of which 84% (11,039) were interviewed and 80% (10,480) completed the health examination component of the survey. For NHANES 2003–2004, 6,410 households had at least one eligible sample person identified for interviewing. A total of 12,761 eligible sample persons were identified, of which 79% (10,115) were interviewed and 76% (9,653) completed the health examination component. For NHANES 2005–2006, a total of 12,862 persons were identified, of which 80% (10,348) were interviewed and 77% (9,950) completed the health examination component. For NHANES 2007–2008, a total of 12,943 persons were identified, of which 78% (10,149) were interviewed and 75% (9,762) completed the health examination component. For more information on unweighted NHANES response rates and response weights using sample size weighted to Current Population Survey population totals, see: http://www.cdc.gov/nchs/nhanes/response_rates_CPS.htm.

Issues Affecting Interpretation. Data elements, laboratory tests performed, and the technological sophistication of medical examination and laboratory equipment have changed over time. Therefore, trend analyses should carefully examine how specific data elements were collected across the various NHES and NHANES surveys.

References:

Gordon T, Miller HW. Cycle I of the Health Examination Survey: Sample and response, United States, 1960–1962. Vital Health Stat 11(1). Hyattsville, MD: NCHS; 1974. Available from: http://www.cdc.gov/nchs/data/series/sr_11/sr11_001.pdf.

NCHS. Plan, operation, and response results of a program of children's examinations. Vital Health Stat 1(5). Hyattsville, MD: NCHS; 1967. Available from: http://www.cdc.gov/nchs/data/series/sr_01/sr01_005.pdf.

Schaible WL. Quality control in a National Health Examination Survey. Vital Health Stat 2(44). Hyattsville, MD: NCHS; 1973. Available from: http://www.cdc.gov/nchs/data/series/sr_02/sr02_044.pdf.

Miller HW. Plan and operation of the Health and Nutrition Examination Survey, United States, 1971–73, part A, Development, plan, and operation. Vital Health Stat 1(10a). Hyattsville, MD: NCHS; 1973. Available from: http://www.cdc.gov/nchs/data/series/sr_01/sr01_010a.pdf.

NCHS. Plan and operation of the Health and Nutrition Examination Survey, United States, 1971–73, part B, Data collection forms of the survey. Vital Health Stat 1(10b). Hyattsville, MD: NCHS; 1977. Available from: http://www.cdc.gov/nchs/data/series/sr_01/sr01_010b.pdf.

Engel A, Murphy RS, Maurer K, Collins E. Plan and operation of the HANES I augmentation survey of adults 25–74 years: United States, 1974–1975. Vital Health Stat 1(14). Hyattsville, MD: NCHS; 1978. Available from: http://www.cdc.gov/nchs/data/series/sr_01/sr01_014.pdf.

McDowell A, Engel A, Massey JT, Maurer K. Plan and operation of the second National Health and Nutrition Examination Survey, 1976–80. Vital Health Stat 1(15). Hyattsville, MD: NCHS; 1981. Available from: http://www.cdc.gov/nchs/data/series/sr_01/sr01_015.pdf.

Maurer KR. Plan and operation of the Hispanic Health and Nutrition Examination Survey, 1982–84. Vital Health Stat 1(19). Hyattsville, MD: NCHS; 1985. Available from: http://www.cdc.gov/nchs/data/series/sr_01/sr01_019.pdf.

Ezzati TM, Massey JT, Waksberg J, Chu A, Maurer KR. Sample design: Third National Health and Nutrition Examination Survey. Vital Health Stat 2(113). Hyattsville, MD: NCHS; 1992. Available from: http://www.cdc.gov/nchs/data/series/sr_02/sr02_113.pdf.

NCHS. Plan and operation of the Third National Health and Nutrition Examination Survey, 1988–94. Vital Health Stat 1(32).Hyattsville, MD: NCHS; 1994. Available from: http://www.cdc.gov/nchs/data/series/sr_01/sr01_032.pdf.

For More Information. See the NHANES website at: http://www.cdc.gov/nchs/nhanes.htm.

National Health Interview Survey (NHIS)

CDC/NCHS

Overview. NHIS monitors the health of the U.S. population through the collection and analysis of data on a broad range of health topics. A major strength of this survey lies in the ability to analyze health measures by many demographic and socioeconomic characteristics.

Selected Content. NHIS obtains information, during household interviews, on illnesses, injuries, activity limitation, chronic conditions, health insurance coverage, utilization of health care, and other health topics. Demographic data gathered include age, sex, education, race/ethnicity (reported by respondent or proxy), place of birth, income, and residence. Other data collected include risk factors such as lack of exercise, smoking, alcohol consumption, and use of prevention services such as vaccinations, mammography, and Pap smears. Special modules and supplements focus on different issues each year and have included topics such as vaccinations, aging, cancer screening, prevention, alternative and complementary medicine, and many other topics.

Data Years. NHIS has been conducted annually since 1957, with a major redesign every 10–15 years.

Coverage. NHIS covers the civilian noninstitutionalized population of the United States. Among those excluded are patients in long-term care facilities, persons on active duty with the Armed Forces (although their dependents are included), incarcerated persons, and U.S. nationals living in foreign countries.

Methodology. NHIS is a cross-sectional household interview survey. Sampling and interviewing are continuous throughout each year. The sampling plan follows a multistage area probability design that permits the representative sampling of households. Traditionally, the sample for NHIS is redesigned and redrawn about every 10 years to better measure the changing U.S. population and to meet new survey objectives. A new sample design was implemented in the 2006 survey. The fundamental structure of the new design is very similar to the previous design for the 1995–2005 surveys. Information is presented only for the current sampling plan covering design years 2006–2014. The first stage of the current sampling plan consists of a sample of 428 primary sampling units (PSUs) drawn from approximately 1,900 geographically defined PSUs that cover the 50 states and the District of Columbia. A PSU consists of a county, a small group of contiguous counties, or a metropolitan statistical area.

Within a PSU, two types of second-stage units are used: area segments and permit segments. Area segments are defined geographically and contain an expected 8, 12, or 16 addresses. Permit segments cover housing units built after the 2000 census. The permit segments are defined using updated lists of building permits issued in the PSU since 2000 and contain an expected four addresses. Within each segment, all occupied households at the sample addresses are targeted for interview.

The total NHIS sample of PSUs is subdivided into four separate panels, or subdesigns, such that each panel is a representative sample of the U.S. population. This design feature has a number of advantages, including flexibility for the total sample size. The households selected for interview each week in NHIS are a probability sample representative of the target population.

In the 2006–2014 redesign, the NHIS sample was reduced by 13% compared with the 1995–2005 design. In addition, the NHIS sample was reduced by approximately 50% during the third quarter of 2006, cutting about 13% of the sample size of the original 2006 sample. In 2007, the NHIS sample was reduced by approximately 50% during July–September. The 2007 sample reduction was implemented in the same way and during the same time of year as the 2006 sample reduction. Overall, about 13% of the households in the 2007 NHIS sample were deleted from interviewers' assignments. The NHIS sample was reduced by approximately 50% during October–December 2008 and by approximately 50% during January–March 2009. The 2009 sample reduction was implemented in the same way as the 2006, 2007, and 2008 sample reductions; however, the timing of the 2009 reduction was different: the 2006 and 2007 reductions occurred during July–September, and the 2008 reduction occurred during October–December. Newly available funding later in 2009 permitted an expansion during October–December to increase that quarter's normal sample size by approximately 50%. The net effect of the January–March cut and the October–December expansion is that the 2009 NHIS sample size is approximately the same as it would have been if the sample had been maintained at a normal level during the entire calendar year.

Oversampling of the black and Hispanic populations was retained in the 2006–2014 design to allow for more precise estimation of health characteristics in these growing minority populations. The new sample design also oversamples the Asian population. In addition, the sample adult selection process was revised so that when black, Hispanic, or Asian persons 65 years of age and over are present, they have an increased chance of being selected as the sample adult.

The NHIS that was fielded from 1982–1996 consisted of two parts: (a) a set of basic health and demographic items (known as the Core questionnaire) and (b) one or more sets of questions on current health topics (known as Supplements). The Core questionnaire remained the same over that time period, whereas the current health topics changed depending on data needs.

The NHIS questionnaire revision, implemented in 1997, has two basic parts: a Basic Module or Core and one or more supplements that vary by year. The Core remains largely unchanged from year to year and allows for trend analysis and for data from more than 1 year to be pooled to increase the sample size for analytic purposes. The Core contains three components: the Family, the Sample Adult, and the Sample Child. The Family component collects information on everyone in the family and allows NHIS to serve as a sampling frame for additional integrated surveys as needed. Information collected in the Family section for all family members includes household composition and sociodemographic characteristics, tracking information, information for matches to administrative databases, health insurance coverage, and basic indicators of health status and utilization of health care services. Information from the Family component is included on the Person file (see the NHIS website, below). From each family in NHIS, one sample adult and, for families with children under 18 years of age, one sample child are randomly selected to participate in the Sample Adult and Sample Child questionnaires. For children, information is provided by a knowledgeable family member 18 years or over residing in the household. Because some health issues are different for children and adults, these two questionnaires differ in some items but both collect basic information on health status, use of health care services, health conditions, and health behaviors.

Sample Size and Response Rates. Between 1997 and 2005, the sample numbered about 100,000 persons with about 30,000–36,000 persons participating in the Sample Adult and about 12,000–14,000 persons in the Sample Child questionnaire. In 2009, the sample numbered 88,446 with 27,731 persons participating in the

Sample Adult and 11,156 persons in the Sample Child questionnaires. In 2009, the total household response rate was 82%. The final response rate for the Sample Adult file was 65% and for the Sample Child file was 73%.

Issues Affecting Interpretation. In 1997, the questionnaire was redesigned; some basic concepts were changed, and other concepts were measured in different ways. For some questions there was a change in the reference period. Also in 1997, the collection methodology changed from paper-and-pencil questionnaires to computer-assisted personal interviewing (CAPI). Because of the major redesign of the questionnaire in 1997, most NHIS trend tables in *Health, United States* begin with 1997 data. Starting with *Health, United States, 2005*, estimates for 2000–2002 were revised to use 2000-based weights and differ from previous editions of *Health, United States* that used 1990-based weights for those data years. The weights available on the public-use NHIS files for 2000–2002 are 1990-based. Data for 2003 and later years use weights derived from the 2000 Census. In 2006 and beyond, the sample size was reduced, and this is associated with slightly larger variance estimates than in previous years when a larger sample was fielded.

References:

Massey JT, Moore TF, Parsons VL, Tadros W. Design and estimation for the National Health Interview Survey, 1985–94. Vital Health Stat 2(110). Hyattsville, MD: NCHS; 1989. Available from: http://www.cdc.gov/nchs/data/series/sr_02/sr02_110.pdf.

NCHS. National Health Interview Survey: Research for the 1995–2004 redesign. Vital Health Stat 2(126). Hyattsville, MD: NCHS; 1999. Available from: http://www.cdc.gov/nchs/data/series/sr_02/sr02_126.pdf.

Botman SL, Moore TF, Moriarity CL, Parsons VL. Design and estimation for the National Health Interview Survey, 1995–2004. Vital Health Stat 2(130). Hyattsville, MD: NCHS; 2000. Available from: http://www.cdc.gov/nchs/data/series/sr_02/sr02_130.pdf.

For More Information. See the NHIS website at: http://www.cdc.gov/nchs/nhis.htm.

National Home and Hospice Care Survey (NHHCS)

CDC/NCHS

Overview. NHHCS is a national probability sample survey of U.S. home health and hospice care agencies. The survey is designed to provide descriptive information on the agencies and their staffs, services, and patients.

Selected Content. NHHCS provides information on home health and hospice care agencies from two perspectives—that of the provider of services and that of the recipient of services. Data about the agencies include characteristics such as ownership; affiliation; services offered; and number, training, and characteristics of staff. Data about the current home health care patients and discharged hospice care patients include demographic characteristics, diagnoses, health status, level of assistance needed with activities of daily living, services received, sources of payment, and discharge disposition (for discharges). The redesigned NHHCS, conducted in 2007, included new agency data items on electronic information systems, cultural competency, end-of-life practices, and special service programs, as well as new patient-level data items on pain assessment and pain relief, medications, family and caregiver services, end-of-life care, and advance directives. The 2007 survey also included a supplemental survey of home health aides employed by home health and/or hospice care agencies, called the National Home Health Aide Survey.

Data Years. NHHCS was first conducted in 1992 and was repeated in 1993, 1994, 1996, 1998, 2000, and most recently in 2007. The 2007 NHHCS, which was reintroduced into the field after a 7-year break that included a redesign, was conducted between August 2007 and February 2008.

Coverage. The survey covers agencies that provide home health and hospice care services in the United States and the care recipients of these agencies. Agencies are freestanding health facilities or units of larger organizations, such as hospitals or nursing homes. Agencies that provide only homemaker services or housekeeping services, assistance with instrumental activities of daily living (IADLs), or durable medical equipment and supplies are excluded from the survey.

Methodology. The survey uses a stratified two-stage probability sample design; the 1992–1994 surveys used a stratified three-stage probability sample design. The first stage of the 2007 survey, carried out by NCHS, was the selection of home health and hospice care agencies from the sample frame of over 15,000 agencies, representing the universe of agencies providing home health and hospice care services in the United States. The primary sampling strata of agencies were defined by agency type (i.e., home health care only, hospice care only, and mixed (provides both home health and hospice care services)) and metropolitan statistical area (MSA) status. Within these sampling strata, agencies were sorted by census region, ownership, certification status, state, county, ZIP code, and size (number of employees).

The second stage of sample selection was completed by the interviewers during the agency interviews. The current home health care patients and hospice care discharges were randomly selected by a computer algorithm, based on a census list provided by each agency director or his or her designee. Up to 10 current home health care patients were randomly selected per home health care agency; up to 10 hospice care discharges were randomly selected per hospice care agency; and a combination of up to 10 current home health care patients and hospice care discharges were randomly selected per mixed agency. Current home health care patients were defined as patients who were on the rolls of the home health care agency as of midnight of the day immediately before the agency interview. The hospice care discharges were defined as patients who were discharged from the hospice care agency during the 3-month period beginning 4 months before the agency interview. Discharges that occurred because of the death of a sampled hospice patient were included.

All data, except for the paper-and-pencil self-administered staffing questionnaire, were collected using a computer-assisted personal interviewing instrument. Agency data, available in agency administrative records, were collected through in-person interviews with agency directors and their designated staff. Data on home health care patients and hospice care discharges, available in medical records, were collected by interviewing the staff member most familiar with the care provided to the sampled patients/discharges. No interviews were conducted directly with patients or their families or friends.

Estimates based on NHHCS take into account the selection procedures of the complete survey design to develop the final sample weight for each sampled agency and each sampled patient/discharge. The final weight for each sampled unit is the product of up to three components: inverse of the probability of selection; nonresponse adjustment; and ratio adjustment. The data from the surveys are adjusted for three types of nonresponse: an in-scope agency did not respond; an in-scope agency did not provide the number of current home health care patients and/or hospice care discharges; and the administrative and medical records of the sampled current home health care patients and/or hospice discharges were not made available to complete the survey.

Sample Size and Response Rates. The sampling frame for the 2007 NHHCS was constructed using three sources: (a) Centers for Medicare & Medicaid Services Provider of Services File of home health care agencies and hospices, (b) state licensing lists of home health care agencies compiled by a private organization, and (c) the National Hospice and Palliative Care Organization file of hospices. The combined files were matched and identified duplicates were removed, resulting in a sampling frame of 15,488 agencies. A sample of 1,545 agencies were selected, of which 1,461 (95%) were considered in scope. Of the in-scope agencies, 1,036 agreed to participate, resulting in a first-stage agency unweighted response rate of 71% and a weighted response rate of 59%. A total of 10,009 current home health care patients and hospice care discharges were sampled from the responding agencies: 5,026 current home health care patients and 4,983 hospice care discharges. Of these, 106 home health care patients and 19 hospice care discharges were considered out of scope. Furthermore, 237 current home health care patients and 231 hospice care discharges were excluded due to one of the following reasons: consent problems, record problems, refusals, ran out of time, and nonresponse. This resulted in 4,683 home health cases and 4,733 hospice cases, for a second-stage unweighted response rate of 95% and a weighted response rate of 96%.

Issues Affecting Interpretation. The current home health care patient sample describes individuals receiving home health care on the night before data collection began and represents home health care utilization on any given day between August 2007 and February 2008. Because frequent short-term users are less likely than long-term users to be enrolled with the agency on any given day, the current home health care patients with a very short length of service may be underestimated. The hospice care discharge sample describes the annual number of discharges from hospice care. Estimates of hospice discharges may underestimate those patients who tend to receive care for longer periods of time. Finally, various survey items were added or modified in the 2007 survey, which may preclude comparisons from previous years or trend analyses.

References:

Haupt BJ. Development of the National Home and Hospice Care Survey. Vital Health Stat 1(33). Hyattsville, MD: NCHS; 1994. Available from: http://www.cdc.gov/nchs/data/series/sr_01/sr01_033acc.pdf.

Haupt B, Hing E, Strahan G. The National Home and Hospice Care Survey: 1992 Summary. Vital Health Stat 13(117). Hyattsville, MD: NCHS; 1994. Available from: http://www.cdc.gov/nchs/data/series/sr_13/sr13_117.pdf.

Jones A, Strahan G. The National Home and Hospice Care Survey: 1994 Summary. Vital Health Stat 13(126). Hyattsville, MD: NCHS; 1997. Available from: http://www.cdc.gov/nchs/data/series/sr_13/sr13_126.pdf.

Haupt BJ, Jones A. The National Home and Hospice Care Survey: 1996 Summary. Vital Health Stat 13(141). Hyattsville, MD: NCHS; 1999. Available from: http://www.cdc.gov/nchs/data/series/sr_13/sr13_141.pdf.

Haupt BJ. Characteristics of hospice care discharges and their length of service: United States, 2000. Vital Health Stat 13(154). Hyattsville, MD: NCHS; 2003. Available from: http://www.cdc.gov/nchs/data/series/sr_13/sr13_154.pdf.

Dwyer LL, Harris-Kojetin LD, Branden L, Shimizu IM. Redesign and operation of the National Home and Hospice Care Survey, 2007. Vital Health Stat 1(53). Hyattsville, MD: NCHS; 2010. Available from: http://www.cdc.gov/nchs/data/series/sr_01/sr01_053.pdf.

For More Information. See the National Health Care Surveys website at: http://www.cdc.gov/nchs/nhcs.htm and the NHHCS website at: http://www.cdc.gov/nchs/NHHCS.htm.

National Hospital Ambulatory Medical Care Survey (NHAMCS)

CDC/NCHS

Overview. NHAMCS collects data on the utilization and provision of medical care services provided in hospital emergency and outpatient departments.

Selected Content. Data are collected from medical records on types of providers seen; reason for visit; diagnoses; drugs ordered, provided, or continued; and selected procedures and tests performed during the visit. Patient data include age, sex, race, and expected source of payment. Data are also collected on selected characteristics of the hospitals included in the survey.

Data Years. Annual data collection began in 1992.

Coverage. The survey is a representative sample of visits to emergency departments (EDs) and outpatient departments (OPDs) of nonfederal, short-stay, or general hospitals. Telephone contacts are excluded.

Methodology. A four-stage probability sample design is used in NHAMCS, involving (a) samples of geographically defined primary sampling units (PSUs), (b) hospitals within PSUs, (c) clinics within OPDs, and (d) patient visits within clinics. EDs are treated as their own stratum, and all service areas within EDs are included. The first-stage sample of NHAMCS consists of 112 PSUs selected from 1,900 such units that make up the United States. Within PSUs, 600 general and short-stay hospitals were sampled and assigned to 1 of 16 panels. In any given year, 13 panels are included. Each panel is assigned to a 4-week reporting period during the calendar year.

In the NHAMCS OPD survey, a clinic is defined as an administrative unit of the OPD in which ambulatory medical care is provided under the supervision of a physician. Clinics where only ancillary services—such as radiology, laboratory services, physical rehabilitation, renal dialysis, and pharmacy—are provided, or other settings in which physician services are not typically provided, are considered out of scope. If a hospital OPD has five or fewer in-scope clinics, all are included in the sample. If an outpatient department has more than five clinics, the clinics are assigned into one of six specialty groups: general medicine, surgery, pediatrics, obstetrics/gynecology, substance abuse, and other. Within these specialty groups, clinics are grouped into clinic sampling units (SUs). A clinic SU is generally one clinic, except when a clinic expects fewer than 30 visits. In that case, it is grouped with one or more other clinics to form a clinic SU. If the grouped SU is selected, all clinics included in that SU are included in the sample. Prior to 2001, a sample of generally five clinic SUs was selected per hospital, based on probability proportional to the total expected number of patient visits to the clinic during the assigned 4-week reporting period. Starting in 2001, clinic sampling within each hospital was stratified. If an OPD had more than five clinics, two clinic SUs were selected from each of the six specialty groups with a probability proportional to the total expected number of visits to the clinic. The change was made

to ensure that at least two SUs were sampled from each of the specialty group strata.

The U.S. Census Bureau acts as the data collection agent for NHAMCS. Census field representatives contact sample hospitals to determine whether they have a 24-hour ED or an OPD that offers physician services. Visits to eligible EDs and OPDs are systematically sampled over the 4-week reporting period such that about 100 ED encounters and about 200 OPD encounters are selected. Hospital staff are asked to complete patient record forms (PRFs) for each sampled visit, but census field representatives typically abstract data for more than one-third of these visits.

Sample data are weighted to produce national estimates. The estimation procedure used in NHAMCS has three basic components: inflation by the reciprocal of the probability of selection, adjustment for nonresponse, and ratio adjustment to fixed totals.

Sample Size and Response Rate. In any given year, the hospital sample consists of approximately 500 hospitals, of which 80% have EDs and about one-half have eligible OPDs. Typically, about 1,000 clinics are selected from participating hospital OPDs. In each sample year from 2002 to 2008, the number of PRFs completed for EDs ranged from 33,000 to 40,000 and for OPDs from 30,000 to 36,000. The hospital response rate was 83%–94% for EDs and 73%–84% for OPDs during this timeframe. In 2008, the number of PRFs completed for EDs was 34,134 and for OPDs was 33,908, and the hospital response rate was 87% for EDs and 75% for OPDs.

Issues Affecting Interpretation. The NHAMCS PRF is modified approximately every 2 to 4 years to reflect changes in physician practice characteristics, patterns of care, and technological innovations. Examples of recent changes are the number of drugs recorded on the PRF form and the number of checkboxes for specific tests or procedures performed.

Reference:

McCaig LF, McLemore T. Plan and operation of the National Hospital Ambulatory Medical Care Survey. Vital Health Stat 1(34). Hyattsville, MD: NCHS; 1994. Available from: http://www.cdc.gov/nchs/data/series/sr_01/sr01_034acc.pdf.

For More Information. See the National Health Care Surveys website at: http://www.cdc.gov/nchs/nhcs.htm and the Ambulatory Health Care Data website at: http://www.cdc.gov/nchs/ahcd.htm.

National Hospital Discharge Survey (NHDS)

CDC/NCHS

Overview. NHDS collects and produces national estimates on characteristics of inpatient stays in nonfederal, short-stay hospitals in the United States.

Selected Content. Patient information collected includes demographics, length of stay, diagnoses, and procedures. Hospital characteristics collected include region, ownership, and bed size.

Data Years. NHDS has been conducted annually since 1965.

Coverage. The survey design covers the 50 states and the District of Columbia. Included in the survey are hospitals with an average length of stay of less than 30 days for all inpatients, general hospitals, and children's general hospitals. Excluded are federal, military, and Department of Veterans Affairs hospitals, as well as hospital units of institutions (such as prison hospitals) and hospitals with fewer than six beds staffed for patient use. All discharged patients from in-scope hospitals are included in the survey; however, data for newborns are not included in *Health, United States.*

Methodology. The NHDS design implemented in 1965 continued through 1987, and a redesign with a new sample of hospitals, fielded in 1988, is currently in place. The sample for the 1965 NHDS was selected in 1964 from a frame of short-stay hospitals listed in the National Master Facility Inventory. A two-stage stratified sample design was used, with hospitals stratified according to bed size and geographic region. Sample hospitals were selected with probabilities ranging from certainty for some hospitals to 1 in 40 for other hospitals. Within each participating hospital, a systematic random sample was selected from a daily listing sheet of discharges. Within-hospital sampling rates for discharges varied inversely with the probability of hospital selection, so the overall probability of selecting a discharge was approximately the same across the sample.

Data collection was conducted by means of manual abstraction of patient information from sampled medical records. Sample selection and transcription of information from inpatient medical records to NHDS survey forms were performed by hospital staff, representatives of NCHS, or both. In 1985, a second data collection procedure was introduced that involved the purchase of computer data tapes from commercial abstracting services that contained automated discharge data for some hospitals

participating in NHDS. This procedure was used in approximately 17% of the sample hospitals for 1985–1987. Discharges on these computer files were subjected to the NHDS sampling specifications as well as the computer edits and estimation procedures. Two data collection methods, manual and automated, continue to be used in NHDS.

A redesign of NHDS was implemented for the 1988 survey. Under the redesign, hospitals were selected using a modified three-stage stratified design. Units selected at the first stage consisted of either hospitals or geographic areas. The geographic areas were the primary sampling units (PSUs) used for the 1985–1994 National Health Interview Survey, which are geographic areas such as counties or townships. Hospitals within PSUs were then selected at the second stage. Strata at this stage were defined by geographic region, PSU size, abstracting service status, and hospital specialty-size groups. Within these strata, hospitals were selected with probabilities proportional to their annual number of discharges. At the third stage, a sample of discharges was selected by a systematic random sampling technique. The sampling rate was determined by the hospital's sampling stratum and the type of data collection system (manual or automated) used. Discharge records from hospitals submitting data from commercial abstracting services and selected state data systems (approximately 45% of sample hospitals in 2007) were arrayed by primary diagnoses, patient sex and age group, and date of discharge, before sampling.

The NHDS hospital sample is updated every 3 years by continuing the sampling process among hospitals that become eligible for the survey during the intervening years and by deleting hospitals that are no longer eligible. This update was conducted in 1991, 1994, 1997, 2000, 2003, and 2006.

The basic unit of estimation for NHDS is a sampled discharge. The basic estimation procedure involves inflation by the reciprocal of the probability of selection. Adjustments are made for nonresponding hospitals and discharges, and a post-ratio adjustment to fixed totals is employed.

Sample Size and Response Rate. In 2007, 501 hospitals were selected: 477 were within scope, 422 participated (88%), and data were collected from medical records for approximately 366,000 discharges.

Issues Affecting Interpretation. NHDS was redesigned in 1988, and caution is required in comparing trend data from before and after the redesign. In addition, annual modifications to the *International*

Classification of Diseases, 9th Revision, Clinical Modification (ICD–9–CM) may affect diagnosis and procedure categories. (See Appendix II, *International Classification of Diseases, 9th Revision, Clinical Modification*; and Tables XI and XII.)

Hospital utilization rates per 10,000 population were computed using estimates of the civilian population of the United States as of July 1 of each year. Rates for 1990–1999 use postcensal estimates of the civilian population based on the 1990 census, adjusted for net underenumeration using the 1990 National Population Adjustment Matrix from the U.S. Census Bureau. The estimates for 2000 and beyond that appear in *Health, United States, 2003* and later editions were calculated using estimates of the civilian population based on Census 2000, and therefore are not strictly comparable with postcensal rates calculated for the 1990s. (See Appendix I, Population Census and Population Estimates.)

References:

Hall MJ, DeFrances CJ, Williams SN, Golosinskiy A, Schwartzman A. National Hospital Discharge Survey: 2007 summary. National health statistics reports; no 29. Hyattsville, MD: NCHS; 2010. Available from: http://www.cdc.gov/nchs/data/nhsr/nhsr029.pdf.

Dennison C, Pokras R. Design and operation of the National Hospital Discharge Survey: 1988 Redesign. Vital Health Stat 1(39). Hyattsville, MD: NCHS; 2000. Available from: http://www.cdc.gov/nchs/data/series/sr_01/sr01_039.pdf.

Haupt BJ, Kozak LJ. Estimates from two survey designs: National Hospital Discharge Survey. Vital Health Stat 13(111). Hyattsville, MD: NCHS; 1992. Available from: http://www.cdc.gov/nchs/data/series/sr_13/sr13_111.pdf.

For More Information. See the National Health Care Surveys website at: http://www.cdc.gov/nchs/nhcs.htm and the National Hospital Discharge Survey website at: http://www.cdc.gov/nchs/nhds.htm.

National Immunization Survey (NIS)

CDC/National Center for Immunization and Respiratory Diseases (NCIRD) and NCHS

Overview. NIS is a continuing nationwide telephone sample survey to monitor vaccination coverage rates among children 19–35 months of age and among teenagers (NIS–Teen) 13–17 years.

Selected Content. Data collected for children include vaccination status and date of vaccinations for diphtheria, tetanus toxoids, and acellular pertussis vaccine (DTP/DT/DTaP); poliovirus vaccine (Polio); measles, mumps, and rubella vaccine (MMR); *Haemophilus influenzae* type b vaccine (Hib); hepatitis B vaccine (Hep B); varicella zoster vaccine; pneumococcal conjugate vaccine (PCV); hepatitis A (Hep A); influenza; and for adolescents meningococcal conjugate vaccine (MCV4) and human papillomavirus vaccine (HPV). Demographic data include age, gender, race and ethnicity, and poverty level. Data are available at a variety of geographic levels, including census regions, state, and selected urban areas.

Data Years. Annual household data collection was initiated beginning with the data year 1994. Data collection for varicella began in July 1996; data collection for PCV began in July 2001. Data collection for adolescents 13–17 years of age began in 2006.

Coverage. Children 19–35 months of age and adolescents 13–17 years in the civilian noninstitutionalized population are represented in this survey. Estimates of vaccine-specific coverage are available for the Nation, states, and selected urban areas.

Methodology. NIS is a nationwide telephone sample survey of households with age-eligible children. NIS uses a two-phase sample design. First, a random-digit-dialing sample of telephone numbers is drawn. When households with age-eligible children are contacted, the interviewer collects information on the vaccinations received by all age-eligible children and obtains permission to contact the children's vaccination providers. Second, identified providers are sent vaccination history questionnaires by mail. Providers' responses are compared with information obtained from households to provide a more accurate estimate of vaccination coverage levels. Final estimates are adjusted for households without telephones and for nonresponse. NIS–Teen followed the same sample design and data collection procedures as NIS except that only one age-eligible adolescent was selected from each household for data collection.

Sample Size and Response Rate. In 2009, vaccination data were collected from providers for 17,313 children 1–35 months of age. The overall interview response rate was 64%. Vaccination information from providers was obtained for 71% of all children who were eligible for provider follow-up in 2009.

In 2009, vaccination data were collected from providers for 20,399 adolescents 13–17 years of age.

The overall interview response rate was 58%. Vaccination information from providers was obtained for 57% of all adolescents who were eligible for provider follow-up in 2009.

Issues Affecting Interpretation. For data years 1998, 2002, 2004, and 2005, slight modifications to the estimation procedure were implemented to obtain vaccination coverage rates from the provider data. Published estimates of vaccination coverage based on NIS data for years prior to 1998 (e.g., estimates published in *Morbidity and Mortality Weekly Report* (MMWR) articles) may differ slightly from estimates published in *Health, United States* and on the NIS website for the same NIS data. All released public-use data files include the sampling weights using the revised estimation procedure. The findings in recent years are subject to at least three limitations. First, NIS is a telephone survey, and statistical adjustments might not compensate fully for nonresponse and for households without landline telephones. Second, underestimates of vaccination coverage might have resulted in exclusive use of provider-reported vaccination histories because completeness of records is unknown. Finally, although national coverage estimates are precise, annual estimates and trends for state and local areas should be interpreted with caution because of smaller sample sizes and wider confidence intervals.

Before January 2009, NIS did not distinguish between Hib vaccine production types; therefore, children who received three doses of a vaccine product that requires four doses were misclassified as fully vaccinated. For more information, see "Changes in Measurement of *Haemophilus influenzae* Serotype b (Hib) Vaccination Coverage—National Immunization Survey, United States, 2009" (2010).

References:

CDC. National, state, and local area vaccination coverage among children aged 19–35 months—United States, 2009. MMWR 2010;59(36):1171–77. Available from: http://www.cdc.gov/mmwr/preview/mmwrhtml/mm5936a2.htm?s_cid=mm5936a2_w.

CDC. National, state, and local area vaccination coverage among adolescents aged 13–17 years—United States, 2009. MMWR 2010;59(32):1018–23. Available from: http://www.cdc.gov/mmwr/preview/mmwrhtml/mm5932a3.htm?s_cid=mm5932a3_w.

Smith PJ, Hoaglin DC, Battaglia MP, Khare M, Barker LE. Statistical methodology of the National Immunization Survey, 1994–2002. Vital Health Stat 2(138). Hyattsville, MD: NCHS; 2005. Available from: http://www.cdc.gov/nchs/data/series/sr_02/sr02_138.pdf.

CDC. Changes in measurement of *Haemophilus influenzae* serotype b (Hib) vaccination coverage—National Immunization Survey, United States, 2009. MMWR 2010; 59(33)1069–72. Available from: http://www.cdc.gov/mmwr/preview/mmwrhtml/mm5933a3.htm?s_cid=mm5933a3_e%0d%0a.

For More Information. See the NIS website at: http://www.cdc.gov/nchs/nis.htm.

National Medical Expenditure Survey (NMES)—See Medical Expenditure Panel Survey

National Notifiable Disease Surveillance System (NNDSS)

CDC

Overview. NNDSS provides weekly provisional information on the occurrence of diseases defined as notifiable by the Council of State and Territorial Epidemiologists (CSTE).

Selected Content. Data include incidence of reportable diseases using uniform case definitions.

Data Years. The first annual summary of the notifiable diseases in 1912 included reports of 10 diseases from 19 states, the District of Columbia (D.C.), and Hawaii. By 1928, all states, D.C., Hawaii, and Puerto Rico were participating in national reporting of 29 specified diseases. At their annual meeting in 1950, State and Territorial Health Officers authorized a conference of state and territorial epidemiologists whose purpose was to determine which diseases should be reported to Public Health Service. In 1961, CDC assumed responsibility for the collection and publication of data concerning nationally notifiable diseases.

Coverage. Notifiable disease reports are received from health departments in the 50 states, five territories, New York City, and D.C. Policies for reporting notifiable disease cases can vary by disease or by reporting jurisdiction, depending on case status classification (i.e., confirmed, probable, or suspect).

Methodology. CDC, in partnership with CSTE, operates NNDSS. Notifiable disease surveillance is conducted by public health practitioners at local, state, and national levels to support disease prevention and control activities. The system also provides annual summaries of the data. CSTE and CDC annually review the status of national infectious disease surveillance and recommend additions or deletions to the list of nationally notifiable diseases, based on the need to respond to emerging priorities. For example, Q fever and tularemia became nationally notifiable in 2000. However, reporting nationally notifiable diseases to CDC is voluntary. Because reporting is currently mandated by law or regulation only at the local and state levels, the list of diseases that are considered notifiable varies slightly by state. For example, reporting of cyclosporiasis to CDC is not done by some states in which this disease is not notifiable to local or state authorities.

State epidemiologists report cases of notifiable diseases to CDC, which tabulates and publishes these data in *Morbidity and Mortality Weekly Report* (MMWR) and in *Summary of Notifiable Diseases, United States* (before 1985, titled *Annual Summary*).

Issues Affecting Interpretation. NNDSS data must be interpreted in light of reporting practices. Some diseases that cause severe clinical illness (for example, plague and rabies) are likely reported accurately if diagnosed by a clinician. However, persons who have diseases that are clinically mild and infrequently associated with serious consequences (e.g., salmonellosis) may not seek medical care from a health care provider. Even if these less severe diseases are diagnosed, they are less likely to be reported.

The degree of completeness of data reporting is also influenced by the diagnostic facilities available, the control measures in effect, public awareness of a specific disease, and the interests, resources, and priorities of state and local officials responsible for disease control and public health surveillance. Finally, factors such as changes in case definitions for public health surveillance, introduction of new diagnostic tests, or discovery of new disease entities can cause changes in disease reporting that are independent of the true incidence of disease.

Reference:

CDC. Summary of notifiable diseases—United States, 2008. MMWR 2010;57(54). Available from: http://www.cdc.gov/mmwr/preview/mmwrhtml/mm5754a1.htm.

For More Information. See the NNDSS website at: http://www.cdc.gov/ncphi/disss/nndss/nndsshis.htm.

National Nursing Home Survey (NNHS)

CDC/NCHS

Overview. NNHS collects and provides national estimates on the characteristics of nursing homes and their residents and staff.

Selected Content. NNHS provides information on nursing homes from two perspectives—that of the provider of services and that of the recipient. Data about the facilities include characteristics such as bed size, ownership, affiliation, Medicare/Medicaid certification, specialty units, services offered, number and characteristics of staff, expenses, and charges. Data about the current residents and discharges include demographic characteristics, health status, level of assistance needed with activities of daily living, vision and hearing impairment, continence, services received, sources of payment, and discharge disposition (for discharges). The redesigned NNHS conducted in 2004 included new facility data items on Joint Commission on Accreditation of Healthcare Organizations (JCAHO) accreditation, electronic information systems, cultural competency, immunization policies and practices, end-of-life practices, and special service programs, as well as new patient-level data items on hospitalizations and emergency department admissions, pain assessment and pain relief, medications, family and caregiver services, end-of-life care and advance directives, pressure ulcers, behavior or mood symptoms, falls, and out-of-pocket charges. In addition to these facility and resident data items, data were also collected on nurse staffing and a supplemental survey was conducted on nursing assistants working in nursing homes.

Data Years. NCHS has conducted seven NNHSs. The first survey was performed August 1973–April 1974; the second, May–December 1977; the third, August 1985–January 1986; the fourth, July–December 1995; the fifth, July–December 1997; and the sixth, July–December 1999. The seventh and most recent NNHS, which had undergone a major redesign, was conducted August 2004–January 2005.

Coverage. The initial NNHS, conducted in 1973–1974, included the universe of nursing homes that provided some level of nursing care and excluded homes providing only personal or domiciliary care. The 1977 NNHS encompassed all types of nursing homes, including personal care and domiciliary care homes. The 1985 NNHS was designed to be similar to the 1973–1974 survey in that it excluded personal or domiciliary care homes; however, in 1985 an unknown number of residential care facilities were present in the sampling frame. These facilities were identified in the 1986 inventory survey and can be removed from the estimate of facilities and beds for 1985. The 1995, 1997, 1999, and 2004 NNHS also included only nursing homes that provided some level of nursing care and excluded homes providing only personal or domiciliary care, similar to the 1985 and 1973–1974 surveys.

Methodology. The survey uses a stratified two-stage probability design. The first stage is the selection of facilities, and the second stage is the selection of residents and discharges. Prior to the 2004 NNHS, up to six current residents and/or six discharges were selected for each facility. The 2004 survey was designed to select only 12 current residents from each facility to participate in the survey. Information on the facility was collected through a personal interview with the administrator or with staff designated by the administrator. Resident data were provided by staff familiar with the care provided to the resident. Staff relied on the medical record and personal knowledge of the resident. In addition to employee data collected during the interview with the administrator, in several years staffing data were collected by means of a self-administered questionnaire. Discharge data, when collected, were based on information recorded in the medical record.

Current residents are those on the facility's roster as of the night before the survey. Included are all residents for whom beds are maintained, even though they may be away on an overnight leave or in the hospital. People residing in personal care or domiciliary care homes are excluded. Discharges are those who are formally discharged from care by the facility during a designated reference period randomly selected for each facility before data collection. Both live and deceased discharges are included. Residents were counted more than once if they were discharged more than once during the reference period. Resident rates are calculated using estimates of the civilian population of the United States, including institutionalized persons. Population data are from unpublished tabulations provided by the U.S. Census Bureau. The 2004 population estimates are postcensal estimates as of July 1, 2004, based on the 2000 census. For more information about the 2004 population estimates, see Technical Notes in: Kozak LJ, DeFrances CJ, Hall MJ. National Hospital Discharge Survey: 2004 annual summary with detailed diagnosis and procedure data. Vital Health Stat 13(162). Hyattsville, MD: NCHS; 2006. Available from: http://www.cdc.gov/nchs/data/series/sr_13/sr13_162acc.pdf.

Statistics for NNHS are derived by a multistage estimation procedure that has three major components: (a) inflation by the reciprocals of the probabilities of sample selection, (b) adjustment for nonresponse, and (c) ratio adjustment to fixed totals. The surveys are adjusted for four types of nonresponse: (a) when an eligible nursing facility did not respond, (b) when the facility failed to complete the sampling lists, (c) when the facility did not complete the facility questionnaire but did complete the questionnaire for residents in the facility, and (d) when the facility did not provide information to complete the questionnaire for the sample resident or discharge.

Sample Size and Response Rates. In 1973–1974, the sample of 2,118 homes was selected from the 1971 National Master Facility Inventory (NMFI) and from those that opened for business in 1972. For the 1977 NNHS, the sample of 1,698 facilities was selected from nursing homes in the sampling frame, which consisted of all homes listed in the 1973 NMFI and those opening for business between 1973 and December 1976. The sample for the 1985 survey consisted of the 1,220 facilities selected from the 1982 NMFI, data for homes identified in the 1982 Complement Survey of the NMFI, data on hospital-based nursing homes obtained from the Health Care Financing Administration (now known as the Centers for Medicare & Medicaid Services), and data on nursing homes open for business between 1982 and June 1, 1984. The 1995 sample of 1,500 homes was selected from a sampling frame consisting of nursing homes from the 1991 National Health Provider Inventory (NHPI) and updated lists from the Agency Reporting System (ARS). The ARS was an ongoing system designed to periodically update the NHPI and consisted primarily of lists or directories of facilities from state agencies, federal agencies, and national voluntary organizations. For the 1997 survey, data were obtained from about 1,488 nursing homes from a sampling frame consisting of nursing homes listed on the 1991 NHPI that was updated with a current listing of nursing facilities supplied by the Health Care Finance Administration and other national organizations. The facility frame for the 1999 NNHS consisted of all nursing homes identified in the 1997 NNHS and updated with current nursing facilities listed by the Centers for Medicare & Medicaid Services and other national organizations. The 1999 sample consisted of 1,496 nursing homes. In 1995, 1997, and 1999, facility-level response rates were over 93%. For the 2004 redesigned and expanded NNHS, 1,500 nursing homes were selected and a facility response rate of 81% was achieved.

Issues Affecting Interpretation. Samples of discharges and residents contain different populations with different characteristics. The resident sample is more likely to contain long-term nursing home residents and, conversely, to underestimate short nursing home stays. Because short-term residents are less likely to be on the nursing home rolls on a given night, they are less likely to be sampled. Estimates of discharges underestimate long nursing home stays. In addition, analysts should ensure that the underlying populations are similar across survey years—for example, whether the survey includes personal or domiciliary care homes.

References:

Meiners MR. Selected operating and financial characteristics of nursing homes, United States: 1973–74 National Nursing Home Survey. Vital Health Stat 13(22). Hyattsville, MD: NCHS; 1975. Available from: http://www.cdc.gov/nchs/data/series/sr_13/sr13_022.pdf.

Van Nostrand JF, Zappolo A, Hing E, Bloom B, Hirsch B, Foley DJ. The National Nursing Home Survey: 1977 summary for the United States. Vital Health Stat 13(43). Hyattsville, MD: NCHS; 1979. Available from: http://www.cdc.gov/nchs/data/series/sr_13/sr13_043.pdf.

Hing E, Sekscenski E, Strahan G. The National Nursing Home Survey: 1985 summary for the United States. Vital Health Stat 13(97). Hyattsville, MD: NCHS; 1989. Available from: http://www.cdc.gov/nchs/data/series/sr_13/sr13_097.pdf.

Strahan GW. An overview of nursing homes and their current residents: Data from the 1995 National Nursing Home Survey. Advance data from vital and health statistics; no 280. Hyattsville, MD: NCHS; 1997. Available from: http://www.cdc.gov/nchs/data/ad/ad280.pdf.

Gabrel CS, Jones A. The National Nursing Home Survey: 1997 summary. Vital Health Stat 13(147). Hyattsville, MD: NCHS; 2000. Available from: http://www.cdc.gov/nchs/data/series/sr_13/sr13_147.pdf.

Jones A. The National Nursing Home Survey: 1999 summary. Vital Health Stat 13(152). Hyattsville, MD: NCHS; 2002. Available from: http://www.cdc.gov/nchs/data/series/sr_13/sr13_152.pdf.

Jones AL, Dwyer LL, Bercovitz AR, Strahan GW. The National Nursing Home Survey: 2004 overview. Vital Health Stat 13(167).

Hyattsville, MD: NCHS; 2009. Available from: http://www.cdc.gov/nchs/data/series/sr_13/sr13_167.pdf.

For More Information. See the National Health Care Surveys website at: http://www.cdc.gov/nchs/dhcs.htm and the NNHS website at: http://www.cdc.gov/nchs/nnhs.htm.

National Survey on Drug Use & Health (NSDUH)

Substance Abuse and Mental Health Services Administration (SAMHSA)

Overview. NSDUH, formerly called the National Household Survey on Drug Abuse (NHSDA), collects data on substance use, abuse, and dependence; mental health problems; and receipt of substance abuse and mental health treatment.

Selected Content. NSDUH reports on the prevalence, incidence, and patterns of drug and alcohol use and abuse in the general U.S. civilian noninstitutionalized population 12 years of age and over. Data are collected primarily on the use of illicit drugs, the nonmedical use of prescription psychotherapeutic drugs, and the use of alcohol and tobacco products; dependence and abuse involving drugs and alcohol; mental health problems; and treatment of substance use and mental health problems. Data are also collected on special topics of interest, such as attitudes about drugs, health conditions, driving under the influence of alcohol and illicit drugs, and criminal behavior.

Data Years. NHSDA has been conducted periodically since 1971 and annually starting in 1990. In 1999, NHSDA underwent a major redesign affecting the method of data collection, sample design, sample size, and oversampling. In 2002, the survey's name was changed to NSDUH, a monetary incentive for participation was introduced, and other improvements were made.

Coverage. The survey is representative of persons 12 years of age and over in the civilian noninstitutionalized population of the United States in each state and the District of Columbia. This includes civilians living on military bases and persons living in noninstitutionalized group quarters, such as college dormitories, rooming houses, and shelters. Persons excluded from the survey include homeless people who do not use shelters, active military personnel, and residents of institutional group quarters such as jails and hospitals.

Methodology. The data collection method is in-person interviews conducted with a sample of individuals at their place of residence. Prior to 1999, NSDUH used a paper-and-pencil interviewing methodology. Since 1999, the interview has been carried out with computer-assisted interviewing methodology. The survey uses a combination of computer-assisted personal interviewing (CAPI), conducted by the interviewer to obtain basic demographic information, and audio computer-assisted self-interviewing (ACASI) for most of the questions. ACASI provides a highly private and confidential means of responding to questions, to increase the level of honest reporting of illicit drug use and other sensitive behaviors.

In 1999, a 50-state sample design was introduced. Eight states (California, Florida, Illinois, Michigan, New York, Ohio, Pennsylvania, and Texas) are designated as large sample states with target sample sizes of 3,600 per year. The remaining states and the District of Columbia have target sample sizes of 900 per year. This approach ensures that there are sufficient samples in every state to support small area estimation, while maintaining efficiency for national estimates. In the 1999–2001 and 2002–2004 surveys, the first-stage sampling units were clusters of census blocks called area segments. In 2005, NSDUH introduced a coordinated 5-year sample design in which the first stage of selection involved census tracts, with sample segments within a single census tract to the extent possible. States were first stratified into a total of 900 state sampling (SS) regions (48 regions in each large sample state and 12 regions in each small sample state). These regions were contiguous geographic areas designed to yield the same number of interviews on average. In the 2005–2009 surveys, a total of 48 census tracts per SS region were selected with probability proportional to size. Within sampled census tracts, adjacent census blocks were combined to form the second-stage sampling units, or area segments. One segment was selected within each sampled census tract with probability proportional to population size to support the 5-year sample and any supplemental studies that SAMHSA may choose to field. Of these segments, 24 were designated for the coordinated 5-year sample and 24 were designated as reserve segments. Eight sample segments per SS region were fielded during the 2005 survey year. These sampled segments were allocated equally into four separate samples, one for each 3-month period (calendar quarter) during the year, so that the survey was essentially continuous in the field.

The design also oversampled youths and young adults, so that each state's sample was approximately equally distributed among three major age groups: 12–17 years, 18–25 years, and 26 years and over.

Sample Size and Response Rate: Nationally, of the 160,133 eligible households sampled, 142,938 addresses were successfully screened for the 2008 survey, and in these screened households, a total of 86,435 sample persons were selected, from which 68,736 completed interviews were obtained. The survey was conducted from January to December 2008. Weighted response rates were 89% for household screening and 74% for interviewing.

Issues Affecting Interpretation. Several improvements to the survey were implemented in 2002. In addition to the name change, respondents were offered a $30 incentive payment for participation in the survey starting in 2002, and quality control procedures for data collection were enhanced in 2001 and 2002. Because of these improvements and modifications, estimates from the NSDUH completed in 2002 and later should not be compared with estimates from the 2001 or earlier versions of the survey. The data collected in 2002 represent a new baseline for tracking trends in substance use and other measures. Special questions on methamphetamine were added in 2005 and 2006. Data for years prior to 2007 were adjusted for comparability. Estimates of substance use for youth based on NSDUH are not directly comparable with estimates based on Monitoring the Future (MTF) and the Youth Risk Behavior Surveillance System (YRBSS). In addition to the fact that MTF excludes dropouts and absentees, rates are not directly comparable across these surveys because of differences in the populations covered, sample design, questionnaires, and interview setting. NSDUH collects data in residences, whereas MTF and YRBSS collect data in school classrooms. In addition, NSDUH estimates are tabulated by age, whereas MTF and YRBSS estimates are tabulated by grade, representing different ages as well as different populations.

References:

Hughes A, Muhuri P, Sathe N, Spagnola K. State estimates of substance use from the 2007–2008 National Surveys on Drug Use and Health. NSDUH series H–37, HHS pub no SMA 10–4472. Rockville, MD: Substance Abuse and Mental Health Services Administration, Office of Applied Studies; 2010. Available from: http://www.oas.samhsa.gov/2k8State/toc.cfm.

Office of Applied Studies. Results from the 2008 National Survey on Drug Use and Health: National findings. NSDUH series H–36; HHS pub no SMA 09–4434. Rockville, MD: Substance Abuse and

Mental Health Services Administration; 2009. Available from: http://www.oas.samhsa.gov/NSDUH/2k8NSDUH/2k8results.cfm.

For More Information. See the NSDUH website at: https://nsduhweb.rti.org and the SAMHSA Office of Applied Studies website at: http://oas.samhsa.gov.

National Survey of Family Growth (NSFG)

CDC/NCHS

Overview. NSFG provides national data on factors affecting birth and pregnancy rates, adoption, and maternal and infant health.

Selected Content. Data elements include sexual activity, marriage, divorce and remarriage, unmarried cohabitation, forced sexual intercourse, contraception and sterilization, infertility, breastfeeding, pregnancy loss, low birthweight, and use of medical care for family planning and infertility.

Data Years. Seven cycles of the survey have been completed: 1973, 1976, 1982, 1988, 1995, 2002, and 2006–2008.

Coverage. The 1973–1995 cycles of NSFG were based on samples of women 15–44 years of age in the civilian noninstitutionalized population of the United States. Cycles 1 and 2 (1973 and 1976) excluded most women who had never been married. Cycles 3–5 (1982, 1988, and 1995) included all women 15–44 years of age in the civilian noninstitutionalized population of the United States. Cycles 6 (2002) and 7 (2006–2008) included men and women 15–44 years of age in the household population of the United States.

Methodology. Interviews are conducted in person by professional female interviewers using a standardized questionnaire. In all cycles, black women were sampled at higher rates than white women so that detailed statistics for black women could be produced. In cycles 5 and 6 (1995 and 2002), Hispanic persons were also oversampled. In cycle 7 (2006–2008), black and Hispanic adults and all 15–19 year olds were oversampled.

To produce national estimates from the sample for the millions of women 15–44 years of age in the United States, data for the interviewed sample women were (a) inflated by the reciprocal of the probability of selection at each stage of sampling (for example, if there was a 1 in 5,000 chance that a woman would be selected for the sample, her sampling weight was 5,000); (b) adjusted for

nonresponse; and (c) poststratified, or forced to agree with benchmark population values based on data from the U.S. Census Bureau.

Sample Size and Response Rates. For cycle 1, from 101 primary sampling units (PSUs), 10,879 women 15–44 years of age were selected; 9,797 of these were interviewed. In cycle 2, from 79 PSUs, 10,202 eligible women were identified; of these, 8,611 were interviewed. In cycle 3, household screener interviews were completed in 29,511 households (95%). Of the 9,964 eligible women identified, 7,969 were interviewed. In cycle 4, 10,566 eligible women 15–44 years of age were sampled. Interviews were completed with 8,450 women. The response rate for the 1990 telephone reinterview was 68% of those responding to the 1988 survey and still eligible for the 1990 survey. In cycle 5, of the 13,795 eligible women in the sample, 10,847 were interviewed. In cycle 6, from 120 PSUs, 7,643 (about 80%) interviews were completed with eligible women and 4,928 (78%) interviews were completed with men. In cycle 7, from 110 PSUs, 7,356 (about 76%) interviews were completed with eligible women and 6,139 (about 73%) interviews were completed with men.

References:

French DK. National Survey of Family Growth, Cycle I: Sample design, estimation procedures, and variance estimation. Vital Health Stat 2(76). Hyattsville, MD: NCHS; 1978. Available from: http://www.cdc.gov/nchs/data/series/sr_02/sr02_076.pdf.

Grady WR. National Survey of Family Growth, Cycle II: Sample design, estimation procedures, and variance estimation. Vital Health Stat 2(87). Hyattsville, MD: NCHS; 1981. Available from: http://www.cdc.gov/nchs/data/series/sr_02/sr02_087.pdf.

Bachrach CA, Horn MC, Mosher WD, Shimizu I. National Survey of Family Growth, Cycle III: Sample design, weighting, and variance estimation. Vital Health Stat 2(98). Hyattsville, MD: NCHS; 1985. Available from: http://www.cdc.gov/nchs/data/series/sr_02/sr02_098.pdf.

Judkins DR, Mosher WD, Botman S. National Survey of Family Growth: Design, estimation, and inference. Vital Health Stat 2(109). Hyattsville, MD: NCHS; 1991. Available from: http://www.cdc.gov/nchs/data/series/sr_02/sr02_109.pdf.

Göksel H, Judkins DR, Mosher WD. Nonresponse adjustments for a telephone follow-up to a national in-person survey. J Off Stat 1992;8(4):417–31.

Kelly JE, Mosher WD, Duffer AP, Kinsey SH. Plan and operation of the 1995 National Survey of Family Growth. Vital Health Stat 1(36). Hyattsville, MD: NCHS; 1997. Available from: http://www.cdc.gov/nchs/data/series/sr_01/sr01_036.pdf.

Potter FJ, Iannacchione VG, Mosher WD, Mason RE, Kavee JD. Sample design, sampling weights, imputation, and variance estimation in the 1995 National Survey of Family Growth. Vital Health Stat 2(124). Hyattsville, MD: NCHS; 1998. Available from: http://www.cdc.gov/nchs/data/series/sr_02/sr02_124.pdf.

Groves RM, Benson G, Mosher WD, Rosenbaum J, Granda P, Axinn W, et al. Plan and operation of cycle 6 of the National Survey of Family Growth. Vital Health Stat 1(42). Hyattsville, MD: NCHS; 2005. Available from: http://www.cdc.gov/nchs/data/series/sr_01/sr01_042.pdf.

Lepkowski JM, Mosher WD, Davis KE, Groves RM, Van Hoewyk J. The 2006–2010 National Survey of Family Growth: Sample design and analysis of a continuous survey. Vital Health Stat 2(150). Hyattsville, MD: NCHS; 2010. Available from: http://www.cdc.gov/nchs/data/series/sr_02/sr02_150.pdf.

For More Information. See the NSFG website at: http://www.cdc.gov/nchs/nsfg.htm.

National Vital Statistics System (NVSS)

CDC/NCHS

Overview. NVSS collects and publishes official national statistics on births, deaths, fetal deaths, and, prior to 1996, marriages and divorces occurring in the United States, based on U.S. Standard Certificates. Fetal deaths are classified and tabulated separately from other deaths. The five vital statistics files—Birth, Mortality, Multiple Cause-of-Death, Linked Birth/Infant Death, and Compressed Mortality—are described in detail below.

Data Years. The death registration area for 1900 consisted of 10 states, the District of Columbia (D.C.), and a number of cities located in nonregistration states; it covered 40% of the continental U.S. population. The birth registration area was established in 1915 with 10 states and D.C. The birth and death registration areas continued to expand until 1933, when they included all 48 states and D.C. Alaska and Hawaii were added to both registration areas in 1959 and 1960, respectively—the years in which they gained statehood.

Coverage. NVSS collects and presents U.S. resident data for the aggregate of 50 states, New York City, and D.C., as well as for each individual state and D.C. Vital events occurring in the United States to non-U.S. residents and vital events occurring abroad to U.S. residents are excluded.

Methodology. NCHS's Division of Vital Statistics obtains information on births and deaths from the registration offices of each of the 50 states, New York City, D.C., Puerto Rico, the U.S. Virgin Islands, Guam, American Samoa, and Northern Mariana Islands. Until 1972, microfilm copies of all death certificates and a 50% sample of birth certificates were received from all registration areas and processed by NCHS. In 1972, some states began sending their data to NCHS through the Cooperative Health Statistics System (CHSS). States that participated in the CHSS program processed 100% of their death and birth records and sent the entire data file to NCHS on computer tapes. Currently, data are sent to NCHS through the Vital Statistics Cooperative Program (VSCP), following the same procedures as with CHSS. The number of participating states grew from 6 in 1972 to 46 in 1984. Starting in 1985, all 50 states and D.C. participated in VSCP.

U.S. Standard Certificates. U.S. Standard Certificates of Live Birth and Death and Fetal Death Reports are revised periodically, allowing evaluation and addition, modification, and deletion of items. Beginning with 1989, revised Standard Certificates replaced the 1978 versions. The 1989 revision of the birth certificate included items to identify the Hispanic parentage of newborns and to expand information about maternal and infant health characteristics. The 1989 revision of the death certificate included items on educational attainment and Hispanic origin of decedents, as well as changes to improve the medical certification of cause of death. Standard Certificates recommended by NCHS are modified in each registration area to serve the area's needs. However, most certificates conform closely in content and arrangement to the Standard Certificate, and all certificates contain a minimum data set specified by NCHS. The 2003 revision of vital records went into effect in some states beginning in 2003, but full implementation in all states will be phased in over several years.

Birth File

Overview. Vital statistics natality data are a fundamental source of demographic, geographic, and medical and health information on all births occurring in the United States. This is one of the few sources of comparable health-related data for small geographic areas over an extended time period. The data are used to present the characteristics of babies and their mothers, track trends such as birth rates for teenagers, and compare natality trends with those in other countries.

Selected Content. The Birth file includes characteristics of the baby, such as sex, birthweight, and weeks of gestation; demographic information about the parents, such as age, race, Hispanic origin, parity, educational attainment, marital status, and state of residence; medical and health information, such as prenatal care, based on hospital records; and behavioral risk factors for the birth, such as mother's tobacco use during pregnancy.

Data Years. The birth registration area began in 1915 with 10 states and the District of Columbia.

Methodology. In the United States, state laws require birth certificates to be completed for all births. The registration of births is the responsibility of the professional attendant at birth, generally a physician or midwife. The birth certificate must be filed with the local registrar of the district in which the birth occurs. Each birth must be reported promptly; the reporting requirements vary from state to state, ranging from 24 hours to as much as 10 days after the birth.

Federal law mandates national collection and publication of birth and other vital statistics data. NVSS is the result of cooperation between NCHS and the states to provide access to statistical information from birth certificates. Standard forms for the collection of the data, and model procedures for the uniform registration of the events, are developed and recommended for state use through cooperative activities of the states and NCHS. NCHS shares the costs incurred by the states in providing vital statistics data for national use.

Issues Affecting Interpretation. Data on mother's educational attainment, tobacco use during pregnancy, and prenatal care based on the 2003 revision of the U.S. Standard Certificate of Live Birth are not comparable with data based on the 1989 revision of the U.S. Standard Certificate of Live Birth. For 2006 and 2007, data on mother's educational attainment, tobacco use during pregnancy, and prenatal care are shown separately for the 17–19 reporting areas that used the 2003 revision in 2006–2007 and for the 28 reporting areas that continued to use the 1989 revision in 2007, in order to provide 2 years of comparable data. Data are not shown for reporting areas that were transitioning from the 1989 revision to the 2003 revision during 2006–2007 or for states that had other comparability

issues with these three items during that timeframe. The states that implemented the 2003 revision of the U.S. Standard Certificate of Live Birth are as follows: starting in 2003, Pennsylvania and Washington; and starting in 2004, Idaho, Kentucky, New York state (excluding New York City), South Carolina, and Tennessee. Starting in 2005, the reporting area using the 2003 revision expanded to 13 states, adding Florida, Kansas, Nebraska, New Hampshire, Texas, and Vermont (midyear). Starting in 2006, the reporting area using the 2003 revision included 19 states, with the addition of California, Delaware, North Dakota, Ohio, South Dakota, and Wyoming. California does not report information on tobacco use during pregnancy. Twenty-two states (California, Colorado, Delaware, Florida, Idaho, Indiana, Iowa, Kansas, Kentucky, Nebraska, New Hampshire, New York state (excluding New York City), North Dakota, Ohio, Pennsylvania, South Carolina, South Dakota, Tennessee, Texas, Vermont, Washington, and Wyoming) reported births using the 2003 revision. Approximately one-half (53%) of all births in 2007 were reported using the 2003 revision. Prior to 2003, the number of states reporting information on maternal education, Hispanic origin, marital status, and tobacco use during pregnancy increased over the years. Interpretation of trend data should take into consideration changes to reporting areas and immigration. For methodological and reporting area changes for the following birth certificate items, see Appendix II: Age (maternal); Cigarette smoking; Education (maternal); Hispanic origin; Marital status; Prenatal care; Race.

References:

Vital Statistics of the United States 2000, vol I: Natality, Technical appendix. Hyattsville, MD: NCHS; 2002. Available from: http://www.cdc.gov/nchs/data/techap00.pdf.

Martin JA, Hamilton BE, Sutton PD, Ventura SJ, Menacker F, Kirmeyer S, Mathews TJ. Births: Final data for 2006. National vital statistics reports; vol 57 no 7. Hyattsville, MD: NCHS; 2009. Available from: http://www.cdc.gov/nchs/data/nvsr/nvsr57/nvsr57_07.pdf.

Martin JA, Hamilton BE, Sutton PD, Ventura SJ, Mathews TJ, Kirmeyer S, Osterman MJK. Births: Final data for 2007. National vital statistics reports; vol 58 no 24. Hyattsville, MD: NCHS; 2010. Available from: http://www.cdc.gov/nchs/data/nvsr/nvsr58/nvsr58_24.pdf.

For More Information. See the Birth Data website at: http://www.cdc.gov/nchs/births.htm.

Mortality File

Overview. Vital statistics mortality data are a fundamental source of demographic, geographic, and cause-of-death information. This is one of the few sources of comparable health-related data for small geographic areas over an extended time period. The data are used to present the characteristics of those dying in the United States, to determine life expectancy, and to compare mortality trends with those in other countries.

Selected Content. The Mortality file includes demographic information on age, sex, race, Hispanic origin, state of residence, and educational attainment, as well as medical information on cause of death.

Data Years. The death registration area began in 1900 with 10 states and the District of Columbia.

Methodology. By law, the registration of deaths is the responsibility of the funeral director. The funeral director obtains demographic data for the death certificate from an informant. The physician in attendance at the death is required to certify the cause of death. Where death is from other than natural causes, a coroner or medical examiner may be required to examine the body and certify the cause of death. Data for the entire United States refer to events occurring within the United States; data for geographic areas are by place of residence. For methodological and reporting area changes for the following death certificate items, see Appendix II: Education; Hispanic origin; Race.

Issues Affecting Interpretation. The *International Classification of Diseases* (ICD), by which cause of death is coded and classified, is revised approximately every 10–20 years. Because revisions of the ICD may cause discontinuities in trend data by cause of death, comparison of death rates by cause of death across ICD revisions should be done with caution and with reference to the comparability ratio. (See Appendix II, Comparability ratio.) Prior to 1999, modifications to the ICD were made only when a new revision of the ICD was implemented. A process for updating the ICD was introduced with the 10th revision (ICD–10) that allows for mid-revision changes. These changes, however, may affect comparability of data between years for select causes of death. Minor changes may be implemented every year, whereas major changes may be implemented every 3 years (e.g., 2003 data year). In data year 2006, major changes were implemented, including the addition and deletion of several ICD codes. For more information, see:

Heron M, Hoyert DL, Murphy SL, Xu JQ, Kochanek KD, Tejada-Vera B. Deaths: Final data for 2006. National vital statistics reports; vol 57 no 14. Hyattsville, MD: NCHS; 2009. Available from: http://www.cdc.gov/nchs/data/nvsr/nvsr57/nvsr57_14.pdf.

The death certificate has been revised periodically. A revised U.S. Standard Certificate of Death was recommended for state use beginning January 1, 1989. Among the changes were the addition of a new item on educational attainment and Hispanic origin of the decedent and changes to improve the medical certification of cause of death. The U.S. Standard Certificate of Death was revised again in 2003; states are adopting this new certificate on a rolling basis. The 2003 revision included significant changes in the way that information on educational attainment, maternal mortality, and race are collected and coded. The educational attainment item was changed to be consistent with the U.S. Census Bureau data and to improve the ability to identify specific types of educational degrees. Educational attainment data collected using the 2003 revision are not comparable with data collected using the 1989 revision. The 2003 revision introduced a standard question on pregnancy status of female decedents. This change, in addition to changes in the classification of maternal death under ICD–10, allows for more complete reporting of deaths associated with pregnancy, childbirth, and the puerperium. These changes may affect trends in maternal mortality. The 2003 revision also permits reporting of more than one race (multiple races). This change was implemented to reflect the increasing diversity of the U.S. population and to be consistent with the decennial census. Many states, however, are still using the 1989 revision of the U.S. Standard Certificate of Death, which allows only a single race to be reported. Until all states adopt the new death certificate, the race data reported using the 2003 revision were "bridged" for those for whom more than one race was reported (multiple race) to one, single race to provide comparability with race data reported on the 1989 revision. For more information on the impact of the 2003 certificate revisions on mortality data presented in *Health, United States*, including a list of states that have adopted the 2003 certificate, see Appendix II: Education; Maternal death; Race.

References:

Grove RD, Hetzel AM. Vital statistics rates in the United States, 1940–1960. Washington, DC: U.S. Government Printing Office; 1968.

Xu JQ, Kochanek KD, Murphy SL, Tejada-Vera B. Deaths: Final data for 2007. National vital statistics reports; vol 58 no 19. Hyattsville, MD: NCHS; 2010. Available from: http://www.cdc.gov/nchs/data/nvsr/nvsr58/nvsr58_19.pdf.

NCHS. Vital Statistics of the United States, vol II: Mortality, part A, Technical appendix. Hyattsville, MD: NCHS; [published annually]. Available from: http://www.cdc.gov/nchs/products/vsus.htm#appendices.

For More Information. See the Mortality Data website at: http://www.cdc.gov/nchs/deaths.htm.

Multiple Cause-of-Death File

Overview. Multiple cause-of-death data reflect all medical information reported on death certificates and complement traditional underlying cause-of-death data. Multiple-cause data give information on diseases that are a factor in death, whether or not they are the underlying cause of death; on associations among diseases; and on injuries leading to death.

Selected Content. In addition to the same demographic variables listed for the Mortality file, the Multiple Cause-of-Death file includes record axis and entity axis cause-of-death data (see Methodology, below).

Data Years. Multiple cause-of-death data files are available for every data year since 1968.

Methodology. NCHS is responsible for compiling and publishing annual national statistics on causes of death. In carrying out this responsibility, NCHS adheres to the World Health Organization (WHO) Nomenclature Regulations. These regulations require (a) that cause of death be coded in accordance with the applicable revision of the *International Classification of Diseases* (ICD) (see Appendix II, *International Classification of Diseases*; and Table IV); and (b) that underlying cause of death be selected in accordance with international rules. Traditionally, national mortality statistics have been based on a count of deaths, with one underlying cause assigned for each death.

Prior to 1968, mortality medical data were based on manual coding of an underlying cause of death for each certificate, in accordance with WHO rules. Starting with 1968, NCHS converted to computerized coding of the underlying cause and manual coding of all causes (multiple causes) on the death certificate. In this system, called Automated Classification of Medical Entities (ACME), multiple cause codes serve as inputs to the computer

software that employs WHO rules to select the underlying cause. All cause-of-death data in this report are coded using ACME. ACME is used to select the underlying cause of death for all death certificates in the United States. In addition, NCHS has developed two computer systems as inputs to ACME. Beginning with 1990 data, the Mortality Medical Indexing, Classification, and Retrieval system (MICAR) was introduced to automate coding multiple causes of death. In addition, MICAR provides more detailed information on the conditions reported on death certificates than is available through the ICD code structure. Then, beginning with data year 1993, SuperMICAR, an enhancement of MICAR, was introduced. SuperMICAR allows for literal entry of the multiple cause-of-death text as reported by the certifier. This information is then processed automatically by the MICAR and ACME computer systems. Records that cannot be processed automatically by MICAR or SuperMICAR are manually multiple-cause coded and then further processed through ACME. In 2006, SuperMICAR was used to process all of the Nation's death records.

Issues Affecting Interpretation. The ICD, by which cause of death is coded and classified, is revised approximately every 10 to 15 years. Revisions of the ICD may cause discontinuities in trend data by cause of death; therefore, comparison of death rates by cause of death across ICD revisions should be done with caution and with reference to the comparability ratio. (See Appendix II, Comparability ratio.) Data were obtained from all certificates for 1968–1971, 1973–1980, and 1983–present. Data were obtained from a 50% sample of certificates for 1972. Multiple-cause data for 1981 and 1982 were obtained from a 50% sample of certificates from 19 registration areas. For the other states, data were obtained from all certificates.

Reference:

NCHS. Multiple causes of death in the United States. Monthly vital statistics report; vol 32 no 10, suppl 2. Hyattsville, MD: NCHS; 1984. Available from: http://www.cdc.gov/nchs/data/mvsr/supp/mv32_10s2.pdf.

For More Information. See the Mortality Multiple Cause-of-Death data file website at: http://www.cdc.gov/nchs/data_access/Vitalstatsonline.htm.

Linked Birth/Infant Death Data Set

Overview. National linked files of live births and infant deaths are used for research on infant mortality.

Selected Content. The Linked Birth/Infant Death data set includes all variables on the natality (Birth) file, including racial and ethnic information, birthweight, and maternal smoking, as well as variables on the Mortality file, including cause of death and age at death.

Data Years. National linked files of live births and infant deaths were first produced for the 1983 birth cohort. Birth cohort linked file data are available for 1983–1991, and both period linked files and birth cohort linked files are available starting with 1995. National linked files do not exist for 1992–1994.

Coverage. To be included in the U.S. linked file, both the birth and death must have occurred in the 50 states or the District of Columbia.

Methodology. Infant mortality rates are based on infant deaths per 100,000 live births. Infant deaths are defined as a death before the infant's first birthday. About 97%–99% of files can be linked. The linkage makes available extensive information about the pregnancy, maternal risk factors, infant characteristics, and health items at birth that can be used in analyses of infant mortality.

Starting with data year 1995, more timely linked file data are produced in a period data format preceding the release of the corresponding birth cohort format. The 2006 period linked file contains a numerator file that consists of all infant deaths occurring in 2006 that have been linked to their corresponding birth certificates, whether the birth occurred in 2005 or 2006. In contrast, the 2006 birth cohort linked file will contain a numerator file that consists of all infant deaths to babies born in 2006, whether the death occurred in 2006 or 2007. Starting with 1995 data, period linked files are used for infant mortality rates tables, using the linked file data in *Health, United States*. For the 2006 file, NCHS accepted birth records that could be linked to infant deaths even if the births were registered after the closure of the 2006 Birth file (fewer than 100 cases). This improved the infant birth/death linkage and made the denominator file distinctly different from the official 2006 Birth file.

Other changes to the data set starting with 1995 include addition of record weights to compensate for the 1%–2% infant death records that could not be linked to their corresponding birth records. In addition, not-stated birthweight was imputed if the period of gestation was known. This imputation was done to improve the accuracy of birthweight-specific infant mortality rates because the percentage of records with not-stated birthweight is generally higher for infant deaths (3.1% in 2006) than for live births (0.1% in 2006). In 2006, not-stated birthweight was imputed for 0.09% of births.

Issues Affecting Interpretation. Period linked file data starting with 1995 are not strictly comparable with birth cohort data for 1983–1991. Although birth cohort linked files have methodological advantages, their production incurs substantial delays in data availability because it is necessary to wait until the close of a second data year to include all infant deaths to the birth cohort. Data on mother's educational attainment, tobacco use during pregnancy, and prenatal care based on the 2003 revision are not comparable with data based on the 1989 revision of the U.S. Standard Certificate of Live Birth and are currently excluded from the *Health, United States* statistics on infant mortality by mother's educational attainment. (See Appendix II, Education.)

Reference:

> Mathews TJ, MacDorman MF. Infant mortality statistics from the 2006 period linked birth/infant death data set. National vital statistics report; vol 58 no 17. Hyattsville, MD: NCHS; 2010. Available from: http://www.cdc.gov/nchs/data/nvsr/nvsr58/nvsr58_17.pdf.

For More Information. See the NCHS Linked Birth and Infant Death Data website at: http://www.cdc.gov/nchs/linked.htm.

Compressed Mortality File (CMF)

Overview. The CMF is a county-level national mortality and population database.

Selected Content. The CMF contains mortality data derived from the detailed Mortality files of the National Vital Statistics System and estimates of U.S. national, state, and county resident populations from the U.S. Census Bureau. For 1968–1998, number of deaths, crude death rates, and age-adjusted death rates can be obtained by place of residence (total U.S., state, and county), age group, race (white, black, and other), sex, year of death, and underlying cause of death. For 1999–2006, mortality statistics can be obtained by place of residence, by age group and expanded race groups (white, black, American Indian or Alaska Native, Asian or Pacific Islander), and by Hispanic origin.

Data Years. The CMF spans the years 1968–2006. On CDC WONDER, data are available starting with 1979.

Methodology. In *Health, United States*, the CMF is used to compute death rates by urbanization level of the decedent's county of residence. Counties are categorized according to level of urbanization based on the 2006 NCHS Urban–Rural Classification Scheme for Counties. This scheme assigns counties and county equivalents to one of six urbanization levels: four metropolitan and two nonmetropolitan.

For More Information. See the CMF website at: http://www.cdc.gov/nchs/data_access/cmf.htm and the CDC WONDER website at: http://wonder.cdc.gov. (Also see Appendix II, Urbanization.)

Occupational Employment Statistics (OES)

Bureau of Labor Statistics (BLS)

Overview. The OES program conducts a semiannual survey designed to produce estimates of employment and wages for specific occupations.

Selected Content. The OES survey produces estimates of occupational employment and wages for most, three-, four-, and selected five-digit North American Industry Classification System (NAICS) levels in these sectors: forestry and logging; mining; utilities; construction; manufacturing; wholesale trade; retail trade; transportation and warehousing; information; finance and insurance; real estate and rental and leasing; professional, scientific, and technical services; management of companies and enterprises; administrative and support and waste management and remediation services; educational services; health care and social assistance; arts, entertainment, and recreation; accommodation and food services; other services (except public administration); and federal, state, and local government.

Data Years. Prior to 1996, the OES program collected only occupational employment data for selected industries in each year of the 3-year survey cycle and produced only industry-specific estimates of occupational employment. The 1996 survey round was the first year that the OES program began collecting occupational employment and wage data in every state. In addition, the program's 3-year survey cycle was modified to collect data from all covered industries each year. The year 1997 is the earliest year available for which the OES program produced estimates of cross-industry as well as industry-specific occupational employment and wages.

Coverage. The OES survey covers all full-time and part-time wage and salary workers in nonfarm establishments. Surveys collect data for the payroll period including the 12th day of May or November, depending on the industry surveyed. The survey does not cover the self-employed, owners and partners in unincorporated firms, household workers, or unpaid family workers.

Methodology. The OES survey is a federal–state cooperative program between the BLS and state workforce agencies (SWAs). The OES program surveys approximately 200,000 establishments per panel (every 6 months), taking 3 years to fully collect the sample of 1.2 million establishments. Mail surveys collect data for the payroll period including the 12th day of May or November, depending on the industry surveyed. The estimates for occupations in nonfarm establishments are based on OES data collected for the reference months of May and November. BLS provides the procedures and technical support, draws the sample, and produces the survey materials, while SWAs collect the data. SWAs from all 50 states plus the District of Columbia (D.C.), Puerto Rico, Guam, and the U.S. Virgin Islands participate in the survey. Occupational employment and wage rate estimates at the national level are produced by BLS using data from the 50 states and D.C. Employers who respond to states' requests to participate in the OES survey make these estimates possible. The nationwide response rate for the May 2009 survey was 78% for establishments, covering 74% of employment. The survey included establishments sampled in the May 2009, November 2008, May 2008, November 2007, May 2007, and November 2006 semiannual panels.

Issues Affecting Interpretation. The OES survey began using NAICS in 2002. Data prior to 2002 are based on the Standard Industrial Classification system. In 1999, the OES survey began using the new Office of Management and Budget (OMB) Standard Occupational Classification (SOC) system. The new SOC system, which will be used by all federal statistical agencies for reporting occupational data, consists of 821 detailed occupations, grouped into 449 broad occupations, 96 minor groups, and 23 major groups. The OES program provides occupational employment and wage estimates at the major group and detailed occupation level. Because of the OES survey's transition to the SOC system, estimates for 1999 and subsequent years are not directly comparable with previous years' OES estimates, which were based on a classification system having seven major occupational groups and 770 detailed occupations. Approximately one-half of the detailed occupations were unchanged under the new SOC system, with the other half being SOC occupations or occupations that are slightly different from similar occupations in the old OES classification system. Guam, Puerto Rico, and the U.S. Virgin Islands were surveyed, but their data were not included in the May 2008 survey.

Reference:

> Bureau of Labor Statistics. Occupational employment and wages, May 2009. Washington, DC: U.S. Department of Labor; May 2010.

For More Information. See the OES website at: http://www.bls.gov/OES.

Online Survey Certification and Reporting Database (OSCAR)

Centers for Medicare & Medicaid Services (CMS)

Overview. OSCAR is an administrative database containing detailed information on all Medicare- and Medicaid-certified institutional health care providers, including all currently and previously certified Medicare and Medicaid nursing homes, short-term hospitals, and intermediate care facilities for the mentally retarded in the United States and territories. (Data for the territories are not shown in *Health, United States*.) The purpose of the facility survey certification process is to ensure that facilities meet the current CMS care requirements and thus can be reimbursed for services furnished to Medicare and Medicaid beneficiaries.

Selected Content. OSCAR contains information on facility and patient characteristics and health deficiencies issued by the government during state surveys.

Data Years. OSCAR has been maintained by CMS, formerly the Health Care Financing Administration (HCFA), since 1992. OSCAR is an updated version of the Medicare and Medicaid Automated Certification System that had been in existence since 1972.

Coverage. Facilities in the United States that receive Medicare or Medicaid payments are included.

Methodology. A facility representative fills out the forms with the required information, and the forms are submitted to CMS. The information provided can be audited at any time.

All certified facilities are inspected periodically by representatives of the state survey agency (generally the department of health). For nursing homes, for

example, the survey cycle is every 15 months. Therefore, a complete census of nursing homes must be based on a 15-month reporting cycle rather than a 12-month cycle. Some nursing homes are inspected twice, or more often, during any given reporting cycle. To avoid overcounting, the data must be edited and duplicates removed. Data editing and compilation of nursing home data were performed by Cowles Research Group and published in the group's *Nursing Home Statistical Yearbook* series. Data editing and compilation for other facilities were performed by NCHS staff.

References:

> Cowles CM, ed. Nursing home statistical yearbooks for 1995, 1996, and 1997. Anacortes, WA: Cowles Research Group (CRG); published 1995, 1997, and 1998, respectively.

> Cowles CM, ed. Nursing home statistical yearbooks for 1998, 1999, 2000, 2001, and 2002. Washington, DC: American Association of Homes and Services for the Aging (AAHSA); published 1999, 2000, 2001, 2002, and 2003, respectively.

> Cowles CM, ed. Nursing home statistical yearbooks for 2003–2009. McMinnville, OR: Cowles Research Group (CRG); published 2004, 2005, 2006, 2007, 2008, 2009, and 2010, respectively.

> *Centers for Medicare & Medicaid Services.* Certification and compliance. 2005. Available from: http://www.cms.gov/Certification andComplianc/01_Overview.asp.

For More Information. See CMS website at: http://www.cms.hhs.gov/NonIdentifiableDataFiles and the CRG website at: http://www.longtermcareinfo.com/index.html.

Population Census and Population Estimates

U.S. Census Bureau Decennial Census

The census of population (decennial census) has been held in the United States every 10 years since 1790. It has enumerated the resident population as of April 1 of the census year since 1930. Data on sex, race, Hispanic origin, age, and marital status are collected from 100% of the enumerated population. More detailed information such as income, education, housing, occupation, and industry are collected from a representative sample of the population.

Race Data on the 1990 Census

The question on race on the 1990 census was based on the Office of Management and Budget's (OMB) 1977 Race and Ethnic Standards for Federal Statistics and Administrative Reporting (Statistical Policy Directive 15). This document specified rules for the collection, tabulation, and reporting of race/ethnicity data within the federal statistical system. The 1977 Standards required federal agencies to report race-specific tabulations using four single-race categories: American Indian or Alaska Native, Asian or Pacific Islander, black, and white. Under the 1977 Standards, race and ethnicity were considered to be two separate and distinct concepts. Thus, persons of Hispanic origin may be of any race.

Race Data on the 2000 Census

The question on race on the 2000 census was based on OMBs 1997 *Revisions to the Standards for the Classification of Federal Data on Race and Ethnicity* (Fed Regist 1997 October 30;62:58781–90). (Also see Appendix II, Race.) The 1997 Standards incorporated two major changes in the collection, tabulation, and presentation of race data. First, the 1997 Standards increased from four to five the minimum set of categories to be used by federal agencies for identification of race: American Indian or Alaska Native, Asian, black or African American, Native Hawaiian or Other Pacific Islander, and white. Second, the 1997 Standards included the requirement that federal data collection programs allow respondents to select one or more race categories when responding to a query on their racial identity. This provision means that there are potentially 31 race groups, depending on whether an individual selects one, two, three, four, or all five of the race categories. The 1997 Standards continue to call for use, when possible, of a separate question on Hispanic or Latino ethnicity and specify that the ethnicity question should appear before the question on race. Thus, under the 1997 Standards, as under the 1977 Standards, Hispanics may be of any race.

Modified Decennial Census Files

For several decades the U.S. Census Bureau has produced Modified Decennial Census files. These modified files incorporate adjustments to the 100% April 1 count data for (a) errors in the census data discovered subsequent to publication, (b) misreported age data, and (c) nonspecified race.

For the 1990 census, the U.S. Census Bureau modified the age, race, and sex data on the census and produced the Modified Age Race Sex (MARS) file. The differences between the population counts in the original census file and the MARS file are primarily due to modification of the race data. Of the 248.7 million persons enumerated in 1990, 9.8 million persons did not specify their race (over 95% were of Hispanic origin). For the 1990 MARS file, these persons were assigned the race reported by a nearby person with an identical response to the Hispanic origin question.

For the 2000 census, the U.S. Census Bureau modified the race data on the census and produced the Modified Race Data Summary file. For this file, persons who reported the category Some Other Race as part of their race response were assigned to one of the 31 race groups, which are the single- and multiple-race combinations of the five race categories specified in the 1997 race and ethnicity standards. Persons who did not specify their race were assigned to one of the 31 race groups by imputation. Of the 18.5 million persons who reported the category Some Other Race as part of their race response, or who did not specify their race, 16.8 million (90.4%) were of Hispanic origin.

Bridged-race Population Estimates for Census 2000

Race data on the 2000 census are not comparable with race data on other data systems that are continuing to collect data using the 1977 Standards on race and ethnicity during the transition to full implementation of the 1997 Standards. For example, states are implementing the revised birth and death certificates, which have race and ethnicity items that are compliant with the 1997 OMB Standards, at different times, and to date, many states are still using the 1989 certificates that collect race and ethnicity data in accordance with the 1977 Standards. Thus, population estimates for 2000 and beyond with race categories comparable to the 1977 categories are needed so that race-specific birth and death rates can be calculated. To meet this need, NCHS, in collaboration with the U.S. Census Bureau, developed methodology to bridge the 31 race groups in Census 2000 to the four single-race categories specified under the 1977 Standards.

The bridging methodology was developed using information from the 1997–2000 National Health Interview Survey (NHIS). The NHIS provides a unique opportunity to investigate multiple-race groups because, since 1982, it has allowed respondents to choose more than one race but has also asked respondents reporting multiple races to choose a primary race. The bridging methodology developed by NCHS involved the application of regression models relating person-level and county-level covariates to the selection of a particular primary race by the multiple-race respondents. Bridging proportions derived from these models were applied by the U.S. Census Bureau to the Census 2000 Modified Race Data Summary file. This application resulted in bridged counts of the April 1, 2000, resident single-race populations for four racial groups: American Indian or Alaska Native, Asian or Pacific Islander, black, and white. As bridged-race population estimates continue to be needed for the calculation of vital rates, the Census Bureau annually produces postcensal bridged-race estimates of the July 1 resident single-race populations.

Reference:

> Ingram DD, Parker JD, Schenker N, Weed JA, Hamilton B, Arias E, Madans JH. United States Census 2000 population with bridged race categories. Vital Health Stat 2(135). Hyattsville, MD: NCHS; 2003. Available from: http://www.cdc.gov/nchs/data/series/sr_02/sr02_135.pdf.

For More Information. See the NCHS website for U.S. Census Populations with Bridged Race Categories: http://www.cdc.gov/nchs/nvss/bridged_race.htm.

Postcensal Population Estimates

Postcensal population estimates are estimates made for the years following a census, before the next census has been taken. National postcensal population estimates are derived annually by updating the resident population enumerated in the decennial census using a components-of-population-change approach. Each annual series includes estimates for the current data year and revised estimates for the earlier years in the decade. The following formula is used to derive the estimates for a given year from those for the previous year, starting with the decennial census enumerated resident population as the base:

> Resident population
>
> + Births to U.S. resident women
>
> − Deaths to U.S. residents
>
> + Net international migration.

The postcensal estimates are consistent with official decennial census figures and do not reflect estimated decennial census underenumeration.

Estimates for the earlier years in a given series are revised to reflect changes in the components-of-change data sets (for example, births to U.S. resident women from a preliminary natality file are replaced with counts from a final natality file). To help users keep track of which postcensal estimate is being used, each annual series is referred to as a vintage and the last year in the series is used to name the series. For example, the Vintage 2001 postcensal series has estimates for July 1, 2000, and July 1, 2001, and the Vintage 2002 postcensal series has revised estimates for July 1, 2000, and July 1, 2001, as well as estimates for July 1, 2002. The estimates for July 1, 2000, and for July 1, 2001, from the Vintage 2001 and Vintage 2002 postcensal series, differ.

The U.S. Census Bureau also produces postcensal estimates of the resident population for each state and county by using a component of population change method at the county level. An additional component of population change, net internal migration, is involved. The state population estimates are produced by summing all county populations within each state.

The Census Bureau has annually produced a postcensal series of estimates of the July 1 resident population of the United States based on Census 2000 by applying the components of change methodology to the Modified Race Data Summary file. These series of postcensal estimates have race data for 31 race groups, in accordance with the 1997 race and ethnicity standards. So that the race data for 2000-based postcensal estimates will be comparable with race data on vital records, the Census Bureau has applied the NHIS bridging methodology to each 31-race-group postcensal series of population estimates to obtain bridged-race postcensal estimates (estimates for the four single-race categories: American Indian or Alaska Native, Asian or Pacific Islander, black, and white). Bridged-race postcensal population estimates are available from: http://www.cdc.gov/nchs/nvss/bridged_race.htm.

Vital rates for 2000 were calculated using the bridged-race April 1, 2000, census counts, and vital rates for 2001 and beyond were calculated using bridged-race estimates of the July 1 population from the corresponding postcensal vintage.

Intercensal Population Estimates

Intercensal population estimates are estimates made for the years between two censuses and are produced once the decennial census at the end of the decade has been completed. They replace the postcensal estimates that were produced prior to the completion of the census at the end of the decade. Intercensal estimates are more accurate than postcensal estimates because they are based on both the census at the beginning and the census at the end of the decade and thus correct for the error of closure (the difference between the estimated population at the end of the decade and the census count for that date). The error of closure at the national level was quite small for the 1960s (379,000). However, for the 1970s it amounted to almost 5 million; for the 1980s, 1.5 million; and for the 1990s, about 6 million. The error of closure affects age, race, sex, and Hispanic origin subgroup populations differently, as well as the rates based on these populations. Vital rates that were calculated using postcensal population estimates are routinely revised when intercensal estimates become available.

Intercensal estimates for the 1990s with race data comparable to the 1977 Standards have been derived so that vital rates for the 1990s could be revised to reflect Census 2000. Calculation of the intercensal population estimates for the 1990s was complicated by the incomparability of the race data on the 1990 and 2000 censuses. The Census Bureau, in collaboration with National Cancer Institute and NCHS, derived race-specific intercensal population estimates for the 1990s using the 1990 MARS file as the beginning population base and the bridged-race population estimates for April 1, 2000, as the ending population base. Bridged-race intercensal population estimates are available from: http://www.cdc.gov/nchs/nvss/bridged_race.htm.

For More Information. See the U.S. Census Bureau website at: http://www.census.gov.

Sexually Transmitted Disease (STD) Surveillance

CDC/National Center for HIV/AIDS, Viral Hepatitis, STD, and TB Prevention (NCHHSTP)

Overview. Surveillance information on the incidence and prevalence of STDs is used to inform public and private health efforts to control these diseases.

Selected Content. Case reporting data are available for nationally notifiable chanchroid, chlamydia, gonorrhea, and syphilis. Surveillance of other STDs, such as genital herpes simplex virus, genital warts or other human papillomavirus infections, and

trichomoniasis are based on estimates of office visits in physicians' office practices provided by the National Disease and Therapeutic Index.

Data Years. STD national surveillance data have been collected since 1941.

Coverage. Case reports of STDs are reported to CDC by STD surveillance systems operated by state and local STD control programs and health departments in 50 states, the District of Columbia, selected cities, 3,141 U.S. counties, and outlying areas consisting of U.S. dependencies, possessions, and independent nations in free association with the United States. Data from outlying areas are not included in *Health, United States.*

Methodology. Information is obtained from the following data sources: (a) case reports from STD project areas; (b) prevalence data from the Regional Infertility Prevention Project, the National Job Training Program (formerly the Job Corps), the Corrections STD Prevalence Monitoring Projects, and the Men Who Have Sex With Men Prevalence Monitoring Project; (c) sentinel surveillance of gonococcal antimicrobial resistance from the Gonococcal Isolate Surveillance Project; and (d) national sample surveys implemented by federal and private organizations. STD data are submitted to CDC on a variety of hard-copy summary reporting forms (monthly, quarterly, and annually) and in electronic summary or individual case-specific (line-listed) formats via the National Electronic Telecommunications System for Surveillance.

Issues Affecting Interpretation. Because of incomplete diagnosis and reporting, the number of STD cases reported to CDC undercounts the actual number of cases occurring among the U.S. population.

Reference:

CDC. Sexually transmitted diseases surveillance 2008. Atlanta, GA: CDC, National Center for HIV/AIDS, Viral Hepatitis, STD, and TB Prevention; 2009. Available from: http://www.cdc.gov/std/stats08/toc.htm.

For More Information. See the STD Surveillance Report website at: http://www.cdc.gov/std/stats and the STD website at: http://www.cdc.gov/std/default.htm.

Surveillance, Epidemiology, and End Results Program (SEER)

National Cancer Institute (NCI)

Overview. SEER tracks the incidence of new cancers each year and collects follow-up information on all previously diagnosed patients until their death.

Selected Content. For each cancer, SEER registries routinely collect data on patient demographics, primary tumor site, morphology, stage at diagnosis, first course of treatment, and follow-up for vital status.

Data Years. Case ascertainment for SEER began January 1, 1973, and has continued for more than 37 years. The most recent data available are for 2007.

Coverage. The SEER 9 registries (Atlanta, Connecticut, Detroit, Hawaii, Iowa, New Mexico, San Francisco–Oakland, Seattle–Puget Sound, and Utah) have been part of the program continuously since 1975. The SEER 13 registries (the SEER 9 registries plus Los Angeles, San Jose–Monterey, rural Georgia, and the Alaska Native Tumor Registry) have been part of the program continuously since 1992. The SEER 17 registries (the SEER 13 plus Kentucky, Greater California, New Jersey, and Louisiana) have been part of the program continuously since 2000. SEER currently collects and publishes cancer incidence and survival data from 17 population-based cancer registries covering approximately 26% of the U.S. population.

To ensure continuity in reporting areas for trend data, the SEER data file is commonly used both for statistical analyses and for analysis of cancer survival rates in *Health, United States*. The SEER 13 data file is commonly used for analysis of cancer incidence by expanded racial and ethnic groups.

Methodology. A cancer registry collects and stores data on cancers diagnosed in a specific hospital or medical facility (hospital-based registry) or in a defined geographic area (population-based registry). A population-based registry includes, but is not limited to, a number of hospital-based registries. In SEER registry areas, trained coders abstract medical records using the *International Classification of Diseases for Oncology, Third Edition* (ICD–O–3), which provides coding systems for site and tumor morphology. The third edition, implemented in 2001, is the first complete review and revision of the text and guidelines since the original publication in 1988. The major staging systems used by cancer registries are American Joint Committee on Cancer TNM (tumor, nodes, metastasis) staging and SEER Summary Stage. The SEER Extent of Disease (EOD) and TNM stages include schemes for all sites and morphologies and are used by NCI to derive SEER Summary Stage and Collaborative Staging.

NCI obtains population counts from the U.S. Census Bureau and uses them to calculate incidence rates. It also uses estimation procedures as needed to obtain estimates for years and races not included in data provided by the U.S. Census Bureau. Life tables used to determine general population life expectancy when calculating relative survival rates were obtained from NCHS and in-house calculations. Separate life tables are used for each race-sex-specific group included in SEER.

Issues Affecting Interpretation. Because of the addition of registries over time, analysis of long-term incidence and survival trends is limited to those registries that have been in SEER for similar lengths of time. Analysis of Hispanic and American Indian and Alaska Native data is limited to shorter trends. Starting with *Health, United States, 2006*, the North American Association of Central Cancer Registries (NAACCR) Hispanic Identification Algorithm was used on a combination of variables to classify cases as Hispanic for analytic purposes. Starting with *Health, United States, 2007*, Hispanic incidence data exclude data for Alaska. Earlier editions of *Health, United States* also excluded Hispanic data for Hawaii and Seattle. Starting with *Health, United States, 2007*, incidence estimates for the American Indian or Alaska Native population are limited to contract health service delivery area (CHSDA) counties within SEER reporting areas. This change is believed to produce estimates that more accurately reflect the incidence rates for this population group. More information on CHSDA is available from: http://www.ihs.gov/NonMedicalPrograms/dqwg/dqwg-section1-home.asp. For more information on SEER estimates by race/ethnicity, see: http://seer.cancer.gov/seerstat/variables/seer/race_ethnicity/index.html. Rates presented in this report may differ somewhat from those reported previously due to changes in population estimates and the addition and deletion of small numbers of incidence cases.

Reference:

Altekruse SF, Kosary CL, Krapcho M, Neyman N, Aminou R, Waldron W, et al., eds. SEER cancer statistics review, 1975–2007. (Based on November 2009 SEER data submission.) Bethesda, MD: National Cancer Institute; 2010. Available from: http://seer.cancer.gov/csr/1975_2007.

For More Information. See the SEER website at: http://seer.cancer.gov.

Survey of Mental Health Organizations (SMHO)

Substance Abuse and Mental Health Services Administration (SAMHSA)

Overview. SMHO/General Hospital Mental Health Services (GHMHS) collects data on the number and characteristics of specialty mental health organizations in the United States.

Selected Content. This inventory collects basic information such as types of mental health organizations, ownership, number of additions and residents, and number of beds. The sample survey is a more detailed questionnaire that covers types of services provided, revenues and expenditures, staffing, and many items relating to managed behavioral health care.

Data Years. The Inventory of Mental Health Organizations (IMHO/GHMHS) was conducted biannually from 1986 until 1994. SMHO replaced IMHO/GHMHS in 1998. SMHO and the inventory used as its sampling frame have been conducted biannually, starting in 1998.

Coverage. Organizations included are state and county mental hospitals, private psychiatric hospitals, nonfederal general hospitals with separate psychiatric services, Department of Veterans Affairs medical centers, residential treatment centers for emotionally disturbed children, freestanding outpatient psychiatric clinics, partial care organizations, freestanding day–night organizations, and multiservice mental health organizations not elsewhere classified.

Methodology. IMHO was an inventory of all mental health organizations. Its core questionnaire included a version designed for specialty mental health organizations and another for nonfederal general hospitals with separate psychiatric services. The data system was based on questionnaires mailed every other year to mental health organizations in the United States. In 1998, IMHO was replaced by SMHO. SMHO is made up of two parts. A complete inventory is done by postcard, gathering a limited amount of information. The inventory is then used as a sampling frame for SMHO, which contains most of the information from the IMHO core questionnaire as well as new items about managed behavioral health care.

Sample Size and Response Rate. In Phase I, all organizations (about 10,000) were inventoried by postcard. A complete enumeration was needed to define the sampling frame for the sample survey. In Phase II, general hospitals without separate mental health units, community residential organizations, and managed behavioral health care organizations are dropped from the sampling frame. From this number, approximately 1,600–2,200 organizations are drawn for the sample survey and are sent a questionnaire, with a response rate of approximately 90%.

Issues Affecting Interpretation. Revisions to definitions of providers include phasing out Community Mental Health Centers as a category after 1981–1982; increasing the number of multiservice mental health organizations from 1981–1986; increasing the number of psychiatric outpatient clinics in 1981–1982 but decreasing the number in 1983–1984, 1986, 1990, and 1992; and increasing the number of partial care services in 1983–1984. These changes should be noted when interyear comparisons for the affected organizations and service types are made. The increase in the number of general hospitals with separate psychiatric services was partially due to a more concerted effort to identify these organizations. Forms had been sent only to those hospitals previously identified as having a separate psychiatric service. Beginning in 1980–1981, a screener form was sent to general hospitals not previously identified as providing a separate psychiatric service, to determine whether they had such a service.

Reference:

> Center for Mental Health Services. Mental Health, United States, 2004. Manderscheid RW, Berry JT, eds. DHHS pub no (SMA) 06–4195. Rockville, MD: Substance Abuse and Mental Health Services Administration; 2006. Available from: https://store.samhsa.gov/shin/content/SMA06-4195/SMA06-4195.pdf.

For More Information. See the Center for Mental Health Services website at: http://mentalhealth.samhsa.gov/cmhs.

Survey of Occupational Injuries and Illnesses (SOII)

Bureau of Labor Statistics (BLS)

Overview. SOII is a federal/state program that collects statistics used to identify problems with workplace safety and to develop programs to improve workplace safety. Occupational Safety and Health Administration (OSHA) regulations require the recording and reporting by employers of occupational fatalities, injures, and illnesses. Each January, a sample of employers is selected by BLS to participate in a mandatory SOII for that calendar year.

Selected Content. Data include the number of new nonfatal injuries and illnesses by industry. The case and demographic data provide additional details on workers injured, the nature of the disabling condition, and the event and source producing that condition for those cases that involve one or more days away from work.

Data Years. BLS has conducted an annual survey since 1971.

Coverage. The data represent persons employed in private industry establishments in the United States. The survey excludes the self-employed, farms with fewer than 11 employees, private households, and federal government agencies. BLS produces annual estimates of injuries and illnesses for many of the two-, three-, four-, five-, and six-digit private-sector industries as defined by the North American Industry Classification System (NAICS).

Methodology. Survey estimates of occupational injuries and illnesses are based on a scientifically selected probability sample of establishments, rather than a census of all establishments. Each January, an independent sample of establishments is selected for each state and the District of Columbia to participate in the mandatory SOII. BLS includes all the state samples in the national sample.

Establishments included in the survey are instructed to maintain lists of injuries and illnesses and to track days away from work, restricted, or transferred for the calendar year, using the OSHA Summary of Work-Related Injuries and Illnesses form (OSHA no 300A). In January following the year of data collection, BLS mails this sample of employers the SOII. An occupational injury is any injury, such as a cut, fracture, sprain, or amputation, that results from a work-related event or from a single instantaneous exposure in the work environment. An occupational illness is any abnormal condition or disorder, other than one resulting from an occupational injury, caused by exposure to factors associated with employment. It includes acute and chronic illnesses or diseases that may be caused by inhalation, absorption, ingestion, or direct contact. Prior to 2002, injury and illness cases involved days away from work, days of restricted work activity, or both (lost workday cases). Starting in 2002, injury and illness cases may involve days away from work, job transfer, or restricted work activity. Restriction may involve shortened hours, a temporary job change, or temporary restrictions on certain duties (for example, no heavy lifting) of a worker's regular job.

Sample Size and Response Rates. Employer reports were collected from about 205,500 private industry establishments in 2008. The survey response rate was 91% in 2008.

Issues Affecting Interpretation. The number of new injuries and illnesses reported in any given year can be influenced by the level of economic activity, working conditions and work practices, worker experience and training, and number of hours worked. Long-term latent illnesses caused by exposure to carcinogens are believed to be understated in the survey's illness measures. In contrast, new illnesses such as contact dermatitis and carpal tunnel syndrome are easier to relate directly to workplace activity.

Effective January 1, 2002, OSHA revised its requirement for recording occupational injuries and illnesses. Because of the revised recordkeeping rule, the estimates from the 2002 survey and beyond are not comparable with those from previous years. See http://www.osha.gov/recordkeeping/index.html for details on the revised recordkeeping requirements.

Data for the mining industry and for railroad activities are provided by the Department of Labor's Mine Safety and Health Administration and the Department of Transportation's Federal Railroad Administration. Neither of these agencies adopted the revised OSHA recordkeeping requirements for 2002. Therefore, estimates for these industries for 2002 and beyond are not comparable with estimates for other industries but are comparable with estimates for prior years. Excluded from the survey are self-employed individuals, farmers with fewer than 11 employees, private households, federal government agencies, and employees in state and local government agencies.

Starting with 2003 data, SOII began using NAICS to classify industries. Prior to 2003, the program used the Standard Industrial Classification (SIC) system and the Bureau of the Census occupational classification system. Although some titles in SIC and NAICS are similar, there is limited compatibility because industry groupings are defined differently in the two systems. (See Appendix II, Industry of employment.)

Reference:

Bureau of Labor Statistics. Workplace injuries and illnesses—2008 [press release]. USDL pub no 09–1302. Washington, DC: U.S. Department of Labor; 2009 October 29. Available from: http://www.bls.gov/iif/oshwc/osh/os/osnr0032.pdf.

For More Information. See the BLS website at: http://www.bls.gov/iif/home.htm.

United States Renal Data System (USRDS)

National Institute of Diabetes and Digestive and Kidney Diseases (NIDDK), in conjunction with the Centers for Medicare & Medicaid Services (CMS) and the Health Resources and Services Administration (HRSA)

Overview. USRDS is a national data system that collects, analyzes, and distributes information about end-stage renal disease (ESRD) in the United States. USRDS staff collaborate with staff from the Centers for Medicare & Medicaid Services (CMS), HRSA, the Organ Procurement and Transplantation Network (OPTN), under the auspices of HRSA, and the ESRD networks, sharing data sets and actively working to improve the accuracy of ESRD patient information. USRDS has five goals: (a) to characterize the ESRD population; (b) to describe the prevalence and incidence of ESRD, along with trends in mortality and disease rates; (c) to investigate relationships among patient demographics, treatment modalities, and morbidity; (d) to identify new areas for special renal studies and support investigator-initiated research; and (e) to provide data sets and samples of national data to support research by the Special Studies Centers.

Selected Content. USRDS maintains a stand-alone database with data on the diagnoses and demographic characteristics of ESRD patients, along with biochemical data, dialysis claims, and information on treatment and payor histories, hospitalization events, deaths, physician/supplier services, and providers.

Data Years. Data have been compiled annually since 1988.

Coverage. The primary source of ESRD identification is the ESRD Medical Evidence form that is used to register patients at the onset of ESRD and must be submitted by dialysis or transplant providers within 45 days of initiation. The form establishes Medicare eligibility for individuals previously not Medicare beneficiaries, reclassifies previously eligible beneficiaries as ESRD patients, and provides demographic and diagnostic information on all new patients. The CMS, USRDS, and renal research communities rely on the form to ascertain patient demographics, primary diagnosis, comorbidities, and biochemical test results at the time of ESRD initiation. Since 1995, providers have been required to complete the form for all new ESRD patients (Medicare and non-Medicare eligible).

Methodology. Data for the USRDS database are compiled from existing data sources including the CMS Renal Management Information System (REMIS), CMS claims data, facility survey data, CDC survey data (NHANES), Standard Information Management System (SIMS), Medicare Evidence form (CMS–2728), ESRD Death Notification form (CMS–274 6), and OPTN transplant and wait-list data. The CMS data files are supplemented by CMS with enrollment, payer history, and other administrative data, to provide utilization and demographic information on ESRD patients.

Sample Size and Response Rate. Response or coverage rates are 100% of people treated for ESRD since May 1995 because the amended ESRD entitlement policy requires a Medicare Evidence form to be submitted for all ESRD patients, regardless of their insurance and eligibility status. However, the payment data for non-Medicare ESRD patients may be absent during the 30-month coordination period. Ascertainment of incident cases may also be incomplete because the data are for persons receiving ESRD treatment as reported to CMS and do not include patients who die of ESRD before receiving treatment and those who are not reported to CMS.

For More Information. See the USRDS website at: http://www.usrds.org.

Youth Risk Behavior Survey (YRBS)

CDC/National Center for Chronic Disease Prevention and Health Promotion (NCCDPHP)

Overview. YRBS monitors health risk behaviors among students in grades 9–12 that contribute to morbidity and mortality in both adolescence and adulthood.

Selected Content. Data are collected on behaviors that contribute to unintentional injuries and violence; tobacco use; alcohol and other drug use; sexual behaviors that contribute to unintended pregnancy and sexually transmitted diseases (STDs), including human immunodeficiency virus (HIV) infection; unhealthy dietary behaviors; and physical inactivity. In addition, YRBS monitors the prevalence of obesity and asthma.

Data Years. The national YRBS of high school students was conducted in 1990, 1991, 1993, 1995, 1997, 1999, 2001, 2003, 2005, 2007, and 2009.

Coverage. Data are representative of high school students in public and private schools in the United States.

Methodology. The national YRBS school-based surveys employ a three-stage cluster sample design to produce a nationally representative sample of students in grades 9–12 attending public and private high schools. The first-stage sampling frame contains primary sampling units (PSUs) consisting of large counties or groups of smaller, adjacent counties. The PSUs are then stratified based on degree of urbanization and relative percentage of black and Hispanic students in the PSU. The PSUs are selected from these strata with probability proportional to school enrollment size. At the second sampling stage, schools are selected with probability proportional to school enrollment size. To enable separate analysis of data for black and Hispanic students, schools with substantial numbers of black and Hispanic students are sampled at higher rates than all other schools. The third stage of sampling consists of randomly selecting one or two intact classes of a required subject from grades 9–12 at each chosen school. All students in the selected classes are eligible to participate in the survey. A weighting factor is applied to each student record to adjust for nonresponse and for the varying probabilities of selection, including those resulting from the oversampling of black and Hispanic students.

Sample Size and Response Rate. The sample size for the 2009 YRBS was 16,460 students in 158 schools. The school response rate was 81%, and the student response rate was 88%, for an overall response rate of 71%.

Issues Affecting Interpretation. National YRBS data are subject to at least two limitations. First, these data apply only to adolescents who attend regular high school. These students may not be representative of all persons in this age group because those who have dropped out of high school or attend an alternative high school are not surveyed. Second, the extent of underreporting or overreporting cannot be determined, although the survey questions demonstrate good test–retest reliability.

Estimates of substance use for youth based on the YRBS differ from the National Survey on Drug Use & Health (NSDUH) and Monitoring the Future (MTF). Rates are not directly comparable across these surveys because of differences in populations covered, sample design, questionnaires, and interview setting. NSDUH collects data in residences, whereas MTF and YRBS collect data in school classrooms. In addition, NSDUH estimates are tabulated by age, whereas MTF and YRBS estimates are tabulated by grade, representing different ages as well as different populations.

References:

Brener ND, Kann L, Kinchen SA, Grunbaum JA, Whalen L, Eaton D, et al. Methodology of the Youth Risk Behavior Surveillance System. MMWR 2004;53(RR–12):1–13. Available from: http://www.cdc.gov/mmwr/PDF/rr/rr5312.pdf.

Eaton DK, Kann L, Kinchen S, Shanklin S, Ross J, Hawkins J, et al. Youth Risk Behavior Surveillance—United States, 2009. In: Surveillance Summaries, 4 June 2010. MMWR 2010;59(SS–05):1–148. Available from: http://www.cdc.gov/mmwr/PDF/ss/ss5905.pdf.

Cowan CD. Coverage, sample design, and weighting in three federal surveys. J Drug Issues 2001;31(3):599–614.

For More Information. See the YRBS website at: http://www.cdc.gov/yrbs.

Private and Global Sources

American Association of Colleges of Osteopathic Medicine (AACOM)

AACOM, founded in 1898, compiles data on various aspects of osteopathic medical education for distribution to the profession, the government, and the public. Questionnaires are sent annually to schools of osteopathic medicine requesting information on characteristics of applicants, students and graduates, faculty, curriculum, contract and grant activity, revenues and expenditures, and clinical facilities. The response rate is 100%.

Reference:

American Association of Colleges of Osteopathic Medicine. 2006 Annual statistical report on osteopathic medical education. Chevy Chase, MD: American Association of Colleges of Osteopathic Medicine; 2007.

For More Information. Contact the American Association of Colleges of Osteopathic Medicine, 5550 Friendship Boulevard, Suite 310, Chevy Chase, MD 20815–7231; or see the AACOM website at: http://www.aacom.org.

American Association of Colleges of Pharmacy (AACP)

AACP compiles data on colleges of pharmacy, including information on student enrollment and types of degrees conferred. Data are collected through an annual survey. In 2007, the response rate was 99%.

Reference:

> American Association of Colleges of Pharmacy. Profile of pharmacy students: Fall 2008. Alexandria, VA: American Association of Colleges of Pharmacy. 2009.

For More Information. Contact the American Association of Colleges of Pharmacy, 1727 King Street, Alexandria, VA 22314; or see the AACP website at: http://www.aacp.org.

American Association of Colleges of Podiatric Medicine (AACPM)

AACPM compiles data on colleges of podiatric medicine, including information on the schools and enrollment. Data are collected annually through written questionnaires. The response rate is 100%.

For More Information. Contact the American Association of Colleges of Podiatric Medicine, 15850 Crabbs Branch Way, Suite 320, Rockville, MD 20855; or see the AACPM website at: http://www.aacpm.org.

American Dental Association (ADA)

ADA's Division of Educational Measurement conducts annual surveys of predoctoral dental educational institutions. A questionnaire, mailed to all dental schools, collects information on academic programs, admissions, enrollment, attrition, graduates, educational expenses and financial assistance, patient care, advanced dental education, and faculty positions.

Reference:

> American Dental Association. 2007–2008 Survey of dental education, vol 1, Academic programs, enrollments, and graduates. Chicago, IL: American Dental Association; 2009.

For More Information. Contact the American Dental Association, 211 East Chicago Avenue, Chicago, IL 60611–2678; or see the ADA website at: http://www.ada.org.

American Hospital Association (AHA) Annual Survey of Hospitals

Data from the AHA's annual survey are based on questionnaires sent to all AHA-registered and nonregistered hospitals in the United States and its associated areas. U.S. government hospitals located outside the United States are excluded. Overall, the average response rate over the past 5 years has been approximately 85%. For nonreporting hospitals and for the survey questionnaires of reporting hospitals on which some information was missing, estimates are made for all data except those on beds, bassinets, and facilities. Data for beds and bassinets of nonreporting hospitals are based on the most recent information available from those hospitals. Data for facilities and services are based only on reporting hospitals. Estimates of other types of missing data are based on data reported the previous year, if available. When unavailable, estimates are based on data furnished by reporting hospitals similar in size, control, major service provided, length of stay, and geographic and demographic characteristics.

For More Information. Contact the AHA Annual Survey of Hospitals, Health Forum, LLC, an American Hospital Association Company, One North Franklin Street, Chicago, IL 60606; or see the AHA website at: http://www.aha.org.

American Medical Association (AMA) Physician Masterfile

A master file of physicians has been maintained by the AMA since 1906. The Physician Masterfile contains data on all physicians in the United States, both members and nonmembers of the AMA, and on those graduates of American medical schools temporarily practicing overseas. The file also includes information on international medical graduates (IMGs), who are graduates of foreign medical schools, who reside in the United States, and who meet U.S. educational standards for primary recognition as physicians.

A file is initiated on each individual upon entry into medical school or, in the case of IMGs, upon entry into the United States. Between 1965 and 1985, a mail questionnaire survey was conducted every 4 years to update the file information on professional activities, self-designated area of specialization, and present employment status. Since 1985, approximately one-fourth of all physicians are surveyed each year.

Reference:

> American Medical Association, Division of Survey and Data Resources. Physician characteristics and distribution in the U.S., 2009. Chicago, IL: American Medical Association; 2009.

For More Information. Contact the American Medical Association, 515 North State Street, Chicago, IL 60654; or see the AMA website at: http://www.ama-assn.org.

American Osteopathic Association (AOA)

AOA was established to promote the public health, to encourage scientific research, and to maintain and improve high standards of medical education in osteopathic colleges. The AOA Department of Educational Affairs sets the standards for and accredits osteopathic medical colleges and hospitals, postdoctoral training, and board certification programs. AOA publishes both professional and public informational materials. Professional publications include information on osteopathic education, accreditation of hospitals and other health care delivery facilities, and physician licensing. Public information materials include introductory materials on osteopathic medicine, brochures on osteopathic physicians and osteopathic medicine, and patient education materials. AOA compiles the number of osteopathic physicians (DOs); the number of active DOs by gender, age, and specialty and by 50 states and the District of Columbia; and the number of osteopathic medical students by selected characteristics. Statistics for 2007 are available from: http://www.osteopathic.org/inside-aoa/about/who-we-are/Pages/aoa-annual-statistics.aspx.

For More Information. Contact the American Osteopathic Association, 142 East Ontario Street, Chicago, IL 60611; or see the AOA website at: http://www.osteopathic.org.

Association of American Medical Colleges (AAMC)

AAMC collects information on student enrollment in medical schools through its annual Liaison Committee on Medical Education questionnaire, the fall enrollment questionnaire, and the American Medical College Application Service (AMCAS) data system. Other data sources are the Medical School Profile System, the Pre-MCAT questionnaire, the Minority Student Opportunities in Medicine

questionnaire, the Faculty Roster system, data from the Medical College Admission Test, and one-time surveys developed for special projects.

The AAMC Data Warehouse (DW) stores two sections of data relevant to applicants and students: AAMC DW: AMF (Applicant Matriculant file) and AAMC DW: Student. From these two source files, AAMC derives summary statistics about applicants, accepted applicants, matriculants, enrollees, and graduates. AAMC DW: AMF compiles applicant and matriculant data from AMCAS and other medical school application processes. AAMC DW: Student compiles enrollee and graduate data from the AAMC Student Records System. Applicant, enrollment, and graduate statistical data are arranged by academic year, which begins July 1 and ends June 30.

Reference:

> Association of American Medical Colleges. Statistical information related to medical schools and teaching hospitals. Washington, DC: Association of American Medical Colleges; 2008.

For More Information. Contact the Association of American Medical Colleges, 2450 N Street, NW, Washington, DC 20037–1126; or see the AAMC website at: http://www.aamc.org.

Association of Schools and Colleges of Optometry (ASCO)

ASCO compiles data on various aspects of optometric education, including data on schools and enrollment. Questionnaires are sent annually to all schools and colleges of optometry. The response rate is 100%.

Reference:

> Association of Schools and Colleges of Optometry. Annual survey of optometric educational institutions: July 1992–June 1993. Rockville, MD: Association of Schools and Colleges of Optometry; 1994.

For More Information. Contact the Association of Schools and Colleges of Optometry, 6110 Executive Boulevard, Suite 420, Rockville, MD 20852; or see the ASCO website at: http://www.opted.org.

Association of Schools of Public Health (ASPH)

ASPH compiles data on schools of public health in the United States and Puerto Rico. Questionnaires are sent annually to all member schools. The response rate is 100%.

Unlike health professional schools that emphasize specific clinical occupations, schools of public health offer study in specialty areas such as biostatistics, epidemiology, environmental health, occupational health, health administration, health planning, nutrition, maternal and child health, social and behavioral sciences, and other population-based sciences.

For More Information. Contact the Association of Schools of Public Health, 1101 15th Street, NW, Suite 910, Washington, DC 20005; or see the ASPH website at: http://www.asph.org.

Computed Tomography (CT) and Magnetic Resonance Imaging (MRI) Census

The CT/MRI Census is a biennial telephone survey that queries all hospital and nonhospital sites in the United States performing CT and MRI procedures. The census details the types of procedures being performed, procedure volumes, staffing and productivity, installed equipment, planned equipment purchases, and annual budgets for consumables, including contrast media.

Candidate sites for MRI/CT procedures are identified in the American Hospital Association's *AHA Guide*. U.S. territories are not included.

References:

> American Hospital Association. AHA guide, 2010. Chicago, IL: American Hospital Association; 2009. IMV, Medical Information Division. 2006 Computed tomography (CT) and magnetic resonance imaging (MRI) census, Benchmark report: Installed base of CT scanners; Installed base of MRI scanners. DesPlaines, IL: IMV Ltd., Medical Information Division; 2007.

For More Information. Contact IMV, 6301 Ivy Lane, Suite 204, Greenbelt, MD 20770; or see the IMV website at: http://www.imvinfo.com/index.aspx?sec=def.

Dartmouth Atlas of Health Care

The Dartmouth Institute

Overview. The Dartmouth Atlas Project (DAP) began in 1993 as a study of health care markets in the United States, measuring variations in health care resources and their utilization by geographic areas: local hospital market areas, regional referral regions, and states. More recently, the research agenda has expanded to reporting on the resources and utilization among patients at specific hospitals. DAP research uses very large claims databases from the Medicare program and other sources to define where Americans seek care, what kind of care they receive, and to correlate increasing expenditures and the supply of health providers and services with health outcomes.

Selected Content. The database contains information on Medicare spending and on Medicare utilization of selected services, providers, and facilities, by state, local, and regional market areas; by selected subpopulations of Medicare beneficiaries, including decedents and chronically ill beneficiaries; and by providers. The database also allows users to compare quality measures across hospitals.

Data Years. Dartmouth Atlas data are available for 1994 onward.

Coverage. Medicare beneficiaries between the ages of 65 and 99 years with full Part A and Part B entitlement are included in the database. Persons enrolled in managed care organizations are excluded from the analysis.

Methodology. Data reported in *Health, United States*, as computed by DAP, use Medicare claims and administrative data (see Appendix I, Medicare Administrative Data). The percentage of Medicare deaths occurring in a hospital was computed using "death in a hospital" (discharge status B in the Medicare Provider Analysis and Review (MEDPAR) file) as the numerator event. For the percentage of Medicare deaths who were admitted to an intensive care unit (ICU) in the last 6 months of life, the numerator event was "death in a hospital with admission to an ICU within 6 months of the death date" using MEDPAR files. Rates were age-, sex-, and race-adjusted and were expressed as a percentage of deaths. Medicare decedents are identified by their ZIP code of residence.

Total ICU days measures intensive care days (which includes medical, surgical, trauma, and burn care) and coronary care days to produce a total ICU days measure. Intermediate care or step-down units are also included.

Sample Size and Response Rate. The data are from the MEDPAR file, a 100% sample of inpatient claims. The file includes one record for each hospital stay by a Medicare beneficiary, including data on dates of admission and discharge, diagnoses, procedures, and Medicare reimbursements to the hospital.

Issues Affecting Interpretation. The data do not include Medicare enrollees enrolled in managed care organizations under Medicare Advantage.

For More Information. Contact Dartmouth Atlas of Health Care, c/o The Dartmouth Institute for Health Policy and Clinical Practice, 35 Centerra Parkway, Suite 202, Lebanon, NH 03766; or see the Dartmouth Atlas of Health Care website at: http://www.dartmouthatlas.org/faq.shtm.

Guttmacher Institute Abortion Provider Census

Overview. The Guttmacher Institute (previously called the Alan Guttmacher Institute, or AGI) is a not-for-profit organization for reproductive health research, policy analysis, and public education. The institute's abortion provider surveillance program documents the number of legal induced abortions, monitors unintended pregnancy, and assists in efforts to identify and reduce preventable causes of morbidity and mortality associated with abortions.

Selected Content. Guttmacher reports the number of induced abortions; number, types, and locations of providers; and types of procedures performed by state and region. *Health, United States* presents the total number of abortions reported by Guttmacher for each data year.

Data Years. Guttmacher has collected or estimated national abortion data since 1973. Fourteen provider surveys have been conducted for selected data years 1973–2005. No data were collected for 1983, 1986, 1989, 1990, 1993, 1994, 1997, 1998, 2001, 2002, and 2003.

Coverage. The abortion data reported to Guttmacher include women of all ages, including adolescents, who obtain legal induced abortions, and includes both surgical and medication (e.g., using mifepristone, misoprostol, or methotrexate) abortion procedures. Data are collected from three major categories of providers that were identified as potential providers of abortion services: clinics, physicians, and hospitals.

Methodology. For 1999–2000 and 2004–2005, a version of the survey questionnaire was created for each of the three major categories of providers, modeled on the survey questionnaire used for Guttmacher's data collection in 1997. Questionnaires were mailed to all potential providers, with two additional mailings and telephone follow-up for nonresponse. All surveys asked the number of induced abortions performed at the provider's location. State health statistics agencies were also contacted, requesting all available data reported by providers to each state health agency on the number of abortions performed in the survey year. For states that provided data to the Guttmacher Institute, the health agency figures were used for providers who did not respond to the survey. Estimates of the number of abortions performed by some providers were ascertained from knowledgeable sources in the community.

To estimate the number of abortions performed in 2001, 2002, and 2003, the Guttmacher Institute first estimated the change in the number of abortions between 2000 and 2001, beginning with the number of abortions occurring in each state, as reported by the CDC, in each of those 2 years (see Appendix I, Abortion Surveillance System). The three states without reporting systems were excluded. Guttmacher also eliminated the states with very incomplete or inconsistent reporting (Arizona, Maryland, Nevada, and the District of Columbia (D.C.)) and summed the number of abortions that took place in the 44 remaining states for each year. The percentage change between 2000 and 2001 was then applied to Guttmacher's more complete nationwide count of 1,312,990 abortions in 2000 to arrive at the national estimate for 2001. The same procedure was used to estimate the change in the number of abortions between 2001 and 2002 and between 2002 and 2003, except that the data for both years were collected directly from state health departments because the CDC abortion surveillance report for the latest year was not yet available. The states without reporting systems were not included, and, as before, Guttmacher excluded states with incomplete or inconsistent reporting. Further adjustments were made after the 2004–2005 Guttmacher survey results became available.

Sample Size and Response Rate. Of the 2,310 potential providers surveyed for 2004–2005 data, 1,552 responded directly or in follow-up; health department data were used for 274 providers; knowledgeable sources were used for 59 providers; and Guttmacher made its own estimates for 330 facilities. The level of internal estimation was higher than in previous years because health department data from New York and California were less complete.

Issues Affecting Interpretation. The drug mifepristone for medical abortion was approved in September 2000 by the U.S. Food and Drug Administration (FDA) for distribution and use in the United States. For the 2004–2005 data, the distributor of mifepristone also mailed surveys to all facilities and medical professionals that had ever purchased mifepristone.

The CDC national count of abortions was 15% lower than the Guttmacher survey in 1977 and 1978, 12% lower in 1987, 11% lower in 1991 and 1992, and 12% lower in 1995. Beginning in 1998, CDC reported totals for only 48 states and D.C.; since then, the total number of abortions reported to CDC has been about 34% less than the total estimated by Guttmacher. The three reporting areas that did not report abortions to CDC in 2005 (the largest of which was California) accounted for 18% of all abortions tallied by Guttmacher's 2005 survey. (See Appendix I, Abortion Surveillance System.)

References:

Finer LB, Henshaw SK. Abortion incidence and services in the United States in 2000. Perspect Sex Reprod Health 2003;35(1):6–15. Available from: http://www.guttmacher.org/pubs/psrh/full/3500603.pdf.

Jones RK, Zolna MRS, Henshaw SK, Finer LB. Abortion in the United States: Incidence and access to services, 2005. Perspect Sex Reprod Health 2008;40(1):6–16. Available from: http://www.guttmacher.org/pubs/journals/4000608.pdf.

For More Information. Contact the Guttmacher Institute, 125 Maiden Lane, 7th floor, New York, NY 10038; or see the Guttmacher Institute website at: http://www.guttmacher.org.

Organisation for Economic Co-operation and Development (OECD) Health Data

OECD provides annual data on statistical indicators for health and health systems collected from 30 member countries, with some time series going back to 1960. The international comparability of health expenditure estimates depends on the quality of national health accounts in OECD member countries. In recent years, an increasing number of countries have adopted the standards for health accounting defined by OECD, greatly increasing the compara-bility of national health expenditure data reporting. Additional limitations in international comparisons include differing boundaries between health care and other social care, particularly for the disabled and elderly, and underestimation of private expenditures on health.

OECD was established in 1961 with a mandate to promote policies to achieve the highest sustainable economic growth and a rising standard of living among member countries. The organization now comprises 30 member countries: Australia, Austria, Belgium, Canada, Czech Republic, Denmark, Finland, France, Germany, Greece, Hungary, Iceland, Ireland, Italy, Japan, Korea, Luxembourg, Mexico, the Netherlands, New Zealand, Norway, Poland, Portugal, Slovak Republic, Spain, Sweden, Switzerland, Turkey, the United Kingdom, and the United States.

As part of its mission, OECD has developed a number of activities related to health and health care systems. The main aim of OECD work on health policy is to conduct cross-national studies of the performance of OECD health systems and to facilitate exchanges between member countries regarding their experiences in financing, delivering, and managing health services. To support this work, each year OECD compiles cross-country data in the OECD Health Data database, one of the most comprehensive sources of comparable health-related statistics. OECD Health Data is an essential tool for conducting comparative analyses and drawing lessons from international comparisons of diverse health care systems. This international database now incorporates the first results arising from implementation of the OECD manual, *A System of Health Accounts*, which provides a standard framework for producing a set of comprehensive, consistent, and internationally comparable data on health spending. OECD collaborates with other international organizations such as the World Health Organization.

Reference

Organisation for Economic Co-operation and Development. A system of health accounts, version 1.0. Paris, France: Organisation for Economic Co-operation and Development; 2000. Available from: http://www.oecd.org/dataoecd/41/4/1841456.pdf.

For More Information. Contact the OECD Washington Center, 2001 L Street, NW, Suite 650, Washington, DC 20036–4922; or see the OECD website at: http://www.oecd.org/health.

Appendix II. Definitions and Methods

This appendix contains an alphabetical listing of terms used in *Health, United States*, and these definitions are specific to the data presented in this report. The methods used for calculating age-adjusted rates, average annual rates of change, relative standard errors, birth rates, death rates, and years of potential life lost are described. Included are standard populations used for age adjustment (Tables I–III); *International Classification of Diseases* (ICD) codes for cause of death from the 6th through 10th revisions of ICD (Table V) and the years when the revisions were in effect (Table IV); comparability ratios between the 9th and 10th revisions (ICD–9 and ICD–10) for selected causes (Table VI); imputed family income percentages from the National Health Interview Survey (NHIS) (Table VII); an analysis of the effect of added probe questions for Medicare and Medicaid coverage on health insurance rates in NHIS (Table VIII); industry codes from the North American Industry Classification System (NAICS) (Table IX); and ICD–9–CM (Clinical Modification) codes for external causes of injury, diagnostic, and procedure categories (Tables X–XII). Standards for presenting federal data on race and ethnicity are described, and sample tabulations of NHIS data comparing the 1977 and 1997 Office of Management and Budget standards for the classification of federal data on race and ethnicity are presented in Tables XIII and XIV.

Acquired immunodeficiency syndrome (AIDS)—Human immunodeficiency virus (HIV) is the pathogen that causes AIDS, and HIV disease is the term that encompasses all the condition's stages—from infection to the deterioration of the immune system and the onset of opportunistic diseases. However, AIDS is still the term most people use to refer to the immune deficiency caused by HIV. An AIDS diagnosis (indicating that the person has reached the late stages of the disease) is given to people with HIV who have CD4$^+$ cell (also known as T cells or T4 cells, which are the main target of HIV) counts below 200 cells per cubic millimeter (less than 200 cells/µL) or less than 14% of total lymphocytes, or who have been diagnosed with at least one of a set of opportunistic diseases. All 50 states and the District of Columbia report AIDS cases to CDC using a uniform surveillance case definition and case report form. The case reporting definitions were expanded in 1985 (see MMWR 1985;34:373–5); 1987 (MMWR 1987;36(SS–01):1S–15S); 1993 for adults and adolescents (MMWR 1992;41(RR–17):1–19); and 1994

for pediatric cases (MMWR 1994;43(RR–12):1–19). The revisions incorporated a broader range of AIDS-indicator diseases and conditions and used HIV diagnostic tests to improve the sensitivity and specificity of the definition. The 1993 expansion of the case definition caused a temporary distortion of AIDS incidence trends.

In 2005, CDC collaborated with the Council of State and Territorial Epidemiologists (CSTE) to recommend a change in the AIDS case definition to require laboratory confirmation of HIV infection in addition to a CD4$^+$ T-lymphocyte count of less than 200 cells/µL, a CD4$^+$ T-lymphocyte percentage of total lymphocytes of less than 14, or diagnosis of an AIDS-defining condition. This CDC/CSTE recommendation has been incorporated into the 2008 HIV infection case definition, which includes AIDS (stage 3) (see MMWR 2008;57(RR–10):1–8). In 1996, regimens of proven combinations of medications, known as highly active antiretroviral therapy (HAART), became the standard of care for HIV and AIDS. These therapies have prevented or delayed the onset of AIDS and premature death among many HIV-infected persons, and this should be considered when interpreting trend data. AIDS surveillance data are published annually by CDC in the *HIV/AIDS Surveillance Report*. Available from: http://www.cdc.gov/hiv/topics/surveillance/resources/reports/index.htm. (Also see Appendix II, Human immunodeficiency virus (HIV) disease.)

Active physician—See Physician.

Activities of daily living (ADLs)—ADLs are activities related to personal care and include bathing or showering, dressing, getting into or out of bed or a chair, using the toilet, and eating. In the National Health Interview Survey, respondents were asked whether they or family members 3 years of age and over need the help of another person with personal care because of a physical, mental, or emotional problem. Persons were considered to have an ADL limitation if any condition(s) causing the respondent to need help with the specific activities was chronic.

In the Medicare Current Beneficiary Survey, if a sample person had any difficulty performing an activity by him- or herself and without special equipment, or did not perform the activity at all because of health problems, the person was

Table I. United States year 2000 standard population and age groups used to age-adjust data

Data system and age	Population
DVS mortality data	
Total	274,633,642
Under 1 year	3,794,901
1–4 years	15,191,619
5–14 years	39,976,619
15–24 years	38,076,743
25–34 years	37,233,437
35–44 years	44,659,185
45–54 years	37,030,152
55–64 years	23,961,506
65–74 years	18,135,514
75–84 years	12,314,793
85 years and over	4,259,173
NHIS, NAMCS, NHAMCS, NNHS, and NHDS	
All ages	274,633,642
18 years and over	203,852,188
25 years and over	177,593,760
40 years and over	118,180,367
65 years and over	34,709,480
Under 18 years	70,781,454
2–17 years	63,227,991
18–44 years	108,151,050
18–24 years	26,258,428
25–34 years	37,233,437
35–44 years	44,659,185
45–64 years	60,991,658
45–54 years	37,030,152
55–64 years	23,961,506
65–74 years	18,135,514
75 years and over	16,573,966
18–49 years	127,956,843
40–64 years:	
40–49 years	42,285,022
50–64 years	41,185,865
NHES and NHANES	
20 years and over	195,850,985
20–74 years	179,277,019
20–34 years	55,490,662
35–44 years	44,659,185
45–54 years	37,030,152
55–64 years	23,961,506
65–74 years	18,135,514
or	
65 years and over	34,709,480
NHANES (Table 69)	
20–39 years	77,670,618
40–59 years	72,816,615
60–74 years	28,789,786
75 years and over	16,573,966

See footnotes at end of table.

Table I. United States year 2000 standard population and age groups used to age-adjust data—Con.

Data system and age	Population
NHANES (Table 50)	
20–44 years	100,149,847
45–64 years	60,991,658
65 years and over	34,709,480
NHANES (Table 94)	
Under 18 years	70,781,454
18–44 years	108,151,050
45–64 years	60,991,658
65 years and over	34,709,480

NOTES: DVS is Division of Vital Statistics.
NHIS is National Health Interview Survey.
NAMCS is National Ambulatory Medical Care Survey.
NHAMCS is National Hospital Ambulatory Medical Care Survey.
NNHS is National Nursing Home Survey.
NHDS is National Hospital Discharge Survey.
NHES is National Health Examination Survey.
NHANES is National Health and Nutrition Examination Survey.

SOURCE: National Institutes of Health, National Cancer Institute. Surveillance, Epidemiology, and End Results (SEER). Standard populations—single ages. Available from: http://seer.cancer.gov/stdpopulations.

categorized as having a limitation in that activity. The limitation may have been temporary or chronic at the time of interview. Sampled people who were administered a community interview answered questions about health status and functioning themselves, if able to do so. For persons in a long-term care facility, a proxy such as a nurse answered questions about the sample person's health status and functioning. Beginning in 1997, interview questions for people residing in long-term care facilities were changed slightly from those administered to people living in the community, to differentiate residents who were independent from those who received supervision or assistance with transferring, locomotion on unit, dressing, eating, toilet use, and bathing. (Also see Appendix II, Complex activity limitation; Condition; Instrumental activities of daily living; Limitation of activity.)

Addition—See Admission.

Admission—The American Hospital Association defines admissions as persons, excluding newborns, accepted for inpatient services during the survey reporting period. (Also see Appendix II, Days of care; Discharge; Inpatient.)

An admission (also sometimes referred to as an addition) to a mental health organization is defined by the Substance Abuse and Mental Health Services Administration's Center for Mental Health Services as a new admission, a readmission, a return from long-term leave, or a transfer from another service of the same organization or another organization. (Also see Appendix II, Mental health organization; Mental health service type.)

Age—Age is reported as age at last birthday (i.e., age in completed years), often calculated by subtracting the date of birth from the reference date, with the reference date being the date of the examination, interview, or other contact with an individual.

Mother's (maternal) age is reported on the birth certificate by all states. Birth statistics are presented for mothers 10–49 years of age through 1996 and 10–54 years of age starting in 1997, based on mother's date of birth or age as reported on the birth certificate. The age of the mother is edited for upper and lower limits. When the age of the mother is computed to be under 10 years or 55 years and over (50 years and over in 1964–1996), it is considered not stated and is imputed according to the age of the mother from the previous birth record of the same race and total birth order (total of fetal deaths and live births). Before 1963, not stated ages were distributed in proportion to the known ages for each racial group. Beginning in 1997, the birth rate for the maternal age group 45–49 years has included data for mothers 50–54 years of age in the numerator and has been based on the population of women 45–49 years of age in the denominator. Beginning in 2003, for births occurring in states using the 2003 revision of the birth certificate (revised), age of mother is imputed for ages 8 years and under and 65 years and over (mother's age 9 years is recoded as 10 years). Starting in 2007, the same procedures are used for states using the unrevised certificate.

Age adjustment—Age adjustment is used to compare risks for two or more populations at one point in time or for one population at two or more points in time. Age-adjusted rates are computed by the direct method by applying age-specific rates in a population of interest to a standardized age distribution, to eliminate differences in observed rates that result from age differences in population composition. Age-adjusted rates should be viewed as relative indexes rather than actual measures of risk.

Age-adjusted rates are calculated by the direct method, as follows:

$$\sum_{i=1}^{n} r_i \times (p_i / P)$$

where r_i = rate in age group i in the population of interest

p_i = standard population in age group i

$$P = \sum_{i=1}^{n} p_i$$

n = total number of age groups over the age range of the age-adjusted rate.

Age adjustment by the direct method requires the use of a standard age distribution. The standard for age-adjusting death rates and estimates from surveys in *Health, United States* is the projected year 2000 U.S. resident population. Starting with *Health, United States, 2000*, the year 2000 U.S. standard population replaced the 1970 civilian non-institutionalized population for age-adjusting estimates from most NCHS surveys; and starting with *Health, United States, 2001*, it was used uniformly and replaced the 1940 U.S. population for age-adjusting mortality statistics and the 1980 U.S. resident population, which previously had been used for age-adjusting estimates from the National Health and Nutrition Examination Survey.

Changing the standard population has implications for racial and ethnic differentials in mortality. For example, the mortality ratio for the black to white populations is reduced from 1.6 using the 1940 standard to 1.4 using the 2000 standard, reflecting the greater weight the 2000 standard gives to the older population, in which race differentials in mortality are smaller.

Age-adjusted estimates from any data source presented in *Health, United States* may differ from age-adjusted estimates based on the same data presented in other reports, if different age groups are used in the adjustment procedure.

For more information on implementing the 2000 population standard for age-adjusting death rates, see: Anderson RN, Rosenberg HM. Age standardization of death rates: Implementation of the year 2000 standard. National vital statistics reports; vol 47 no 3. Hyattsville, MD: NCHS; 1998. Available from: http://www.cdc.gov/nchs/data/nvsr/nvsr47/nvs47_03.pdf. For more information on the derivation of age-adjustment weights for use with NCHS survey data, see: Klein RJ, Schoenborn CA. Age adjustment using the 2000 projected

Table II. United States year 2000 standard population and proportion distribution by age, for age-adjusting death rates prior to 2003

Age	Population	Proportion distribution (weight)	Standard million
Total	274,634,000	1.000000	1,000,000
Under 1 year	3,795,000	0.013818	13,818
1–4 years	15,192,000	0.055317	55,317
5–14 years	39,977,000	0.145565	145,565
15–24 years	38,077,000	0.138646	138,646
25–34 years	37,233,000	0.135573	135,573
35–44 years	44,659,000	0.162613	162,613
45–54 years	37,030,000	0.134834	134,834
55–64 years	23,961,000	0.087247	87,247
65–74 years	18,136,000	0.066037	66,037
75–84 years	12,315,000	*0.044842	44,842
85 years and over	4,259,000	0.015508	15,508

* Figure is rounded up instead of down to force total to 1.0.

SOURCE: CDC/NCHS. Anderson RN, Rosenberg HM. Age standardization of death rates: Implementation of the year 2000 standard. National vital statistics reports; vol 47 no 3. Hyattsville, MD: NCHS; 1998. Available from: http://www.cdc.gov/nchs/data/nvsr/nvsr47/nvs47_03.pdf.

U.S. population. Healthy People 2010 statistical notes, no 20. Hyattsville, MD: NCHS; 2001. Available from: http://www.cdc.gov/nchs/data/statnt/statnt20.pdf. The year 2000 U.S. standard population is available from the National Cancer Institute's Surveillance, Epidemiology, and End Results (SEER) Program: http://seer.cancer.gov/stdpopulations/stdpop. singleages.html.

Mortality data—Death rates are age-adjusted to the year 2000 U.S. standard population (Table I). Prior to 2003 data, age-adjusted rates were calculated using standard million proportions based on rounded population numbers (Table II). Starting with 2003 data, unrounded population numbers are used to age-adjust. Adjustment is based on 11 age groups, with two exceptions. First, age-adjusted death rates for black males and black females in 1950 are based on nine age groups, with under 1 year and 1–4 years of age combined as one group and 75–84 years and 85 years of age and over combined as one group. Second, age-adjusted death rates by educational attainment for the age group 25–64 years are based on four 10-year age groups (25–34 years, 35–44 years, 45–54 years, and 55–64 years).

Age-adjusted rates for years of potential life lost before 75 years of age also use the year 2000 standard population and are based on eight age groups: under 1 year, 1–14 years, 15–24 years, and 10-year age groups through 65–74 years.

Maternal mortality rates for pregnancy, childbirth, and the puerperium are calculated as the number of maternal deaths per 100,000 live births. Maternal deaths are those with ICD–10 codes A34, O00–O95, and O98–O99. These rates are age-adjusted to the 1970 distribution of live births by mother's age in the United States, as shown in Table III. (Also see Appendix II, Rate: Death and related rates.)

National Health and Nutrition Examination Survey (NHANES)—Estimates based on the National Health Examination Survey and NHANES are generally age-adjusted to the year 2000 U.S. standard population by using five age groups: 20–34 years, 35–44 years, 45–54 years, 55–64 years, and 65–74 years or 65 years and over (see Table I). Prior to *Health, United States, 2001*, these estimates were age-adjusted to the 1980 U.S. resident population.

National Health Care Surveys—Estimates based on the National Hospital Discharge Survey, the National Ambulatory Medical Care Survey, the National Hospital Ambulatory Medical Care Survey, and the National Nursing Home Survey are age-adjusted to the year 2000 U.S. standard population (Table I). Information on the age groups used in the age-adjustment procedure is contained in the footnotes to the specific tables.

National Health Interview Survey (NHIS)—Estimates based on NHIS are age-adjusted to the year 2000 U.S. standard population (Table I).

Table III. Number of live births and mother's age group used to adjust maternal mortality rates to live births: United States, 1970

Mother's age	Live births
All ages....................	3,731,386
Under 20 years..............	656,460
20–24 years.................	1,418,874
25–29 years.................	994,904
30–34 years.................	427,806
35 years and over...........	233,342

SOURCE: CDC/NCHS. Summary report: Final natality statistics, 1970. Monthly vital statistics report; vol 22 no 12 suppl. Hyattsville, MD: NCHS; 1974. Available from: http://www.cdc.gov/nchs/data/mvsr/supp/mv22_12sacc.pdf.

Prior to *Health, United States, 2000*, NHIS estimates were age-adjusted to the 1970 civilian noninstitutionalized population. Information on the age groups used in the age-adjustment procedure is contained in the footnotes to the specific tables.

AIDS—See Acquired immunodeficiency syndrome.

Alcohol consumption—Alcohol consumption is measured differently in the following data systems. (Also see Appendix II, Binge drinking.)

Monitoring the Future (MTF)—This school-based survey of secondary school students collects information on alcohol use by using self-completed questionnaires. Students are asked a preliminary alcohol consumption (defined as beer, wine, liquor, and any other beverage that contains alcohol) screening question, "Have you ever had any alcoholic beverage to drink—more than just a few sips?" Students who reply in the affirmative are then asked additional questions on alcohol consumption: "On how many occasions (if any) have you had alcohol to drink—more than just a few sips—in the last 30 days?" and "How many times have you had five or more drinks in a row in the last 2 weeks?" For this question, a drink is defined as a bottle of beer, a glass of wine, a wine cooler, a shot glass of liquor, a mixed drink, etc.

National Health Interview Survey (NHIS)—Starting with the 1997 NHIS, information on alcohol consumption has been collected in the sample adult questionnaire. Adult respondents are asked two screening questions about their lifetime alcohol consumption: "In any one year, have you had at least 12 drinks of any type of alcoholic beverage?" and "In your entire life, have you had at least 12 drinks of any type of alcoholic beverage?" Persons who report at least 12 drinks in a lifetime are then asked several questions about alcohol consumption in the past year: "In the past year, how often did you drink any type of alcoholic beverage?" and "In the past year, on those days that you drank alcoholic beverages, on the average, how many drinks did you have?" Adults who had at least one drink in the past year were also asked, "In the past year, on how many days did you have five or more drinks of any alcoholic beverage?"

Levels of alcohol consumption are defined as follows: light drinkers, three drinks or fewer per week; moderate drinkers, more than three drinks and up to 14 drinks per week for men and more than three drinks and up to seven drinks per week for women; heavier drinkers, more than 14 drinks per week for men and more than seven drinks per week for women, on average.

National Survey on Drug Use & Health (NSDUH)—Starting in 1999, NSDUH information about the frequency of the consumption of alcoholic beverages in the past 30 days has been obtained for all persons surveyed who are 12 years of age and over. An extensive list of examples of the kinds of beverages covered is given to respondents prior to question administration. A drink is defined as a can or bottle of beer, a glass of wine or a wine cooler, a shot of liquor, or a mixed drink with liquor in it. Those times when the respondent had only a sip or two from a drink are not considered consumption. Alcohol use is based on the following questions: "During the past 30 days, on how many days did you drink one or more drinks of an alcoholic beverage?", "On the days that you drank during the past 30 days, how many drinks did you usually have?", and "During the past 30 days, on how many days did you have five or more drinks on the same occasion?"

Any-listed diagnosis—See Diagnosis.

Average annual rate of change (percent change)—In *Health, United States*, average annual rates of change, or growth rates, are calculated as follows:

$$[(P_n / P_o)^{1/N} - 1] \times 100$$

where P_n = later time period

P_o = earlier time period

N = number of years in interval.

This geometric rate of change assumes that a variable increases or decreases at the same rate during each year between the two time periods.

Average length of stay—In the National Hospital Discharge Survey, average length of stay is computed by dividing the total number of hospital days of care (counting the date of admission but not the date of discharge) by the number of patients discharged. The American Hospital Association computes average length of stay by dividing the number of inpatient days by the number of admissions. (Also see Appendix II, Days of care; Discharge; Inpatient.)

Basic actions difficulty—Basic actions difficulty captures limitations or difficulties in movement, emotional, sensory, or cognitive functioning associated with a health problem. Persons with more than one of these difficulties are counted only once in the estimates. The full range of functional areas cannot be assessed on the basis of National Health Interview Survey (NHIS) questions; however, the available questions can identify difficulty in the following core areas of functioning:

■ Movement (walking, standing, sitting, bending or kneeling, reaching overhead, grasping objects with fingers, and lifting).

■ Selected elements of emotional functioning, in particular, feelings that interfere with accomplishing daily activities. Respondents were classified based on responses to a series of questions that measure psychological distress.

■ Sensory functioning, based on difficulties seeing or hearing.

■ Selected elements in cognitive functioning, specifically difficulties with remembering or experiencing confusion.

For many measures of disability, only disabilities resulting from an underlying condition that is chronic (based on nature and duration) are considered. However, whether the underlying conditions related to the core areas of basic actions difficulty were chronic was not a requirement in classifying persons. For more information on how this measure was constructed using NHIS data, including the specific questions asked, see: Altman B, Bernstein A. Disability and Health in the United States, 2001–2005. Hyattsville, MD: NCHS; 2008. Available from: http://www.cdc.gov/nchs/data/misc/disability2001-2005.pdf.

(Also see Appendix II, Complex activity limitation; Hearing trouble.)

Bed, health facility—The American Hospital Association defines bed count as the number of beds, cribs, and pediatric bassinets that are set up and staffed for use by inpatients on the last day of the reporting period. In the Center for Medicare & Medicaid Service's Online Survey Certification and Reporting (OSCAR) database, all beds in certified facilities are counted on the day of certification inspection. The Center for Mental Health Services within the Substance Abuse and Mental Health Services Administration counts the number of beds set up and staffed for use in inpatient and residential treatment services on the last day of the survey reporting period. (Also see Appendix II, Hospital; Mental health organization; Mental health service type; Occupancy rate.)

Binge drinking—Binge drinking is measured in the following data systems. (Also see Appendix II, Alcohol consumption.)

Monitoring the Future (MTF)—This school-based survey of secondary school students collects information on alcohol use by using self-completed questionnaires. To determine whether they have tried alcohol in the past year, students are asked: "On how many occasions (if any) have you had alcohol to drink—more than just a few sips—in the last 30 days?" Alcoholic beverages are defined as beer, wine, liquor, and any other beverage that contains alcohol. Among students who answer in the affirmative, information on binge drinking is obtained for high school seniors (starting in 1975) and for 8th and 10th graders (starting in 1991) based on the following question referring to the prior 2-week period: "How many times have you had five or more drinks in a row?" For this question, a drink means a 12-oz can (or bottle) of beer, a 4-oz glass of wine, a 12-oz bottle or can of wine cooler, a mixed drink, a shot of liquor, or the equivalent.

National Survey on Drug Use & Health (NSDUH)—In NSDUH, binge alcohol use is defined as "Five or more drinks on the same occasion (i.e., at the same time or within a couple of hours of each other) at least once in the past 30 days." Heavy alcohol use is defined as "Five or more drinks on the same occasion (binge drinking) on at least 5 different days in the past 30 days." (Also see Appendix II, Alcohol consumption.)

Birth cohort—A birth cohort consists of all persons born within a given period of time, such as a calendar year.

Birth rate—See Rate: Birth and related rates.

Birthweight—Birthweight is the first weight of the newborn obtained after birth. Low birthweight is defined as weighing less than 2,500 grams (5 lb 8 oz). Very low birthweight is defined as weighing less than 1,500 grams (3 lb 4 oz). Before 1979, low birthweight was defined as weighing 2,500 grams or less, and very low birthweight as 1,500 grams or less.

Blood pressure, high—In *Health, United States*, uncontrolled blood pressure is defined as having an average systolic blood pressure reading of at least 140 mmHg or diastolic reading of at least 90 mmHg, among those with hypertension. These blood pressure standards are consistent with the following: National Heart, Lung, and Blood Institute. Seventh report of the Joint National Committee on Prevention, Detection, Evaluation, and Treatment of High Blood Pressure. NIH pub no 04–5230. Bethesda, MD: National Institutes of Health; 2004. Available from: http://www.nhlbi.nih.gov/guidelines/ hypertension/jnc7full.pdf.

Those with elevated blood pressure also may be taking prescribed medicine for high blood pressure. Data on hypertension also are presented in *Health, United States*. People are considered to have hypertension if they have measured elevated blood pressure or if they report that they are taking a prescription medicine for high blood pressure, even if their blood pressure readings are within the normal range.

Blood pressure is measured by averaging the blood pressure readings taken. Blood pressure readings of 0 mmHg are assumed to be in error and are not included in the estimates. The methods used to measure the blood pressure of National Health and Nutrition Examination Survey (NHANES) participants have changed over the different NHANES survey years. Changes include the following:

■ Number of blood pressure measurements taken (increased from one to four).

■ Equipment maintenance procedures.

■ Training of persons taking readings (physician, nurse, interviewer).

■ Proportion zero end digits for systolic and diastolic readings.

■ Published diastolic definition.

■ Location where the measurements were taken (mobile examination center (MEC) or home).

In 1999 and subsequent years, blood pressure has been measured in the NHANES MEC by one of the MEC physicians. For people 20 years of age and over,

three consecutive blood pressure readings are obtained using the same arm. If a blood pressure measurement was interrupted or the measurer was unable to get one or more of the readings, a fourth attempt may be made. Both systolic and diastolic measurements are recorded to the nearest even number.

In NHANES III, three sets of blood pressure measurements were taken in the MEC for examinees 5 years of age and over. Blood pressure measurements were also taken by trained interviewers during the household interview, on sample persons 17 years of age and over. Systolic and diastolic average blood pressures were computed as the arithmetic mean of six or fewer measurements obtained at the household interview (maximum of three) and the MEC examination (maximum of three). If the examinee did not have blood pressure measurements taken in the MEC, this variable was calculated from measurements taken at the household interview. Both systolic and diastolic measurements were recorded to the nearest even number.

For more information on changes in blood pressure measurement in NHANES up to 1991, see: Burt VL, Cutler JA, Higgings M, Horan MJ, Labarthe D, Whelton P, et al. Trends in the prevalence, awareness, treatment, and control of hypertension in the adult US population: Data from the health examination surveys, 1960 to 1991. Hypertension 1995;26(1):60–9.

Body mass index (BMI)—BMI is a measure that adjusts bodyweight for height. It is calculated as weight in kilograms divided by height in meters squared.

Healthy weight for adults is defined as a BMI of 18.5 to less than 25; overweight (including obese), as a BMI greater than or equal to 25; and obesity, as a BMI greater than or equal to 30. BMI cut points are defined in the following: U.S. Department of Health and Human Services and U.S. Department of Agriculture. Dietary guidelines for Americans, 2005, 6th ed. Washington, DC: U.S. Government Printing Office, January 2005. Available from: http://www.health.gov/dietaryguidelines/dga2005/ document/default.htm; National Heart, Lung, and Blood Institute. Clinical guidelines on the identification, evaluation, and treatment of overweight and obesity in adults: The evidence report. NIH pub no 98–4083. Bethesda, MD: National Institutes of Health; 1998. Available from: http://www.nhlbi.nih.gov/guidelines/obesity/ ob_gdlns.htm; and U.S. Department of Health and Human Services. Tracking healthy people 2010, Part B, Operational definitions, ch 19, Nutrition and

Table IV. Revision of the *International Classification of Diseases* (ICD), by year of conference by which adopted and years in use in the United States

ICD revision	Year of conference by which adopted	Years in use in United States
1st	1900	1900–1909
2nd	1909	1910–1920
3rd	1920	1921–1929
4th	1929	1930–1938
5th	1938	1939–1948
6th	1948	1949–1957
7th	1955	1958–1967
8th	1965	1968–1978
9th	1975	1979–1998
10th	1990	1999–present

SOURCE: CDC/NCHS. Available from: http://www.cdc.gov/nchs/icd.htm.

overweight, Objectives 19–1 to 19–3. Washington, DC: U.S. Government Printing Office; 2000. Available from: ftp://ftp.cdc.gov/pub/Health_Statistics/NCHS/Datasets/DATA2010/Focusarea19.

Obesity for children and adolescents is defined as a BMI at or above the sex- and age-specific 95th percentile BMI cut points from the 2000 CDC Growth Charts (http://www.cdc.gov/growthcharts/). Starting with *Health United States, 2010*, the terminology describing excess weight among children changed from previous editions. The term obesity now refers to children who were formerly labeled as overweight. This is a change in terminology only and not a change in measurement. For more information, see: Ogden CL, Flegal KM. Changes in terminology for childhood overweight and obesity. National health statistics report; no 25. Hyattsville, MD: NCHS; 2010. Available from: http://www.cdc.gov/nchs/data/nhsr/nhsr025.pdf.

Cause of death—For the purpose of national mortality statistics, every death is attributed to one underlying condition, based on information reported on the death certificate and using the international rules for selecting the underlying cause of death from the conditions stated on the certificate. The underlying cause is defined by the World Health Organization (WHO) as "the disease or injury that initiated the train of events leading directly to death, or the circumstances of the accident or violence that produced the fatal injury." Generally, more medical information is reported on death certificates than is directly reflected in the underlying cause of death. Conditions that are not selected as underlying cause of death constitute the nonunderlying causes of death, also known as multiple cause of death.

Cause of death is coded according to the appropriate revision of the *International Classification of Diseases* (ICD) (see Table IV). Effective with deaths occurring in 1999, the United States began using the 10th revision of the ICD (ICD–10); during the period 1979–1998, causes of death were coded and classified according to the 9th revision (ICD–9). Table V lists ICD codes for the 6th through 10th revisions for causes of death shown in *Health, United States*.

Each ICD revision has produced discontinuities in cause-of-death trends. These discontinuities are measured by using comparability ratios that are essential to the interpretation of mortality trends. For further discussion, see: http://www.cdc.gov/nchs/nvss/mortality/comparability_icd.htm.

(Also see Appendix II, Comparability ratio; *International Classification of Diseases*; and Appendix I, National Vital Statistics System; Multiple Cause-of-Death File.)

Cause-of-death ranking—Selected causes of death of public health and medical importance are compiled into tabulation lists and are ranked according to the number of deaths assigned to these causes. The top-ranking causes determine the leading causes of death. Certain causes on the tabulation lists are not ranked if, for example, the category title represents a group title (such as "Major cardiovascular diseases" and "Symptoms, signs, and abnormal clinical and laboratory findings, not elsewhere classified") or the category title begins with the words "Other" or "All other." In addition, when one of the titles that represents a subtotal (such as malignant neoplasms) is ranked, its component parts are not ranked. The tabulation lists used for ranking in the 10th revision of the

Table V. Cause-of-death codes, by applicable revision of the *International Classification of Diseases* (ICD)

Cause of death (10th Revision titles)	6th and 7th Revisions	8th Revision	9th Revision	10th Revision
Communicable diseases	. . .	. . .	001–139, 460–466, 480–487, 771.3	A00–B99, J00–J22
Chronic and noncommunicable diseases . . .	. . .	. . .	140–459, 470–478, 490–799	C00–I99, J30–R99
Meningococcal infection	. . .	. . .	036	A39
Septicemia	. . .	. . .	038	A40–A41
Human immunodeficiency virus (HIV) disease[1]	. . .	. . .	*042–*044	B20–B24
Malignant neoplasms	140–205	140–209	140–208	C00–C97
Colon, rectum, and anus	153–154	153–154	153, 154	C18–C21
Trachea, bronchus, and lung	162–163	162	162	C33–C34
Breast	170	174	174–175	C50
Prostate	177	185	185	C61
In situ neoplasms and benign neoplasms . . .	. . .	. . .	210–239	D00–D48
Diabetes mellitus	260	250	250	E10–E14
Anemias	. . .	. . .	280–285	D50–D64
Meningitis	. . .	. . .	320–322	G00, G03
Alzheimer's disease	. . .	. . .	331	G30
Diseases of heart	400–402, 410–443	390–398, 402, 404, 410–429	390–398, 402, 404, 410–429	I00–I09, I11, I13, I20–I51
Ischemic heart disease	. . .	. . .	410–414, 429.2	I20–I25
Cerebrovascular diseases	330–334	430–438	430–434, 436–438	I60–I69
Atherosclerosis	. . .	. . .	440	I70
Influenza and pneumonia[2]	480–483, 490–493	470–474, 480–486	480–487	J09–J18
Chronic lower respiratory diseases	241, 501, 502, 527.1	490–493, 519.3	490–494, 496	J40–J47
Chronic liver disease and cirrhosis	581	571	571	K70, K73–K74
Nephritis, nephrotic syndrome, and nephrosis	. . .	. . .	580–589	N00–N07, N17–N19, N25–N27
Pregnancy, childbirth, and the puerperium	640–689	630–678	630–676	A34, O00–O95, O98–O99
Congenital malformations, deformations, and chromosomal abnormalities	. . .	. . .	740–759	Q00–Q99
Certain conditions originating in the perinatal period	. . .	. . .	760–779	P00–P96
Newborn affected by maternal complications of pregnancy	. . .	. . .	761	P01
Newborn affected by complications of placenta, cord, and membranes	. . .	. . .	762	P02
Disorders related to short gestation and low birthweight, not elsewhere classified	. . .	. . .	765	P07
Birth trauma	. . .	. . .	767	P10–P15
Intrauterine hypoxia and birth asphyxia . . .	. . .	. . .	768	P20–P21
Respiratory distress of newborn	. . .	. . .	769	P22
Sudden infant death syndrome	. . .	. . .	798.0	R95

See footnotes at end of table.

Table V. Cause-of-death codes, by applicable revision of the *International Classification of Diseases* (ICD)—Con.

Cause of death (10th Revision titles)	6th and 7th Revisions	8th Revision	9th Revision	10th Revision
Occupational diseases:				
Angiosarcoma of liver................	. . .	. . .	. . .	C22.3
Malignant mesothelioma..............	. . .	. . .	158.8, 158.9, 163	C45
Pneumoconiosis	. . .	. . .	500–505	J60–J66
Coal workers' pneumoconiosis	. . .	. . .	500	J60
Asbestosis......................	. . .	. . .	501	J61
Silicosis.......................	. . .	. . .	502	J62
Other (including unspecified)	. . .	. . .	503–505	J63–J66
Injuries[2]	. . .	. . .	E800–E869, E880–E929, E950–E999	*U01–*U03, V01–Y36, Y85–Y87, Y89
Unintentional injuries[3]	E800–E936, E960–E965	E800–E929, E940–E946	E800–E869, E880–E929	V01–X59, Y85–Y86
Motor vehicle-related injuries[3]	E810–E835	E810–E823	E810–E825	V02–V04, V09.0, V09.2, V12–V14, V19.0–V19.2, V19.4–V19.6, V20–V79, V80.3–V80.5, V81.0–V81.1, V82.0–V82.1, V83–V86, V87.0–V87.8, V88.0–V88.8, V89.0, V89.2
Poisoning	E870–E888, E890–E895	E850–E877	E850–E869	X40–X49
Suicide[2]	E963, E970–E979	E950–E959	E950–E959	*U03, X60–X84, Y87.0
Homicide[2]	E964, E980–E983	E960–E969	E960–E969	*U01–*U02, X85–Y09, Y87.1
Injury by firearms	. . .	E922, E955, E965, E970, E985	E922, E955.0–E955.4, E965.0–E965.4, E970, E985.0–E985.4	*U01.4, W32–W34, X72–X74, X93–X95, Y22–Y24, Y35.0

. . . Cause-of-death codes are not provided for causes not shown in *Health, United States.*

[1]Categories for coding human immunodeficiency virus (HIV) infection were introduced in 1987. The asterisk (*) indicates codes that are not part of ICD–9.

[2]Starting with 2001 data, NCHS introduced categories *U01–*U03 for classifying and coding deaths due to acts of terrorism. The asterisk (*) indicates codes that are not part of ICD–10. Starting with 2007 data, NCHS introduced the category J09 for coding avian influenza virus.

[3]In the public health community, the term unintentional injuries is preferred to accidents, and the term motor vehicle-related injuries is preferred to motor vehicle accidents.

SOURCE: CDC/NCHS. Advance report: Final mortality statistics, 1974. Monthly vital statistics report; vol 24 no 11 suppl. Hyattsville, MD: NCHS; 1976. Available from: http://www.cdc.gov/nchs/data/mvsr/supp/mv24_11sacc.pdf.

Hoyert DL, Kochanek KD, Murphy SL. Deaths: Final data for 1997. National vital statistics reports; vol 47 no 19. Hyattsville, MD: NCHS; 1999. Available from: http://www.cdc.gov/nchs/data/nvsr/nvsr47/nvsr47_19.pdf.

Hoyert DL, Heron MP, Murphy SL, Kung H-C. Deaths: Final data for 2003. National vital statistics reports; vol 54 no 13. Hyattsville, MD: NCHS; 2006. Available from: http://www.cdc.gov/nchs/data/nvsr/nvsr54/nvsr54_13.pdf.

Xu JQ, Kochanek KD, Murphy SL, Tejada-Vera B. Deaths: Final data for 2007. National vital statistics reports; vol 58 no 19. Hyattsville, MD: NCHS; 2010. Available from: http://www.cdc.gov/nchs/data/nvsr/nvsr58/nvsr58_19.pdf.

International Classification of Diseases (ICD) include the List of 113 Selected Causes of Death, which replaces the ICD–9 List of 72 Selected Causes, HIV Infection, and Alzheimer's Disease; and the ICD–10 List of 130 Selected Causes of Infant Death, which replaces the ICD–9 List of 60 Selected Causes of Infant Death and HIV Infection. Causes that are tied receive the same rank; the next cause is assigned the rank it would have received had the lower-ranked causes not been tied, that is, a rank is skipped. For more information, see: Xu JQ, Kochanek KD, Murphy SL, Tejada-Vera B. Deaths: Final data for 2007. National vital statistics reports; vol 58 no 19. Hyattsville, MD: NCHS; 2010. Available from: http://www.cdc.gov/nchs/data/nvsr/nvsr58/nvsr58_19.pdf. (Also see Appendix II, *International Classification of Diseases*.)

Children's Health Insurance Program (CHIP)—Title XXI of the Social Security Act, sometimes referred to as the Children's Health Insurance Program (CHIP), is a program originally enacted by the Balanced Budget Act of 1997 (BBA). The Children's Health Insurance Program Reauthorization Act of 2009 (CHIPRA, P.L. 111–3) reauthorized CHIP. CHIPRA appropriated funding for CHIP through FY 2013. CHIP provides federal funds for states to provide health care coverage to eligible low-income, uninsured children who do not qualify for Medicaid. CHIP gives states broad flexibility in program design within a federal framework that includes important beneficiary protections. Funds from CHIP may be used for a separate child health program or to expand Medicaid. Although CHIP is not part of Medicaid, in some instances in *Health, United States*, data on CHIP and Medicaid are presented together. For additional information, see: http://www.cms.hhs.gov/chipra/. (Also see Appendix II, Health insurance coverage; Medicaid.)

Cholesterol—Serum total cholesterol is a combination of high-density lipoproteins (HDLs), low-density lipoproteins (LDLs), and very-low-density lipoproteins (VLDLs). High serum total cholesterol is a risk factor for cardiovascular disease. According to the National Cholesterol Education Program, high serum total cholesterol is defined as being greater than or equal to 240 mg/dL (6.20 mmol/L). Borderline high serum total cholesterol is defined as greater than or equal to 200 mg/dL and less than 240 mg/dL. Assessments of the components of total cholesterol, or lower thresholds for high total cholesterol, may be used for individuals with other risk factors for cardiovascular disease. For more information on high cholesterol guidelines, see: National Cholesterol Education Program (NCEP). Third report of the NCEP

Expert Panel on Detection, Evaluation, and Treatment of High Blood Cholesterol in Adults (Adult Treatment Panel III): Final report. NIH pub no 02–5215. Bethesda, MD: National Institutes of Health, National Heart, Lung, and Blood Institute; 2002. Available from: http://www.nhlbi.nih.gov/guidelines/cholesterol/atp3full.pdf.

In *Health, United States*, three measures of total cholesterol are presented: high total cholesterol, high serum total cholesterol, and mean serum total cholesterol level. High total cholesterol is based on both laboratory testing and self-reported medication use. It is defined as measured serum total cholesterol greater than or equal to 240 mg/dL or reporting taking cholesterol-lowering medications. Respondents answering "yes" to the question, "Are you now following this advice [from a doctor of health professional] to take prescribed medicine [to lower your cholesterol]?" were classified as taking cholesterol-lowering medications. High serum total cholesterol is defined as measured serum total cholesterol greater than or equal to 240 mg/dL (6.20 mmol/L). Mean serum total cholesterol level is based on serum samples collected during the National Health and Nutrition Examination Survey (NHANES) examination.

Venous blood serum samples collected from NHANES participants at mobile examination centers were frozen and shipped on dry ice to the laboratory conducting the lipid analyses. Serum total cholesterol was measured on all examined adults regardless of whether they had fasted, and data were analyzed regardless of fasting status. Cholesterol measurements are standardized according to the criteria of the CDC—and later the CDC–National Heart, Lung, and Blood Institute Cholesterol Standardization Program—to ensure comparable and accurate measurements. For more information, see: Myers GL, Cooper GR, Winn CL, Smith SJ. The Centers for Disease Control–National Heart, Lung, and Blood Institute Lipid Standardization Program: An approach to accurate and precise lipid measurements. Clin Lab Med 1989;9(1):105–35. A detailed summary of the procedures used for measurement of total cholesterol in the earlier NHANES survey years has been published in: Johnson CL, Rifkind BM, Sempos CT, Carroll MD, Bachorik PS, Briefel RR, et al. Declining serum total cholesterol levels among U.S. adults: The National Health and Nutrition Examination Surveys. JAMA 1993;269(23):3002–8. A description of the laboratory procedures for the total cholesterol measurement for different NHANES survey years is published by NCHS. Available from: http://www.cdc.gov/nchs/nhanes.htm.

Chronic condition—See Condition.

Cigarette smoking—Cigarette smoking and related tobacco use are measured in the following data systems.

Birth file—With the 1989 revision of the U.S. Standard Certificate of Live Birth, information on cigarette smoking by the mother during pregnancy became available for the first time. Data from the 1989 revision are based on "yes/no" responses to the birth certificate item: "Other risk factors for this pregnancy: Tobacco use during pregnancy" and the average number of cigarettes per day with no specificity on timing during pregnancy. In 1989, 43 states and the District of Columbia (D.C.) collected data on tobacco use. The following states did not require the reporting of tobacco use in the standard format on the birth certificate: California, Indiana, Louisiana, Nebraska, New York, Oklahoma, and South Dakota. In 1990, information on tobacco use became available from Louisiana and Nebraska, increasing the number of reporting states to 45 and D.C. In 1991–1993, with the addition of Oklahoma to the reporting area, information on tobacco use was available for 46 states and D.C.; in 1994–1998, 46 states, D.C., and New York City reported tobacco use. In 1999, information on tobacco use became available from Indiana and New York, increasing the number of reporting states to 48 and D.C.; starting in 2000, with the addition of South Dakota, the reporting area included 49 states and D.C. During 1989–2006, California did not require the reporting of tobacco use. The area reporting tobacco use encompassed 87% of U.S. births in 1999–2002.

Starting in 2003, some states implemented the 2003 revision of the U.S. Standard Certificate of Live Birth, which asked for the number of cigarettes smoked at different intervals before and during pregnancy. Data on mother's tobacco use during pregnancy from the 2003 revision of the birth certificate are not comparable with data from the 1989 revision. Therefore, 2006 and 2007 data on smoking are shown separately for the 28 reporting areas that used the 1989 revision in 2006 and 2007 and for the reporting areas that used the 2003 revision in 2006 and 2007, in order to provide 2 years of comparable data. The 28 reporting areas using the 1989 certificate are Alabama, Alaska, Arizona, Arkansas, Connecticut, Hawaii, Illinois, Louisiana, Maine, Massachusetts, Maryland, Minnesota, Mississippi, Missouri, Montana, Nevada, New Jersey, New Mexico, North Carolina, Oklahoma, Oregon, Rhode Island,

Utah, Virginia, West Virginia, Wisconsin, D.C., and New York City. The states that used the 2003 revision of the U.S. Standard Certificate of Live Birth for data on smoking in 2006 and 2007 were Delaware, Idaho, Kansas, Kentucky, Nebraska, New Hampshire, New York state (excluding New York City), North Dakota, Ohio, Pennsylvania, South Carolina, South Dakota, Tennessee, Texas, Vermont, Washington state, and Wyoming. In *Health, United States*, data were not shown for the five states (Colorado, Georgia, Iowa, Indiana, and Michigan) that implemented the 2003 revision sometime during 2007 and therefore do not have consistent smoking data for 2006–2007. California did not report smoking data in 2006; therefore, data for California are not presented. Florida collected smoking data, but these data are not comparable and therefore are not presented.

Monitoring the Future (MTF)—Information on current cigarette smoking was obtained for high school seniors (starting in 1975) and for 8th and 10th graders (starting in 1991), based on the following question: "How frequently have you smoked cigarettes during the past 30 days?"

National Health Interview Survey (NHIS)—Information about cigarette smoking is obtained for adults 18 years of age and over. Starting in 1993, current smokers are identified by asking the following two questions: "Have you smoked at least 100 cigarettes in your entire life?" and "Do you now smoke cigarettes every day, some days, or not at all?" Persons who smoked 100 cigarettes and who now smoke every day or some days were defined as current smokers. Before 1992, current smokers were identified based on positive responses to the following two questions: "Have you smoked 100 cigarettes in your entire life?" and "Do you smoke now?" (traditional definition). In 1992, the definition of current smoker in NHIS was modified to specifically include persons who smoked on some days (revised definition). In 1992, cigarette smoking data were collected for a half-sample with half the respondents (one-quarter sample) using the traditional smoking questions and the other half of respondents (one-quarter sample) using the revised smoking question ("Do you smoke every day, some days, or not at all?"). An unpublished analysis of the 1992 traditional smoking measure revealed that the crude percentage of current smokers 18 years of age and over remained the same as for 1991. The estimates for 1992 shown in *Health, United States* combine data collected using both the traditional and revised questions.

In 1993–1995, estimates of cigarette smoking prevalence were based on a half-sample. Smoking data were not collected in 1996. Starting in 1997, smoking data were collected in the sample adult questionnaire. For further information on survey methodology and sample sizes pertaining to NHIS cigarette smoking data, see the NHIS tobacco information website at: http://www.cdc.gov/nchs/nhis/tobacco.htm.

National Survey on Drug Use & Health (NSDUH)— Information on current cigarette smoking is obtained for all persons surveyed who were 12 years of age and over, based on the following question: "During the past 30 days, have you smoked part or all of a cigarette?"

Civilian noninstitutionalized population; Civilian population—See Population.

Community hospital—See Hospital.

Comparability ratio—About every 10 to 20 years, the *International Classification of Diseases* (ICD) is revised to stay abreast of advances in medical science and changes in medical terminology. Each of these revisions produces breaks in the continuity of cause-of-death statistics because of changes in classification and in the rules for selecting an underlying cause of death. Classification and rule changes affect cause-of-death trend data by shifting deaths away from some cause-of-death categories and into others. Comparability ratios measure the effect of changes in classification and coding rules. For the causes shown in Table VI, comparability ratios range between 0.6974 and 1.0365. Influenza and pneumonia had the lowest comparability ratio (0.6974), indicating that this cause is about 30% less likely to be selected as the underlying cause of death in ICD–10 than in ICD–9. Unintentional poisoning had the highest comparability ratio (1.0365), indicating that unintentional poisoning was more than 3% more likely to be selected as the underlying cause when ICD–10 coding is used.

For selected causes of death, the ICD–9 codes used to calculate death rates for 1980–1998 differ from the ICD–9 codes most nearly comparable with the corresponding ICD–10 cause-of-death category, which also affects the ability to compare death rates across ICD revisions. Examples of these causes are ischemic heart disease; cerebrovascular diseases; trachea, bronchus, and lung cancer; unintentional injuries; and homicide. To address this source of discontinuity, mortality trends for 1980–1998 were

Table VI. Comparability of selected causes of death between the 9th and 10th revisions of the *International Classification of Diseases* (ICD)

Cause of death[1]	Final comparability ratio[2]
Human immunodeficiency virus (HIV) disease	1.0821
Malignant neoplasms	1.0093
Colon, rectum, and anus	0.9988
Trachea, bronchus, and lung	0.9844
Breast	1.0073
Prostate	1.0144
Diabetes mellitus	1.0193
Alzheimer's disease	1.5812
Diseases of heart	0.9852
Ischemic heart diseases	1.0006
Essential (primary) hypertension and hypertensive renal disease	1.1162
Cerebrovascular diseases	1.0502
Influenza and pneumonia	0.6974
Chronic lower respiratory diseases	1.0411
Chronic liver disease and cirrhosis	1.0321
Nephritis, nephrotic syndrome, and nephrosis	1.2555
Pregnancy, childbirth, and the puerperium . . .	1.1404
Unintentional injuries	1.0251
Motor vehicle-related injuries	0.9527
Poisoning	1.0365
Suicide	1.0022
Homicide	1.0020
Injury by firearms	1.0012
Chronic and noncommunicable diseases . . .	1.0100
Injuries	1.0159

[1]See Table V for ICD–9 and ICD–10 cause-of-death codes.
[2]Ratio of number of deaths classified by ICD–10 to number of deaths classified by ICD–9.

SOURCE: CDC/NCHS. Final comparability ratios for 113 selected causes of death. Available from: ftp://ftp.cdc.gov/pub/Health_Statistics/NCHS/Datasets/Comparability/icd9_icd10/Comparability_Ratio_tables.xls. Miniño M, Anderson RN, Fingerhut LA, Boudreault MA, Warner M. Deaths: Injuries, 2002. National vital statistics reports; vol 54 no 10. Hyattsville, MD: NCHS; 2006. Available from: http://www.cdc.gov/nchs/data/nvsr/nvsr54/nvsr54_10.pdf.

recalculated using ICD–9 codes that are more comparable with codes for corresponding ICD–10 categories. Table V shows the ICD–9 codes used for these causes. This modification may lessen the discontinuity between the 9th and 10th revisions, but the effect on the discontinuity between the 8th and 9th revisions is not measured.

Comparability ratios shown in Table VI are based on a comparability study in which the same deaths were coded using both the 9th and 10th revisions. The comparability ratio was calculated by dividing the number of deaths classified by ICD–10 by the number of deaths classified by ICD–9. The resulting ratios represent the net effect of the 10th revision on cause-of-death statistics and can be used to adjust mortality statistics for causes of death classified by the 9th revision to be comparable with cause-specific mortality statistics classified by the 10th revision.

The application of comparability ratios to mortality statistics helps make the analysis of change between 1998 and 1999 more accurate and complete. The 1998 comparability-modified death rate is calculated by multiplying the comparability ratio by the 1998 death rate. Comparability-modified rates should be used to estimate mortality change between 1998 and 1999.

Caution should be used when applying the comparability ratios presented in Table VI to age-, race-, and sex-specific mortality data. Demographic subgroups may sometimes differ with regard to their cause-of-death distribution, and this would result in demographic variation in cause-specific comparability ratios.

For more information, see: Anderson RN, Miniño AM, Hoyert DL, Rosenberg HM. Comparability of cause of death between ICD–9 and ICD–10: Preliminary estimates. National vital statistics reports; vol 49 no 2. Hyattsville, MD: NCHS; 2001; and Kochanek KD, Smith BL, Anderson RN. Deaths: Preliminary data for 1999. National vital statistics reports; vol 49 no 3. Hyattsville, MD: NCHS; 2001. Final ratios for 113 selected causes of death. Available from: ftp://ftp.cdc.gov/pub/Health_Statistics/NCHS/ Datasets/Comparability/icd9_icd10/ and the ICD comparability ratio website at: http://www.cdc.gov/ nchs/nvss/mortality/comparability_icd.htm. (Also see Appendix II, Cause of death; *International Classification of Diseases*.)

Compensation—See Employer costs for employee compensation.

Complex activity limitation—Complex activity limitation is a construct used to measure disability as defined by the inability to function successfully in certain social roles. Complex activities consist of the tasks and organized activity that make up numerous social roles like working, maintaining a household, living independently, or participating in community activities. Complex activity performance requires the execution of a combination of core areas of functioning. Complex activity limitation describes limitations or restrictions in an individual's ability to participate fully in social role activities. Complex activities include the following:

■ Maintaining independence, including self care and the ability to carry out activities associated with maintaining a household, such as shopping, cooking, and taking care of bills (measures are based on questions commonly known as activities of daily living (ADLs) and instrumental activities of daily living (IADLs)). Limitations in these activities usually reflect severe restrictions and are associated with limitations in other complex activities.

■ Difficulties experienced with social and leisure activities—represented in this measure by using questions about attending movies or sporting events, visiting with friends, or pursuing hobbies or relaxation activities.

■ Perceived limitation in the ability to work (a core aspect of social participation for the majority of the U.S. population)—represented by the respondent's self-defined limitation in the kind or amount of work they can do or their inability to work at a job or business.

For many measures of disability, only disabilities resulting from an underlying condition that is chronic (based on nature and duration) are considered. However, whether the underlying conditions related to the complex activities were chronic was not a requirement in classifying persons as having a complex activity limitation. For more information on how this measure was constructed using data from the National Health Interview Survey, including the specific questions asked, see: Altman B, Bernstein A. Disability and health in the United States, 2001–2005. Hyattsville, MD: NCHS; 2008. Available from: http://www.cdc.gov/nchs/data/misc/disability2001-2005.pdf. (Also see Appendix II, Activities of daily living; Basic actions difficulty; Instrumental activities of daily living.)

Computed tomography (CT) scanner—A CT, or computed axial tomography (CAT), scanner is an x-ray machine that combines many x-ray images, with the aid of a computer, to generate cross-sectional views and, if needed, three-dimensional images of the internal organs and structures of the body.

Condition—A health condition is a departure from a state of physical or mental well-being. In the National Health Interview Survey, each condition reported as a cause of an individual's activity limitation has been classified as chronic, not chronic, or unknown if chronic, based on the nature and duration of the condition. Conditions that are not cured once acquired (such as heart disease, diabetes, and birth defects in the original response categories, and amputee and old age in the ad hoc categories) are considered chronic, whereas conditions related to pregnancy are never considered chronic. Other conditions must have been present for 3 months or longer to be considered chronic. An exception is made for children less than 1 year of age who have had a condition since birth because such conditions are always considered chronic.

Consumer Price Index (CPI)—The CPI, prepared by the U.S. Bureau of Labor Statistics, is a monthly measure of the average change in the prices paid by urban consumers for a fixed market basket of goods and services. The medical care component of the CPI shows trends in medical care prices based on specific indicators of hospital, medical, and drug prices. A revision of the definition of the CPI has been in use since January 1988. (Also see Appendix II, Gross domestic product; Health expenditures, national; and Appendix I, Consumer Price Index.)

Contraception—The National Survey of Family Growth collects information on contraceptive use during heterosexual vaginal intercourse, as reported by women 15–44 years of age. For current contraceptive use, women were asked about contraceptive use during the month of interview. Women were classified by whether they reported using any of 19 methods of contraception at any time in the month of interview. Contraceptive methods listed as "other methods" in 2006–2008 included the contraceptive ring, female condom/vaginal pouch, foam, cervical cap, Today sponge, suppository or insert, jelly or cream (without diaphragm), and other methods. Previously, contraceptive methods listed as "other methods" included the following: for 2002, the female condom, foam, cervical cap, Today sponge, suppository or insert, jelly or cream (without diaphragm), or other method; for 1995, the female condom or vaginal pouch, foam, cervical cap, Today sponge, suppository or insert, jelly or cream, or other method; for 1988, foam, douche, Today sponge, suppository or insert, jelly or cream, or other method; and for 1982, foam, douche, suppository or insert, or other method.

Critical access hospital—See Hospital.

Crude birth rate; Crude death rate—See Rate: Birth and related rates; Rate: Death and related rates.

Days of care—Days of care is defined similarly in several data systems, as discussed below. (Also see Appendix II, Admission; Average length of stay; Discharge; Hospital; Hospital utilization; Inpatient.)

American Hospital Association—Days, hospital days, or inpatient days are the number of adult and pediatric days of care rendered during the entire reporting period. Days of care for newborns are excluded.

National Health Interview Survey (NHIS)—Hospital days during the year refer to the total number of hospital days occurring in the 12-month period before the interview week. A hospital day is a night spent in the hospital (excluding a night spent in the emergency department) for persons admitted as inpatients. Starting in 1997, hospitalization data from NHIS are for all inpatient stays, whereas estimates for prior years published in previous editions of *Health, United States* excluded hospitalizations for deliveries and newborns.

National Hospital Discharge Survey (NHDS)—Days of care refers to the total number of patient days accumulated by inpatients at the time of discharge from nonfederal short-stay hospitals during a reporting period. All days from and including the date of admission, but not including the date of discharge, are counted.

Death rate—See Rate: Death and related rates.

Dental caries—Dental caries is evidence of dental decay on any surface of a tooth. Untreated dental caries was determined by an oral examination as part of the National Health and Nutrition Examination Survey (NHANES). In *Health, United States*, data on dental caries for 2001–2004 and earlier are based on an examination conducted by a trained dentist. Untreated dental caries refers to coronal caries, that is, caries on the crown or enamel surface of the tooth. Treated dental caries and root caries are not included. Study participants 2 years of age and over were eligible for the examination, as long as they did not meet other exclusion criteria. Both permanent and primary (baby) teeth were evaluated, depending on the age of the participant. For children 2–5 years of age, only caries in primary teeth was included. For children 6–11 years of age, caries in both primary and permanent teeth was included. For children 12 years of age and over, and for adults, only caries in permanent teeth was included. Starting with 2005–2006 NHANES data, data on dental caries were collected using the Basic Screening Examination (BSE), a simplified screening process to collect information on untreated caries, dental restorations, and dental sealants. BSE differs from previous NHANES oral health protocols because it does not assess each tooth surface, the assessments are not made by a dentist, and the presence of dental caries on primary or permanent teeth cannot be distinguished in the dataset. Dental caries and other oral health surveillance data are collected by a health technologist on examined persons 5 years of age and older. Because of this change in the examination process and because 2005–2008 dental caries data are based on both primary and permanent teeth, regardless of age, data for 2005–2008 need to be interpreted with caution, especially when comparing with earlier data. For more information, see: Dye BA, Barker LK, Li X, Lewis BG, Beltran-Aguilar ED. Overview and quality assurance for the Oral Health Component of the National Health and Nutrition Examination Survey (NHANES), 2005–08. J Public Health Dent. In press.

For more information, see: http://www.cdc.gov/nchs/data/nhanes/nhanes_05_06/ohx_d.pdf and http://www.cdc.gov/nchs/nhanes/nhanes2007-2008/OHX_E.htm.

Dental visit—Starting in 1997, National Health Interview Survey respondents were asked "About how long has it been since you last saw or talked to a dentist? Include all types of dentists, such as orthodontists, oral surgeons, and all other dental specialists as well as hygienists." Starting in 2001, the question was modified slightly to ask respondents how long it had been since they last saw a dentist. Questions about dental visits were not asked for children under 2 years of age for years 1997–1999 and under 1 year of age for years 2000 and beyond. Starting with 1997 data, estimates are presented for people with a dental visit in the past year. Prior to 1997, dental visit estimates were based on a 2-week recall period.

Diabetes—Diabetes is a group of conditions in which insulin is not adequately secreted or utilized. Diabetes is a leading cause of disease and death in the United States. Eight million Americans are known to have diabetes, and an estimated equal number have undiagnosed diabetes. Using data from National Health and Nutrition Examination Survey (NHANES), three measures of diabetes are presented in *Health, United States*—physician-diagnosed diabetes, undiagnosed diabetes, and total diabetes. Physician-diagnosed diabetes was obtained by self-report and excludes women who reported having diabetes only during pregnancy. Respondents who answered "yes" to the question, "Other than during pregnancy, have you ever been told by a doctor or health professional that you have diabetes or sugar diabetes?" were classified as having physician-diagnosed diabetes.

Only respondents who were not classified as having physician-diagnosed diabetes were evaluated to determine if they had undiagnosed diabetes. Undiagnosed diabetes was based on the results of laboratory testing of venous blood (plasma) serum samples collected from NHANES participants at mobile examination centers. Undiagnosed diabetes was defined as a fasting blood glucose (FBG) of at least 126 mg/dL or a hemoglobin A1c of at least 6.5% and no reported physician diagnosis. Respondents had fasted for at least 8 hours and less than 24 hours. Fasting is not necessary for accurate testing of hemoglobin A1c. However, to be consistent with the subsample of fasting respondents used for FBG, assessment of undiagnosed diabetes in *Health, United States* is limited to the fasting subsample. In 2005–2006 and 2007–2008, testing was performed at a different laboratory and using different instruments than testing in earlier years. NHANES conducted a crossover study to evaluate the impact of these changes on FBG and A1c measurements, and thus their impact on evaluation of data over time. As a result of that study, NHANES recommended that 2005–2008 data on FBG and A1c measurements be adjusted to be compatible with earlier years. Undiagnosed diabetes estimates in *Health, United States* were produced after adjusting the 2005–2008 laboratory data as recommended. For more information, see: http://www.cdc.gov/nchs/data/nhanes/nhanes_05_06/glu_d.pdf, http://www.cdc.gov/nchs/nhanes/nhanes2007-2008/GLU_E.htm, http://www.cdc.gov/nchs/data/nhanes/nhanes_05_06/ghb_d.pdf, and http://www.cdc.gov/nchs/nhanes/nhanes2007-2008/GHB_E.htm.

Starting with *Health, United States, 2010*, an elevated hemoglobin A1c (greater than or equal to 6.5%) was included as a component of the definition of undiagnosed diabetes, along with FBG. Previous editions of *Health, United States* did not evaluate hemoglobin A1c to classify respondents as having undiagnosed diabetes; undiagnosed diabetes was solely based on elevated FBG (greater than or equal to 126 mg/dL) among those without physician-diagnosed diabetes. The revised definition of undiagnosed diabetes was based on recommendations from the American Diabetes Association. Hemoglobin A1c testing is a preferred indicator of diabetes because it measures average blood glucose over several months, thus yielding more reliable results, and is more convenient because patients do not need to fast prior to testing. Hemoglobin A1c was recommended as a component in diagnosing diabetes because recent improvements in assay standardization make A1c results more reliable. In addition, recent research has provided evidence linking elevated A1c levels with diabetic complications, thus allowing for a threshold to be set above which patients would be diagnosed as having diabetes. For more information, see: Standards of medical care in diabetes—2010. Diabetes Care 2010;33(suppl 1):S11–S61 and International expert committee report on the role of the A1c assay in the diagnosis of diabetes. Diabetes Care 2009;32(7): 1327–34. As expected, this revised definition increased the percentage of respondents classified as having undiagnosed diabetes.

Prevalence estimates of undiagnosed diabetes among those 20 years of age and over in 1988–1994 increased from 2.7% to 3.3% using the new definition, and total diabetes prevalence increased from 7.8% to 8.4%. Among men, the prevalence using the new definition increased from 3.0% to 3.7%, and among women it increased to from 2.4% to 3.0%. The prevalence for non-Hispanic white persons increased from 2.5% to 2.8%, for non-Hispanic black persons from 3.4% to 6.0%, and for Mexican persons from 3.4% to 4.1%. Increases in the prevalence of undiagnosed diabetes by age group were from 0.8% to 1.0% among those 20–44 years of age, from 5.0% to 6.0% among those 45–64 years, and from 5.6% to 6.7% among those 65 years and over. For 2005–2008, the prevalence of undiagnosed diabetes among those 20 years and over increased from 2.4% to 3.1% using the new definition, and total diabetes prevalence increased from 10.6% to 11.3%. Among men, the prevalence increased from 3.2% to 3.9%, and among women it increased from 1.7% to 2.3%. The prevalence for non-Hispanic white persons increased from 2.4% to 2.9%, for non-Hispanic black persons from 3.5% to 5.0%, and for Mexican persons from 3.4% to 3.7%. Increases by age group were from 2.3% to 3.2% among those 45–64 years and from 6.8% to 8.6% among those 65 and over. There was no increase in the prevalence of undiagnosed diabetes among those 20–44 years of age using the new definition.

Total diabetes includes those who were classified as having either physician-diagnosed or undiagnosed diabetes. Prevalence estimates of total diabetes increased using the new definition of undiagnosed diabetes.

Diagnosis—Diagnosis is the act or process of identifying or determining the nature and cause of a disease or injury through evaluation of patient history, examination, and review of laboratory data. Diagnoses in the National Hospital Discharge Survey, the National Ambulatory Medical Care Survey, the National Hospital Ambulatory Medical Care Survey, and the National Nursing Home Survey are abstracted from medical records and coded to the *International Classification of Diseases, 9th Revision, Clinical Modification* (ICD–9–CM). For a given medical care encounter, the first-listed diagnosis can be used to categorize the visit, or, if more than one diagnosis is recorded on the medical record, the visit can be categorized based on all diagnoses recorded. Analyzing first-listed diagnoses avoids double-counting events such as visits or hospitalizations; the first-listed diagnosis is often, but not always, considered the most important or dominant condition among all comorbid conditions. However, the choice of the first-listed diagnosis by the medical facility may be influenced by reimbursement or other factors. A hospital discharge would be considered a first-listed stroke discharge if the ICD–9–CM diagnosis code for stroke was recorded in the first diagnosis field on the hospital record. An any-listed stroke discharge would classify all diagnoses of stroke recorded on the hospital face sheet, regardless of the order in which they are listed. Any-listed diagnoses double-count events such as visits or hospitalizations with more than one recorded diagnosis but provide information on the burden a specific diagnosis presents to the health care system. (Also see Appendix II, External cause of injury; Injury; Injury-related visit.)

Diagnostic and other nonsurgical procedure—See Procedure.

Dietary supplement—A dietary supplement is a product that contains one or more dietary ingredients, such as vitamins, minerals, botanicals, or amino acids. Data on dietary supplement use come from the National Health and Nutrition Examination Survey (NHANES). During the in-person household interviews, participants were asked about their use of vitamins, minerals, herbals, or other dietary supplements (including prescription and nonprescription products) in the past 30 days. Participants reporting supplement use were asked to show the supplement containers to the interviewer. If no container was available, the interviewer asked the participant for a detailed name of the supplement. For each supplement reported, the interviewer recorded the supplement's name and manufacturer. Trained nutritionists at NCHS matched the product names entered by the interviewer to a known dietary supplement product. NCHS attempts to obtain a label for each supplement reported by a participant from sources such as the manufacturer or retailer, the Internet, company catalogs, and the *Physician's Desk Reference*. In *Health, United States*, three measures of dietary supplement use are included: (a) taking any supplement, (b) taking any supplement containing folic acid, and (c) taking any supplement containing vitamin D (or cholecalciferol, calciferol, ergocalciferol, or calcitriol).

For more information on dietary supplement data in NHANES, see: http://www.cdc.gov/nchs/nhanes.htm and http://www.cdc.gov/nchs/nhanes/nhanes2007-2008/DSQ3_E.htm.

For more information on dietary supplements, see the web page for the National Institutes of Health Office of Dietary Supplements at: http://ods.od.nih.gov/index.aspx.

Discharge—The National Health Interview Survey defines a hospital discharge as the completion of any continuous period of stay of one night or more in a hospital as an inpatient. According to the National Hospital Discharge Survey, a discharge is a completed inpatient hospitalization. A hospitalization may be completed by death or by releasing the patient to the customary place of residence, a nursing home, another hospital, or other locations. In the 2007 National Home and Hospice Care Survey, a hospice discharge is a patient who was discharged from the hospice care agency during the 3-month period beginning 4 months before the agency interview. Discharges that occurred because of the death of a sampled hospice care patient were included. (Also see Appendix II, Admission; Average length of stay; Days of care; Inpatient.)

Domiciliary care home—See Long-term care facility; Nursing home.

Drug—Drugs are pharmaceutical agents, by any route of administration, for the prevention, diagnosis, or treatment of medical conditions or diseases. Data on specific drug use are collected in three NCHS surveys. (Also see Appendix II, Multum Lexicon Plus therapeutic class.)

National Ambulatory Medical Care Survey (NAMCS) and *National Hospital Ambulatory Medical Care Survey (NHAMCS)*—In the NAMCS and NHAMCS outpatient and emergency department components, data are collected from the medical record of an in-person physician office visit or a hospital outpatient or emergency department visit, rather than from the patient. Information on generic or brand name drugs is abstracted from the medical record, including prescription and over-the-counter drugs, immunizations, allergy shots, and anesthetics that were prescribed, ordered, supplied, administered, or continued during the visit. Prior to 1995, up to five drugs per

visit could be reported on the patient record form; in data years 1995 and beyond, up to six drugs could be reported. Starting with data year 2003, up to eight drugs could be reported, as well as a count of the total number of drugs prescribed, ordered, supplied, administered, or continued during the visit.

For more information on drugs collected by NAMCS and NHAMCS, see the NAMCS website and the drug database. For more information on how data on drugs were collected and classified into therapeutic use categories, see: http://www.cdc.gov/nchs/ahcd.htm or http://www.cdc.gov/nchs/ahcd/ahcd_database.htm. (Also see Appendix I, National Ambulatory Medical Care Survey and National Hospital Ambulatory Medical Care Survey.)

National Health and Nutrition Examination Survey (NHANES)—Drug information from NHANES III and from NHANES from 1999 onward was collected during an in-person interview conducted in the participant's home. Participants were asked whether they had taken a medication in the past month for which they needed a prescription. Those who answered "yes" were asked to produce the prescription medication containers for the interviewer. For each medication reported, the interviewer entered the product's complete name from the container. If no container was available, the interviewer asked the participant to verbally report the name of the medication. In addition, participants were asked how long they had been taking the medication and the main reason for use.

All reported medication names were converted to their standard generic ingredient name. For multi-ingredient products, the ingredients were listed in alphabetical order and counted as one drug (e.g., Tylenol #3 was listed as aceta-minophen; codeine). No trade or proprietary names were provided on the data file.

Drug data from NHANES provide a snapshot of all prescribed drugs reported by a sample of the civilian noninstitutionalized population for a 1-month period. Drugs taken on an irregular basis, such as every other day, once per week, or for a 10-day period, were captured in the 1-month recall period. Data shown in *Health, United States* for the percentage of the population reporting three or more prescription drugs during the past month include a range of drug utilization patterns—for example, persons who took three or more drugs daily during the past month or persons who took a different drug three separate times—as long as at least three different drugs were taken during the past month.

For more information on prescription drug data collection and coding in NHANES, see: http://www.cdc.gov/nchs/nhanes/nhanes2007-2008/RXQ_DRUG.htm. For more information on NHANES III prescription drug data collection and coding, see: ftp://ftp.cdc.gov/pub/Health_Statistics/NCHS/nhanes/nhanes3/2A/pupremed.pdf. (Also see Appendix I, National Health and Nutrition Examination Survey.)

Drug abuse—See Illicit drug use.

Education—Several approaches to defining educational categories are used in *Health, United States*.

Birth file—Information on educational attainment of mother is based on number of years of school completed, as reported by the mother on the birth certificate. Between 1970 and 1992, the reporting area for maternal education expanded.

Mother's education was reported on the birth certificate by 38 states in 1970. Data were not available from Alabama, Arkansas, California, Connecticut, Delaware, the District of Columbia (D.C.), Georgia, Idaho, Maryland, New Mexico, Pennsylvania, Texas, and Washington state. In 1975, these data became available from Connecticut, Delaware, Georgia, Maryland, and D.C., increasing the number of states reporting mother's education to 42 and D.C. Between 1980 and 1988, only three states—California, Texas, and Washington—did not report mother's education. In 1988, mother's education was also missing for New York state outside New York City. In 1989–1991, mother's education was missing only from Washington state and New York state outside New York City. During 1992–2002, mother's education was reported by all 50 states and D.C.

Starting in 2003, some states implemented the 2003 revision of the U.S. Standard Certificate of Live Birth. The education item on the 2003 revision asks for the highest degree or level of school completed, whereas the education item on the 1989 revision asks for highest grade completed. Data on mother's education from the 2003 revision of the birth certificate are not comparable with data from the 1989 revision. Therefore, 2006 and 2007 data on mother's education are shown separately for the 28 reporting areas that used the 1989 revision in 2006 and 2007 and for the 19 reporting areas that used the 2003 revision in 2005 and 2006, in order to provide 2 years of comparable data. The 28 reporting areas using the 1989 certificate are Alabama, Alaska, Arizona, Arkansas, Connecticut, Hawaii, Illinois, Louisiana, Maine, Massachusetts, Maryland, Minnesota, Mississippi, Missouri, Montana, Nevada, New Jersey, New Mexico, North Carolina, Oklahoma, Oregon, Rhode Island, Utah, Virginia, West Virginia, Wisconsin, D.C., and New York City. The states that used the 2003 revision of the U.S. Standard Certificate of Live Birth for data on mother's education were California, Delaware, Florida, Idaho, Kansas, Kentucky, Nebraska, New Hampshire, New York state (excluding New York City), North Dakota, Ohio, Pennsylvania, South Carolina, South Dakota, Tennessee, Texas, Vermont, Washington, and Wyoming. Data are not shown in *Health, United States* for states that were transitioning to the 2003 revision during 2006 and 2007.

National Health Interview Survey (NHIS)—Starting in 1997, the NHIS questionnaire was changed to ask "What is the highest level of school [person] has completed or the highest degree received?" Responses were used to categorize adults according to educational credentials (e.g., no high school diploma or general educational development high school equivalency diploma (GED); high school diploma or GED; some college, no bachelor's degree; bachelor's degree or higher).

Prior to 1997, the education variable in NHIS was measured by asking, "What is the highest grade or year of regular school [person] has ever attended?" and "Did [person] finish the grade/year?" Responses were used to categorize adults according to years of education completed (e.g., less than 12 years, 12 years, 13–15 years, and 16 or more years).

Data from the 1996 and 1997 NHIS were used to compare distributions of educational attainment for adults 25 years of age and over, using categories based on educational credentials (1997) and categories based on years of education completed (1996). A larger percentage of persons reported some college than 13–15 years of education, and a correspondingly smaller percentage reported a high school diploma or GED than 12 years of education. In 1997, 19% of adults reported no high school diploma, 31% a high school diploma or GED, 26% some college, and 24% a bachelor's degree or higher. In 1996, 18% of adults reported less than 12 years of education, 37% 12 years of education, 20% 13–15 years, and 25% 16 or more years of education.

Emergency department—According to the National Hospital Ambulatory Medical Care Survey, an emergency department is a hospital facility that is staffed 24 hours a day and provides unscheduled outpatient services to patients whose condition requires immediate care. Off-site emergency departments open fewer than 24 hours are included if staffed by the hospital's emergency department. (Also see Appendix II, Emergency department or emergency room visit; Outpatient department.)

Emergency department or emergency room visit—Starting with the 1997 National Health Interview Survey, respondents to the sample adult and sample child questionnaires (generally a parent) were asked about the number of visits to hospital emergency rooms during the past 12 months, including visits that resulted in hospitalization. In the National Hospital Ambulatory Medical Care Survey, an emergency department visit is a direct personal exchange between a patient and a physician or other health care providers working under the physician's supervision, for the purpose of seeking care and receiving personal health services. (Also see Appendix II, Emergency department; Injury-related visit.)

Employer costs for employee compensation—Employer costs for employee compensation is a measure of the average cost per employee hour worked to employers for wages, salaries, and benefits. Wages and salaries are defined as the hourly straight-time wage rate or, for workers not paid on an hourly basis, straight-time earnings divided by the corresponding hours. Straight-time wage and salary rates are total earnings before payroll deductions, excluding premium pay for overtime and for work on weekends and holidays, shift differentials, nonproduction bonuses, and lump-sum payments provided in lieu of wage increases. Production bonuses, incentive earnings, commission payments, and cost-of-living adjustments are included in straight-time wage and salary rates. Benefits covered are paid leave (paid vacations, holidays, sick leave, and other leave), supplemental pay (premium pay for overtime and work on weekends and holidays, shift differentials, nonproduction bonuses, and lump-sum payments provided in lieu of wage increases), insurance benefits (life, health, and short- and long-term disability), retirement and savings benefits (pension and other retirement plans and savings and thrift plans), legally required benefits (Social Security, Medicare, federal and state unemployment insurance, workers' compensation, and other benefits required by law, such as state temporary disability insurance), and other benefits (severance pay and supplemental unemployment plans). As of June 2008, other leave benefit includes only paid personal leave. (Also see Appendix I, National Compensation Survey.)

End-stage renal disease (ESRD)—ESRD is a complete or near complete failure of the kidneys to function to excrete wastes, concentrate urine, and regulate electrolytes. ESRD occurs when the kidneys are no longer able to function at the level necessary for day-to-day life. It usually occurs as chronic renal failure worsens to the point where kidney function is less than 10% of normal. At that point, kidney function is so low that without dialysis or kidney transplantation, complications are multiple and severe, and death will occur from accumulation of fluids and waste products in the body. Without treatment, the loss of kidney function in ESRD is usually irreversible and permanent, and death follows.

Although the Medicare program covers the majority of ESRD-certified patients, not all individuals with ESRD are eligible for Medicare. In addition to being medically determined to have ESRD, filing an application, and meeting any applicable waiting period, an individual must meet one of the following criteria:

■ The individual has earned the required work credits under Social Security, Railroad Retirement, or as a government employee.

■ The individual is receiving Social Security or Railroad Retirement benefits.

■ The individual is the spouse or dependent child of a person who has earned the required work credits or is receiving Social Security or Railroad Retirement benefit.

The United States Renal Data Network has tracked both Medicare-eligible and -ineligible ESRD patients since May 1995. See Appendix I, United States Renal Data System.

Ethnicity—See Hispanic origin.

Exercise—See Physical activity, leisure-time.

Expenditures—See Health expenditures, national. (Also see Appendix I, National Health Expenditure Accounts.)

External cause of injury—The external cause of injury is used for classifying the circumstances in which injuries occur. The *International Classification of Diseases, 9th Revision* (ICD–9), External Cause of Injury Matrix is a two-dimensional array describing both the mechanism or external cause of the injury (e.g., fall, motor vehicle traffic) and the manner or intent of the injury (e.g., unintentional, self-inflicted, or assault). Although this matrix was originally developed for mortality, it has been adapted for use with the ICD–9 Clinical Modification (ICD–9–CM). For more information, see the NCHS website at: http://www.cdc.gov/nchs/injury/injury_tools.htm; and see: Bergen G, Chen LH, Warner M, Fingerhut LA. Injury in the United States: 2007 chartbook. Hyattsville, MD: NCHS; 2008. Available from: http://www.cdc.gov/nchs/data/misc/injury2007.pdf.

Family income—For the National Health Interview Survey and the National Health and Nutrition Examination Survey, all people within a household who are related to each other by blood, marriage, or adoption constitute a family. Each member of a family is classified according to the total income of the family. Unrelated individuals are classified according to their own income.

National Health Interview Survey (NHIS)—Prior to 1997, family income was the total income received by members of a family (or by an unrelated individual) in the 12 months before interview. Family income included wages, salaries, rents from property, interest, dividends, profits and fees from their own businesses, pensions, and help from relatives. Starting in 1997, NHIS collected family income data for the calendar year prior to interview (e.g., 2009 family income data were based on calendar year 2008 information). The 1997–2006 instrument allowed the respondent to supply a specific dollar amount (up to $999,995). Any family income responses greater than $999,995 were entered as $999,996. Respondents who did not know or refused to give a dollar amount in response to this question were asked if their total combined family income for the previous year was $20,000 or more, or less than $20,000. If the respondent answered this question, he/she was then given one of two flash cards and asked to indicate which income group listed on the card best represented the family's combined income during the previous calendar year. One flash card listed incomes that were $20,000 or more, and the other flash card listed incomes that were less than $20,000. Starting with the 2007 NHIS, the income amount follow-up questions that had been in place since 1997 were replaced with a series of unfolding bracket questions. The unfolding bracket method asked a series of closed-ended income range questions (e.g., "Is it less than $50,000?") if the respondent did not provide an answer to the exact income amount question. The closed-ended income

range questions were constructed so that each successive question establishes a smaller range for the amount of the family's income. For more information on the current income questions, see: 2009 NHIS public-use data release [online]. NCHS. 2010. Available from: ftp://ftp.cdc.gov/pub/Health_Statistics/NCHS/Dataset_Documentation/NHIS/2009/srvydesc.pdf.

Also see: Pleis JR, Cohen RA. Impact of income bracketing on poverty measures used in the National Health Interview Survey's Early Release Program: Preliminary data from the 2007 NHIS [online]. NCHS. 2007. Available from: http://www.cdc.gov/nchs/data/nhis/income.pdf.

Family income data are used in the computation of poverty level. Starting with *Health, United States, 2004*, a new methodology for imputing family income data for NHIS was implemented for data years 1997 and beyond. Multiple imputations were performed for survey years 1997 and beyond, with five sets of imputed values created to allow for the assessment of variability caused by imputation. A detailed description of the multiple imputation procedure, and data files for 1997 and beyond, are available from: http://www.cdc.gov/nchs/nhis/quest_data_related_1997_forward.htm through the data release or the imputed income files link under that year. For data years 1990–1996, about 16%–18% of persons had missing data for family income. In those years, missing values were imputed for family income by using a sequential hot deck within matrix cells imputation approach. A detailed description of the imputation procedure and data files, with imputed annual family income for 1990–1996, is available from: ftp://ftp.cdc.gov/pub/Health_Statistics/NCHS/Datasets/NHIS/1990-96_Family_Income/ and http://www.cdc.gov/nchs/nhis/quest_data_related_1996_prior.htm. (Also see Appendix II, Table VII.)

National Health and Nutrition Examination Survey (NHANES)—In NHANES 1999 and onward, family income is asked in a series of questions about possible sources of income, including wages, salaries, interest and dividends, federal programs, child support, rents, royalties, and other possible sources. After the information about sources of income was obtained in the family interview income section of the questionnaire, the respondent was asked to report total combined family income for themselves and the other members of their family, in dollars. If the respondent did not provide an answer or did not

Table VII. Imputed poverty in the National Health Interview Survey, by age: United States, 1990–2009

Year	All ages	Under 18 years	18 years and over	18–64 years	Under 65 years	1–64 years	65 years and over	Females 18 years and over	Females 40 years and over	2 years and over	45 years and over
						Percent					
1990	16	14	18	16	15	15	24	18	21	17	22
1991	18	15	19	17	17	17	26	19	23	18	23
1992	18	16	19	18	17	17	27	20	23	18	23
1993	16	14	17	16	15	15	23	17	19	16	20
1994	17	15	18	17	16	16	25	18	21	17	21
1995	16	14	16	15	15	15	22	17	19	16	19
1996	17	14	17	16	16	16	24	18	20	17	20
1997	24	21	26	24	23	23	34	26	30	17	30
1998	29	25	30	28	27	27	39	30	34	29	34
1999	31	27	32	30	29	29	43	33	37	31	37
2000	32	28	33	31	30	31	45	34	38	32	38
2001	32	27	33	30	30	30	44	34	37	32	38
2002	32	28	33	31	30	30	44	33	37	32	37
2003	33	30	35	33	32	32	44	35	38	34	38
2004	33	29	34	32	31	31	41	34	36	33	37
2005	33	29	34	32	31	31	44	35	37	33	38
2006	34	31	35	33	33	33	45	36	39	34	39
2007	33	29	34	32	31	31	43	35	38	33	37
2008	30	27	31	29	29	29	40	32	34	30	34
2009	25	21	26	24	23	23	34	26	29	25	29

NOTES: Weighted percentages. See Appendix II, Family income.

SOURCE: CDC/NCHS, National Health Interview Survey.

know the total combined family income, he or she was asked if the total family income was less than $20,000 or $20,000 or more. If the respondent answered, a follow-up question asked the respondent to select an income range from a list on a printed hand card. The midpoint of the income range was then used as the total family income value. Family income values were used to calculate the poverty income ratio. NHANES II did include questions on components of income. NHANES III did not ask the detailed components of income questions but asked respondents to identify their income based on a set of ranges provided on a flash card. Family income was not imputed for individuals or families with no reported income information in any of the NHANES survey years. (Also see Appendix II, Poverty.)

Federal hospital—See Hospital.

Fee-for-service health insurance—Fee-for-service health insurance is private (commercial) health insurance that reimburses health care providers on the basis of a fee for each health service provided to the insured person. It is also known as indemnity health insurance. In addition, fee-for-service is a term often applied to original Medicare, before Medicare

managed care plans or other new payment systems were introduced. (Also see Appendix II, Health insurance coverage; Managed care; Medicare.)

Fertility rate—See Rate: Birth and related rates.

General hospital—See Hospital.

General hospital providing separate psychiatric services—See Mental health organization.

Geographic region—The U.S. Census Bureau groups the 50 states and the District of Columbia, for statistical purposes, into four geographic regions—Northeast, Midwest, South, and West—and nine divisions, based on geographic proximity. (See Figure I.)

Gestation—For the National Vital Statistics System and CDC's Abortion Surveillance, the period of gestation is defined as beginning with the first day of the last normal menstrual period and ending with the day of birth or day of termination of pregnancy. Data on gestational age are subject to error for several reasons, including imperfect maternal recall or misidentification of the last menstrual period because of post-conception bleeding, delayed ovulation, or intervening early miscarriage.

Figure I. U.S. Census Bureau: Four geographic regions and nine divisions of the United States

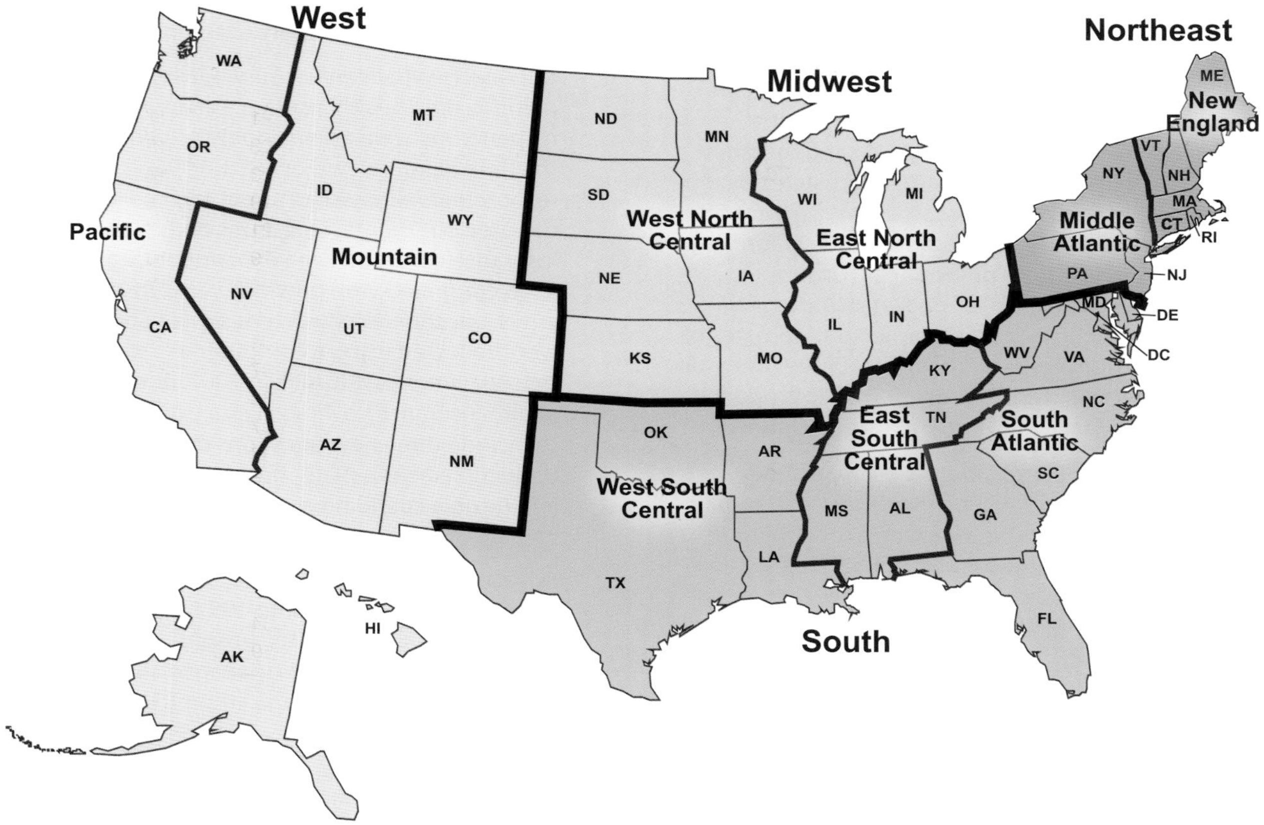

SOURCE: U.S. Census Bureau.

Gross domestic product (GDP)—The GDP is the market value of the goods and services produced by labor and property located in the United States. As long as the labor and property are located in the United States, the suppliers (i.e., the workers and, for property, the owners) may be U.S. residents or residents of other countries. (Also see Appendix II, Consumer Price Index; Health expenditures, national.)

Health care contact—Starting in 1997, the National Health Interview Survey has collected information on health care contacts with doctors and other health care professionals by using the following questions: "During the past 12 months, how many times have you gone to a hospital emergency room about your own health?", "During the past 12 months, did you receive care at home from a nurse or other health care professional? What was the total number of home visits received?", and "During the past 12 months, how many times have you seen a doctor or other health care professional about your own health at a doctor's office, a clinic, or some other place? Do not include times you were hospitalized overnight, visits to hospital emergency rooms, home

visits, or telephone calls." Starting with 2000 data, this question was amended to exclude dental visits. For 1997–1999, for each question, respondents were shown a flash card with response categories of 0, 1, 2–3, 4–9, 10–12, or 13 or more visits. Starting with 2000 data, response categories were expanded to 0, 1, 2–3, 4–5, 6–7, 8–9, 10–12, 13–15, or 16 or more. Analyses of the percentage of persons with health care visits were conducted as follows: For tabulation of the 1997–1999 data, responses of 2–3 were recoded to 2, and responses of 4–9 were recoded to 6. Starting with 2000 data, tabulation of responses of 2–3 were recoded to 2, and other responses were recoded to the midpoint of the range. A summary measure of health care visits was constructed by adding recoded responses for these questions and categorizing the sum as none, 1–3, 4–9, or 10 or more health care visits in the past 12 months.

Analyses of the percentage of children without a health care visit are based on the following question: "During the past 12 months, how many times has [person] seen a doctor or other health care professional about (his/her) health at a doctor's office, a clinic, or some other place? Do not include times [person] was hospitalized overnight, visits to hospital emergency rooms, home visits, or telephone calls." (Also see Appendix II, Emergency department or emergency room visit; Home visit.)

Health expenditures, national—National health expenditures are estimated by the Centers for Medicare & Medicaid Services (CMS) and measure spending for health care in the United States by type of service delivered (e.g., hospital care, physician services, nursing home care) and source of funding for those services (e.g., private health insurance, Medicare, Medicaid, out-of-pocket spending). CMS produces both historical and projected estimates of health expenditures by category. (Also see Appendix II, Consumer Price Index; Gross domestic product.) Types of national health expenditures include:

National health expenditures estimates the amount spent for all health services and supplies, and health-related research and construction activities, consumed in the United States during the calendar year. Detailed estimates are available by source of expenditure (e.g., out-of-pocket payments, private health insurance, and government programs) and by type of expenditure (e.g., hospital care, physician services, and prescription drugs) and are in current dollars for the year of report. Data are compiled from a variety of sources.

Health services and supplies expenditures are outlays for goods and services relating directly to patient care, plus expenses for administering health insurance programs and government public health activities. This category is equivalent to total national health expenditures minus expenditures for research and construction.

Personal health care expenditures are outlays for goods and services relating directly to patient care. The expenditures in this category are total national health expenditures minus expenditures for research and construction, health insurance program administration, and government public health activities.

Private expenditures are outlays for services provided or paid for by nongovernmental sources: consumers, insurance companies, private industry, and philanthropic and other nonpatient care sources.

Public expenditures are outlays for services provided or paid for by federal, state, and local government agencies or expenditures required by governmental mandate (such as worker's compensation insurance payments).

Health insurance coverage—Health insurance is broadly defined to include both public and private payors who cover medical expenditures incurred by a defined population in a variety of settings.

National Health Interview Survey (NHIS)—For point-in-time health insurance estimates, NHIS respondents were asked about their coverage at the time of interview. For 1993–1996, respondents were asked about their coverage in the previous month. Questions on health insurance coverage were expanded starting in 1993 compared with previous years. In 1997, the entire questionnaire was redesigned and data were collected using a computer-assisted personal interview (CAPI). In 2007, questions on health insurance coverage were expanded again to include three new questions on high deductible health plans, health savings accounts, and flexible spending accounts.

Respondents were considered to be covered by private health insurance if they indicated private health insurance or, prior to 1997, if they were covered by a single-service hospital plan. Private health insurance includes managed care such as health maintenance organizations (HMOs).

Private insurance obtained through the workplace was defined as any private insurance that was originally obtained through a present or former employer or union, or, starting in 1997, through the workplace, self-employment, or a professional association.

Until 1996, persons were defined as having Medicaid or other public assistance coverage if they indicated that they had either Medicaid or other public assistance or if they reported receiving Aid to Families with Dependent Children (AFDC) or Supplemental Security Income (SSI). After welfare reform in late 1996, Medicaid was delinked from AFDC and SSI. Starting in 1997, persons were considered to be covered by Medicaid if they reported Medicaid or a state-sponsored health program. Starting in 1999, persons were considered covered by Medicaid if they reported coverage by the Children's Health Insurance Program (CHIP). Medicare or military health plan coverage was also determined in the interview, and, starting in 1997 other government-sponsored program coverage was determined as well.

If respondents did not report coverage under one of the above types of plans and they had unknown coverage under either private health insurance or Medicaid, they were considered to have unknown coverage.

The remaining respondents without any indicated coverage were considered uninsured. The uninsured were persons who did not have coverage under private health insurance, Medicare, Medicaid, public assistance, a state-sponsored health plan, other government-sponsored programs, or a military health plan. Persons with only Indian Health Service coverage were considered uninsured. Estimates of the percentage of persons who were uninsured based on NHIS may differ slightly from those based on the March Current Population Survey (CPS) because of differences in survey questions, recall period, and other aspects of survey methodology.

In NHIS, on average, fewer than 2% of people 65 years of age and over reported no current health insurance coverage, but the small sample size precludes the presentation of separate estimates for this population. Therefore, the term uninsured refers only to the population under age 65.

Two additional questions were added to the health insurance section of NHIS beginning with the third quarter of 2004 (Table VIII). One question was asked of persons 65 years of age and over who had not indicated that they had Medicare: "People covered by Medicare have a card which looks like this. [Are/Is] [person] covered by Medicare?" The other question was asked of persons under 65 years of age who had not indicated any type of coverage: "There is a program called Medicaid that pays for health care for persons in need. In this state it is also called [state name]. [Are/Is] [person] covered by Medicaid?"

Respondents who originally classified themselves as uninsured, but whose classification was changed to Medicare or Medicaid on the basis of a "yes" response to either question, subsequently received appropriate follow-up questions concerning periods of noncoverage for insured respondents. Of the 892 people (unweighted) who were eligible to receive the Medicare probe question in the third and fourth quarters of 2004, 55% indicated that they were covered by Medicare. Of the 9,146 people (unweighted) who were eligible to receive the Medicaid probe question in the third and fourth quarters of 2004, 3% indicated that they were covered by Medicaid. Estimates in *Health, United States* were calculated using the responses to the two additional probe questions. For a complete discussion of the effect of the addition of these two probe questions on the estimates for insurance coverage, see: Cohen RA, Martinez ME. Impact of Medicare and Medicaid probe questions on health insurance estimates from the National Health Interview Survey, 2004 [online]. Health E-Stats. NCHS. 2005. Available from: http://www.cdc.gov/nchs/data/hestat/impact04/impact04.htm.

Survey respondents may be covered by health insurance at the time of interview but may have experienced one or more lapses in coverage during the 12 months prior to interview. Starting with *Health, United States, 2006*, NHIS estimates have been presented for the following three exhaustive categories: (a) people with health insurance continuously for the full 12 months prior to interview, (b) those who had a period of up to 12 months prior to interview without coverage, and (c) those who were uninsured for more than 12 months prior to interview. This stub variable has been added to selected tables. Two additional NHIS questions were used to determine the appropriate category for the survey respondents: (a) all persons without known comprehensive health insurance plan were asked, "About how long has it been since [person] last had health care coverage?", and (b) all persons with known health insurance coverage were asked, "In the past 12 months, was there any time when [person] did NOT have ANY health insurance coverage?"

(Also see Appendix II, Fee-for-service health insurance; Health maintenance organization; Managed care; Medicaid; Medicare; Children's Health Insurance Program; Uninsured.)

Health maintenance organization (HMO)—An HMO is a health care system that assumes or shares both the financial risks and the delivery risks associated with providing comprehensive medical services to a voluntarily enrolled population in a particular geographic area, usually in return for a fixed, prepaid fee. Pure HMO enrollees use only the prepaid, capitated health services of the HMO panel of medical care providers. Open-ended HMO enrollees use the prepaid HMO health services but may also receive medical care from providers who are not part of the HMO panel. There is usually a substantial deductible, copayment, or coinsurance associated with use of nonpanel providers. HMO model types are as follows:

Group model HMO is an HMO that contracts with a single multispecialty medical group to provide care to the HMO's membership. The group practice may work exclusively with the HMO, or it may provide services to non-HMO patients as

Table VIII. Percentage of persons under 65 years of age with Medicaid or who are uninsured, by selected demographic characteristics, using Method 1 and Method 2 estimation procedures: United States, 2004

Characteristic	Medicaid[1]		Uninsured[2]	
	Method 2[3]	Method 1[3]	Method 2[3]	Method 1[3]
	Percent (standard error)			
Age				
Under 65 years	12.0 (0.24)	11.8 (0.24)	16.4 (0.23)	16.6 (0.23)
Under 18 years	25.4 (0.49)	24.9 (0.49)	9.2 (0.30)	9.7 (0.29)
18–64 years	6.6 (0.17)	6.5 (0.17)	19.3 (0.26)	19.4 (0.26)
Percent of poverty level[4]				
Below 100%........................	47.5 (1.03)	46.6 (1.03)	29.6 (0.89)	30.5 (0.92)
100%–less than 200%................	22.0 (0.59)	21.5 (0.60)	28.9 (0.66)	29.4 (0.66)
200% or more	2.9 (0.13)	2.8 (0.13)	9.4 (0.23)	9.5 (0.23)
Age and percent of poverty level[4]				
Under 18 years:				
Below 100%	71.9 (1.35)	70.2 (1.35)	14.5 (1.15)	16.2 (1.22)
100%–less than 200%...............	39.2 (1.13)	38.4 (1.14)	15.0 (0.81)	15.8 (0.82)
200% or more.....................	6.2 (0.33)	6.1 (0.33)	4.9 (0.30)	4.9 (0.30)
18–64 years:				
Below 100%	31.2 (1.02)	30.8 (1.02)	39.7 (1.09)	40.1 (1.09)
100%–less than 200%...............	12.0 (0.48)	11.8 (0.48)	37.0 (0.72)	37.2 (0.72)
200% or more.....................	1.7 (0.11)	1.7 (0.10)	11.0 (0.26)	11.1 (0.26)
Hispanic origin and race[5]				
Hispanic or Latino....................	22.2 (0.55)	21.5 (0.55)	34.4 (0.64)	35.1 (0.65)
Mexican	22.0 (0.63)	21.5 (0.63)	37.6 (0.82)	38.1 (0.83)
Not Hispanic or Latino................	10.2 (0.25)	10.1 (0.25)	13.2 (0.23)	13.3 (0.23)
White only	7.4 (0.26)	7.4 (0.26)	12.0 (0.25)	12.1 (0.25)
Black or African American only	23.9 (0.80)	23.5 (0.79)	17.3 (0.58)	17.8 (0.58)

[1]The category Medicaid includes persons who do not have private coverage, but who have Medicaid or other state-sponsored health plans, including the Children's Health Insurance Program (CHIP).

[2]The category uninsured includes persons who have not indicated that they are covered at the time of interview under private health insurance, Medicare, Medicaid, CHIP, a state-sponsored health plan, other government programs, or military health plan (includes VA, TRICARE, and CHAMP–VA). This category includes persons who are only covered by Indian Health Service (IHS) or only have a plan that pays for one type of service, such as accidents or dental care.

[3]Starting with the third quarter of 2004, two additional questions were added to the National Health Interview Survey (NHIS) insurance section to reduce potential errors in reporting of Medicare and Medicaid status. Persons 65 years of age and over not reporting Medicare coverage were asked explicitly about Medicare coverage, and persons under 65 years of age with no reported coverage were asked explicitly about Medicaid coverage. Estimates calculated without using the additional information from these questions are noted as Method 1. Estimates calculated using the additional information from these questions are noted as Method 2.

[4]Percent of poverty level is based on family income and family size and composition, using the U.S. Census Bureau's poverty thresholds. The percentage of respondents with unknown poverty level was 28.2% in 2004. See the NHIS Survey Description Document for 2004. Available from: http://www.cdc.gov/nchs/data/nhis/srvydesc.pdf.

[5]Persons of Hispanic origin may be of any race or combination of races. Similarly, the category Not Hispanic or Latino refers to all persons who are not of Hispanic or Latino origin, regardless of race.

SOURCE: CDC/NCHS, National Health Interview Survey, 2004, Family Core Component. Data are based on household interviews of a sample of the civilian noninstitutionalized population. Available from: http://www.cdc.gov/nchs/data/hestat/impact04/impact04.htm.

well. The HMO pays the medical group a negotiated per capita rate, which the group distributes among its physicians, usually on a salaried basis.

Staff model HMO is a closed-panel HMO (where patients can receive services only through a limited number of providers) in which physicians are HMO employees. The providers see members in the HMO's own facilities.

Network model HMO is an HMO that contracts with multiple physician groups to provide services to HMO members. It may include single or multispecialty groups.

Individual practice association (IPA) is a health care provider organization composed of a group of independent practicing physicians who maintain their own offices and band together for the purpose of contracting their services to HMOs, preferred provider organizations, and insurance companies. An IPA may contract with and provide services to both HMO and non-HMO plan participants.

Mixed model HMO is an HMO that combines features of more than one HMO model.

(Also see Appendix II, Managed care; Preferred provider organization.)

Health services and supplies expenditures—See Health expenditures, national.

Health status, respondent-assessed—Health status was measured in the National Health Interview Survey by asking the family respondent about his or her health or the health of a family member: "Would you say [person's] health in general is excellent, very good, good, fair, or poor?"

Hearing trouble—In the National Health Interview Survey, information about hearing trouble is obtained by asking respondents how well they hear without the use of hearing aids. Prior to 2007 data, respondents were asked, "Which statement best describes your hearing without a hearing aid: good, a little trouble, a lot of trouble, or deaf?" In *Health, United States*, a lot of trouble and deaf are combined into one category: hearing trouble. Starting with 2007 data, the question was revised to expand the response categories. Respondents were asked, "These next questions are about your hearing WITHOUT the use of hearing aids or other listening devices. Is your hearing excellent, good, a little trouble hearing, moderate trouble, a lot of trouble, or are you deaf?" For 2007 and subsequent data, a lot of trouble and deaf are still combined into the one

category, hearing trouble, in *Health, United States*. However, because of the expanded response categories, 2007 and subsequent data are not strictly comparable with earlier years and caution is urged when interpreting trends. For example, in 2006, 3.5% of adults (18 years of age and over) were classified as having hearing difficulty (response categories: a lot of trouble or deaf). In 2007, 2.3% of adults (18 years and over) were classified as having hearing difficulty (response categories: a lot of trouble or deaf). This more than 30% decline from 2006 to 2007 in the estimate of those with hearing trouble is likely attributable to the addition of the moderate trouble response category, rather than changes in the prevalence of hearing trouble. Although all age groups saw a decline in the percentage reporting hearing trouble between 2006 and 2007, the amount of the decline varied. There was a 50% decline in reported hearing trouble among adults 18–44 years of age (from 0.8% in 2006 to 0.4% in 2007). Among adults 45–64 years, the percentage that reported hearing trouble declined 43%, from 3.5% in 2006 to 2.0% in 2007. Among adults 65 years and over, reported hearing trouble declined 24%, from 11.4% in 2006 to 8.7% in 2007. For all age groups, these declines are likely attributable to the additional response categories in the revised hearing question.

For more information, see: Pleis JR, Lucas JW. Summary health statistics for U.S. adults: National Health Interview Survey, 2007. Vital Health Stat 10(240). Hyattsville, MD: NCHS; 2009. Available from: http://www.cdc.gov/nchs/data/series/sr_10/sr10_240.pdf.

Hispanic origin—Hispanic or Latino origin includes persons of Mexican, Puerto Rican, Cuban, Central and South American, and other or unknown Latin American or Spanish origins. Persons of Hispanic origin may be of any race.

Birth file—The reporting area for an Hispanic-origin item on the birth certificate expanded between 1980 and 1993 (when the Hispanic item was included on the birth certificate in all states and the District of Columbia (D.C.)). Trend data on births of Hispanic and non-Hispanic parentage in *Health, United States* are affected by expansion of the reporting area and by immigration. These two factors affect numbers of events, composition of the Hispanic population, and maternal and infant health characteristics.

In 1980 and 1981, information on births of Hispanic parentage was reported on the birth certificate by the following 22 states: Arizona,

Arkansas, California, Colorado, Florida, Georgia, Hawaii, Illinois, Indiana, Kansas, Maine, Mississippi, Nebraska, Nevada, New Jersey, New Mexico, New York, North Dakota, Ohio, Texas, Utah, and Wyoming. In 1982 Tennessee, and in 1983 D.C., began reporting this information. Between 1983 and 1987, information on births of Hispanic parentage was available for 23 states and D.C. In 1988, this information became available for Alabama, Connecticut, Kentucky, Massachusetts, Montana, North Carolina, and Washington state, increasing the number of states reporting information on births of Hispanic parentage to 30 states and D.C. In 1989, this information became available from an additional 17 states, increasing the number of Hispanic-reporting states to 47 and D.C. In 1989, only Louisiana, New Hampshire, and Oklahoma did not report Hispanic parentage on the birth certificate. With the inclusion of Louisiana in 1989 and Oklahoma in 1990 as Hispanic-reporting states, 99% of birth records included information on mother's origin. Hispanic origin of the mother was reported on the birth certificates of 49 states and D.C. in 1991 and 1992; only New Hampshire did not provide this information. Starting in 1993, Hispanic origin of mother was reported by all 50 states and D.C.

Mortality file—The reporting area for an Hispanic-origin item on the death certificate expanded between 1985 and 1997. In 1985, mortality data by Hispanic origin of decedent were based on deaths of residents of the following 17 states and D.C. whose data on the death certificate were at least 90% complete on a place-of-occurrence basis and of comparable format: Arizona, Arkansas, California, Colorado, Georgia, Hawaii, Illinois, Indiana, Kansas, Mississippi, Nebraska, New York, North Dakota, Ohio, Texas, Utah, and Wyoming. In 1986, New Jersey began reporting Hispanic origin of decedent, increasing the number of reporting states to 18 and D.C. in 1986 and 1987. In 1988, Alabama, Kentucky, Maine, Montana, North Carolina, Oregon, Rhode Island, and Washington state were added to the reporting area, increasing the number of states to 26 and D.C. In 1989, an additional 18 states were added, increasing the Hispanic reporting area to 44 states and D.C.; only Connecticut, Louisiana, Maryland, New Hampshire, Oklahoma, and Virginia were not included in the reporting area. Starting with 1990 data in *Health, United States*, the criterion was changed to include states whose data were at least 80% complete. In 1990, Maryland, Virginia, and Connecticut; in 1991

Louisiana; and in 1993 New Hampshire were added, increasing the reporting area for Hispanic origin of decedent to 47 states and D.C. in 1990; 48 states and D.C. in 1991 and 1992; and 49 states and D.C. in 1993–1996. Only Oklahoma did not provide this information in 1993–1996. Starting in 1997, Hispanic origin of decedent was reported by all 50 states and D.C. Based on data from the U.S. Census Bureau, the 1990 reporting area encompassed 99.6% of the U.S. Hispanic population. In 1990, more than 96% of death records included information on Hispanic origin of the decedent.

Starting with 2003 data, some states began using the 2003 revision of the U.S. Standard Certificate of Death, which allows the reporting of more than one race (multiple races) and includes some revisions in the item reporting Hispanic origin. In 2003, 7 states reported multiple-race data; in 2004, 15 states reported multiple-race data; in 2005, 21 states and D.C. reported multiple-race data; in 2006, 25 states and D.C. reported multiple-race data; and in 2007, 27 states and D.C. reported multiple-race data. The effect of the 2003 revision of the Hispanic origin item on the reporting of Hispanic origin on death certificates is presumed to be minor. For more information, see Appendix II, Race. Also see: Xu JQ, Kochanek KD, Murphy SL, Tejada-Vera B. Deaths: Final data for 2007. National vital statistics reports; vol 58 no 19. Hyattsville, MD: NCHS; 2010. Available from: http://www.cdc.gov/nchs/data/nvsr/nvsr58/nvsr58_19.pdf; and NCHS procedures for multiple-race and Hispanic origin data: Collection, coding, editing, and transmitting. Hyattsville, MD: NCHS; 2004. Available from: http://www.cdc.gov/nchs/data/dvs/Multiple_race_docu_5-10-04.pdf.

National Health Interview Survey (NHIS) and *National Health and Nutrition Examination Survey (NHANES)*—Questions on Hispanic origin are self-reported in NHANES III and subsequent years, and since 1976 in NHIS, and precede questions on race. For 1999–2006 data, the NHANES sample was designed to provide estimates specifically for persons of Mexican origin and not for all Hispanic-origin persons in the United States. Persons of Hispanic origin other than Mexican were entered into the sample with different selection probabilities that are not nationally representative of the total U.S. Hispanic population. Starting with 2007–2008 data collection, all Hispanic persons were oversampled, not just Mexican American persons. For more information on the sampling methodology changes, see http://www.cdc.gov/nchs/nhanes/nhanes2007-2008/sampling_0708.htm. For more information on race and Hispanic origin in NHIS, see the NHIS Race and Hispanic Origin Information home page. Available from: http://www.cdc.gov/nchs/nhis/rhoi.htm.

Surveillance, Epidemiology, and End Results (SEER) Program—SEER data are available from the National Institutes of Health, National Cancer Institute. SEER Hispanic data used in *Health, United States* tables exclude data from Alaska. The North American Association of Central Cancer Registries, Inc. (NAACCR) Hispanic Identification Algorithm was used on a combination of variables to classify incidence cases as Hispanic for analytic purposes. See: NAACCR Guideline for Enhancing Hispanic–Latino Identification. Bethesda, MD: National Cancer Institute; 2003. Available from: http://seer.cancer.gov/seerstat/variables/seer/yr1973_2004/race_ethnicity/.

Youth Risk Behavior Survey (YRBS)—Prior to 1999, a single question was asked about race and Hispanic origin, with the option of selecting one of the following categories: white not Hispanic, black not Hispanic, Hispanic or Latino, Asian or Other Pacific Islander, American Indian or Alaska Native, or other. Between 1999 and 2003, respondents were asked a single question about race and Hispanic origin with the option of choosing one or more of the following categories: white, black or African American, Hispanic or Latino, Asian, Native Hawaiian or Other Pacific Islander, or American Indian or Alaska Native. In 2005, 2007, and 2009, respondents were asked a question about Hispanic origin ("Are you Hispanic or Latino?") and a second separate question about race that included the option of selecting one or more of the following categories: American Indian or Alaska Native, Asian, black or African American, Native Hawaiian or Other Pacific Islander, or white. Because of the differences between questions, the data about race and Hispanic ethnicity for the years prior to 1999 are not strictly comparable with estimates for the subsequent years. However, analyses of data collected between 1991 and 2003 have indicated that the data are comparable across years and can be used to study trends. See Appendix II, Race; and see: Brener ND, Kann L, McManus T. A comparison of two survey questions on race and ethnicity among high school students. Public Opin Q 2003;67(2): 227–36.

HIV—See Human immunodeficiency virus disease.

Home visit—Starting in 1997, the National Health Interview Survey has been collecting information on home visits received during the 12 months prior to interview. Respondents are asked "During the past 12 months, did you receive care at home from a nurse or other health care professional? What was the total number of home visits received?" These data are combined with data on visits to doctors' offices, clinics, and emergency departments to provide a summary measure of health care visits. (Also see Appendix II, Emergency department or emergency room visit; Health care contact.)

Hospital—According to the American Hospital Association (AHA), hospitals are licensed institutions with at least six beds whose primary function is to provide diagnostic and therapeutic patient services for medical conditions; they have an organized physician staff and provide continuous nursing services under the supervision of registered nurses. The World Health Organization (WHO) considers an establishment to be a hospital if it is permanently staffed by at least one physician, can offer inpatient accommodation, and can provide active medical and nursing care. Hospitals may be classified by type of service, ownership, size in terms of number of beds, and length of stay. In the National Hospital Ambulatory Medical Care Survey, hospitals include all those with an average length of stay for all patients of less than 30 days (short-stay) or hospitals whose specialty is general (medical or surgical) or children's general. Federal hospitals and hospital units of institutions and hospitals with fewer than six beds staffed for patient use are excluded. (Also see Appendix II, Average length of stay; Bed, health facility; Days of care; Emergency department; Inpatient; Outpatient department.)

Community hospital—Community hospitals, based on the AHA definition, include all nonfederal short-term general and special hospitals whose facilities and services are available to the public. Special hospitals include obstetrics and gynecology; eye, ear, nose, and throat; rehabilitation; orthopedic; and other specialty services. Short-term general and special children's hospitals are also considered to be community hospitals. A hospital may include a nursing-home-type unit and still be classified as short-term, provided the majority of its patients are admitted to units where the average length of stay is less than 30 days. Hospital units of institutions such as prisons and college infirmaries that are not open to the public and are contained within a nonhospital facility are not included in the category of community hospitals.

Traditionally, the definition included all nonfederal short-stay hospitals except facilities for the mentally retarded. In a revised definition, the following additional sites were excluded: hospital units of institutions, and alcoholism and chemical dependency facilities.

Critical access hospital—The designation critical access hospital (CAH) was created as part of the Balanced Budget Act of 1997. A CAH is a hospital that is certified to receive cost-based reimbursement from Medicare. The general requirements for CAHs are that they (a) be located in a rural area, (b) be more than 35 miles from another hospital (or 15 miles in mountainous terrain), (c) maintain 25 or fewer inpatient beds, and (d) have an annual average length of stay of 96 hours or less per patient for acute inpatient care. For more information, see: https://www.cms.gov/CertificationandComplianc/04_CAHs.asp.

Federal hospital—Federal hospitals are those operated by the federal government.

For-profit hospital—For-profit hospitals are operated for profit by individuals, partnerships, or corporations.

General hospital—General hospitals provide diagnostic, treatment, and surgical services for patients with a variety of medical conditions. According to WHO, these hospitals provide medical and nursing care for more than one category of medical discipline (e.g., general medicine, specialized medicine, general surgery, specialized surgery, and obstetrics). Excluded are hospitals, usually in rural areas, that provide a more limited range of care.

Nonprofit hospital—Nonprofit hospitals are those controlled by nonprofit organizations, such as religious organizations and fraternal societies.

Psychiatric hospital—Psychiatric hospitals are those whose major type of service is psychiatric care. (Also see Appendix II, Mental health organization.)

Registered hospital—Registered hospitals are those registered with the AHA. About 98% of U.S. hospitals are registered.

Short-stay hospital—In the National Hospital Discharge Survey, short-stay hospitals are those in which the average length of stay is less than 30 days. The National Health Interview Survey defines short-stay hospitals as any hospital or hospital department in which the type of service provided is general; maternity; eye, ear, nose, and throat; children's; or osteopathic.

Specialty hospital—Specialty hospitals are those, such as psychiatric, tuberculosis, chronic disease, rehabilitation, maternity, and alcoholic or narcotic dependency facilities, that provide a particular type of service to the majority of their patients.

Hospital-based physician—See Physician.

Hospital day—See Days of care.

Hospital utilization—Estimates of hospital utilization (such as hospital discharge rate, days of care rate, average length of stay, and percentage of the population with a hospitalization) presented in *Health, United States* are based on data from three sources: the National Health Interview Survey (NHIS), the National Hospital Discharge Survey (NHDS), and the American Hospital Association (AHA). NHIS data are based on household interviews of the civilian noninstitutionalized population and thus exclude hospitalizations for institutionalized persons and those who died while hospitalized. NHDS data are based on hospital discharge records of persons who had an inpatient stay in a nonfederal, short-stay hospital. NHDS includes hospital discharge records for persons discharged alive or deceased and for institutionalized persons. NHDS tables shown in *Health, United States* exclude data for newborns. Estimates for average length of stay between the NHDS and AHA data presented in *Health, United States* differ because of different methods for counting days of care. (Also see Appendix II, Average length of stay; Days of care; Discharge; and Appendix I, National Health Interview Survey; National Hospital Discharge Survey.)

Human immunodeficiency virus (HIV) disease—HIV disease is caused by infection with a cytopathic retrovirus, which in turn leads to destruction of parts of the immune system. A surveillance case for HIV requires laboratory-confirmed evidence of infection, including a positive result on a screening test for HIV antibody, followed by a positive result on a confirmatory test, or a positive result or detectable quantity on an HIV virologic test (see MMWR 2008;57(RR–10):1–8).

Since 1985, many states and U.S. dependent areas have implemented HIV case reporting as part of their comprehensive HIV and AIDS surveillance programs. As of April 2008, all states, the District of Columbia, and five U.S. independent areas had implemented HIV case surveillance using a confidential system for name-based case reporting for both HIV infection and AIDS. To better capture and characterize populations in which HIV infection has been newly diagnosed, including persons with evidence of recent HIV infection, many states report the prevalence of those living with a diagnosis of HIV infection, including those living with AIDS. In 2008, changes were made to the case definition for HIV infection. The new case definition combined the two previous case definitions for HIV and AIDS and established a new disease staging classification. The term "HIV/AIDS" was replaced with the term "diagnosis of HIV infection" (see MMWR 2008;57(RR–10):1–8). Mortality and morbidity coding for HIV disease are similar and have evolved over time.

Mortality coding—Starting with 1999 data and the introduction of the 10th revision of the *International Classification of Diseases* (ICD–10), the title for this cause of death was changed from HIV infection to HIV disease, and the ICD codes were changed to B20–B24. Starting with 1987 data, the National Center for Health Statistics (NCHS) introduced category numbers *042–*044 for classifying and coding HIV infection as a cause of death in ICD, 9th revision (ICD–9). The asterisks before the category numbers indicate that these codes were not part of the original ICD–9. HIV infection was formerly referred to as human T-cell lymphotropic virus-III/lymphadenopathy-associated virus (HTLV–III/LAV) infection. Before 1987, deaths involving HIV infection were classified to Deficiency of cell-mediated immunity (ICD–9 code 279.1) contained in the title All other diseases; to Pneumocystosis (ICD–9 code 136.3) contained in the title All other infectious and parasitic diseases; to Malignant neoplasms, including neoplasms of lymphatic and hematopoietic tissues; and to a number of other causes. Therefore, before 1987, death statistics for HIV infection are not strictly comparable with data for 1987 and subsequent years and are not shown in *Health, United States*.

Morbidity coding—The National Hospital Discharge Survey codes diagnosis data using the *International Classification of Diseases, 9th Revision, Clinical Modification* (ICD–9–CM). During 1984 and 1985, only data for AIDS (ICD–9–CM 279.19) were included. In 1986–1994, discharges with the following diagnoses were included: AIDS, HIV infection and associated conditions, and positive serological or viral culture findings for HIV (ICD–9–CM 042–044, 279.19, and 795.8). Beginning in 1995, discharges with the following diagnoses were included: HIV disease and asymptomatic HIV infection status (ICD–9–CM 042 and V08).

(Also see Appendix II, Acquired immunodeficiency syndrome; Cause of death; *International Classification of Diseases*; *International Classification of Diseases, 9th Revision, Clinical Modification*; Tables V and XI.)

Hypertension—See Blood pressure, high.

ICD; ICD codes—See Cause of death; *International Classification of Diseases*.

Illicit drug use—Illicit drug use refers to the use and misuse of illegal and controlled drugs.

Monitoring the Future (MTF)—In this school-based survey of secondary school students, information on illicit drug use is collected using self-completed questionnaires. The information is based on the following questions: "On how many occasions (if any) have you used marijuana in the last 30 days?" and "On how many occasions (if any) have you used hashish in the last 30 days?" Questions on cocaine use include the following: "On how many occasions (if any) have you taken crack (cocaine in chunk or rock form) during the last 30 days?" and "On how many occasions (if any) have you taken cocaine in any other form during the last 30 days?"

National Survey on Drug Use & Health (NSDUH)—Information on illicit drug use is collected for survey participants 12 years of age and over. Information on any illicit drug use includes any use of marijuana or hashish, cocaine, heroin, hallucinogens, or inhalants, as well as nonmedical use of prescription psychotherapeutic drugs. Current use (within the past month) is based on the question: "How long has it been since you last used (drug name)?" (Also see Appendix II, Substance use.)

Immunization—See Vaccination.

Incidence—Incidence is the number of cases of disease having their onset during a prescribed period of time. It is often expressed as a rate (e.g., the incidence of measles per 1,000 children 5–15 years of age during a specified year). Measuring incidence may be complicated because the population at risk for the disease may change during the period of interest, for example, due to births, deaths, or migration. In addition, determining whether a case is new—that is, whether its onset occurred during the prescribed period of time—may be difficult. Because of these difficulties in measuring incidence, many health statistics are instead measured in terms of prevalence. (Also see Appendix II, Prevalence.)

Income—See Family income.

Individual practice association (IPA)—See Health maintenance organization.

Industry of employment—For the presentation of data in *Health, United States*, industries are classified according to the North American Industry Classification System (NAICS). For each year of data presented, the most recent version of NAICS was used. NAICS groups establishments into industries based on their production or supply function: establishments using similar raw material inputs, capital equipment, and labor are classified in the same industry. This approach creates homogeneous categories well suited for economic analysis. NAICS uses a six-digit hierarchical coding system to classify all economic activity into 20 industry sectors. The first two digits of the six-digit code designate the highest level of aggregation, into the government and 19 private industry sectors (Table IX). With the exception of the agriculture, forestry, farming, and hunting sector, private industry sectors are classified as goods- or service-producing. Mining, construction, and manufacturing are primarily goods-producing sectors, and the remaining 15 are entirely service-providing sectors. NAICS allows for the classification of 1,170 industries. For more information on NAICS, see: http://www.census.gov/epcd/www/naics.html.

NAICS replaces the Standard Industrial Classification (SIC) system, originally designed in the 1930s and revised and updated periodically to reflect changes in the U.S. economy. The last SIC revision was in 1987. The SIC system focused on the manufacturing sector of the economy and provided significantly less detail for the now-dominant service sector, including newly developed industries in information services, health care delivery, and high-tech manufacturing. Although some titles in SIC and NAICS are similar, there is little comparability between the two systems because industry groupings are defined differently. Estimates of deaths, injuries, and illnesses classified by NAICS should not be compared with earlier estimates that used SIC.

Starting with *Health United States, 2005*, health data by industry from the Bureau of Labor Statistics' Census of Fatal Occupational Injuries (CFOI) and Survey of Occupational Injuries and Illnesses (SOII) data systems are classified using the NAICS system and replace trends in occupational health data based on the SIC system in previous editions of *Health, United States*.

Infant death—An infant death is the death of a live-born child before his or her first birthday. Age at

Table IX. Codes for industries, based on the North American Industry Classification System (NAICS)

Private Industry	Code
Agriculture, forestry, fishing and hunting.	11
Mining, quarrying, and oil and gas extraction	21
Utilities.	22
Construction	23
Manufacturing.	31–33
Wholesale trade	42
Retail trade.	44–45
Transportation and warehousing.	48–49
Information	51
Finance and insurance.	52
Real estate and rental and leasing	53
Professional, scientific, and technical services	54
Management of companies and enterprises	55
Administrative and support and waste management and remediation services	56
Educational services	61
Health care and social assistance.	62
Arts, entertainment, and recreation	71
Accommodation and food services	72
Other services, except public administration	81

SOURCE: Bureau of Labor Statistics. Available from: http://www.census.gov/eos/www/naics/.

death may be further classified as neonatal or postneonatal. Neonatal deaths are those that occur before the 28th day of life; postneonatal deaths are those that occur between 28 and 365 days of age. (Also see Appendix II, Rate: Death and related rates.)

Injury—The International Classification of External Causes of Injuries (ICECI) Coordination and Maintenance Group defines injury as a (suspected) bodily lesion resulting from acute overexposure to energy (this can be mechanical, thermal, electrical, chemical, or radiant) interacting with the body in amounts or rates that exceed the threshold of physiological tolerance. The time between exposure to the energy and the appearance of an injury is short. In some cases, an injury results from an insufficiency of any of the vital elements (i.e., air, water, or warmth), as in strangulation, drowning, or freezing. Acute poisonings and toxic effects, including overdoses of substances and wrong substances given or taken in error, are included, as are adverse effects and complications of therapeutic, surgical, and medical care. Psychological harm is excluded. Injuries can be intentional or unintentional (i.e., accidental). In NCHS data systems, external causes of nonfatal injuries are coded to the *International Classification of Diseases, 9th Revision, Clinical Modification, Supplementary Classification of External Causes of Injury and Poisoning,* and the codes are often referred to as E codes. See Table X for a list of external causes of injury categories and E codes used in *Health, United States.* See the NCHS injury website at: http://www.cdc.gov/nchs/injury.htm; and see: ICECI Coordination and Maintenance Group. International Classification of External Causes of Injuries (ICECI), version 1.2. Amsterdam, The Netherlands: Consumer Safety Institute; and Adelaide, Australia: Australian Institute of Health and Welfare National Injury Surveillance Unit. Flinders University; 2004. Available from: http://www.who.int/classifications/icd/adaptations/iceci/en/index.html. (Also see Appendix II, Diagnosis; Injury-related visit.)

Injury-related visit—In the National Hospital Ambulatory Medical Care Survey (NHAMCS), an emergency department visit was considered injury-related if the physician's diagnosis was injury-related *(International Classification of Diseases, 9th Revision, Clinical Modification* (ICD–9–CM, code 800–999)), an external cause-of-injury code was present (ICD–9–CM E800–E999), or the patient's reason for visit code was injury-related. Starting with *Health, United States, 2008,* the definition of an injury-related visit was redefined as an initial injury visit. In the 2001–2005 NHAMCS, an initial injury visit was the first visit to an emergency department for an injury that was characterized by either the first-listed diagnosis being a valid injury diagnosis or by a valid first-listed external cause of injury code, regardless of the diagnosis code. Visits for which the first-listed diagnosis or the first-listed external-cause code was for a complication of medical care or for an adverse event were not counted as injury visits. For 2001–2004 data, the patient record form had a specific question on whether or not the visit was the initial one for that condition. In the 2005 and 2006 surveys, this variable was dropped, and in its place an imputed variable indicating that the visit was or was not the initial visit was included on the public-use file. For an explanation of the methodology used to create the initial visit variable, see: http://www.cdc.gov/nchs/data/ahcd/initialvisit.pdf. In the 2007 and 2008 surveys, the patient record form had a specific question on whether the visit was the initial one for that condition. For more information, see: the CDC/NCHS Injury Data and resources website at: http://www.cdc.gov/nchs/injury.htm; and Fingerhut LA. Recommended definition of initial injury visits to emergency departments for use with the NHAMCS–ED data [online].

Table X. Codes for first-listed external causes of injury, from the *International Classification of Diseases, 9th Revision, Clinical Modification*

External cause of injury category	E code
Unintentional	E800–E869, E880–E929
Motor vehicle traffic	E810–E819
Falls	E880–E886, E888
Struck by or against objects or persons	E916–E917
Caused by cutting and piercing instruments or objects	E920
Intentional (suicide and homicide) . . .	E950–E969, E979, E999.1

Health E-Stats. NCHS. 2006. Available from: http://www.cdc.gov/nchs/data/hestat/injury/injury.htm. (Also see Appendix II, Emergency department or emergency room visit; External cause of injury; Injury.)

Inpatient—An inpatient is a person who is formally admitted to the inpatient service of a hospital for observation, care, diagnosis, or treatment. (Also see Appendix II, Admission; Average length of stay; Days of care; Discharge; Hospital.)

Inpatient care—See Hospital utilization; Mental health service type.

Inpatient day—See Days of care.

Instrumental activities of daily living (IADLs)— IADLs are activities related to independent living and include preparing meals, managing money, shopping for groceries or personal items, performing light or heavy housework, and using a telephone. In the National Health Interview Survey (NHIS), respondents are asked whether they or family members 18 years of age and over need the help of another person for handling routine IADL needs because of a physical, mental, or emotional problem. Persons are considered to have an IADL limitation in NHIS if any causal condition is chronic.

In the Medicare Current Beneficiary Survey, if a sample person had any difficulty performing an activity by him- or herself and without special equipment, or did not perform the activity at all because of health problems, the person was categorized as having a limitation in that activity. The limitation may have been temporary or chronic at the time of interview. Sample persons in the community answered health status and functioning questions themselves, if able to do so. For sample persons in a long-term care facility, a proxy such as a nurse answered questions about the sample person's health status and functioning.

(Also see Appendix II, Activities of daily living; Complex activity limitation; Limitation of activity.)

Insurance—See Health insurance coverage.

Intermediate care facility—See Nursing home.

International Classification of Diseases (ICD)—The ICD is used to code and classify cause-of-death data. The ICD is developed collaboratively by the World Health Organization and 10 international centers, one of which is housed at NCHS. The purpose of the ICD is to promote international comparability in the collection, classification, processing, and presentation of health statistics. Since 1900, the ICD has been modified about once every 10 years, except for the 20-year interval between the 9th and 10th revisions (ICD–9 and ICD–10) (see Table IV). The purpose of the revisions is to stay abreast of advances in medical science. New revisions usually introduce major disruptions in time series of mortality statistics (see Tables V and VI). For more information, see the NCHS ICD–10 website at: http://www.cdc.gov/nchs/icd/icd10.htm. (Also see Appendix II, Cause of death; Comparability ratio; *International Classification of Diseases, 9th Revision, Clinical Modification.*)

International Classification of Diseases, 9th Revision, Clinical Modification (ICD–9–CM)—ICD–9–CM is based on, and is compatible with, the World Health Organization's ICD–9. The United States currently uses ICD–9–CM to code morbidity diagnoses and inpatient procedures. ICD–9–CM consists of three volumes. Volumes 1 and 2 contain the diagnosis tabular list and index; Volume 3 contains the procedure classification (tabular list and index combined).

ICD–9–CM is divided into 17 chapters and two supplemental classifications. The chapters are arranged primarily by body system. In addition, there are chapters for Infectious and parasitic diseases; Neoplasms; Endocrine, nutritional, and metabolic diseases; Mental disorders; Complications of pregnancy, childbirth, and puerperium; Certain conditions originating in the perinatal period; Congenital anomalies; and Symptoms, signs, and ill-defined conditions. The two supplemental classifications are for factors influencing health status and contact with health services (V codes), and for external causes of injury and poisoning (E codes).

In *Health, United States*, morbidity data are classified using ICD–9–CM. Diagnostic categories and codes for ICD–9–CM are shown in Table XI; ICD–9–CM procedure categories and codes are shown in Table XII. For additional information about ICD–9–

CM, see the NCHS Classifications of Diseases, Functioning, and Disability website at: http://www.cdc.gov/nchs/icd.htm. (Also see Appendix II, *International Classification of Diseases.*)

Late fetal death rate—See Rate: Death and related rates.

Leading causes of death—See Cause-of-death ranking.

Length of stay—See Average length of stay.

Life expectancy—Life expectancy is the average number of years of life remaining to a person at a particular age and is based on a given set of age-specific death rates, generally the mortality conditions existing in the period mentioned. Life expectancy may be determined by race, sex, or other characteristics by using age-specific death rates for the population with that characteristic. (Also see Appendix II, Rate: Death and related rates.)

Starting with 2000 data, a revised methodology that uses vital statistics death rates for ages under 66 and modeled probabilities of death for ages 66–100 based on blended vital statistics and Medicare probabilities of dying was implemented. As a result, data post-2000 may differ from figures published previously. The revised methodology is similar to that developed for the 1999–2001 decennial life tables. For more information, see: Xu JQ, Kochanek KD, Murphy SL, Tejada-Vera B. Deaths: Final data for 2007. National vital statistics reports; vol 58 no 19. Hyattsville, MD: NCHS; 2010. Available from: http://www.cdc.gov/nchs/data/nvsr/nvsr58/nvsr58_19.pdf.

Limitation of activity—Limitation of activity may be defined in different ways, depending on the conceptual framework. In the National Health Interview Survey, limitation of activity refers to a long-term reduction in a person's capacity to perform the usual kind or amount of activities associated with his or her age group as a result of a chronic condition. Limitation of activity is assessed by asking persons a series of questions about limitations in their or a household member's ability to perform activities usual for their age group because of a physical, mental, or emotional problem. Persons are asked about limitations in activities of daily living, instrumental activities of daily living, play, school, work, difficulty walking or remembering, and any other activity limitations. For reported limitations, the causal health conditions are determined, and persons are considered limited if one or more of these conditions is chronic. Children under 18 years of age who receive special education or early intervention services are considered to have

Table XI. Codes for diagnostic categories, from the *International Classification of Diseases, 9th Revision, Clinical Modification*

Diagnostic category	Code
Childbirth	V27
Septicemia	038
Human immunodeficiency virus (HIV/AIDS) (1990–1994 data)	042–044, 279.19, 795.8
(Starting with 1995 data)	042, V08
Cancer, all	140–208, 230–234
Colorectal cancer	153–154, 197.5, 230.3–230.6
Lung/bronchus/tracheal cancer	162, 176.4, 197.0, 197.3, 231.1–231.2
Breast	174–175, 198.81, 233.0
Prostate	185, 233.4
Uterine fibroids	218
Diabetes	250
Dehydration	276.5
(Starting with 2006 data)	276.50–276.52
Alcohol and drug	291–292, 303–304, 305.0, 305.2–305.9
Schizophrenia, mood disorders, delusional disorders, nonorganic psychoses	295–298
Schizophrenia	295
Mood disorders	296
Dementia and Alzheimer's disease	290, 294, 331.0
Heart disease	391–392.0, 393–398, 402, 404, 410–416, 420–429
Ischemic heart disease	410–414
Heart attack	410
Arrhythmias	427
Heart failure	428
Hypertension	401
Stroke	430–438
Acute bronchitis and bronchiolitis	466
Pneumonia	480–486, 487.0
Chronic obstructive pulmonary disease	490–492, 496
Asthma	493
Appendicitis	540–543
Gallstones	574
Kidney disease	580–589
Urinary tract infection	599.0
Hyperplasia of the prostate	600
Osteoarthritis	715, 721
Intervertebral disc disorders	722
Injury	800–909.2, 909.4, 909.9, 910–994.9, 995.5, 995.80–995.85
Fracture	800–829
Hip fracture	820
Internal organ injury	850–854, 860–869, 952, 995.55
Poisoning and toxic effects	960–989
Complications of care and adverse effects	996–999, 909.3, 909.5, 995.0–995.4, 995.6–995.7, 995.86, 995.89

a limitation of activity. (Also see Appendix II, Activities of daily living; Condition; Instrumental activities of daily living.)

Long-term care facility—A long-term care facility is a residence that provides a specific level of personal or medical care or supervision to residents. In the Medicare Current Beneficiary Survey, a residence is considered a long-term care facility if it has three or more long-term care beds and answers affirmatively to at least one of three questions: "Does this facility (a) provide personal care services to residents, (b) provide continuous supervision of residents, (c) provide any long-term care?" Types of long-term care facilities include licensed nursing homes, skilled nursing homes, intermediate care facilities, retirement homes (that provide services), domiciliary or personal care facilities, distinct long-term care units in a hospital complex, mental health facilities and centers, assisted and foster

Table XII. Codes for procedure categories, from the *International Classification of Diseases, 9th Revision, Clinical Modification*

Procedure category	Code
Operations on vessels of heart (Through 2005 data)	36
Operations on vessels of heart (Starting with 2006 data)	36, 00.66
Coronary angioplasty or arthrectomy (Through 2005 data)	36.01, 36.02, 36.05
(Starting with 2006 data)	00.66
Coronary artery stent insertion	36.06, 36.07
Drug-eluting stent insertion	36.07
Coronary artery bypass graft (CABG)	36.1
Cardiac catheterization	37.21–37.23
Pacemaker	37.7–37.8
(Starting with 2003 data)	37.7–37.8, 00.50, 00.52, 00.53
Carotid (neck arteries) endarterectomy	38.12
Endoscopy of small intestine	45.11–45.14, 45.16
Endoscopy of large intestine	45.21–45.25
Gall bladder removal	51.2
Laparoscopic gall bladder removal	51.23, 51.24
Treatment of intra-abdominal scar tissue	54.5
Removal of prostate	60.2–60.6
Transurethral prostatectomy	60.2
Hysterectomy	68.3–68.5
Abdominal hysterectomy	68.4
Vaginal hysterectomy	68.5
Forceps, vacuum, and breech delivery	72
Episiotomy	72.1, 72.21, 72.31, 72.71, 73.6
Other procedures inducing or assisting delivery	73
Medical induction of labor	73.4
Cesarean section	74.0–74.2, 74.4, 74.99
Reduction of fracture	79.0–79.5, 76.7, 21.7, 02.02, 03.53
Excision of intervertebral disc and spinal fusion	80.5 and 81.0
Total hip replacement	81.51
Partial hip replacement	81.52
Total knee replacement	81.54
Mastectomy	85.4
CT scan	87.03, 87.41, 87.71, 88.01, 88.38
Arteriography and angiocardiography with contrast	88.4–88.5
Diagnostic ultrasound	00.2, 37.28, 88.7, 95.13
Magnetic resonance imaging	88.91–88.97
Mechanical ventilation (1990–1991 data)	93.92
(Starting with 1992 data)	96.7

care homes, and institutions for the mentally retarded and developmentally disabled. (Also see Appendix II, Nursing home.)

Low birthweight—See Birthweight.

Magnetic resonance imaging (MRI) unit—MRI is an imaging technique designed to visualize internal structures of the body by using magnetic and electromagnetic fields that induce a resonance effect of hydrogen atoms. The electromagnetic emission created by these atoms is registered and processed by a dedicated computer to produce the images of the body structures.

Mammography—A mammogram is an x-ray image of the breast used to detect irregularities in breast tissue. In the National Health Interview Survey, questions concerning use of mammography were asked on an intermittent schedule, and question content differed across years. In 1987 and 1990, women were asked to report when they had their last mammogram. In 1991, women were asked whether they had a mammogram in the past 2 years. In 1993 and 1994, women were asked whether they had a mammogram within the past year, between 1 and 2 years ago, or over 2 years ago. In 1998, women were asked whether they had a mammogram a year ago or less, more than 1 year but not more than 2 years, or more than 2 years ago.

In 1999, women were asked when they had their most recent mammogram, in days, weeks, months, or years. In 1999, 10% of women in the sample responded 2 years ago, and in this analysis these women were coded as within the past 2 years, although a response of 2 years ago may include women whose last mammogram was more than 2 but less than 3 years ago. Thus, estimates for 1999 are overestimated to some degree in comparison with estimates in previous years.

In 2000 and 2003, women were asked when they had their most recent mammogram (give month and year). Women who did not respond were given a follow-up question that used the 1999 wording, and women who did not answer the question with the 1999 wording were asked a second follow-up question that used the 1998 wording. In 2000 and 2003, 2% of women in the sample answered 2 years ago using the 1999 wording, and they were coded as within the past 2 years. Thus, estimates for 2000 and 2003 may be slightly overestimated in comparison with estimates for years prior to 1999.

In 2005, women were asked the same series of mammography questions as in the 2000 and 2003 surveys but the skip pattern was modified so that more women were asked the follow-up question using the 1998 wording. Because additional information was available for women who replied that their last mammogram was 2 years ago, these women were not uniformly coded as having had a mammogram within the past 2 years. Thus, estimates for 2005 are more precise than estimates for 1999, 2000, and 2003 and are slightly lower than they would have been without this additional information. For example, using the improved methodology instituted in 2005, 66.8% of women 40 years of age and over reported a mammogram in the past 2 years, compared with an estimate of 68.7% in 2005 using the method employed in 2000 and 2003. SAS code to categorize mammography data for 2000 and beyond is available from: http://www.cdc.gov/nchs/nhis/nhis_2005_data_release.htm.

In 2008, the mammography questions were identical to those asked in 2005.

Mammography screening recommendations have changed over time and vary in the recommended age to begin screening and the interval for screening. For a summary of the current and historic recommendations see: U.S. Preventive Services Task Force. Screening for breast cancer. Rockville, MD: Agency for Healthcare Research and Quality; 2009. Available from: http://www.uspreventiveservicestaskforce.org/uspstf/uspsbrca.htm; and see: U.S. Preventive Services Task Force. Guide to clinical preventive services, 2009. Rockville, MD: Agency for Healthcare Research and Quality; 2009. Available from: http://www.ahrq.gov/clinic/pocketgd1011/.

Managed care—Managed care is a term originally used to refer to prepaid health plans (generally, health maintenance organizations, or HMOs) under which care is provided through a network of providers under a fixed budget and costs are "managed." Increasingly, the term is also being used to include preferred provider organizations (PPOs) and even forms of indemnity insurance coverage (i.e., "fee-for-service" insurance) that incorporate preadmission certification and other utilization controls.

Medicare managed care has included a combination of risk-based and cost-based plans. Risk-based plans receive a fixed prepayment per beneficiary per month to cover the cost of all covered services that a beneficiary may receive. The Centers for Medicare & Medicaid Services (CMS) announces a "benchmark" amount each year for each county for coverage of Medicare Part A and B services. A managed care plan contracting with Medicare then submits a "bid" representing its revenue needs to cover such services. If the bid is above the benchmark, this amount must be charged in a premium to the enrollees of the plan. If the bid is below the benchmark, then 75% of the difference must be used to provide additional benefits to enrollees, with the Medicare trust funds receiving the remaining 25%. Cost-based plans are offered by an HMO or a Competitive Medical Plan and receive reimbursement for their "reasonable costs" in providing Medicare services to enrollees, based on annual cost reports filed with CMS. For current definitions of the various Medicare managed care plans, see: Centers for Medicare & Medicaid Services. Medicare managed care manual, ch 1, sec 30, Types of MA plans. Baltimore, MD: CMS; 2007. Available from: http://www.cms.hhs.gov/manuals/downloads/mc86c01.pdf.

Medicare enrollees have the choice to enroll in a managed care program (if available) or to receive services on a fee-for-service basis.

The two major Medicaid managed care categories are risk-based plans (managed care organizations (MCOs)) and primary care case management (PCCM) arrangements. In risk-based plans, MCOs are paid a fixed monthly fee per enrollee. The MCOs assume some or all of the financial risk for providing the services covered under the contract. PCCM providers are usually physicians, physician group practices, or entities employing or having other arrangements with such physicians but sometimes also including nurse practitioners, nurse midwives, or physician assistants. These PCCM providers, sometimes called gatekeepers, contract directly with the state to locate, coordinate, and monitor covered primary care (and sometimes additional services). PCCM providers are paid a per-patient case management fee and usually do not assume financial risk for the provision of services. Some states allow Medicaid enrollees to voluntarily enroll in managed care plans; most states require that at least certain categories of Medicaid beneficiaries join managed care plans. Within both risk-based plans and PCCM arrangements there are plans that provide specialized services to certain categories of Medicaid beneficiaries. For more information on state Medicaid managed care plans, see: http://www.cms.hhs.gov/home/medicaid.asp. (Also see Appendix II, Health maintenance organization; Medicare; Medicaid; Preferred provider organization.)

Marital status—Marital status is classified through self-reporting into the categories married and unmarried. The term married encompasses all married people, including those separated from their spouses. Unmarried includes those who are single (never married), divorced, or widowed. Prior to 1978, abortion data collected by the Centers for Disease Control and Prevention's Abortion Surveillance Program included separated women with unmarried women.

Birth file—In 1970, 39 states and the District of Columbia (D.C.), and in 1975, 38 states and D.C., included a direct question about mother's marital status on the birth certificate. Since 1980, national estimates of births to unmarried women have been based on two methods for determining marital status: a direct question in the birth registration process and inferential procedures. In 1980–1996, marital status was reported on the birth certificates of 41–45 states and D.C.; with the addition of California in 1997, 46 states and D.C.; and in 1998–2001, 48 states and D.C. In 1997, all but four states (Connecticut, Michigan, Nevada, and New York), and in 1998, all but two states (Michigan and New York), included a direct question about mother's marital status on their birth certificates. In 1998–2007, marital status was imputed as married on birth records with missing information in the 48 states and D.C. where this information was obtained by a direct question.

For states lacking a direct question, marital status was inferred. Before 1980, the incidence of births to unmarried women in states with no direct question on marital status was assumed to be the same as the incidence in reporting states in the same geographic division. Starting in 1980, for states without a direct question, marital status was inferred by comparing the parents' and child's surnames. For 1994–1996, birth certificates in 45 states and the D.C. included a question about the mother's marital status. Beginning in 1997, the marital status of women giving birth in California and Nevada has been determined by a direct question in the birth registration process. Beginning June 15, 1998, Connecticut discontinued inferring the mother's marital status and added a direct question regarding mother's marital status to the state's birth certificate.

For 2006 and 2007 data, inferential procedures were used to compile birth statistics by marital status, in full or in part, for New York and Michigan, respectively. In 2005, Michigan added a direct question to the birth registration process but uses inferential procedures to update information collected using the direct question. In both Michigan and New York, a birth is inferred as nonmarital if either of these factors, listed in priority-of-use order, is present: (a) a paternity acknowledgment was received or (b) the father's name is missing.

National Health Interview Survey (NHIS)—In NHIS, marital status is asked of, or about, all persons 14 years of age and over. Respondents are asked: "Are you now married, widowed, divorced, separated, never married, or living with a partner?"

National Home and Hospice Care Survey (NHHCS)—In NHHCS, data were collected through interviews with agency directors and their designated staffs; no interviews were conducted directly with patients or their families or friends. Agency staff were asked to answer the following question about hospice care discharged patients and current home health care patients: "Is/was [patient] married, widowed, divorced, separated, never married, or living with a partner in a marriage-like relationship?"

Maternal age—See Age.

Maternal death—Maternal death is defined by the World Health Organization as the death of a woman while pregnant or within 42 days of termination of pregnancy, irrespective of the duration and site of the pregnancy, from any cause related to or aggravated by the pregnancy or its management, but not from accidental or incidental causes. A maternal death is one for which the certifying physician has designated a maternal condition as the underlying cause of death. Maternal conditions are those assigned to pregnancy, childbirth, and the puerperium: *International Classification of Diseases, 10th Revision* (ICD–10) codes A34, O00–O95, O98–O99 (Table V). Changes were made in the classification and coding of maternal deaths between ICD–9 and ICD–10, effective with mortality data for 1999. ICD–10 changes pertain to indirect maternal causes and timing of death relative to pregnancy. If only indirect maternal causes of death (i.e., a previously existing disease or a disease that developed during pregnancy that was not due to direct obstetric causes but was aggravated by physiologic effects of pregnancy) are reported in Part I of the death certificate and pregnancy is reported in either Part I or Part II, ICD–10 classifies this as a maternal death. ICD–9 only classified the death as maternal if pregnancy was reported in Part I. Some state death certificates include a separate question regarding pregnancy status. A positive response to the question is interpreted as "pregnant" being reported in Part II of the cause-of-death section of the death certificate. If the medical certifier did not specify when death occurred relative to the pregnancy, it is assumed that the pregnancy terminated 42 days or less prior to death.

The 2003 revision of the U.S. Standard Certificate of Death introduced a standard question format with categories designed to utilize additional codes available in ICD–10 for deaths associated with pregnancy, childbirth, and the puerperium. As states revise their certificates, most states are expected to introduce the standard item or replace preexisting questions with the standard item, so that there will be wider adoption of a pregnancy status item across the country and greater standardization of the particular item used. As of 2007, 34 states and the District of Columbia have a separate question related to pregnancy status of female decedents around the time of their death, and two states have a prompt encouraging certifiers to report recent pregnancies on the death certificate. However, at least six different questions were used in the 34 states, reflecting the mix of states using the 2003 standard format and states with preexisting questions. (Also see Appendix II, Rate: Death and related rates.)

Maternal education—See Education.

Maternal mortality rate—See Rate: Death and related rates.

Medicaid—Medicaid was authorized by Title XIX of the Social Security Act in 1965 as a jointly funded cooperative venture between the federal and state governments to assist states in the provision of adequate medical care to eligible needy persons. Within broad federal guidelines, each state establishes its own eligibility standards; determines the type, amount, duration, and scope of services; sets the rate of payment for services; and administers its own program.

Medicaid is the largest program providing medical and health-related services to America's poorest people. However, Medicaid does not provide medical assistance to all persons with limited income and resources. Under the broadest provisions of the federal statute, Medicaid does not provide health care services for very poor childless adults under 65 years of age unless they are disabled. The major eligibility groups covered by most states include

■ Individuals who meet the requirements for the Aid to Families with Dependent Children (AFDC) program that were in effect in their state on July 16, 1996, or, at state option, more liberal criteria (with some exceptions).

■ Children under age 6 whose family income is at or below 133% of the federal poverty level.

■ Infants born to Medicaid-eligible women.

■ Pregnant women whose family income is at or below 133% of the federal poverty level (services to these women are limited to those related to pregnancy, complications of pregnancy, delivery, and postpartum care).

■ Supplemental Security Income (SSI) recipients in most states (some states use more restrictive Medicaid eligibility requirements that predate SSI).

■ Recipients of adoption or foster care assistance under Title IV of the Social Security Act.

■ Special protected groups (typically individuals who lose their cash assistance because of earnings from work or from increased Social Security benefits but who may keep Medicaid for a period of time).

■ Children (born after September 30, 1983) who are at least 6 years of age, but under 19 years, in families with incomes at or below the federal poverty level.

States also have the option of providing Medicaid coverage for other groups.

Medicaid operates as a vendor payment program. States may pay health care providers directly on a fee-for-service basis, or states may pay for Medicaid services through various prepayment arrangements, such as through health maintenance organizations or other forms of managed care. Within federally imposed upper limits and specific restrictions, each state for the most part has broad discretion in determining the payment methodology and payment rate for services. Thus, the Medicaid program varies considerably from state to state, as well as within each state over time. For more information see: http://www.cms.hhs.gov/home/medicaid.asp and http://www.cms.hhs.gov/MedicaidEligibility/. (Also see Appendix II, Health expenditures, national; Health insurance coverage; Health maintenance organization; Managed care; and Appendix I, Medicaid Statistical Information System.)

Medicaid payments—Under the Medicaid program, medical vendor payments are payments (expenditures) to medical vendors from the state through a fiscal agent or to a health insurance plan. Adjustments are made for Indian Health Service payments to Medicaid, cost settlements, third-party recoupments, refunds, voided checks, and other financial settlements that cannot be related to specific provided claims. Excluded are payments made for medical care under the emergency assistance provisions; payments made from state medical assistance funds that are not federally matchable; disproportionate-share hospital payments, cost sharing, or enrollment fees collected from recipients or a third-party; and administration and training costs. Medicaid payment data presented in *Health, United States* are from the Medical Statistical Information System (MSIS). MSIS payment data are from electronic Medicaid data submitted to the Centers for Medicare & Medicaid Services by each state. Payment data are based on adjudicated claims for medical services reimbursed with Title XIX funds.

Medical specialty—See Physician specialty.

Medicare—Medicare is a nationwide health insurance program providing health insurance protection to people 65 years of age and over, people entitled to Social Security disability payments for 2 years or more (with limited exceptions for people with specific diagnoses), and people with end-stage renal disease, regardless of income. The program was enacted July 30, 1965, as Title XVIII, Health Insurance for the Aged of the Social Security Act, and became effective July 1, 1966. From its inception, it has included two separate but coordinated programs: hospital insurance (Part A) and supplementary medical insurance (Part B). In 1999, additional choices were allowed for delivering Medicare Part A and Part B benefits. Medicare Advantage (previously Medicare+Choice) (Part C) is an expanded set of options for the delivery of health care under Medicare, created in the Balanced Budget Act passed by Congress in 1997. The term Medicare Advantage refers to options other than those in original Medicare. Although all Medicare beneficiaries can receive their benefits through the original fee-for-service program, most beneficiaries enrolled in both Part A and Part B can choose to participate in a Medicare Advantage plan instead. Organizations that seek to contract as Medicare Advantage plans must meet specific organizational, financial, and other requirements. Most Medicare Advantage plans are coordinated care plans, which include health maintenance organizations, preferred provider organizations, private fee-for-service plans, medical savings account (MSA) plans—which provide benefits after a single high deductible is met—and special needs plans. These programs are available in only a limited number of states. For those providers who agree to accept the plan's payment terms and conditions, this option does not place the providers at risk, nor does it vary payment rates based on utilization. Only the coordinated care plans are considered managed care plans. Except for MSA plans, all Medicare Advantage plans are required to provide at least the current Medicare benefit package, excluding hospice services. Plans may offer additional covered services and are required to do so (or return excess payments) if plan costs are lower than the Medicare payments received by the plan.

The Medicare Prescription Drug, Improvement, and Modernization Act (also called the Medicare Modernization Act, or MMA) was passed December 8, 2003. The MMA established a voluntary drug benefit for Medicare beneficiaries and created a new Medicare Part D. People eligible for Medicare could begin to enroll in Part D beginning in January 2006. For more information see: http://www.medicare.gov/publications/pubs/pdf/10050.pdf. (Also see Appendix II, Fee-for-service health insurance; Health insurance coverage; Health maintenance organization; Managed care; and Appendix I, Medicare Administrative Data.)

Mental health organization—The Center for Mental Health Services of the Substance Abuse and Mental Health Services Administration defines a mental health organization as an administratively distinct public or private agency or institution whose primary concern is provision of direct mental health services to the mentally ill or emotionally disturbed. Excluded are private office-based practices of psychiatrists, psychologists, and other mental health providers; psychiatric services of all types of hospitals or outpatient clinics operated by federal agencies other than the Department of Veterans Affairs (e.g., Public Health Service, Indian Health Service, Department of Defense, and Bureau of Prisons); general hospitals that have no separate psychiatric services but admit psychiatric patients to nonpsychiatric units; and psychiatric services of schools, colleges, halfway houses, community residential organizations, local and county jails, state prisons, and other human services providers. The major types of mental health organizations are described below.

Freestanding psychiatric outpatient clinic—These clinics provide only outpatient mental health services on either a regular or emergency basis. A psychiatrist generally assumes the medical responsibility for services.

Psychiatric hospital—These hospitals primarily provide 24-hour inpatient care and treatment in a hospital setting to persons with mental illnesses. Psychiatric hospitals may be under state, county, private for-profit, or private nonprofit auspices.

General hospital psychiatric service—These are organizations that provide psychiatric services with assigned staff for 24-hour inpatient or residential care and/or less than 24-hour outpatient care in a separate ward, unit, floor, or wing of the hospital.

Department of Veterans Affairs medical center—These are hospitals operated by the Department of Veterans Affairs (formerly Veterans Administration) that include general hospital psychiatric services (including large neuro-psychiatric units) and psychiatric outpatient clinics.

Residential treatment center for emotionally disturbed children—These centers must meet all of the following criteria: (a) provide 24-hour residential services; (b) are not licensed as a psychiatric hospital and have the primary purpose of providing individually planned mental health treatment services in conjunction with residential care; (c) include a clinical program directed by a psychiatrist, psychologist, social worker, or psychiatric nurse with a graduate degree; (d) serve children and youth primarily under the age of 18; and (e) have the primary diagnosis as mental illness, classified as other than mental retardation, developmental disability, or substance-related disorders, according to the *Diagnostic and Statistical Manual of Mental Disorders* (DSM), 2nd edition *International Classification of Diseases* adapted for use in the United States (ICDA), 8th revision (DSM–II/ICDA–8); or DSM, 3rd edition, revised/ICD, 9th revision, Clinical Modification (DSM–IIIR/ICD–9–CM) codes, for the majority of admissions.

Multiservice mental health organization—These organizations provide services in both 24-hour and less-than-24-hour settings and are not classifiable as a psychiatric hospital, general hospital, or residential treatment center for emotionally disturbed children. (The classification of a psychiatric or general hospital or residential treatment center for emotionally disturbed children takes precedence over a multiservice classification, even if two or more services are offered.)

Partial care organization—These organizations provide a program of ambulatory mental health services or rehabilitation, habitation, or education programs.

(Also see Appendix II, Admission; Mental health service type.)

Mental health service type—This term refers to the following types of mental health services:

24-hour mental health care, formerly called inpatient care, provides care in a mental health hospital setting.

Less-than-24-hour care, formerly called outpatient or partial care treatment, provides mental health services on an ambulatory basis.

Residential treatment care, provides overnight mental health care in conjunction with an intensive treatment program in a setting other than a hospital. Facilities may offer care to emotionally disturbed children or mentally ill adults.

(Also see Appendix II, Admission; Mental health organization.)

Metropolitan statistical area (MSA)—The Office of Management and Budget (OMB) defines MSAs according to published standards that are applied to U.S. Census Bureau data. The standards are revised periodically, generally prior to the decennial census. The most recent standards were released in June 2010 (available from: http://www.whitehouse.gov/sites/default/files/omb/assets/fedreg_2010/06282010_metro_standards-Complete.pdf) but have not yet been applied to data presented in *Health, United States*. In the 2000 standards, an MSA is a county or group of contiguous counties that contains at least one urbanized area of 50,000 or more population. In addition to the county or counties that contain all or part of the urbanized area, an MSA may contain other counties if there are strong economic ties with the central county or counties, as measured by commuting. Counties that are not within an MSA are considered to be nonmetropolitan. For additional information, see: http://www.census.gov/population/www/metroareas/metroarea.html and http://www.whitehouse.gov/omb/bulletins_fy05_b05-02. (Also see Appendix II, Urbanization.)

For respondents to the National Health Interview Survey (NHIS), designation of place of residence as metropolitan or nonmetropolitan is based on the following MSA definitions: for 2006 and beyond, on the June 2003 OMB definitions (2000 OMB standards applied to 2000 census data); for 1995–2005, on the June 1993 OMB definitions (1990 OMB standards applied to 1990 census data); for 1985–1994, on the June 1983 OMB definitions (1980 OMB standards applied to 1980 census data); and for years prior to 1985 shown in *Health, United States*, on April 1973 definitions (1971 OMB standards applied to 1970 census data). For estimates based on 2006 NHIS data combined with earlier years of NHIS, metropolitan status of residence for all years involved is based on the June 2003 definitions. Introduction of each set of standards may create a discontinuity in trends. For example, when coding is based on the 2000 census data and the 2000 standards, the percentage of the population under 65 years of age obtaining private insurance through the workplace in 2005 was 64.3% for persons residing within MSAs and 59.7% for persons living outside MSAs; when coding is based on the 1990 standards and 1990 census data, the percentages are 64.5% and 59.6%, respectively.

Designation of place of residence as metropolitan or nonmetropolitan for respondents to the National Immunization Survey (NIS) is based on 2000 census data and 2000 standards and the following versions and revisions of MSA definitions: for quarter 1 of 2009, on the November 2007 definitions; for 2008, on the December 2006 definitions; for quarter 4 of 2007, on the December 2006 definitions; for quarters 1–3 of 2007, on the December 2005 definitions; for 2006, on the November 2004 definitions; for 2005, on the December 2003 definitions; for quarters 3 and 4 of 2004, on the December 2003 definitions; and for quarters 1 and 2 of 2004 and quarter 4 of 2003, on the June 2003 definitions. For more information see: http://www.census.gov/population/www/metroareas/metroarea.html.

Micropolitan statistical area—The Office of Management and Budget (OMB) defines micropolitan statistical areas based on published standards that are applied to U.S. Census Bureau data. A micropolitan statistical area is a nonmetropolitan county or group of contiguous nonmetropolitan counties that contains an urban cluster of 10,000–49,999 persons. A micropolitan statistical area may include surrounding counties if there are strong economic ties with the central county or counties as measured by commuting. Nonmetropolitan counties that are not classified as part of a micropolitan statistical area are considered nonmicropolitan. For additional information about micropolitan statistical areas, see http://www.census.gov/population/www/metroareas/metroarea.html. (Also see Appendix II, Urbanization.)

Multiservice mental health organization—See Mental health organization.

Multum Lexicon Plus therapeutic class—Starting with 2003 data, NCHS used Lexicon Plus, a proprietary database (Cerner Multum, Inc.) to assist with data editing and classification of human drugs. Starting with 2005 data, Multum Lexicon Drug Database has also been used to assist with data collection. Data collected before 2003 were updated by adding a generic drug code from Multum Lexicon Drug Database. The Lexicon Plus is a comprehensive database of all prescription and some non-prescription drug products available in the U.S. drug market. It uses a three-level nested category system to assign a therapeutic classification to each drug (e.g., for atenolol: cardiovascular agents [level 1]; beta-adrenergic blocking agents [level 2]; cardioselective beta blockers [level 3]). Not all drugs have three classification levels; some may only have two [e.g., for diltiazem: cardiovascular agents [level 1]; calcium channel blocking agents [level 2]). Other drugs may have only one classification level.

All drugs in NCHS surveys were assigned into a Multum drug category, even those drugs not found in Multum's drug database. "Unspecified" drugs were assigned to their respective therapeutic category (e.g., hormones–unspecified: category id = 97, category name = hormones).

Data presented in *Health, United States* using Lexicon Plus are based on the second level of the nested category system (e.g., calcium channel blocking agents). A drug may have up to four drug therapeutic categories; drugs classified into more than one class were counted in each class. For example, if a person reported taking lorazepam, that respondent was classified as taking an anticonvulsant and an anxiolytics, sedatives, and hypnotics drug.

For more information, see: http://www.cdc.gov/nchs/nhanes/nhanes2007-2008/RXQ_DRUG.htm.

Neonatal mortality rate—See Rate: Death and related rates.

Nonprofit hospital—See Hospital.

North American Industry Classification System (NAICS)—See Industry of employment.

Notifiable disease—A notifiable disease is one that, when diagnosed, health providers are required, usually by law, to report to state or local public health officials. Notifiable diseases are those of public interest by reason of their contagiousness, severity, or frequency. For more information, see: http://www.cdc.gov/ncphi/disss/nndss/phs/infdis.htm.

Nursing home—In the Online Survey Certification and Reporting (OSCAR) database, a nursing home is a facility that is certified and meets the Centers for Medicare & Medicaid Services' long-term care requirements for Medicare and Medicaid eligibility.

In the National Master Facility Inventory (NMFI), which provided the sampling frame for the 1973–1974, 1977, and 1985 National Nursing Home Surveys, a nursing home was an establishment with three or more beds that provided nursing or personal care services to the aged, infirm, or chronically ill. The 1977 National Nursing Home Survey included personal care homes and domiciliary care homes, whereas the National Nursing Home Surveys of 1973–1974, 1985, 1995, 1997, 1999, and 2004 excluded them. The following definitions of nursing home types applied to facilities listed in the NMFI:

Nursing care home—These homes employ one or more full-time registered or licensed practical nurses and provide nursing care to at least one-half of residents.

Personal care home with nursing—These homes have fewer than one-half of residents receiving nursing care. In addition, such homes employ one or more registered or licensed practical nurses or provide administration of medications and treatments in accordance with physicians' orders, supervision of self-administered medications, or three or more personal services.

Personal care home without nursing—These homes have no residents who receive nursing care. The homes provide administration of medications and treatments in accordance with physicians' orders, supervise self-administered medications, or provide three or more personal services.

Domiciliary care home—These homes primarily provide supervisory care and one or two personal services.

The following definitions of certification levels apply to data collected in the National Nursing Home Surveys of 1973–1974, 1977, and 1985:

Skilled nursing facility—These facilities provide the most intensive nursing care available outside a hospital. Facilities certified by Medicare provide posthospital care to eligible Medicare enrollees. Facilities certified by Medicaid as skilled nursing facilities provide skilled nursing services on a daily basis to individuals eligible for Medicaid benefits.

Intermediate care facility—These facilities are certified by Medicaid to provide health-related services on a regular basis to Medicaid eligibles who do not require hospital or skilled nursing facility care but do require institutional care above the level of room and board.

Not certified facility—These facilities are not certified by Medicare or Medicaid as providers of care.

Beginning with the 1995 National Nursing Home Survey, nursing homes have been defined as facilities that routinely provide nursing care services and have three or more beds set up for residents. Facilities may be certified by Medicare or Medicaid or not certified but licensed by the state as a nursing home. The facilities may be freestanding or a distinct unit of a larger facility.

After October 1, 1990, long-term care facilities that met the Omnibus Budget Reconciliation Act of 1987 (OBRA 87) nursing home reform requirements and were formerly certified under Medicaid as skilled nursing, nursing home, or intermediate care facilities were reclassified as nursing facilities. Medicare continues to certify skilled nursing facilities but not intermediate care facilities. State Medicaid programs can certify intermediate care facilities for the mentally retarded or developmentally disabled. In order to be certified for participation in Medicaid, nursing facilities must also be certified to participate in Medicare (except those facilities that have obtained waivers). Thus, most nursing home care is now provided in skilled care facilities. (Also see Appendix II, Long-term care facility; Nursing home; Resident, health facility.)

Nursing home expenditures—See Health expenditures, national.

Obesity—See Body mass index.

Occupancy rate—In American Hospital Association statistics, hospital occupancy rate is calculated as the average daily census divided by the number of hospital beds, cribs, and pediatric bassinets set up and staffed on the last day of the reporting period, expressed as a percentage. Average daily census is calculated by dividing the total annual number of inpatients, excluding newborns, by 365 days to derive the number of inpatients receiving care on an average day during the annual reporting period. The occupancy rate for facilities other than hospitals is calculated as the number of residents at the facility reported on the day of interview, divided by the number of reported beds. In the Online Survey Certification and Reporting (OSCAR) database, occupancy is determined as of the day of certification inspection as the total number of residents on that day divided by the total number of beds on that day.

Office-based physician—See Physician.

Office visit—In the National Ambulatory Medical Care Survey, a physician's ambulatory practice (office) can be in any location other than in a hospital, nursing home, other extended care facility, patient's home, industrial clinic, college clinic, or family planning clinic. Offices in health maintenance organizations and private offices in hospitals are included. An office visit is any direct personal exchange between an ambulatory patient and a physician or members of his or her staff for the purposes of seeking care and rendering health services. (Also see Appendix II, Outpatient visit.)

Operation—See Procedure.

Outpatient department—According to the National Hospital Ambulatory Medical Care Survey (NHAMCS), an outpatient department (OPD) is a hospital facility where nonurgent ambulatory medical care is provided. The following types of OPDs are excluded from the NHAMCS: ambulatory surgical centers, chemotherapy, employee health services, renal dialysis, methadone maintenance, and radiology. (Also see Appendix II, Emergency department; Outpatient visit.)

Outpatient surgery—According to the American Hospital Association, outpatient surgery is a surgical operation, whether major or minor, performed on patients who do not remain in the hospital overnight. Outpatient surgery may be performed in inpatient operating suites, outpatient surgery suites, or procedure rooms within an outpatient care facility. A surgical operation involving more than one surgical procedure is considered one surgical operation. (Also see Appendix II, Procedure.)

Outpatient visit—The American Hospital Association defines outpatient visits as visits for receipt of medical, dental, or other services at a hospital by patients who are not lodged in the hospital. Each appearance by an outpatient to each unit of the hospital is counted individually as an outpatient visit, including all clinic visits, referred

visits, observation services, outpatient surgeries, and emergency department visits. In the National Hospital Ambulatory Medical Care Survey, an outpatient department visit is a direct personal exchange between a patient and a physician or other health care provider working under the physician's supervision for the purpose of seeking care and receiving personal health services. (Also see Appendix II, Emergency department or emergency room visit; Outpatient department.)

Overweight—See Body mass index.

Pap smear—A Pap smear (also known as a Papanicolaou smear or Pap test) is a microscopic examination of cells scraped from the cervix that is used to detect cancerous or precancerous conditions of the cervix or other medical conditions.

In the National Health Interview Survey, questions concerning Pap smear use were asked on an intermittent schedule, and the question content differed slightly across years. In 1987, women were asked to report when they had their most recent Pap smear, in days, weeks, months, or years. Women who did not respond were asked a follow-up question, "Was it 3 years ago or less, between 3 and 5 years, or 5 years or more ago?" Pap smear data in the past 3 years were not available in 1990 and 1991. In 1993 and 1994, women were asked whether they had a Pap smear within the past year, between 1 and 3 years ago, or more than 3 years ago. In 1998, women were asked whether they had a Pap smear 1 year ago or less, more than 1 year but not more than 2 years, more than 2 years but not more than 3 years, more than 3 years but not more than 5 years, or more than 5 years ago.

In 1999, women were asked when they had their most recent Pap smear, in days, weeks, months, or years. In 1999, 4% of women in the sample responded 3 years ago. In *Health, United States*, these women were coded as within the past 3 years, although a response of 3 years ago may include women whose last Pap smear was more than 3 but less than 4 years ago. Thus, estimates for 1999 may be overestimated to some degree in comparison with estimates for previous years.

In 2000 and 2003, women were asked when they had their most recent Pap smear (give month and year). Women who did not respond were given a follow-up question that used the 1999 wording, and women who did not answer the follow-up question were asked a second follow-up question that used the 1998 wording. In 2000 and 2003, less than 1% of women in the sample answered 3 years ago using the 1999 wording, and they were coded as within the past 3 years. Therefore, estimates for 2000 and 2003 may be slightly overestimated in comparison with estimates for years prior to 1999.

In 2005, women were asked the same series of questions about Pap smear use as in the 2000 and 2003 surveys, but the skip pattern was modified so that more women were asked the follow-up question using the 1998 wording. Because additional information was available for women who replied that their last Pap smear was 3 years ago, these women were not uniformly coded as having had a Pap smear within the past 3 years. Thus, estimates for 2005 are more precise than estimates for 1999, 2000, and 2003 and are slightly lower than they would have been without this additional information. For example, using the improved methodology instituted in 2005, 77.7% of women 18 years of age and over reported a Pap smear in the past 3 years, compared with an estimate of 78.3% in 2005 using the method employed in 2000 and 2003. SAS code to categorize Pap smear data for 2000 and beyond is available from: http://www.cdc.gov/nchs/nhis/nhis_2005_data_release.htm.

In 2008, Pap smear questions were identical to those asked in 2005.

All women 18 years of age and over are asked the Pap smear question(s). In some data years, a series of questions was asked that also included information about hysterectomy. Women who reported having had a hysterectomy (removal of the uterus, with or without removal of the ovaries and cervix) were still asked the Pap smear questions because a woman who has had a hysterectomy may still have Pap smear testing.

The U.S. Preventive Services Task Force recommends against routine Pap smear screening in women who have had a total hysterectomy for benign disease. Therefore, two measures of Pap smear screening are presented in *Health, United States*: one among all women and one among women who did not report having a hysterectomy. Questions about whether the respondent had a hysterectomy were not asked in 2003. For other survey years, questions about hysterectomy in the National Health Interview Survey differed slightly. In 1987, women who reported that they had not had a recent Pap smear were asked the most important reason they had not had a Pap smear. One reason women could select was because they had had a hysterectomy. In 1993, 1994, 1998, and 1999, women were asked, "Have you had a hysterectomy?" In 2000, 2005, and 2008, two questions were used to determine if women had had a hysterectomy. Women were asked, "Have you had a hysterectomy?" In addition, women who reported

that they had not had a recent Pap smear were asked the most important reason they had not had a Pap smear. One reason women could select was because they had had a hysterectomy. Women indicating in either of these questions that they had had a hysterectomy were excluded from the Pap smear screening estimates.

Pap smear screening recommendations have changed over time and vary in the recommended age to begin and end screening and the interval for screening. For a summary of the current and historic recommendations see: U.S. Preventive Services Task Force. Screening for cervical cancer: Recommendations and rationale. Rockville, MD: Agency for Healthcare Research and Quality; 2003. Available from: http://www.ahrq.gov/clinic/3rduspstf/cervcan/cervcanrr.pdf; and see: U.S. Preventive Services Task Force. The guide to clinical preventive services, 2008. Rockville, MD: Agency for Healthcare Research and Quality; 2008. Available from: http://www.ahrq.gov/clinic/pocketgd.htm.

Partial care organization—See Mental health organization.

Partial care treatment—See Mental health service type.

Patient—See Inpatient; Office visit; Outpatient visit.

Percent change/percentage change—See Average annual rate of change (percent change).

Perinatal mortality rate; ratio—See Rate: Death and related rates.

Personal care home with or without nursing—See Nursing home.

Personal health care expenditures—See Health expenditures, national.

Physical activity, leisure-time—Starting with *Health, United States, 2010*, estimates on leisure-time physical activity changed to reflect the 2008 Federal Physical Activity Guidelines for Americans (available from: http://www.health.gov/PAGuidelines/guidelines/default.aspx. Adults who met the 2008 guidelines reported at least 150 minutes per week of moderate-intensity or 75 minutes per week of vigorous-intensity aerobic physical activity (or an equivalent combination of moderate- and vigorous-intensity aerobic activity) and muscle-strengthening activities at least twice a week. The estimates for the percentage of Americans who met the 2008 guidelines for aerobic and muscle strengthening are not comparable to estimates shown in previous editions of *Health, United States* that showed the percentage of Americans with regular leisure-time physical activity. For more information, see: Carlson SA, Fulton JE, Schoenborn CA, Loustalot F. Trend and prevalence estimates based on the 2008 Physical Activity Guidelines for Americans. Am J Prev Med 2010;39(4)305–13.

Starting with 1998 data, leisure-time physical activity has been assessed in the National Health Interview Survey (NHIS) by asking adults a series of questions about how often they do vigorous or light/moderate physical activity of at least 10 minutes duration and about how long these sessions generally last. All questions related to leisure-time physical activity were phrased in terms of current behavior and lack a specific reference period. Vigorous physical activity is described as causing heavy sweating or a large increase in breathing or heart rate, and light/moderate as causing light sweating or a slight to moderate increase in breathing or heart rate. Adults were also asked about how often they did leisure-time physical activities specifically designed to strengthen their muscles, such as lifting weights or doing calisthenics. For more information see the NHIS physical activity website at: http://www.cdc.gov/nchs/nhis/physical_activity.htm.

Physician—Data on physician characteristics are obtained through physician self-report from the American Medical Association's (AMA) Physician Masterfile. The AMA tabulates data only for doctors of medicine (MDs), but some tables in *Health, United States* include data for both MDs and doctors of osteopathy (DOs).

Active (or professionally active) physician—These physicians are currently engaged in patient care or other professional activity for a minimum of 20 hours per week. Other professional activity includes administration, medical teaching, research, and other activities such as employment with insurance carriers, pharmaceutical companies, corporations, voluntary organizations, and medical societies. Physicians who are retired, semiretired, working part-time, or not practicing are classified as inactive and are excluded. Also excluded are physicians with unknown address and physicians who did not provide information on type of practice or present employment (not classified).

Hospital-based physician—These physicians are employed under contract with hospitals to provide direct patient care and include physicians in residency training (including clinical fellows) and full-time members of the hospital staff.

Office-based physician—These physicians are engaged in seeing patients in solo practice, group practice, two-physician practice, other patient care employment, or in providing inpatient services such as those offered by pathologists and radiologists.

Data for physicians are presented by type of education (doctors of medicine and doctors of osteopathy); place of education (U.S. medical graduates and international medical graduates); activity status (professionally active and inactive); area of specialty; and geographic area. (Also see Appendix II, Physician specialty.)

Physician specialty—A physician specialty is any specific branch of medicine in which a physician may concentrate. Data are based on physician self-reports of their primary area of specialty. Physician data are broadly categorized into two areas of practice: those who provide primary care and those who provide specialty care.

Primary care generalist—These physicians practice in the general fields of family medicine, general practice, internal medicine, obstetrics and gynecology, and pediatrics. Specifically excluded are primary care specialists associated with these generalist fields.

Primary care specialist—These specialists practice in the primary care subspecialties of family medicine, internal medicine, obstetrics and gynecology, and pediatrics. Family medicine subspecialties include geriatric medicine and sports medicine. Internal medicine subspecialties include adolescent medicine, critical care medicine, diabetes, endocrinology, diabetes and metabolism, hematology, hepatology, hematology/oncology, cardiac electrophysiology, infectious diseases, clinical and laboratory immunology, geriatric medicine, sports medicine, nephrology, nutrition, medical oncology, pulmonary critical care medicine, and rheumatology. Obstetrics and gynecology subspecialties include gynecological oncology, gynecology, maternal and fetal medicine, obstetrics, critical care medicine, and reproductive endocrinology. Pediatric subspecialties include adolescent medicine, pediatric critical care medicine, pediatrics/internal medicine, neonatal–perinatal medicine, pediatric allergy, pediatric cardiology, pediatric endocrinology, pediatric infectious disease, pediatric pulmonology, medical toxicology (pediatrics), pediatric emergency medicine, pediatric gastroenterology, pediatric hematology/oncology, clinical and laboratory immunology (pediatrics), pediatric nephrology, pediatric rheumatology, and sports medicine (pediatrics).

Specialty care physician—These physicians are sometimes called specialists and include primary care specialists listed above in addition to all other physicians not included in the generalist definition. Specialty fields include allergy and immunology, aerospace medicine, anesthesiology, cardiovascular diseases, child and adolescent psychiatry, colon and rectal surgery, dermatology, diagnostic radiology, forensic pathology, gastroenterology, general surgery, medical genetics, neurology, nuclear medicine, neurological surgery, occupational medicine, ophthalmology, orthopedic surgery, otolaryngology, psychiatry, public health and general preventive medicine, physical medicine and rehabilitation, plastic surgery, anatomic and clinical pathology, pulmonary diseases, radiation oncology, thoracic surgery, urology, addiction medicine, critical care medicine, legal medicine, and clinical pharmacology.

(Also see Appendix II, Physician.)

Population—The U.S. Census Bureau collects and publishes data on populations in the United States according to several different definitions. Various statistical systems then use the appropriate population for calculating rates. (Also see Appendix I, Population Census and Population Estimates.)

Resident population includes persons whose usual place of residence (i.e., the place where one usually lives and sleeps) is in one of the 50 states or the District of Columbia. It includes members of the Armed Forces stationed in the United States and their families. It excludes members of the Armed Forces stationed outside the United States and civilian U.S. citizens whose usual place of residence is outside the United States. The resident population is the denominator for calculating birth and death rates and incidence of disease.

Civilian population is the resident population excluding members of the Armed Forces, although families of members of the Armed Forces are included. The civilian population is the denominator in rates calculated for the National Home and Hospice Care Survey, the National Hospital Discharge Survey, and the National Nursing Home Survey, and for emergency department visit rates using the National Hospital

Ambulatory Medical Care Survey—Emergency Department Component.

Civilian noninstitutionalized population is the civilian population excluding persons residing in institutions (such as nursing homes, prisons, jails, mental hospitals, and juvenile correctional facilities). U.S. Census Bureau estimates of the civilian noninstitutionalized population are used to calculate sample weights for the National Health Interview Survey, the National Health and Nutrition Examination Survey, and the National Survey of Family Growth, and as denominators in rates calculated for the National Ambulatory Medical Care Survey and the National Hospital Ambulatory Medical Care Survey—Outpatient Department Component.

Postneonatal mortality rate—See Rate: Death and related rates.

Poverty—Poverty statistics are based on definitions originally developed by the Social Security Administration. These include a set of money income thresholds that vary by family size and composition. Families or individuals with income below the appropriate threshold are classified as below poverty. These thresholds are updated annually by the U.S. Census Bureau using the change in the average annual Consumer Price Index for all urban consumers (CPI–U). For example, the average poverty threshold for a family of four was $22,128 in 2009, $22,025 in 2008, $17,603 in 2000, and $13,359 in 1990. For more information, see: DeNavas-Walt C, Proctor BD, Smith JC. Income, poverty, and health insurance coverage in the United States: 2008. U.S. Census Bureau Current Population Report, P60–236. Washington, DC: U.S. Government Printing Office; 2009. Available from: http://www.census.gov/prod/2009pubs/p60-236.pdf.

Also see the U.S. Census Bureau's poverty website at: http://www.census.gov/hhes/www/poverty/poverty.html.

National Health Interview Survey (NHIS) and *National Health and Nutrition Examination Survey (NHANES)*—Percent of poverty level, for years prior to 1997, was based on family income and family size using U.S. Census Bureau poverty thresholds. Starting with 1997 data, percent of poverty level has been based on family income, family size, number of children in the family, and for families with two or fewer adults, the age of the adults in the family. Percent of poverty level in NHANES is also based on family income and family size and composition. (Also see Appendix II, Consumer Price Index; Family income; and

Appendix I, Current Population Survey; National Health Interview Survey; National Health and Nutrition Examination Survey.)

Preferred provider organization (PPO)—A PPO is a type of medical plan in which coverage is provided to participants through a network of selected health care providers, such as hospitals and physicians. Enrollees may seek care outside the network but pay a greater percentage of the cost of coverage than within the network. (Also see Appendix II, Health maintenance organization; Managed care.)

Prenatal care—Prenatal care is medical care provided to a pregnant woman to prevent complications and decrease the incidence of maternal and prenatal mortality. Information on when pregnancy care began is recorded on the birth certificate. Between 1970 and 1980, the reporting area for prenatal care expanded. In 1970, 39 states and the District of Columbia (D.C.) reported prenatal care on the birth certificate. Data were not available from Alabama, Alaska, Arkansas, Connecticut, Delaware, Georgia, Idaho, Massachusetts, New Mexico, Pennsylvania, and Virginia. In 1975, data were available from three additional states (Connecticut, Delaware, and Georgia), increasing the number of states reporting prenatal care to 42 and D.C. During 1980–2002, prenatal care information was available for the entire United States.

Starting in 2003, some states began implementation of the 2003 revision of the U.S. Standard Certificate of Live Birth. The prenatal care item on the 2003 revision of the certificate asks for the date of first prenatal visit, whereas the prenatal care item on the 1989 revision asks for the month prenatal care began. In addition, the 2003 revision recommends that information on prenatal care be gathered from prenatal care or medical records, whereas the 1989 revision did not recommend a source for these data. Data on prenatal care from the 2003 revision of the birth certificate are not comparable with data from the 1989 revision. Therefore, 2006 and 2007 data on prenatal care are shown separately for the 28 reporting areas (26 states, D.C., and New York City) that used the 1989 revision for data on prenatal care in 2006 and 2007 and for the 18 reporting areas that used the 2003 revision in 2006 and 2007, in order to provide 2 years of comparable data. The 28 reporting areas using the 1989 certificate are Alabama, Alaska, Arizona, Arkansas, Connecticut, Hawaii, Illinois, Louisiana, Maine, Massachusetts, Maryland, Minnesota, Mississippi, Missouri, Montana, Nevada, New Jersey, New Mexico, North Carolina, Oklahoma, Oregon, Rhode Island, Utah, Virginia, West Virginia, Wisconsin, D.C., and New York City. The states that used the 2003 revision of the U.S. Standard Certificate of Live Birth for data on prenatal care in 2006 and 2007 are Delaware, Florida, Idaho, Kansas, Kentucky, Nebraska, New Hampshire, New York state (excluding New York City), North Dakota, Ohio, Pennsylvania, South Carolina, South Dakota, Tennessee, Texas, Vermont, Washington state, and Wyoming. Data are not shown in *Health, United States* for states that were transitioning to the 2003 revision during 2006 and 2007. Although California implemented the 2003 revision in 2006, the state did not revise the prenatal care question; therefore, prenatal care data for California are included with data for the states that used the 1989 revision in 2006 and 2007.

Prevalence—Prevalence is the number of cases of a disease, number of infected persons, or number of persons with some other attribute present during a particular interval of time. It is often expressed as a rate (e.g., the prevalence of diabetes per 1,000 persons during a year). (Also see Appendix II, Incidence.)

Primary care specialty—See Physician specialty.

Private expenditures—See Health expenditures, national.

Procedure—The National Hospital Discharge Survey (NHDS) used to classify a procedure as a surgical or nonsurgical operation, diagnostic procedure, or therapeutic procedure (such as respiratory therapy); however, the distinction between types of procedures has become less meaningful because of the development of minimally invasive and noninvasive surgery. Thus, the practice of classifying the type of procedure has been discontinued. Procedures are coded according to the *International Classification of Diseases, 9th Revision, Clinical Modification* (see Table XII). Up to four different procedures are coded in the NHDS. Procedures per hospital stay can be classified as any-listed—that is, if more than one procedure with the same code is performed it is counted only once—or all-listed, where multiple occurrences of the same procedure are counted each time they appear on the medical record, up to the maximum of four available codes. Because all-listed procedures overcount the number of procedures of a given type that are performed, all-listed procedure counts are greater than the number of hospital stays that occurred. Any-listed procedure counts approximate the number of hospital stays where a procedure was performed at any time during the stay. (Also see Appendix II, Outpatient surgery.)

Proprietary hospital—See Hospital.

Psychiatric hospital—See Hospital; Mental health organization.

Public expenditures—See Health expenditures, national.

Purchasing power parities (PPPs)—PPPs are calculated rates of currency conversion that equalize the purchasing power of different currencies by eliminating the differences in price levels between countries. PPPs show the ratio of prices in national currencies for the same good or service in different countries. PPPs can be used to make intercountry comparisons of the gross domestic product (GDP) and its component expenditures. (Also see Appendix II, Gross domestic product.)

Race—In 1977, the Office of Management and Budget (OMB) issued Race and Ethnic Standards for Federal Statistics and Administrative Reporting (Statistical Policy Directive 15) to promote comparability of data among federal data systems. The 1977 Standards called for the federal government's data systems to classify individuals into the following four racial groups: American Indian or Alaska Native, Asian or Pacific Islander, black, and white. Depending on the data source, the classification by race was based on self-classification or on observation by an interviewer or other person filling out the questionnaire.

In 1997, revisions were announced for classification of individuals by race within the federal government's data systems. [See: Revisions to the Standards for the Classification of Federal Data on Race and Ethnicity. Fed Regist 1997 October 30;62(210):58781–90.] The 1997 Standards specify five racial groups: American Indian or Alaska Native, Asian, black or African American, Native Hawaiian or Other Pacific Islander, and white. These five categories are the minimum set for data on race in federal statistics. The 1997 Standards also offer an opportunity for respondents to select more than one of the five groups, leading to many possible multiple-race categories. As with the single-race groups, data for the multiple-race groups are to be reported when estimates meet agency requirements for reliability and confidentiality. The 1997 Standards allow for observer or proxy identification of race but clearly state a preference for self-classification. The federal government considers race and Hispanic origin to be two separate and distinct concepts. Thus, Hispanics may be of any race. Federal data systems were required to comply with the 1997 Standards by 2003.

National Health Interview Survey (NHIS)—Starting with *Health, United States, 2002*, race-specific estimates based on NHIS were tabulated using the 1997 Standards for data year 1999 and beyond and are not strictly comparable with estimates for earlier years. The 1997 Standards specify five single-race categories plus multiple-race categories. Estimates for specific race groups are shown when they meet requirements for statistical reliability and confidentiality. The race categories white only, black or African American only, American Indian or Alaska Native only, Asian only, and Native Hawaiian or Other Pacific Islander only include persons who reported only one racial group; the category 2 or more races includes persons who reported more than one of the five racial groups in the 1997 Standards or one of the five racial groups and "some other race." Prior to data year 1999, data were tabulated according to the 1977 Standards, with four racial groups, and the Asian only category included Native Hawaiian or Other Pacific Islander. Estimates for single-race categories prior to 1999 included persons who reported one race or, if they reported more than one race, identified one race as best representing their race. Differences between estimates tabulated using the two standards for data year 1999 are discussed in the footnotes for each NHIS table in the *Health, United States* 2002, 2003, and 2004 editions. Available from: http://www.cdc.gov/nchs/hus/previous.htm#editions.

Tables XIII and XIV illustrate NHIS data tabulated by race and Hispanic origin according to the 1997 and 1977 Standards for two health statistics (cigarette smoking and private health insurance coverage). In these examples, three separate tabulations using the 1997 Standards are shown: (a) Race: mutually exclusive race groups, including several multiple-race combinations; (b) Race, any mention: race groups that are not mutually exclusive because each race category includes all persons who mention that race; and (c) Hispanic origin and race: detailed race and Hispanic origin with a multiple-race total category. Where applicable, comparison tabulations by race and Hispanic origin are shown based on the 1977 Standards. Because there are more race groups with the 1997 Standards, the sample size of each race group under the 1997 Standards is slightly smaller than the sample size under the 1977 Standards. Only those few multiple-race groups with sufficient numbers of observations to meet standards of statistical reliability are shown. Tables XIII and XIV also illustrate changes in labels and group categories resulting from the 1997 Standards. The race

Table XIII. Current cigarette smoking among persons 18 years of age and over, by race and Hispanic origin under the 1997 and 1977 Standards for federal data on race and ethnicity: United States, average annual 1993–1995

1997 Standards	Sample size	Percent	Standard error	1977 Standards	Sample size	Percent	Standard error
White only.	46,228	25.2	0.26	White	46,664	25.3	0.26
Black or African American only . . .	7,208	26.6	0.64	Black.	7,334	26.5	0.63
American Indian or Alaska Native only.	416	32.9	2.53	American Indian or Alaska Native	480	33.9	2.38
Asian only	1,370	15.0	1.19	Asian or Pacific Islander	1,411	15.5	1.22
2 or more races total.	786	34.5	2.00				
Black or African American; white	83	*21.7	6.05				
American Indian or Alaska Native; white.	461	40.0	2.58				
			Race, any mention				
White, any mention	46,882	25.3	0.26				
Black or African American, any mention.	7,382	26.6	0.63				
American Indian or Alaska Native, any mention.	965	36.3	1.71				
Asian, any mention	1,458	15.7	1.20				
Native Hawaiian or Other Pacific Islander, any mention	53	*17.5	5.10				
			Hispanic origin and race				
Not Hispanic or Latino:				Non-Hispanic:			
White only	42,421	25.8	0.27	White	42,976	25.9	0.27
Black or African American only.	7,053	26.7	0.65	Black	7,203	26.7	0.64
American Indian or Alaska Native only	358	33.5	2.69	American Indian or Alaska Native.	407	35.4	2.53
Asian only	1,320	14.8	1.21	Asian or Pacific Islander	1,397	15.3	1.24
2 or more races total	687	35.6	2.15				
Hispanic or Latino.	5,175	17.8	0.65	Hispanic.	5,175	17.8	0.65

* Estimates are considered unreliable. Data preceded by an asterisk have a relative standard error of 20%–30%.

NOTES: The Office of Management and Budget's (OMB) 1997 Revisions to the Standards for the Classification of Federal Data on Race and Ethnicity specifies five race groups (white, black or African American, American Indian or Alaska Native, Asian, and Native Hawaiian or Other Pacific Islander) and allows respondents to report one or more race groups. Estimates for single-race and multiple-race groups not shown above do not meet standards for statistical reliability or confidentiality (relative standard error greater than 30%). Race groups under the 1997 Standards were based on the question, "What is the group or groups which represents [person's] race?" For persons who selected multiple groups, race groups under the OMB's 1977 Race and Ethnic Standards for Federal Statistics and Administrative Reporting were based on the additional question, "Which of those groups would you say best represents [person's] race?" Race-specific estimates in this table were calculated after excluding respondents of other and unknown race. Other published race-specific estimates are based on files in which such responses have been edited. Estimates are age-adjusted to the year 2000 standard population using five age groups: 18–24 years, 25–34 years, 35–44 years, 45–64 years, and 65 years and over. See Appendix II, Age adjustment.

SOURCE: CDC/NCHS, National Health Interview Survey.

Table XIV. Private health care coverage among persons under 65 years of age, by race and Hispanic origin under the 1997 and 1977 Standards for federal data on race and ethnicity: United States, average annual 1993–1995

1997 Standards	Sample size	Percent	Standard error	1977 Standards	Sample size	Percent	Standard error
White only.	168,256	76.1	0.28	White	170,472	75.9	0.28
Black or African American only . . .	30,048	53.5	0.63	Black.	30,690	53.6	0.63
American Indian or Alaska Native only.	2,003	44.2	1.97	American Indian or Alaska Native	2,316	43.5	1.85
Asian only	6,896	68.0	1.39	Asian and Pacific Islander.	7,146	68.2	1.34
Native Hawaiian or Other Pacific Islander only	173	75.0	7.43				
2 or more races total.	4,203	60.9	1.17				
Black or African American; white	686	59.5	3.21				
American Indian or Alaska Native; white.	2,022	60.0	1.71				
Asian; white	590	71.9	3.39				
Native Hawaiian or Other Pacific Islander; white	56	59.2	10.65				

Race, any mention

1997 Standards	Sample size	Percent	Standard error
White, any mention	171,817	75.8	0.28
Black or African American, any mention.	31,147	53.6	0.62
American Indian or Alaska Native, any mention	4,365	52.4	1.40
Asian, any mention	7,639	68.4	1.27
Native Hawaiian or Other Pacific Islander, any mention	283	68.7	6.23

Hispanic origin and race

1997 Standards	Sample size	Percent	Standard error	1977 Standards	Sample size	Percent	Standard error
Not Hispanic or Latino:				Non-Hispanic:			
White only	146,109	78.9	0.27	White	149,057	78.6	0.27
Black or African American only.	29,250	53.9	0.64	Black	29,877	54.0	0.63
American Indian or Alaska Native only	1,620	45.2	2.15	American Indian or Alaska Native.	1,859	44.6	2.05
Asian only	6,623	68.2	1.43	Asian and Pacific Islander	6,999	68.4	1.40
Native Hawaiian or Other Pacific Islander only	145	76.4	7.79				
2 or more races total	3,365	62.6	1.18				
Hispanic or Latino.	31,040	48.8	0.74	Hispanic	31,040	48.8	0.74

NOTES: The Office of Management and Budget's (OMB) 1997 Revisions to the Standards for the Classification of Federal Data on Race and Ethnicity specifies five race groups (white, black or African American, American Indian or Alaska Native, Asian, and Native Hawaiian or Other Pacific Islander) and allows respondents to report one or more race groups. Estimates for single-race and multiple-race groups not shown above do not meet standards for statistical reliability or confidentiality (relative standard error greater than 30%). Race groups under the 1997 Standards were based on the question, "What is the group or groups which represents [person's] race?" For persons who selected multiple groups, race groups under the OMB's 1977 Race and Ethnic Standards for Federal Statistics and Administrative Reporting were based on the additional question, "Which of those groups would you say best represents [person's] race?" Race-specific estimates in this table were calculated after excluding respondents of other and unknown race. Other published race-specific estimates are based on files in which such responses have been edited. Estimates are age-adjusted to the year 2000 standard population using three age groups: under 18 years, 18–44 years, and 45–64 years. See Appendix II, Age adjustment.

SOURCE: CDC/NCHS, National Health Interview Survey.

designation black was changed to black or African American, and the ethnicity designation Hispanic was changed to Hispanic or Latino.

Data systems included in *Health, United States*, other than NHIS, the National Survey of Drug Use & Health (NSDUH), and the National Health and Nutrition Examination Survey (NHANES), generally do not permit tabulation of estimates for the detailed race and ethnicity categories shown in Tables XIII and XIV, either because race data based on the 1997 Standards categories are not yet available or because there are insufficient numbers of observations in certain subpopulation groups to meet statistical reliability or confidentiality requirements.

To improve the quality of data on ethnicity and race in NHIS, hot-deck imputation of selected race and ethnicity variables was done for the first time in the 2000 NHIS and continued to be used for subsequent data years. Starting with 2003 data, records for persons for whom "other race" was the only race response were treated as having missing data on race and were added to the pool of records for which selected race and ethnicity variables were imputed. Prior to the 2000 NHIS, a crude imputation method that assigned a race to persons with missing values for the variable MAINRACE (the respondent's classification of the race he or she most identified with) was used. Under these procedures, if an observed race was recorded by the interviewer, it was used to code a race value. If there was no observed race value, all persons who had a missing value for MAINRACE and were identified as Hispanic on the Hispanic origin question were coded as white. In all other cases, non-Hispanic persons were coded as "other race." Additional information on the NHIS methodology for imputing race and ethnicity is available from the survey documentation at: http://www.cdc.gov/nchs/nhis/quest_data_related_1997_forward.htm and from the NHIS race and Hispanic origin home page at: http://www.cdc.gov/nchs/nhis/rhoi.htm.

National Health and Nutrition Examination Survey (NHANES)—Starting with *Health, United States, 2003*, race-specific estimates based on NHANES were tabulated using the 1997 Standards for data years 1999 and beyond. Prior to data year 1999, the 1977 Standards were used. Because of the differences between the two standards, the race-specific estimates shown in trend tables based on NHANES for 1999–2004 are not strictly comparable with estimates for earlier years. Race in NHANES I and II was determined primarily by

interviewer observation; starting with NHANES III, race was self-reported by survey participants.

The NHANES sample for data years 1999–2006 was designed to provide estimates specifically for persons of Mexican origin and not for all Hispanic-origin persons in the United States. Persons of Hispanic origin other than Mexican were entered into the sample with different selection probabilities that are not nationally representative of the total U.S. Hispanic population. Starting with 2007–2008 data collection, all Hispanics were oversampled, not just Mexican Americans. Estimates are shown for non-Hispanic white, non-Hispanic black, and Mexican-origin persons. Although data were collected according to the 1997 Standards, there are insufficient numbers of observations to meet statistical reliability or confidentiality requirements for reporting estimates for additional race categories.

National Survey on Drug Use & Health (NSDUH)— Race-specific estimates based on NSDUH are tabulated using the 1997 Standards. Estimates in the NSDUH trend table begin with data year 2002. Estimates for specific race groups are shown when they meet requirements for statistical reliability and confidentiality. The race categories white only, black or African American only, American Indian or Alaska Native only, Asian only, and Native Hawaiian or Other Pacific Islander only include persons who reported only one racial group; the category 2 or more races includes persons who reported more than one of the five racial groups in the 1997 Standards or one of the five racial groups and "some other race."

National Vital Statistics System (NVSS)—Most of the states in the Vital Statistics Cooperative Program are still revising their birth and death records to conform to the 1997 Standards on race and ethnicity. During the transition to full implementation of the 1997 Standards, vital statistics data will continue to be presented for four major race groups—white, black or African American, American Indian or Alaska Native, and Asian or Pacific Islander—in accordance with the 1977 Standards.

Birth file—Information about the race and Hispanic ethnicity of the mother and father are provided by the mother at the time of birth and are recorded on the birth certificate and fetal death record. Since 1980, birth rates, birth characteristics, and death rates for live-born infants and fetal deaths are presented in *Health,*

United States according to race of mother. Before 1980, data were tabulated by race of the newborn and fetus, taking into account the race of both parents. If the parents were of different races and one parent was white, the child was classified according to the race of the other parent. When neither parent was white, the child was classified according to father's race, with one exception: if either parent was Hawaiian, the child was classified Hawaiian. Before 1964, if race was unknown, the birth was classified as white. Starting in 1964, unknown race was classified according to information on the birth record. Starting with the 2000 census, the race and ethnicity data used for denominators (population) to calculate birth and fertility rates have been collected in accordance with 1997 revised OMB standards for race and ethnicity. However, the numerators (births) will not be compatible with the denominators until all the states revise their birth certificates to reflect the new standards. To compute rates, it is currently necessary to bridge population data for multiple-race persons to single-race categories. (Also see Appendix I, Population Census and Population Estimates, Bridged-Race Population Estimates for Census 2000.)

Starting with 2003 data, multiple-race data were reported by both Pennsylvania and Washington state, which used the 2003 revision of the U.S. Standard Certificate of Live Birth, as well as by California, Hawaii, Ohio (for births occurring in December only), and Utah, which used the 1989 revision of the U.S. Standard Certificate of Live Birth. In 2004, multiple race was reported on the revised birth certificates of Florida (for births occurring after March 19, 2004, only), Idaho, Kentucky, New Hampshire (for births occurring after July 19, 2004, only), New York state (excluding New York City), Pennsylvania, South Carolina, Tennessee, and Washington state, as well as on the unrevised certificates of California, Hawaii, Michigan (for births at selected facilities only), Minnesota, Ohio, and Utah (a total of 15 states). For the 2005 data year, multiple race was also reported by those 15 states that reported multiple-race data in 2004 and additionally by Kansas, Nebraska, Texas, and Vermont (for births occurring from July 1, 2005, only) using the 2003 revision. In 2006, multiple race was additionally reported by Delaware, North Dakota, South Dakota, and Wyoming, which used the 2003 revision of the U.S. Standard Certificate of Live Birth. The 27 states reporting multiple race in 2007 represent 63% of all U.S. resident births.

More than one race was reported for 1.7% of mothers in the states that reported multiple race. Data from the vital records of the remaining 25 states, the District of Columbia (D.C.), and New York City followed the 1977 OMB Standards. In addition, these areas also report the minimum set of four race categories as stipulated in the 1977 Standards, compared with the minimum of five race categories for the 1997 Standards. To provide uniformity and comparability of the data during the transition period, before multiple-race data are available for all reporting areas, the responses of those who reported more than one race must be bridged to a single race. See: Martin JA, Hamilton BE, Sutton PD, Ventura SJ, Mathews TJ, Kirmeyer S, Osterman, MJK. Births: Final data for 2007. National vital statistics reports; vol 58 no 24. Hyattsville, MD: NCHS; 2010. Available from: http://www.cdc.gov/nchs/data/nvsr/nvsr58/nvsr58_24.pdf.

Although the bridging procedure imputes multiple race of mothers to one of the four minimum races stipulated in the 1977 Standards, mothers of a specified Asian or Pacific Islander (API) subgroup (Chinese, Japanese, Hawaiian, or Filipino) in combination with another race (American Indian or Alaska Native, black, and/or white) or another API subgroup cannot be imputed to a single API subgroup. API mothers are slightly overrepresented in the 27 states with complete reporting of multiple race for 2007 (which account for 66% of API births in the United States), compared with the remaining 23 states, New York City, and D.C. Data for the API subgroups are available in the 2007 Natality public-use data file at: http://www.cdc.gov/nchs/births.htm.

Mortality file—Information about the race and Hispanic ethnicity of a decedent is reported by the funeral director as provided by an informant, often the surviving next of kin, or in the absence of an informant, on the basis of observation. Death rates by race and Hispanic origin are based on information from death certificates (numerators of the rates) and on population estimates from the Census Bureau (denominators). Race and ethnicity information from the census is by self-report. To the extent that race and Hispanic origin are inconsistent between these two data sources, death rates will be biased. Studies have shown that persons self-reported as American Indian, Asian, or Hispanic on census and survey records may sometimes be reported as white or non-Hispanic on the death certificate, resulting in an underestimation of deaths and death rates for the American Indian, Asian, and Hispanic groups. Bias also results from undercounts of some population groups in the census, particularly young black males, young white males, and elderly persons, resulting in an overestimation of death rates. The net effects of misclassification and undercoverage result in overstated death rates for the white population and the black population estimated to be 1% and 5%, respectively. Understated death rates for other population groups are estimated as follows: American Indians, 21%; Asian or Pacific Islanders, 11%; and Hispanics, 2%. For more information, see: Rosenberg HM, Maurer JD, Sorlie PD, Johnson NJ, MacDorman MF, Hoyert DL, et al. Quality of death rates by race and Hispanic origin: A summary of current research, 1999. Vital Health Stat 2(128). Hyattsville, MD: NCHS; 1999; and see: Arias E, Schauman WS, Eschbach K, Sorlie PD, Backlund E. The validity of race and Hispanic origin reporting on death certificates in the United States. Vital Health Stat 2(148). Hyattsville, MD: NCHS; 2008.

Denominators for infant and maternal mortality rates are based on the number of live births, rather than on population estimates. Race information for the denominator is supplied from the birth certificate. Before 1980, race of child for the denominator took into account the races of both parents. Starting in 1980, race information for the denominator has been based solely on the race of the mother. Race information for the numerator is supplied from the death certificate. For the infant mortality rate, race information for the numerator is race of the deceased child; for the maternal mortality rate, it is race of the mother.

Issues affecting the interpretation of vital event rates for the American Indian or Alaska Native population include (a) the presence of two enumeration techniques for estimating the American Indian or Alaska Native population, (b) changes in the classification or self-identification of American Indian or Alaska Native heritage over time, and (c) misclassification of American Indian or Alaska Native persons on death certificates. Vital event rates for the American Indian or Alaska Native population shown in Health, United States are based on the total U.S. resident population of American Indians and Alaska Natives, as enumerated by the U.S. Census Bureau. In contrast, the Indian Health Service calculates vital event rates for this population based on U.S. Census Bureau county

data for American Indians and Alaska Natives who reside on or near reservations. Interpretation of trends for the American Indian and Alaska Native population should take into account that population estimates for these groups increased by 45% between 1980 and 1990, partly because of better enumeration techniques in the 1990 decennial census and the increased tendency for people to identify themselves as American Indian in 1990. Because of misclassification of American Indian or Alaska Native persons on death certificates (for some states, estimated at greater than 10%), or no information on misclassification, American Indian or Alaska Native state-specific mortality estimates published in Health, United States should be interpreted with caution.

Interpretation of trends for the Asian population in the United States should take into account that this population more than doubled between 1980 and 1990, primarily because of immigration. Between 1990 and 2000, the increase in the Asian population was 48% for persons reporting that they were Asian alone and 72% for persons who reported they were either Asian alone or Asian in combination with another race.

For more information on coding race by using vital statistics, see: NCHS. Vital statistics of the United States, vol I, Natality, and vol II, Mortality, part A, Technical appendix. Hyattsville, MD: NCHS; published annually. Available from: http://www.cdc.gov/nchs/nvss.htm.

Starting with 2003 data, some states began using the 2003 revision of the U.S. Standard Certificate of Death, which allows the reporting of more than one race (multiple races). This change was implemented to reflect the increasing diversity of the U.S. population and to be consistent with the decennial census. Most states, however, are still using the 1989 revision of the U.S. Standard Certificate of Death, which allows only a single race to be reported.

To provide uniformity and comparability of data until all states are reporting multiple-race data, it has been necessary to "bridge" the responses of those for whom more than one race is reported (multiple race) to one single race. The states using the 2003 death certificate and reporting multiple-race data from 2003 onward were California, Idaho, Montana, and New York; in addition, Hawaii, Maine, and Wisconsin reported multiple-race data using the 1989 revision of the death certificate. Starting with 2004, multiple-race data were reported for those seven states, plus Michigan, Minnesota, New Hampshire, New

Jersey, Oklahoma, South Dakota, Washington, and Wyoming. Starting with 2005, the seven additional reporting areas providing multiple-race data were Connecticut, D.C., Florida, Kansas, Nebraska, South Carolina, and Utah. Starting with 2006, the four additional states providing multiple-race data were New Mexico, Oregon, Rhode Island, and Texas; and starting in 2007, Delaware and Ohio provided multiple-race data. For more information on coding race by using vital statistics, see: Xu JQ, Kochanek, KD, Murphy SL, Tejada-Vera B. Deaths: Final data for 2007. National vital statistics reports; vol 58 no 19. Hyattsville, MD: NCHS; 2009. Available from: http://www.cdc.gov/nchs/data/nvsr/nvsr58/nvsr58_19.pdf; see: NCHS procedures for multiple-race and Hispanic origin data: Collection, coding, editing, and transmitting. Hyattsville, MD: NCHS; 2004. Available from: http://www.cdc.gov/nchs/data/dvs/Multiple_race_docu_5-10-04.pdf; and see: NCHS. Vital statistics of the United States, vol I, Natality, and vol II, Mortality, part A, Technical appendix. Hyattsville, MD: NCHS; published annually. Available from: http://www.cdc.gov/nchs/nvss.htm.

Youth Risk Behavior Survey (YRBS)—Prior to 1999, the 1977 OMB Standards were used. Respondents could select only one of the following categories: white (not Hispanic), black (not Hispanic), Hispanic or Latino, Asian or Pacific Islander, American Indian or Alaska Native, or other. Beginning in 1999, the 1997 OMB Standards were used for race-specific estimates, and respondents were given the option of selecting more than one category to describe their race/ethnicity. Between 1999 and 2003, students were asked a single question about race and Hispanic origin, with the option of choosing more than one of the following responses: white, black or African American, Hispanic or Latino, Asian, Native Hawaiian or Other Pacific Islander, or American Indian or Alaska Native. In 2005, students were asked a question about Hispanic origin ("Are you Hispanic or Latino?") and a second separate question about race that included the option of selecting more than one of the following categories: American Indian or Alaska Native, Asian, black or African American, Native Hawaiian or Other Pacific Islander, or white. Because of the differences between questions, data about race and Hispanic ethnicity for the years prior to 1999 are not strictly comparable with estimates for the later years. However,

analyses of data collected between 1991 and 2003 have indicated that the data are comparable across years and can be used to study trends.

See: Brener ND, Kann L, McManus T. A comparison of two survey questions on race and ethnicity among high school students. Public Opin Q 2003;67(2):227–36.

(Also see Appendix II, Hispanic origin; and Appendix I, Population Census and Population Estimates.)

Rate—A rate is a measure of some event, disease, or condition in relation to a unit of population, along with some specification of time. (Also see Appendix II, Age adjustment; Population.)

■ *Birth and related rates*

Birth rate is calculated by dividing the number of live births in a population in a year by the resident population. For census years, rates are based on unrounded census counts of the resident population as of April 1. For the noncensus years 1981–1989, rates were based on national estimates of the resident population as of July 1, rounded to thousands. Rounded population estimates for 5-year age groups were calculated by summing unrounded population estimates before rounding to thousands. Starting in 1991, rates were based on unrounded national population estimates. Birth rates for 1991–1999 were revised based on the April 1, 2000, census. The rates for 1990 and 2000 were based on populations from the censuses in those years as of April 1. Birth rates for 2001–2006 are based on populations estimated from the 2000 census as of July 1 each year. The population estimates have been provided by the U.S. Census Bureau and are based on the 2000 census counts by age, race, and sex, which have been modified to be consistent with OMB racial categories as of 1977 and historical categories for birth data. Beginning in 1997, the birth rate for the maternal age group 45–49 years includes data for mothers 50–54 years of age in the numerator and is based on the population of women 45–49 years of age in the denominator. Birth rates are expressed as the number of live births per 1,000 population. The rate may be restricted to births to women of specific age, race, marital status, or geographic location (specific rate), or it may be related to the entire population (crude rate).

Fertility rate is the total number of live births, regardless of the age of the mother, per 1,000 women of reproductive age (15–44 years).

Beginning in 1997, the birth rate for the maternal age group 45–49 years includes data for mothers 50–54 years of age in the numerator and is based on the population of women 45–49 years in the denominator.

■ *Death and related rates*

Death rate is calculated by dividing the number of deaths in a population in a year by the midyear resident population. For census years, rates are based on unrounded census counts of the resident population as of April 1. For the noncensus years 1981–1989, rates were based on national estimates of the resident population as of July 1, rounded to thousands. Rounded population estimates for 10-year age groups were calculated by summing unrounded population estimates before rounding to thousands. Starting in 1991, rates were based on unrounded national population estimates. Rates for the Hispanic and non-Hispanic white populations in each year are based on unrounded state population estimates for states in the Hispanic reporting area. Death rates are expressed as the number of deaths per 100,000 population. The rate may be restricted to deaths in specific age, race, sex, or geographic groups or from specific causes of death (specific rate), or it may be related to the entire population (crude rate).

Birth cohort infant mortality rates are based on linked birth and infant death files. In contrast to period rates in which the births and infant deaths occur in the same period or calendar year, infant deaths constituting the numerator of a birth cohort rate may have occurred in the same year as, or in the year following, the year of birth. The birth cohort infant mortality rate is expressed as the number of infant deaths per 1,000 live births. (Also see Appendix II, Birth cohort.)

Fetal death rate is the number of fetal deaths with stated or presumed gestation of 20 weeks or more, divided by the sum of live births plus fetal deaths, per 1,000 live births plus fetal deaths.

Infant mortality rate is based on period files and is calculated by dividing the number of infant deaths during a calendar year by the number of live births reported in the same year. It is expressed as the number of infant deaths per 1,000 live births. *Neonatal mortality rate* is the number of deaths of children under 28 days of age per 1,000 live births. *Postneonatal mortality rate* is the number of deaths of children that occur between 28 days and 365 days after birth,

per 1,000 live births. (Also see Appendix II, Infant death.)

Late fetal death rate is the number of fetal deaths with stated or presumed gestation of 28 weeks or more, divided by the sum of live births plus late fetal deaths per 1,000 live births plus late fetal deaths. (Also see Appendix II, Gestation.)

Maternal mortality rate is the number of maternal deaths per 100,000 live births. The maternal mortality rate is a measure of the likelihood that a pregnant woman will die from maternal causes. The number of live births used in the denominator is a proxy for the population of pregnant women who are at risk of a maternal death. (Also see Appendix II, Maternal death.)

Perinatal mortality rates and ratios relate to the period surrounding the birth event. Rates and ratios are based on events reported in a calendar year. *Perinatal mortality rate* is the sum of late fetal deaths plus infant deaths within 7 days of birth, divided by the sum of live births plus late fetal deaths per 1,000 live births plus late fetal deaths. *Perinatal mortality ratio* is the sum of late fetal deaths plus infant deaths within 7 days of birth, divided by the number of live births per 1,000 live births.

Visit rate is a basic measure of service utilization for event-based data. Examples of events include physician office visits with drugs provided or hospital discharges. In the visit rate calculation, the numerator is the number of estimated events, and the denominator is the corresponding U.S. population estimate for those who possibly could have had events during a given period of time. The interpretation is that for every person in the population there were, on average, *x* events. It does not mean that *x* of the population had events, because some persons in the population had no events while others had multiple events. The only exception is when an event can occur just once for a person (e.g., if an appendectomy is performed during a hospital stay). The visit rate is best used to compare utilization across various subgroups of interest, such as age or race groups or geographic regions.

Region—See Geographic region.

Registered hospital—See Hospital.

Registration area—The United States has separate registration areas for birth, death, marriage, and divorce statistics. In general, registration areas correspond to states and include two separate registration areas for the District of Columbia (D.C.) and New York City. The term reporting area may be used interchangeably with the term registration area. All states have adopted laws that require registration of births and deaths and the reporting of fetal deaths. It is believed that more than 99% of births and deaths occurring in this country are registered.

The death registration area was established in 1900 with 10 states and D.C., and the birth registration area was established in 1915, also with 10 states and D.C. Beginning in 1933, all states were included in the birth and death registration areas. The specific states added year by year are shown in: Hetzel AM. History and organization of the vital statistics system. Hyattsville, MD: NCHS; 1997. Available from: http://www.cdc.gov/nchs/data/misc/usvss.pdf. Currently, Puerto Rico, the U.S. Virgin Islands, and Guam each constitute a separate registration area, although their data are not included in statistical tabulations of U.S. resident data. (Also see Appendix II, Reporting area.)

Relative standard error (RSE)—RSE is a measure of an estimate's reliability. The RSE of an estimate is obtained by dividing the standard error of the estimate (SE (r)) by the estimate itself (r). This quantity is expressed as a percentage of the estimate and is calculated as follows:

$$RSE = 100 \times (SE\,(r)\,/\,(r)).$$

Estimates with large RSE are considered unreliable. In *Health, United States*, most statistics with large RSE are preceded by an asterisk or are not presented.

Relative survival rate—The relative survival rate is the ratio of the observed survival rate for the patient group to the expected survival rate for persons in the general population similar to the patient group with respect to age, sex, race, and calendar year of observation. The 5-year relative survival rate is used to estimate the proportion of cancer patients potentially curable. Because over one-half of all cancers occur in persons 65 years of age and over, many of these individuals die of other causes with no evidence of recurrence of their cancer. Thus, because it is obtained by adjusting observed survival for the normal life expectancy of the general population of the same age, the relative survival rate is an estimate of the chance of surviving the effects of cancer.

Reporting area—In the National Vital Statistics System, the reporting area for such basic items on the birth and death certificates as age, race, and sex is based on data from residents of all 50 states in the United States, the District of Columbia, and New York City. The term reporting area may be used interchangeably with the term registration area. (Also see Appendix II, Registration area; and Appendix I, National Vital Statistics System.)

Resident, health facility—In the Online Survey Certification and Reporting (OSCAR) database, all residents in certified facilities are counted on the day of certification inspection. In the National Nursing Home Survey, a resident is a person on the roster of the nursing home as of the night before the survey. Included are all residents for whom beds are maintained, even though they may be on overnight leave or in a hospital. (Also see Appendix II, Nursing home.)

Resident population—See Population.

Residential treatment care—See Mental health service type.

Residential treatment center for emotionally disturbed children—See Mental health organization.

Rural—See Urbanization.

Self-assessment of health—See Health status, respondent-assessed.

Serious psychological distress—The K6 instrument is a measure of psychological distress associated with unspecified but potentially diagnosable mental illness that may result in a higher risk for disability and higher utilization of health services. In the National Health Interview Survey (NHIS), the K6 was asked of adults 18 years of age and older. The K6 is designed to identify persons with serious psychological distress, using as few questions as possible. The six items included in the K6 are presented as follows:

During the past 30 days, how often did you feel:

- So sad that nothing could cheer you up?
- Nervous?
- Restless or fidgety?
- Hopeless?
- That everything was an effort?
- Worthless?

Possible answers are "All of the time" (4 points), "Most of the time" (3 points), "Some of the time" (2 points), "A little of the time" (1 point), and "None of the time" (0 points).

To score the K6, the points are added together, yielding a possible total of 0–24 points. A threshold of 13 points or more is used to define serious psychological distress. Persons answering "Some of the time" to all six questions would not reach the threshold for serious psychological distress because to achieve a score of 13 they would need to answer "Most of the time" to at least one item. The version of the K6 used in the NHIS provides 1-month prevalence rates because the reference period is the past 30 days. For more information, see: Kessler RC, Barker PR, Colpe LJ, Epstein JF, Gfroerer JC, Hiripi E, et al. Screening for serious mental illness in the general population. Arch Gen Psychiatry 2003;60(2):184–9. (Also see Appendix II, Basic actions difficulty.)

Short-stay hospital—See Hospital.

Skilled nursing facility—See Nursing home.

Smoker—See Cigarette smoking.

Specialty hospital—See Hospital.

State mental health agency—Refers to the agency or department within state government, headed by the state or territorial health official, that deals with mental health issues. Generally, the state mental health agency is responsible for setting statewide mental health priorities, carrying out national and state mandates, responding to mental health hazards, and ensuring access to mental health care for underserved state residents.

Substance use—Substance use refers to the use of selected substances, including alcohol, tobacco products, drugs, inhalants, and other substances that can be consumed, inhaled, injected, or otherwise absorbed into the body with possible dependence and other detrimental effects. (Also see Appendix II, Illicit drug use.)

Monitoring the Future (MTF)—MTF collects information on the use of selected substances by using self-completed questionnaires in a school-based survey of secondary school students. MTF has tracked 12th graders' illicit drug use and attitudes toward drugs since 1975. In 1991, 8th and 10th graders were added to the study. The survey includes questions on abuse of substances including (but not limited to) marijuana, inhalants, other illegal drugs, alcohol, cigarettes, and other tobacco products. (Also see Appendix I, Monitoring the Future.)

National Survey on Drug Use & Health (NSDUH)—NSDUH conducts in-person, computer-assisted interviews of a sample of individuals 12 years of age and older at their place of residence. For illicit drug use, alcohol use, and tobacco use, information is collected about use in the lifetime, past year, and past month. However, only estimates of use in the past month are presented in *Health, United States*. For illicit drug use, respondents in NSDUH are asked about use of marijuana/hashish, cocaine (including crack), inhalants, hallucinogens, heroin, and prescription-type psychotherapeutic drugs (pain relievers, tranquilizers, stimulants, and sedatives) used nonmedically. A series of questions is asked about each substance: "Have you ever, even once, used [substance]?" "How long has it been since you last used [substance]?" Numerous probes and checks are included in the computer-assisted interview system. Nonprescription medications and legitimate use of prescription drugs under a doctor's supervision are not included in the survey. Summary measures, such as current illicit drug use, are produced. (Also see Appendix II, Alcohol consumption; Cigarette smoking; Illicit drug use; and Appendix I, National Survey on Drug Use & Health.)

Suicidal ideation—Suicidal ideation means having thoughts of suicide or of taking action to end one's own life. Suicidal ideation includes all thoughts of suicide, both when the thoughts include a plan to commit suicide and when they do not include a plan. Suicidal ideation is measured in the Youth Risk Behavior Survey by the following three questions: "During the past 12 months, did you ever seriously consider attempting suicide?", "During the past 12 months, how many times did you actually attempt suicide?", and "If you attempted suicide during the past 12 months, did any attempt result in an injury, poisoning, or overdose that had to be treated by a doctor or nurse?" For more information, see: http://www.cdc.gov/HealthyYouth/yrbs/index.htm.

Surgery—See Outpatient surgery; Procedure.

Surgical specialty—See Physician specialty.

Tobacco use—See Cigarette smoking.

Uninsured—In the Current Population Survey (CPS), persons are considered uninsured if they do not have coverage through private health insurance, Medicare, Medicaid, Children's Health Insurance Program, military or veterans coverage, another government program, a plan of someone outside the household, or other insurance. Persons with only Indian Health Service coverage are considered uninsured. In addition, if the respondent has missing Medicaid information but has income from certain low-income public programs, then Medicaid coverage is imputed. The questions on health insurance are administered in March and refer to the previous calendar year.

In the National Health Interview Survey (NHIS), the uninsured are persons who do not have coverage under private health insurance, Medicare, Medicaid, public assistance, a state-sponsored health plan, other government-sponsored programs, or a military health plan. Persons with only Indian Health Service coverage are considered uninsured. Estimates of the percentage of persons who are uninsured based on NHIS (Table 138) may differ slightly from those based on the March CPS (Table 148) because of differences in survey questions, recall period, and other aspects of survey methodology. Estimates for the uninsured are shown only for the population under 65 years of age.

Survey respondents may be covered by health insurance at the time of interview but may have experienced one or more lapses in coverage during the year prior to interview. Starting with *Health, United States, 2006*, NHIS estimates for people with health insurance coverage for all 12 months prior to interview, for those who were uninsured for any period up to 12 months, and for those who were uninsured for more than 12 months were added as stub variables to selected tables. (Also see Appendix II, Health insurance coverage; and Appendix I, Current Population Survey.)

Urbanization—Urbanization is the degree of urban (city-like) character of a particular geographic area. Urbanization can be measured in a variety of ways. In *Health United States*, the two measures used to categorize counties by urbanization level are the Office of Management and Budget's (OMB) metropolitan statistical area (MSA) classification and the 2006 NCHS Urban–Rural Classification Scheme for Counties. For more information on the OMB classification of counties, see Appendix II, Metropolitan statistical area (MSA); Micropolitan statistical area.

The 2006 NCHS Urban–Rural Classification Scheme for Counties is a six-level classification scheme developed by NCHS to categorize the 3,141 U.S. counties and county equivalents based on their urban and rural characteristics. The classification scheme includes four metropolitan (or urban) categories and two nonmetropolitan (or rural) categories. The county classifications are based on the following information: (a) the 2003 OMB definitions of metropolitan and micropolitan counties (with revisions through 2005); (b) the 2004 postcensal county population estimates; and (c) county-level data on several settlement density, socioeconomic, and demographic variables from Census 2000. The six categories of the 2006 NCHS Urban–Rural Classification Scheme for Counties are

large central metro (central counties of metro areas of 1 million or more population), large fringe metro (outlying counties of metro areas of 1 million or more population), medium metro (metro areas of 250,000–999,999 population), small metro (metro areas with less than 250,000 population), nonmetropolitan micropolitan, and nonmetropolitan noncore. For more information on this classification scheme, see: http://www.cdc.gov/nchs/data_access/urban_rural.htm.

Usual source of care—Usual source of care was measured in the National Health Interview Survey (NHIS) in 1993 and 1994 by asking the respondent "Is there a particular person or place that [person] usually goes to when [person] is sick or needs advice about [person's] health?" In the 1995 and 1996 NHIS, the respondent was asked "Is there one doctor, person, or place that [person] usually goes to when [person] is sick or needs advice about health?" Starting in 1997, the respondent was asked "Is there a place that [person] usually goes when he/she is sick or you need advice about [his/her] health?" Persons who report the emergency department as their usual source of care are defined as having no usual source of care in *Health, United States*.

Vaccination—Vaccinations, or immunizations, work by stimulating the immune system—the natural disease-fighting system of the body. A healthy immune system is able to recognize invading bacteria and viruses and produce substances (antibodies) to destroy or disable these invaders. Vaccinations prepare the immune system to ward off a disease. In addition to the initial immunization process, the effectiveness of some immunizations can be improved by periodic repeat injections or "boosters." Vaccines are among the most successful and cost-effective public health tools available for reducing morbidity and mortality from vaccine-preventable diseases. For a comprehensive list of vaccine-preventable diseases, see: http://www.cdc.gov/vaccines/vpd-vac/vpd-list.htm and http://www.cdc.gov/vaccines/spec-grps/default.htm.

The currently recommended childhood vaccination schedule includes vaccines that prevent infectious diseases including hepatitis A, diphtheria, tetanus toxoids, acellular pertussis (whooping cough), measles, mumps, rubella (German measles), polio, varicella (chicken pox), and some forms of meningitis, influenza, and pneumonia. In February 2006, a rotavirus vaccine (RotaTeq) was licensed for use among U.S. infants.

A vaccine that protects against the four types of human papillomavirus (HPV) that cause most cervical cancers and genital warts began to be marketed in

2006 and is now available for females and males. The vaccine is recommended for 11- and 12-year-old girls. It is also recommended for girls and women 13–26 years of age who have not yet been vaccinated or completed the vaccine series.

Boosters (revaccination) of vaccinations received during childhood or adulthood are necessary for some vaccines. In addition to keeping current with the vaccines listed above, and annual influenza vaccination, some additional vaccinations are recommended for older adults, persons with specific health conditions, or health care workers who are likely to be exposed to infectious persons. Herpes zoster vaccination is recommended one time for adults 60 years of age and over, and pneumococcal vaccination is recommended one time for adults 65 years of age and over.

For a full discussion of recommended vaccination schedules by age or population, see CDC's vaccination and immunization website at: http://www.cdc.gov/vaccines/recs/schedules/default.htm.

Wages and salaries—See Employer costs for employee compensation.

Years of potential life lost (YPLL)—YPLL is a measure of premature mortality. Starting with *Health, United States*, 1996, YPLL has been presented for persons under 75 years of age because the average life expectancy in the United States is over 75 years. YPLL–75 is calculated using the following eight age groups: under 1 year, 1–14 years, 15–24 years, 25–34 years, 35–44 years, 45–54 years, 55–64 years, and 65–74 years. The number of deaths for each age group is multiplied by years of life lost, calculated as the difference between age 75 years and the midpoint of the age group. For the eight age groups, the midpoints are 0.5, 7.5, 19.5, 29.5, 39.5, 49.5, 59.5, and 69.5 years. For example, the death of a person 15–24 years of age counts as 55.5 years of life lost. Years of potential life lost is derived by summing years of life lost over all age groups. In *Health, United States, 1995* and earlier editions, YPLL was presented for persons under 65 years of age. For more information, see: CDC. Premature mortality in the United States: Public health issues in the use of years of potential life lost. MMWR 1986;35(SS–02):1S–11S. Available from: http://www.cdc.gov/mmwr/preview/mmwrhtml/00001773.htm.

Appendix III. Additional Data Years Available

For Trend Tables spanning long periods, only selected data years are shown, to highlight major trends. Additional years of data for some of these tables are available in electronic spreadsheet form on the *Health, United States, 2010* website at:

http://www.cdc.gov/nchs/hus.htm. Standard errors are included in the spreadsheet files for tables that are based on the National Health Interview Survey, the National Health and Nutrition Examination Survey, and the National Survey of Family Growth.

Table number	Table topic	Additional data years available
1	Resident population	2001–2005
2	Poverty	1986–1989, 1991–1994, 1996–1999, 2001–2003, 2005–2006
3	Fertility rates and birth rates	1981–1984, 1986–1989, 1991–1994, 1996–1999, 2001–2004
4	Live births	1972–1974, 1976–1979, 1981–1984, 1986–1989, 1991–1994, 1996–1999, 2001–2005
5	Prenatal care	1975, 1981–1989, 1991–1999, 2001–2002
6	Teenage childbearing	1981–1984, 1986–1989, 1991–1994, 1996–1999, 2001–2003
7	Nonmarital childbearing	1981–1984, 1986–1989, 1991–1994, 1996–1999, 2001–2003
8	Maternal smoking	1991–1994, 1996–1999, 2001–2002
9	Low birthweight	1981–1984, 1986–1989, 1991–1994, 1996–1998, 2001–2004
10	Low birthweight	1991–1999, 2001
12	Abortions	1981–1984, 1986–1989, 1991–1994, 1996–1998, 2001–2002, 2005
13	Contraceptive use	1998
15	Infant mortality rates	1996–1999, 2001–2003
16	Infant mortality rates	1984, 1986–1989, 1991, 1996–1999, 2001–2003
17	Infant mortality rates	1981–1989, 1991–1994, 1996–1999
20	International mortality rates and rankings	2001, 2002–2005; ranking 2005–2006
21	International life expectancy	1999, 2001–2003, 2005–2006
22	Life expectancy	1975, 1981–1989, 1991–1994, 1996–1998
24	Age-adjusted death rates for selected causes	1981–1989, 1991–1999, 2001–2004
25	Years of potential life lost	1991–1999, 2001–2006; crude 1999–2006
28	Urbanization level	2002–2004, 2003–2005, 2004–2006
29	Death rates for all causes	1981–1989, 1991–1999, 2001–2005
30	Diseases of heart	1981–1989, 1991–1999, 2001–2005
31	Cerebrovascular diseases	1981–1989, 1991–1999, 2001–2005
32	Malignant neoplasms	1981–1989, 1991–1999, 2001–2005
33	Malignant neoplasms of trachea, bronchus, and lung	1981–1989, 1991–1999, 2001–2005
34	Malignant neoplasm of breast	1981–1989, 1991–1999, 2001–2005
35	Human immunodeficiency virus (HIV) disease	1988–1989, 1991–1994, 2001–2004
36	Maternal mortality	1981–1989, 1991–1999, 2001–2004
37	Motor vehicle-related injuries	1981–1989, 1991–1999, 2001–2005
38	Homicide	1981–1989, 1991–1999, 2001–2005
39	Suicide	1981–1989, 1991–1999, 2001–2005
40	Firearm-related injuries	1981–1989, 1991–1994, 1996–1999, 2001–2004
41	Occupational diseases	1981–1984, 1986–1989, 1991–1994, 1996–1999, 2001–2004

Table number	Table topic	Additional data years available
43	Nonfatal occupational injuries and illnesses	2004–2005
44	Notifiable diseases	1985, 1988–1989, 1991–1999, 2001–2004
46	Health conditions among children	2006–2008
47	Cancer incidence rates	1991–1994, 1996–1999, 2001
48	Five-year relative cancer survival rates	1978–1980, 1984–1986, 1990–1992, 1993–1995
49	Respondent-reported prevalence of heart disease, cancer, and stroke	2001–2002, 2003–2004, 2007–2008
50	Diabetes	2001–2004
51	End-stage renal disease	1985, 1995, 2001–2005
52	Severe headache or migraine, low back pain, and neck pain	1998–2007
53	Joint pain	2003–2007
54	Basic actions difficulty and complex activity limitation	1998–1999, 2000–2006
55	Vision and hearing limitations	1998–1999, 2001–2006
56	Respondent-assessed health status	1998–1999, 2001–2004, 2006
57	Serious psychological distress	2000–2001, 2002–2003, 2003–2004, 2006–2007
58	Cigarette smoking	1983, 1987–1988, 1991–1994, 1997–1999, 2001–2004, 2006
59	Cigarette smoking	1983, 1987–1988, 1991–1994, 1997–1999, 2001–2004, 2006
60	Cigarette smoking	1993–1995, 2006–2008
61	Use of selected substances	2003–2005
62	Use of selected substances	1981–1984, 1986–1989, 1992–1994, 1996–1999, 2001–2005
63	Health risk behaviors among students	1993, 1995, 1997, 1999, 2001, 2003, 2005
64	Lifetime alcohol drinking status	1998–1999, 2001–2007
65	Heavier drinking and drinking five or more drinks in a day	1998–1999, 2001–2007
67	Hypertension (high blood pressure)	2001–2004
68	Cholesterol	2001–2004, 2003–2006
69	Mean energy and macronutrient intake	2003–2006
70	Leisure-time aerobic/muscle-strengthing physical activity	1999, 2001–2008
71	Overweight, obesity, and healthy weight	2001–2004
72	Overweight among children and adolescents	2001–2004, 2003–2006
73	Untreated dental caries	1999–2002
74	No usual source of health care	1995–1996, 1997–1998, 2001–2002, 2003–2004, 2004–2005, 2005–2006, 2006–2007, 2007–2008
75	No usual source of health care	2003–2004, 2004–2005, 2005–2006, 2006–2007
76	Reduced access to medical care	1998–2007
77	Reduced access to medical care	19981999, 1999–2000, 2000–2001, 2002–2003, 2003–2004, 2004–2005, 2005–2006, 2006–2007, 2007–2008
78	No heath care visits	1999–2000, 2003–2004, 2004–2005, 2005–2006, 2006–2007
79	Health care visits	1998–2007
81	Vaccinations	1996–1999, 2001–2003
82	Vaccinations	2003
84	Influenza vaccination	1991, 1993–1994, 1997–1999, 2001–2004
85	Pneumococcal vaccination	1991, 1993–1994, 1997–1999, 2001–2004
86	Mammography	1991, 1998
87	Pap smears	1998
88	Emergency department visits for children	1998–2007

Table number	Table topic	Additional data years available
89	Emergency department visits for adults	1998–1999, 2001–2007
90	Injury-related visits to hospital emergency departments	2005–2006, 2006–2007
91	Ambulatory care visits	1997–1999, 2001–2006
92	Ambulatory care visits	1997–1999, 2001–2007
93	Dental visits	1998–2007
94	Prescription drug use	1999–2000, 1999–2002, 2001–2004, 2003–2006
96	Dietary supplement use	2001–2004, 2003–2005
97	Additions to mental health organizations	1992, 1994, 1998, 2000
98	Discharges	1998–1999, 2001–2007
99	Discharges	1991–1994, 1996–1999, 2001–2004
100	Days of care	1991–1999, 2001–2006
101	Diagnoses	1991–1999, 2001–2006
102	Average length of stay	1991–1999, 2001–2006
103	Procedures	1991–1999, 2001–2006
105	Persons employed in health service sites	2001–2002
110	Employees and wages	2002, 2004–2005, 2007–2008
114	Mental health organizations	1992
117	Nursing homes	1996–1999, 2001–2007
118	Certified intermediate care facilities	2000, 2007
119	Medicare-certified providers and suppliers	1997–1998, 2002, 2004, 2006
120	Magnetic Resonance Imaging (MRI) units and Computed Tomography (CT) scanners	2001–2002
121	Total health expenditures as a percent of gross domestic product	1961–1969, 1971–1979, 1981–1989, 1991–1994, 1996–1999, 2001–2002
122	Gross domestic product	2005
126	Personal health care expenditures	2005
128	Expenditures for mental health services	1987–1989, 1991–1994, 1996–1999, 2001–2003
129	Expenditures for substance abuse treatment	1987–1989, 1991–1994, 1996–1999, 2001
130	Expenditures for health care	1996, 1998–1999, 2001–2006
131	Sources of payment for health care	1996, 1998–1999, 2001–2006
132	Out-of-pocket health care expenses	1997–1999, 2001–2003
133	Expenditures for health services and supplies	2003
134	Employers' costs and health insurance	1992–1993, 1995, 1997–1999, 2001–2005
135	Private health insurance	1994, 1998–1999, 2001–2004
136	Private health insurance	1994, 1999, 2001–2004, 2006
137	Medicaid coverage	1994, 1998–1999, 2001–2003, 2005–2006
138	No health insurance coverage	1994, 1998–1999, 2001–2003, 2005–2006
139	Health care coverage	1993–1994, 1996–1999, 2001–2005
141	Medicare	1996–1998, 2001, 2003–2004
142	Medicare	All: 1999–2002; 1993–2003
143	Medicaid	2001
144	Medicaid	2001
145	Department of Veterans Affairs	1985, 1988–1989, 1991–1994, 1996–1999, 2001–2004
146	Medicare	1995–2006
147	Medicaid	2001–2007
148	Persons without health insurance coverage	2004–2006, 2005–2007

Index

(Numbers refer to tables and figures)

Table/Figure

Table/Figure

P—Con.

R

S

T